Joint Structure and Function:
A Comprehensive Analysis

Fourth Edition

Joint Structure and Function:
A Comprehensive Analysis

Fourth Edition

Pamela K. Levangie, PT, DSc
Professor
Physical Therapy Program
Sacred Heart University
Fairfield, CT

Cynthia C. Norkin, PT, EdD
Former Director and Associate Professor
School of Physical Therapy
Ohio University
Athens, OH

F. A. Davis Company • Philadelphia

F. A. Davis Company
1915 Arch Street
Philadelphia, PA 19103
www.fadavis.com

Printed in the United States of America

Last digit indicates print number: 10 9 8 7 6 5 4 3 2 1

Acquisitions Editor: Margaret M. Biblis
Development Editor: Jennifer Pine
Design Manager: Carolyn O'Brien

As new scientific information becomes available through basic and clinical research, recommended treatments and drug therapies undergo changes. The author(s) and publisher have done everything possible to make this book accurate, up to date, and in accord with accepted standards at the time of publication. The author(s), editors, and publisher are not responsible for errors or omissions or for consequences from application of the book, and make no warranty, expressed or implied, in regard to the contents of the book. Any practice described in this book should be applied by the reader in accordance with professional standards of care used in regard to the unique circumstances that may apply in each situation. The reader is advised always to check product information (package inserts) for changes and new information regarding dose and contraindications before administering any drug. Caution is especially urged when using new or infrequently ordered drugs.

Library of Congress Cataloging-in-Publication Data

Levangie, Pamela K.
  Joint structure and function : a comprehensive analysis / Pamela K. Levangie, Cindy Norkin.— 4th ed.
    p. ; cm.
  Includes bibliographical references and index.
  ISBN 0–8036–1191–9 (hardcover : alk. paper)
  1. Human mechanics. 2. Joints.
  [DNLM: 1. Joints—anatomy & histology. 2. Joints—physiology. WE 399 L655j 2005] I.Norkin, Cynthia C. II. Title.
QP303.N59 2005
    612.7′5—dc22

                                                                                    2004021449

Dedication for the Fourth Edition

For more than 20 years, we have been privileged to contribute to the professional development of students and practitioners . The four editions of *Joint Structure and Function* have been shaped as much by the faculty and students who use this text as by the changes in evidence and technology. Therefore , we dedicate this 4th edition of *Joint Structure and Function* to the faculty, the students, and the health care professionals who are both our consumers and our partners.

Preface to the Fourth Edition

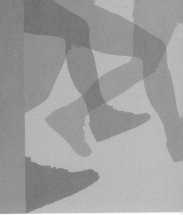

With the 4th edition of *Joint Structure and Function*, we continue a tradition of excellence in education that began more than 20 years ago. Although we entered the market when there were few resource options for our readers, we are now in an era of increasingly numerous choices in a variety of media. We continue with this edition to respond to the ever-accelerating changes taking place in media and research technology as well as in the education of individuals who assess human function. In the move toward what many believe will be a "paperless" society, the role of textbooks is evolving rapidly; learners demand changes but are not ready to give up the textbook as an educational modality. With the 4th edition, we attempt to meet the challenges before us and our learners by taking advantage of new technologies, current evidence, the expertise of colleagues, and a more integrated approach to preparing those who wish to understand human kinesiology and pathokinesiology.

Use of digital imaging technology allows us to substantially change the visual support for our readers. Line drawings (many taking advantage of our two-color format) have been added or modified because these often work best to display complex concepts. However, we now include in this edition a greater variety of image options, including photographs, medical imaging, and three-dimensional computer output that should better support learning and better prepare the reader for negotiating published research. Changes in size, layout, and two-color format provide a more reader-friendly page and enhance the reader's ability to move around within each chapter.

Recognizing the increasing challenge of remaining current in published research across many areas, we now take advantage of the expertise of a greater number of respected colleagues as chapter contributors. Our contributors straddle the environs largely of research, practice, and teaching—grounding their chapters in best evidence and in clinical relevance. A key change in our educational approach is in use of patient cases, not as adjuncts to the text but as integrated elements within the text of each chapter. Patient cases (in both highlighted *Patient Case* and *Patient Application* boxes) substantially facilitate an understanding of the continuum between normal and impaired function, making use of emerging case-based and problem-based learning educational strategies. We have maintained highlighted summary boxes (now called *Concept Cornerstones*) while also adding highlighted *Continuing Exploration* boxes that provide the reader or the instructor additional flexibility in setting learning objectives.

What is unchanged in this edition of *Joint Structure and Function* is our commitment to maintaining a text that provides a strong foundation in the principles that underlie an understanding of human structure and function while also being readable and as concise as possible. We hope that our years of experience in contributing to the education of health care professionals allow us to strike a unique balance. We cannot fail to recognize the increased educational demands placed on many entry-level health care professionals and hope that the changes to the 4th edition help students meet that demand. However, *Joint Structure and Function*, while growing with its readers, continues to recognize that the new reader requires elementary and interlinked building blocks that lay a strong but flexible foundation to best support continued learning and growth in a complex and changing world.

We continue to appreciate our opportunity to contribute to health care by assisting in the professional development of the students and practitioners who are our readers.

Pamela K. Levangie
Cynthia C. Norkin

Acknowledgments

No endeavor as labor-intensive as updating a science and research-based textbook such as *Joint Structure and Function* can be accomplished without the expertise and support of many committed individuals. We appreciate the very considerable investment of our continuing contributors, as well as the willingness of our new group of clinical and academic professionals to also lend their names and expertise to this project. Our thanks, therefore, to Drs. Borstad, Chleboun, Curwin, Hoover, Lewik, Ludewig, Mueller, Olney, Ritzline, and Snyder-Mackler as well as to Mss. Austin, Dalton, and Starr. All brought from their various institutions, states, and countries their enthusiasm and a wealth of new knowledge and ideas. We also would like to thank the reviewers, listed on pages xiii and xiv, who provided us with many helpful suggestions for improving the text.

We further extend our gratitude to FA Davis for their investment in this book's future. Margaret Biblis, Publisher, brought new energy and a contemporary vision to this project; Jennifer Pine, Developmental Editor, managed the project in a manner that merged Margaret's vision with Jennifer's own unique contributions. We credit our artist, Anne Raines, with many new clear images that appear in the book. We are grateful to artists Joe Farnum and Timothy Malone, whose creative contributions to previous editions also appear in the 4th edition.

Of course, none of us would be able to would be able to make such large investment of time and energy to a project like this without the support of our colleagues and the ongoing loving support of families. We can only thank them for giving up countless hours of our time and attention to yet another edition of *Joint Structure and Function*.

Contributors

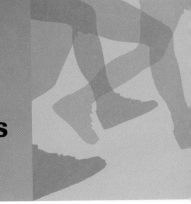

Noelle M. Austin, PT, MS, CHT
CJ Education and Consulting, LLC
Woodbridge CT
cj-education.com &
The Orthopaedic Group
Hamden, Connecticut

John D. Borstead, PT, PhD
Assistant Professor
Physical Therapy Division
Ohio State University
Columbus, Ohio

Gary Chleboun, PT, PhD
Professor
School of Physical Therapy
Ohio University
Athens, Ohio

Sandra Curwin, PT, PhD
Associate Professor
Department of Physical Therapy
University of Alberta
Edmonton, Alberta
Canada

Diane Dalton, PT, MS, OCS
Clinical Assistant Professor of Physical Therapy
Physical Therapy Program
Boston University
Boston, Massachusetts

Don Hoover, PT, PhD
Assistant Professor
Krannert School of Physical Therapy
University of Indianapolis
Indianapolis, Indiana

Michael Lewek, PT, PhD
Post Doctoral Fellow, Sensory Motor Performance
Program
Rehabilitation Institute of Chicago
Northwestern University
Chicago, Illinois

Paula M. Ludewig, PT, PhD
Associate Professor
Program in Physical Therapy
University of Minnesota
Minneapolis, Minnesota

Michael J. Mueller, PT, PhD, FAPTA
Associate Professor
Program in Physical Therapy
Washington University School of Medicine
St. Louis, Missouri

Sandra J. Olney, PT, OT, PhD
Director, School of Rehabilitation Therapy
Associate Dean of Health Sciences
Queens University
Kingston, Ontario
Canada

Pamela Ritzline, PT, EdD
Associate Professor
Krannert School of Physical Therapy
University of Indianapolis
Indianapolis, Indiana

Lynn Snyder-Macker, PT, ScD, SCS, ATC, FAPTA
Professor
Department of Physical Therapy
University of Delaware
Newark, Delaware

Julie Starr, PT, MS, CCS
Clinical Associate Professor of Physical Therapy
Physical Therapy Program
Boston University
Boston, Massachusetts

Reviewers

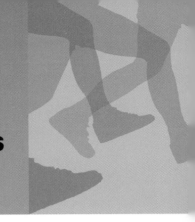

Thomas Abelew, PhD
Assistant Professor
Department of Rehabilitation Medicine
Emory University
Atlanta, Georgia

Gordon Alderink, PT, PhD
Assistant Professor
Physical Therapy Department
Grand Valley State University
Allendale, Michigan

Mary Brown, PT, MEd
Physical Therapist
Department of Rehabilitation
Morristown Memorial Hospital, Atlantic Health System
West Orange, New Jersey

John A. Buford, PT, PhD
Assistant Professor of Physical Therapy
Division of Physical Therapy
School of Allied Medical Professions
The Ohio State University
Columbus, Ohio

Margaret Carton, MSPT
Assistant Professor
Allied Health, Nursing, and HPE Department
Black Hawk College
Moline, Illinois

Gary Chleboun, PT, PhD
Professor
School of Physical Therapy
Ohio University
Athens, Ohio

Deborah Edmondson, PT, EdD
Assistant Professor/Academic Coordinator of Clinical Education
Department of Physical Therapy
Tennessee State University
Nashville, Tennessee

Ricardo Fernandez, PT, MHS, OCS, CSCS
Assistant Professor/Clinician
Department of Physical Therapy and Human Movement Sciences
Northwestern University Feinberg School of Medicine
Chicago, Illinois

Jason Gauvin, PT, SCS, ATC, CSCS
Physical Therapist
Departments of Occupational Therapy and Physical Therapy
Duke University
Durham, North Carolina

Barbara Hahn, PT, MA
Director, Physical Therapist Assistant Program
University of Evansville
Evansville, Indiana

John Hollman, PT, PhD
Assistant Professor and Director
Program in Physical Therapy
Mayo School of Health Sciences
Rochester, MN

Birgid Hopkins, MS, L.ATC
Director
Department of Sports Medicine
Merrimack College
North Andover, Massachusetts

Edmund Kosmahl, PT, EdD
Professor
Department of Physical Therapy
University of Scranton
Scranton, Pennsylvania

Gary Lentell, PT, MS, DPT
Professor
Department of Physical Therapy
University of California, Fresno
Fresno, California

Robin Marcus, PT, PhD, OCS
Clinical Associate Professor
Division of Physical Therapy
University of Utah
Salt Lake City, Utah

R. Daniel Martin, EdD, ATC
Associate Professor and Director, Athletic Training
Program
Exercise Science, Sport, and Recreation
Marshall University
Huntingdon, West Virginia

Matthew C. Morrissey, PT, ScD
Department of Physiotherapy
King's College London, KCL
London, England

Suzanne Reese, PT, MS
Director, Physical Therapist Assistant Program
Allied Health Department
Tulsa Community College
Tulsa, Oklahoma

Claire Safran-Norton, PT, PhD-ABD, MS, MS, OCS
Assistant Professor
Department of Physical Therapy
Simmons College
Boston, Massachusetts

Contents

SECTION 4 Hip Joint   354

Chapter 10 The Hip Complex   355
Pamela K. Levangie, PT, DSc

Chapter 11 The Knee
Lynn Snyder-Macker, PT, ScD, SCS, ATC, FAPTA
Michael Lewek, PT, PhD

Chapter 12 The Ankle and Foot Complex   437
Michael J. Mueller, PT, PhD, FAPTA

Joint Structure and Function:
A Comprehensive Analysis
Fourth Edition

Joint Structure and Function: Foundational Concepts

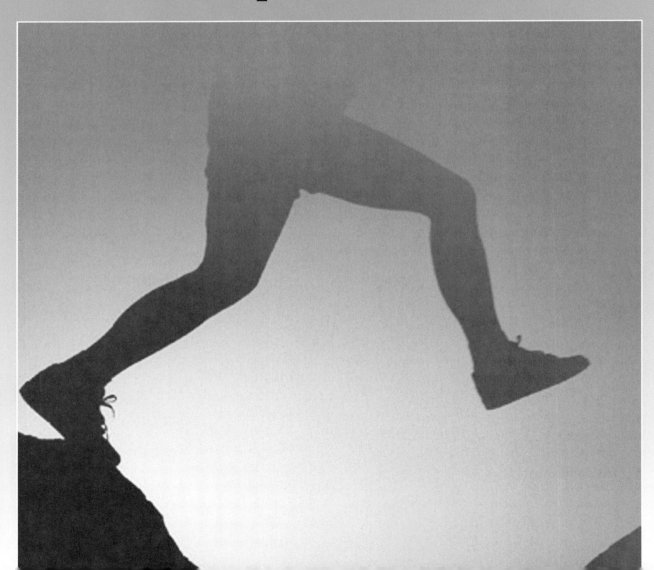

Chapter 1

Biomechanical Applications to Joint Structure and Function

Pamela K. Levangie, PT, DSc

"HUMANS HAVE THE CAPACITY TO PRODUCE A NEARLY INFINITE VARIETY OF POSTURES AND MOVEMENTS THAT REQUIRE THE TISSUES OF THE BODY TO BOTH GENERATE AND RESPOND TO FORCES THAT PRODUCE AND CONTROL MOVEMENT."

◆ Introduction

Humans have the capacity to produce a nearly infinite variety of postures and movements that require the structures of the human body to both generate and respond to forces that produce and control movement at the body's joints. Although it is impossible to capture all the kinesiologic elements that contribute to human musculoskeletal function at a given point in time, a knowledge of at least some of the physical principles that govern the body's response to active and passive stresses on its segments is prerequisite to an understanding of both human function and dysfunction.

We will examine some of the complexity of human musculoskeletal function by examining the role of the bony segments, joint-related connective tissue structure, muscles, and the external forces applied to those structures. We will develop a conceptual framework that provides a basis for understanding the stresses on the body's major joint complexes and the responses to those stresses. Case examples will be used to ground the reader's understanding in clinically relevant applications of the presented principles. The objective is to provide comprehensive coverage of foundational kinesiologic principles necessary to understand individual joint complexes and their interdependent composite functions in posture and locomotion. Although we acknowledge the role of the neurological system in motor control, we leave it to others to develop an understanding of the theories that govern the role of the controller and feedback mechanisms.

The goal of this first chapter is lay the biomechanical foundation for the principles used in subsequent chapters. This chapter will explore the biomechanical principles that must be considered to examine the internal and external forces that produce or control movement. The focus will be largely on rigid body analysis; subsequent chapters explore how forces affect deformable connective tissues (Chapter 2) and how muscles create and are affected by forces (Chapter 3). Subsequent chapters then examine the interactive nature of force, stress, tissue behaviors, and function through a regional exploration of the joint complexes

of the body. The final two chapters integrate the function of the joint complexes into the comprehensive tasks of posture and gait.

In order to maintain our focus on clinically relevant applications of the biomechanical principles presented in this chapter, the following case example will provide a framework within which to explore the relevant principles of biomechanics.

| 1-1 | Patient Case |

Sam Alexander is 20 years old, is 5 feet, 9 inches (1.75 m) in height, and weighs 165 pounds (~75 kg or 734 N). Sam is a member of the university's golf team. He sustained an injury to his right knee as he fell when his foot went through a gopher hole on a slope. Physical examination and magnetic resonance imaging (MRI) resulted in a diagnosis of a tear of the medial collateral ligament, a partial tear of the anterior cruciate ligament (ACL), and a partial tear of the medial meniscus. Sam agreed with the orthopedist's recommendation that a program of knee muscle strengthening was in order before moving to more aggressive options. The initial focus will be on strengthening the quadriceps muscle. The fitness center at the university has a leg-press machine (Fig. 1-1A) and a free weight boot (see Fig. 1-1B) that Sam can use.

As we move through this chapter, we will consider the biomechanics of each of these rehabilitative options in relation to Sam's injury and strengthening goals. [*Side-bar:* The case in this chapter provides a background for presentation of biomechanical principles. The values and angles chosen for the forces in the various examples used in this case are representative but are not intended to correspond to values derived from sophisticated instrumentation and mathematical modeling, in which different experimental conditions, instrumentation, and modeling can provide substantially different and often contradictory findings.]

Human motion is inherently complex, involving multiple segments (bony levers) and forces that are most often applied to two or more segments simultaneously. In order to develop a conceptual model that can be understood and applied clinically, the common

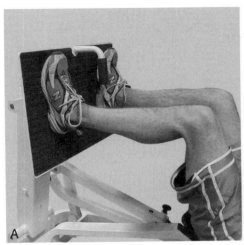
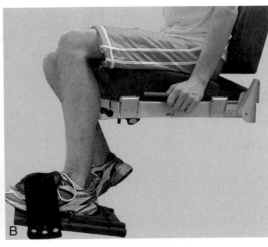

◀ **Figure 1-1** ▪ **A.** Leg-press exercise apparatus for strengthening hip and knee extensor muscles. **B.** Free weight boot for strengthening knee extensor muscles.

strategy is to focus on one segment at a time. For the purposes of analyzing Sam Alexander's issues, the focus will be on the leg-foot segment, treated as if it were one rigid unit acting at the knee joint. Figure 1-2A and B is a schematic representation of the leg-foot segment in the leg-press and free weight boot situations. The leg-foot segment is the focus of the figure, although the contiguous components (distal femur, footplate of the leg-press machine, and weight boot) are maintained to give context. In some subsequent figures, the femur, footplate, and weight boot are omitted for clarity, although the forces produced by these segments and objects will be shown. This limited visualization of a segment (or a selected few segments) is referred to as a free body diagram or a space diagram. If proportional representation of all forces is maintained as the forces are added to the segment under consideration, it is known as a free body diagram. If the forces are shown but a simplified understanding rather than graphic accuracy is the goal, then the figure is referred to as a space diagram.[1] We will use space diagrams in this chapter and text because the forces are generally not drawn in proportion to their magnitudes.

As we begin to examine the leg-foot segment in either exercise situation, the first step is to describe the motion of the segment that is or will be occurring. This involves the area of biomechanics known as **kinematics.**

Part 1: *Kinematics and Introduction to Kinetics*

✦ Descriptions of Motion

Kinematics includes the set of concepts that allows us to describe the motion (or **displacement**) of a segment without regard to the forces that cause that movement. The human skeleton is, quite literally, a system of segments or levers. Although bones are not truly rigid, we

A

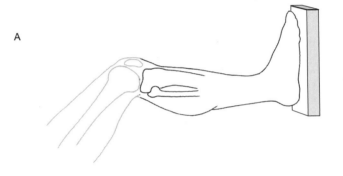

B

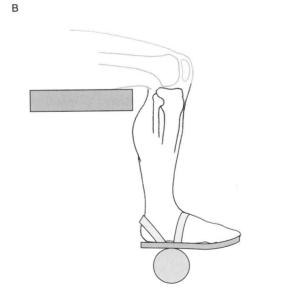

▲ **Figure 1-2** ▪ **A.** Schematic representation of the leg-foot segment in the leg-press exercise, with the leg-foot segment highlighted for emphasis. **B.** Schematic representation of the leg-foot segment in the weight boot exercise, with the leg-foot segment highlighted for emphasis.

will assume that bones behave as rigid levers. There are five kinematic variables that fully describe motion or displacement of a segment: (1) the type of displacement (motion), (2) the location in space of the displacement, (3) the direction of displacement of the segment, (4) the magnitude of the displacement, and (5) the rate of displacement or rate of change of displacement (velocity or acceleration).

Types of Displacement

Translatory and rotatory motions are the two basic types of movement that can be attributed to any rigid segment. Additional types of movement are achieved by combinations of these two.

■ Translatory Motion

Translatory motion (linear displacement) is the movement of a segment in a straight line. In true translatory motion, each point on the segment moves through the same distance, at the same time, in parallel paths. In human movement, translatory movements are generally approximations of this definition. An example of translatory motion of a body segment is the movement of the combined forearm-hand segment as it moves forward to grasp an object (Fig. 1-3). This example assumes, however, that the forearm-hand segment is free and unconstrained—that is, that the forearm-hand segment is not linked to the humerus. Although it is easiest to describe pure translatory motion by using the example of an isolated and unconstrained segment,

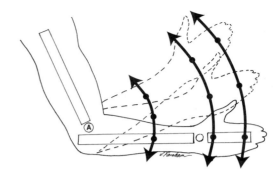

▲ **Figure 1-4** ■ Rotatory motion. Each point in the forearm-hand segment moves through the same angle, in the same time, at a constant distance from the center of rotation or axis (A).

segments of the body are neither isolated nor unconstrained. Every segment is linked to at least one other segment, and most human motion occurs as movement of more than one segment at a time. The translation of the forearm-hand segment in Figure 1-3 is actually produced by motion of the humerus, with rotation occurring at both the shoulder and the elbow joints. In fact, translation of a body segment rarely occurs in human motion without some concomitant rotation of that segment (even if the rotation is barely visible).

■ Rotatory Motion

Rotatory motion (angular displacement) is movement of a segment around a fixed axis (**center of rotation [CoR]**) in a curved path. In true rotatory motion, each point on the segment moves through the same angle, at the same time, at a constant distance from the CoR. True rotatory motion can occur only if the segment is prevented from translating and is forced to rotate about a fixed axis. This does not happen in human movement. In the example in Figure 1-4, all points on the forearm-hand segment appear to move through the same distance at the same time around what appears to be a fixed axis. In actuality, none of the body segments move around truly fixed axes; all joint axes shift at least slightly during motion because segments are not sufficiently constrained to produce pure rotation.

■ General Motion

When nonsegmented objects are moved, combinations of rotation and translation (**general motion**) are common and can be very evident. If someone were to attempt to push a treatment table across the room by using one hand, it would be difficult to get the table to go straight (translatory motion); it would be more likely to both translate and rotate. When rotatory and translatory motions are combined, a number of terms can be used to describe the result.

Curvilinear (plane or **planar) motion** designates a combination of translation and rotation of a segment in *two dimensions* (parallel to a plane with a maximum of three degrees of freedom).[2-4] When this type of motion occurs, the axis about which the segment moves is not fixed but, rather, shifts in space as the object moves.

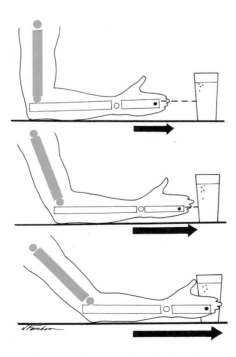

▲ **Figure 1-3** ■ Translatory motion. Each point on the forearm-hand segment moves through the same distance, at the same time, in parallel paths.

The axis around which the segment appears to move in any part of its path is referred to as the **instantaneous center of rotation (ICoR)**, or **instantaneous axis of rotation (IaR)**. An object or segment that travels in a curvilinear path may be considered to be undergoing rotatory motion around a fixed but quite distant CoR[3,4]; that is, the curvilinear path can be considered a segment of a much larger circle with a distant center.

Three-dimensional motion is a general motion in which the segment moves across all three dimensions. Just as curvilinear motion can be considered to occur around a single distant CoR, three-dimensional motion can be considered to be occurring around a **helical axis of motion (HaM)**, or **screw axis of motion**.[3]

As already noted, motion of a body segment is rarely sufficiently constrained by the ligamentous, muscular, or other bony forces acting on it to produce pure rotatory motion. Instead, there is typically at least a small amount of translation (and often a secondary rotation) that accompanies the primary rotatory motion of a segment at a joint. Most joint rotations, therefore, take place around a series of ICoRs. The "axis" that is generally ascribed to a given joint motion (e.g., knee flexion) is typically a midpoint among these ICoRs rather than the true CoR. Because most body segments actually follow a curvilinear path, the true CoR is the point around which true rotatory motion of the segment would occur and is generally quite distant from the joint.[3,4]

Location of Displacement in Space

The rotatory or translatory displacement of a segment is commonly located in space by using the three-dimensional Cartesian coordinate system, borrowed from mathematics, as a useful frame of reference. The origin of the x-axis, y-axis, and z-axis of the coordinate system is traditionally located at the **center of mass (CoM)** of the human body, assuming that the body is in **anatomic position** (standing facing forward, with palms forward) (Fig. 1-5). According to the common system described by Panjabi and White, the x-axis runs side to side in the body and is labeled in the body as the **coronal axis;** the y-axis runs up and down in the body and is labeled in the body as the **vertical axis;** the z-axis runs front to back in the body and is labeled in the body as the **anteroposterior (A-P) axis**.[3] Motion of a segment can occur either *around* an axis (rotation) or *along* an axis (translation). An unconstrained segment can either rotate or translate around each of the three axes, which results in six potential options for motion of that segment. The options for movement of a segment are also referred to as **degrees of freedom.** A completely unconstrained segment, therefore, always has six degrees of freedom. Segments of the body, of course, are not unconstrained. A segment may appear to be limited to only one degree of freedom (although, as already pointed out, this rarely is strictly true), or all six degrees of freedom may be available to it.

Rotation of a body segment is described not only as occurring around one of three possible axes but also as

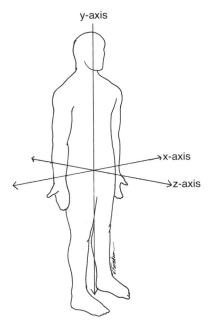

▲ **Figure 1-5** ■ Body in anatomic position showing the x-axis, y-axis, and z-axis of the Cartesian coordinate system (the coronal, vertical, and anteroposterior axes, respectively).

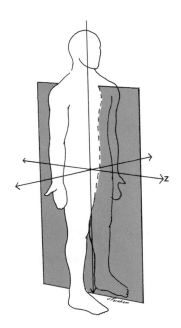

▲ **Figure 1-6** ■ The sagittal plane.

moving in or parallel to one of three possible **cardinal planes.** As a segment rotates *around* a particular axis, the segment also moves in a plane that is both perpendicular to that axis of rotation and parallel to another axis. Rotation of a body segment *around* the x-axis or coronal axis occurs in the **sagittal plane** (Fig. 1-6). Sagittal plane motions are most easily visualized as front-to-back motions of a segment (e.g., flexion/extension of the upper extremity at the glenohumeral joint).

Rotation of a body segment *around* the y-axis or vertical axis occurs in the **transverse plane** (Fig. 1-7).

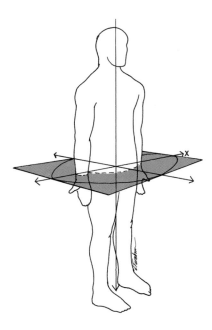

▲ **Figure 1-7** ■ The transverse plane.

Transverse plane motions are most easily visualized as motions of a segment parallel to the ground (medial/lateral rotation of the lower extremity at the hip joint). Transverse plane motions often occur around axes that pass through the length of long bones that are not truly vertically oriented. Consequently, the term **longitudinal** (or **long**) **axis** is often used instead of vertical axis. Rotation of a body segment *around* the z-axis or A-P axis occurs in the **frontal plane** (Fig. 1-8). Frontal plane motions are most easily visualized as side-to-side motions

of the segment (e.g., abduction/adduction of the upper extremity at the glenohumeral joint).

Rotation and translation of body segments are not limited to motion along or around cardinal axes or within cardinal planes. In fact, cardinal plane motions are the exception rather than the rule and, although useful, are an oversimplification of human motion. If a motion (whether in or around a cardinal axis or plane) is limited to rotation around a single axis *or* translatory motion along a single axis, the motion is considered to have one degree of freedom. Much more commonly, a segment moves in three dimensions with two or more degrees of freedom. The following examples demonstrate three of the many different ways in which rotatory and translatory motions along or around one or more axes can combine in human movement to produce two- and three-dimensional segmental motion.

Example 1-1

When the forearm-hand segment and a glass (all considered as one rigid segment) are brought to the mouth (Fig. 1-9), rotation of the segment around an axis and translation of that segment through space occur simultaneously. As the forearm-hand segment and glass rotate around a coronal axis at the elbow joint (one degree of freedom), the shoulder joint also rotates to translate the forearm-hand segment forward in space along the forearm-hand segment's A-P axis (one degree of freedom). By combining the two degrees of freedom, the elbow joint axis (the ICoR for flexion of the forearm-hand segment) does not remain fixed but moves in space; the glass attached to the forearm-hand segment moves through a curvilinear path.

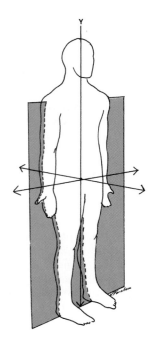

▲ **Figure 1-8** ■ The frontal plane.

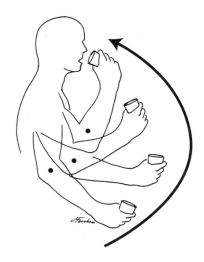

▲ **Figure 1-9** ■ The forearm-hand segment rotates around a coronal axis at the elbow joint and along A-P axis (through rotation at the shoulder joint), using two degrees of freedom that result in a moving axis of rotation and produce curvilinear motion of the fprearm-hand segment.

Example 1-2

With the forearm-hand and glass still being considered as one rigid segment, the glass is now taken away from the mouth while also being turned over and emptied. This combined motion involves pronation of the forearm-hand segment as an additional degree of freedom while the forearm-hand segment rotates (extends) around a coronal axis at the elbow joint, and the segment again translates backward in space. The three-dimensional motion could be described by a single helical axis of rotation but is more commonly thought of as having sequential ICoRs.

Example 1-3

Continuing to use the forearm-hand segment and glass example, assume that the glass begins in the same position as in Figure 1-9. This time, however, the forearm-hand segment is moved *exclusively* by the biceps brachii; the humerus is *fixed in space,* thus eliminating the translatory component of forearm-hand motion. The biceps brachii both flexes the forearm-hand around a coronal axis and simultaneously supinates the forearm-hand segment around a longitudinal axis. The three-dimensional nature of the motion would be evident because the glass would miss the mouth and, instead, empty onto the shoulder. Panjabi and White[3] used the term main (or primary) motion to refer to the motion of forearm-hand flexion and the term **coupled** (or secondary) **motion** to refer to the motion of forearm-hand supination.

Direction of Displacement

Even if displacement of a segment is confined to a single axis, the rotatory or translatory motion of a segment around or along that axis can occur in two different directions. For rotatory motions, the direction of movement of a segment around an axis can be described as occurring in a clockwise or counterclockwise direction. Clockwise and counterclockwise rotations are generally assigned negative and positive signs, respectively.[5] However, these terms are dependent on the perspective of the viewer (viewed from the left side, flexing the forearm is a clockwise movement; if the subject turns around and faces the opposite direction, the same movement is now seen by the viewer as a counterclockwise movement). Anatomic terms describing human movement are independent of viewer perspective and, therefore, more useful clinically. Because there are two directions of rotation (positive and negative) around each of the three cardinal axes, we can describe three pairs of (or six different) anatomic rotations available to body segments.

Flexion and **extension** are motions of a segment occurring around the same axis and in the same plane (uniaxial or uniplanar) but in opposite directions. Flexion and extension generally occur in the sagittal plane around a coronal axis, although exceptions exist (carpometacarpal flexion and extension of the thumb). Anatomically, flexion is the direction of segmental rotation that brings ventral surfaces of adjacent segments closer together, whereas extension is the direction of segmental rotation that brings dorsal surfaces closer together. [*Side-bar:* Defining flexion and extension by ventral and dorsal surfaces makes use of the true embryologic origin of the words ventral and dorsal, rather than using these terms as synonymous with anterior and posterior, respectively.]

Abduction and **adduction** of a segment occur around the same axis and in the same plane but in opposite directions. Abduction/adduction and lateral flexion generally occur in the frontal plane around an A-P axis, although carpometacarpal abduction and adduction of the thumb again serve as an exception. Anatomically, abduction is the direction of segmental rotation that brings the segment away from the midline of the body, whereas adduction brings the segment toward the midline of the body. When the moving segment *is* part of the midline of the body (e.g., the trunk and the head), the rotatory movement is commonly termed **lateral flexion** (to the right or to the left).

Medial (or **internal**) **rotation** and **lateral** (or **external**) **rotation** are opposite motions of a segment that generally occur around a vertical (or longitudinal) axis in the transverse plane. Anatomically, medial rotation occurs as the segment moves parallel to the ground and toward the midline, whereas lateral rotation occurs opposite to that. When the segment is part of the midline (e.g., the head or trunk), rotation in the transverse plane is simply called rotation to the right or rotation to the left. The exceptions to the general rules for naming motions must be learned on a joint-by-joint basis.

As is true for rotatory motions, translatory motions of a segment can occur in one of two directions along any of the three axes. Again by convention, linear displacement of a segment along the x-axis is considered positive when displacement is to the right and negative when to the left. Linear displacement of a segment up along the y-axis is considered positive, and such displacement down along the y-axis is negative. Linear displacement of a segment forward (anterior) along the z-axis is positive, and such displacement backward (posterior) is negative.[1]

Magnitude of Displacement

The magnitude of rotatory motion (or angular displacement) of a segment can be given either in degrees (**United States [US]** units) or in radians (**International System of Units [SI units]**). If an object rotates through a complete circle, it has moved through 360°, or 6.28 radians. A radian is literally the ratio of an arc to the radius of its circle (Fig. 1-10). One radian is equal to 57.3°; 1° is equal to 0.01745 radians. The magnitude of rotatory motion that a body segment moves through or

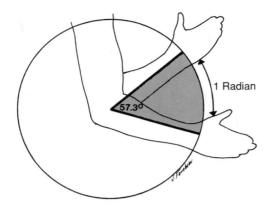

▲ **Figure 1-10** ■ An angle of 57.3° describes an arc of 1 radian.

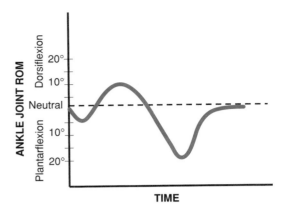

▲ **Figure 1-11** ■ When a joint's range of motion is plotted on the y-axis (vertical axis) and time is plotted on the x-axis (horizontal axis), the resulting time-series plot portrays the change in joint position over time. The slope of the plotted line reflects the velocity of the joint change.

can move through is known as its **range of motion** (**ROM**). The most widely used standardized clinical method of measuring available joint ROM is goniometry, with units given in degrees. Consequently, we typically will use degrees in this text to identify angular displacements (rotatory motions). ROM may be measured and stored on computer for analysis by an electrogoniometer or a three-dimensional motion analysis system, but these are available predominantly in research environments. Although we will not be addressing instruments, procedures, technologic capabilities, or limitations of these systems, data collected by these sophisticated instrumentation systems are often the basis of research cited through the text.

Translatory motion or displacement of a segment is quantified by the linear distance through which the object or segment is displaced. The units for describing translatory motions are the same as those for length. The SI system's unit is the meter (or millimeter or centimeter); the corresponding unit in the US system is the foot (or inch). This text will use the SI system but includes a US conversion when this appears to facilitate understanding. Linear displacements of the entire body are often measured clinically. For example, the 6-minute walk[6] (a test of functional status in individuals with cardiorespiratory problems) measures the distance (in feet or meters) someone walks in 6 minutes. Smaller full body or segment displacements can also be measured by three-dimensional motion analysis systems.

Rate of Displacement

Although the magnitude of displacement is important, the rate of change in position of the segment (the displacement per unit time) is equally important. Displacement per unit time regardless of direction is known as **speed**, whereas displacement per unit time in a given direction is known as **velocity**. If the velocity is changing over time, the change in velocity per unit time is **acceleration**. Linear velocity (velocity of a translating segment) is expressed as meters per second (m/sec) in SI units or feet per second (ft/sec) in US units; the corresponding units for acceleration are

meters per second squared (m/sec^2) and feet per second squared (ft/sec^2). Angular velocity (velocity of a rotating segment) is expressed as degrees per second (deg/sec), whereas angular acceleration is given as degrees per second squared (deg/sec^2).

An electrogoniometer or a three-dimensional motion analysis system allows documentation of the changes in displacement over time. The outputs of such systems are increasingly encountered when summaries of displacement information are presented. A computer-generated time-series plot such as that in Figure 1-11 graphically portrays not only the angle between two bony segments (or the rotation of one segment in space) at each point in time but also the direction of motion. The steepness of the slope of the graphed line represents the angular velocity. Figure 1-12 shows a plot of the change in linear acceleration of a body segment (or a point on the body segment) over time without regard to changes in joint angle.

◆ Introduction to Forces

Definition of Forces

Kinematic descriptions of human movement permit us to visualize motion but do not give us an understanding of why the motion is occurring. This requires a study of forces. Whether a body or body segment is in motion or at rest depends on the forces exerted on that body. A **force,** simplistically speaking, is a push or a pull exerted by one object or substance on another. Any time two objects make contact, they will either push on each other or pull on each other with some magnitude of force (although the magnitude may be small enough to be disregarded). The unit for a force (a push or a pull) in the SI system is the **newton** (**N**); the unit in the US system is the **pound** (**lb**). The concept of a force as a push or pull can readily be used to describe the forces encountered in evaluating human motion.

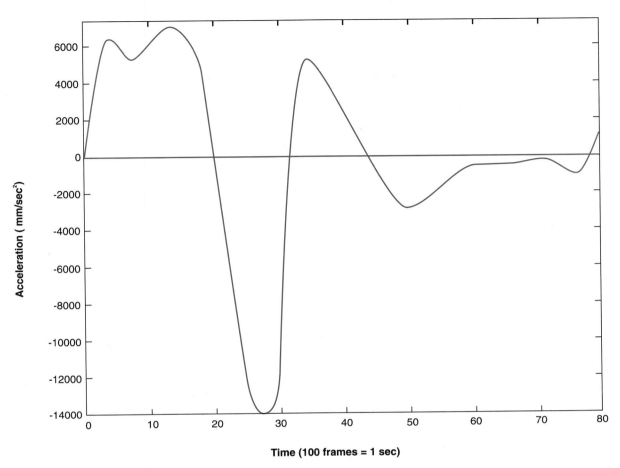

Acceleration (mm/sec²)

Time (100 frames = 1 sec)

▲ **Figure 1-12** ■ Movement of a point on a segment can be displayed by plotting acceleration of the segment (y-axis) over time (x-axis). The slope and trend of the line represent increases or decreases in magnitude of acceleration as the movement continues. [Courtesy of Fetters, L: Boston University, 2003.]

Continuing Exploration: **A Force**

Although a force is most simply described as a push or a pull, it is also described as a "theoretical concept" because only its effects (acceleration) can be measured.[4] Consequently, a force (F) is described by the acceleration (a) of the object to which the force is applied, with the acceleration being directly proportional to the mass (m) of that object; that is,

$$\text{force} = (\text{mass})(\text{acceleration})$$

$$\text{or } F = (m)(a)$$

Because mass is measured in kilograms (kg) and acceleration in m/sec^2, the unit for force is actually $kg\text{-}m/sec^2$ or, more simply, the newton; that is, a newton is the force required to accelerate 1 kg at 1 m/sec^2 (the pound is correspondingly the amount of force required to accelerate a mass of 1 slug [to be described] at 1 ft/sec^2).

External forces are pushes or pulls on the body that arise from sources outside the body. **Gravity (g)**, the attraction of the Earth's mass to another mass, is an external force that under normal conditions constantly affects all objects. The weight (W) of an object is the pull of gravity on the object's mass with an acceleration of 9.8 m/sec^2 (or 32.2 ft/sec^2) in the absence of any resistance:

$$\text{weight} = (\text{mass})(\text{gravity})$$

$$\text{or } W = (m)(g)$$

Because weight is a force, the appropriate unit is the newton (or pound). However, it is not uncommon to see weight given in **kilograms (kg)**, although the kilogram is more correctly a unit of mass. In the US system, the pound is commonly used to designate mass when it is appropriately a force unit. The correct unit for mass in the US system is the infrequently used **slug** (1 slug = 14.59 kg).

Continuing Exploration: **Force and Mass Unit Terminology**

Force and mass units are often used incorrectly in the vernacular. The average person using the metric system expects a produce scale to show weight in kilograms, rather than in newtons. In the United States, the average person appropriately thinks of weight in pounds but also considers the pound to be a unit of mass. Because people commonly tend to think of mass in terms of weight (the force of gravity acting on the mass of an object) and because the slug is an unfamiliar unit to most people, the pound is often used to represent the mass of an object in the US system.

One attempt to maintain common usage but to clearly differentiate force units from mass units for scientific purposes is to designate lb and kg as mass units and to designate the corresponding force units as lbf (pound-force) and kgf (kilogram-force).[3,4] When the kilogram is used as a force unit:

$$1 \text{ kgf} = 9.8 \text{ N}$$

When the pound is used as a mass unit:

$$1 \text{ pound} = 0.031 \text{ slugs}$$

These conversions assume an unresisted acceleration of gravity of 9.8 m/sec^2 or 32.2 ft/sec^2, respectively.

The distinction between a measure of mass and a measure of force is important because mass is a scalar quantity (without action line or direction), whereas the newton and pound are measures of force and have vector characteristics. In this text, we will consistently use the terms "newton" and "pound" as force units and will use the terms "kilogram" and "slug" as the corresponding mass units.

Because gravity is the most consistent of the forces encountered by the body, gravity should be the first force to be considered when the potential forces acting on a body segment are identified. However, gravity is only one of an infinite number of external forces that can affect the body and its segments. Examples of other external forces that may exert a push or pull on the human body or its segments are wind (push of air on the body), water (push of water on the body), other people (the push or pull of an examiner on Sam Alexander's leg), and other objects (the push of floor on the feet, the pull of a weight boot on the leg). A critical point is that the forces on the body or any one segment must come from something that is touching the body or segment. The major exception to this rule is the force of gravity. However, if permitted the conceit that gravity (the pull of the earth) "contacts" all objects on earth, we can circumvent this exception and make it a standing rule that *all forces on a segment must come from something that is contacting that segment* (including gravity). The obverse also holds true: that *anything that contacts a segment must create a force on that segment*, although the magnitude may be small enough to disregard.

Concept Cornerstone 1-1: *Primary Rule of Forces*

- All forces on a segment *must* come from something that is contacting that segment.
- Anything that contacts a segment *must* create a force on that segment (although the magnitude may be small enough to disregard).
- Gravity can be considered to be "touching" all objects.

Internal forces are forces that act on structures of the body and arise from the body's own structures (that is, the contact of two structures within the body). A few common examples are the forces produced by the muscles (pull of the biceps brachii on the radius), the ligaments (pull of a ligament on bone), and the bones (the push of one bone on another bone at a joint). Some forces, such as atmospheric pressure (the push of air pressure), work both inside and outside the body, but—in our definition—are considered external forces because the source is not a body structure.

External forces can either facilitate or restrict movement. Internal forces are most readily recognized as essential for *initiation* of movement. However, it should be apparent that internal forces also control or counteract movement produced by external forces, as well as counteracting other internal forces. Much of the presentation and discussion in subsequent chapters of this text relate to the interactive role of internal forces, not just in causing movement but also in maintaining the integrity of joint structures against the effects of external forces and other internal forces.

Force Vectors

All forces, despite the source or the object acted on, are **vector** quantities. A force is represented by an arrow that (1) has its base on the object being acted on (the point of application), (2) has a shaft and arrowhead in the direction of the force being exerted and at an angle to the object acted on (direction/orientation), and (3) has a length drawn to represent the amount of force being exerted (magnitude). As we begin to examine force vectors (and at least throughout this chapter), the *point of application* (*base*) of each vector in each figure will be placed on the segment or object to which the force is applied—which is generally also the object under discussion.

Figure 1-13 shows Sam Alexander's leg-foot segment. The weight boot is shaded in lightly for context but is not really part of the space diagram. Because the weight boot makes contact with the leg-foot segment, the weight boot must exert a force (in this case, a pull) on the segment. The force, called weightboot-on-legfoot, is represented by vector WbLf. The point of application is on the leg (closest to where the weight boot exerts its pull); the action line and direction indicate the direction of the pull and the angle of pull in relation to the leg; and the length is drawn to represent the magnitude of the pull. The force weightboot-on-legfoot is an external force because the weight boot is not part of the body, although it contacts the body. Figure 1-14 shows the force of a muscle (e.g., the brachialis) pulling on the forearm-hand segment. The point of application is at the attachment of the muscle, and the orientation and direction are toward the muscle (pulls are toward the source of the force) and at an angle to the segment. The force is called muscle-on-forearmhand (represented by the vector MFh). Although the designation of a force as "external" or "internal" may be useful in some contexts, the rules for drawing (or visualizing) forces

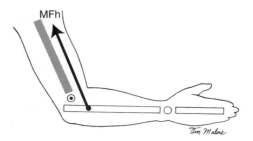

▲ **Figure 1-14** ■ Vector MFh represents the pull of a muscle on the forearm-hand segment.

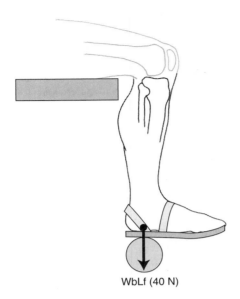

WbLf (40 N)

▲ **Figure 1-13** ■ Vector representation of the pull of the weight boot on the leg-foot segment (weightboot-on-legfoot [WbLf]), with a magnitude proportional to the mass and equivalent to the weight of the apparatus.

are the same for external forces such as the weight boot and for internal forces such as the muscle.

The length of a vector is usually drawn proportional to the magnitude of the force according to a given scale. For example, if the scale is specified as 5 mm = 20 N of force, an arrow of 10 mm would represent 40 N of force. The length of a vector, however, does not necessarily need to be drawn to scale (unless a graphic solution is desired) as long as its magnitude is labeled (as is done in Fig. 1-13). Graphically, the action line of any vector can be considered infinitely long; that is, any vector can be extended in either direction (at the base or at the arrowhead) if this is useful in determining the relationship of the vector to other vectors or objects. The length of a vector should not be arbitrarily drawn, however, if a scale has been specified.

Continuing Exploration: **Pounds and Newtons**

Although SI units are commonly used mostly in scientific writing, the SI unit of force—the newton—does not have much of a context for those of us habituated to the US system. It is useful, therefore, to understand that 1 lb = 4.448 N. Vector WbLf in Figure 1-13 is labeled as 40 N. This converts to 8.99 lb. To get a gross idea of the pound equivalent of any figure given in newtons, you can divide the number of newtons by 5, understanding that you will be *underestimating* the actual number of pound equivalents.

Figure 1-15A shows Sam Alexander's leg-foot segment on the leg-press machine. The footplate is shaded in lightly for context but is not really part of the space diagram. Because the footplate is contacting the leg-

foot segment, it must exert—in this case—a *push* on the segment. The force, footplate-on-legfoot, is represented by vector FpLf with a point of application on the leg-foot segment and in a direction away from the source. The magnitude of FpLf will remain unspecified until we have more information. However, the presence of the vector in the space diagram means that the force does, in fact, have some magnitude. Although the force is applied at the point where the footplate makes contact with the foot, the point of application can also be drawn anywhere *along the action of the vector* as long as the point of application (for purposes of visualization) remains on the object under consideration. Just as a vector can be extended to any length, the point of application can appear anywhere along the line of push or pull of the force (as long as it is on the same object) without changing the represented effect of the force (see Fig. 1-15B). In this text, the point of application will be placed as close to the actual point of contact as possible but may be shifted slightly along the action line for clarity when several forces are drawn together.

It is common to see in other physics and biomechanics texts a "push"' force represented as shown in Figure 1-15C. However, this chapter will consistently use the convention that the *base* of the vector will be at the point of application, with the "push" being away from that point of application (see Fig. 1-15A). This convention maintains the focus on the *point of application* on the segment and will enhance visualization later when we begin to resolve a vector into components. When the "push" of "footplate-on-legfoot" is drawn with its base (point of application) on the object (see Fig. 1–15A), the representation is similar in all respects (except name) to the force "strap-on-legfoot," shown as vector SLf in Figure 1-16. Vector SLf, however, is the *pull* of the strap connected to either side of the leg-foot segment. It is reasonable for vector FpLf in Figure 1-15A and vector SLf in Figure 1-16 to look the same because the two forces "footplate-on-legfoot" and "strap-on-legfoot" will have an identical effect as long on the rigid leg-foot segment as the point of application, direction/orientation, and magnitude are similar—as they are here. The magnitude and direction/orientation of a force are what affect the object to which the force is applied, without consideration of whether the force is, in fact, a push or a pull.

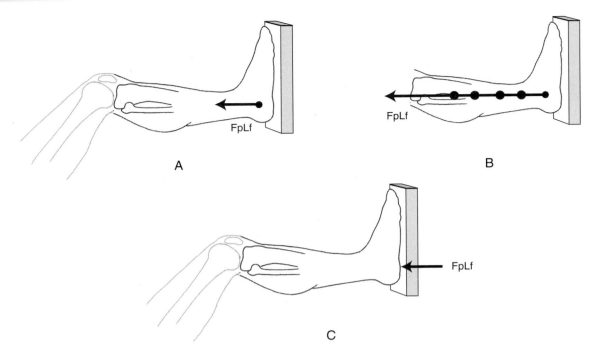

FpLf

A

FpLf

B

FpLf

C

▲ **Figure 1-15** ■ **A.** Vector representation of the force of the footplate of the leg-press machine on the leg-foot segment (footplate-on-leg-foot [FpLf]). **B.** The vector footplate-on-legfoot (FpLf) may be drawn with any length and with a point of application anywhere along the line of pull of the vector as long as the point of application remains on the leg-foot segment. **C.** The push of the footplate on the leg-foot segment is commonly shown elsewhere by placing the arrowhead of vector FpLf at the point of application.

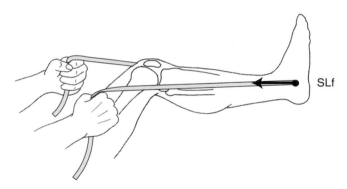

SLf

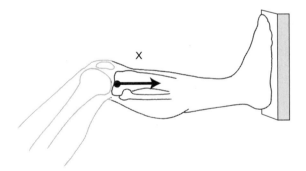

X

▲ **Figure 1-16** ■ The vector representing the pull of a strap connected to each side of the legfoot (strap-on-legfoot [SLf]) will look the same as the push of the footplate on the leg-foot segment (Fig. 1-15A) because both have identical effects on the leg-foot segment as long as the direction and magnitude are the same.

▲ **Figure 1-17** ■ An unknown vector (X) can be named by identifying the segment to which it is applied and the source of the force (something that must be touching the segment).

 CONCEPT CORNERSTONE 1-2: *Force Vectors Are Characterized By:*

■ a point of application *on the object acted upon.*
■ an action line and direction/orientation indicating a *pull toward* the source object or a *push away from* the source object, at a given angle to the object acted upon.
■ length that represents and may be drawn proportional to its magnitude (the quantity of push or pull).
■ a length that may be extended to assess the relation between two or more vectors or to assess the relation of the vector to adjacent objects or points.

 CONCEPT CORNERSTONE 1-3: *Naming Forces*

We have already begun to establish the naming convention of *"something-on-something"* to identify forces and label vectors. The first part of the force name will always identify the *source* of the force; the second part of the force name will always identify the object or segment that is *being acted on.*

Figure 1-17 shows Sam Alexander's leg-foot segment on the leg-press machine. A new vector is shown in this figure. Because vector X is applied to the leg-foot segment, the vector is named *"blank-on-legfoot."* The name of the vector is completed by identifying the source of the force. The leg-foot segment is being contacted by gravity, by the footplate, and by the femur. We can eliminate gravity as the source because gravity is always in a downward direction. The footplate can only push on the leg-foot segment, and so the vector is in the wrong direction. The femur will also push on the leg-foot segment because a bone cannot pull. Because vector X is directed away from the femur, the femur appears to be the source of vector X in Figure 1-17. Therefore, vector X is named femur-on-legfoot and can be labeled vector FLf.

Force of Gravity

As already noted, gravity is one of the most consistent and influential forces that the human body encounters in posture and movement. For that reason, it is useful to consider gravity first when examining the properties of forces. As a vector quantity, the force of gravity can be fully described by point of application, action line/direction/orientation, and magnitude. Unlike other forces that may act on point or limited area of contact, gravity acts on each unit of mass that composes an object. For simplicity, however, the force of gravity acting on an object or segment is considered to have its point of application at the CoM or **center of gravity** (**CoG**) of that object or segment—the hypothetical point at which all the mass of the object or segment appear to be concentrated. Every object or segment can be considered to have a single CoM.

In a symmetrical object, the CoM is located in the geometric center of the object (Fig. 1-18A). In an asymmetrical object, the CoM will be located toward the heavier end because the mass must be evenly distributed around the CoM (see Fig. 1-18B). The crutch in Figure 1-18C demonstrates that the CoM is only a hypothetical point; it need not lie within the object being acted on. Even when the CoM lies outside the object, it

is still the point from which the force of gravity *appears* to act. The actual location of the CoM of any object can be determined experimentally by a number of methods not within the scope of this text. However, the CoM of an object can be approximated by thinking of the CoM as the balance point of the object (assuming you could balance the object on one finger) as shown in Figure 1-18A to C.

Although the direction and orientation of most forces vary with the source of the force, the force of gravity acting on an object is *always* vertically downward toward the center of the earth. The gravitational vector is commonly referred to as the **line of gravity** (**LoG**). The length of the LoG can be drawn to scale (as in a free body diagram, in which the length is determined by its magnitude) or it may be extended (like any vector) when the relationship of the vector to other forces, points, or objects is being explored. The LoG can best be visualized as a string with a weight on the end (a plumb line), with the string tied or attached to the CoM of the object. A plumb line applied to the CoM of an object gives an accurate representation of the point of application, direction, and orientation of the force of gravity on an object or segment, although not its magnitude.

■ Segmental Centers of Mass and Composition of Gravitational Forces

Each segment in the body can be considered to have its own CoM and LoG. Figure 1-19A shows the gravitational vectors (LoGs) acting at the CoMs of the arm, the forearm, and the hand segments (vectors GA, GF, and GH, respectively). The CoMs in Figure 1-19A approximate those identified in studies done on cadavers and on *in vivo* body segments that have yielded standardized data on centers of mass and weights of individual and combined body segments.[1] It is often useful, however, to consider two or more segments as if they were a single segment or object and to treat them as if they are

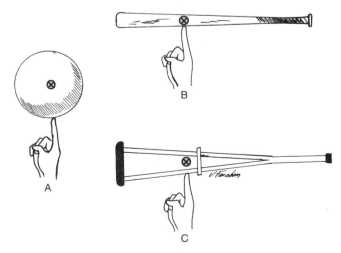

▲ **Figure 1-18** ■ **A.** Center of mass of a symmetrical object. **B.** Center of mass of an asymmetrical object. **C.** The center of mass may lie outside the object.

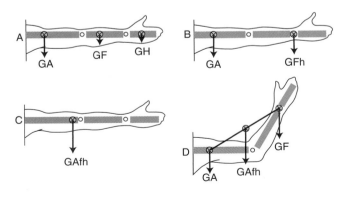

▲ **Figure 1-19** ■ **A.** Gravity acting on the arm segment (GA), the forearm segment (GF), and the hand segment (GH). **B.** Gravity acting on the arm and forearm-hand segments (GFh). **C.** Gravity acting on the arm-forearm-hand segment (GAfh). **D.** The CoM of the arm-forearm-hand segment shifts when segments are rearranged.

going to move together as a single rigid segment (such as the leg-foot segment in the patient case). When two gravity vectors acting on the same (now larger) rigid object are composed into one gravitational vector, the new common point of application (the new CoM) is located between and in line with the original two segmental CoMs. When the linked segments are not equal in mass, the new CoM will lie closer to the heavier segment. The new vector will have the same effect on the combined forearm-hand segment as the original two vectors and is known as the **resultant force**. The process of combining two or more forces into a single resultant force is known as **composition of forces.**

Example 1-4

If we wish to treat two adjacent segments (e.g., the forearm and the hand segments) as if these were one rigid segment, the two gravitational vectors (GH and GF) acting on the new larger segment (forearm-hand) can be combined into a single gravitational vector (GFh) applied at the new CoM. Figure 1-19B shows vector GA on the arm and new vector GFh on the now combined forearm-hand segment. Vector GFh is applied at the new CoM for the combined forearm-hand segment (on a line between the original CoMs), is directed vertically downward (as were both GF and GH), and has a magnitude equal to the sum of the magnitudes of GF and GH. Figure 1-19C shows the force of gravity (GAfh) acting on the rigid arm-forearm-hand segment. Vector GAfh is applied at the new CoM located between and in line with the CoMs of vectors GA and GFh; the magnitude of GAfh is equal to the sum of the magnitudes of GA and GFh; the direction of GAfh is vertically downward because it is still the pull of gravity and because that is the direction of the original vectors.

The CoM for any one object or rigid series of segments will remain unchanged regardless of the position of that object in space. However, when an object is composed of two or more linked and movable segments, the location of the CoM of the combined unit will change if the segments are rearranged in relation to each other. The *magnitude* of the force of gravity will not change because the mass of the combined segments is unchanged, but the point of application of the resultant force will be different. A more precise method for mathematically composing two gravitational forces into a single resultant force will be addressed later when other attributes of the forces (the torque that each generates) are used to identify the exact position of the new CoM between the original two CoMs.

■ Center of Mass of the Human Body

When all the segments of the body are combined and considered as a single rigid object in anatomic position, the CoM of the body lies approximately anterior to the second sacral vertebra (S2) (Fig. 1-20). The precise

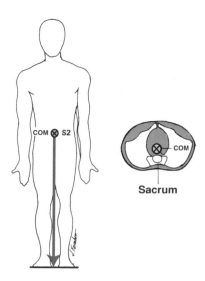

▲ **Figure 1-20** ■ The CoM of the human body lies approximately at S2, anterior to the sacrum (inset). The extended LoG lies within the BoS.

location of the CoM for a person in anatomic position depends on the proportions (weight distribution) of that person. If a person really were a rigid object, the CoM would not change its position in the body, regardless of whether the person was standing up, lying down, or leaning forward. Although the CoM does not change its location in the rigid body as the body moves in space, the LoG changes its *relative* position or alignment within the body. In Figure 1-20, the LoG is between the person's feet (**base of support [BoS]**) as the person stands in anatomic position; the LoG is parallel to the trunk and limbs. If the person is lying down (still in anatomic position), the LoG projecting from the CoM of the body lies perpendicular to the trunk and limbs, rather than parallel as it does in the standing position. In reality, of course, a person is not rigid and does not remain in anatomic position. Rather, a person is constantly rearranging segments in relation to each other as the person moves. With each rearrangement of body segments, the location of the individual's CoM will potentially change. The amount of change in the location of the CoM depends on how disproportionately the segments are rearranged.

Example 1-5

If a person is considered to be composed of a rigid upper body (head-arms-trunk [HAT]) and a rigid lower limb segment, the CoMs for each of these two segments will typically be located approximately as shown in Figure 1-21A. The combined CoM for these two segments in anatomic position remains at S2 because the position of the body is the same as in Figure 1-20. When the trunk is inclined forward, however, the point at which the mass of the body appears to be concentrated shifts forward. The new CoM is on a line between the original two CoMs and is located toward the heavier

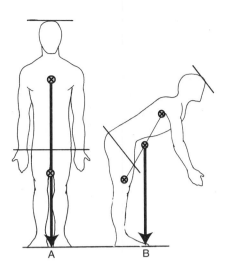

▲ **Figure 1-21** ■ **A.** Location of the CoMs of the head-arms-trunk (HAT) segment and lower limb segment. **B.** Rearrangement of segments produces a new combined CoM and a new location for the LoG in relation to the base of support.

upper body segment (Fig. 1-21B). This new CoM is physically located outside the body, with the LoG correspondingly shifted forward. Figure 1-22 shows a more disproportionate rearrangement of body segments. The CoMs of the two lower limb segments (segment A and segment B) and the CoM of the HAT segment (segment C) are composed into a new CoM located at point ABC, the point of application for the gravitational vector for the entire body (LoG = GABC).

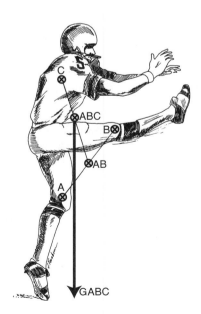

▲ **Figure 1-22** ■ CoM of the football player's left leg (A) and the right leg (B) combine to form the CoM for the lower limbs (AB). The CoM (AB) combines with the upper trunk CoM (C) to produce the CoM for the entire body (ABC). The LoG from the combined CoM falls well outside the football player's BoS. He is unstable and cannot maintain this position.

■ **Center of Mass, Line of Gravity, and Stability**

In Figure 1-22, the LoG (GABC) falls outside the football player's left toes, which serve as his BoS. The LoG has been extended (lengthened) to indicate its relationship to the football player's BoS. It must be noted that the extended vector is no longer proportional to the magnitude of the force. However, the point of application, action line, and direction remain accurate. By extending the football player's LoG in Figure 1-22, we can see that the LoG is anterior to his BoS; it would be impossible for the player to hold this pose. For an object to be stable, the *LoG must fall within the BoS*. When the LoG is outside the BoS, the object will fall. As the football player moved from a starting position of standing on both feet with his arms at his sides, two factors changed as he moved to the position in Figure 1-22. He reduced his BoS from the area between and including his two feet to the much smaller area of the toes of one foot. His CoM, with his rearrangement of segments, also has moved from S2 to above S2. Each of these two factors, combined with a slight forward lean, influenced the shift in his LoG and contributed to his instability.

When the BoS of an object is large, the LoG is less likely to be displaced outside the BoS, and the object, consequently, is more stable. When a person stands with his or her legs spread apart, the base is large side to side, and the trunk can move a good deal in that plane without displacing the LoG from the BoS and without falling over (Fig. 1-23). Whereas the CoM remains in approximately the same place as the trunk shifts to each side, the LoG moves within the wide BoS. Once again, it is useful here to think of the LoG as a plumb line. As long as the plumb line does not leave the BoS, the person should not fall over.

Figure 1-24 shows the same football player in exactly the same position as previously shown (see Fig. 1-22), with vector GABC still in front of his toes. However, it now appears that the football player can

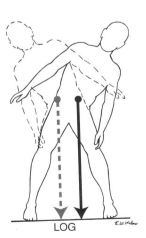

▲ **Figure 1-23** ■ A wide base of support permits a wide excursion of the line of gravity (LoG) without the LoG's falling outside the base of support.

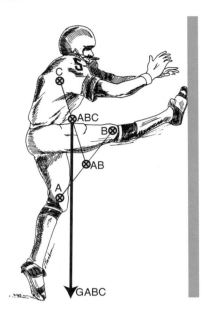

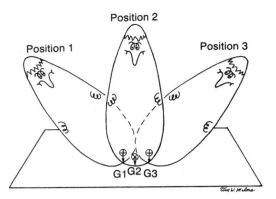

▲ **Figure 1-24** ■ The football player's segments are arranged identically to those in Figure 1-22, but by fixing his foot against the wall, he has expanded his BoS and is now stable.

▲ **Figure 1-25** ■ Given the very low CoM of the punching bag, the LoG remains within the base of support, regardless of the tipping of the bag from one position to another.

maintain the pose. This is not a violation of the rule that the LoG must fall within the BoS. Rather, the BoS has been expanded. When a person grasps or leans on another object (or another person), that object (or person) becomes part of the BoS. In Figure 1-24, the football player's BoS now includes not only his left toes but also all the space between his supporting foot and the wall he is leaning against. If the football player moves his head, arms, and trunk around, he will shift the location of the CoM as these segments are rearranged. However, he will remain stable as long as the LoG projecting from the CoM remains somewhere within the extended BoS.

When the CoM of an object is close to the supporting surface, movement of the object in space is less likely to cause the LoG to fall outside the BoS. If you hold a plumb line that is 100 cm (~3 ft) long in your hand with the weight at the end just above the ground, the plumb line can be made to swing through a wide arc over the floor with very little side-to-side movement of your hand. Conversely, a plumb line that is only 10 cm (~4 inches) long and held just above the ground will move through a much smaller arc with the same amount of side-to-side motion of your hand. If the BoS is the same size, an object with a higher CoM will be less stable than an object with a lower CoM because the longer LoG (projecting from the higher the CoM) is more likely to be displaced outside the BoS.

Figure 1-25 shows a punching bag as it moves from side to side. The base of the punching bag is filled with sand; everything above the base is air. This distribution of mass creates a CoM that nearly lies on the ground. Because the punching bag is not a segmented object, the position of the CoM within the punching bag is the same regardless of how tipped the bag might be. Even though the BoS of the punching bag is much smaller

than that of the man leaning from side to side in Figure 1-23, the punching bag can "lean" farther without falling over because it is nearly impossible to get the very short LoG in the punching bag to displace outside the BoS. With a very low CoM and a very short LoG, the punching bag is extremely stable.

 CONCEPT CORNERSTONE 1-4: *Stability of an Object or the Human Body*

- The larger the BoS of an object is, the greater is the stability of that object.
- The closer the CoM of the object is to the BoS, the more stable is the object.
- An object cannot be stable unless its LoG is located within its BoS.

■ **Alterations in Mass of an Object or Segment**

The location of the CoM of an object or the body depends on the distribution of mass of the object. The mass can be redistributed not only by rearranging linked segments in space but also by adding or taking away mass. People certainly gain weight and may gain it disproportionately in the body (thus shifting the CoM). However, the most common way conceptually (as opposed to literally) to redistribute mass in the body is to add external mass. Every time we add an object to the body by wearing it (a backpack), carrying it (a box), or using it (a power drill), the new CoM for the combined body and external mass will shift toward the additional weight; the shift will be proportional to the weight added.

Example 1-6

The man in Figure 1-26 has a cast applied to the right lower limb. Assuming the cast is now part of his mass,

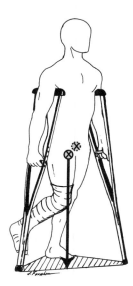

▲ **Figure 1-26** ■ The addition of the weight of the cast has shifted the CoM. The addition of crutches enlarges the base of support to the shaded area between the weight-bearing foot and crutches to improve stability.

the new CoM is located down and to the right of the original CoM at S2. Because his CoM with the cast is now lower, he is theoretically more stable. However, if he could not bear weight on his right leg, his BoS would consist only of the left foot. The patient will be stable only if he can lean to the left to swing his LoG into his left foot. However, he remains relatively unstable because of the very small BoS (it would take very little inadvertent leaning to displace the LoG outside the foot, causing the man to fall). To improve his stability, crutches have been added. The crutches and the left foot combine to form a much larger BoS, adding to the patient's stability and avoiding a large compensatory weight shift to the left.

Example 1-7

In Figure 1-27, the man is carrying a heavy box on his right shoulder. The push of the weight of the box on this shoulder girdle moves the new CoM up and to the right of S2. A LoG projecting vertically downward from the new CoM will move into the right foot (and potentially to the lateral aspect of the right foot if the box is of sufficient weight). Because this is a relatively unstable position (even a small shift of the LoG to the right will cause the LoG to be displaced outside the BoS), the man will lean to the left to "compensate." The small rearrangement of segments caused by the left leaning of the trunk does relatively little to relocate the CoM. The goal of the body shift is not to relocate the CoM but to swing the LoG back into the center of the BoS; with the LoG in the center of the BoS, any new shifts in the CoM or LoG from disturbances in position (perturbations) are less likely to displace the LoG to outside the BoS.

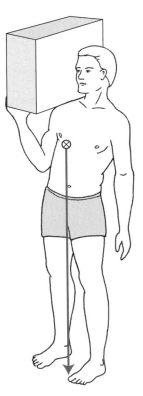

▲ **Figure 1-27** ■ The weight of the box added to the shoulder girdle causes the CoM to shift up and to the right. The man laterally leans to the left to bring the LoG back to the middle of his base of support.

◆ Introduction to Statics and Dynamics

The primary concern when looking at forces that act on the body or a particular segment is the effect that the forces will have on the body or segment. If all the forces acting on a segment are "balanced" (a state known as **equilibrium**), the segment will remain at rest or in uniform motion. If the forces are not "balanced," the segment will accelerate. **Statics** is the study of the conditions under which objects remain at rest. **Dynamics** is the study of the conditions under which objects move. Isaac Newton's first two laws will govern whether an object is static or dynamic.

Newton's Law of Inertia

Newton's first law, the **law of inertia,** identifies the conditions under which an object will be in equilibrium. **Inertia** is the property of an object that resists both the initiation of motion and a change in motion and is directly proportional to its mass. The law of inertia states that an object will remain at rest or in uniform (unchanging) motion unless acted on by an unbalanced (net or resultant) force. An object that is acted upon by balanced forces and remains motionless is in **static equilibrium.** However, an object acted upon by balanced forces may also be in uniform motion, moving with a given speed and direction. **Velocity** is a vector quantity that describes both speed and direction/orientation. An object in equilibrium can have a velocity of any magnitude (≥ 0), but that velocity remains constant. When velocity of an object is greater than 0, the object is in constant motion (**dynamic equilibrium**) that can be linear (as for translatory motion), angular (as for rotatory motion), or a combination of both (as for general motion). With regard to motion at joints of the body, dynamic equilibrium (constant velocity) of segments of the body occurs infrequently. Therefore, within the scope of this text, equilibrium will be simplified to mean an object at rest (in static equilibrium) unless otherwise specified.

Newton's law of inertia (or law of equilibrium) can be restated thus: For an object to be in equilibrium, the sum of all the forces *applied to that object* must be zero.

$$\Sigma F = 0$$

The equilibrium of an object is determined *only by forces applied to (with points of application on) that object.* There is no restriction on the number of forces that can be applied to an object in equilibrium as long as there is more than one force. If one (and only one) force is applied to an object, the sum of the forces cannot be 0. Any time the sum of the forces acting on an object is not zero ($\Sigma F \neq 0$), the object cannot be in equilibrium and must be accelerating.

Newton's Law of Acceleration

The magnitude of acceleration of a moving object is defined by Newton's second law, the **law of acceleration.** Newton's second law states that the acceleration (a) of an object is proportional to the net unbalanced (resultant) forces acting on it (F_{unbal}) and is inversely proportional to the mass (m) of that object:

$$a = \frac{F_{unbal}}{m}$$

Because an object acted upon by a net unbalanced force *must* be accelerating, it is invariably in motion or in a *dynamic state.* The acceleration of an object will be in the direction of the net unbalanced force. A net unbalanced force can produce translatory, rotatory, or general motion.

CONCEPT CORNERSTONE 1-5: *Applying the Law of Acceleration (Inertia)*

To put the law of acceleration into simple words: A large unbalanced push or pull (F_{unbal}) applied to an object of a given mass (m) will produce more acceleration (a) than an unbalanced small push or pull. Similarly, a given magnitude of unbalanced push or pull on an object of large mass will produce less acceleration than that same push or pull on an object of smaller mass. From the law of acceleration, it can be seen that inertia (a body's or object's resistance to change in velocity) is resistance to acceleration and is proportional to the mass of the body or object. The greater the mass

of an object, the greater the magnitude of net unbalanced force needed either to get the object moving or to change its motion. A very large woman in a wheelchair has more inertia than does a small woman in a wheelchair; an aide must exert a greater push on a wheelchair with a large woman in it to get the chair in motion than on the wheelchair with a small woman in it.

◆ Translatory Motion in Linear and Concurrent Force Systems

The process of composition of forces is used to determine whether a net unbalanced force (or forces) exists on a segment, because this will determine whether the segment is at rest or in motion. Furthermore, the direction/orientation and location of the net unbalanced force or forces determine the type and direction of motion of the segment. The process of composition of forces was oversimplified in Examples 1-4 and 1-5 (see Figs. 1-19 and 1-21). The process of composition depends on the relationship of the forces to each other: that is, whether the forces are in a linear, concurrent, or parallel force system.

Let us return to our case example of Sam Alexander and the weight boot. In Figure 1-13, we identified the force of weightboot-on-legfoot (WbLf) on Sam's leg-foot segment. However, Figure 1-13 must be incomplete because WbLf cannot exist alone; otherwise, the leg-foot segment would accelerate downward. We also have not yet accounted for the force of gravity. Figure 1-28 is the same figure but with the addition of a new vector: gravity-on-legfoot (GLf). Vector GLf is applied at the CoM of the leg-foot segment, is directed vertically downward, and has a magnitude proportional to the mass of the segment. The leg-foot segment typically has approximately 6.5% of the mass of the body.[1]

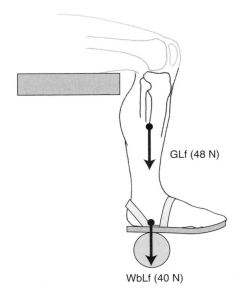

GLf (48 N)

WbLf (40 N)

▲ **Figure 1-28** ■ The forces of gravity-on-legfoot (GLf) and weightboot-on-legfoot (WbLf) are in the same linear force system when the leg-foot segment is at 90° of knee flexion.

Because Sam weighs 734 N (165 lb), his leg-foot segment will weigh about 48 N (10.8 lb). Because vectors WbLf and GLf are applied to the same segment, have action lines that lie in the same plane, and act in the same line (co-linear and coplanar), these two vectors are part of a **linear force system.**

Linear Force System

A linear force system exists whenever two or more forces act *on the same segment*, in the same plane, and in the same line (their action lines, if extended, overlap). Forces in a linear force system are assigned positive or negative signs. We will use the same convention previously described for translatory forces. Forces applied up (y-axis), forward or anterior (z-axis), or to the right (x-axis) will be assigned positive signs, whereas forces applied down, back or posterior, or to the left will be assigned negative signs. The magnitudes of vectors in opposite directions should always be assigned opposite signs.

Determining Resultant Forces in a Linear Force System

The net effect, or resultant, of all forces that are part of the same linear force system is determined by finding the arithmetic sum of the magnitudes of each of the forces in that force system (considering its positive or negative value). All forces in the *same* linear force system can be composed into a single resultant vector. The resultant vector has an action line in the same line as that of the original composing vectors, with a magnitude and direction equivalent to the arithmetic sum of the composing vectors. Because the vectors in a linear force system are all co-linear and coplanar, the point of application of the resultant vector will lie along the common action line of the composing vectors, and the resultant will have the same orientation in space as the composing vectors.

We previously assigned vector WbLf a magnitude of 40 N (~8 lb). Vectors WbLf and GLf are in the same linear force system. The resultant of the two forces, therefore, can be found by adding their magnitudes. Because both WbLf and GLf are directed down, they are assigned negative values of -40 N and -48 N, respectively. The sum of these forces is -88 N. The two forces WbLf and GLf can be represented graphically as a single resultant vector of -88 N. If Sam is not trying to lift the weight boot yet, there should be no motion of the leg-foot segment. If there is no motion (static equilibrium), the sum of the forces acting on the leg-foot segment must total zero. Instead, there is (in Fig. 1-28) a net unbalance force of -88 N; the leg-foot segment appears to be accelerating downward. In order to "balance" the net downward force, we must identify something touching the leg-foot segment that will be part of the same linear force system.

Figure 1-28 indicates that the femur is potentially touching the leg-foot segment. However, the contact of the femur would be a *push* on the leg-foot segment and, in the position shown in Figure 1-28, would be away from the femur and in the *same* direction as WbLf and GLf. Also, the net downward force of WbLf and GLf would tend to move the leg-foot segment *away* from the femur, minimizing or eliminating the contact of the femur with the leg-foot segment. A net force that moves a bony segment away from its adjacent bony segment is known as a **distraction force.** A distraction force tends to cause a separation between the bones that make up a joint. In this case, however, we still need to account for a force of 88 N acting upward on the leg-foot segment to have equilibrium.

In the human body, the two bones of a synovial joint (e.g., the knee joint) are connected by a joint capsule and ligaments made of connective tissue. Until we explore connective tissue behavior in detail in Chapter 2, capsuloligamentous structures are best visualized as string or cords with some elasticity that can "pull" (not "push") on the bones to which they attach. Figure 1-29A shows a schematic representation of the capsuloligamentous structures that join the femur and the tibia. [*Side-bar:* In reality, the capsule *surrounds* the adjacent bones, and the ligamentous connections are more complex.] We will nickname the structures "Acapsule" (anterior capsule) and "Pcapsule" (posterior capsule), understanding that these two forces are representing the pull of both the capsule and the capsular ligaments at the knee. Because capsules and ligaments can only pull, the forces that are created by the contact of Acapsule and Pcapsule in Figure 1-29A–C are directed upward toward the capsuloligamentous structures (positive). Under the assumption that the pull of the capsule anteriorly and posteriorly in this example are likely to be symmetrical, the vectors are given the same length in Figure 1-29A.

The vectors for Acapsule-on-legfoot (AcLf) and Pcapsule-on-legfoot (PcLf) are drawn in Figure 1-29A so that the point of application is at the point on the leg-foot segment where the fibers of the capsular segments converge (or in the center of the area where the fibers converge). [*Side-bar:* Although the anterior and posterior segments of the capsule also touch the femur, we are considering only the leg-foot segment at this time.] The vector arrows for the pulls of AcLf and PcLf must follow the fibers *at the point of application* and *continue in a straight line.* A vector, for any given snapshot of time, is always a straight line. The vector for the pull of the capsule does not change direction even if the fibers of the capsule change direction after the fibers emerge from their attachment to the bone.

In a linear force system, vectors must be co-linear and coplanar. Vectors AcLf and PcLf are not co-linear or coplanar with vectors WbLf and GLf. Therefore, they cannot be part of the same linear force system. If vectors AcLf and PcLf are extended slightly at their bases, the two vectors will converge (see Fig. 1-29B). When two or more vectors *applied to the same object* are not co-linear but converge (intersect), the vectors are part of a **concurrent force system.**

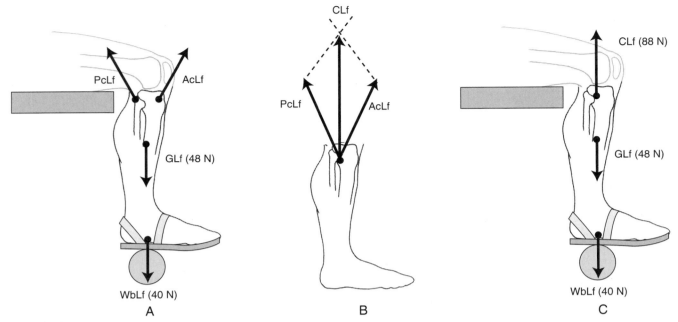

▲ **Figure 1–29** ■ **A.** Schematic representation of the pull of the anterior capsule (AcLf) and posterior capsule (PcLf) on the leg-foot segment. **B.** Determination of the direction and relative magnitude of the resultant (capsule-on-legfoot [CLf]) of concurrent forces AcLf and PcLf, through the process of composition by parallelogram. **C.** The resultant force CLf has been added to the leg-foot segment, with a magnitude equivalent to that of GLf + WbLf.

Concurrent Force System

It is quite common (and perhaps most common in the human body) for forces applied to an object to have action lines that lie at angles to each other. A common point of application may mean that the forces are literally applied to the same point on the object or that forces applied to the same object have vectors that intersect when extended in length (even if the intersection is outside the actual segment or object as we saw with the CoM). The net effect, or resultant, of concurrent forces *appears* to occur at the common point of application (or point of intersection). Any two forces in a concurrent force system can be composed into a single resultant force with a graphic process known as **composition by parallelogram.**

■ **Determining Resultant Forces in a Concurrent Force System**

In composition by parallelogram, two vectors are taken at a time. The two vectors and their common point of application or point of intersection form two sides of a parallelogram. The parallelogram is completed by drawing two additional lines at the arrowheads of the original two vectors (with each new line parallel to one of the original two). The resultant has the same point of application as the original vectors and is the diagonal of the parallelogram. If there are more than two vectors in a concurrent force system, a third vector is added to the resultant of the original two through the same process. The sequential use of the resultant and one of the original vectors continues until all the vectors in the original concurrent force system are accounted for.

In Figure 1-29B, vectors AcLf and PcLf are composed into a single resultant vector (CLf). Vectors AcLf and PcLf are extended to identify the point of application of the new resultant vector that represents the combined action of AcLf and PcLf. A parallelogram is constructed by starting at the arrowhead of one vector (AcLf) and drawing a line of relatively arbitrary length that is *parallel* to the adjacent vector (PcLf). The process is repeated by starting at the arrowhead of PcLf and drawing a line of relatively arbitrary length *parallel* to AcLf. Both the lengths of the two new lines should be long enough that the two new lines intersect. Because the two new lines are drawn parallel to the original two and intersect (thus closing the figure), a parallelogram is created (see Fig. 1-29B). The resultant of AcLf and PcLf is a new vector ("capsule-on-legfoot" [CLf]) that has a shared point of application with the original two vectors and has a magnitude that is equal to the length of the diagonal of the parallelogram. If the vectors were drawn to scale, the length of CLf would represent +88 N.

Vector CLf in Figure 1-29C is the resultant of vectors PcLf and AcLf in Figure 1-29B. Presuming nothing else is touching the leg-foot segment, vector CLf must be equal in magnitude and opposite in direction to the sum of GLf and WbLf because these three vectors are co-linear, coplanar, and applied to the same object. The arithmetic sum of the three forces must be 0 because (1) these vectors are part of the same linear force system, (2) nothing else is touching the leg-foot segment, and (3) the leg-foot segment is not moving.

The magnitude of the resultant of two concurrent forces has a fixed proportional relationship to the original two vectors. The relationship between the two composing vectors and the resultant is dependent on both the magnitudes of the composing vectors *and* the angle between (orientation of) the composing vectors. In composition of forces by parallelogram, the *relative* lengths (the scale) of the concurrent forces being composed must be appropriately represented to obtain the correct relative magnitude of the resultant force. Although the magnitude and direction of the resultant force are related to both the magnitude and the angle between the composing forces, it is always true that the magnitude of the resultant will be less than the sum of the magnitudes of the composing forces. In Figure 1-29B, the sum of the lengths of PcLf and AcLf (if measured) is greater than the length of CLf; that is, pulling directly up on the leg-foot segment (as seen with CLf) is more efficient than pulling up and anteriorly and pulling up and posteriorly, as AcLf and PcLf, respectively, do.

Trigonometric functions can also be used to determine the magnitude of the resultant of two concurrent forces. The trigonometric solution is presented below. The trigonometric solution, however, requires knowledge both of the actual magnitudes of the two composing vectors and of the angle between them; that is, we would need to know the magnitudes of vectors AcLf and PcLf, as well as the angle between the vectors. These values are rarely known in a clinical situation. [*Side-bar:* Once sufficiently comfortable with the graphic composition of forces by parallelogram, the reader should be able to transfer this skill to visualize the resultant of any two concurrent forces that can be "seen" as acting on an object or body segment.]

Continuing Exploration: **Trigonometric Solution**

Let us assume that PcLf and AcLf each have a magnitude of 51 N and that the vectors are at a 60° angle (α) to each other. As done for the graphic solution, the parallelogram is completed by drawing AcLf′ and PcLf′ parallel to and the same lengths as AcLf and PcLf, respectively (Fig. 1-30). The cosine law for triangles can be used to find the length of the side opposite a known angle once we identify the triangle of interest and the angle of interest

The reference triangle (shaded) is that formed by PcLf, AcLf′, and CLf (see Fig. 1-30). To apply the law of cosines, angle β must be known because vector CLf (whose length we are solving for) is the "side opposite" that angle. The known angle (α) in Figure 1-30 is 60°. If PcLf is extended (as shown by the dotted line in Fig. 1-30), angle α is replicated because it is the angle between PcLf and AcLf′ (given AcLf′ is parallel to AcLf). Angle β, then, is the complement of angle α, or:

$$\beta = 180° - 60° = 120°$$

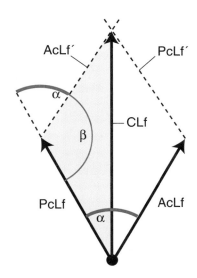

▲ **Figure 1-30** ■ The cosine law for triangles is used to compute the magnitude of CLf, given the magnitudes of AcLf and PcLf, as well as the angle of application (α) between them. The relevant angle (β) is the complement of angle α (180 − α).

By substituting the variables given in the example, the magnitude of the resultant, CLf, can be solved for using the following equation[1]:

$$CLf = PcLf^2 + AcLf^2 - 2(PcLf)(AcLf)(\cos \beta)$$

If the value of 51 N is entered into the equation for both PcLf and AcLf and an angle of 120° is used, vector CLf = 88 N. As we shall see, the trigonometric solution is simpler when the triangle has one 90° angle (right triangle).

When there are more than two forces in the concurrent force system, the process is the same whether a graphic or trigonometric solution is used. The first two vectors are composed into a resultant vector, the resultant and a third vector are then composed to create a second resultant vector, and so on until all vectors are accounted for. Regardless of the order in which the vectors are taken, the solution will be the same. Although we could show this sequential process by using the four vectors in Figure 1-29A, the procedure is generally useful only for graphic solutions. It is unlikely that you will be able to (or need to) compose *multiple* concurrent vectors into a single resultant vector in a clinical situation (other than as a very gross estimate).

Returning to Sam Alexander's weight boot, we have established that vectors GLf and WbLf have a net force of −88 N and that CLf has a magnitude of +88 N. Although a space diagram considers only one segment at a time (the leg-foot segment in this case), an occasional departure from that view is necessary to establish clinical relevance. In Sam's case, we must consider not only the pull of the capsule *on his leg-foot segment* but also the pull of his leg-foot segment *on his capsule,* because Sam has injured his medial collateral ligament (part of that capsule). We can segue to consideration of this new "object" (the capsule) by examining the principle

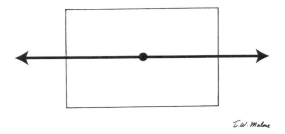

T.W. Malone

▲ **Figure 1-31** ■ Newton's third law ("for every action there is an equal and opposite reaction") is commonly *but incorrectly* represented by two vectors acting on the same object.

in **Newton's law of reaction.** We will present a discussion of the law of reaction before returning to its application to the joint capsule of Sam Alexander's knee.

Newton's Law of Reaction

Every force on an object comes from another object that touches or is contacting that object (acknowledging again our conceit that gravity "touches" an object). When two objects touch, both must touch *each other* and touch *with the same magnitude*. Isaac Newton noted this compulsory phenomenon and concluded that all forces come in pairs that are applied to contacting objects, are equal in magnitude, and are opposite in direction. This is known as **Newton's third law**, or the law of reaction.

Newton's third law is commonly stated as follows: For every action, there is an equal and opposite reaction. This statement is misleading because it seems to result in the *incorrect* interpretation shown in Figure 1-31. Newton's third law can be more clearly restated as follows: When one object applies a force to the second object, the second object *must* simultaneously apply a force equal in magnitude and opposite in direction to that of the first object. These two forces that are applied to the two contacting objects are an **interaction pair** and can also be called **action-reaction** (or simply **reaction**) **forces.**

Continuing Exploration: **Reactions to Leg-Foot Segment Forces**

Figure 1-29C showed the force vector of weightboot-on-legfoot (WbLf). WbLf arises from the contact of the weight boot with the leg-foot segment. If the weight boot contacts the leg-foot segment, then the leg-foot segment must also contact the weight boot. Legfoot-on-weightboot (LfWb) is a reaction force that is equal in magnitude and opposite in direction to WbLf (Fig. 1-32). We did not examine LfWb initially because it is not part of the space diagram under consideration. It is presented here simply as an example of a reaction force. [*Side-bar:* In Figure 1-32, the points of application and action lines of the reaction forces are shifted slightly so that the two vectors can be seen as distinctly different and as applied to different but touching objects.] The force of gravity-on-legfoot in Figure 1-29A also has a reaction

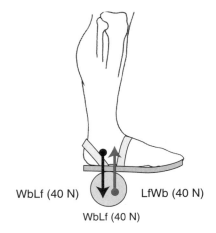

WbLf (40 N)   LfWb (40 N)

WbLf (40 N)

▲ **Figure 1-32** ■ Weightboot-on-legfoot (WbLf) and legfoot-on-weightboot (LfWb) are reaction forces or an interaction pair. Both forces exist by virtue of the contact between the two objects. Although separated for clarity, these two vectors will be in line with each other.

force. If we consider that gravity-on-legfoot might more properly be named earth-on-legfoot (ELf), we can appreciate that the reaction force, legfoot-on-earth (LfE) actually represents that attraction that the mass of the leg-foot segment has for the earth (that is, the earth and the leg-foot segment pull on each other). Vector LfE is a force applied to the CoM of the earth, acting vertically upward toward the leg-foot segment with a magnitude equivalent to the weight of the leg-foot segment.

Reaction forces are *always* in the same line and applied to the *different* but contacting objects. The directions of reaction forces are always *opposite* to each other because the two touching objects either pull on each other or push on each other. Because the points of application of reaction forces are never on the same object, reaction forces are never part of the same force system and typically are not part of the same space diagram. However, we will see that reaction forces can be an important consideration in human function, because one segment never exists in isolation (as in a space diagram).

■ Gravitational and Contact Forces

A different scenario can be used to demonstrate the sometimes subtle but potentially important distinction between (and relevance of) a force applied to an object and its reaction. We generally assume when we get on a scale that the scale shows our weight (Fig. 1-33). A person's weight (gravity-on-person [GP]), however, is not applied to the scale and thus cannot act on the scale. What is actually being recorded on the scale is the *contact* (push) of the "person-on-scale" (PS) and not "gravity-on-person." The distinction between the forces GP and PS and the relation between these two forces can be established by using both Newton's first and third laws.

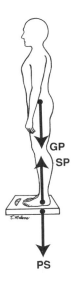

▲ **Figure 1-33** ■ Although a scale is commonly thought to measure the weight of the person (gravity-on-person [GP]), it is actually recording the contact of the person-on-scale (PS). Vectors GP and PS are equal in magnitude as long as nothing else is touching the person.

The person standing on the scale must be in equilibrium ($\Sigma F = 0$). If vector GP is acting down with a magnitude of -734 N (Sam Alexander's weight), there must also be a force of equal magnitude acting up on the person for the person to remain motionless. The only other object besides gravity that appears to be contacting the person in Figure 1-33 is the scale. The scale, therefore, must be exerting an upward push on the person (scale-on-person [SP]) with magnitude equal to that of GP ($+734$ N). The force of scale-on-person, of course, has a reaction force of person-on-scale (PS) that is equal in magnitude (734 N) and opposite in direction (down) but applied to the scale. Consequently, in this instance, the magnitude of the person's weight and the person's contact with the scale are equivalent in magnitude *although applied to different objects*. The vectors person-on-scale and scale-on-person occur as a result of a push by the contacting objects. When reaction forces arise from the *push* of one object on another, they are often referred to as **contact forces** ($\mathbf{F_C}$). When contact forces are perpendicular to the surfaces that produce them, the term **normal force** ($\mathbf{F_N}$) is also used.[5,7] Contact forces, therefore, are a subset of reaction forces.

Under usual conditions of weighing oneself, little or no attention is paid to whether the scale is recording the person's weight or the person's contact with the scale. The distinction between GP and the reaction force PS, however, can be very important if something else is touching the person or the scale. If the person is holding something while on the scale, the person's weight (GP) does not change, but the contact forces (PS and SP) will increase. Similarly, a gentle pressure down on the bathroom countertop as a person stands on the scale will result in an apparent weight reduction. The pressure of the fingers down on the countertop

creates an upward reaction of countertop-on-person (CP). The contact between the person and the countertop create an additional contact force acting on the person, resulting in what appears to be a weight reduction. It is not a decrease in GP, of course, but a decrease in PS. In the example of measuring someone's weight, the reaction force (PS) to GP *cannot* be ignored because it is the variable of interest.

Situations are frequently encountered when the contact of an object with a supporting surface and its weight are used interchangeably. Care should be taken to assess the situation to determine whether the magnitudes are, in fact, equivalent. The recognition of weight and contact as separate forces permits more flexibility in understanding how to modify these forces if necessary.

■ CONCEPT CORNERSTONE 1-6: *Action-Reaction Forces*

- Whenever two objects or segments touch, the two objects or segments exert a force *on each other*. Consequently, every force has a reaction or is part of an action-reaction pair.
- The term contact force or contact forces is commonly used to indicate one or both of a set of reaction forces in which the "touch" is a push rather than a pull.
- Reaction forces are *never part of the same force system* and cannot be composed (cannot either be additive or offset each other) because the two forces are, by definition, applied to different objects.
- The static or dynamic state (equilibrium or motion) of an object cannot be affected by another object that is not touching it or by a force that is not applied to it.
- The reaction to a force should be acknowledged but may be ignored graphically and conceptually *if* the object to which it is applied and the other forces on that object are not of interest.

◆ Additional Linear Force Considerations

The equilibrium established in Sam Alexander's leg-foot segment as he sits with the dangling weight boot is dependent on the capsule (and ligaments) to pull upward on the leg-foot segment with the same magnitude as that with which gravity and the weight boot pull downward (see Fig. 1-29C). Because the capsuloligamentous structures are injured in Sam's case, we need to explore the forces *applied to the capsule*. If the capsule pulls on the leg-foot segment with a magnitude of 88 N, the law of reaction stipulates that the leg-foot segment must also be pulling on the capsule with an equivalent force. If the capsule cannot withstand an 88-N pull, then it cannot pull on the leg-foot segment with an 88-N force; that is, the ability of the capsule to pull on the leg-foot segment is dependent on the amount of **tension** that the capsule can withstand. This requires an understanding of tensile forces and the forces that produce them.

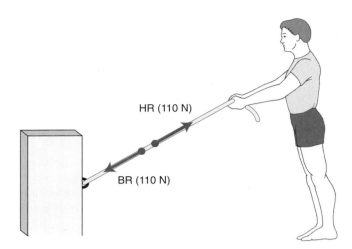

▲ **Figure 1-34** ■ The tensile forces of the pull of hand-on-rope (HR) and the pull of the cement block on the rope (BR) produce two forces of equal magnitude (110 N) that result in 110 N of tension within and throughout the rope.

Tensile Forces

Tension in the joint capsule, just like tension in any passive structure (including relatively solid materials such as bone), is created by opposite pulls on the object. If there are not two opposite pulls on the object (each of which is a **tensile force**), there cannot be tension in the object. Remembering that the connective tissue capsule and ligaments are best analogized to slightly elasticized cord, we first examine tension in a cord or rope.

If a man pulls on a rope that is not attached to anything, no tension will develop in the rope, regardless of how hard or lightly he pulls, because there is no counterforce. The rope will simply accelerate in the direction of the man's pull (with a magnitude equivalent to the force of pull [F_{unbal}] divided by the mass [m] of the rope). If the rope is tied to an immovable block of cement, there will be two forces applied to the rope. The two forces are created by the only two things contacting the rope: the man's hands and the block (Fig. 1-

34). If "hands-on-rope" (HR) has a magnitude of +110 N (~25 lb), then "block-on-rope" (BR) must have a magnitude of −110 N because the rope is in equilibrium. If it is assumed that rope has a homogenous composition (unlike most biological tissues), the tension will be the same throughout the rope (as long as there is no friction on the rope), and the tension in the rope will be equivalent to the magnitude of the two tensile forces acting on the rope.[5] In Figure 1-34, both hands-on-rope (+110 N) and block-on-rope (−110 N) can be designated as tensile forces.

Assume for the moment that the rope is slack before the man begins to pull on the rope. As the man initiates his pull, the man's hands will accelerate away from the block because the force pulling his hands toward his body ("muscles-on-hands" [MsH]) will be greater than the pull of the rope on the hands ("rope-on-hands" [RH]). As the man's hands get farther from the block, the rope will get tighter, and the force of rope-on-hands (RH) will increase. The acceleration of the hands will gradually slow down as the resultant of MsH and RH diminishes. When MsH and RH are equal, the man will be in equilibrium. Because RH and HR are reaction forces (and always equal in magnitude), the tension in the rope (HR) will eventually be equivalent to the magnitude of the man's pull (MsH) (Fig. 1-35).

■ Tensile Forces and Their Reaction Forces

The interactive nature of reaction forces and net forces on an object can be seen as we continue our example. Hands-on-rope (HR) is a tensile vector and, therefore, must be equivalent in magnitude and opposite in direction to the other tensile vector, block-on-rope (BR). Not only is the tensile vector block-on-rope (BR) equal to the other tensile vector (HR), but tensile vector BR is also equivalent in magnitude and opposite in direction to its *reaction force,* rope-on-block (RB) (see Fig. 1-35). Consequently, as long as the rope can structurally withstand the tension, the pull of hands-on-rope (HR) will be transmitted through the rope to an equivalent pull on the block (RB).

The example of the man pulling on the rope and

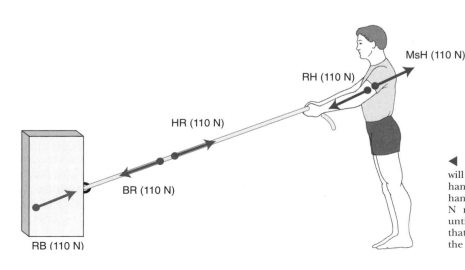

◀ **Figure 1-35** ■ Equilibrium of the man will be achieved when the force of the rope-on-hand (RH) reaches the magnitude of muscles-on-hand (MsH). Rope-on-hand will not reach the 110 N magnitude needed to establish equilibrium until the tension in the initially slack rope reaches that magnitude as the man accelerates away from the block.

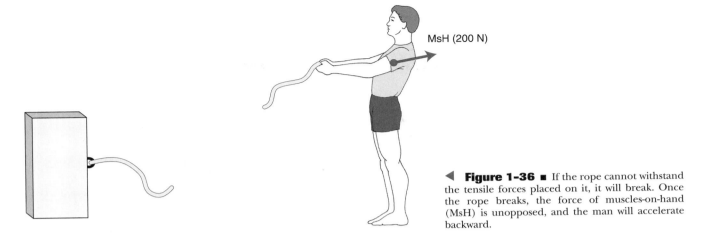

MsH (200 N)

◀ **Figure 1-36** ■ If the rope cannot withstand the tensile forces placed on it, it will break. Once the rope breaks, the force of muscles-on-hand (MsH) is unopposed, and the man will accelerate backward.

cement block assumed so far that the rope could withstand whatever tension was required of it. If the rope is damaged, it may be able to withstand *no more than* 110 N of tension. If, however, the man in our example pulls on the rope (HR) with a magnitude of 200 N (45 lb), the rope will break. Once the rope breaks, there is no longer tension in the rope. The man pulling on the rope (HR) with a magnitude of 200 N will have a net unbalanced force that will accelerate the hands (or the man) backwards (Fig. 1-36) until his muscles stop pulling (which will, it is hoped, happen before he punches himself in the stomach or falls over!).

Let us go back to Sam Alexander to determine how the tension example is applied to Sam's use of the weight boot. The equilibrium of Sam's leg-foot segment was based on the ability of the capsule (CLf) to pull on the leg-foot segment with a magnitude equivalent to GLf + WbLf. If the capsule pulls on the leg-foot segment with a magnitude of +88 N (as we established earlier), the leg-foot segment must pull on the capsule (legfoot-on-capsule [LfC]) with an equivalent force of −88 N (Fig. 1-37). Two questions can be raised around

the assumption that there is 88 N of tension in the capsule: (1) Does the magnitude of tension reach 88 N in the capsule immediately, and (2) can the injured capsule (and ligaments) withstand 88 N of tension? Case Application 1-1 applies the concepts from the example of tension in the rope to Sam's joint capsule.

Case Application 1-1: **Tension in the Knee Joint Capsule**

The reaction forces of capsule-on-legfoot (CLf) and legfoot-on-capsule (LfC) have a magnitude of 88 N (see Fig. 1-37). [*Side-bar:* Vectors LfC and CLf should be co-linear in the figure but are separated for clarity.] Legfoot-on-capsule is a tensile vector. Tension can occur in a passive structure only if there are two pulls on the object. Therefore, there must be a second tensile vector (of +88 N) applied to the capsule from something touching the capsule at the other end. The second tensile vector, therefore, must be femur-on-capsule (FC) (Fig. 1-38), where the tensile vectors are effectively co-linear but separated for clarity. The magnitudes of CLf,

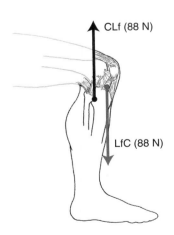

CLf (88 N)

LfC (88 N)

▲ **Figure 1-37** ■ The pull of the capsule-on-legfoot (CLf) must have a concomitant reaction force of legfoot-on-capsule (LfC) that is an 88-N tensile force on the joint capsule.

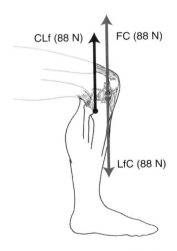

CLf (88 N)   FC (88 N)

LfC (88 N)

▲ **Figure 1-38** ■ The tensile forces of legfoot-on-capsule (LfC) and femur-on-capsule (FC) are shown with their interaction pairs, capsule-on-legfoot (CLf) and capsule-on-femur (CF), respectively.

LfC, and FC are equivalent because vector CLf is part of the same linear force system with WbLf and GLf (see Fig. 1-29C) and vectors LfC and FC are part of the same linear force system. The sum of the forces in both linear force systems is 0 because it is assumed that no movement is occurring.

 CONCEPT CORNERSTONE 1-7: *Tension and Tensile Forces*

- Tensile forces (or the resultants of tensile forces) on an object are always equal in magnitude, opposite in direction, and applied parallel to the long axis of the object.
- Tensile forces are co-linear, coplanar, and applied to the same object; therefore, tensile vectors are part of the same linear force system.
- Tensile forces applied to a flexible or rigid structure of homogenous composition create the same tension at all points along the long axis of the structure in the absence of friction; that is, tensile forces are transmitted along the length (long axis) of the object.

Joint Distraction

Joint capsule and ligaments are not necessarily in a constant state of tension. In fact, if Sam started out with his leg-foot segment on the treatment table, there would effectively be no tension in his capsule or ligaments because the sum of the forces on the leg-foot segment from the "contacts" of gravity (gravity-on-legfoot) and the treatment table (table-on-legfoot) (Fig. 1-39) would be sufficient for equilibrium ($\Sigma F = 0$). Although both the capsule and the weight boot are still attached to the leg-foot segment, the magnitudes of pull would be negligible (too small to include in the space diagram).

A situation similar to the leg-foot segment on the treatment table would exist if Sam's foot were supported by someone's hand if his leg-foot segment and weight boot were moved off the treatment table to the vertical position. In Figure 1-40, the hand is pushing up (+88 N) on the leg-foot segment (hand-on-legfoot segment [HLf]) with a magnitude equivalent to the pull of gravity and the weight boot (−88 N). [*Side-bar:* Vector

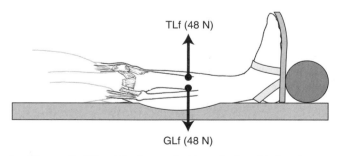

▲ **Figure 1-39** ■ The forces of table-on-legfoot (TLf) and gravity-on-legfoot (GLf) in this position are sufficient for equilibrium of the leg-foot segment, with zero (or negligible) tension in the knee joint capsule.

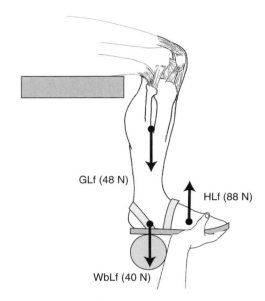

▲ **Figure 1-40** ■ As long as the 88 N force on the leg-foot segment from gravity (GLf) and the weight boot (WbLf) are supported by an equal upward force from the hand (HLf), the tension in the capsule and ligaments will be zero (or negligible).

HLf is shown to one side of GLf and WbLf for clarity, but assume that the supporting hand is directly below the weight boot.] The magnitude of pull of the capsule (and ligaments) on the leg-foot segment would be negligible as long as HLf had a magnitude equal and opposite to that of GLf and WbLf. As the upward support of the hand is taken away, however, there would be a net unbalanced force down on the leg-foot segment that would cause the leg-foot segment to accelerate away from the femur. The pull or movement of one bony segment away from another is known as **joint distraction.**[8] As the upward push of the hand decreases and the leg-foot segment moves away from the femur, the capsule will become increasingly tensed. The magnitude of acceleration of the leg-foot segment will be directly proportional to the unbalanced force and indirectly proportional to the mass of the leg-foot segment and weight boot combined ($a = F_{unbal} \div m$). However, the unbalanced force is difficult to quantify because it is constantly changing. Although the increase in capsular tension occurs concomitantly with the reduction in hand support, the two forces are not equivalent in magnitude because the leg-foot segment must move away from the femur for the capsule to get tighter; that is, there must be a net unbalanced force on the leg-foot segment to create the movement that causes the capsule to get tighter.

The Continuing Exploration: Reactions to Leg-Foot Segment Forces presented calculation of acceleration of the leg-foot segment at one point in time (a static rather than dynamic analysis). However, the concepts are more important than the calculations, given that the weight of a limb, the support of the hand, and the tension in the capsule in a true clinical situation are generally unknown.

Continuing Exploration: **Acceleration in Joint Distraction**

The leg-foot segment and weight boot together weigh 88 N. To calculate acceleration ($a = F_{unbal} \div m$), however, the mass (not just the weight) of the leg-foot segment and weight boot must be known. Recalling that 1 N is the amount of force needed to accelerate 1 kg at 1 m/sec^2, weight (in newtons or equivalently in kg-m/sec^2) is mass (in kilograms) multiplied by the acceleration of gravity, or:

$$W = (m)(9.8 \text{ m/sec}^2)$$

Solving for mass, a weight of 88 N is equivalent to 88 kg-m/sec^2 ÷ 9.8 m/sec^2 = 8.97 kg. Consequently, the leg-foot segment and weight boot together have a mass of approximately 9 kg. Assigning some arbitrary values, assume that a downward force of −88 N is offset in this static example by an upward push of the supporting hand of +50 N and capsular tensile force of +10 N. The net unbalanced force on the leg-foot segment (−88 + 50 + 10) is −28 N. Therefore:

$$a = \frac{-28 \text{ kg-m/sec}^2}{9 \text{ kg}}$$

$$a = -3.11 \text{ m/sec}^2$$

When the hand in Figure 1-40 is no longer in contact with the leg-foot segment and the tension in the capsule reaches 88 N, the leg-foot segment will stop accelerating away from the femur and will reach equilibrium.

■ Distraction Forces

The resultant pull of gravity and the weight boot on the leg-foot segment (composed into a single vector) can be referred to as a **distraction force**[3] or **joint distraction force.** A distraction force is directed away from the joint surface to which it is applied, is perpendicular to its joint surface, and leads to the separation of the joint surfaces. [*Side-bar:* It is important to note that the term "distraction" here refers to separation of rigid nondeformable bones. Distraction across or within a deformable body is more complex and will be considered in Chapter 2.]

A joint distraction force cannot exist in isolation; joint surfaces will not separate unless there is a distraction force applied to the adjacent segment in the opposite direction. As the leg-foot segment is pulled away from the femur, any tension in the capsule created by the pull of the leg-foot segment on the capsule results in a second tensile vector in the capsule (femur-on-capsule). If the femur pulls on the capsule, then the capsule must concomitantly pull on the femur (see Fig. 1-38). If there is no opposing force on the femur, the net unbalanced downward force on the leg-foot segment will be transmitted through the capsule to the femur; the femur will also accelerate downward as soon as any appreciable tension is developed in the capsule. If the femur accelerates downward with the same mag-

nitude of acceleration as the leg-foot segment, the joint surfaces will not separate any farther than was required to initiate movement of the femur. Although we did not set the *femur* in equilibrium (did not stabilize the femur) in Case Application 1-1, there must be a force applied to the femur that is opposite in direction to capsule-on-femur for there to be effective joint distraction. Joint distraction can occur only when the acceleration of one segment is less than (or in a direction opposite to) the acceleration of the adjacent segment, resulting in a separation of joint surfaces.

In the human body, the acceleration of one or both segments away from each other in joint distraction (the dynamic phase) is very brief unless the capsule and ligaments (or muscles crossing the joint) fail. Sam's leg-foot segment will not accelerate away from the femur for very long before the distraction forces applied to the adjacent joint segments (leg-foot and femur) are balanced by the tensile forces in the capsule. Given that Sam is still relaxed as the weight boot hangs on his leg-foot segment (we have not asked him to do anything yet), the check to joint distraction (the pull of gravity and the weight boot) is the tension in the capsule (and ligaments). Sam presumably has a ligamentous injury that is likely to cause pain with tension in these pain-sensitive connective tissues. If the distraction force remains, the capsule and ligaments may fail either microscopically or macroscopically (see Chapter 2). In the short term, we can prevent this problem by putting the supporting hand back under the weight boot. If the upward push of the hand is sufficient, the tensile forces on the ligaments can be completely eliminated.

Continuing Exploration: **Stabilization of the Femur**

Because our primary interest is in Sam Alexander's leg-foot segment and secondarily in the injured knee joint capsule, the source of stabilization of the femur (the other joint distraction force) was not a necessary component of our exploration. However, the principles established thus far will allow us to identify that distraction force.

In Figure 1-41, WbLf and GLf are composed in-to a single resultant distraction force (GWbLf) of −88 N, with the leg-foot segment once again unsupported. Vector GWbLf creates an 88 N tensile force in the capsule that creates a pull of the capsule on the femur (CF) with an equal magnitude of 88 N (see Fig. 1-41). A net distractive force of +88 N applied to the femur is necessary to stabilize the femur and create tension in the capsule.

The femur is contacted both by gravity (GF) and by the treatment table (TF) (see Fig. 1-41). To determine the net force acting on the femur, we must estimate the mass or weight of that segment. Sam weighs approximately 734 N, and his thigh constitutes approximately 10.7% of his body weight.[1] Consequently, his thigh is estimated to weigh approximately 78 N. With the magnitudes of CF (−88 N) and GF (−78 N) known, it appears that the magnitude of TF

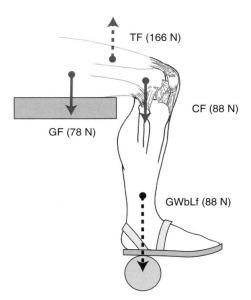

▲ **Figure 1-41** ■ Distraction of the joint and tensile forces in the knee joint capsule occurs when there is a net distractive force directed away from the joint surfaces applied to *each* of the adjacent joint segments (dashed vectors). The distractive force on the femur is provided by the force of table-on-femur (TF), whereas the distractive force on the leg-foot segment is provided by GWbLf.

should be the sum of the magnitudes of CF and GF (but opposite in direction). However, vectors CF, GF, and TF are not in a linear force system because they are not co-linear. Rather, they are parallel forces. Although we will tackle composition (and the effects) of parallel forces in more detail later, we can use the same shorthand system here that we used to compose two gravitational vectors earlier in the chapter.

Because both GF and CF (see Fig. 1-41) are vertically downward, the resultant of these two forces would be a new downward force with the combined magnitudes of the original two (88 N + 78 N), with a point of application along a line drawn between the original two points and located slightly toward the vector with the greater magnitude. Because this new resultant vector will lie approximately in line with vector TF, we now have two forces in a linear force system on an object in equilibrium. Therefore, vector TF must have a magnitude of +166 N. Vector TF must be the second distraction force because it is applied perpendicular to and away from the joint surface. In Figure 1-41, the two distraction forces (GWbLf and TF) are shown as dashed vectors.

 CONCEPT CORNERSTONE 1-8: *Joint Distraction and Distraction Forces*

- Distraction forces create separation of joint surfaces.
- There must be a minimum of one (or one resultant) distraction force on each joint segment, with each distraction force perpendicular to the joint surfaces, opposite in direction to the distraction force on the adjacent segment, and directed away from its joint surface.
- Joint distraction can be dynamic (through unequal or oppo-

site acceleration of segments) or static (when the tensile forces in the tissues that join the segments are balanced by distraction forces of equal or greater magnitude).

■ Joint Compression and Joint Reaction Forces

Supporting Sam Alexander's leg-foot segment can minimize or eliminate the tension in his injured capsuloligamentous structures. In Figure 1-42, the supporting upward push of the hand on the leg-foot segment has been increased to +90 N. Given that the magnitude of GWbLf (resultant of gravity and weight boot) is still −88 N, these two forces will result in a net unbalanced force on the leg-foot segment of +2 N. The leg-foot segment will accelerate upward until a new force is encountered. This new force cannot come from the capsule that is now becoming increasingly slack, but it will arise once the leg-foot segment makes contact with the femur. The upward acceleration of the leg-foot segment will stop when the contact force, femur-on-legfoot (FLf), reaches a magnitude of −2 N (see Fig. 1-42), at which point equilibrium of the leg-foot segment is restored.

When the two segments of a joint are pushed together and "touch," as occurs with the upward support of the hand in Figure 1-42 (legfoot-on-femur and femur-on-legfoot), the resulting reaction (contact) forces are also referred to as **joint reaction forces**.[3] Joint reaction forces are contact forces that result whenever two or more forces cause contact between contiguous joint surfaces. Joint reaction forces are dependent on the existence of one force on each of the adjacent joint segments that is perpendicular to and directed *toward* its joint surface. The two forces that *cause* joint reactions forces are known as **compression forces**. Compression forces are required to push joint surfaces together to produce joint reaction forces in the same way that distraction forces are required to produce capsuloligamentous or muscular tension across separating (or separated) joint surfaces. [*Side-bar:* It is important to note that the term "compression" here refers to pushing together rigid nondeformable bones to close a joint space. Compression across or within a deformable body is more complex and will be considered in Chapter 2.]

In Figure 1-42, one of the forces causing joint compression at the knee joint is hand-on-legfoot (HLf) because HLf is applied toward the articulating surface of the leg-foot segment and is perpendicular to that surface. If, however, the +2 N push of the leg-foot segment *on the femur* is not offset by a downward force of at least 2 N *on the femur,* the femur will also accelerate upward. If the femur and leg-foot segment were to accelerate upward at the same rate (and in the same direction), the contact between the joint surfaces might be maintained but could not be greater than 2 N. [*Side-bar:* Although the leg-foot segment is our focus, rather than the femur, it is worth noting that the femur is not likely to move because gravity is acting downward on the femur to stabilize it with a force of 78 N (see Fig. 1-42). Gravity-on-femur is the second joint compression force because it is the only force on the femur that is applied

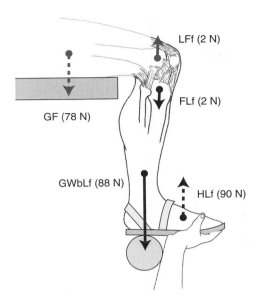

▲ **Figure 1-42** ■ Joint compression results in joint reaction forces (FLf and LfF) when there is a net compression force applied to *each* of the adjacent joint segments (dashed vectors) toward the joint surfaces, in this case provided by hand-on-legfoot (HLf) and gravity-on-femur (GF).

perpendicular to and toward the joint surface. In Figure 1-42, the two joint compression forces are shown as dashed vectors.]

Whenever there is a net compression of joint surfaces (resulting in joint reaction forces), the capsule and ligaments at the joint are generally not under tension (as long as all forces are perpendicular to contacting surfaces). The pull of capsule-on-legfoot segment is not shown in Figure 1-42 because the tension in the capsule has effectively been eliminated (or reduced to imperceptible magnitude). Equilibrium between two bony segments with net joint compression and equal and opposite joint reaction forces also assumes that the push of one bony segment on another does not result in failure of the bone (that is, that one bone does not accelerate through the other).

Continuing Exploration: **Close-Packing of a Joint**

Although capsuloligamentous structures are typically not under tension when there are *net* compressive forces (with no shear forces) across a joint, there is an important exception. With sufficient twisting of the capsuloligamentous structures of a joint, the adjacent articular surfaces are drawn into contact by the pull of the capsule on the bony segments. This is called "close-packing" of the joint. This concept will be elaborated upon in Chapter 2 and in examination of the individual joint complexes.

 CONCEPT CORNERSTONE 1-9: *Joint Compression and Joint Compression Forces*

■ Joint compression forces create contact between joint surfaces.

■ There must be a minimum of one (or one resultant) compression force on each contiguous joint segment, with each compression force perpendicular to and directed toward the segment's joint surface, and opposite in direction to the compression force on the adjacent segment.

Revisiting Newton's Law of Inertia

It would appear that the weight boot is a poor option for Sam, given the potential tensile forces created in his injured joint capsule (and ligaments), unless we plan to continue supporting his leg-foot segment with a hand (or, perhaps, a bench). However, it has been assumed thus far that Sam is relaxed. As soon as Sam initiates a contraction of his quadriceps muscle, the balance of forces will change. Before we add the muscle force to the weight boot exercise, however, let us return to the leg-press exercise to identify what effect, if any, the forces from the leg press will have on the leg-foot segment or Sam's injured capsuloligamentous structures.

In the leg-press exercise, Sam Alexander's leg-foot segment is contacting the footplate of the leg-press machine, creating the force of footplate-on-legfoot (FpLf). The magnitude of vector FpLf is not yet known. There are also other forces acting on the leg-foot segment because other things are touching the leg-foot segment. One of these is gravity. Two other options are contacts of femur-on-legfoot or capsule-on-legfoot. Whether the push of the femur on the leg-foot segment or the pull of the capsule on the leg-foot segment is a factor in this space diagram requires further exploration. We will begin with the known force, gravity-on-legfoot (GLf).

The magnitude of the weight of the leg-foot segment remains the same as in the weight boot example (−88 N), but the orientation to the leg-foot segment differs. Consequently, the orientation of gravity to the leg-foot segment differs (Fig. 1-43). The force of footplate-on-legfoot (FpLf) is also shown in the figure but has no designated magnitude because the magnitude is not yet unknown. Vectors GLf and FpLf cannot be summed to find their resultant effect because the two

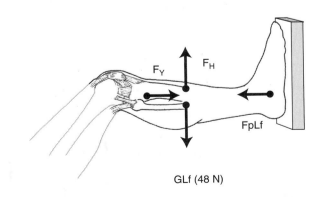

▲ **Figure 1-43** ■ The known forces of footplate-on-legfoot (FpLf) and gravity-on-legfoot (GLf) must be balanced by another horizontal (F_H) and vertical (F_V) force, respectively.

forces are not in the same linear force system (they are not co-linear). It is theoretically possible to find the resultant of these two forces through composition by parallelogram because these two vectors are part of a concurrent force system (the vectors will intersect if the vectors are extended). That solution, however, requires that we know at least the relative magnitudes of FpLf and GLf. A second option is to consider the two different linear force systems of which vectors GLf and FpLf are a part and determine the magnitudes of the vectors within each linear force system.

■ Vertical and Horizontal Linear Force Systems

Newton's law of inertia (or law of equilibrium) can be broken down into component parts: The sum of the **vertical forces** (F_V) acting on an object in equilibrium must total zero ($\sum F_V = 0$), *and, independently*, the sum of the **horizontal forces** (F_H) acting on an object in equilibrium must total zero ($\sum F_H = 0$). Consequently, there must be at least two additional forces acting on the leg-foot segment that are equal in magnitude and opposite in direction to GLf and FpLf because the leg-foot segment cannot be at rest unless the sum of forces in both linear forces systems equals zero. Forces F_V and F_H are drawn in Figure 1-43, but the source of each force is not yet established.

We know that the femur and the capsule are both contacting and potentially creating forces on the leg-foot segment. Given these options, it appears that vector F_H is likely to be the push of the femur on the leg-foot segment (FLf) because the pull of capsule-on-legfoot would be in the opposite direction. The magnitude of FLf and FpLf can be estimated to be fairly small if Sam is relaxed and the footplate is locked in position. Before attempting to determine the magnitude of FLf and FpLf, we will examine the source and magnitude of F_V because it will be seen that, in this example, F_V and F_H are related.

The source of the F_V is difficult to ascertain because it appears that we have accounted for all objects contacting the leg-foot segment, including gravity, with none that appear to act in the direction of F_V. To identify F_V, we must acknowledge an additional property of all contact forces. Whenever there is contact between two objects (or surfaces of objects), the potential exists for friction forces on both contacting surfaces. The friction forces will have magnitude, however, only if there are concomitant opposing shear forces on the contacting objects.

Shear and Friction Forces

A force (regardless of its source) that moves or attempts to move one object on another is known as a **shear force** (F_S). A shear force is any force (or the component of a force) that is parallel to contacting surfaces (or tangential to curved surfaces) and has an action line in the direction of attempted movement. [*Side-bar:* The discussion here is on shear forces *between* two

rigid (nondeformable) structures (e.g., bones). Shear within deformable structures will be considered in Chapter 2.]

A **friction force** (**Fr**) *potentially exists* on an object whenever there is a contact force on that object. Friction forces are always parallel to contacting surfaces (or tangential to curved surfaces) and have a direction that is opposite to potential movement. For friction to have magnitude, some other force (a shear force) must be moving or attempting to move one or both of the contacting objects on each other. The force of friction can be considered a special case of a shear force because both are forces parallel to contacting surfaces, but friction is a shear force that is *always* in the direction opposite to movement or potential movement.

Whenever a shear force (F_{S1}) is present on an object, there will always be *at least one* opposing shear force (F_{S2}) on that object. In the absence of an opposing shear force created by the contact of a new object, the opposing shear force (F_{S2}) will be friction (Fr). If the magnitude of an opposing shear force (F_{S2}) created by a contact of a new object is inadequate to prevent movement by F_{S1}, friction (F_{S3}) will also oppose F_{S1}.

Sam Alexander's leg-foot segment is contacting the footplate. Because FpLf is a contact (or normal) force, it can also be labeled F_C (Fig. 1-44). The force of gravity-on-legfoot is parallel to the foot and footplate and has the potential to slide the foot down the footplate. Consequently, gravity-on-legfoot (GLf) may also be referred to as a shear force. In the absence of another other opposing shear, there will be a concomitant opposing force of friction-on-legfoot (FrLf) that is parallel to the foot and footplate surfaces and is in a direction opposite to the potential slide of the foot (see Fig. 1-44). To understand the magnitude of FrLf, we need to further explore the force of friction.

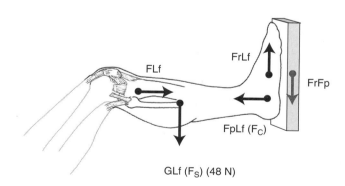

▲ **Figure 1-44** ■ Footplate-on-legfoot (FpLf) is a contact force (F_C) that will result in friction-on-legfoot (FrLf) between the foot and footplate, given the shear force (F_S), GLf. Femur-on-legfoot (FLf) is also a contact force, but the low coefficient of friction for articular cartilage makes the value of friction between the femur and leg-foot segment negligible. Shown in a shaded vector that is not part of the space diagram is the reaction force to FrLf, friction-on-footplate (FrFp).

■ Static Friction and Kinetic Friction

The magnitude of a friction force on an object is always a function of the magnitude of contact between the objects and the slipperiness or roughness of the contacting surfaces. When two contacting objects with shear forces applied to each are *not moving*, the magnitude of friction on each object is also proportional to the magnitude of the shear forces. If the two objects are *not* moving (objects are static), the *maximum* magnitude of the **force of static friction** (**Fr$_s$**) on each object is the product of a constant value known as the **coefficient of static friction** (μ_s) and the magnitude of the contact force (F$_C$) on each object; that is,

$$Fr_s \leq \mu_s F_C$$

The coefficient of static friction is a constant value for given materials. For example, μ_s for ice on ice is approximately 0.05; the value of μ_s for wood on wood is as little as 0.25.[5] As the contacting surfaces become softer or rougher, μ_s increases. As the magnitude of contact (F$_C$) between objects increases, so too does the magnitude of potential friction. The greater the contact force on an object is and the rougher the contacting surfaces are, the greater the maximum potential force of friction is. When using friction to warm your hands, the contact of the hands warms both of them (friction forces exist on both the right and the left hands). If you wish to increase the friction, you press your hands together harder (increase the contact force) as you rub. Increasing the pressure increases the contact force between the hands and increases the maximum value of friction (the coefficient of friction remains unchanged because the surface remains skin on skin). [*Side-bar:* It is commonly thought that the magnitude of friction between two surfaces is related to the amount of surface area in contact (pressure or force per unit area). However, the only contributing factors are the magnitude of contact and the coefficient of the contacting surfaces. The area of contact does not affect the magnitude of friction.[2]]

In Figure 1-45A, a large box weighing 445 N (~45 kg or 100 lb) is resting on the floor. The floor must push on the box (FB) with a magnitude equal to the weight of the box (GB) because the box is not moving ($\sum F_V = 0$). Because nothing is attempting to move the box parallel to the contacting surfaces (bottom of the box and the floor), there will be no friction on either the box or the floor. However, as soon as the man begins to push on the box (see Fig. 1-45B), the man's force (man-on-box [MB]) creates a shear force, with a concomitant resulting force of friction-on-box (FrB). (Note that Fig. 1-45B is oversimplified because the FrB is shown acting in line with MB, rather than at the bottom of the box as would actually be the case.) Assuming that the man's initial push is not sufficient to move the box, we can begin by calculating the *maximum* possible magnitude of friction-on-box.

The maximum friction force on the box when the box is not moving is a product of the coefficient of static friction of wooden box on wood floor (0.25) and the magnitude (445 N) of the contact of floor-on-box (FB):

$$FrB \leq (0.25)(445 \text{ N})$$

$$FrB \leq 111.25 \text{ N}$$

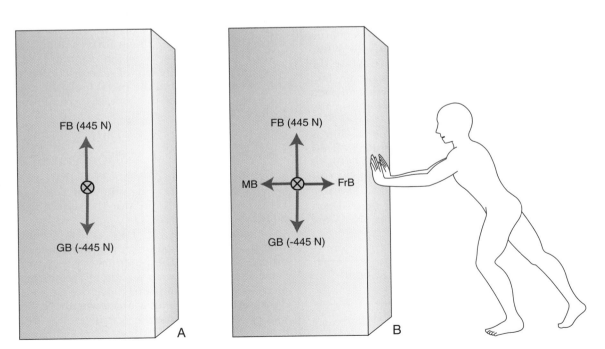

▲ **Figure 1-45** ■ **A.** The box is acted on by the forces of gravity (GB) and the contact of floor-on-box (FB). The force of friction has no magnitude (so is not shown) because there is no attempted movement. **B.** The force of the man-on-box (MB) causes an opposing friction force (FrB).

The magnitude of FrB will be equal to the MB as long as the box is not moving ($\Sigma F_H = 0$). No matter how much the man increases the magnitude of his push on the box (up to a maximum of 111.25 N), the magnitude of FrB will increase by the same amount. The magnitude of static friction, therefore, might be considered to be "dynamic"—with the magnitude of static friction changing to meet the changing magnitude of the shear force (or shear forces) applied to the object. However, *the magnitude of the force of friction can never exceed the magnitude of the shear force or forces*. Friction can oppose movement of a segment, but it cannot create movement.

If the push of the man on the box exceeds 111.25 N, the box will begin to move because FrB cannot be more than 111.25 N and there will be a net unbalanced force of some magnitude to the left. Once an object is moving, the magnitude of the **force of kinetic friction** ($\mathbf{Fr_K}$) on the contacting objects is a constant value, equal to the product of the contact force (F_C) and the **coefficient of kinetic friction** (μ_K):

$$Fr_K = (\mu_K)(F_C)$$

The coefficient of kinetic friction (μ_K) is always smaller in magnitude than the coefficient of static friction (μ_S) for any set of contacting surfaces. Consequently, the magnitude of the force of friction is always greatest immediately before the object is about to move (when the shear force has the same magnitude as the maximum value of static friction). Once the shear force exceeds the maximum value of static friction, the object will move because there will be a net unbalanced force ($\Sigma F_H \neq 0$). However, as soon as movement is initiated, the value of friction drops from its maximum static value to its smaller kinetic value, resulting in a sudden increase in the net unbalanced force on the object even if the magnitude of the shear force remains the same. The sudden drop in magnitude of friction results in the classic situation in which the man pushes harder and harder to get the box moving along the floor and then suddenly finds himself and the box accelerating too rapidly.

The box example provides evidence that two linear force systems applied to the same object are effectively independent. Once the box is moving, the box is not in horizontal equilibrium (MB > FrB), but the box remains in vertical equilibrium (GB = FB). The balance of forces in any force system must be assessed independently of other force systems on the same object.

CONCEPT CORNERSTONE 1-10: *Friction and Shear Forces*

■ Shear and friction forces potentially exist whenever two objects touch.
■ A shear force is any force (or force component) that lies parallel to the contacting surfaces (or tangential to curved surfaces) of an object and causes or attempts to cause movement between the surfaces.

■ Friction is a special case of a shear force in which the direction is always opposite to the direction of potential or relative movement of the objects (opposite in direction to the shear force on that object).
■ Friction has magnitude only when there is a *net* shear force applied to an object; that is, friction has magnitude only when two contacting objects move or attempt to move on each other after all potential shear forces are accounted for.
■ The magnitude of static friction can change with a change in the net shear force that friction opposes; the magnitude of kinetic friction remains the same regardless of the shear force or forces it opposes or the speed of the moving object.
■ The magnitude of friction can never exceed the magnitude of the shear force or forces it opposes.
■ Shear and friction forces are always parallel to contacting surfaces, whereas the contact force (or contact force component) that must exist concomitantly is perpendicular (normal) to the contacting surfaces. Consequently, shear and friction forces are perpendicular to a contact force (or, more correctly, the component of a contact force that is "normal" to the contacting surfaces).[3]

■ **Considering Vertical and Horizontal Linear Equilibrium**

We can now return to Sam and the leg-press example and use our understanding of shear and friction forces to calculate the contact between the leg-foot segment and the footplate. Because the leg-foot segment is in equilibrium and there are only two vertical forces, the magnitude of the friction force, FrLf, must be the same as the magnitude of the shear force, GLf (48 N) (see Fig. 1-44). [*Side-bar:* Although vector FrLf is appropriately drawn on the leg-foot segment where the contact with the footplate takes place, we will treat it for now as if it is part of the same linear force system as shown for F_H in Fig. 1-43.] If we know the magnitude of FrLf and we estimate the coefficient of static friction between the sole of Sam's shoe and the metal footplate at $\mu_S = 0.6$,[5] then we can solve for the contact force of footplate-on-legfoot (FpLf):

$$48\ N = (0.6)(F_C)$$
$$F_C = 80\ N$$

If the magnitude of vector FpLf (F_C) (see Fig. 1-44) is −80 N, then the magnitude of femur-on-legfoot (FLf) must be +80 N, because the sum of the horizontal forces must be zero.

Vector FLf (see Fig. 1-44) is also a contact force (the push of the leg-foot segment and femur on each other). Therefore, the potential for a vertical friction force also exists between the femur and the leg-foot segment as gravity attempts to move the leg-foot segment downward on the femur. However, the coefficient of friction between articular cartilage has been determined to be extremely low, with estimates such as 0.016[7] or 0.005.[3] Even if the higher of these two values is used, the magnitude of friction for an 80 N contact force cannot be greater than 1.28 N (~0.28 lb). Given this negligible magnitude, the force of friction on the leg-foot segment arising from the contact of the femur cannot be an important factor contributing to the vertical equilibrium of the leg-foot segment.

Continuing Exploration: **Friction and Reaction Forces**

The shear force in Figure 1-44 is gravity-on-legfoot. Although this is not part of what we need to consider, gravity-on-legfoot has a reaction force of legfoot-on-earth. Friction-on-legfoot also has a reaction force, although the name and location are not intuitive. Friction forces are directly related to contact forces, and contact forces must exist on both touching objects; therefore, friction also exists on both touching objects. In Figure 1-44, friction-on-leg-foot has a reaction force of friction-on-footplate (FrFp). Friction-on-footplate is a different color than the other vectors in Figure 1-44 because it is not part of the space diagram (and not a force we need to account for in our consideration of the leg-foot segment). Vectors FrFp and FrLf are equal in magnitude and opposite in direction and are applied to different but touching objects (Newton's law of reaction). Vector FrFp is directed down because any movement of the foot downward is a *relative* movement of the footplate up, and friction is always in the direction opposite to potential movement of the object to which the force is applied.

It appears that Figure 1-44 accounts for all the forces acting on the static leg-foot segment in the leg-press exercise. That assessment, however, is based on the supposition that vectors FrLf and GLf are part of the same linear force system, even though it is evident that these two forces are parallel and not co-linear. Thus far, not only have we treated all forces as part of one or more linear force systems, but all unbalanced forces have resulted in linear displacement (translatory motion). This is a substantial oversimplification and

rarely true in human motion. A fuller understanding of human motion requires consideration of the forces that produce rotatory motion.

Part 2: *Kinetics—Considering Rotatory and Translatory Forces and Motions*

When an object is completely unconstrained (not attached to anything), a single force applied *at or through the CoM* of the object will produce linear displacement regardless of the angle at which the force is applied (Fig. 1-46A to C). In the previous examples used in this chapter, it has essentially been assumed that linear displacement is occurring. As we begin exploring rotatory and general plane (curvilinear) motion that is more commonly part of human motion, the reader is cautioned that discussion and examples are largely confined to two-dimensional analyses. Although human motion occurs in a three-dimensional environment, it is, in general, sufficiently challenging for the novice to understand a two-dimensional approach. Subsequent chapters will superimpose the third dimension conceptually, although rarely mathematically. Readers who wish to pursue three-dimensional mathematical analyses are encouraged to access more advanced resources.

◆ **Torque, or Moment of Force**

When the force applied to an unattached object does not pass through the CoM, a combination of rotation and translation will result (Fig. 1-47). To produce pure rotatory motion (angular displacement), a *second force* that is parallel to the original force must be applied to

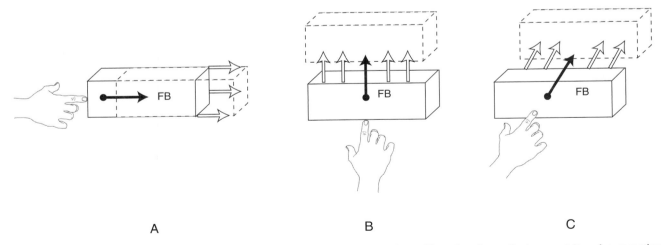

A   B   C

▲ **Figure 1-46** ■ An isolated force applied to the block that passes through its CoM will produce linear displacement (translatory motion) of the block in the direction of the unbalanced force.

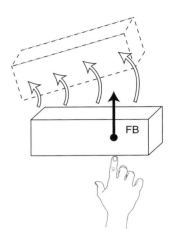

▲ **Figure 1-47** ■ When an isolated force that does not pass through its CoM is applied to the block, a combination of rotatory and translatory motion of the block will occur (general motion).

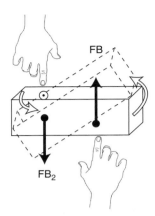

▲ **Figure 1-49** ■ Two forces of equal magnitude applied to the block in opposite directions constitute a force couple and will create rotation around the point of application of one of the forces if that point is fixed.

the object or segment. When a second force (FB₂) equal in magnitude and opposite in direction to FB (Fig. 1-48) is applied parallel to FB (applied to the same object at any other point), the translatory motions of FB and FB₂ will offset each other (as they do in a linear force system), and pure rotatory motion will occur. If the object is unconstrained as it is in Figure 1-48, the rotation of the segment will occur around a point (⊙) midway between vectors FB and FB₂, If the object is constrained by one of the forces (if the second finger cannot move from its point of contact), the rotation will occur around the point of application (⊙) of the constrained force (Fig. 1-49). Two forces that are equal in magnitude, opposite in direction, and applied to the same object at different points are known as a **force couple**. A force couple will always produce pure rotatory motion of an object (if there are no other forces on the object). The strength of rotation produced by a force couple is known as **torque** (**T**), or **moment of**

force, and is a product of the magnitude of one of the forces and the shortest distance (which always will be the perpendicular distance) between the forces:

$$T = (F)(d)$$

The perpendicular distance between forces that produce a torque, or moment of force, is also known as the **moment arm** (**MA**). Consequently, we can also say that:

$$T = (F)(MA)$$

Presuming that force is measured in newtons and distance in meters, the unit for torque is the newton-meter (Nm). In the US system, the torque unit is the foot-pound (ftlb). As already noted under this chapter's section on kinematics, a torque that tends to produce a clockwise rotatory motion is generally given a negative sign, whereas a torque that tends to produce counter-clockwise motion is given a positive sign. Of course, the direction of potential rotation or torque at a joint segment can also be labeled by using the terms flexion/extension, medial/lateral rotation, or abduction/adduction. The terms torque and moment of force are synonymous as they are used in this text (although there is no unanimity on equivalence of these terms). Consequently, a torque in the direction of joint flexion, for example, may also be referred to as a **flexion moment,** or as a flexion torque.

Because the terms "torque" and "moment of force" are often unfamiliar or intimidating to readers, the best simplistic translation we might use here is that torque, or moment of force, is the "strength of rotation" of a segment. Torque is directly proportional to both magnitude of applied force and the distance between the force couple. The greater the magnitude of the force couple is (remember that the forces in a force couple have equivalent magnitudes), the greater the strength of rotation is. The farther apart the forces of a force couple are (the greater the MA), the greater the strength of rotation is.

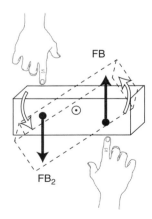

▲ **Figure 1-48** ■ Two forces of equal magnitude applied to the block in opposite directions constitute a force couple and will create rotation about a point midway between the forces if both points of application are free to move.

Angular Acceleration and Angular Equilibrium

If the torque created by the force couple is unopposed (there are no other forces on the segment), the result will be rotatory (or angular) acceleration of the segment. Linear (translatory) acceleration (a), as already noted, is a function of net unbalanced force and the mass (m) of the object ($a = F_{unbal} \div m$). Angular acceleration (α) is given in deg/sec^2 and is a function of net unbalanced *torque* and the mass (m) of the object:

$$\alpha = T_{unbal} \div m$$

When the torques on an object are balanced ($\Sigma T = 0$), the object must be in angular (rotatory) equilibrium (no resultant angular acceleration).

We can now identify three conditions that are *independently* necessary for an object or segment to be completely at rest:

$$\Sigma F_V = 0$$
$$\Sigma F_H = 0$$
$$\Sigma T = 0$$

If one or more of the three conditions are not met, the object will be in motion. In Figure 1-46A, the sum of the horizontal forces is unequal to zero, which results in a net positive horizontal linear acceleration. In Figure 1-46B, the sum of the vertical forces is unequal to zero, which results in a net positive vertical linear acceleration. In Figure 1-48 and 1-49, the sum of the torque in each figure is unequal to zero, which results in a net positive (counterclockwise) angular acceleration. In Figure 1-47, there is both a net unbalanced vertical force and a net unbalanced torque, which results both in a positive angular acceleration and in a positive vertical linear acceleration (general motion). Every time we consider whether a segment is at rest or, alternatively, the type and direction of motion that is occurring, *each* of the three conditions for equilibrium of that segment must be considered separately.

The concept of torque is not as intuitive as the concept of magnitude of a force or weight. Nevertheless, we use the principle of maximizing torque on a regular basis.

Example 1-9

The doors of commercial buildings have a mechanism built into the hinges that generates a "closing" torque (or a resistance to opening). If the person is to succeed in opening the door, the "opening" torque must be greater than the "closing" torque. The "opening" torque generated by the force of person-on-door (PD) (Fig. 1-50) is a product of the magnitude of PD and the distance (MA) that PD is applied from the axis of rotation (the door hinges). Let us assume that the "closing" torque of the door is set at 5 Nm. The person would have to generate a torque greater than 5 Nm to open the door. If the person pushed at a distance of 0.25 m from the door hinge (vector PD1 in the top view of the door in Fig. 1-50), the person would have to push with a force of more than 20 N (~4.5 lb) to open the door. At 0.5 m from the hinge (vector PD2), the person could open the door with a push of slightly more than 10 N (~2.2 lb). A push at the far edge of the 1-m–wide door would require a push (PD3) of only a little over 5 N (~1+ lb). Because it is easiest to open the door (requires the least force) when the distance from the axis of rotation (the MA) is maximized, we have automatically learned to place our hand as far from the axis as possible, thus generating the most torque with the least effort. If a large force is applied far from the axis, it will generate a large amount of unbalanced torque and greater angular acceleration (that is, the door will open faster!). [*Side-bar:* In Fig. 1-50, only the force PD is

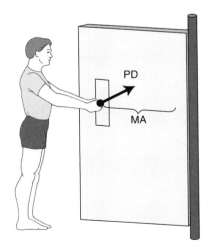
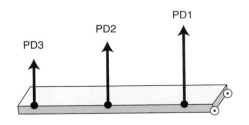

▲ **Figure 1-50** ■ The force of person-on-door (PD) creates a torque at the axis (hinges) of the door because the force is applied at a distance (MA) from the hinge. **Inset.** Three different magnitudes of force (PD1, PD2, and PD3) can produce the same "opening" torque only if the magnitudes of force are inversely proportional to their distance from the door hinge.

shown acting on the door. However, there must be at least one other force opposite in direction and of equal magnitude applied to the door (creating a force couple) to permit pure rotation. That counterforce will come from the hinge but is somewhat more complicated because of the "closing" torque created by the mechanism in the hinge. We will not stop to analyze this.]

Parallel Force Systems

Because the forces in a force couple are parallel to each other, the two forces are part of a **parallel force system.** A parallel force system exists whenever two *or more* forces applied to the same object are parallel to each other. The torque generated by each force is determined by multiplying the magnitude of that force by its distance (MA) either from the point of constraint of the segment or from an arbitrarily chosen point on the segment (as long as the same point is used for all forces). Consequently, the torque generated by a force of constant magnitude may change if the force is moved closer to or farther from the point of constraint. The torque attributed to a force of constant magnitude with a *fixed* point of application on an object can change if the reference point (axis or point of constraint) is changed.

■ Determining Resultant Forces in a Parallel Force System

The net or resultant torque produced by forces in the same parallel force system can be determined by adding the torques contributed by each force (with their appropriate signs). Three forces are applied to an unconstrained segment (Fig. 1-51). The magnitudes of F1, F2, and F3 are 5 N, 3 N, and 7 N, respectively. The MAs between F1, F2, and F3 and an arbitrarily chosen point (⊙) are 0.25 m, 0.12 m, and 0.12 m, respectively. F1 and F2 are applied in a clockwise direction, whereas F3 is applied in a counterclockwise direction (in relation to the chosen point of rotation). The resultant torque (T) would be:

$$T_{unbal} = (0.25 \text{ m})(-5 \text{ N}) + (0.12 \text{ m})(-3 \text{ N})$$
$$+ (0.12 \text{ m})(+7 \text{ N})$$

$$T_{unbal} = -0.77 \text{ Nm}$$

That is, there will be a net rotation of the segment in a clockwise direction with a magnitude of 0.77 Nm.

In Figure 1-52, forces F1, F2, and F3 have the same magnitude and points of application as they did in Figure 1-51. However, the reference point (the point of potential rotation) has been moved. The new MAs for F1, F2, and F3 are 0.6 m, 0.7 m, and 0.31 m, respectively. Force F2 is now on the other side of the reference point, thus creating a counterclockwise (instead of clockwise) torque. The new torques around the new reference point and their resultant torque are found in the following equation:

$$T_{unbal} = (0.6 \text{ m})(-5 \text{ N}) + (0.7 \text{ m})(+3 \text{ N}) +$$
$$(0.31\text{m})(+7 \text{ N})$$

$$T_{unbal} = +1.27 \text{ Nm}$$

Because the relatively small net torques in Figures 1-51 and 1-52 are calculated around a point that is *not* at the CoM of the segment, the segment will not only rotate but will also translate. This is particularly evident if we consider sum of the vertical forces, as well as the sum of the torques. Because all the vertical forces are upward in both figures, there is a concomitant net upward translatory force of 15 N. Consequently, the linear acceleration ($F_{unbal} \div m$) will substantially exceed the angular acceleration ($T_{unbal} \div m$), although both angular and linear acceleration will occur in each instance.

If the goal in Figure 1-51 is to rotate rather than translate the segment (as it is at joints in the human body), then the unwanted translation of the segment must be eliminated by the addition of a new force. However, let us first simplify the figure by composing F1 and F2 into a single resultant force, given both producing clockwise rotation of the lever.

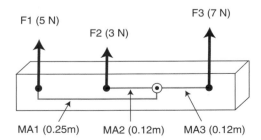

▲ **Figure 1-51** ■ The resultant of three parallel forces is found by the sum of the torques produced by the product of each force (F1, F2, and F3) and its MA (distance from the specified point of rotation).

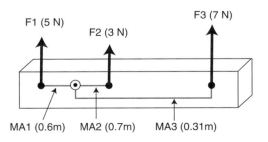

▲ **Figure 1-52** ■ The same forces shown in Fig. 1-51 produce different torques around a new point of rotation because the MAs of each force will differ from those in Figure 1-51.

CONCEPT CORNERSTONE 1-11: *Composition of Forces in a Parallel Force System*

When two parallel forces create torques in the same direction, the forces may be composed into a single resultant force whereby (1) the resultant force will have the same magnitude as the sum of the original two forces and (2) the resultant force will create the same torque as the sum of the torques of the two composing forces. If F1 (5 N) and F2 (3 N) are composed into a new force, F1-2, the new resultant will have a magnitude of 8 N (3 N + 5 N). The torque of F1-2 would be the sum of the torques of F1 and F2:

$$T_{F1\text{-}2} = (0.25\ m)(+5\ N) + (0.12\ m)(+3\ N) = 1.61\ Nm$$

The point of application of F1-2 can be determined by solving for its MA now that we know the torque and the force:

$$MA_{F1\text{-}2} = \frac{1.61\ Nm}{8\ N} = 0.20\ m$$

Consequently, F1 and F2 can be represented by force F1-2 that has a magnitude of 8 N and is located 0.20 m from the point of rotation.

In Figure 1-53, vectors F1 and F2 have been resolved into vector F1-2, and a new vector (F4) has been added. [*Side-bar:* Vector F4 might be easier in this particular figure to visualize as a push downward as shown by the dotted gray arrow. However, we will continue to use the convention that the base of the arrow is on the point of application, as shown for the vector labeled F4.] Vector F4 has a magnitude of -15 N. With the introduction of this force on the object, $\Sigma F_V = 0$. Vector F4 is applied at 0 m from the designated point (⊙), so the torque produced by this force is zero. Any force applied *through* a reference point or point of rotation will not produce torque. Although the addition of vector F4 results in vertical equilibrium, the net torque is still −0.77 Nm. The effect produced by the addition of F4 is what happens in the human body. A body segment will translate (with or without a concomitant rotation) until an equal and opposite constraint is encountered, at which point the forces on the segment produce pure rotation.

■ **Bending Moments and Torsional Moments**

When parallel forces are applied to an unsegmented object (assumed to be rigid) in a way that results in equilibrium (neither rotation nor translation of the segment), the torques, or moments of force, applied to a particular point on the object are considered to be **bending moments.**[3,4] Although a bending moment can also be defined as the torque between two forces that compose a force couple[3] (e.g., vectors F1 and F2 in 1–54A), the segment will rotate (rather than tend to bend) unless a third force is introduced (F3) to prevent this. For this reason, bending moments on a segment that is not rotating are also known as **three-point bending** because three parallel forces are required. If the segment is in both rotatory and translatory equilibrium (Fig. 1-54A), the sum of the vertical forces and the sum of the torques must be zero. In order to meet the conditions for translatory equilibrium, the magnitudes of F2 and F3 must each be half the magnitude of F1 (F2 + F3 = F1). Similarly, the torques (bending moments) of F2 and F3 around the point of application of F1 must be equal in magnitude and opposite in direction (the force of F1 does not create a torque). If the torques of F2 and F3 are equal and the magnitudes of F2 and F3 are equal, then the MAs of F2 and F3 must be equivalent as well. Although the segment is neither rotating nor translating, the bending force around the point of application of F1 could result in deformation (bending) of the segment *if the segment was nonrigid.* As long as a body segment can rotate, three-point bending forces on the segment are minimized.

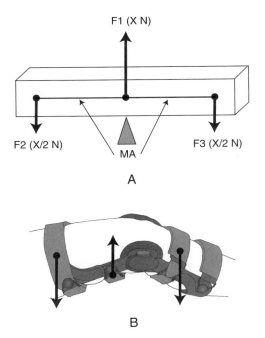

▲ **Figure 1-54** ■ **A.** A bending moment is created when a third force is added to a force couple, resulting in rotatory and translatory equilibrium but tending to "bend" the object around the center force. **B.** The principle of bending moments (or three-point bending) is often used in orthoses either to control motion or to "bend" a restricted joint.

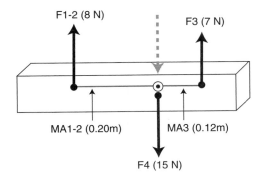

▲ **Figure 1-53** ■ Forces F1 and F2 (Fig. 1-51) have been composed into vector F1-2. The addition of F4, applied through the point of rotation, will produce vertical equilibrium without producing any additional torque. The block will now rotate around a fixed axis in the direction of unbalanced torque.

Continuing Exploration: **Three-Point Bending and Orthoses**

The principle of three-point bending is used in many orthoses either to limit motion (such as the knee brace intended to limit knee hyperextension in Figure 1-54B) or to "bend" (produce tissue deformation) in a stiff joint. We already know that the two forces applied in one direction (F2 and F3) will be equivalent in magnitude to the force in the opposite direction (F1). The implication of this is that the pressure (force per unit area) under F1 has the potential to be much greater. It is common, therefore, to use a larger contact area for the F1 force so that the pressure for that contact is reduced.

A **torsional moment** is sometimes considered a special case (or subcategory) of a torque, or moment of force, whereby a so-called torsional force creates (or tends to create) a rotation of a segment *around its long axis* (Fig. 1-55). The magnitude of the moment is still the product of the magnitude of the force and its shortest distance (MA) from the axis of rotation. When a force creates a rotation of a body segment around its longitudinal (or long) joint axis (typically but not always the y-axis in anatomic position; see Fig. 1-7), the resulting torque produces a medial or lateral rotatory moment that is similar to the flexion or abduction moment produced by a force around, respectively, a coronal or A-P axis. Because most muscles are attached at the periphery of somewhat cylindrically shaped long bones, most muscles create torques (moments) around two or more axes. In Example 1-3 in this chapter, the biceps brachii both flexed the forearm around a coronal axis and simultaneously supinated the forearm around a longitudinal axis. Although the magnitude of force for both motions (flexion and supination) would be the same, the magnitude of the flexion *moment* and the magnitude of the supination *moment* would be different because the line of pull of the biceps lies at a different distance from the two axes about which the motions occur.

Continuing Exploration: **Torsional Moments versus Torque**

In this text, the terms torque and moment of force will be used whenever there is rotation between two segments around any one of three joint axes. The term **torsion** (or torsional moment) will be used (and is probably used most often) to describe a torsional force applied to a single object (rather than between two objects); that is, a torsion creates a "twist" within the structure of the segment. Torsional forces certainly exist in rigid structures. However, torsional forces are a consideration primarily when the force has the potential to deform or damage the structure. Torsional forces, therefore, will be a more significant consideration when we examine deformable structures such as connective tissue (bone, cartilage, tendon, and ligament) in Chapter 2.

■ Identifying the Joint Axis about which Body Segments Rotate

In the human body, the motion of a segment at a joint is ultimately constrained by the articular structures, either by joint reaction forces (bony contact) or by capsuloligamentous forces. Any translatory motion of a segment produced by a force (e.g., gravity) will be checked before too long (we hope!) by the application of a new force (the push of a joint reaction force or the pull of a joint capsule or ligaments). The joint reaction or capsuloligamentous force that constrains further translation of the segment becomes one part of a force couple, resulting in continued movement of the segment as rotation around the point of constraint. The net effect of the translation (to the point of constraint) followed by rotation (around the point of constraint) is a subtle curvilinear motion of the segment with a very small translatory component. However, the implication is that the pivot point, or axis of rotation, for the segment is not fixed as is generally assumed to be the case. The axis shifts slightly during the motion, with the rotation point for any increment of the motion (if it were plotted) serving as the ICoR. The longer it takes for the articular constraints to limit translation of the segment, the greater will be the shift in the ICoR as the motion proceeds. Because of differences in bony configuration and behavior of connective tissues in individuals without impairments, the point or points of constraint can be expected to differ slightly. If the normal articular constraints are inadequate, there will be excessive translatory motion and shift of the joint axis before rotation can occur.

In order to assess the net rotation of a body segment around a joint, a common point needs to be iden-

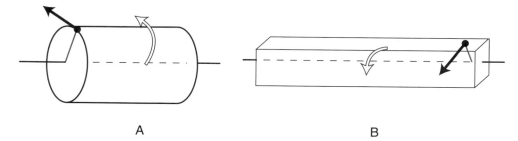

A   B

▲ **Figure 1-55 ■** A force applied to the periphery of a long segment (through which an axis passes longitudinally) produces a "torsional moment" that is directly proportional to the magnitude of the force and its distance from the longitudinal axis.

tified from which the torque of each force acting on the segment will be calculated. For human motion, we are interested in the rotation of a segment at a joint. Although it is acknowledged that the ICoR of a joint moves (and that the true CoR may lie at a considerable distance from the joint), common practice is to identify a point about which the joint rotation *appears* to occur. This is most often assumed to be approximately in the center of the sequential ICoRs and is referred to as the joint axis. It must be acknowledged, however, that this practice oversimplifies assessment of torques on a body segment.

In Figure 1-56, Sam's leg-foot segment is shown in the same position as in the leg-press exercise but without the contact of the footplate. If Sam is still relaxed in Figure 1-56, his leg-foot segment cannot remain in equilibrium. Initially, the leg-foot segment would translate downward linearly because of the downward force of gravity (vector GLf, 48 N). Vector GLf in this instance is a shear force because it lies parallel to the contacting surfaces of the femur and the leg-foot segment. A shear force has the potential to generate an opposing friction force (which would be vertically upward in this example). However, the contact between the femur and leg-foot segment would be minimal at the point in time shown in Figure 1-56 and the coefficient of friction would be small, resulting in a negligible upward friction force on the leg-foot segment. The leg-foot segment, therefore, would translate downward until the knee joint capsule became tensed. Once the magnitude of tension in the capsule and the concomitant pull of capsule-on-legfoot (CLf) reached 48 N, CLf would form a force couple with GLf, and the motion of the leg-foot segment would continue as a nearly pure rotation around the central point (⊙) of the attachments of the knee joint capsule.

If, in Figure 1-56, the CoM of Sam's leg-foot segment was located 20 cm (0.20 m) from the pivot point in the capsule that serves as the axis for the movement of the leg-foot segment, the torque (strength of rotation) of the leg-foot segment that weighs 48 N would be 9.6 Nm (or ~7 ftlb) around the pivot point of the capsule. Note in Figure 1-56 that the axis around which the

rotatory motion ultimately occurred is shifted down slightly from the original point of application of the capsular force because of the downward translation of the segment that preceded the pure rotatory motion.

The example presented in Figure 1-56 demonstrates why calculating torques as if there were a fixed joint axis can introduce at least some error in that calculation. Shifts in the point of constraint (or ICoR) during a motion can, by itself, result in slight differences in the MA for a given force and, therefore, slight differences in the torque even if all other factors remained constant. As we will see, however, other factors do not remain constant; there are other more influential factors that will also cause the torque of a force to vary as the segment moves at the joint. We begin to acknowledge here how complex even a simple joint rotation truly is.

Meeting the Three Conditions for Equilibrium

We have now established that everything that contacts a segment of the body creates a force on that segment and that each force has the potential to create translatory motion (vertical or horizontal), rotatory motion (torque), or both. We cannot possibly think about or account for the effects of all forces in a clinical environment. However, it is useful to understand the complexity of the potential effect of forces because it helps us understand why a small change in the balance of forces can result in a substantive change in the static or dynamic state of the segment. Before we increase the complexity by adding muscle forces to a segment, let us return to a previously oversimplified example to now consider all three conditions needed for equilibrium.

The magnitude of the contact force of the footplate on the leg-foot segment was initially calculated by assuming that the force of gravity and the force of friction were part of a linear force system and were equal in magnitude (see Fig. 1-44). Figure 1-57 shows the same four forces—gravity (GLf), friction (FrLf), footplate (FpLf), and femur (FLf)—each acting on the static leg-foot segment. Vectors FLf and FpLf are part of a horizontal linear force system and, in the absence of any other horizontal forces, must be equal in magnitude. It can now be appreciated that the action lines of FLf and FpLf pass approximately through the knee joint axis; therefore, FLf and FpLf will not create a torque around the knee joint (MA ≈ 0). Because these two forces balance each other out linearly ($\sum F_H = 0$) and create no other torque, FLf and FpLf have been shaded in Figure 1-57 as a way of removing them from further consideration.

The forces of gravity (a shear force) and friction (a response to the shear force) in Figure 1-57 are not co-linear (as we simplistically considered them in Fig. 1-44) but are both vertical and parallel. *If* these two forces are equal in magnitude (a working assumption only), the sum of the vertical forces would be zero. However, GLf and FrLf also constitute a force couple that would rotate the leg-foot segment counterclockwise with a

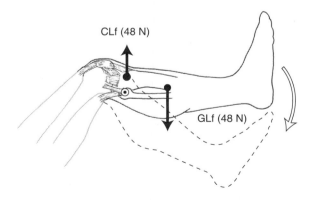

▲ **Figure 1-56** ■ The force of gravity (GLf) would translate the leg-foot segment down until tension in the capsule (CLf) reached an equivalent magnitude, at which point GLf and CLf would form a force couple to rotate the leg-foot segment around the point of application of CLf.

CLf (48 N)

GLf (48 N)

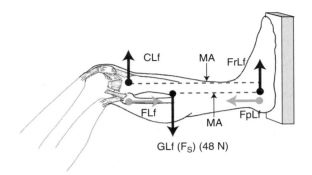

▲ **Figure 1-57** ■ Vectors FLf and FpLf are shaded because they produce horizontal equilibrium and do not contribute to torque. The sum of horizontal vectors (CLf, GLf, and FpLf) must be zero. Assuming that friction-on-legfoot (FrLf) is fixing the foot to the footplate, the torques are computed as the product of the magnitudes of gravity-on-legfoot (GLf) and capsule-on-legfoot (CLf) and their distances (MA and MA[1], respectively) from the point of application of FrLf. The sum of the torques will be zero.

torque equivalent to the magnitude of 48 N (GLf) multiplied by the distance (MA) between GLf and FrLf. Because friction can resist clockwise rotation but cannot actually move the leg-foot segment in a counterclockwise direction. The force of friction will effectively act as the constraint (its point of application being the point of potential rotation for the force couple) because friction can resist clockwise rotation but cannot actually move the leg-foot segment in a counterclockwise direction.

Given that GLf is not rotating the leg-foot segment around the point of application of FrLf, there must be at least one other force acting on the leg-foot segment that is creating a clockwise torque with a magnitude equal to that of the torque of GLf. The only other contact on the leg-foot segment in Figure 1-57 is that of the joint capsule. If the leg-foot segment started to rotate clockwise around the point of application of FrLf, the proximal articular surface of the leg-foot segment would slide down the femur, as we saw in Figure 1-56. Although the motion of the leg-foot segment is actually rotatory, it would look very similar to the downward slide that we saw in Figure 1-56 and would have the same effect: the capsule would become tight, and the force of capsule-on-legfoot (CLf) would be reintroduced.

To create a torque equivalent to the torque of GLf, the magnitude of CLf would have to be only about half the magnitude of GLf because CLf lies approximately twice as far (2 × MA) from the point of application of FrLf (the presumed point of constraint). If the magnitude of CLf is 24 N (48 N/2), then the magnitude of FrLf must also be 24 N in order for $\Sigma F_V = 0$. We have now met all three conditions for equilibrium of the leg-foot segment:

$$\Sigma F_H = (+FLf) + (-FpLf) = 0$$

$$\Sigma F_V = (+CLf) + (-GLf) + (+FrLf) = 0$$

$$\Sigma T = (+CLf)(2MA) + (-GLf)(MA) + (FrLf)(0) = 0$$

We used the magnitude of FrLf to calculate the contact force (FpLf) in Figure 1-44. Because it is now

evident that we overestimated the magnitude of friction in that example, we also overestimated the magnitude of FpLf in that example. However, the magnitudes of FpLf and FLf will continue to be equivalent (both less than originally estimated) because they are the only horizontal forces on the leg-foot segment.

Thus far, we have considered that Sam Alexander is relaxed and that the leg-foot segment is in equilibrium in both the weight boot example and in the leg-press example. If the goal is to strengthen Sam's quadriceps muscle, it is time to introduce a muscle force.

◆ Muscle Forces

Total Muscle Force Vector

The force applied by a muscle to a bony segment is actually the resultant of the pull on a common point of attachment of all the fibers that compose the muscle. Because each muscle fiber can be represented by a vector that has a common point of application (Fig. 1-58), the fibers taken together form a concurrent force system with a resultant that represents the total muscle force vector (Fms). Vector Fms can be approximated by putting the point of application at the muscle's attachment on the segment under consideration and then drawing an action line symmetrically toward the middle of the muscle's fibers that is also parallel to the tendon or fibers at that attachment. The direction of pull for any muscle is *always* toward the center of the muscle. The magnitude or length of Fms may be drawn arbitrarily unless a hypothetical magnitude is specified. The actual magnitude of the total force muscle (the pull of a muscle on its attachment) cannot be determined in the living person.

Continuing Exploration: **Measuring Muscle Force**

Electromyography (EMG) can measure the electrical activity of a muscle. The electrical activity is directly proportional to the motor unit activity that is, in turn, directly proportional to the muscle force (see Chapter 3). However, neither electrical activity nor number of motor units is a measure of absolute force generated by a muscle, because different motor units produce different tension under different con-

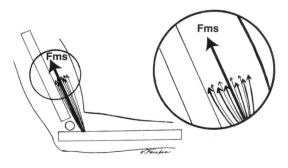

▲ **Figure 1-58** ■ The total muscle force (F_{TOT} or Fms) is the resultant of all the fiber pulls taken together.

ditions. When "strength" of a muscle is measured by using weights, force transducers, or isokinetic devices, what is actually being measured directly or indirectly is the torque on the segment being created by the internal forces in relation to the torque of the external force (measurement device). Although the net (resultant) internal *torque* on the segment can be estimated if the MAs of the known forces (gravity and the external force) can be estimated, the magnitudes of internal forces contributing to the net internal force are difficult, if not impossible, to identify. Even if a single muscle were active (which is almost never the case), it would be impossible to separate out the influence of forces such as joint reaction forces, capsuloligamentous forces, and small friction forces. The result is that the actual magnitude of pull of a single muscle cannot be assessed in a living person (*in vivo*) without surgical implantation of a device—which may itself alter the force normally produced by a muscle.

Every muscle pulls on each of its attachments every time the muscle exerts a force. Therefore, every muscle creates a minimum of two force vectors, one on each of the two (or more) segments to which the muscle is attached; each of the two (or more) vectors is directed toward the middle of the muscle. The type and direction of motion that results from an active muscle contraction depends on the net forces and net torques acting on each of its levers. The muscle will move a segment in its direction of pull only when the torque of the muscle exceeds the potential opposing torques.

In a space diagram (e.g., Sam Alexander's leg-foot segment), we will often identify only the pull of the muscle on the segment under consideration. However, it should be recognized that we are purposefully ignoring that same muscle's concomitant pull on one or more *other* segments—at least until we move on to considering that segment.

■ **Anatomic Pulleys**

Frequently, the fibers of a muscle or a muscle tendon wrap around a bone or are deflected by a bony prominence. When the direction of pull of a muscle is altered, the bone or bony prominence causing the deflection forms an anatomic pulley. Pulleys (if they are

frictionless) change the direction without changing the magnitude of the applied force. As we will see, the change in action line produced by an anatomic pulley (even without affecting force) will have implications for the ability of the muscle to produce torque.

Figure 1-59A is a schematic representation of what the middle deltoid muscle might look like if the muscle were attached to two straight levers. The muscle force vector is shown acting on the humerus (at the point of application of the deltoid muscle on the humerus), directed toward the center of the muscle, with the vector parallel to and in the middle of the fibers at the point of attachment. Figure 1-59B shows the middle deltoid muscle as it crosses the actual glenohumeral joint, wrapping around the acromion and the rounded head of the humerus and its tubercles. The humeral head and acromion change the direction of the fibers at both ends of the muscle and function, therefore, as an anatomic pulley. The action line of the middle deltoid muscle acting on the humerus is no longer parallel to the humerus because the action line follows the muscle fibers at the point of attachment on the humerus. Because vectors are always straight lines, the effect of the pull of a muscle on a bony segment is governed by the direction of pull of the muscle *at the point of attachment* and is not changed by subsequent shifts in fiber direction. The action line and direction of Fms are significantly different between parts A and B of Figure 1-59, although the point of application and magnitude of the force are the same in each figure part.

■ **Anatomic Pulleys, Action Lines, and Moment Arms**

The function of any pulley is to redirect a force to make a task easier. The "task" in human movement is to rotate a body segment. Anatomic pulleys (in the majority of instances) make this task easier by deflecting the action line of the muscle *away* from the joint axis, thus increasing the MA of the muscle force. By increasing the MA for a muscle force, a force of the same magnitude (with no extra energy expenditure) produces greater torque. If the middle deltoid muscle had the action line shown in Figure 1-59A, the MA would be quite small. The MA is substantially greater when the humeral head and overhanging acromion result in a shift of the action line of the muscle away from the joint

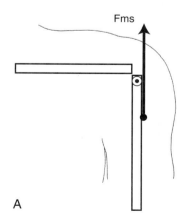

Fms

A

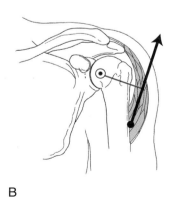

B

◀ **Figure 1-59** ■ **A.** A schematic representation of the muscle and muscle force produced by the middle deltoid muscle *if* the muscle crosses two straight levers. **B.** A more anatomic representation of the bony levers to which the middle deltoid muscle is attached, showing its line of pull deflected away from the joint axis by the anatomic pulley of the humeral head.

axis (see Fig. 1-59B). Consequently, the deltoid muscle will be able to produce an equivalent abduction moment on the humerus with less force in Figure 1-59B than in Figure 1-59A.

Example 1-11

The Patella as an Anatomic Pulley

The classic example of an anatomic pulley is that formed by the patella. The quadriceps muscle belly lies parallel to the femur. The tendon of the muscle passes over the knee joint and attaches to the leg (tibia) via the patellar tendon at the tibial tubercle. For knee joint extension, the joint axis is considered to be located through the femoral condyles. The MA for the quadriceps muscle force (QLf) lies in space between the vector and the joint axis. Without the patella, the line of pull of the quadriceps muscle on the leg-foot segment would follow the patellar tendon at the tibial tubercle and would lie parallel to the leg-foot segment (Fig. 1-60A). However, the patella lies between the quadriceps tendon and the femur, changing the angle that the patellar tendon makes with the leg (tibia) and changing the line of pull of the quadriceps muscle away from the knee joint axis (see Fig. 1-60B). The effect of changing the line of pull of the quadriceps muscle on the tibia (QLf) is to increase the MA in Figure 1-60B. Given the increased MA, the same magnitude of force from QLf would produce greater torque (and a greater angular acceleration as the only force) in Figure 1-60B than in Figure 1-60A with the same energy expenditure.

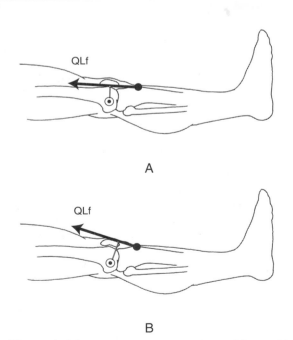

▲ **Figure 1-60** ■ **A.** The line of pull and MA of the quadriceps muscle without the patella. **B.** With the patella's pulley effect, the line of pull of the muscle is deflected away from the joint axis, increasing the MA of the muscle force.

There are other sesamoid bones in the human body (although the patella is by far the largest), each of which has a similar function and effect of changing the direction of the action line of the muscle or tendon that passes over it and, as a result, increasing the ability of the muscle to produce torque around one or more joint axes.

 CONCEPT CORNERSTONE 1-12: *Moment Arm and Lever Arm*

The MA for any force vector will always be the length of a line that is perpendicular to the force vector and intersects the joint axis (presuming a two-dimensional perspective). The MA will *always* be the shortest distance between the vector and the axis of rotation. For a force that is perpendicular to the long axis of a segment (as the forces were for Figs. 1-49 through 1-54), the MA will be parallel to and lie along the lever. In this instance, the term lever arm (LA) may also be used to describe this distance; that is, a LA is simply a special case of a MA in which the MA lies *along the lever* and is also the distance between the point of application of the force and the joint axis. Although it is not necessary to employ the term "lever arm" (because MA covers all situations), there are some instances in which the term serves as a convenient reminder that the force is perpendicular to the lever.

 CONCEPT CORNERSTONE 1-13: *Muscle Force Vectors*

- Active or passive tension in a muscle creates a force (a pull) on all segments to which the muscle is attached, although one may choose to consider only one segment at a time.
- The point of application of a muscle force vector is located at the point of attachment of the muscle on the segment under consideration.
- The muscle action line is in the direction of pull that the fibers or tendons of the muscle create *at the point of application*.
- Muscle vectors (like all vectors) continue in a straight line from the point of application, regardless of any change in direction of muscle fiber or tendon after the point of application.
- The magnitude of a muscle force is generally a hypothetical or theoretical value because the absolute force of a muscle's pull on its attachments cannot be measured in most living subjects.

◆ Torque Revisited

We are now ready to add the quadriceps muscle force to Sam Alexander's leg-foot segment at the point at which knee extension is to be initiated in the weight boot example. Figure 1-61 shows the pull of the quadriceps muscle on the leg-foot segment (QLf). In the figure, the force of gravity (GLf) and the force of the weight boot (WbLf) are represented as a single resultant force, GWbLf, as was done in Figure 1-41. Case Application 1-2 shows the calculation for the point of application of resultant vector GWbLf for Sam.

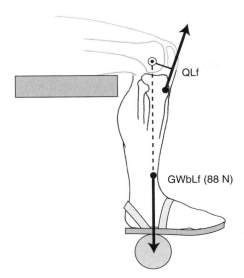

▲ **Figure 1-61** ■ The resultant force for gravity and the weight boot (GWbLf) and the force of the quadriceps muscle (QLf) are shown with their respective MAs when the knee is at 90° of flexion. Vector GWbLf must be extended to ascertain its shortest distance to the joint axis.

Case Application 1-2: **Composition of GLf and WbLf**

The magnitude of the resultant force (GWbLf) is the sum of the magnitudes of the composing forces (GLf + WbLf). The torques contributed by each of the composing forces can be determined if the MA for each force is known. Using segmental lengths from LeVeau,[1] we will estimate (1) that Sam's CoM for his leg-foot segment lies 0.25 m from his knee joint axis and (2) that the weight boot (at the end of his leg-foot segment) is 0.5 m from his knee joint axis. These values are the distances from each point of application of the force to the knee joint axis. This distance is the MA of the force *only* if the force is perpendicular to the lever (when MA = LA), and so we will compute the torques for the point at which GLf and WbLf are perpendicular to the leg-foot segment (or when the leg-foot segment is parallel to the ground). Using the values for Sam and recognizing that both the forces that are being composed are downward, we find that the torques for GLf and WbLf are:

$$T_{GLf} = (48 \text{ N})(0.25 \text{ m}) = -12 \text{ Nm}$$

$$T_{WbLf} = (40 \text{ N})(0.5 \text{ m}) = -20 \text{ Nm}$$

If the resultant (GWbLf) has a magnitude of 88 N (the magnitudes of GLf + WbLf) and a torque of –32 Nm, then the MA for GWbLf must be T ÷ F, or 0.36 m.

The magnitude of QLf (see Fig. 1-61) is currently unknown. The net effect of QLf and the downward pull on the leg-foot segment at the moment in time captured in the figure may be approached several ways. Vectors GWbLf and QLf could be treated as concurrent forces, allowing determination of the resultant using composition of forces by parallelogram. Alternatively,

the torque produced by each force can be determined separately, with the understanding that there needs to be an unbalanced torque in the direction of knee extension if Sam is to lift his leg.

Changes to Moment Arm of a Force

For some vectors, as for GWbLf, finding the shortest (or perpendicular) distance between a vector and a joint axis (MA) requires that the vector be extended. The effect of a vector is not changed by extending it graphically—nor should it be considered to change the magnitude of the force. When vector GWbLf is extended in Figure 1-61, GWbLf still has a magnitude of −88 N, but its MA is effectively zero because the extended vector lies so close to the knee joint axis. GWbLf in this position of the leg-foot segment creates negligible torque on the segment. Given that GWbLf produces no torque in this knee joint position, a relatively small force by the quadriceps muscle (QLf) applied through its relatively larger MA (0.03 m) will yield a net resultant torque in the direction of knee extension. This will not continue to be the case for very long, because as soon as the position of the leg-foot segment changes, so too do the torques created by the forces applied to the leg-foot segment.

In Figure 1-62, the leg-foot segment has been brought farther into the knee extension (~45°of knee flexion). As the segment moves in space, the relation between the forces applied to the segment and the segment itself change. The extended vector GWbLf now lies at a substantially greater distance from the knee joint axis. Vector QLf has a larger MA (increasing from 0.03 m to 0.05 m), but the increase is minimal in comparison with the increase in the moment of GWbLf, which has increased from 0 m to 0.27 m. The magnitude of QLf necessary to continue knee extension from this point in the ROM can now be estimated.

If the MA for GWbLf is 0.27 m in Figure 1-62, then

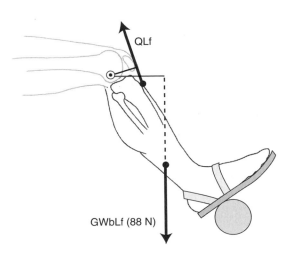

▲ **Figure 1-62** ■ As the leg-foot segment moves to 45° of knee flexion, the relative sizes of the MAs for both QLf and GWbLf increase.

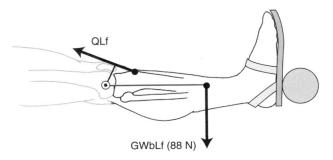

▲ **Figure 1-63** ■ At full knee extension, the MA of vector GWbLf is as large as it can be, whereas the MA for QLf is now at its smallest.

a force of 88 N would create a clockwise (knee flexion) torque of 23.76 Nm. The quadriceps muscle would have to create a counterclockwise (extension) torque of 23.76 Nm to maintain rotatory equilibrium. If the MA for QLf in Figure 1-62 is 0.05 m, then QLf would have to have a magnitude of 475.2 N (~107 lb) just to maintain the leg-foot segment at 45°. The force of QLf would have to be greater than 475.2 N for a net unbalanced torque in the direction of knee extension.

Figure 1-63 shows the leg-foot segment at the end of knee extension (0° of knee flexion). Vector GWbLf is now perpendicular to the leg-foot segment, and its MA has further increased (0.36 m). The MA for QLf in Figure 1-63 has gotten smaller from that seen in the previous figure. The magnitude of the GWbLf remains unchanged at 88 N. However, GWbLf now creates a clockwise (flexion) torque of 31.68 Nm. If the MA for QLf is now 0.01 m, the quadriceps muscle will have to generate a force of 3168 N (712 lb) to maintain this position (rotatory equilibrium).

Whenever any force is applied at 90° to the long axis of a segment (as GWbLf is in Fig. 1-63), the length of the MA of the force is maximal. The MA will lie parallel to the long axis of the segment (the lever) and, under these conditions (as noted earlier), can also be referred to as the LA of the force. Because the MA of a force is greatest when that force is at 90° to the segment, the torque *for a given magnitude of force* will also be greatest at this point. When lifting the weight boot, Sam will find the position in Figure 1-63 hardest to maintain. Although Sam is working against the consistent 88-N weight of the leg-foot segment and weight boot, the flexion torque generated by the combined force (GWbLf) is greatest when the leg-foot segment is horizontal (parallel to the ground). At this point, it requires the greatest contraction of the quadriceps muscle to offset the torque of GWbLf.

◫ CONCEPT CORNERSTONE 1-14: *Moment Arms and Torque*

- As the angle of application of a force increases, the MA of the force increases.
- As the MA of a force increases, its potential to produce torque increases.

- The MA of a force is maximal when the force is applied at 90° to its segment.
- The MA of a force is minimal (0.0) when the action line of the force passes through the CoR of the segment to which the force is applied.

Angular Acceleration with Changing Torques

We have approached Sam's weight boot example as a series of freeze-frames or single points in time (see Figs. 1-61 through 1-63). We have also established that Sam will have to contract his quadriceps muscle with a force of approximately 3168 N to maintain full knee extension against the flexion torque of gravity and the weight boot. If Sam *initiated* the exercise at 90° of knee flexion (see Fig. 1-61) with a quadriceps muscle contraction of 3168 N, almost all the torque generated by the muscle contraction would be unopposed, and the unbalanced torque would result in a substantial angular acceleration of the leg-foot segment in the direction of extension with the initiation of the muscle contraction. As the leg-foot segment moves from 90° of flexion toward increased extension, the flexion torque generated by GWbLf gradually increases until it is maximal in full knee extension (see Fig. 1-63). Consequently, the net unbalanced torque and acceleration of the segment must be changing as the knee extends. If knee extension proceeded through the series of freeze-frames from 90° of knee flexion to full knee extension, and *if the force of quadriceps muscle contraction is constant*, the leg-foot segment would generally accelerate less as extension continues until equilibrium is reached in full knee extension (when posterior knee structures would, along with gravity and the weight boot, contribute to checking further knee extension). The decrease in acceleration of the segment, however, is not consistent through the ROM. Whereas the torque produced by GWbLf will continually increase as the force's MA increases, the torque of QLf (even with a constant contraction of 3168 N) varies with the change in MA of the quadriceps muscle. It is a characteristic of the quadriceps muscle that its MA is greatest in the middle of the motion and less at either end (being least in full knee extension). [*Side-bar:* The change in MA of a muscle through the range of the joint it crosses is somewhat unique to each muscle and not predictable.]

Moment Arm and Angle of Application of a Force

We have seen that the MA of a force can change as a segment rotates around its joint axis and as the segment changes its orientation in space. The length of the MA is directly related to the **angle of application of the force** on the segment. The angle of application of a vector is the angle made by the intersection of the force vector and the segment to which it applied, *on the side of the joint axis under consideration.* Any time a vector is

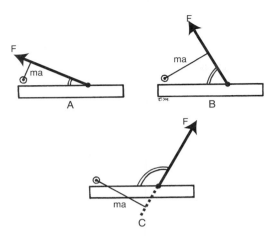

▲ **Figure 1-64** ■ Changes in the angle of application of the force (the angle between the force vector and lever *on the side of the axis*) result in changes to the MA of the force, with the MA maximal when the force is at 90° to the lever.

applied to a lever (segment), a minimum of two angles are formed. The viewer's eye will automatically tend to find the acute (rather than obtuse) angle. To identify the angle of application of a force, the angle *on the side of the joint axis* is the angle of interest, regardless of whether that angle is acute or obtuse (>90°).

Figure 1-64 shows a force vector at three different angles in relation to a segment. We can see in those three depictions how the angle of application affects the size of the MA. When the angle of application of a force is small, the MA will be small (see Fig. 1-64A). As the angle of application for the force increases, the MA increases because the vector lies farther from the joint axis (see Fig. 1-64B). As the angle of application of the force moves beyond 90° (see Fig. 1-64C), the MA is measured from the extended tail of the vector; the extended tail swings closer to the joint axis as the angle of application of the force increases beyond 90°. For all forces (internal or external), the MA of a force is smallest when the vector is parallel to the segment (whether at 0° or at 180°) and greatest when the vector is perpendicular to the segment.

Figure 1-65 shows the force of gravity (G) acting on the forearm-hand segment in four different positions of the elbow joint. Figure 1-66 shows a muscle force (Fms) of constant magnitude acting on the forearm-hand segment at the same elbow joint angles as shown in Figure 1-65. As the forearm segment rotates around the elbow joint axis, the angles of application for gravity and for Fms change *in relation to the forearm segment*. As the angle of application of the force changes, the MA must also change. Although the magnitudes of forces G (see Fig. 1-65) and Fms (see Fig. 1-66) do not change from position to position, the *torque* generated by each force changes in direct proportion to the change in length of the MA. The MAs are maximal when the force is applied perpendicularly to the segment and smallest when the forces lie closest to being parallel to the segment.

Although Figures 1-65 and 1-66 show that torques forces change as a segment moves through a ROM, the basis for the change in angle of application is somewhat different for the gravitation force than for the muscle force. A gravitational force is always vertically downward. Consequently, it is the position of the *segment in space* that causes a change in the angle of application of a gravitational vector, not a change in the joint angle. Figure 1-67 shows the force of gravity (G) applied to the forearm-hand segment at two different orientations in space. Although the elbow joint angle is the same in Figure 1-67A and B, the MAs are quite different. The angle of application of a gravitational force is dependent exclusively on the position of the segment of interest in space. Because the *magnitude* of the gravitational force does not change as the segment moves through space (as long as its mass is not rearranged), the torque produced by the weight (G) of a segment is directly a function of the position of the segment in space.

External forces, such as gravity, are more commonly affected by the *position of the segment* than by the angle the segment makes with its adjacent segment (*joint angle*). Unlike gravity, however, external forces (e.g., a manual resistance, mechanical resistance, or applied load) can change the point of application of the force to different points on the body segment.

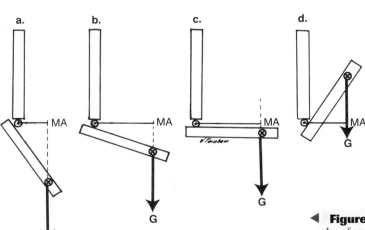

◀ **Figure 1-65** ■ Gravity (G) acting on the forearm-hand segment at angles of application of 35° (**A**), 70° (**B**), 90° (**C**), and 145° (**D**) of elbow flexion. The MA of gravity changes with the position of the forearm in space.

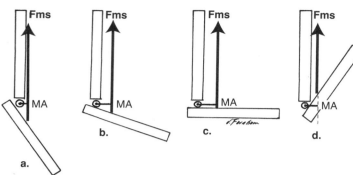

◄ **Figure 1-66** ■ A muscle force (Fms) acting on the forearm-hand segment at angles of application of 35° (**A**), 70° (**B**), 90° (**C**), and 145° (**D**). As the joint crossed by the muscles moves through its range of motion, the MA of the muscle changes.

When the point of application on the segment changes, so too does the MA. This can be observed in Figure 1-50 as the person moved his hand farther from the door hinge. With the increase in MA as the hand moved away from the hinge (the axis), production of the same torque required less force. The point of application of a gravitational force (CoM) can be relocated *only* if the segments that compose the object are rearranged. However, such rearrangement of segments is often done to change the effects of gravity.

Example 1-12

Changing the Gravitation Moment Arm by Changing the CoM

Figure 1-68 shows three graded exercises for the abdominal muscles. The vertebral interspace of L5 to S1 is considered here to be a hypothetical axis about which **HAT** rotates. In each figure, the arms are positioned slightly differently, which results in a rearrangement of mass and a shift in the CoM. In Figure 1-68A, the arms are raised above the head. As a result, the CoM of HAT is located closer to the head (cephalad), with a LoG that is farther from the axis of rotation (greater MA) than when the arms are in the other two positions. The torque generated by gravity is counterclockwise (a trunk extension moment). To maintain this position (rotational equilibrium), the abdominal muscles must generate an equal torque in the opposite direction (an equivalent flexion moment). In Figure 1-68B and C, the CoMs move caudally as the arms are lowered. The relocation of the CoM of HAT (through rearrangement of the segments) brings the LoG closer to the axis. Because the weight of the upper body does not change when the arms are lowered, the magnitude of torque applied by gravity to the upper body diminishes in proportion to the reduction in the MA. The decreased gravitational torque requires less opposing torque by the abdominal muscles to maintain equilibrium. Consequently, it is easiest to maintain the position in Figure 1-68C and hardest to maintain the position in Figure 1-68A.

The angle of application and MAs of internal forces such as active or passive muscle forces, capsuloligamentous forces, and joint reaction forces (unlike gravity and most other external forces) are directly affected by the relationship between the two adjacent segments and minimally affected by the position of the segment in space. The angle of application of Fms in Figure 1-66 would be the same at each elbow joint angle, regardless of where the adjacent segments are in space (whether you turned the figures right side up, upside down, or sideways). Another distinction to be made between internal forces and most external forces is that the points of application of internal forces typically cannot change but are anatomically fixed. Lastly, the *magnitude* of an internal force (unlike the magnitudes of a gravitational force and many external forces) is rarely consistent as a joint rotates. The magnitude of an internal force is dependent on and responsive to a substantial number of factors (e.g., passive stretch or active contraction) that will be explored further in Chapters 2 and 3.

◆ Lever Systems, or Classes of Levers

One perspective used to assess the relative torques of internal and external forces is that of **lever systems,** or **classes of levers.** Although applying the terminology of lever systems to human movement requires some important oversimplifications, the terms (like those of

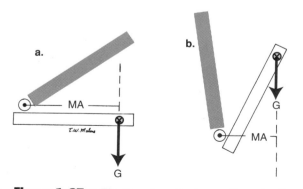

▲ **Figure 1-67** ■ The line of gravity changes its angle of application to the forearm-hand segment and its MA when the forearm-hand segment moves in space, although the elbow joint angle remains unchanged.

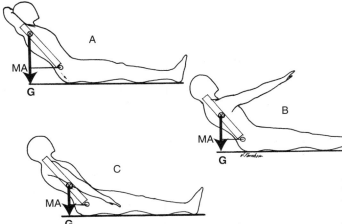

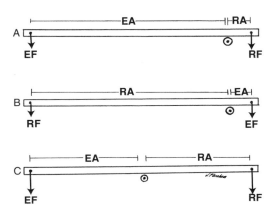

▲ **Figure 1-68** ■ Changes in arm position in a sit-up cause the CoM of the upper body segment to move, the MA to change, and the torque of gravity (G) to decrease from **A** to **C.** Although vector G (weight of HAT) varies in length from A to C, the *magnitude* of G is actually unchanged regardless of arm position.

the cardinal planes and axes) provide a useful frame of reference and common language that permit us to break complex kinetics into describable component parts.

A lever is any rigid segment that rotates around a fulcrum. A lever system exists whenever two forces are applied to a lever in a way that produces opposing torques. We have used the terms segment and lever essentially interchangeably when referencing the body, while acknowledging that bones are not, strictly speaking, rigid. In order to apply concepts of levers to a bony segment, we must also consider the joint axis of the bony segment to be relatively fixed (a problematic assumption, as we have already discussed). However, it is common to apply the concepts of levers to bony segments when looking at the net rotation produced by (1) a muscle force and (2) a gravitational and/or external force.

In a lever system, the force that is producing the resultant torque (the force acting in the direction of rotation) is called the **effort force** (**EF**). Because the other force must be creating an opposing torque, it is known as the **resistance force** (**RF**). Another way to think of effort and resistance forces acting on a lever is that the effort force *is always the winner* in the torque game, and the resistance *force is always the loser* in producing rotation of the segment. The MA for the EF is referred to as the **effort arm** (**EA**), whereas the MA for the RF is referred to as the **resistance arm** (**RA**). Once the effort and resistance forces are identified and labeled, the position of the axis and relative sizes of the effort and resistance arms determine the class of the lever.

A **first-class lever** is a lever system in which the axis lies between the point of application of the effort force and the point of application of the resistance force, without regard to the size of EA or RA. As long as the axis lies between the points of application of the EF and RF, EA can be bigger than RA (Fig. 1-69A), smaller than RA (see Fig. 1-69B), or the same size as RA (see Fig. 1-69C). A **second-class lever** is a lever system in which the resistance force has a point of application

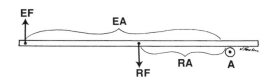

▲ **Figure 1-69** ■ In a first-class lever system, EA may be greater than RA (**A**), smaller than RA (**B**), or equal to RA (**C**).

▲ **Figure 1-70** ■ A second-class lever system. The effort arm (EA) is always larger than the resistance arm (RA).

between the axis and the point of application of the effort force, which always results in EA being larger than RA (Fig. 1-70). A **third-class lever** is a lever system in which the effort force has a point of application between the axis and the point of application of the resistance force, which always results in RA being larger than EA (Fig. 1-71). [*Side-bar:* The class of lever is most easily and most often described, as is done here, by considering a muscle force acting on the muscle's *distal* segment. When a muscle is contracting during movement of its *proximal* segment, the analysis becomes more complex, typically involves *more* than two forces, and is probably not clarified by reference to lever systems.]

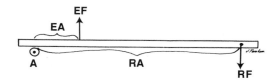

▲ **Figure 1-71** ■ A third-class lever system. The effort arm (EA) is always smaller than the resistance arm (RA).

Muscles in Third–Class Lever System

In the human body, a muscle creating joint rotation of its *distal segment* in the direction of its pull (making the muscle the EF) is most often part of third-class lever system. The action of the quadriceps muscle on the leg-foot segment against the resistance of gravity and the weight boot serves as a typical example. Figure 1-72A shows Sam contracting his quadriceps muscle in the weight boot exercise. If the magnitude of QLf is at least 3169 N, the leg-foot segment will extend (regardless of

position) because the $T_{QLf} > T_{GWbLf}$ (as was determined in the section Angular Acceleration with Changing Torques). As long as the net rotation is in the direction of extension in Figure 1-72A, QLf must be the effort force (EF) and GWbLf must be the resistance force (RF). Because QLf lies closer to the joint axis than does GWbLf (MAs are 0.05 m and 0.27 m, respectively), the lever must be third class (EA < RA).

The example shown in Figure 1-72A is typical because the point of attachment of a muscle on its distal segment is almost always closer to the joint axis than an external force is likely to be. Consequently, when the muscle is the effort force, EA is most likely to be smaller than RA, with the muscle acting on a third-class lever. It is also important to note that whenever a muscle is the effort force, the muscle must be moving the segment in its direction of pull. This means that the muscle must be performing a shortening contraction, also known as a **concentric contraction.** In fact, any time a muscle is the effort force, the muscle must be contracting concentrically because it is "winning."

Muscles in Second-Class Lever System

Muscles most commonly act on second-class levers when gravity or another external force is the effort force and the muscle is the resistance force (acting on the muscle's distal segment). Figure 1-72B is identical to 1-72A except for the magnitude of QLf. If QLf exerted a force of 450 N (less force than is required to maintain equilibrium in this position), the net torque would now be in the direction of flexion. If the net torque is in the direction of flexion, GWbLf would be the EF and QLf would become RF. Because the MA (EA) for GWbLf (0.27 m) is larger than the MA (RA) for QLf (0.05 m), the quadriceps muscle is now working in a second-class lever system.

It is important to notice that even when the quadriceps muscle is the resistance force, its force vector remains unchanged except in magnitude (see Fig. 1-72B). The quadriceps muscle is *still* creating an extension moment. If a muscle that creates rotation of a segment in one direction is actively contracting while the *opposite motion* occurs, the muscle must be actively lengthening. Active lengthening of a muscle is referred to as an **eccentric contraction** and always indicates that the muscle is serving as a resistance force (creating torque in a direction opposite to the observed rotation). A muscle that is working eccentrically is generally providing *control* (resistance) by minimizing the acceleration produced by the EF. The switching of a muscle's role from effort to resistance also shows why a kinematic description of motion cannot be used in isolation to identify muscle action. In Figure 1-72B, the knee joint is flexing despite the fact that there are no active *knee joint flexors.* In fact, the only active muscle is a knee extensor! An understanding of the muscles and other forces involved in any movement can be achieved only through a kinetic analysis of the motion and not simply from a description of the location, direction, or magnitude of motion.

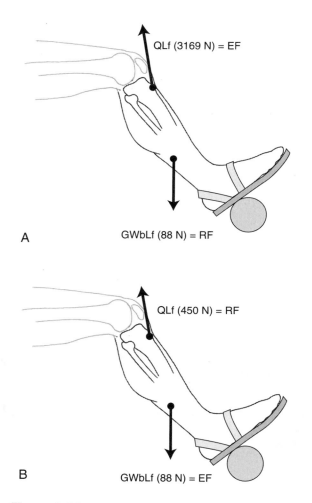

QLf (3169 N) = EF

GWbLf (88 N) = RF

A

QLf (450 N) = RF

GWbLf (88 N) = EF

B

▲ **Figure 1-72** ■ **A.** When $T_{QLf} > T_{GWbLf}$, then QLf is contracting concentrically as the effort force (EF) and GWbLf is the resistance force (RF) in a third-class lever system. **B.** If $T_{QLf} < T_{GWbLf}$, then GWbLf is the effort force (EF) and QLf is contracting eccentrically as the resistance force (RF) in a second-class lever system.

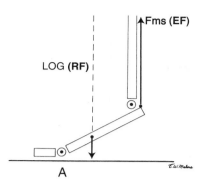

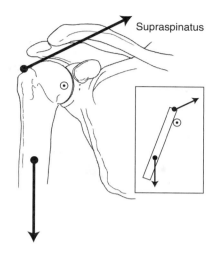

▲ **Figure 1-73** ▪ As the triceps surae (Fms) contracts concentrically, the weight of the body (LoG) is lifted around the metatarsophalangeal joint axis (A) of the toes. The triceps surae force (Fms = EF) and the force of gravity (LoG = RF) are part of a second-class lever.

▲ **Figure 1-74** ▪ The supraspinatus is attached to the humerus on one side of the joint axis, and the point of application of gravity (CoM) lies on the other side of the axis (inset). Regardless of whether the muscle is working concentrically (EF) or eccentrically (RF), the muscle is part of a first-class lever.

When a muscle works in a second-class lever system on its distal lever, the muscle is most often going to be the resistance force. There are a limited number of examples in which a muscle is the *effort force* acting on its distal segment in a second-class lever system, but this is most likely to occur when the distal segment to which the muscle is attached is weight bearing. Figure 1-73 shows the calf muscles (triceps surae muscle group, or Fms) acting on the foot segment (the foot being considered as a rigid lever), lifting the body around the axis of the toes (metatarsophalangeal [MTP] joints). The superimposed body weight acting at the point of application of the LoG on the foot is the resistance force (RF). Because the effort force (Fms) is farther from the MTP axis than the point of application of the body weight on the foot segment, Fms is contracting concentrically in a second-class lever system.

Muscles in First-Class Lever System

There are a limited number of muscles in the human body that work in first-class lever systems because the point of application of the muscle must be on the opposite side of the joint axis from the external force. This is infrequently the case. One example of a muscle working on a first-class lever is the pull of the supraspinatus on the humerus (Fig. 1-74). The attachment of the supraspinatus on the greater tubercle of the humerus is on the opposite side of the composite axis of rotation for the glenohumeral joint from the CoM of the upper extremity, which is just above the elbow (see inset). Because the muscle and the gravitational force lie on either side of the joint axis, this remains a first-class lever whether the supraspinatus is contracting concentrically (as the EF) or eccentrically (as the RF).

For second- and third-class levers, the classification of a lever is dependent on the designation of the muscle as either the effort or resistance force. The designation is based on the net rotation of the lever. When a lever is in rotational equilibrium, there is no net torque (no winner); the muscle will be performing an **isometric contraction** because the length is not changing if the

segment is not rotating. When a muscle is acting on a lever in equilibrium, it is common to designate the active muscle as the effort force. The designation of the active muscle as the effort force in an equilibrium situation makes conceptual sense because the muscle contraction uses energy (requires "effort"). However, the EF and RF labels are arbitrary in a lever that is in rotational equilibrium and could just as easily be reversed. It is also true that a muscle uses energy (requires "effort" to resist a force during an eccentric contraction), and so designation of the effort force on the basis of energy requirements cannot be done and still maintain the principles that we have established.

🪨 CONCEPT CORNERSTONE 1-15: *Muscles in Lever Systems*

■ When a muscle is contracting concentrically (actively shortening), the muscle must be moving the segment to which it is attached in the direction of its pull. Therefore, the muscle will be the effort force (EF).

■ When a muscle is contracting eccentrically (actively lengthening), the muscle must be acting in a direction opposite to the motion of the segment; that is, the muscle must be the resistance force (RF). When a muscle is contracting eccentrically, it generally serves to control (slow down) the acceleration of the segment produced by the effort force.

■ When a lever is in rotational equilibrium, the muscle acting on the lever is contracting isometrically. In such a case, labeling the muscle as the effort or resistance force is arbitrary.

Mechanical Advantage

Mechanical advantage (M Ad) is a measure of the mechanical efficiency of the lever (the relative effectiveness of the effort force in comparison with the resistance force). Mechanical advantage is related to the classification of a lever and provides an understanding of the relationship between the torque of an external force (that we can roughly estimate) and the torque of a muscular force (that we can estimate only in relation to the external torque). Mechanical advantage of a lever is the ratio of the effort arm (MA of the effort force) to the resistance arm (MA of the resistance force), or:

$$M\,Ad = \frac{EA}{RA}$$

When EA is larger than RA, the M Ad will be greater than 1. The "advantage" of a lever with a mechanical advantage greater than 1 is simply that the effort force can be (but is not necessarily) smaller than the resistance force and yet will nonetheless create more torque to "win." The torque of the effort force is *always* greater than the torque of the resistance force; that is, (EF)(EA) > (RF)(RA). If EA is greater than RA, then the effort torque can still be greater than the resistance torque if EF is smaller in magnitude than RF.

In the example shown in Figure 1-72B, the effort force is GWbLf, and the EA is 0.27 m. The resistance force is QLf, and the RA is 0.05 m. Therefore, for the freeze-frame in Figure 1-72B:

$$M\,Ad = 0.27\,m \div 0.05\,m = 5.4$$

The leg-foot segment, a second-class lever in this situation, is mechanically efficient because the 88-N force of GWbLf creates more torque than the 450-N force of QLf. Because it is always true in a second-class lever that EA > RA, the M Ad of a second-class lever will always be greater than 1.

Continuing Exploration: **Mechanical Advantage and the Effort Force**

The mechanical advantage of a lever is determined by the lengths of the MAs and not by the *magnitudes* of the effort and resistance forces. An effort force with a magnitude smaller than the resistance force *must* be working through a larger MA; otherwise, it cannot produce a larger torque (cannot be the "winner"). However, EF is *not necessarily* smaller than RF. If we added 400 N to Sam's weight boot in Figure 1-

72B, GWbLf (now 488 N) would still be the effort force (although larger than the 450-N force of QLf) and the M Ad would still be 5.4. However, the angular acceleration of the flexing leg-foot segment would be extremely large because there would be a large increase in the net unbalanced torque. The "advantage" remains with GWbLf.

In third-class levers, the M Ad will always be less than 1 because EA is always smaller than RA (the effort force lies closer to the axis than the resistance force). A third-class lever is "mechanically inefficient" or is working at a "disadvantage" because the magnitude of the effort force *must* always be *greater* than the magnitude of the resistance force in order for the torque of the EF to exceed the torque of the RF (as it must for the force to "win"). In a first-class lever system, the EA can be larger than, smaller than, or equal to the RA. However, because the distal attachment of a muscle tends to be closer to the joint axis than is the point of application of an external force even when muscles are working on first-class levers, muscles working in first-class lever systems (like those in third-class systems) tend to be at a mechanical *disadvantage*.

Trade-Offs of Mechanical Advantage

It has already been observed that the majority of the muscles in the human body, when contracting concentrically and distal lever free, work over a shorter MA than does the external force on that lever. To move a lever, a muscle must exert a proportionally very large force to produce a "winning" torque. It appears, then, that the human body is structured inefficiently. In fact, the muscles of the body are structured to take on the burden of "mechanical disadvantage" to achieve the goal of rotating the segment through space.

Figure 1-75A shows the forearm-hand segment being flexed (rotated counterclockwise) through space by a concentrically contracting muscle (Fms) against the resistance of gravity (G). The segment is moving in the direction of the pull of Fms. Consequently, this is a third-class lever because EA < RA. The magnitude of Fms must be much larger than the magnitude of G for Fms to "win," and so the lever is, indeed, mechanically inefficient. However, as Fms pulls its point of application (on the proximal forearm-hand segment) through

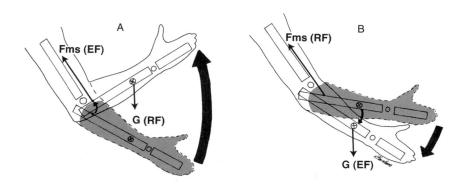

Figure 1-75 ■ A. In a mechanically inefficient third-class lever, movement of the point of application of EF (Fms) through a small arc produces a large arc of movement of the lever distally. **B.** In a mechanically efficient second-class lever, movement of the point of application of EF (G) through a small arc produces little increase in the arc distally.

a very small arc, the distal portion of the segment is displaced through a much greater arc. Although the magnitude of force needed to create the rotation is large in comparison with the magnitude of the resistance force, the result is that minimal shortening of the muscle is required to produce a large angular displacement and angular velocity for the distal portion of the segment. Because the goal in human function is to maximize angular displacement of a distal segment through space (even at the expense of energy cost), third-class lever systems achieve the desired goal. In fact, the shorter the MA of the effort force is (resulting in a diminishing mechanical advantage), the greater will be the angular displacement and angular velocity of the distal end of the lever for a given amount of shortening of the muscular EF.

In second-class levers in the human body, the effort force is usually (but not always) the external force. Although the effort force in a second-class lever can be smaller in magnitude than the resistance (and still "win"), less is gained in angular displacement and velocity at the distal end of the segment (per unit displacement of the EF). In Figure 1-75B, a small arc of movement at the point of application of the effort force (G) results in only a small increase in angular displacement of the more distal segment. In any second-class lever (and in a first-class lever in which EA > RA), the lever is mechanically efficient in terms of the ratio of force output to torque production, but relatively less is gained in terms of angular displacement of the distal end of the segment through space.

CONCEPT CORNERSTONE 1-16: *Mechanical Advantage and Classes of Levers*

- In all second-class levers, the mechanical advantage (M Ad) of the lever will always be greater than 1. The magnitude of the effort force can be (but is not necessarily) less than the magnitude of the resistance.
- In all third-class levers, the M Ad of the lever will always be less than 1. The magnitude of the effort force *must* be *greater* than the magnitude of the resistance for the effort to produce greater torque.
- The M Ad of a first-class lever can be greater than, less than, or equal to 1. However, it is often true of first-class levers in the body that the MA of the muscle will be shorter than the MA of the external force.
- When the muscle is the effort force in a lever with a M Ad of less than 1, the necessary expenditure of energy to produce sufficient muscle force to "win" is offset by the need for minimal shortening of the muscle to produce proportionally greater angular displacement and angular velocity of the distal portions of the segment.
- When an external force is the effort force in a lever with a M Ad greater than 1 (e.g., a second-class lever), the magnitude of the effort can be small in comparison with the resistance, but less is gained in angular displacement and velocity.

The basis for examining classes of levers is to gain perspective on the implications for muscle function and the ability of muscles to rotate or control the rotation of a segment. When EA is greater than RA (as it is in a second-class lever), the "advantage" tends to belong to the external effort force. The muscle will still have to generate a large eccentric resistance force if the rotational acceleration of the segment needs to be minimized (as is true, for example, when lowering a glass from the mouth or sitting in a chair without falling into it). When EA is smaller than RA (as it is in a third-class lever when the muscle is the EF), the muscle overcomes the external resistance only by generating a large concentric force. Consequently, the muscle must be able to create large forces regardless of the class of the lever. As shall be shown in Chapter 3, the muscle is structured to optimize production of the large forces required both to produce large angular displacements of the distal segments of the body in mechanically inefficient lever systems and to resist the external forces in mechanically efficient lever systems.

Limitations to Analysis of Forces by Lever Systems

Although the conceptual framework of lever systems described here provides useful terms and some additional insights into rotation of segments and muscle function, there are distinct limitations to this approach. Our discussion of lever systems ignored the fact that rotation of a lever requires at least one force couple. An effort force and resistance force are *not* a force couple because the effort and resistance forces produce rotation in the opposite (rather than the same) direction. Consequently, in an analysis of a simple two-force lever system that includes an effort force and a resistance force, at least one force that forms the second part of the force couple for the effort force is missing. The second force in the "couple" is generally an articular constraint (a joint reaction force or capsuloligamentous force) that may serve as the pivot point for the rotation (see Figs. 1-49 and 1-56). Consequently, a simple lever system approach to analyzing human motion requires oversimplification that fails to take into consideration key elements that affect function and structural integrity. Torques of human segments are not simply produced by muscles and external forces; they result both from additional internal forces *and* from the vertical and horizontal forces produced by muscles and external forces that are often ignored in a simple lever approach.

◆ Force Components

In the analysis of Sam's leg-foot segment in Figure 1-61, only the *torques* produced by the forces applied to the segment were considered. The substantial vertical force of GWbLf was ignored in that analysis because the force produced very little torque. In identifying QLf as the force that created rotation of the leg-foot segment, we did not identify the other force (the second part of the force couple) that QLf required to produce an extension torque. We also did not identify the mechanism by which translatory equilibrium ($\Sigma F_V = 0$ and $\Sigma F_H = 0$) of the leg-foot segment was established—a necessary condition for rotation of a joint around a relatively fixed axis. To examine the degree to which these conditions are met (net extension torque and translatory equilibrium), we need to understand how to resolve forces into their component parts.

A force applied to a lever produces its greatest torque when the force is applied at 90° to the lever (presuming a second part to the force couple). If the *same* magnitude of force produces *less* torque when the angle of application is not 90°, some of that force must be doing something other than producing rotation. Torque, in fact, is typically considered to be produced only by that *portion* of the force that is directed toward rotation. When the force is applied to a lever at some other angle (>90° or <90°), the component of force that *is* applied at 90° to the lever will contribute to rotation. Consequently, the portion of a force that is applied at 90° to the segment is known as the **perpendicular** (**rotatory** or **y**) **component** of the force (**Fy**). The rotatory component is the "y" component because the long axis of the body segment is usually the reference line or essentially the x-axis. Consequently, the component that is perpendicular to the segment is the y-axis.

The magnitude of Fy can be found graphically by the process of **resolution of forces.** In resolution of forces, the original (or **total**) force ($\mathbf{F_{TOT}}$) is broken down into two components. Just as two concurrent forces can be composed into a single resultant vector, a single vector ($\mathbf{F_{TOT}}$) can be resolved into two concurrent components. In this instance, the components will be specifically constructed so that one component (Fy) lies perpendicular to the segment. The second component is the so-called **parallel** (**translatory,** or **x**) **component** and is drawn parallel to the lever. The abbreviation **Fx** is used because, again, the body segment is always the reference or x-axis, and a line drawn parallel to the segment will be along or parallel to that x-axis. The process of resolution of forces is essentially the reverse of composition of forces by parallelogram. With resolution of forces, the parallelogram will always be a rectangle because the sides (Fx and Fy) are perpendicular to each other.

Resolving Forces into Perpendicular and Parallel Components

In Figure 1-76, three steps are shown to resolve QLf into its perpendicular (Fy_{QLf}) and parallel (Fx_{QLf}) components:

Step 1 (see Fig. 1-76A). A line with the *same point of application* as the original force is drawn *perpendicular* to the long axis of the lever in the direction of the original force (this is the draft line of component Fy). A second line with the *same point of application* as the original force is drawn *parallel* to the long axis of the lever in the direction of the original force (this is the draft line of

component Fx). The draft Fx and Fy component lines should reach or go past the arrowhead of the original vector.

Step 2 (see Fig. 1-76B). The rectangle is completed (closed) by drawing (from the arrowhead of the F_{TOT} vector) lines that are parallel to each of the draft Fx and Fy components.

Step 3 (see Fig. 1-76C). All the lines are "trimmed," leaving only the completed rectangle. Components Fy (the rotatory component) and Fx (the translatory component) each form one side of the rectangle, have a common point of application, and have arrowheads at the corners of the rectangle; F_{TOT} is now the diagonal of the rectangle. It is important that the lengths of vectors Fy and Fx are "trimmed" to the confines of the rectangle to maintain the proportional relation among Fx, Fy, and F_{TOT}. This proportional relation will permit determination of the predominant and relative effects of F_{TOT}.

Perpendicular and Parallel Force Effects

Once QLf is resolved into its components, it will be more evident that components Fy_{QLf} and Fx_{QLf} (see Fig. 1-76C) have the potential to create three different motions of the leg-foot segment: vertical motion, horizontal motion, and rotatory motion. Component Fx will tend to create vertical translatory motion in Figure 1-76C. However, component Fy will both create rotation and tend to create horizontal translation. Because a force component (e.g., Fy) may create both rotation and translation, labeling components as "rotatory" and "translatory" can be confusing. We will, therefore, proceed in the remainder of this chapter to refer to Fy exclusively as the perpendicular component and to Fx exclusively as the parallel component, with their effects (rotation or translation) determined by the situation.

We have already established that determining the state of motion of a segment requires assessment of ΣF_V, ΣF_H, and ΣT. We have also established that the Fx and Fy components of a force (e.g., QLf) will tend to create both translatory (F_V and F_H) and rotatory (T) motion. [*Side-bar:* We continue with a two-dimensional analysis, with three rather than six degrees of freedom available.] In order to reduce terms, consider that a force or force component that is both perpendicular to the segment and horizontally oriented in space (e.g., Fy_{QLf} in Figure 1-76C) may become vertically oriented in space, although still remaining perpendicular to the segment, if the segment moves in space. Consequently, we will proceed from this point to assess the net translatory motion of a segment by looking at the sum of the parallel (ΣFx) and the sum of the perpendicular (ΣFy) forces in lieu of the position-dependent corollaries: ΣF_V and ΣF_H. The rotatory equilibrium of the body segment will be assessed by determining the sums of the torques contributed by the forces (or force components) that are perpendicular to the long axis of the segment (ΣT). Although it is not feasible to attempt to quantify the forces or torques in a clinical environment, determin-

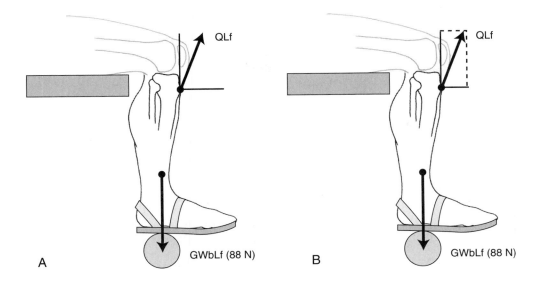

A

GWbLf (88 N)

B

GWbLf (88 N)

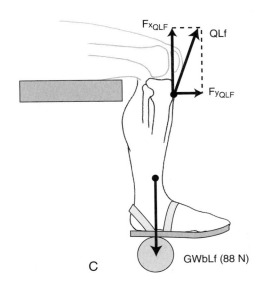

C

GWbLf (88 N)

◀ **Figure 1-76** ■ When a force is resolved into its components, (**A**) two lines that are perpendicular and parallel to the long axis of the bone are drawn from the point of application of the original force; (**B**) a rectangle is completed by drawing parallel lines from the arrowhead of the original force; and (**C**) the perpendicular (Fy) and parallel (Fx) component vectors are the adjacent sides of the rectangle that have a common point of application with the original force.

ing the magnitudes of the forces and torques in a sample situation will facilitate understanding of the additional forces or torques that are necessary to accomplish the functional demands of stabilization and/or rotation of a segment in space.

■ **Determining Magnitudes of Component Forces**

In a figure drawn to scale, the relative vectors lengths can be used to ascertain the net unbalanced forces. Because the vectors are not drawn to scale in Figure 1-76C, the relative magnitudes of Fy and Fx must be determined by using trigonometric functions of sines (sin) and cosines (cos) that are based on fixed relationships for right (90°) triangles.

It must first be recognized that the Fx and Fy are always part of a right triangle in relation to F_{TOT}. In Figure 1-77A, vector QLf and its components have been pulled out and enlarged. As the diagonal of a rectangle,

QLf divides the rectangle into two right triangles. The shaded half of the rectangle is the triangle of interest because the angle of application (as previously defined) for QLf is the angle between the vector and the segment on the side of the knee joint (θ in Fig. 1-77A). In the shaded triangle, vector QLf is the hypotenuse (side opposite the 90° angle) and is now assigned a magnitude of 1000 N. The angle of application θ is, in this example, presumed to be 25°. Vector Fx is the side adjacent to angle θ, and vector Fy is the side opposite to angle θ. Because the orientation of this triangle in Figure 1-77A is visually a little different than the reader might be used to (given the position of the leg-foot segment in Fig. 1-76), the force components have been replicated in a more "typical" orientation in Figure 1-77B. It should be noted that the "side opposite" the angle θ is not *literally* the perpendicular component (Fy) as we initially labeled it but is identical in magnitude (see Fig. 1-77B) because these are opposite

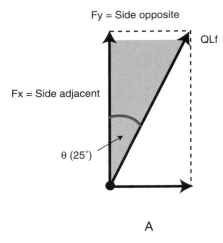

Fy = Side opposite

QLf

Fx = Side adjacent

θ (25°)

A

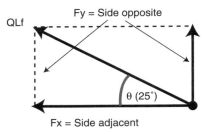

QLf

Fy = Side opposite

θ (25°)

Fx = Side adjacent

B

▲ **Figure 1-77** ■ **A.** Vector QLf and its Fx and Fy components are replicated (although enlarged) in the same orientation shown in Figure 1-76C. The reference triangle (shaded) shows that QLf is the hypotenuse, Fx is the side adjacent to angle θ, and Fy (or its equivalent length) is the side opposite to angle θ. **B.** The same figure is reoriented in space to provide an alternative visualization.

sides of a rectangle and, therefore, equivalent in length.

The Pythagorean theorem (trigonometry) is now used to solve for the magnitudes of Fx and Fy, where the angle of application θ is given as 25° and F_{TOT} (or QLf) is assigned a value of 1000 N.

Continuing Exploration: **Trigonometric Resolution of Forces**

The relation between the lengths of the three sides in a right (90°) triangle is given by the Pythagorean theorem: $A^2 + B^2 = C^2$, where C is the length of the hypotenuse of the triangle (the side opposite the 90° angle) and A and B are, respectively, the lengths of the sides adjacent to and opposite to the angle θ (Fig. 1-78A). According to the theorem, it will hold that:

$$\sin \theta = \frac{\text{side opposite}}{\text{hypotenuse}}$$

$$\cos \theta = \frac{\text{side adjacent}}{\text{hypotenuse}}$$

The formulas may be used to solve for the length of the adjacent side (Fx) or opposite side (Fy) when angle θ (the angle of application of the force) and the hypotenuse (the magnitude of the force) are known:

$$\text{side opposite} = (\sin \theta)(\text{hypotenuse})$$

$$\text{side adjacent} = (\cos \theta)(\text{hypotenuse})$$

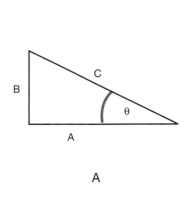

C

B

θ

A

A

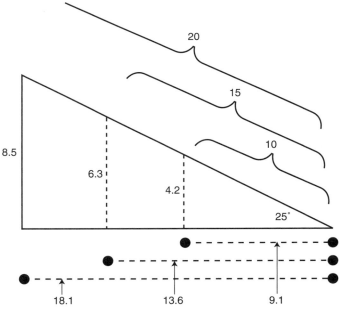

20

15

10

8.5

6.3

4.2

25°

18.1   13.6   9.1

B

▲ **Figure 1-78** ■ **A.** The Pythagorean theorem states that $A^2 + B^2 = C^2$, where A, B, and C are the lengths of the sides of the right triangle. **B.** For a given angle θ (e.g., 25°), the lengths of the side opposite and side adjacent to the angle will have a fixed relationship to each other and to the original force, regardless of the size of the triangle.

The values of the sine and cosine functions in trigonometry are not arbitrary numbers. The sine and cosine values represent that fact that there is a fixed relationship between the lengths of the sides for a given angle. In Figure 1-78B, a right triangle with an angle θ of 25° is drawn. The triangle is divided so that there are sides of three different lengths, whereby the hypotenuses are assigned scaled values of 10 cm, 15 cm, and 20 cm for the smallest to largest triangles, respectively. On the same scale, the values of Fy (side opposite) will be 4.2 cm, 6.3 cm, and 8.5 cm, respectively; the values of Fx (side adjacent) will be 9.1 cm, 13.6 cm, and 18.1 cm, respectively. The ratio of any two sides of one of these 25° triangles will be the same, regardless of size, and *that ratio will be the value of the trigonometric function for that angle.*

1. For the (side opposite/hypotenuse) for each of the three triangles: (4.2/10 = 0.42); (6.3/15 = 0.42); and (8.5/20 = 0.42). The value of sin 25° is 0.42.
2. For the (side adjacent/hypotenuse) for each of the three triangles: (9.1/10 = 0.91); (13.6/15 = 0.91); and (18.1/20 = 0.91). The value of cos 25° is 0.91.
3. For the (side opposite/side adjacent) for each of the three right triangles: (4.2/9.1 = 0.46); (6.3 /13.6 = 0.46); and (8.5/18.1 = 0.46). The value of the tangent (tan, or sin/cos) 25° is 0.46.

This is the "proof" that, for a given angle of application of F_{TOT}, Fx and Fy have a fixed proportional relation to F_{TOT} *and* a fixed relation to each other, regardless of the magnitude of F_{TOT} (and regardless of the orientation of the segment in space or whether the force is internal or external).

The magnitudes of Fx_{QLf} and Fy_{QLf} can be computed by using the Pythagorean theorem (see Continuing Exploration: Trigonometric Resolution). If it is given that QLf has a magnitude of 1000 N and is applied at 25° to the leg-foot segment then:

$$Fx_{QLf} = (\cos 25°)(1000\ N) = (0.91)(1000\ N) = 910\ N$$

$$Fy_{QLf} = (\sin 25°)(1000\ N) = (0.42)(1000\ N) = 420\ N$$

It should be noted that the sum of the magnitudes of the Fx and Fy components will always be greater than the magnitude of the resultant force (F_{TOT}). As with composition of forces, the resultant is more "efficient." However, analysis of the translatory or rotatory effects of any set of forces will produce mathematically equivalent results whether the total force or the force components are used in appropriate analyses.

 CONCEPT CORNERSTONE 1-17: *Angles of Application Greater than 90°*

We have identified that the magnitudes of Fx and Fy are calculated by using the *angle of application of the F_{TOT}*. However, there is a variation of this rule. When the angle of application of F_{TOT} is greater than 90° (an obtuse angle) as in the schematic in Figure 1-79, the complement of θ ($\theta^1 = 180° - \theta$) must be used. This makes sense both in looking at Figure 1-79 and because none of the three angles in a right triangle can be greater than 90°. Note in

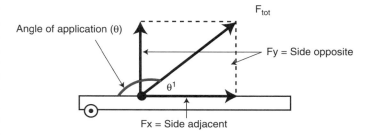

▲ **Figure 1-79** ■ When the angle of application (θ) is greater than 90° (an obtuse angle), the angle (θ^1) used to compute Fx, and Fy will be the complement ($180° - \theta$) of the angle of application.

Figure 1-79, however, that Fx remains the side adjacent to θ^1 and that the magnitude of Fy remains the side opposite to θ^1. Figure 1-80 shows gravity (G) acting on the leg-foot segment at 45° (see Fig. 1-80A) and at 135° (see Fig. 1-80B). The magnitudes of Fx and Fy are identical in both figures because both the sides of the rectangle (in this case, a square) are based on a 45° angle. The angle used to compute the components for the force applied at 135° is the complement of the angle (180° − 135°, or 45°.]

It may seem like the definition of angle of application of a vector should be changed to define the *acute angle* between the segment and the vector, rather than the *angle on the side of the joint axis*. However, allowing the angle of application (θ) to be any size from 0° to

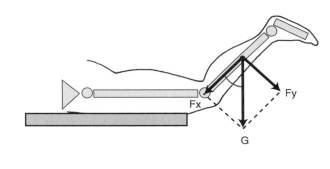

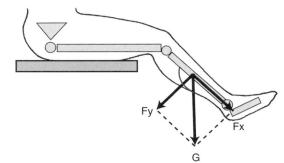

▲ **Figure 1-80** ■ Vector G is applied to the leg-foot segment at 45° (**A**) and at 135° (**B**). The magnitudes of Fx and Fy are the same in both **A** and **B** because the angle used to compute the components for a force applied at 135° is the complement of the angle (180° - 135°) or 45°. However, Fx is compressive in **A** and distractive in **B**.

180° permits a useful general statement to be made: Whenever the angle of application of a force is less than 90°, the Fx component will be directed toward the joint axis and will be a compressive force (see Fig. 1-80A), and whenever the angle of application is greater than 90°, the Fx component will be a distractive force (see Fig. 1-80B).

■ Force Components and the Angle of Application of the Force

When a force of constant magnitude is applied to a segment as the segment rotates around its joint axis (see Figs. 1-65 and 1-66), there is a change in the MA and, therefore, in the torque produced by the force at different joint angles. The change in the MA is a function of the change in angle of application of the force to the segment. Because the perpendicular component (Fy) of a force is effectively the portion of the total force that produces torque, a change in torque produced by a force of constant magnitude must mean that the magnitude of Fy is changing. This is quite logical because it has just been established that the magnitude of Fy is a function of the angle of application of the force [Fy = (sin θ)(hypotenuse)].

Figure 1-81 shows a muscle force (Fms) of constant magnitude acting on the forearm-hand segment at the same four positions of the elbow (and same angles of application for the force) as were shown in Figure 1-66. In Figure 1-81, the changes in the magnitudes of the Fx and Fy components of the force are shown, rather than the changes in the MAs. Given that the changes in torque produced by Fms were a function of the changes in MA in Figure 1-66 and a function of the changes in angle of application or Fy in Figure 1-81, MA and Fy must be directly proportional to each other. We have established that when a force is applied at 90° to the segment (e.g., Fig. 1-81C), the MA is as large as it can be for this force. When a force is applied at 90° to the segment, Fy is equivalent in magnitude to the total force (F_{TOT}). [*Side-bar:* Fy = (sin θ)(hypotenuse). If hypotenuse = F_{TOT}, and the sine of 90° = 1, then Fy = (1)(F_{TOT}), and Fy = F_{TOT}.] Consequently, both MA and Fy have their greatest magnitude when a force is applied at 90° to a segment, with any other angle of application that results in a proportional

reduction in both MA and Fy. There will also be a proportional increase in Fx because Fx is inversely proportional to Fy.

Example 1-13

Changes in Force Components with Changes in Angle of Application

Component Fx is larger than Fy at an angle of application of Fms of 35° (see Fig. 1-81A). Component Fx is also larger than Fy when Fms is applied at 145° to the segment (see Fig. 1-81D). As the action line of Fms moves closer to the segment (closer to being parallel to the segment), Fx increases in magnitude. When vector Fms is applied to the segment at an angle of application of 70° (see Fig. 1-81B), Fms lies farther from the axis and Fx gets smaller. As Fms changes its angle of pull, component Fx not only changes in magnitude but also changes in direction. When Fms is at an angle of application of 35° to the segment (see Fig. 1-81A), Fx is toward the joint (compression); when Fms has an angle of application of 145° (see Fig. 1-81D), the translatory component is away from the joint (distraction).

The change of the parallel component from compression to distraction shown in Figure 1-81D is unusual for a muscle force. In fact, the majority of muscles lie nearly parallel to the segment, have relatively small angles of pull (Fx > Fy) regardless of the position in the joint ROM, and almost always pull in the direction of the joint axis. The effect of this arrangement of muscles is that a muscle force generally has a relatively small perpendicular component contributing to rotation, with a larger parallel component that is nearly always compressive. Therefore, most of the force generated by a muscle contributes to joint *compression,* rather than joint *rotation!* This arrangement enhances joint stability but means that a muscle must generate a large total force to produce the sufficient torque to move the lever through space.

We can now expand a bit on our earlier observation

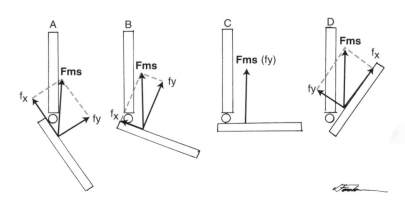

◀ **Figure 1-81** ■ Resolution of the muscle force (Fms) into perpendicular (Fy) and parallel (Fx) components at angles of application of 35° (**A**), 70° (**B**), 90° (**C**), and 145° (**D**) of elbow flexion produces changes in the magnitudes of the components and in the direction of Fx.

that muscles (contracting concentrically, distal lever free) most often work at a mechanical disadvantage and are mechanically "inefficient." The trade-off is that a large arc of motion of the distal end of the segment is produced, although it requires a large force of muscle contraction. Similarly, the large force of muscle contraction needed to produce rotation (large Fy) also has the beneficial effect of producing substantial joint compression (stabilization) because of the even larger Fx component of the muscle force.

CONCEPT CORNERSTONE 1-18: *Components of Muscle Forces*

- The angle of pull of the majority of muscles is small, with an action line more parallel to the lever than perpendicular to the lever.
- The parallel (Fx) component of a muscle force most often is larger than the perpendicular (Fy) component.
- The parallel component of most muscle forces contributes to joint compression, making muscles important joint stabilizers.

The constraints that exist on muscle forces in the body (and, therefore, the generalizations identified in Concept Cornerstone 1-18) do not apply to external forces. We have already seen examples in which gravity is compressive in one instance or distractive in another, depending on the location of the segment in space (see Fig. 1-80). Gravity is constrained in its direction (always vertically downward) and, therefore, has some predictability (the torque of gravity is always greatest with the limb segment is parallel to the ground). Other external forces (e.g., a manual resistance) have few if any constraints and, therefore, most often do not have predictable effects on a segment. However, the *principles* of forces in relation to angle of application and the consequential magnitudes of the MA, Fy, and Fx components apply to any and all forces, including those commonly encountered in clinical situations.

Example 1-14

Manipulating External Forces to Maximize Torque

In Figure 1-82, a manual external force (hand-on-leg-foot [HLf]) of the same magnitude is applied to a leg-foot segment in two different positions. If the goal is to obtain a maximum *isometric* quadriceps muscle contraction ($\Sigma T = 0$) with minimum effort on the part of the person applying the resistance, the position of the manual force in Figure 1-82B provides a distinct advantage to that person. Vector HLf in Figure 1-82A has a substantially smaller MA than that in Figure 1-82B because the resisting hand is placed more proximally on the leg-foot segment. Vector HLf is also applied at an angle to the segment that leads to a potentially undesirable parallel component (Fx) that, in this instance, constitutes a "wasted" force on the part of the person applying the resistance. Because the angle of application of HLf is greater than 90°, the "wasted" force is distractive. By moving the resisting hand down the leg-foot segment and changing the angle of application of the force to 90° to the segment, the MA is maximized and all the force contributes to rotation (HLf = Fy). In Figure 1-82B, the resisting hand placement requires the quadriceps muscle to contract with substantially greater force than in Figure 1-82A to maintain the same knee joint position. The muscle must offset the greater torque produced by the resisting hand. Because the angle of pull of the muscle has not changed, the muscle can change its torque only by changing its force of contraction. An understanding of the ability to manipulate both MA and angle of application by the person providing the resistance will allow that person to either increase or decrease the challenge to the quadriceps muscle, depending on the goal of the exercise.

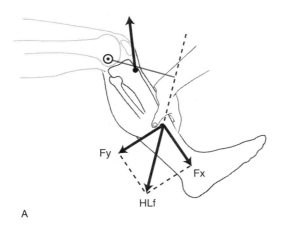
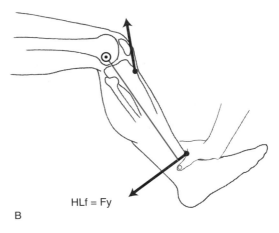

▲ **Figure 1-82** ■ **A.** A manual force is applied at an angle to the leg-foot segment, with about half the force distracting the joint rather than rotating. **B.** A manual resistance of the same magnitude produces substantially greater torque because all the force is directed toward rotation (Fy) and the point of application is farther from the joint axis (MA for HLf in **B** is greater than the MA for HLf in **A**).

CONCEPT CORNERSTONE 1-19: *Manipulating External Forces to Maximize Torque Production*

- The torque of an external force can be increased by increasing the magnitude of the applied force.
- The torque of an external force can be increased by applying the force perpendicular to (or closer to perpendicular to) the lever.
- The torque of an external force can be increased by increasing the distance of the point of application of the force from the joint axis.

◆ Translatory Effects of Force Components

Let us return once again to Sam and the weight boot exercise. The goal as Sam attempts to lift the weight boot (and the goal in all purposeful joint motions) is to have the segment in translatory equilibrium (ΣFx = 0; ΣFy = 0) while having a net torque in the direction of desired motion. Before the torque can rotate the segment, however, we must identify the translatory effects of the forces already applied to the leg-foot segment, as well as determine what additional forces, if any, are necessary to create translatory equilibrium

In Figure 1-83, vectors GWbLf (−88 N) and Fx_{QLf} (+910 N) are both parallel to the leg-foot segment and in opposite directions. Vector GWbLf is a joint distraction force because it is away from the joint, whereas vector Fx_{QLf} is a joint compression force because it is toward the joint. [*Side-bar:* Because vector GWbLf is parallel to the leg-foot segment, we do not need to resolve it into its perpendicular (Fy) and parallel (Fx) components. All of the force of GWbLf is parallel ($F_{TOT} = Fx$).] Given the magnitudes of GWbLf and Fx_{QLf}, there appears to be a net unbalanced force parallel to the leg-foot segment, or a net compression force of +822 N. As is true whenever there is a net compression force, the segment will translate until it contacts the adjacent segment (femur), at which point a new force (femur-on-legfoot [FLf]) is introduced. When FLf reaches a magnitude of 822 N, the leg-foot segment will reach translatory equilibrium parallel to its long axis. If, rather than compression, the resultant of GWbLf and Fx_{QLf} was a net distraction force, the segment would translate away from the adjacent articular surface until sufficient capsuloligamentous tension was developed to check further motion.

Vector Fy_{QLf} has a magnitude of 420 N to the right (see Fig. 1-83). There must be another force (or forces) of 420 N to the left before Fy_{QLf} can cause torque rather than translation. The force will not come from bony contact in this example because of the shape of the articular surfaces; rather, it would presumably come from one or more internal forces because there is nothing else "touching" the leg-foot segment that would produce an external force. The most obvious source of the internal force is capsuloligamentous tension. It is possible that muscles such as the hamstrings may also

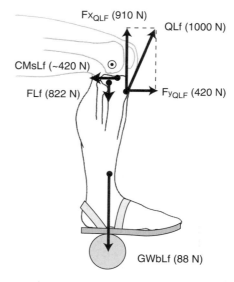

▲ **Figure 1-83** ■ The leg-foot segment in the weight boot exercise with all forces and force components identified for 90° of knee flexion as knee extension is initiated.

be contributing. Although it is unlikely that posterior knee joint muscles such as the hamstrings are *actively contracting* in this activity, muscles have connective tissue elements that can generate *passive* tension (see Chapter 3), but such tension at the posterior knee should be minimal with the knee at 90° of flexion. Because vector Fy_{QLf} is parallel to the articular surfaces (tibial plateau and tangent of femoral condyles), Fy_{QLf} would create an anterior shear between articular surfaces. The shear force would generate a corresponding friction force. The resulting friction force (FrLf) is unlikely to be of sufficient magnitude to check the anterior shear, given the low coefficient of friction for articular cartilage. [*Side-bar:* Given $Fr_S \leq \mu_S F_C$ (and given $\mu_S \approx 0.016$), then $Fr_S \leq (0.016)(822 \text{ N})$.] The most likely explanation in Figure 1-83 is that the Fy_{QLf} will translate the leg-foot segment to the right (anteriorly) until a new force from the joint capsule and passive muscles (CMsLf) reaches the necessary estimated force (tension) of approximately 420 N to the left (posteriorly).

Continuing Exploration: **Tendon Friction**

Vector QLf has been assigned a value of 1000 N. It seems reasonable to presume that the quadriceps femoris muscle is contracting with a force of 1000 N, but this may not be the case. *If* the quadriceps tendon (above the patella) and the patellar ligament (below the patella) were a continuous structure that passed over a frictionless pulley, the tension above and below the patella would be equivalent (1000 N each). However, it appears that this is not the case. As is true for the majority of tendons that pass around bony prominences (such as the femoral condyles) or over sesamoid bones (such as the patella), some friction exists even if accompanying bursae or tendon sheaths minimize that friction.

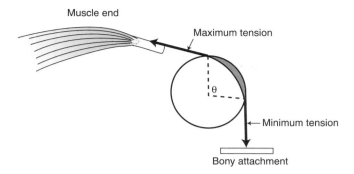

▲ **Figure 1-84** ■ If there is friction between a tendon passing over an anatomic pulley and the anatomic pulley, the tension above and below the pulley will be different. The loss of tension in the tendon distal to the pulley is a function of the angle (θ) of contact and the coefficient of friction.

Figure 1-84 shows the schematic relation between a flexible structure and a rigid "pulley" that is similar to what the quadriceps muscle would look like passing over the patella and/or femoral condyles (because the femoral condyles also deflect the pull of the quadriceps muscle when the knee is flexed, independent of the patella). The maximum tension is generated by the pull of the quadriceps muscle. As the tendon passes over the patella and femoral condyles, however, the tension on the patellar ligament is reduced. Although the mathematical analysis is beyond the scope of the text, the reduction in tension is a function of the angle of contact between the surfaces (θ in Fig. 1-84) and a function of μ_S or μ_K.[1] As the angle of contact increases, there will be a greater differential between the pull of the muscle on the tendon and the tension in the tendon at its bony attachment. As the coefficient of friction is reduced (as it will be with an interposed bursa or tendon sheath), the differential in tension proximal and distal to the pulley is reduced. Given the structure of the quadriceps muscle and its associated elements, one study found an 8:5 ratio between quadriceps tendon tension above the patella and patellar ligament tension below the patella.[9]

Rotatory Effects of Force Components

■ **Rotation Produced by Perpendicular Force Components**

In Figure 1-83, the force (CMsLf) and force component (Fy_{QLf}) are perpendicular to the leg-foot segment. We know that these two forces (as is true for forces perpendicular to a segment) will contribute to rotation of the segment if translation is prevented. These two force vectors have been isolated in Figure 1-85, and it can now be seen that CMsLf and Fy_{QLf} are a force couple. These two forces are applied to the same segment, in opposite directions, with equal magnitudes—both producing counterclockwise rotation of the leg-foot segment (extension). Remember, however, that CMsLf

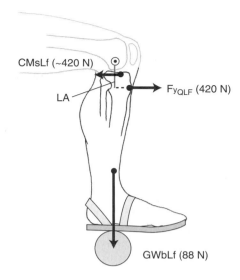

▲ **Figure 1-85** ■ The forces (or force components) applied perpendicular to the leg-foot segment in Figure 1-83 have been isolated in this figure to facilitate assessment of their effect.

does not reach 420 N until the leg-foot segment has already translated anteriorly (to the right) by a small amount. Consequently, rotation will be initiated around the pivot point of the capsular attachment at the particular freeze frame shown in Figure 1-85 (similar to what was seen in Fig. 1-56). Overall, however, it is more correct to think of the motion of the leg-foot segment as a combination of rotation and translation (curvilinear motion of the segment) around a point that is the center of some larger circle. This is why the joint axis (CoR) in Figure 1-85 appears to be at a slight distance from, although close to, the point of application of CMsLf.

The torque produced by a force couple is calculated either as (1) the product of the magnitude of one force (given that the magnitudes are the same for both forces) and the distance between the forces or (2) the product of the magnitude of each force and its distance from a common point between the forces. Although in the particular freeze frame shown in Figure 1-85 the distance between vectors CMsLf and Fy_{QLf} can be used, it is accepted practice to use the joint axis (CoR) as the common reference point for the MA of both forces because this is the point about which *composite* rotation (rotation throughout the knee extension ROM) appears to occur.

Torque has thus far in the text been computed as the product of F_{TOT} and MA. When a force is *not* applied at 90° to the segment (as is true for QLf), the torque can alternatively be computed as the product of the perpendicular component (Fy) of that force and *its* MA (LA) (see Fig. 1-85). Recall that LA is simply a special case of the MA when the force is at 90° to the segment. The distinction is made between MA and LA because the distance (MA) for vector QLf will be different (and shorter) than the distance (LA) for the perpendicular component of QLf (Fy_{QLf}); that is, the

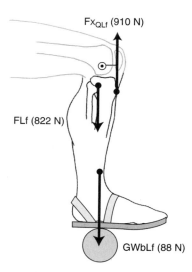

Fx$_{QLf}$ (910 N)

FLf (822 N)

GWbLf (88 N)

▲ **Figure 1-86 ■** The forces (or force components) applied parallel to the leg-foot segment in Figure 1-83 have been isolated in this figure to facilitate assessment of their effect.

shortest distance between the joint axis and QLf is different from the shortest distance between the joint axis and Fy$_{QLf}$. Consequently, the torque of QLf can also be computed as:

$$T_{FyQLf} = (Fy_{QLf})(LA)$$

If the magnitude of Fy$_{QLf}$ is 420 N (see Fig. 1-85) and if the LA for Fy$_{QLf}$ is given as 0.06 m, the torque (T$_{FyQLf}$) would be 25.2 Nm. We will assume (as is most often done) that CMsLf (the force closest to the joint axis) is sufficiently close to the joint axis that its torque is inconsequential (that the attachment of the capsule and the joint axis nearly coincide). This theoretically means that the torque produced by the force couple can be quantified by knowing the torque of Fy$_{QLf}$ alone.

■ **Rotation Produced by Parallel Force Components**

Most often, only the total forces (F$_{TOT}$) or components of the total forces that are perpendicular to the segment (Fy) are considered to produce torques. However, any force that lies at some distance from an axis will produce rotation around that axis, regardless of orientation to the segment. In Figure 1-86, the forces and force components (Fx) that are parallel to the segment in Figure 1-83 are now isolated. Vectors FLf and GWbLf, if extended, will pass approximately through the knee joint axis. Consequently, neither force will create a torque at the joint. However, Fx$_{QLf}$ does not pass through the joint axis and will produce a torque.

Any force that produces torque must be part of a force couple. In Figure 1-86, vectors GWbLf and FLf are part of a linear force system. These two vectors can readily be composed into a single vector (FGWbLf) with a magnitude of −910 N and a point of application that lies between the two forces, very close to the point of application of FLf (given its substantially greater magnitude). Now there are two forces (FGWbLf and Fx$_{QLf}$) that are applied to the same object, equal in

magnitude and opposite in direction, that will together produce a counterclockwise (extension) torque on the leg-foot segment (a force couple!). The torque produced by these forces can be computed as the product of the magnitude (910 N) and the distance between the two forces. Alternatively, we can again assume that the point of application of FGWbLf (see Fig. 1-86) is sufficiently close to the joint axis that the product of Fx$_{QLf}$ and its MA will give a good estimate of the torque of the force couple:

$$T_{FxQLf} = (Fx_{QLf})(MA)$$

If the MA of Fx$_{QLf}$ were less than half that of Fy$_{QLf}$ (~0.005 m), Fx$_{QLf}$ would contribute 4.8 Nm of torque (910 N * 0.005 m) to knee extension. The total torque of QLf would then be the sum of the torque produced by Fy$_{QLf}$ (25.2 Nm) and the torque produced by Fx$_{QLf}$ (4.8 Nm), for a total torque of 30 Nm.

⬧➤ Total Rotation Produced by a Force

Levers in the human body are generally treated as if the axis of rotation not only is fixed but also lies in a direct line with the long axis of the lever. When this is the case, parallel components (Fx) will not contribute to torque, and torque for each force can be equivalently found by:

$$T = (F_{TOT})(MA)$$

$$T = (Fy)(LA)$$

However, using the quadriceps muscle and leg-foot segment example, we have demonstrated that the parallel components of both internal and external forces often do *not* pass through the CoR of the joint. If the torque of a force acting on a segment is estimated only on the basis of the Fy component of that force, the net torque is likely to be underestimated. It would be an underestimation because the sum of the torques produced by the components Fx$_{QLf}$ and Fy$_{QLf}$ cannot be any greater than the torque produced by the original force (F$_{TOT}$); that is:

$$T_{TOT} = [(F_{TOT})(MA_{TOT})]$$
$$= [(Fy)(MA_{Fy})] + [(Fx)(MA_{Fx})].$$

Given that the magnitude of QLf is 1000 N and the MA of QLf (see Fig. 1-61) is 0.03 N, the product of F$_{TOT}$ and its MA is 30 Nm. Of that 30 Nm-torque, the majority (25.2 Nm) is contributed by Fy$_{QLf}$, with an additional 4.8 Nm contributed by Fx$_{QLf}$. Because the contribution of component Fx to torque (as opposed to translation) for any given force is generally small (or smaller than that of Fy), estimating torque based on Fy alone is generally a reasonable (albeit conservative) estimate of torque produce by the total force. The net torque of all forces on a segment, however, may be substantially influenced by the resultant contributions of the Fx components to resultant torque.

CONCEPT CORNERSTONE 1-20: *Force Components and Joint Motion*

- Rotation around a joint axis requires that $\Sigma Fx = 0$. If $\Sigma Fx \neq 0$ initially, translatory motion of the segment will continue (alone or in combination with rotation) until checked either by a capsuloligamentous force or by a joint reaction force (depending on the articular configuration), if the effects of external and muscular forces have already been accounted for.

- Rotation around a joint axis requires that the $\Sigma Fy = 0$. If $\Sigma Fy \neq 0$ initially, translatory motion of the segment will continue (alone or in combination with rotation) until checked either by a capsuloligamentous force or by a joint reaction force (depending on the articular configuration), if the effects of external and muscular forces have already been accounted for.

- The majority of torque on a segment will be produced by forces or force components (Fy) that are applied at 90° to the segment and at some distance from the joint axis.

- Parallel force components (Fx) will produce limited amounts of torque if the action line does not pass through the CoR of the segment.

- Whenever the goal is rotation of a joint, a net unbalanced torque in the direction of movement ($\Sigma T \neq 0$) is necessary to reach the goal. [*Side-bar:* There are circumstances in which moving rotational equilibrium ($\Sigma T = 0$) can be produced with special equipment to produce the external force or a very skilled practitioner providing manual resistance.]

- The greater the net unbalanced torque, the greater the angular acceleration of the segment.

Before we conclude the chapter, let us return to our original question as to whether Sam Alexander should strengthen his quadriceps muscle by using the weight boot exercise or the leg-press exercise.

Case Application 1-3: **Summary of Weight Boot Exercise at 90° of Knee Flexion**

We analyzed the weight boot at 90° of knee flexion (where the exercise begins) and found that there is a potentially problematic net distraction force at the knee joint before the initiation of the quadriceps muscle contraction (see Fig. 1-29C). With the initiation of an active quadriceps muscle contraction, the joint capsule (with the assistance of passive muscle forces) is required to offset the anterior shear of Fy_{QLf} (see Fig. 1-83), although the magnitude of capsuloligamentous tension at 90° is likely to be minimal.[10] Just as the MAs and magnitudes of QLf changed as the leg-foot segment moved through the knee joint ROM in Figures 1-61 through 1-63, there will be corresponding changes in the other forces with a change in position of the leg-foot segment. Although the specific changes to forces on Sam Alexander's leg-foot segment at knee joint positions other than 90° could be examined, no biomechanical principles would be introduced, so we will not pursue those analyses.

We now need to examine the forces produced by the leg-press exercise at the equivalent 90° knee flexion angle (and with an equivalent small weight or resistance of 40 N) to determine the comparative effects of this exercise on Sam's knee joint structures, as well as to introduce a new level of complexity to a segmental force analysis.

◆ Multisegment (Closed-Chain) Force Analysis

The primary difference between the weight boot and leg-press exercise is that the leg-foot segment is "fixed" or weight-bearing at both ends. The distal end of the leg-foot segment is constrained by its contact with the footplate and is not free to move in space; the proximal end is connected to or contacting the femur and is also not free to move in space. Whenever one end of a segment or set of segments is free to move in space, this is referred to as an **open chain.** When *both* ends of a segment or set of segments are constrained in some way (and not free to move in space), this is referred to as a **closed chain.**

Continuing Exploration: **Open and Closed Chains**

The adjectives "kinetic" or "kinematic" are often used to modify the terms "open chain" and "closed chain." Although either might be justified, there is no consensus about which is preferred. At this juncture, the terms "open chain" and "closed chain" are now in such common use that the modifiers no longer seem necessary. What is necessary, however, is to avoid *misuse* of the term "closed chain" as equivalent to "weight-bearing" (unfortunately, a commonly used but inappropriate synonym). Although a segment *may* be fixed at both ends by proximal joint attachments and distal weight-bearing, a segment or set of segments can be weight-bearing *without* being fixed at both ends and without being subjected to the constraints of a closed chain. The effects of open and closed chains on segments will be encountered in subsequent chapters.

With the leg-foot segment in a closed chain in the leg-press exercise, the analysis of forces becomes substantially more complex. In a closed chain, motion of one segment of a joint can be produced by forces applied to the adjacent segment. Figure 1-87 is an oversimplified representation of the leg-press exercise, showing *only* the force of the gluteus maximus muscle extending the hip. The femur (like the leg-foot segment) is in a closed chain because it is fixed to both the pelvis and the leg-foot segment. Consequently, the force of the gluteus maximus on the femur has the potential to produce motion of the femur that will result in extension *at both the hip joint and the knee joint.* [*Side-bar:* If the concomitant hip and knee joint extension are not obvious to you, visualize the femur rotating clockwise (in the direction of Fy_{GM}) around its mid-

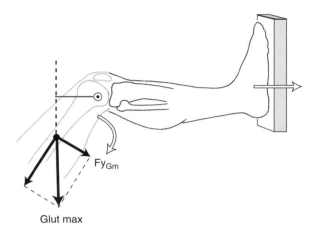

▲ **Figure 1-87** ■ The force of the gluteus maximus muscle (Glut max) is applied to the femur in a closed chain. The resulting extension of the hip from Fy_{Gm} will push the leg-foot segment to the right against the footplate and create an extension torque at the knee joint.

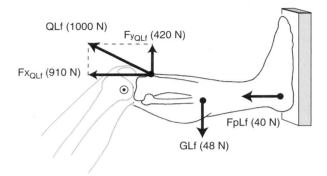

▲ **Figure 1-88** ■ The forces of quadriceps muscle (QLf), gravity (GLf), and the footplate (FpLf) on the leg-foot segment in the leg-press exercise at 90° of knee flexion.

point (the CoM of the femur) . Although this would be an exaggeration of what actually is occurring, the motion of the femoral head on the acetabulum and of the femoral condyles on the tibial plateau is more conceptually obvious.]

In Figure 1-87, the very substantial force that can be generated by the large gluteus maximus on the femur (although substantially underestimated by the length of the vectors in the figure) creates an extension torque at the knee joint. The muscle also acts through a large MA at the knee joint (again underestimated because the actual point of application of the gluteus maximus on the proximal femur is beyond the limits of the figure). The clockwise torque on the femur will cause the femur to contact the leg-foot segment and potentially push the leg-foot segment to the right. [*Side-bar:* At first glance, it might appear that the leg-foot segment is being acted upon by a force (the gluteus maximus) that does not contact the segment, thus violating a basic tenet that we have set. However, the extension (clockwise) torque on the femur initiates a sequence of forces that *are* applied to the leg-foot segment, including femur-on-legfoot.]

Because the leg-press exercise involves forces on the femur as well as forces on the leg-foot segment, a complete analysis would involve (at a minimum) identification of the sources, magnitudes, and effects (ΣFy, Σx, ΣT) of all forces on both the leg-foot and femur segments—a task beyond the scope or intent of this chapter. A simple example of the complex interrelationships is that the magnitude of torque generated by the quadriceps muscle is likely to be indirectly proportional to the torque generated by the gluteus maximus because both are extending the knee; more torque generation by one muscle would mean that less would be needed by the other. The superior mechanical advantage (larger MA) and large force-generating capability of the gluteus maximus would make the gluteus maximus more likely to be the primary "effort force." Consequently, the forces acting on the leg-foot segment

in the leg-press exercise are presented with the understanding that principles rather than actual quantitative analyses are being presented.

Figure 1-88 shows the knee at 90° in the leg-press exercise. Gravity (the first force to consider because it is consistently present) is shown at the CoM of the leg-foot segment (more proximally located than when forces of gravity and the weight boot were combined) with the previously identified magnitude of 48 N (the weight of the leg-foot segment has not changed). The quadriceps muscle (QLf) is shown generating the same 1000-N contraction given for our weight boot exercise analysis (to keep that variable constant and comparable) and has the same force components because the angle of application of QLf will be the same whenever the knee joint is at 90° (regardless of the position of the segment in space). The footplate is contacting and creating a force (FpLf) on the leg-foot segment. A 40-N weight has been placed on the machine (the same weight as used in the weight boot exercise). The footplate cannot push back on the leg-foot segment with more than a 40-N force, and so vector FpLf has been assigned that value. We will identify the remaining forces by looking at the "need" generated by the forces already in place.

With the forces in place in Figure 1-88, there is a net compressive force (ΣFx) of 950 N (Fx_{QLf} = –910 N and FpLf = -40 N). There is a net upward shear (ΣFy) of 372 N (Fy_{QLf} = 420 N, and GLf = -48 N). The quadriceps muscle is generating the same extension torque of 25.2 Nm [(Fy_{QLf})(LA), or (420 N)(0.06)] as it did in the weight boot exercise, but gravity now creates a flexion torque of 9.6 Nm [(40 N)(0.20 m)]. Therefore, the net torque in Figure 1-88 is 15.6 Nm in the direction of extension. The effect of the gluteus maximus must now be added.

The gluteus maximus force (shaded as a vector applied to the femur) has been added to Figure 1-89, along with its concomitant effects on the leg-foot segment. The gluteus maximus creates a push of the femur on the leg-foot segment (FLf) that is at an angle to the tibial plateau (and, more importantly, at an angle to the long axis of the leg-foot segment) because the femur is being rotating clockwise by the muscle. Vector FLf has

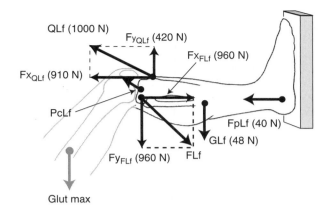

▲ **Figure 1-89** ■ The contact of the femur with the leg-foot segment (FLf) and its components have been added to the force analysis, along with the force of the posterior cruciate ligament on the leg-foot segment (PcLf). The force of the gluteus maximus (Glut Max) on the femur is shaded and remains only as a reminder of one of the potential sources of FLf.

been resolved into its parallel (Fx) and perpendicular (Fy) components. The magnitude of vector Fx_{FLf} will have to exceed +950 N in order to push the footplate to the right, given the resultant –950 N force of Fx_{QLf} and FpLf. If Fx_{FLf} is assigned a value of 960 N, it appears that Fy_{FLf} has the same magnitude because the components are approximately equivalent in size (at least in Figure 1-89).

Case Application 1-4: **Calculation of the Magnitude of FLf**

If the Fx and Fy components (see Fig. 1-89) have equal magnitude, the angle of application of F_{TOT} (or FLf in this instance) must be either 45° or 135° (180° − 45°). Here we can see that FLf is applied at a 45° angle to the long axis of the leg-foot segment. The estimated magnitude of Fx_{FLf} can be used to calculate the magnitude of FLf. The formula cos θ = side adjacent ÷ hypotenuse can be used to solve for the hypotenuse, where hypotenuse = side adjacent ÷ cos θ. The "side adjacent" is Fx_{FLf} (960 N), and the cosine of 45° is 0.707 (according to a scientific or math calculator). The hypotenuse (FLf) has a calculated value of approximately 1359 N. Although the magnitude of FLf is not the same as the force of the gluteus maximus, it should be proportional to the perpendicular (Fy) component of the gluteus maximus. Because the Fy component for most muscles is substantially smaller than the Fx component, we can assume that the resultant gluteus maximus force on the femur is substantially greater than 1359 N (and substantially greater than the 1000-N quadriceps force that has already been factored into this analysis).

If Fy_{FLf} has a magnitude of 960 N, there will be a net downward (posterior) shear force of 588 N (Fy_{FLf} + Fy_{QLf} + GLf). Assuming again that friction, although present, will be a minimal restraint, we must now identify a structure that will prevent this posterior displace-

ment. The likely source is a capsuloligamentous force—more specifically, tension in the anterior capsule or in the posterior cruciate ligament (PCL). Instrumented measurements and mathematical modeling indicate that a closed-chain leg press at 90° of flexion results in peak PCL tension.[10,11] Consequently, the force of posteriorcruciate-on-legfoot (PcLf) has been added to the figure. Although no attempt has been made to resolve PcLf into its components, its Fy component (anterior displacement) should be approximately 588 N. There will also be an Fx component of PcLf, with a magnitude that will depend on the angle of pull but will contribute further to the 950-N joint compression force already created by Fx_{QLf} and FpLf. The joint compression in the leg-press exercise, therefore, will exceed the 822-N compression estimated for the weight boot exercise at the same knee joint position and same magnitude of quadriceps muscle contraction.

Our oversimplified analysis of the leg-press exercise demonstrates the increased complexity of a closed-chain analysis over open-chain analysis. It should also demonstrate, however, that the strategy for understanding and analyzing the forces remains similar. In spite of very rough estimates of angles of application of forces (and concomitant Fy components and MAs), our findings with regard to net effects for both the weight boot and leg press are fairly in line with findings from at least one group of researchers (although we used a minimum resistance in both the weight boot and leg-press exercises, in comparison with their substantially heavier loads).[10,11] This group of researchers also demonstrated the imprecise nature of biomechanical analyses (even using sophisticated instrumentation) because they found differing results (e.g., magnitudes of joint compression and joint shear forces), using the same data from the same subjects, on the basis of different mathematical modeling variables. Their results also contradicted some of the findings in at least one previous study.[12]

Case Application 1-5: **Case Summary**

For those of you who do not wish to leave Sam Alexander without an "answer," we must first grant that our analyses of the weight boot and leg-press exercises are subject to the many limitations that have been acknowledged throughout the chapter. The most important of these—even using our simplistic approach—is that we compared the exercises in detail at only one knee joint angle, but it must be understood that the relative merits change through the ROM. From what we have done, however, we can draw a couple of tentative conclusions. One is that Sam should not be permitted to let the weight boot hang freely (if the weight boot is used) because the direct tensile stresses placed on the capsuloligamentous structures of the knee may further damage his injured ligaments. The other conclusion is that the final choice of exercise may be dependent on further information about his injury. If Sam's PCL is injured, the leg press has a distinct disadvantage, especially in the more flexed knee positions.[10] With ACL injury, the evidence shows increased stress on this ligament in the weight boot exercise but only as the knee approaches full extension.[10] Because the ACL is the more commonly injured of these ligaments, we can recommend the leg-press exercise. If joint compressive forces need to be avoided for some reason (e.g., joint cartilage damage), the weight boot might be a better choice while avoiding completing the extension ROM that might stress the ACL.

Summary

The goal of this chapter was to use Sam Alexander to present the biomechanical principles necessary to establish a conceptual framework for looking at the forces and effects of those forces on joints at various points in a joint ROM (using a predominantly simplistic two-dimensional approach that was based on sequential static rather than dynamic analyses). We identified many (but not all) of the limitations of this conceptual framework when attempting to understand or explain the extremely complex phenomena of human function and dysfunction. We paid particular attention to the interdependence of muscular forces, gravitational forces (or other external forces), and articular constraints. The need for articular constraint (joint reaction forces or capsuloligamentous forces) to accomplish joint rotation is too often under appreciated, assessed only when there are problems with these constraints and ignored when they are effective in their function. To avoid this omission, we will next explore the structural composition and properties of the articular constraints (bone, cartilage, capsule/ligament/fascia), as well as those of the muscles and their tendons (Chapters 2 and 3). The composition and behavior of various tissues is key to understanding the stresses (force per unit area) that these tissues may create on other tissues or to which the tissues must characteristically respond. With that information in hand, the reader is then prepared to understand the basis of both normal and abnormal function at each of the presented joint complexes.

Study Questions

1. Name three types of motion, and provide examples of each.
2. In what plane and around what axis does rotation of the head occur?
3. Is naming the plane of motion considered part of kinetics or kinematics? Why?
4. How does a CoR differ from a fixed axis? How does the distinction apply to motion at human joints?
5. What is the definition of a force, what are the units of measure for force, and how are forces applied to a segment?
6. What characteristics apply to all force vectors? What characteristics apply to all gravitational vectors?
7. What generalizations can be made about the LoG (gravity vector) of all stable objects?
8. What happens to the CoM of a rigid object when the object is moved around in space?
9. What happens to the CoM of the body when the body segments are rearranged? What happens to the CoM if the right upper extremity is amputated?
10. A student is carrying all of her books for the fall semester courses in her right arm. What does the additional weight do to her CoM? To her LoG? How will her body most likely respond to this change?
11. Why did your Superman punching bag always pop up again?
12. Describe the typical gait of a child just learning to walk. Why does the child walk this way?
13. Give the name, point of application, magnitude, and direction of the *contact* force applied to a man weighing 90 kg as he lies on a bed.
14. Are the two forces of an action-reaction pair (reaction forces) part of the same linear force system? Defend your answer.
15. What conditions must exist for friction on an object to have magnitude? When is the magnitude of the force of friction always greatest?
16. How do a contact force, shear force, and friction force differ?
17. A man who weights 90 kg (882 N, or ~198 lb) is lying on a bed in cervical traction with a weight of 5 kg (49 N, or ~12 lb) suspended from a horizontal rope. Assuming that the entire body is a single unsegmented object and that the body is in equilibrium, identify all the forces acting on the body (assuming that μ_S for skin on bed is 0.25).

(Continued on following page)

18. The man in Question 17 is no longer in cervical traction. A nurse standing at the foot of his bed has grasped his right foot and is pulling him down toward the foot of the bed. Again treating the man as a single unsegmented object, determine the minimum force that the nurse must have applied to the man to initiate the movement.

19. Assuming now that the leg-foot segment of the man in Question 18 is joined to the rest of his unsegmented body by capsuloligamentous structures at his knee, what must be the magnitude of tension in the knee joint capsuloligamentous structures just as the man begins to be pulled toward the foot of the bed? What are the names of the forces causing tension in the capsuloligamentous structures? What are the names of the forces causing distraction of the knee joint segments?

20. How do you graphically determine the net (resultant) effect of two forces applied to the same segment and lie at angles to each other? What is this process called?

21. What is the *minimum* requirement to produce rotation of a segment? What are the terms used to refer to the "strength" of rotation? How is the "strength" of rotation computed when the minimal conditions for rotation of a segment exist?

22. Define moment arm. How does moment arm affect the ability of a force to rotate a segment?

23. If two forces exist on a body segment on the same side of the joint axis but in opposite directions, how does one determine which is the effort force and which is the resistance force?

24. How do anatomic pulleys affect the magnitude and direction of a muscle force (Fms)?

25. What factors may cause the torque created by a force on a segment to change?

26. A 2-year-old has difficulty pushing open the door into MacDonald's. What advice will you give him as to how to perform the task independently? What is the rationale for your advice?

27. What kind of contraction is a muscle performing when it is the effort force on a rotating segment? What kind of contraction is a muscle performing when it is the resistance force on a rotating segment?

28. What is the "advantage" of a force acting on a lever with a mechanical advantage greater than 1?

29. Most muscles in the body (contracting concentrically, distal lever free) do *not* work at a mechanical advantage. Why is this true? What do muscles gain by working at a mechanical disadvantage?

30. Using the values below, identify the class of the lever, its mechanical advantage, what kind of contraction the muscle is performing, and the point of application of the resultant force of gravity-on-forearm and ball-on-forearm (the hand will be considered part of the forearm). Here Fms = muscle force, LA = lever arm, G = gravity-on-forearm, and B = ball-on-forearm (assume that all forces are applied perpendicular to the forearm lever):

$$Fms = 500 \text{ N (counterclockwise), LA} = 2 \text{ cm}$$

$$G = 32 \text{ N (clockwise), LA} = 18 \text{ cm}$$

$$B = 20 \text{ N (clockwise), LA} = 28 \text{ cm}$$

31. Describe how the perpendicular component of a force and the MA of that force are related. When is the MA potentially greatest?

32. Describe how you would position a limb in space so that gravity exerts the least torque on the limb. How would you position the limb to have gravity exert the greatest torque?

33. A muscle (Fms) is rotating a segment around a joint against the resistance of gravity (G). Identify a name for at least one other force other than Fms and G that *must* be applied to the segment in order for rotation to occur.

34. If not all a muscle's force is contributing to rotation, what happens to the "wasted" force?

35. What effects at a joint may a perpendicular force have on a segment other than rotation?

36. Under what circumstances may a force or force component that is parallel to a segment create a torque at a joint?

37. When a force is applied at 135° to a segment, what proportion of the force will rotate the segment? What proportion of the force will translate the segment, and will the direction of that force be compressive or distractive?

38. The quadriceps muscle is acting on the free leg-foot segment with a force of 500 N at an angle of 45° (unrealistic, but simplified). Identify the names (not the magnitudes or locations) of the other forces that would be required for the leg-foot segment to successfully extend at the knee joint.

♦ References

1. LeVeau B: Williams and Lissner's Biomechanics of Human Motion (3rd ed). Philadelphia, WB Saunders, 1992.
2. Hall S: Basic Biomechanics (3rd ed). Boston, WCB/McGraw-Hill, 1999.
3. Panjabi M, White AI: Biomechanics in the Musculoskeletal System. Philadelphia, Churchill Livingstone, 2001.
4. Brinckmann P, Frobin W, Leivseth G: Musculoskeletal Biomechanics. New York, Thieme, 2002.
5. Cromer A: Physics for the Life Science (2nd ed). New York, McGraw-Hill, 1994.
6. Hamilton D, Haennel R: Validity and reliability of the 6-minute walk test in a cardiac rehabilitation population. J Cardiopulm Rehabil 20:156–164, 2000.
7. Urone P: Physics with Health Science Applications. New York, John Wiley & Sons, 1986.
8. Venes D, Thomas C: Taber's Cyclopedic Medical Dictionary (19th ed). Philadelphia, F. A. Davis, 2001.
9. Evans E, Benjamin M, Pemberton DJ: Fibrocartilage in the attachment zones of the quadriceps tendon and patellar ligament in man. J Anat 171:155–162, 1990.
10. Escamilla R, Fleisig G, Zheng N, et al: Biomechanics of the knee during closed kinetic chain and open kinetic chain exercises. Med Sci Sports Exerc 30:556–569, 1998.
11. Zheng N, Fleisig G, Escamilla R, et al: An analytical model of the knee for estimation of internal forces during exercise. J Biomech 31:963–967, 1998.
12. Lutz G, Palmitier R, An K, et al: Comparison of tibiofemoral joint forces during open–kinetic-chain and closed–kinetic-chain exercises. J Bone Joint Surg Am 75:732–739, 1993.

Chapter 2

Joint Structure and Function

Sandra Curwin, PT, PhD

"HUMAN JOINTS MUST SERVE MANY FUNCTIONS; THEY ARE MORE COMPLEX THAN MOST MANMADE DESIGNS."

◆ Introduction

Joint Design

■ Form Follows Function

The joints of the human body serve functions similar to those of joints used in the construction of buildings, furniture, and machines. Joints connect different segments together and may allow movement between those segments. The design of the joint will reflect these demands. The dictum *form follows function*, coined by the American architect Louis Sullivan and promoted by the Bauhaus school of design of post-World War I Germany,[1] suggests that the appearance of an object or building should allow the observer to determine its function. The form of a chair, for example, with a seat, arms, and back at appropriate heights and angles, tells us that its function is to support a sitting person. In fact, most forms of successful design require knowledge of a structure's function. The function of the joint between a table top and legs is support, and therefore the components form a stable union. If one also wished the legs of the table to fold, the joint would have to provide mobility in one situation and stability in another situation and would require a different design. One possible method of designing a folding table joint would be by using a metal brace fitted with a locking device. The table leg would be free to move when the brace is unlocked: when the brace is locked, the joint would be stable (Fig. 2-1). We should, therefore, be able to ascertain the function of different joints in the body by examining their structure. Indeed, we do exactly this by studying the anatomy (structure) of joints.

The concept of form following function extends further than the appearance of a structure. Form refers not only to an object's appearance but also to its composition. Conversely, the materials chosen for a structure help determine its function. We are all familiar with the functional limitations of the house made of straw when the Big Bad Wolf came huffing and puffing! A modification of either structure or materials, or both, can affect function. The amputee foot shown in Figure 2-2 reflects this principle. The design of the curved foot allows the structure to flex as body weight is applied, and the heel extension provides stable support. Flexing the material stretches it, creating an elastic recoil that contributes to the subsequent movement as the amputee moves forward. Alterations in the material (usually a carbon fiber composite) affect the amount of

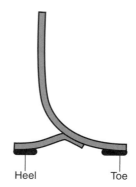

▲ **Figure 2–2** ■ The "Flex foot" facilitates gait by its design and composition. The curved blade bends during loading and then assists with propulsion. A change in material affects how much the structure bends and how much energy it provides to subsequent forward movement.

elastic recoil, and amputees can order limbs made of different materials, depending on their functional demands. Springier materials, which are harder to stretch and which recoil more, are used for activities with large loads and high speeds (e.g., running, jumping), whereas materials with less elastic recoil are used for walking.

Human joints have consistent designs that appear to be determined by a number of factors, including genetic expression, cell-cell interaction during development, and function. Function not only is the end point of joint structure but also appears to play a much larger part in human form than in other forms of design (although use will always affect appearance). For example, the structural elements of the hip joint develop before birth, but the mature shape of the head of the femur and the acetabulum is determined by functional interaction between these two structures. Human connective tissues and joints, in fact, depend on function to assume their final form (Fig. 2-3).

Once joints and tissues have assumed their final structural form, they can still be influenced by changes in functional demands. All components of human joints—bone, muscles, ligaments, cartilage, tendon—can adapt to functional demands. Frequently, for the therapist, this involves interventions aimed at restoring changes that have occurred as a result of inactivity or immobilization. Knowledge of the amount and types of loads that occur during normal loading conditions may allow the therapist to tailor the rehabilitation process to optimize tissue structure and function.

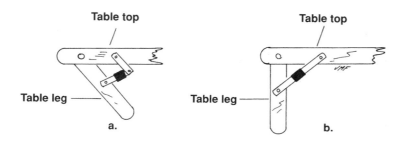

a.

b.

◀ **Figure 2-1** ■ Folding table joint. **A.** The table leg is free to move, and the joint provides mobility when the brace is unlocked. **B.** The table leg is prevented from moving, and the joint provides stability when the brace is locked.

Tissue Structure-Function

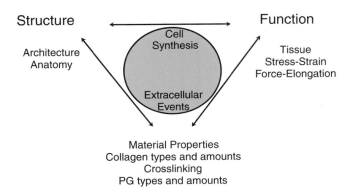

▲ **Figure 2-3** ■ Form determines the overall structure of connective tissues, but the characteristics of the tissue are affected by functional use. Collagen type, crosslinks, and PG type and amount all can be affected by the type and amount of stress applied to the tissue. Alternatively, the tissue may adapt to altered function by becoming larger, longer, or shorter. The size of the tissue and its composition will determine the types of loads the tissue can bear; these loads will likewise signal the cells to synthesize the appropriate type and amount of tissue and either dictate or facilitate extracellular events (such as crosslinking) that enhance tissue function.

2-1	Patient Case

George Chen is a 40-year-old male electrician and business owner who suffered a trimalleolar ankle fracture 2 weeks ago while playing hockey. The fractures were treated with open reduction and internal fixation (ORIF) and he is now non–weight-bearing (NWB), with crutches with his leg and foot immobilized in a cast. Naturally, he has many questions. Does his ankle really need to be in a cast? Why does it still swell and hurt so much? What can he do now to shorten his recovery time? Is it really necessary to be NWB for 8 weeks? When can he drive?

You, as a therapist, also are likely to have many additional questions. What structures are likely to have been damaged with this type of injury? What changes will take place as the structures heal, and how will these changes affect lower extremity function? What are the ideal stimuli to preserve cartilage, bone, muscle, and tendon and ligament structure and function? Does the treatment scenario for this injury create negative consequences for uninjured structures? Is there a way to offset possible changes? What types of exercise should be used in the rehabilitation process, and what are their effects on the tissues that haven't been injured or immobilized?

■ **Basic Principles**

A joint (articulation) connects one component of a structure with one or more other components. The design of a joint and the materials used in its construction depend partly on the function of the joint and partly on the nature of the components. If the function of a joint is to provide stability or static support, the joint will have a different design than when the desired function is mobility. In general, design becomes more complex as functional demands increase. Joints that serve a single function are less complex than joints that serve multiple functions. Because human joints must serve many functions, they are far more complex than most synthetic designs.

Materials used in joint construction also may influence design, and vice versa. Table legs made of particleboard would need to be larger than legs made of steel, to achieve the same function. The reverse also may be true: design constraints may dictate materials. A car tire that must have certain dimensions but needs to last for 40,000 miles will require a change in materials, rather than appearance. Changes also occur in joint structures that allow them to match functional demands. Julius Wolff described the adaptation of bone to increased demands (Wolff's law) and similar changes can occur in tendons and ligaments.[2]

CONCEPT CORNERSTONE 2-1: *Relationships between Function, Structure, and Composition*

Joint function both depends on and affects

- ■ structure (design)
- ■ composition (materials)

◆ Materials Found in Human Joints

The fact that the materials used in human joints are composed of living tissue makes human joints unique. Living tissue can change its structure in response to changing environmental or functional demands. It requires nourishment to survive and is subject to disease processes, injury, and the effects of aging. It can adapt to meet imposed demands and become injured if the adaptation is unsuccessful or if the demands are too great. Therefore, to understand the structure and function of the human joints, it is necessary to have some knowledge of the nature of the materials that are used in joint construction and the forces that are acting at the joints. Although the nervous and muscular systems are integrally involved in overall joint function, this chapter focuses on the tissues that comprise the actual joint structures; that is, the connective tissues.

Case Application 2-1: **Materials (Living Tissues) Affected by the Fracture**

The materials likely to have been affected in George Chen include bone, ligaments, blood vessels, nerves, and the joint capsule. Muscles, tendons, and cartilage may also be involved. Because all of these tissues will be affected by immobilization, a number of structures will undergo a change in size and/or composition.

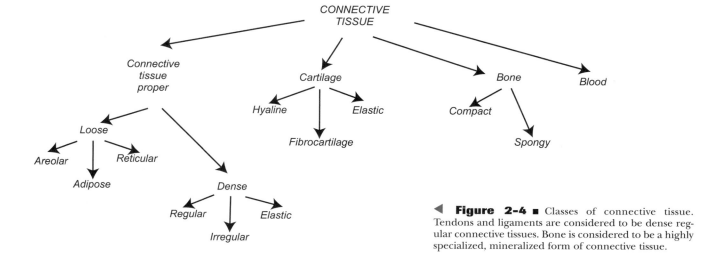

◀ **Figure 2-4** ■ Classes of connective tissue. Tendons and ligaments are considered to be dense regular connective tissues. Bone is considered to be a highly specialized, mineralized form of connective tissue.

Structure of Connective Tissue

The living material comprising human joint components is connective tissue in the form of bones, bursae, capsules, cartilage, disks, fat pads, labra, menisci, plates, ligaments, and tendons. The gross anatomic structure and microarchitecture of these connective tissue structures are extremely varied, and the biomechanical behaviors and composition of capsules, cartilage, specific ligaments, menisci, and tendons are still being investigated.[2–27] There are four classes of connective tissues (Fig. 2-4). In general, the structure of the connective tissue is characterized by a wide dispersion of cells (cellular component) and the presence of a large volume of **extracellular matrix (ECM)**. At the microscopic level, the ECM has both **interfibrillar** (previously referred to as the ground substance) and **fibrillar**

(fibrous) components. Connective tissues are unique among body structures in that their function is primarily determined by the extracellular component, unlike other tissues such as muscle and nerve, in which cell behavior largely determines function (Table 2-1).

■ Cells

The cells of connective tissues derive from mesenchymal precursors that differentiate into the different connective tissue cells. The cells are either **fixed** in specific tissues or **transient** within the circulatory system (see Table 2-1). The **fibroblast** is the "basic" cell of most connective tissues. Depending on its environment, the fibroblast may specialize to become a **chondroblast** or **osteoblast.** As the tissue matures and synthetic activity declines, the cells are referred to as **fibrocytes, chon-**

Table 2-1	Connective Tissue Cell Types	
Type	Name	Location and Function
Fixed	Fibroblast	Found in tendon, ligament, skin, bone, etc.
		Creates mostly type I collagen
	Chondroblast	Differentiated fibroblast found in cartilage
		Produces mostly type II collagen
	Osteoblast	Differentiated fibroblast found in bone
		Produces type I collagen and hydroxyapatite
	Osteoclast	Monocyte-derived, found in bone
		Responsible for bone resorption
	Mast cells	Found in various connective tissues
		Inflammatory mediators
	Adipose cells	Found in adipose tissue
		Produce and store fat
	Mesenchyme cells	Undifferentiated cells found primarily in embryo and in bone marrow
		Can differentiate into any connective tissue cell
Transient	Lymphocytes	White blood cells that have surface proteins specific for antigens
	Neutrophils	White blood cells involved in fighting infection
	Macrophages	Derived from monocytes, move into specific tissues, involved in immune response
	Plasma cells	B lymphocytes producing antibodies

drocytes, and **osteocytes.** This distinction is based primarily on appearance, which reflects cell synthetic activity, and the same cell can go through several cycles as a fibroblast/fibrocyte. The terms **tenoblast** and **tenocyte** refer to fibroblasts and fibrocytes found within tendon. It is possible that the cells of any of the specific connective tissues may "de-differentiate" and change their synthetic output, given the appropriate environment and stimuli. For example, tendon cells can produce cartilage-like tissue when subjected to compressive forces. Such findings suggest that connective tissue structure can be modified by changes in loading conditions. Also, it may be possible for the mechanical environment to be manipulated to cause connective tissues to synthesize materials that will enhance their function.

■ **Extracellular Matrix**

Interfibrillar Component

The interfibrillar component of connective tissue is composed of hydrated networks of proteins: primarily **glycoproteins** and **proteoglycans** (**PGs**).[28] A glycoprotein is a compound containing a carbohydrate (sugar-type molecule) covalently linked to protein. There are

thousands of glycoproteins in the body. The term "glycoprotein" really should include PGs, which in the past were considered as a separate class of compounds because their carbohydrate (a repeating disaccharide unit) seemed to differ so greatly from the carbohydrates found in other glycoproteins. Another reason was their unique distribution: the PGs are found mainly in connective tissues, where they contribute to the organization and physical properties of the ECM. However, PGs are synthesized in the same manner as other glycoproteins, and repeating disaccharide units are present in typical glycoproteins as well. Therefore, PGs are considered to be a subclass of glycoproteins.

It appears that, in describing connective tissues, the term glycoprotein is generally used for proteins with smaller numbers of typical carbohydrates attached, whereas PG refers to proteins with larger numbers of disaccharide units attached. In the past, PGs also were called **mucopolysaccharides,** and the interfibrillar matrix was referred to as the **ground substance.** An overview of some of the PGs found in connective tissues is shown in Table 2-2.

The carbohydrate portion of PGs consists of long chains of repeating disaccharide units called **glycosaminoglycans** (**GAGs**).[27–30] The disaccharide units

Table 2-2	Proteoglycans	
Classification	**Name**	**Location, Composition, and Function**
Large extracellular aggregating	Versican	Found in smooth muscle cells, fibroblasts; function unknown
	Aggrecan	Found in numerous chains of KS and CS Binds to hyaluronan Creates osmotic swelling pressure in cartilage by attracting water
	Brevican	Found in nervous system; cell adhesion and migration
	Neurocan	Found in nervous system; cell adhesion and migration
Small leucine-rich proteoglycans (SLRPs)	Decorin	One or two CS or DS chains Binds and regulates growth factors, modulates cell functions, regulates collagen fibrillogenesis, interacts with collagen types I, II, III, V, VI, XII, XIV
	Biglycan	Two GAG chains containing CS or DS Directs type VI collagen network assembly Binds to complement and transforming growth factor beta (TGF-β)
	Fibromodulin	One KS GAG chain Interacts with type I and II collagen, binds to growth factors
	Lumican	Similar to fibromodulin, found in cornea, muscle, intestine, cartilage
	Epiphycan	Found in epiphyseal cartilage
Cell-associated PGs	Serglycins	Protein core of heparin: PGs regulate enzyme activities in secretory granules
	Syndecans	Cell transmembrane PG containing HS acts as a receptor for heparin-binding factors
	Betaglycan	Contains HS and CS Binds TGF-β
	CD44 family	Cell surface receptor for hyaluronan
	Thrombomodulin	Binds to thrombin
Basement membrane PGs	Perlecan	Found in all tissues; function uncertain
	HS and CS PGs	Found in all tissues; function uncertain
	Bamacan	Found in various tissues; function uncertain
Nervous tissue PGs	Phosphacan	Nervous tissue cell adhesion
	Agrin	Aggregates acetylcholine receptors
	NG2 PG	Found in developing cells

CS, chondroitin sulfate; DS, dermatan sulfate; GAG, glycosaminoglycan; HS, heparan sulfate; KS, keratan sulfate; PG, proteoglycan.

contain either of two modified sugars: *N*-acetylgalactosamine (**GalNAc**) or *N*-acetylglucosamine (**GlcNAc**) and a uronic acid such as **glucuronate** or **iduronate**. The GAGs are all very similar to glucose in structure and are distinguished by the number and location of the amine and sulfate groups that are attached (Table 2-3). The major types of sulfated GAGs include **chondroitin 4** and **chondroitin 6 sulfate, keratan sulfate, heparin, heparan sulfate,** and **dermatan sulfate.** A PG can contain one or more (up to about 100) GAGs, which extend perpendicularly from the protein core in a brushlike structure. GAGs are linked to the protein core by a specific trisaccharide composed of two galactose residues and a xyluose residue (GAG-Gal-Gal-Xyl-O-CH2-protein core). Additional saccharide units are enzymatically added to the growing GAG chain once it has been attached to its protein core. **Hyaluronan** (**HA**) differs from the other GAGs because it is not sulfated and does not attach to a protein core. Rather, HA exists as a free GAG chain of variable length or as a core molecule to which large numbers of PGs are attached. Some PGs can attach to HA through interaction between a globular region at the end of their protein core and a separate **link protein.** The most common of these is **aggrecan,** found in articular cartilage (Fig. 2-5). These PGs can form large aggregating structures with HA.

The proportion of PGs in the ECM of a particular structure (bone, cartilage, tendon, or ligament) affects its hydration through the affects of the attached GAGs.[30] The GAG chains are negatively charged and attract water, creating an osmotic swelling pressure, which causes water to flow into the ECM. The water flow swells the interfibrillar matrix, creating a tensile stress on the surrounding collagen network. The collagen fibers resist and contain the swelling, thus increasing the rigidity of the ECM and its ability to resist compressive forces, as well as supporting the cells. In addition to their water-binding function, the PGs form a reservoir for nutrients and growth factors bound to the PG molecules. The PGs attach to collagen fibers and contribute to the strength of the collagen and also may play a role in directing or limiting the size of collagen fibrils. Tissues that are subjected to high compressive forces have a larger PG content than tissues that resist tensile forces.[30–32] The type of GAG also may change, depending on whether the tissue is subjected to tensile or compressive forces.[33,34] Tissues subjected to compression have larger amounts of chondroitin sulfate, whereas tissues subjected to tension contain more dermatan sulfate.[32–35]

CONCEPT CORNERSTONE 2-2: *Proteoglycan Characteristics*

Proteoglycans:

- are distinguished by their protein core and by their attached GAGs
- attract water through their attached GAGs
- regulate collagen fibril size
- may attach to hyaluronate (a GAG) to form large aggregating structures
- are increased in tissues subjected to alternating cycles of compression

Glycoproteins such as **fibronectin, laminin, chondronectin, osteonectin, tenascin,** and **entactin** play an important role in fastening the various components of the ECM together and in the adhesion between collagen and integrin molecules in the cell membranes of the resident cells of the tissue (Table 2-4). Collagen also is a glycoprotein but is considered separately because of the structural role it plays.

Fibrillar Component

The fibrillar, or fibrous, component of the ECM contains two major classes of structural proteins: collagen and elastin.[2] **Collagen** is the main substance of connective

Table 2-3	Glycosaminoglycans (GAGs)		
GAG	Localization	Comments	Compositon
Hyaluronan	Synovial fluid, vitreous humor, loose CT, healing CT, cartilage	Forms large PG aggregates	Glucuronate uronic acid Glucosamine
Chondroitin sulfate	Cartilage, bone, heart valves, tendons, ligaments	Most abundant GAG, increased with compression	Glucuronate Galactosamine with 4-sulfate or 6-sulfate
Heparan sulfate	Basement membranes, cell surfaces	Interacts with numerous proteins	Glucuronate Glucosamine Variable sulfation
Heparin	Intracellular granules in mast cells lining arteries	Key structural unit is 3-glucosamine + 2-glucuronate	Glucuronate, iduronate Glucosamine Variable sulfation
Dermatan sulfate	Skin, blood vessels, tendons, ligaments	Increased with tensile stress	Iduronate Galactosamine
Keratan sulfate	Cornea, bone, cartilage	Forms part of large PG aggregates in cartilage	Galactose Glucosamine

CT, connective tissue; PG, proteoglycan.

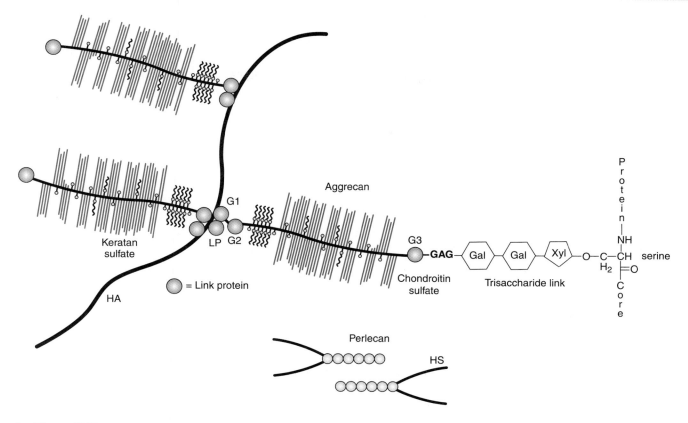

▲ **Figure 2–5** ■ In the extracellular matrix, large complexes of PGs with other matrix molecules are found. Aggrecan is the largest of these PGs. Aggrecan is covalently modified by both chondroitin sulfate (CS) and keratan sulfate (KS) chains and noncovalently associated to a hyaluronan (HA) chain.

tissue and is found in all multicellular organisms. It is the most abundant protein in the human body and accounts for 25% to 30% of all protein in mammals.[36] The word collagen is derived from the Greek word

meaning to produce glue, and in the past the collagen of animal bones and tendons was used in industry to produce glue. Collagen has a tensile strength that approaches that of steel and is responsible for the

Table 2-4	Glycoproteins	
Classification	Name	Comments
Cartilage	Asporin	Related to decorin and biglycan, found in cartilage
		Increases in osteoarthritis
	Chondronectin	Attaches chondrocytes to type II collagen
	Chondroadherin (CHAD)	Found in cartilage
		Binds to cells via integrin
		Function unknown
Bone	Osteoadherin	Found in bone trabeculae
		Binds to cells via integrin
	Osteonectin	Binds to hydroxyapatite, collagens, growth factors, osteoadherin; inhibits cell spreading
	Osteopontin	Binds to osteoclast via integrin
		Assists osteoclast function
	Osteocalcin (BGP)	Thought to be involved in bone formation
Basement membrane	Laminin	Binds type IV collagen, HS, integrin (cell membrane)
	Entactin	Interacts with laminin
Multiple sites	Collagen	Structural component
	Fibronectin	Interacts with cell-surface receptors, blood-clotting components, denatured collagen, cytoskeleton, GAGs
	Tenascin	Function unclear; increases in developing or healing tissue
Synovial fluid	Lubricin	Adheres to articular surface to provide boundary lubrication

GAG, glycosaminoglycan; HS, heparan sulfate.

Table 2-5	Collagen Types	
Classification	Type	Common Locations
Fibrillar	I	Tendons, bone, ligaments, skin, anulus fibrosis, menisci, fibrocartilage, joint capsules, cornea Accounts for 90% of body collagen
	II	Hyaline articular cartilage, nucleus pulposus, vitreous humor
	III	Skin, blood vessels, tendons ligaments
	V	Cartilage, tendons
	XI	Cartilage, other tissues (associated with type V)
	IX	Cartilage, cornea (found with type II)
Fibril-associated	XII	Tendons, ligaments (found with type I)
	XIV	Fetal skin and tendons
	IV	Basement membrane
Network forming	X	Hypertrophic cartilage
	VIII	Unknown
Filamentous	VI	Blood vessels, skin
Anchoring	VII	Anchoring filaments

functional integrity of connective tissue structures and their resistance to tensile forces.[36-44]

Collagens are composed of three alpha chains which have a repeating Gly-X-Y amino acid pattern that allows folding into a triple helix. Although more than 30 distinct alpha chains are known and 15 to 19 types of collagen have been identified, the functions of all of these types have not been determined.[38-40] Some of the types of collagen and their distribution in joint structures are presented in Table 2-5. The Roman numerals that designate each type of collagen—for example, type

I, type II—reflect the order in which each type of collagen was discovered.[2] The fibril-forming collagens (types I, II, III, V, and XI) are the most common. Type I collagen, comprising 90% of the total collagen in the body, is found in almost all connective tissue, including tendons, ligaments, menisci, fibrocartilage, joint capsules, synovium, bones, labra, and skin.[42-44] It appears to be the major load-bearing element in tissues subjected to tensile forces. Type II collagen is found mainly in hyaline articular cartilage and in the nucleus pulposus in the center of the intervertebral disks.[37,38] Type III collagen is found in the skin, in the stratum synovium of joint capsules, in the sheaths within muscle and tendons, and in healing tissues.[38,43]

The basic building block of collagen is the triple helix of three polypeptide chains that is called the **tropocollagen molecule.** Like the protein portion of PGs and other glycoproteins, it is synthesized in the rough endoplasmic reticulum of the fibroblasts. The tropocollagen molecules are attracted to one another and aggregate to form microfibrils. The microfibrils form subfibrils that, in turn, combine to form **fibrils**[44-46] (Fig. 2-6). Intramolecular and intermolecular **crosslinks** stabilize and strengthen the enlarging fibrils.[45] The fibrils form a **fascicle,** and the fascicles combine to form fibers. Collagen fibers may be arranged in many different ways and may also vary in size and length. The relaxed fibers in some structures have a wavy configuration called a **crimp.** When collagen fibers are stretched, the crimp disappears.

Elastin polypeptide chains, like collagen, contain a Gly-X-Y amino acid repeat and a considerable amount of the amino acid **proline,** but, unlike collagen, the molecule consists of single alpha-like strands without the triple helix. The alpha-like strands are crosslinked to each other to form rubber-like, elastic fibers. Each elastin molecule uncoils into a more extended conformation when the fiber is stretched and will recoil spontaneously as soon as the stretching force is relaxed. Elastin fibers are usually yellowish in color, branch freely, and are found in all joint structures, as well in

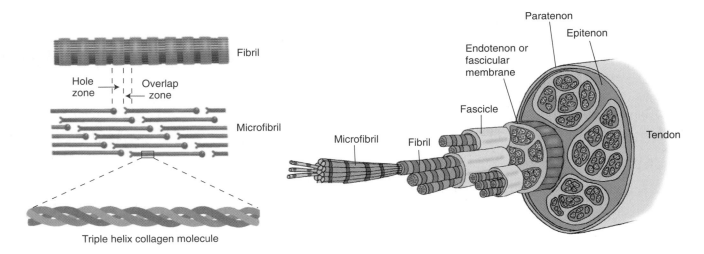

▲ **Figure 2-6** ■ Dense connective tissues such as tendon have a hierarchical structure from the molecule to the entire tissue.

the skin, the tracheobronchial tree, and the walls of arteries. However, the relative proportion of fibers varies considerably, and, in general, elastin fibers make up a much smaller portion of the fibrous component in the ECM than do collagen fibers in most of the load-bearing tissues. The aorta contains approximately 30% elastin and 20% collagen (percentage of dry weight of the tissue), the ligamentum nuchae has 75% elastin and 15% collagen, and the Achilles tendon contains only 4.4.% elastin and 86% collagen.

 CONCEPT CORNERSTONE 2-3: *Extracellular Matrix Function and Structure*

The ECM of connective tissue determines its function, and vice versa. The type and proportions of the components create the different tissues:

- interfibrillar component: PGs (protein + GAGs), glycoproteins
- fibrillar component: collagen (mainly type I or II), elastin

---

Case Application 2-2: **Materials Involved in the Fracture Healing Process**

The early callus of fracture healing in our patient consists largely of fibrocartilage material containing a high proportion of PGs, GAGs and glycoproteins. Undifferentiated mesenchymal cells migrate to the fracture site and have the ability to form cells, which in turn form cartilage, bone, or fibrous tissue. The fracture hematoma is organized, fibroblasts and chondroblasts appear between the bone ends, and cartilage is formed (type II collagen). Later, cells begin to form type I collagen that becomes mineralized to form bone. The amount of callus formed is inversely proportional to the amount of immobilization of the fracture. In fractures that are fixed with rigid compression plates, there can be primary bone healing with little or no visible callus formation. These fractures will tend to heal a bit more slowly, because it takes longer for primary bone formation. This explains why our patient must be nonweight (NWB) for 8 weeks, even though the fracture fragments have been rejoined. Because he fractured his ankle only 2 weeks ago, there is probably very little bone at the fracture site.

Specific Connective Tissue Structures

∎ Ligaments

Ligaments connect one bone to another, usually at or near a joint. Some ligaments blend with the joint capsules and may be difficult to identify because they appear as thickenings in the capsule (e.g., anterior band of the inferior glenohumeral ligament). Other ligaments are distinct, easily recognizable structures often appearing as dense white bands or cords of connective tissue (e.g., anterior cruciate ligament [ACL]).

Ligaments, like other connective tissue structures, are heterogeneous structures containing a small amount of cells (about 10% to 20% of the tissue volume, mainly fibroblasts) and a large ECM (about 80% to 90%). The PGs, which constitute only about 0.2% of the tissue dry weight (after all water has been removed), contain primarily dermatan sulfate GAG. The fibrillar component of the ECM in most ligaments is composed mainly of type I collagen, with lesser amounts of type III, type IV, and type V collagen, and varying amounts of elastin. One notable exception is the **ligamentum flavum,** which has a distinctly yellowish color and contains a large amount of elastin (75% of the tissue's dry weight).

The type I collagen fibrils in ligaments are densely packed, and the fiber bundles are arranged in the direction of applied tensile forces. The arrangement of the collagen fibers and the collagen/elastin fiber ratio in various ligaments determines the relative abilities of these structures to provide stability and allow mobility for a particular joint.[47] Because ligaments are subjected to varying directions of tensile force, depending on joint angle, the collagen fibers in ligaments have a varied arrangement that enables the ligament to resist forces from more than one direction. For example, the posterior fibers of the medial collateral ligament (MCL) of the knee may be under tension in joint extension, whereas the middle fibers may be under tension when a varus stress is applied. The fibers that are aligned in a direction parallel to the imposed forces (due to motion between body segments) resist tensile force applied to the ligament. This is in contrast to a tendon, in which the tensile forces are created by muscle force and so tend to be in one direction.

The cellular appearance and matrix architecture change as the ligament approaches bone. Collagen fibers appear to be cemented into bone during growth and development, forming Sharpey fibers (perforations of fibrous tissue into bone) at the ligamentous bony insertion sites (the **entheses**). The stiffening of the ligament-bone interface decreases the likelihood that the ligament will give way at the enthesis; however, it is a common site for degenerative change, usually in the underlying bone.[48]

Ligaments are usually named descriptively according to their location, shape, bony attachments, and relationship to one another. The anterior longitudinal ligament, which covers most of the anterior surface of the vertebral column, is an example of a ligament that appears to be named both for location (anterior) and shape (longitudinal). The medial and lateral collateral ligaments of the elbow and knee joints are examples of ligaments named for location. Ligaments such as the coracohumeral, which connects the coracoid process of the scapula with the humerus at the shoulder, and the radioulnar ligaments, which connect the radius to the ulna at the distal radioulnar joint, are examples of naming by bony attachment. A ligament named according to shape is the deltoid ligament at the ankle joint. Occasionally, ligaments are given the name of the individual who first identified the ligament. The Y ligament of Bigelow at the hip joint is named both for its inverted

Y shape and for an individual. The cruciate ligaments at the knee are so named because they cross each other.

Case Application 2-3: **Mechanism of Injury**

In the case of George Chen, the mechanism of injury involved an external rotation twist of the ankle and foot. It is likely that both the deltoid ligament and ankle joint capsule were damaged.

■ **Tendons**

Tendons connect muscle to bone and transmit forces developed by muscles to bones to move or stabilize joints. Each muscle has tendinous material interspersed between it and bone, although the attachments may vary widely in configuration, and one tendon may be much more prominent than another. These prominent tendons are usually named for the muscle to which they are attached: for example, biceps tendon for the biceps brachii and the triceps tendon for the triceps. Occasionally, they are named differently; for example, the Achilles tendon at the ankle is named after a Greek warrior in the Trojan War who was killed by an arrow that struck his heel, the only vulnerable spot on his body.

Tendons have approximately the same composition and basic structure as ligaments.[47,49,50] The fibrillar component is composed primarily of type I collagen, with lesser amounts of type III and type V collagen and of type IV collagen associated with the basal lamina of the fibroblasts. Tendons contain slightly more type I collagen and slightly less type III collagen than do ligaments (Table 2-6). This composition suggests that they

are adapted to larger tensile forces, inasmuch as type I collagen is considered stronger than type III collagen. The interfibrillar component of the ECM in tendons contains water, PGs that contain dermatan sulfate GAG, and other glycoproteins. Dermatan sulfate GAG appears to be more prevalent under conditions of tensile loading.

The collagen fibrils of tendon, group in successively larger subunits, to form primary bundles known as fibers[44–46] (see Fig. 2-6). The diameter of these fibers, which contain almost entirely type I collagen, seems to increase in proportion to the tensile loads applied to the tendon. Groups of fiber bundles, enclosed by a loose connective tissue sheath called the **endotendon,** form a secondary bundle called a fascicle. The endotendon, containing a higher proportion of type III collagen fibrils, also encloses nerves, lymphatic vessels, and blood vessels supplying the tendon. Individual fascicles are associated with discrete groups of muscle fibers or motor units at the muscle-tendon insertion. Several fascicles may form a larger group (tertiary bundle) that also is enclosed in endotendon. The sheath that covers the entire tendon is called the **epitenon.** The **paratenon** is a double-layered sheath of areolar tissue that is loosely attached to the outer surface of the epitenon. The epitenon and paratenon together are sometimes called the **peritendon.** The peritendon may become a synovium-filled sheath called the **tenosynovium** (or **tendon sheath**) in tendons that are subjected to high levels of friction. The paratenon protects the tendon, enhances movement of the tendon on adjacent structures, and provides a source of cells if the tendon is injured. Like ligaments, the collagen fibers in tendons align parallel to the loads applied to the tissue. Because these loads are applied by the attached muscle, the col-

---

Table 2-6	**Composition of Dense Connective Tissues**			
Tissue	Water Content*	Collagen†	PG/GAGs†	Comment
Bone	25%	25%–30% Mainly type I	Mainly CS	65%–70% dry weight is inorganic
Cartilage	60%–85%	10%–30% >90% type II	8%–10% aggregating PGs	Cells are 10% of total weight
Ligament	70%	75% 90% type I 10% type III	< 1% Mainly DS	20% dry weight unknown
Tendon	60%–75%	80% 95% type I <5% type III	0.2%–1% Mainly DS	More linear collagen fibrils than ligament
Capsule	70%	90% Mainly type I	CS, DS	Some elastin
Menisci	70%–78%	60%–90% Mainly type I	<10%	Fibrocartilage
Anulus	65%–70%	50%–60% Types I and II	20% CS, KS	
Nucleus	65%–90%	20%–30% Mainly type II	65% aggregating PGs	

*Water content is percentage of total tissue weight.
† Collagen and PG content is percentage of tissue dry weight after water has been removed.
CS, chrondroitin sulfate; DS, dermatan sulfate; GAG, glycosaminoglycan; KS, keratan sulfate; PG, proteoglycan.

lagen fibers in tendons have a largely unidirectional alignment parallel to these tensile forces, although there are also crossed and spiral arrangements.[46,48] The relaxed fibers appear crimped, a feature that appears to be maintained by PG interaction with the collagen fibrils.

There are two types of tendon attachments to bone: **fibrocartilaginous** and **fibrous.**[49] The fibrocartilaginous attachment of tendon to bone (**enthesis**) involves gradual changes in the tendon structure that occur over a length of about 1 mm and can be divided into four zones on the basis of histological observation (Fig. 2-7). The first zone consists of tendon proper and is similar to the tendon midsubstance. The second zone contains fibrocartilage and marks the beginning of the transition from tendon to bone. The third zone contains mineralized fibrocartilage, and the fourth zone consists of bone. The changes in tissue are gradual and continuous, a feature that is presumed to aid in effective load transfer between two very different materials. A tidemark frequently appears between the calcified and uncalcified parts of the enthesis, representing the mechanical boundary between hard and soft tissues. However, the tidemark does not serve as a barrier, and collagen fibers pass through it to the mineralized fibrocartilage. Dramatic changes in gene expression and composition occur in the different zones. Collagen types II, IX, and X and aggrecan are localized to the bony insertion, whereas decorin and biglycan are localized to the tendon side of the insertion.[49] Collagen types I, III, and XII have been found at both locations. These findings suggest that the tendon insertion is subjected to both compressive and tensile forces.

The fibrous entheses may be subdivided into two categories: **periosteal** and **bony.**[49] At the former, the tendon fibers attach to the periosteum, which thus indirectly attaches the tendon to the bone, whereas in the latter, the tendon attaches directly to bone. There can be a mixture of the two types of attachment, and the periosteal attachments sometimes convert to bony attachments with age. Examples of these types of attachment include the attachments of the deltoid muscle to the humerus and to the scapula and clavicle. Interestingly, the new enthesis formed after surgical reattachment of a tendon to bone is initially fibrous, although fibrocartilage may be re-formed with time.

The attachment of tendon to muscle at the **myotendinous junction** (**MTJ**) comprises interdigitation between collagen fibers and muscle cells.[51–53] Surface friction and direct connections between collagen and PGs and the basal lamina and integrins in the muscle cell membrane create a strong interaction (Fig. 2-8). The interdigitating form of the MTJ, essential for normal function of the muscle-tendon unit, is very sensitive

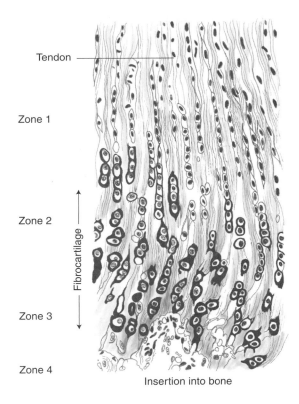

▲ **Figure 2-7** ■ The bone-tendon (or ligament) junction. There are four zones, from pure tendon (zone 1) to bone (zone 4). In between, the material gradually transitions from fibrocartilage (zone 2) to mineralized fibrocartilage (zone 3).

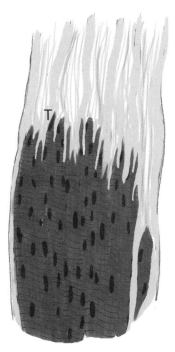

Muscle-tendon junction

▲ **Figure 2-8** ■ The muscle-tendon junction. The muscle cells interdigitate with the tendon (T). There are direct connections between the muscle cell membrane and fibroblasts, PGs, and collagen. The endotenon blends into the endomysium, and the epitenon blends into the epimysium, which forms a meshwork of connective tissue around the muscle fibers.

to decreased loading conditions and tends to become flatter and less infolded when loads are decreased. This weakens the junction and may make it more susceptible to injury. Thus, when muscle-tendon loading begins after a period of immobilization, loads should begin at a lower level and progress gradually.

 CONCEPT CORNERSTONE 2-4: *Gradual Transition between Tissues Serves to Diffuse Load*

Attachments of tendon and ligament to bone reflect a gradual transition between tissue subjected primarily to tensile force, and tissue subjected to compressive and tensile forces. This transition "diffuses" the load at the osseous tendon junction (OTJ) and helps prevent injury. The differences in composition suggest that tension increases collagen type I concentration, whereas alternating compression increases PG concentration.

■ Bursae

Bursae, which are similar in structure and function to tendon sheaths, are flat sacs of synovial membrane in which the inner sides of the sacs are separated by a fluid film. Bursae are located where moving structures are in tight approximation: that is, between tendon and bone, bone and skin, muscle and bone, or ligament and bone. Bursae located between the skin and bone, such as those found between the patella and the skin and between the olecranon process of the ulna and the skin, are called **subcutaneous bursae.**[2] **Subtendinous bursae** lie between tendon and bone, and **submuscular bursae** lie between muscle and bone.

■ Cartilage

Cartilage is usually divided into the following types: (white) **fibrocartilage,** (yellow) **elastic cartilage,** and (articular) **hyaline cartilage.**[7] Cartilage is characterized by containing mainly type II collagen and large amounts of aggregating PGs. White fibrocartilage forms the bonding cement in joints that permit little motion. This type of cartilage also forms the intervertebral disks and is found in the glenoid and acetabular labra and in one surface of the temperomandibular and sacroiliac joints. Unlike other cartilage, which contains almost exclusively type II collagen, white fibrocartilage contains type I collagen in the fibrous component of the ECM. Yellow elastic fibrocartilage is found in the ears and epiglottis and differs from white fibrocartilage in that it has a higher ratio of elastin to collagen fibers than the white variety, which consists primarily of collagen fibers.[2]

Hyaline articular cartilage, from the Greek word "hyalos," meaning glass, forms a relatively thin (1 to 7 mm) covering on the ends of the bones in the majority of joints. It provides a smooth, resilient, low-friction surface for the articulation of one bone with another. These cartilaginous surfaces are capable of bearing and distributing weight over a person's lifetime. However, once hyaline articular cartilage is injured, it has limited and imperfect mechanisms for repair.[7,9,53] Articular cartilage has the same general structure as other connective tissues in that it is characterized by a small cellular component and a large ECM. In contrast to ligaments and tendons, however, the ECM contains a much larger volume of interfibrillar material. The cells of articular cartilage are **chondrocytes** and **chondroblasts.** Chondroblasts are differentiated mesenchymal cells that produce collagen, aggrecan, link protein, and HA, which are extruded into the ECM and aggregate spontaneously. Chondrocytes are the less synthetically active cells observed in nongrowing tissues. The fibrillar component of the articular cartilage ECM includes elastin and type II and other types of collagen, but type II collagen accounts for about 90% to 95% of the collagen content.[54] Type XI collagen regulates the fibril size, and type IX facilitates fibril interaction with PG molecules. Collagen is dispersed throughout the interfibrillar component of the ECM[28] and also forms a meshwork at the joint surface that attaches to bone at the articular cartilage margins.[28,54]

Articular cartilage contains much more PG than do other joint structures, and the major PG is aggrecan, bound with HA to form large PG aggregates.[28] Aggrecan contains the GAGs chondroitin sulfate and keratan sulfate. The ratio of chondroitin sulfate to keratan sulfate shows variations among individuals, as well as age and site variations. The higher the chondroitin sulfate concentration is, the better the tissue can resist compressive forces. Keratan sulfate concentration increases in aging and in joints with arthritic changes, and it decreases in immobilization.[54] If the proportion of keratan sulfate exceeds the chondroitin sulfate portion, the ability of the cartilage to bear loads is compromised. **Chondronectin,** a cartilage glycoprotein, plays an important role in the adhesion of chondroblasts to type II collagen fibers in the presence of chondroitin sulfate.[54,55]

Three distinct layers or zones of articular cartilage are found on the ends of the bony components of synovial joints[7] (Fig. 2-9). In the outermost layer (zone 1), the radially oriented type II collagen fibers are arranged

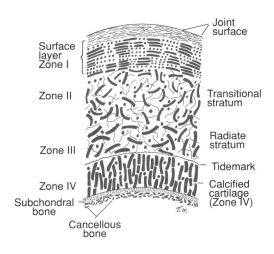

▲ **Figure 2-9** ■ Structure of hyaline cartilage.

parallel to the surface. This smooth outermost layer of the cartilage helps to reduce friction between the opposing joint surfaces and to distribute forces over the joint surface. In the second and third zones, type II collagen fibers are randomly arranged and form an open latticework. The second layer with its loose-coiled collagen fiber network permits deformation and helps to absorb some of the force imposed on the joint surfaces. In the third layer (radiate stratum), some collagen fibers lie perpendicular to the surface and extend across the interface between uncalcified and calcified cartilage to find a secure hold in the calcified cartilage.[2,28] The calcified layer of cartilage, sometimes referred to as the fourth zone, lies adjacent to subchondral bone and anchors the cartilage securely to the bone.[56] The interface between the calcified and uncalcified cartilage is called the **tidemark**.[7,57] The tidemark area of the cartilage is important because of its relation to growth, aging,[57] injury,[54] and healing.[55] Normally, replacement of the calcified layer of articular cartilage by bone occurs by **endochondral ossification.** The calcification front advances to the noncalcified area of cartilage at a slow rate, which is in equilibrium with the rate of absorption of calcified cartilage by endochondral ossification.[57,58] In aging, replacement of the calcified layer of cartilage by bone and subsequent advancement of the tidemark area results in the thinning of the hyaline articular cartilage. In injuries that involve microfractures to the subchondral bone, the secondary ossification center in the bone may be activated to produce new bone growth. A process similar to that which occurs in aging ensues. Bone growth expands into the calcified layer, the tidemark advances, and the noncalcified layer thins.[59]

The design of articular cartilage is a remarkable example of the interaction between form and function. The aggregating PGs attract a large volume of water, creating an osmotic swelling pressure in the cartilage. As the interfibrillar matrix expands, tension is created in the superficial collagen network, creating an opposing force. An equilibrium is reached between the swelling pressure and the load on the joint, and no further deformation takes place. The ability of cartilage to resist compressive force thus depends on two features: (1) a large volume of aggregating PGs and (2) an intact collagen network.

 CONCEPT CORNERSTONE 2-5: *Proteoglycan Type Related to Types of Loading in Tendon, Ligament, and Cartilage*

The types of PGs found in tendon, ligament and cartilage suggest that:

- PGs containing dermatan sulfate are associated with tensile loading.
- PGs containing chondroitin sulfate are associated with compressive loading.
- aggregating PG structures are associated with compressive loading.
- PGs increase with compressive loading.

During joint motion or when the cartilage is compressed, some of the fluid content of the cartilage exudes through pores in the outermost collagen layer.[60–63] The fluid flows back into the cartilage through osmotic pressure after the load is removed. The moving fluid carries nutrients that supply the chondrocytes. The rate of fluid flow is affected by the magnitude and duration of the applied force.[63] When the applied force is sustained over a long period, the equilibrium between swelling pressure and external load reduces fluid flow.[60] Because hyaline cartilage is devoid of blood vessels and nerves in the adult, its nourishment is derived solely from the back and forth flow of fluid; thus, the free flow of fluid is essential for the survival of articular cartilage. Diminished flow also occurs with decreased loading. The absence of compressive forces on the cartilage surface reduces the movement of fluid, which remains immobilized in the ECM. Hyaline articular cartilage can thus undergo degenerative changes after prolonged loading or unloading, presumably as a consequence of interference with the nutrition of the cartilage as fluid flow is diminished.[61] Cartilage formation and health appear to depend on alternating cycles of moderate compressive forces.[64]

Damage to the superficial collagen layer, usually through excessive frictional forces or trauma, removes its ability to resist the swelling pressure of the PGs. Initially, the articular cartilage will swell and become thicker as the PG aggregates attract more water without the opposing force of the now-absent superficial collagen network. Fluid movement in and out of the cartilage is decreased, reducing cell nutrition and synthetic ability. Eventually, without the containment of the superficial collagen meshwork, PGs will begin to escape into the synovial fluid, eroding and thinning the cartilage. This is the sequence that occurs during the development of osteoarthritis.[65]

Case Application 2-4: **Effects of Immobilization on Our Patient's Cartilage and Protection of Cartilage after Immobilization**

While George's ankle and foot are immobilized, the joints encounter decreased loading forces. The cartilage will swell, straining the superficial collagen network, and reducing nutrient diffusion into the cartilage. The early period after immobilization ends is thus a precarious one for articular cartilage, and loading should be resumed gradually. Some loading can be produced during immobilization via isometric muscle contraction (which compresses joint surfaces). A better scenario would involve avoiding immobilization of the joint and reducing weight-bearing. This would allow joint motion and loading of the entire cartilage surface of the joint. A removable brace would be preferable to a cast, but the patient must be fully compliant.

■ Bone

Bone is the hardest of all the connective tissues, because the organic fibrillar ECM is impregnated with inorganic materials, primarily hydroxyapatite. The organic material, primarily type I collagen, gives bone its flexibility, whereas the inorganic material gives bone its compressive strength. The cellular component consists of fibroblasts, fibrocytes, osteoblasts, osteocytes, osteoclasts, and osteoprogenitor cells that can differentiate into osteoblasts. The **fibroblasts** and **fibrocytes** produce type I collagen and other ECM components. The **osteoblasts** are the primary bone-forming cells that are responsible not only for the synthesis of bone but also for its deposition and mineralization. Osteoblasts also secrete **procollagen** (the precursor of type I collagen) into the surrounding matrix. When osteoblasts cease their bone-making activity, they are called **osteocytes. Osteoclasts,** monocyte-derived large polymorphous cells with multiple nuclei, are responsible for bone resorption. Homeostasis between synthesis and deposition is fine-tuned by nutrition, hormonal status, and mechanical loading.[66]

There are numerous terms used to describe the complex architecture of the highly calcified ECM in bones. The innermost layer is called **cancellous** (also **trabecular** or **spongy**) **bone,** and the outer layer is called **compact, or cortical, bone.** In cancellous bone, the calcified tissue forms thin plates called **trabeculae** that are laid down in response to stresses placed on the bone. The trabeculae undergo self-regulated modeling that not only maintains the shaft and other portions of the bone but also maintains an articular surface shape that is capable of distributing the load optimally. The loading history of the trabeculae, including loading from multiple directions, has been suggested to influence the distribution of bone density and trabecular orientation.[67] Increases in bone density in some areas and decreases in density in other areas occur in response to the loads placed on bone. The cancellous bone is covered by a thin layer of dense compact bone called **cortical bone,** which is laid down in concentric layers.

The fibrous layer covering all bones is the **periosteum.** This membrane covers the entire bone except the articular surfaces. The terminal collagen fibers of ligaments and tendons blend into and link with the periosteum and are often embedded in the matrix of cortical bone. The periosteum is well vascularized and contains many capillaries that provide nourishment for the bones. The periosteum contains an osteogenic layer that contains cells that are precursors to osteoblasts and osteoclasts, and it thus acts as a reservoir for cells needed for growth and repair. Damage to the periosteum as a result of trauma or surgery will decrease the healing capacity of the bone.

At the microscopic level, both cortical and cancellous bone may contain two distinct types of bone architecture: **woven bone** and **lamellar bone.** In woven (primary) bone, collagen fibers are irregularly arranged to form a pattern of alternating coarse and fine fibers that resemble woven material. Woven bone is young bone and able to form rapidly without a scaffolding or underlying framework and is often found in newborns and in callous and metaphyseal regions. Lamellar bone requires a framework to form, is organized into parallel layers, and is older bone that constitutes most of the adult skeleton.

Bone remodels throughout life, as it responds to external forces (or loads), such as the pull of tendons and the weight of the body during functional activities. This change in form to match function is known as Wolff's law. Application of external forces (or loads) repetitively or over time causes osteoblast activity to increase, and, as a result, bone mass increases. Without these forces, osteoclast activity predominates and bone mass decreases. Internal influences such as aging, nutritional, metabolic, and disease processes also may affect bone remodeling.

An imbalance between bone synthesis and resorption, in which osteoclasts break down or absorb the bone at a faster rate than the osteoblasts can remodel or rebuild the bone, results in a condition called **osteoporosis.**[68] In osteoporosis, the bones have a decreased mineral density (mass per unit volume) in comparison with normal bone and thus are weaker (more susceptible to fracture) than bones with normal density.

The preceding paragraphs provided a brief overview of the composition of the various connective tissue structures that are associated with the joints. The composition of bones, capsules, cartilage, intervertebral disks, menisci, ligaments, and tendons are summarized in Table 2-6.

 CONCEPT CORNERSTONE 2-6: *Dense Connective Tissue Function*

The function of dense connective tissues is characterized by:

- cell type
- collagen: type, amount, and arrangement
- interfibrillar matrix: PG type, amount, and arrangement

Case Application 2-5: **Status of Fracture Healing, Articular Cartilage, and Bone: Types of Appropriate Exercise and Activity**

The early callus of fracture healing in our patient is primarily fibrocartilage that will later become woven and lamellar bone. Meanwhile, articular cartilage has swelled and softened and will need to be gradually reloaded after cast removal. The unloaded bones will have tipped toward the resorption end of the scale and also will need to be gradually reloaded to resume their original strength.

Safe exercises include active range of motion (ROM) (excellent for cartilage nutrition) and low-level physiological loading such as walking. Joint mobilizations can be used to increase joint ROM (if required) to facilitate normal motion during walking and a larger articular cartilage contact area during movement. Impact-type loading (e.g., running, jumping) and high-load resisted exercise (including isometric exercise) should be avoided early after cast removal. Although the time period for cartilage recovery is unknown, loading should probably be progressed over a period of weeks or months.

General Properties of Connective Tissue

Homogeneous materials, such as steel, display the same mechanical behavior no matter from what direction forces are applied. These are **isotropic** materials. In contrast, heterogeneous connective tissues display very different behavior, depending on the nature and direction of applied forces, and are called **anisotropic.** Connective tissues are described as **heterogeneous** because they are composed of a variety of solid and semisolid components. The function of the structure as a whole depends on a combination of the properties of the different components, the varying proportions of each component in the structure, and the interactions among these components.[14,25,26]

Example 2–1

In the case of a tendon, which is a heterogeneous composite material, the mechanical response by the tendon will vary, depending on whether compressive or tensile forces are applied to the tendon. The tendon can withstand large tensile forces but very little compression or shear.

Connective tissues can change their structure and/or composition (and thus their function) in response to either externally or internally applied forces; that is, they can adapt.[49,69–72] Although this is not a novel concept,[70] the nature and extent of these adaptations is still largely unknown and is an area of active research.[73,74] Connective tissues such as tendon respond to changes in applied compression forces by altering the composition of the ECM (PG content and type). For example, an increase in tensile forces will cause an increase in type I collagen in ligaments and tendons. This adaptive behavior illustrates the dynamic nature of connective tissue and the strong relationships among structure, composition, and function. Muscle response to training is said to exhibit specific adaptation to imposed demand,[71] and a "physical stress theory" has been proposed to guide intervention during rehabilitation.[72]

Mechanical Behavior

The materials used in the construction of human joints are subjected to continually changing forces during activities of daily living, and the ability of these materials to withstand these forces and thus provide support and protection for the joints of the body is extremely important. To understand how different materials and structures are able to provide support (the mechanical behavior of these structures), the reader must be familiar with the concepts and terminology used to describe their behavior for example, **stress, strain, failure,** and **stiffness,** among others. The types of tests that are used to determine the mechanical behavior of human building materials are the same as the types of tests used for nonhuman building materials, although viscoelastic materials may respond differently.

Force and Elongation

The term **load** refers to an external force or forces applied to a structure. Many examples of externally applied loads are given in Chapter 1, including the forces exerted by the weight boot, the leg press footplate, and gravity on Sam Alexander's leg-foot segment. The magnitude, direction, and rate of force application, as well as the size and composition of the tissue, will all affect the tissue's response to load. Connective tissues can be subjected to a variety of forces.

When a force acts on an object, it will produce a **deformation.** A tensile load will produce **elongation.** The **load-deformation curve** is the result of plotting the applied load (external force) against the deformation and provides information regarding the strength properties of a particular material or structure.[12,13,17,48] The load-deformation curve (Fig. 2-10) provides information about the elasticity, plasticity, ultimate strength, and stiffness of the material, as well as the amount of energy that the material can store before failure. The region of the curve between point A and point B is the **elastic region.** In this region, deformation of the material will not be permanent, and the structure will return to its original dimensions immediately after removal of the load. Point B, the **yield point,** signifies the end of the elastic region. After this point, the material will no longer immediately return to its original state when the load is removed, although it may recover in time. The next region on the curve from B to C is the **plastic region.** In this region, deformation of the material will be permanent when the load is removed, although the structure is still intact. Presumably, recovery of original structure after load removal would depend on the synthesis and reorganization of new tissue components. If loading continues into the plastic range, the material will continue to deform until it reaches the **ultimate failure point, C.** The load being applied when this point is reached is the **failure load.**

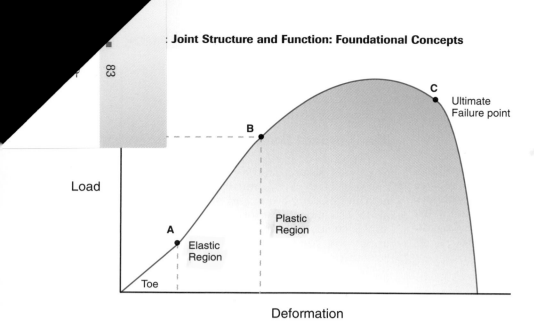

◀ **Figure 2-10** ■ Load-deformation curve for a connective tissue tested in tension. Initially, the crimp straightens with little force (toe region). Then, collagen fibers are stretched as the elastic region begins at A. After the elastic region ends (B), further force application causes a residual change in tissue structure (plastic region). Continuation of load may cause the tissue to rupture at its ultimate failure point (C). (From Butler DL, Grood ES, Noyes FR, et al.: Biomechanics of ligaments and tendons. Exerc Sport Sci Rev 6:144, 1978, with permission from Lippincott William and Wilkins.)

The force values in the load-deformation curve depend on both the size of the structure and its composition[47] (Fig. 2-11). A larger structure (cross-sectional area) will be able to withstand more force, and a longer structure will elongate further when a force is applied. Thus, if two tissues are composed of the same material, a larger tissue will have greater tensile strength, and a longer tissue will have less stiffness. Because the forces and deformations measured during testing are so dependent on the structural features of the tissue, the load-deformation curve is said to reflect the **structural properties** of the structure being tested.[47] Tensile force is measured in newtons (N), compressive force (pressure) is measured in pascals (Pa), and elongation or compression is measured in units of length.

■ **Stress and Strain**

When loads (forces) are applied to a structure or material, an internal resistance to that deformation is produced in the structure or material. The internal reaction to the applied force is called **stress**. Stress is defined as the force per unit of cross-sectional material and can be expressed mathematically in the following formula, where S = stress, F = applied force, and A = area:

$$S = F/A$$

Stress cannot be measured directly but is calculated from the measured forces applied to the material. Stress is expressed in units of pascals (N/m^2).

The relative deformation (change in shape, length, or width) of the structure or material that accompanies the stress is referred to as **strain**.[15] Strain is the amount of deformation that takes place relative to the original length of the material. It cannot be measured directly but is calculated mathematically in the following formula, where L1 = original length and L2 = final length:

$$Strain = L2 - L1/L1$$

Strain is a relative measure expressed as a percentage and thus has no units.

The type of stress and strain that develops in human structures, as we have already discussed, depends on the nature of the material, type of load that is applied, the point of application of the load, direction, magnitude of the load, and the rate and duration of loading.[47] When a structure can no longer support a load (i.e., force drops to zero), the structure is said to have failed. **Ultimate stress** is the stress at the point of failure of the material; **ultimate strain** is the strain at the point of failure.

If two externally applied forces are equal and act along the same line and in opposite directions, they constitute a distractive or **tensile load** and will create **tensile stress** and **tensile strain** in the structure or material (Fig. 2-12A).[26] If two externally applied forces are equal and act in a line toward each other on opposite sides of a structure, they constitute **compressive loading** and **compressive stress** and, as a result, **compressive strain** will develop in the structure (see Fig. 2-12B). If two externally applied forces are equal, parallel, and applied in opposite directions but are not in line with one another, they constitute **shear loading** (see Fig. 2-12C). If two equal, parallel, and opposite forces are applied perpendicular to the long axis of a structure, they constitute **torsional loading**. When combined or **bending forces** are applied to a structure, both tensile and compressive stresses and strains are created. For example, when a longitudinal force is applied to a long bone, tensile stress and strain develop on the convex side and compressive stress and strain develop on the concave side of the long axis of the bone (Fig. 2-13).

Because stress and strain are independent of the size of the structure being tested, the stress-strain curve is said to reflect the **material properties** of the tissue.[47] Only changes in the material constituting the tissue will alter the stress-strain curve. The reason for calculating stresses and strains is to compare these material properties. The stress-strain curve, in which stress is expressed

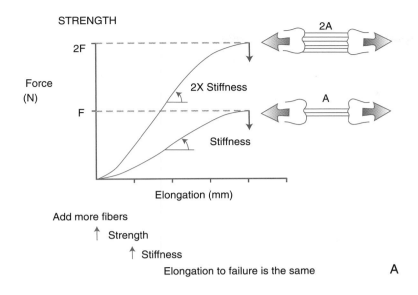

STRENGTH

Add more fibers

↑ Strength

↑ Stiffness

Elongation to failure is the same

A

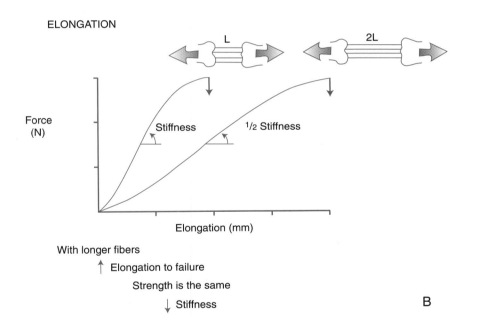

ELONGATION

With longer fibers

↑ Elongation to failure

Strength is the same

↓ Stiffness

B

◄ **Figure 2-11** ■ The size of a tissue (cross-sectional area and length) will affect its overall response to load. **A.** Increasing cross-sectional area means the tissues can withstand more force at any given length (i.e., more stiff). **B.** Increasing tissue length means it can elongate further under the same loading conditions (i.e., less stiff). (From Butler DL, Grood ES, Noyes FR, et al.: Biomechanics of ligaments and tendons. Exerc Sport Sci Rev 6:144, 1978, with permission from Lippincott Williams & Wilkins.)

in load per unit area and strain is expressed in deformation per unit length (or percentage of deformation), can be used to compare the strength properties of one material with another material or to compare the same tissue under different conditions (e.g., ligaments before and after immobilization). The stress-strain curve will contain the same defining features (A, B, and C) no matter what material is being tested, but the shape of the curve and the amount of stress and strain may vary (Fig. 2-14). The curve will be flatter in more elastic materials and steeper in stiffer materials. Weaker materials will resist less stress but will elongate further; thus, the values on the x-axis will be less, and the values on the y-axis more, than those shown in

Figure 2-14. For stronger materials, the reverse would be true.

■ Young's Modulus

Young's modulus or **modulus of elasticity** of a material under compressive or tensile loading is represented by the slope of the linear portion of the curve between point A and point B in Figure 2-14. The modulus of elasticity defines the mechanical behavior of the material and is a measure of the material's stiffness (resistance offered by the material to external loads). A value for **stiffness** can be found by dividing the load by the deformation for any two successive sets of points in the

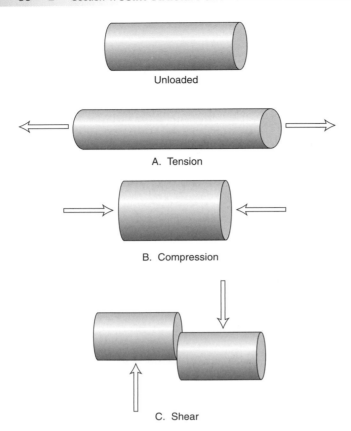

▲ **Figure 2-12** ■ The various types of loads to which connective tissues can be subjected. **A.** Tensile loading. **B.** Compressive loading. **C.** Shear loading.

elastic range of the curve. The inverse of resistance is called **compliance.** If the slope of the curve is steep and the modulus of elasticity is high, the material will exhibit a high degree of stiffness and low compliance. If the

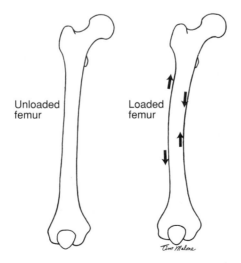

▲ **Figure 2-13** ■ Stress and strain in a long bone. The arrows that point away from each other on the convex side of the bone indicate tensile stress and strain. The arrows that point toward each other on the concave side of the bone indicate compressive stress and strain in the structure.

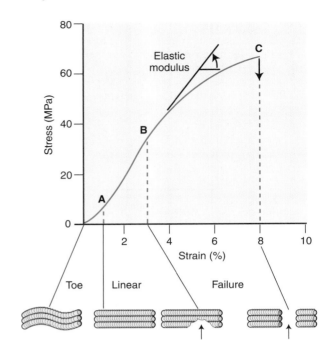

▲ **Figure 2-14** ■ An example of a stress-strain curve for collagenous materials. The results are independent of tissue dimensions and thus reflect the material of which the tissue is made. A-B is the elastic region, and B-C the plastic region. Failure usually occurs at about 8% to 10% strain.

slope of the curve is gradual and the modulus of elasticity is low, the material will exhibit a low degree of stiffness and a large compliance.

Example 2-2

Cortical bone has a high modulus of elasticity, whereas subcutaneous fat has a low modulus of elasticity.

■ **Load Deformation and Stress-Strain Curves**

Each type of material has its own unique curve, but a typical stress-strain curve for tendons and extremity ligaments with a constant rate of loading is presented in Figure 2-14.[47] The first region of the curve from 0 to A is called the **toe region.** Very little force is required to deform the tissue as the wavy crimp pattern is straightened out and PGs and GAGs allow interfibrillar sliding. In this region, a minimal amount of force produces a relatively large amount of deformation (elongation); stress is low, and the strain is typically in the 1% to 2% range. The toe region may be equated to the area in which an evaluator clinically tests the integrity of a ligament by the application of a tensile force or the slack in a tendon that must be taken up by the muscle before the tendon begins to move a bone.

The second region of the curve A to B is the elastic region in which elongation (strain) has a linear relationship with the stress. Each additional unit of applied force creates an equal stress and strain in the tissue. In this region of the curve, the collagen fibrils are being elongated and are resisting the applied force. Thus, the linear region of the stress-strain curve reflects the type of collagen, the fibril size, and the crosslinking among collagen molecules. When the load is removed, the ligament or tendon returns to its prestressed dimensions (although this return is time-dependent). This region includes the stresses and strains that occur during the lower and upper limits of normal physiologic motion and typically extends to about 4% strain.

In the third region, B to C (the plastic range) progressive failure of collagen fibers begins, and the ligament or tendon is no longer capable of returning to its original length. Plasticity may be considered to indicate a form of microfailure. Recovery from this level of loading will require considerable time because it involves, among others, such aspects of healing as synthesis of new tissue and crosslinking of collagen molecules.

As the plastic range is exceeded and force continues to be applied, the remaining collagen fibrils rapidly experience increased stress and fail sequentially, creating overt **failure** or macrofailure of the tissue. In the case of a ligament or tendon, the failure may occur in the middle of the structures through tearing and disruption of the connective tissue fibers; this is called a **rupture.** If the failure occurs through a tearing off of the bony attachment of the ligament or tendon. it is called an **avulsion.** When failure occurs in bony tissue, it is called a **fracture.** Low loading rates tend to create avulsions or fractures, whereas fast loading rates create midsubstance tears.

Each type of connective tissue is able to undergo a different percentage of strain before failure. This percentage varies not only among the types of connective tissue but also within the various types. In general, ligaments and tendons are able to deform more than cartilage. and cartilage is able to deform more than bone. However, the total deformation also will depend on the size (length, width, or depth) of the structure.

Case Application 2-6: **Immobilization Alters Patient's Mechanical Properties**

After immobilization, all George Chen's connective tissues will have altered mechanical properties. Therefore, it may be easier to reinjure the tissues, even under previously normal loading conditions.

Continuing Exploration: **Can You Find the Correct Location on the Stress-Strain Curve?**

Where in the stress-strain curve do you think a ligament may have been loaded to create the following injuries?

■ Grade I sprain: injury to a few fibers of the ligament

■ Grade II sprain: injury to a variable amount of fibers, a partial tear

■ Grade III sprain: complete rupture of the ligament

Viscoelasticity

All connective tissues are viscoelastic materials.[26,47,56, 61,75,76] Their behavior is time and history dependent and is a combination of the properties of elasticity and viscosity. **Elasticity** refers to the material's ability to return to its original state after deformation (change in dimensions, i.e., length or shape) after removal of the deforming load. When a material is stretched, work is done (work = force × distance) and energy increases. An elastic material stores this energy and readily returns it as work so that the stretched elastic material can recoil immediately to its original dimensions after removal of the distractive force. For example, during many functional activities (e.g., walking, running, jumping), a lengthening (**eccentric**) muscle contraction stretches the attached tendon, and this elastic energy is returned during the subsequent shortening (**concentric**) contraction of the muscle-tendon unit.[77-79] The term elasticity implies that length changes or deformations are directly proportional to the applied forces or loads. Elastic materials do not exhibit time-dependent behavior. The elastic qualities in connective tissues primarily depend on collagen and elastin content and organization.

Viscosity refers to a material's resistance to flow. It is a fluid property and depends on the PG and water composition of the tissue. A tissue with high viscosity will exhibit high resistance to deformation, whereas a less viscous fluid will deform more readily. When forces are applied to viscous materials, the tissues exhibit time-dependent and rate-dependent properties. Viscosity diminishes as temperature rises and increases as pressure increases.

Example 2-3

Motor oils with different viscosities are used when more or less resistance to deformation is required. When temperatures are high, the oil's resistance will be lower, and a more viscous type of oil (10-W-30) may be used. During winter, a less viscous oil (5-W-30) will allow the oil to deform more readily and coat the engine surfaces.

Time-Dependent and Rate-Dependent Properties

Viscoelastic materials are capable of undergoing deformation under either a tensile (distractive) or compressive force and of returning to their original state after removal of the force. However, their viscous qualities make the deformation and return time dependent. A viscoelastic material possesses characteristics of creep, stress-relaxation, strain-rate sensitivity, and hysteresis.[76]

■ Creep

If a fixed force is applied to a tissue and maintained, and the deformation produced by this force is measured, the deformation will increase over time. Force remains constant while length changes. For a tendon or ligament, the tissue will gradually elongate under the constant tensile load (creep) and gradually return to its original length when the load is removed (recovery). For cartilage and bone, compressive loading is used, and so the depth of indentation represents creep and recovery (Fig. 2-15A).

■ Stress-Relaxation

If a tissue is stretched to a fixed length while the force required to maintain this length is measured, the force

needed will decrease over time. Length remains constant while force decreases. In a clinical setting, this might apply to a stretch applied to shortened tissue, in which the clinician applies a constant force and the tissue gradually elongates (see Fig. 2-15B).

■ Strain-Rate Sensitivity

Most tissues behave differently if loaded rapidly in comparison with slowly. If connective tissues have a load applied *rapidly,* a larger peak force can be applied to the tissue than if the load was applied *slowly.* The subsequent force relaxation will be larger than if the load

A

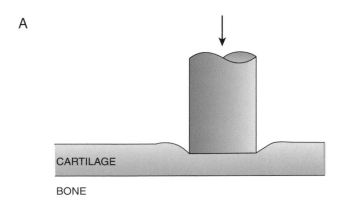

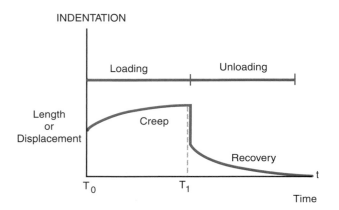

C

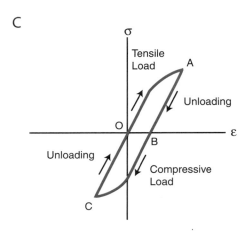

D

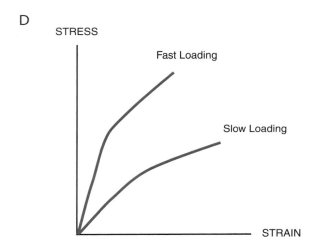

B

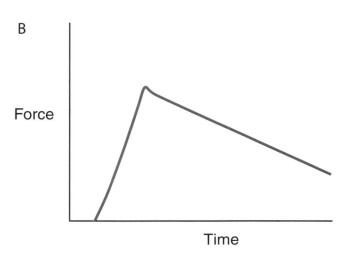

▲ **Figure 2-15** ■ Time- and rate-dependent properties of dense connective tissues. **A.** Creep: when the tissue is loaded to a fixed force level, and length is measured, the latter increases with time (T_0 to T_1) and the tissue recovers its original length in a nonlinear manner (T_1 to T_0). **B.** Force or stress-relaxation: if the tissue is stretched to a fixed length and held there, the force needed to maintain this length will decrease with time. **C.** Hysteresis: as the tissue is loaded and unloaded, some energy is dissipated through tissue elongation and heat release. **D.** If the tissue is loaded rapidly, more energy (force or stress) is required to deform the tissue. (From Oskaya N, Nordin M: Fundamentals of Biomechanics, Equilibrium Motion and Deformation, 2nd ed. New York, Springer-Verlag, 1999, with permission from the publisher as well as the author, Margarita Nordin.)

is applied slowly. Creep will take longer to occur under conditions of rapid loading (see Fig. 2–15D).

■ Hysteresis

When the force and length of the tissues are measured as force is applied (loaded) and removed (unloaded), the resulting load-deformation curves do not follow the same path. The energy gained as a result of the lengthening work (force × distance) is not recovered 100% during the exchange from energy to shortening work. Some energy is lost, usually as heat (see Fig. 2-15C).

Example 2-4

To increase the length of a connective tissue structure, with minimal risk of injury, a load should be applied slowly to a maximum tolerable level and then maintained while creep occurs. As stress-relaxation occurs, the force can be returned to the original level and maintained as further creep occurs. To avoid injury, the total length change should probably be in the range of 2% to 6% strain.

Properties of Specific Tissues

■ Bone

Stress-strain curves for bone demonstrate that cortical bone is stiffer than cancellous (trabecular) bone, meaning that cortical bone can withstand greater stress but less strain than can cancellous bone. Cancellous bone can sustain strains of 75% before failing *in vivo,* but cortical bone will fail if strain exceeds 2%. When cortical bone is loaded in compression, longitudinal sections of the bone show the greatest strength. In tensile testing of the femur, longitudinal sections display twice the modulus of elasticity of transverse sections. The compressive stress and strain that cortical bone can withstand before failure are greater than the tensile stress and strain. Like cortical bone, the compressive strength of trabecular bone is greater than the tensile strength, whereas the modulus of elasticity is higher with tensile loads than with compressive loads. In other words, bone can withstand greater stress, and will undergo less strain, in compression than in tension.[75]

The application of high loads over a short period of time will produce high stresses, whereas lower loads held for a long period of time will produce high strain. The physiologic response of trabecular bone to an increase in loading is hypertrophy. If loading is decreased or absent, the trabeculae become smaller and weaker. The rate, frequency, duration, magnitude, and type of loading affect bone. Repeated loadings, either high repetition coupled with low load or low repetition with high load, can cause permanent strain and lead to bone failure. Bone loses stiffness and strength with repetitive loading as a result of creep strain. **Creep strain** occurs when a tissue is loaded repetitively during the time the material is undergoing creep.

■ Tendons

Tendons exhibit creep when subjected to either constant or uninterrupted cyclic tensile loading. In human subjects, this most likely occurs when a stress is applied to a tendon through muscle contraction, but the overall length of the muscle-tendon unit either is held constant or lengthens (i.e., isometric or eccentric contractions). As the length changes (creep), less tension is required to maintain the overall tissue length.

If the muscle to which the tendon is attached contracts with a force of sufficient magnitude to just straighten out the crimp in the tendon, the tendon will be loaded in the toe region of the stress-strain curve. In this region, there is little increase in stress with elongation and less than 2% strain.[46] A force that stretches the already straightened fibers brings the tendon into the linear region of the curve, in which there is a linear relationship between the applied force and resulting tissue deformation. In this region, the collagen fibrils are loaded directly. As the loading increases higher into the linear region, the first damage is intrafibrillar slippage between molecules, then interfibrillar slippage between fibrils, and finally gross disruption of collagen fibers. The fibers are not perfectly parallel and therefore are not equally straightened as the load is increased. The fibers that become straightened first may be the first to fail, or the smaller, weaker fibrils may rupture. Most normal activities load tendons in the toe region and in the first part of the linear region.

The cross-sectional area, the composition of the tendon, and the length of the tendon determine the amount of force that a tendon can resist and the amount of elongation that it can undergo.[47,51] Under normal conditions, larger tendons should be able to withstand larger forces than smaller tendons, unless they are composed of weaker material; thus, the Achilles tendon can probably be assumed to be stronger than the palmaris longus tendon. Under unusual conditions, this relationship may not be true. For example, a healing tendon may be much larger in diameter than its uninjured opposite, but because it contains less collagen, smaller fibrils, and fewer crosslinks, it may actually be weaker than it smaller counterpart.[51]

The physiologic response of tendons to intermittent tension (application and release of a tensile force) is a moderate increase in thickness and strength.[80] Differences in stress-strain curves among different tendons reflect differences in the proportion of type I and type III collagen, differences in crosslinking, maturity of collagen fibers, organization of fibrils, variations in ground substance concentration, and level of hydration. Because of the change in composition as the tendon inserts into bone, such that stresses are not uniformly distributed, the enthesis is a common site of degenerative changes and injury. The MTJ appears to be stronger, so that although this a common site for muscle strains and pulls, the injury is typically on the muscle side of the normal MTJ.[81] However, because the

MTJ depends on interdigitation of muscle and tendon for its strength, any injury that distorts the form of the MTJ may decrease its tensile strength and predispose it to further injury.

Under normal conditions, the tendon is most vulnerable at either end rather than in the midsubstance. Tendons rarely rupture under normal conditions and are able to withstand large tensile forces without injury.[82] However, if tendons are weakened, they are more likely to be injured. Tendons subject to immobilization show atrophy at the MTJ, with a loss of infolding, and a decrease in collagen concentration and crosslinking.[81–83] Exposure to corticosteroids, nutritional deficiencies, hormonal imbalance, dialysis, chronic loading into the high linear region of the stress-strain curve with inadequate time for recovery, and sudden large loads may predispose the tendon to injury at previously physiological levels of loading. In other words, the same load now produces more deformation in the tendon.

Tendons adapt readily to changes in the magnitude and direction of loading. Tendons subject to continual compressive forces will alter their composition to resemble cartilage, and their tensile strength may decline.[84] Conversely, tendons subjected to tensile loads, especially physiological loads over long periods of time, will increase in size, collagen concentration, and collagen crosslinking.[85–87] Progressive loading programs are successfully used to treat tendon dysfunction, presumably through inducing changes in tendon composition.[50,70]

■ Ligaments

Because tendons are so difficult to test mechanically (it is hard to get a solid grip on the ends), most of our knowledge of connective tissue response to tensile loading comes from ligament testing. Tendons and ligament are very similar mechanically, although the more variable orientation of collagen fibrils in ligament makes them slightly less resistant to tensile stress but more able to function within a range of load directions without being damaged.[17,87–89] This is another example of form (in this case, collagen fibril orientation) following function.

The physiologic response of ligaments to intermittent tension (application and release of a tensile force) is an increase in thickness and strength. Immobilized ligaments become weaker rapidly and can take over 12 months to recover their mechanical properties.[12,13] Ligaments are more variable than tendons in that they are designed to withstand both compressive and shear forces, as well as tensile forces.

■ Cartilage

Three forces interact in cartilage act to resist applied load: (1) stress developed in the fibrillar portion of ECM (type II collagen), (2) swelling pressures developed in the fluid phase (PGs and water), and (3) frictional drag resulting from fluid flow through the ECM.[28] Compression of cartilage reduces the volume of the cartilage and increases the pressure, causing outward flow of interstitial fluid. Fluid flow through the ECM creates frictional resistance to the flow within the tissues (frictional drag). Exudation of fluid occurs rapidly at first, causing a concomitant rapid rate of deformation. Subsequently, fluid flow and deformation gradually diminish and cease when compressive stress in cartilage balances the applied load.[55,59,60] Magnetic resonance imaging (MRI) has made it possible to study changes in cartilage volume and thickness in joints in living subjects. In an MRI study of the knee joints of eight volunteers, Eckstein et al.[90] found that up to 13% of the fluid was displaced from the patellar cartilage 3 to 7 minutes after exercise (50 knee bends).

Tensile stresses called **hoop stresses** are created in the superficial collagen network of cartilage as the compressed PGs and water push against the collagen fibers.[56] Although the tensile behavior of cartilage is similar to that of ligaments and tendons in that all of these tissues exhibit nonlinear tensile behavior, the cause of that behavior is slightly different in cartilage. The nonlinear tensile load-deformation behavior of cartilage in the toe region of the curve is thought to be caused by the drag force between the collagen meshwork and the PGs. In ligaments and tendons, the nonlinear behavior in the toe region is attributed to the straightening of collagen fibers. In cartilage, as in ligaments and tendons, collagen fibers become taut in the linear region of the curve and demonstrate linear behavior. However, cartilage specimens taken from the different zones of cartilage (1, 2, and 3) have shown differences in tensile behavior. These differences have been attributed to differences in orientation of the collagen fibers among the zones and can be considered to represent anisotropic effects.[56] Cartilage resistance to shear depends on the amount of collagen that is present because PGs provide little resistance to shear. Shear stresses are apt to develop at the interface between the calcified cartilage layer and the subchondral bone.

 CONCEPT CORNERSTONE 2-7: *Resistance of Tissues to Compression and Tension*

Resistance of connective tissues to compression and tension depends on an intact collagen network that can resist tensile stress. In tendons and ligaments, the tensile stress is directly caused by the applied load. In cartilage, the tensile stress is created by the fluid pressure of the water and PGs in the interfibrillar part of the ECM pushing against the collagen meshwork. Bone depends on both organic and inorganic components to resist tension and compression.

The properties of the connective tissue structures described in the preceding section are designed to provide the reader with an introduction to the nature of the joint components and should help the reader to understand basic joint structure and function. The following two sections, Complexity of Human Joint Design and Joint Function, include the traditional classification system for human joints, as well as a detailed description of synovial joint structure and function.

Complexity of Human Joint Design

An appreciation of the complexities that are involved in human joint design may be gained by considering the nature of the bony components and the functions that the joints must serve. The human skeleton has about 200 bones that must be connected by joints. These bones vary in size from the pea-sized distal phalanx of the little toe to the long femur of the thigh. The shape of the bones varies from round to flat, and the contours of the ends of the bones vary from convex to concave. The task of designing a series of joints to connect these varied bony components to form stable structures would be difficult. The task of designing joints that are capable of working together to provide both mobility and stability for the total structure represents an engineering problem of considerable magnitude.

Joint designs in the human body vary from simple to complex. Simple human joints usually have stability as a primary function; the more complex joints usually have mobility as a primary function. However, most joints in the human body have to serve a dual mobility-stability function and must also provide dynamic stability. The human stability joints are similar in design to the table joints in that the ends of the bones may be contoured either to fit into each other or to lie flat against each other. Bracing of human joints is accomplished through the use of joint capsules, ligaments, and tendons. Joints designed primarily for human mobility are called **synovial joints.** These joints are constructed so that the ends of the bony components are covered by hyaline cartilage and enclosed in a **synovial sheath** (joint capsule). The capsules, ligaments, and tendons located around mobility (synovial) joints not only help to provide stability for the joint but also guide, limit, and permit motion. Wedges of cartilage, called **menisci, disks, plates,** and **labra** in synovial joints serve to increase stability, to provide shock absorption, and to facilitate motion. In addition, a lubricating fluid, called **synovial fluid,** is secreted at all mobility (synovial) joints to help reduce friction between the articulating surfaces.

In the traditional method of joint classification, the joints (**arthroses** or **articulations**) of the human body are divided into two broad categories on the basis of the type of materials and the methods used to unite the bony components. Subdivisions of joint categories are based on materials used, the shape and contours of the articulating surfaces, and the type of motion allowed. The two broad categories of arthroses are **synarthroses** (nonsynovial joints) and **diarthroses** (synovial joints).[2,25]

Synarthroses

The material used to connect the bony components in synarthrodial joints is interosseus connective tissue (fibrous and/or cartilaginous). Synarthroses are grouped into two divisions according to the type of connective tissue used in the union of bone to bone: **fibrous joints** and **cartilaginous joints.** The connective tissue directly unites one bone to another creating a bone-solid connective tissue-bone interface.

■ Fibrous Joints

In fibrous joints, the fibrous tissue directly unites bone to bone. Three different types of fibrous joints are found in the human body: **sutures, gomphoses,** and **syndesmoses.** A suture joint is one in which two bony components are united by a collagenous sutural ligament or membrane. The ends of the bony components are shaped so that the edges interlock or overlap one another. This type of joint is found only in the skull and, early in life, allows a small amount of movement. Fusion of the two opposing bones in suture joints occurs later in life and leads to the formation of a bony union called a **synostosis.**

Example 2-5

Coronal Suture

The serrated edges of the parietal and frontal bones of the skull are connected by a thin fibrous membrane (the sutural ligament) to form the coronal suture (Fig. 2-16). At birth, the fibrous membrane allows some motion for ease of passage through the birth canal. Also, during infancy, slight motion is possible for growth of the brain and skull. In adulthood, the bones grow together to form a synostosis and little or no motion is possible.

A **gomphosis joint** is a joint in which the surfaces of bony components are adapted to each other like a peg in a hole. In this type of joint, the component parts are connected by fibrous tissue. The only gomphosis joint

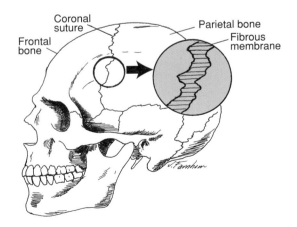

▲ **Figure 2-16** ■ The coronal suture. The frontal and parietal bones of the skull are joined directly by fibrous tissue to form a synarthrodial suture joint.

that exists in the human body is the joint that is found between a tooth and either the mandible or maxilla.

Example 2-6

The conical process of a tooth is inserted into the bony socket of the mandible or maxilla. In the adult, the loss of teeth is, for the most part, caused by disease processes affecting the connective tissue that cements or holds the teeth in approximation to the bone. Under normal conditions in the adult, these joints do not permit motion between the components.

A **syndesmosis** is a type of fibrous joint in which two bony components are joined directly by an interosseous ligament, a fibrous cord, or an aponeurotic membrane. These joints usually allow a small amount of motion.

Example 2-7

The shaft of the tibia is joined directly to the shaft of the fibula by an interosseous membrane (Fig. 2-17). A

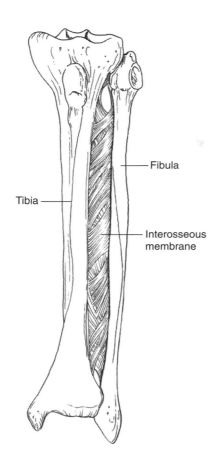

Tibia

Fibula

Interosseous membrane

▲ **Figure 2-17** ■ The shafts of the fibula and tibia are joined directly by a membrane to form a synarthrodial syndesmosis.

slight amount of motion at this joint accompanies movement at the ankle joint.

Case Application 2-7: **Disruption of the Interosseous Membrane**

In our patient's trimalleolar fracture, the interosseous membrane was disrupted, allowing some separation of the tibia and fibula. Restoration of normal talocrural anatomy is crucial after such injuries, and the surgeon must be careful to leave enough space to accommodate the talus in full dorsiflexion. The "give" of the joint may be lost, however.

■ Cartilaginous Joints

The materials used to connect the bony components in cartilaginous joints are **fibrocartilage** and/or **hyaline cartilage.** These materials are used to directly unite one bony surface to another, creating a bone-cartilage-bone interface. The two types of cartilaginous joints are **symphyses** and **synchondroses.**

In a **symphysis joint** (**secondary cartilaginous joint**), the two bony components are covered with a thin lamina of hyaline cartilage and directly joined by fibrocartilage in the form of disks or pads. Examples of symphysis joints include the intervertebral joints between the bodies of the vertebrae, the joint between the manubrium and the sternal body, and the symphysis pubis in the pelvis.

Example 2-8

The Symphysis Pubis

The two pubic bones of the pelvis are joined by fibrocartilage. This joint must serve as a weight-bearing joint and is responsible for withstanding and transmitting forces; therefore, under normal conditions, very little motion is permissible or desirable. During pregnancy, when the connective tissues are softened, some slight separation of the joint surfaces occurs to ease the passage of the baby through the birth canal. However, the symphysis pubis is considered to be primarily a stability joint with the thick fibrocartilage disk forming a stable union between the two bony components (Fig. 2-18A).

Synchondrosis (**primary cartilaginous joint**) is a type of joint in which the material used for connecting the two components is hyaline cartilage. The cartilage forms a bond between two ossifying centers of bone. The function of this type of joint is to permit bone growth while also providing stability and allowing a small amount of mobility. Some of these joints are found in the skull and in other areas of the body at sites of bone growth. When bone growth is complete, some of these joints ossify and convert to bony unions (synostoses).

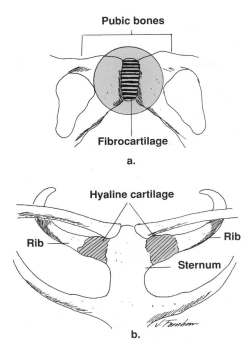

Pubic bones

Fibrocartilage

a.

Hyaline cartilage

Rib

Rib

Sternum

b.

▲ **Figure 2-18** ■ Cartilaginous joints. **A.** The two pubic bones of the pelvis are joined directly by fibrocartilage to form a symphysis joint called the **symphysis pubis. B.** The first rib and the sternum are connected directly by hyaline cartilage to form a synchondrosis joint called the **first chondrosternal joint.**

Example 2-9

The First Chondrosternal Joint

The adjacent surfaces of the first rib and sternum are connected directly by articular cartilage (see Fig. 2-18B).

Diarthroses

The joint construction in diarthrodial or synovial joints differs from that found in synarthrodial joints. In synovial joints, the ends of the bony components are free to move in relation to one another because no connective tissue directly connects adjacent bony surfaces. The bony components are *indirectly connected to one another by means of a joint capsule that encloses the joint.* All synovial joints are constructed in a similar manner and have the following features: (1) a joint capsule that is composed of two layers[4]; (2) a joint cavity that is enclosed by the joint capsule; (3) synovial tissue that lines the inner surface of the capsule; (4) synovial fluid that forms a film over the joint surfaces; and (5) hyaline cartilage that covers the surfaces of the enclosed contiguous bones[9] (Fig. 2-19). Synovial joints may be associated with accessory structures such as fibrocartilaginous disks, plates or menisci, labra, fat pads, and ligaments and tendons. Articular disks, menisci, and the synovial fluid help to prevent excessive compression of opposing joint surfaces. Articular disks and menisci often occur between articular surfaces, where congruity is low. Articular disks may extend all the way across a joint and actually divide it into two separate cavities, such as the articular disk at the distal radioulnar joint. Menisci usually do not divide a joint but provide lubrication and increase congruity. Ligaments and tendons associated with synovial joints play an important role in keeping joint surfaces together and guiding motion. Excessive separation of joint surfaces is limited by passive tension in ligaments, the fibrous joint capsule, and tendons (passive stability).[5] Active tension in muscles (dynamic stability) also limits the separation of joint surfaces.

Case Application 2-8: **Joints Affected by Our Patient's Injury**

Which joints are affected in the case of George Chen? Talocrural, subtalar, midtarsal (talonavicular and calcaneocuboid), and first metatarsophalangeal (MTP) joint.

■ Joint Capsule

Joint capsules vary considerably both in thickness and in composition. Capsules such as the one enclosing the shoulder joint are thin, loose, and redundant and therefore sacrifice stability for mobility. Other capsules such as the hip joint capsule are thick and dense and thus favor stability over mobility. The fact that the thickness, fiber orientation, and even composition of the capsule depend to a large extent on the stresses that are placed on the joint illustrates the dynamic nature of the joint capsule. For example, in portions of the capsule that are subjected to compression forces, the capsule may become fibrocartilagenous.[3,4] Shoulder capsules in patients with shoulder instability in which the capsules are subjected to repeated tensile deformation have significantly larger mean collagen fibril diameters and increased density of elastin fibers in comparison with normal capsules. These changes in collagen fibrils and elastin density are interpreted as capsular adaptations oriented toward increasing capsular strength and resistance to stretching deformation.[5]

The fibrous capsule may be reinforced by and, in some instances, actually incorporate ligaments or tendons as a part of the capsule. For example, the capsule of the proximal interphalangeal joint of the fingers is reinforced by collateral ligaments superficially and a central slip of the extensor tendon superficially and posteriorly.[6]

The joint capsule is composed of two layers: an outer layer called the **stratum fibrosum** and an inner layer called the **stratum synovium** (see Fig. 2-19). The stratum fibrosum, which is sometimes referred to as the fibrous capsule, is composed of dense fibrous tissue. Collagen and elastin account for about 90% of the dry weight and water for about 70% of the wet weight.[4,6] The predominant type of collagen is type I, which is usually arranged in parallel bundles. As the capsule nears its insertion to bone, the tissue changes to

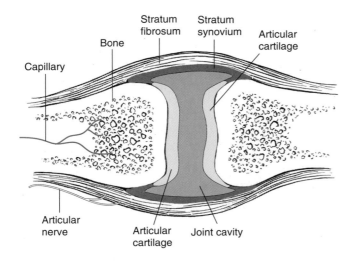

Capillary

Bone

Stratum
fibrosum

Stratum
synovium

Articular
cartilage

Articular
nerve

Articular
cartilage

Joint cavity

▲ **Figure 2-19** ■ A typical diarthrodial joint.

fibrocartilage and then mineralized fibrocartilage and bone. The stratum fibrosum is poorly vascularized but richly innervated by joint receptors. The receptors are located in and around the capsule.[8]

The inner layer (stratum synovium) is the lining tissue of the capsule. It also consists of two layers: the **intima** and the **subsynovial tissue.** The intima is the layer of cells that lines the joint space. It is composed of a layer of specialized fibroblasts known as synoviocytes that are arranged one to three cells deep and set in a fiber-free intercellular matrix.[7] Two types of **synoviocytes** are generally recognized: type A and type B.[2] Type A synoviocytes are macrophage-like cells with prominent Golgi apparatus but sparse granular endoplasmic reticulum. Type A cells are primarily responsible for the removal of debris from the joint cavity. During phagocytosis, type A cells synthesize and release lytic enzymes that have the potential for damaging joint tissues.

Type B synoviocytes have abundant granular endoplasmic reticulum and are twice as numerous as type A cells in normal synovium.[9] Type B cells synthesize and release enzyme inhibitors that inhibit the lytic enzymes and are responsible for initiating an immune response through the secretion of antigens. As part of their function in joint maintenance, both types of cells synthesize

the hyaluronic acid component of the synovial fluid, as well as constituents of the matrix in which the cells are embedded. Type A and B cells also secrete a wide range of cytokines, including multiple growth factors. The interplay of the cytokines acting as stimulators or inhibitors of synoviocytes results in structural repair of synovium, response to foreign or autologous antigens, and tissue destruction.[9]

The subsynovial tissue lies outside the intima as a loose network of highly vascularized fibrous connective tissue. It attaches to the margins of the articular cartilage through a transitional zone of fibrocartilage and joins with the periosteum covering the bones that lie within the confines of the capsule. Its cells are slightly different from the intima cells in that they are more spindle-shaped and more widely dispersed between collagen fibrils than are the intimal cells. Also, they produce matrix collagen.[10] The subsynovial tissue provides support for the intima and merges with the fibrous capsule on its external surface. The intima is richly endowed with capillary vessels, lymphatic vessels, and nerve fibers. The blood vessels in the subsynovial tissue transport oxygen, nutrients, and immunologic cells to the joint.

Branches of adjacent peripheral nerves and branches of nerves from muscles near the joint penetrate the fibrous joint capsule. Large-diameter sensory efferent nerves and thinly myelinated nerves are present in the fibrous capsule; nonmyelinated C-type fibers are found in the synovium. The joint receptors found in the fibrous joint capsule are sensitive to stretching or compression of the capsule, as well as to an increase in internal pressure as a result of increased production of synovial fluid.

For example, most of the joint receptors in the knee are located in the subsynovial layer of the capsule close to the insertions of the ACL. Mechanoreceptors (predominantly Ruffini receptors) in the subsynovial capsule and ACL respond primarily to the stretch involved in terminal knee extension. Pacini receptors are reported less frequently and are thought to be activated by compression. Free nerve endings are more numerous than mechanoreceptors and function as nociceptors that react to inflammation and pain stimuli. Afferent free nerve endings in joints not only transfer information but also serve a local effector role by releasing neuropeptides.[8,11] Table 2-7 summarizes the receptors found in the joint capsule.

Table 2-7	Joint Receptors		
Type	Name	Sensitivity	Location
I	Ruffini	Stretch—usually at extremes of extension	Fibrous layer of joint capsules on flexion side of joints, periosteum, ligaments, and tendons[10]
II	Pacini or pacini-form	Compression or changes in hydrostatic pressure and joint movement[1]	Located throughout joint capsule, particularly in deeper layers and in fat pads
III	Golgi, Golgi-Mazzoni	Pressure and forceful joint motion into extremes of motion	Inner layer (synovium) of joint capsules, ligaments, and tendons[10]
IV	Unmyelinated free nerve endings	Non-noxious and noxious mechanical stress or biomechanical stress	Located around blood vessels in synovial layer of capsule and in adjacent fat pads and collateral ligaments, tendons, and the periosteum

■ Synovial Fluid

The thin film of synovial fluid that covers the surfaces of the inner layer of the joint capsule and articular cartilage helps to keep the joint surfaces lubricated and reduces friction between the bony components. The fluid also provides nourishment for the hyaline cartilage covering the articular surfaces, as fluid moves in and out of the cartilage. The composition of synovial fluid is similar to blood plasma except that synovial fluid contains hyaluronate (hyaluronic acid) and a glycoprotein called **lubricin.**[22] The hyaluronate component of synovial fluid is responsible for the viscosity of the fluid and is essential for lubrication of the synovium. Hyaluronate reduces the friction between the synovial folds of the capsule and the articular surfaces.[22] Lubricin is the component of synovial fluid that is thought to be responsible for cartilage-on-cartilage lubrication.[7] Changes in the concentration of hyaluronate or lubricin in the synovial fluid will affect the overall lubrication and the amount of friction that is present. Many experiments have confirmed that articular coefficients of friction (COFs) in synovial joints are lower than those that can be produced with manufactured lubricants.[22] The lower the COF is, the lower the resistance to sliding is. Hyaluronate is sometimes used to alleviate symptoms of osteoarthritis and is injected into the joint cavity.

Normal synovial fluid appears as a clear, pale yellow viscous fluid that is present in small amounts at all synovial joints.[23] There is a direct exchange between the vasculature of the stratum synovium and the intracapsular space, where nutrients can be supplied and waste products can be taken away from the joint by diffusion.[22] Usually, less than 0.5 mL of synovial fluid can be removed from large joints such as the knee.[2] However, when a joint is injured or diseased, the volume of the fluid may increase.[22] The synovial fluid exhibits properties common to all viscous substances in that it has the ability to resist loads that produce shear.[23] The viscosity of the fluid *varies inversely* with the joint velocity or rate of shear. Thus, the synovial fluid is referred to as **thixotropic.** When the bony components of a joint are moving rapidly, the viscosity of the fluid decreases and provides less resistance to motion.[8] When the bony components of a joint are moving slowly, the viscosity increases and provides more resistance to motion. Viscosity also is sensitive to changes in temperature. High temperatures decrease the viscosity, whereas low temperatures increase the viscosity.[2]

■ Joint Lubrication

The minimal wear of normal cartilage despite the varied loads that synovial joints experience depends on the structure of the cartilage matrix and the presence of lubricating fluid. A number of models have been proposed to explain how diarthrodial joints are lubricated under varying loading conditions. The general consensus is that no single model is adequate to explain human joint lubrication and that human joints are lubricated by two or more of the following types of

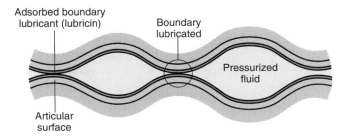

▲ **Figure 2-20** ■ Joint lubrication models. Lubricin molecules coat the joint surfaces in boundary lubrication. The fluid film keeps joint surfaces apart in hydrostatic lubrication.

lubrication used in engineering. The two basic types of lubrication thought to account for joint lubrication are boundary lubrication and fluid-film lubrication.[24]

Boundary lubrication occurs when each load-bearing surface is coated with a thin layer of large molecules that form a gel that keeps the opposing surfaces from touching each other[91] (Fig. 2-20). The layers slide on each other more readily than they are sheared off the underlying surface. In human diarthrodial joints, these molecules are composed of the lubricin molecules that adhere to the articular surfaces.[24] This type of lubrication is considered to be most effective at low loads.[8]

Fluid-film lubrication involves a thin fluid-film that provides separation of the joint surfaces. Surfaces lubricated by a fluid-film typically have a lower COF than do boundary-lubricated surfaces, and because the COF is very low in synovial joints, this suggests that some sort of fluid-film lubrication exists. Several models of fluid-film lubrication exist, including hydrostatic (weeping) lubrication; hydrodynamic, squeeze-film lubrication; and elastohydrodynamic (a combination of hydrodynamic and squeeze-film) and boosted lubrication.

Hydrostatic or **weeping lubrication** is a form of fluid lubrication in which the load-bearing surfaces are held apart by a film of lubricant that is maintained under pressure (see Fig. 2-20). In engineering, the pressure is usually supplied by an external pump. In the human body, the pump action can be supplied by contractions of muscles around the joint or by compression from weight-bearing. Compression of articular cartilage causes the cartilage to deform and to "weep" fluid, which forms a fluid film over the articular surfaces. This is possible because the impervious layer of calcified cartilage keeps the fluid from being forced into the subchondral bone.[19] When the load is removed, the fluid flows back into the articular cartilage. This type of lubrication is most effective under conditions of high loading, but it can be effective under most conditions.[6]

Hydrodynamic lubrication is a form of fluid lubrication in which a wedge of fluid is created when nonparallel opposing surfaces slide on one another. The resulting lifting pressure generated in the wedge of fluid and by the fluid's viscosity keeps the joint surfaces apart. In **squeeze-film lubrication,** pressure is created in the fluid film by the movement of articular surfaces that are perpendicular to one another.[24] As the opposing articular surfaces move closer together, they squeeze the fluid film out of the area of impending contact. The resulting pressure that is created by the fluid's viscosity keeps the surfaces separated. This type of lubrication is suitable for high loads maintained for a short duration.

In the **elastohydrodynamic model,** the protective fluid film is maintained at an appropriate thickness by the elastic deformation of the articular surfaces. In other words, the elastic cartilage deforms slightly to maintain an adequate layer of fluid between the opposing joint surfaces. The **boosted lubrication model** suggests that pools of concentrated hyaluronate molecules are filtered out of the synovial fluid and are trapped in the natural undulations and areas of elastic deformation on the articular surface just as the opposing surfaces meet.[24]

The joint lubrication models presented provide a number of possible options for explaining how diarthrodial joints are lubricated. The variety of conditions under which human joints function make it likely that more than one of the lubrication models are operating. Until a unified model of joint lubrication is proposed, proved, and accepted, the exact mechanisms involved in human joint lubrication will be subject to speculation.[91]

 CONCEPT CORNERSTONE 2-8: *Essentials of Joint Lubrication*

Lubrication depends on

- light irregularities in the joint surface that "trap" hyaluronate.
- lubricin molecules to create a fluid film over the cartilage surfaces.
- elastic deformation of the cartilage to maintain a layer of fluid between opposing cartilage surfaces.
- fluid being squeezed out of cartilage into the joint space as loading increases.

■ **Subclassifications**

Traditionally, synovial joints have been divided into three main categories on the basis of the number of axes about which "gross visible" motion occurs.[25–27] A further subdivision of the joints is made on the basis of the shape and configuration of the ends of the bony components. The three main traditional categories are uniaxial, biaxial, and triaxial. A **uniaxial joint** is constructed so that visible motion of the bony components is allowed in one plane around a single axis. The axis of motion usually is located near or in the center of the joint or in one of the bony components. Because uniaxial joints permit visible motion in only one plane or around only one axis, they are described as having one degree of freedom of motion. The two types of **uniaxial diarthrodial joints** found in the human body are hinge joints and pivot (trochoid) joints. A **hinge joint** is a type of joint that resembles a door hinge.

Interphalangeal Joints of the Fingers

These hinge joints are formed between the distal end of one phalanx and proximal end of another phalanx (Fig. 2-21A). The joint surfaces are contoured so that motion can occur only in the sagittal plane (flexion and extension) around a coronal axis (see Fig. 2-21B).

A **pivot (trochoid) joint** is a type of joint constructed so that one component is shaped like a ring and the other component is shaped so that it can rotate within the ring.

The Median Atlantoaxial Joint

The ring portion of the joint is formed by the atlas and the transverse ligament (Fig. 2-22). The odontoid process (dens) of the axis, which is enclosed in the ring, rotates within the osteoligamentous ring. Motion occurs in the transverse plane around a longitudinal axis.

Biaxial diarthrodial joints are joints in which the bony components are free to move in two planes around two axes. Therefore, these joints have two degrees of freedom. There are two types of biaxial joints in the body: **condyloid** and **saddle.** The joint surfaces in a

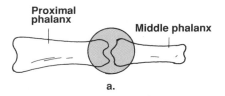

a.

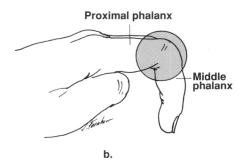

b.

▲ **Figure 2-21** ■ A uniaxial hinge joint. **A.** The interphalangeal joints of the fingers are examples of simple hinge joints. The joint capsule and accessory joint structures have been removed to show the bony components in the superior view of the joint. **B.** Motion occurs in one plane around one axis.

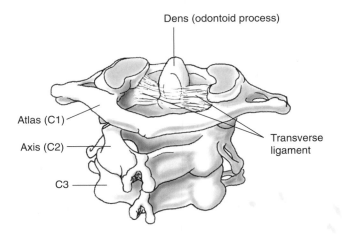

▲ **Figure 2-22** ■ A pivot joint. The joint between the atlas, transverse ligament, and the dens of the axis is a uniaxial diarthrodial pivot joint called the **median atlantoaxial** joint. Rotation occurs in the transverse plane around a vertical axis.

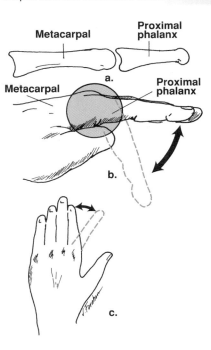

▲ **Figure 2-23** ■ A condyloid joint. **A.** The metacarpophalangeal joints of the fingers are biaxial condyloid joints. The joint capsule and accessory structures have been removed to show the bony components. Motion at these joints occurs in two planes around two axes. **B.** Flexion and extension occur in the sagittal plane around a coronal axis. **C.** Abduction and adduction occur in the frontal plane around an A-P axis.

condyloid joint are shaped so that the concave surface of one bony component is allowed to slide over the convex surface of another component in two directions.

Example 2-12

Metacarpophalangeal Joint

The metacarpophalangeal joint is formed by the convex distal end of a metacarpal bone and the concave proximal end of the proximal phalanx (Fig. 2-23A). Flexion and extension at this joint occur in the sagittal plane around a coronal axis (see Fig. 2-23B). Abduction is movement away from the middle finger, whereas adduction is movement toward the middle finger. Adduction and abduction occur in the frontal plane around an anteroposterior (A-P) axis (see Fig. 2-23C).

A **saddle joint** is a joint in which each joint surface is both convex in one plane and concave in the other, and these surfaces fit together like a rider on a saddle.

Example 2-13

Carpometacarpal Joint of the Thumb

The carpometacarpal joint of the thumb is formed by the distal end of the carpal bone and the proximal end of the metacarpal. The motions available are flexion/extension and abduction/adduction.

Triaxial or **multiaxial diarthrodial joints** are joints in which the bony components are free to move in three planes around three axes. These joints have three degrees of freedom. Motion at these joints also may

occur in oblique planes. The two types of joints in this category are **plane joints** and **ball-and-socket joints**. **Plane** joints have a variety of surface configurations and permit gliding between two or more bones.

Example 2-14

Carpal Joints

These joints are found between the adjacent surfaces of the carpal bones. The adjacent surfaces may glide on one another or rotate with regard to one another in any plane.

Ball-and-socket joints are formed by a ball-like convex surface being fitted into a concave socket. The motions permitted are flexion/extension, abduction/adduction, rotation, and combinations of these movements.

Example 2-15

Hip Joint

The hip joint is formed by the head of the femur and a socket called the acetabulum (Fig. 2-24A). The motions

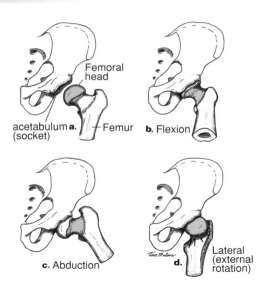

▲ **Figure 2-24** ■ A ball-and-socket joint. **A.** The joint between the femoral head and the acetabulum is a triaxial diarthrodial joint called the **hip joint.** Motion may occur in three planes around three axes. **B.** Flexion/extension occurs in the sagittal plane around a coronal axis. **C.** Abduction/adduction occurs in the frontal plane around an A-P axis. **D.** Rotation occurs in the transverse plane around a longitudinal axis.

of the flexion/extension occur in the sagittal plane around a coronal axis (see Fig. 2-24B). Abduction/adduction occurs in the frontal plane around an A-P axis (see Fig. 2-24C), whereas rotation of the femur occurs in the transverse plane around a longitudinal axis (see Fig. 2-24D).

Case Application 2-9: **Classification of Affected Joints**

Consider the classification of the joints affected after George Chen's fracture:

- uniaxial: talocrural
- biaxial: first MTP, calcaneocuboid (sellar), talonavicular, subtalar

---

◆ Joint Function

The structure of the joints of the human body reflects the functions that the joints are designed to serve. The synarthrodial joints are relatively simple in design and function primarily as stability joints, although some motion does occur. The diarthrodial joints are complex and are designed primarily for mobility, although all of these joints must also provide some variable measure of stability. Effective human functioning depends on the integrated action of many joints, some providing stability and some providing mobility. In general, the ability to stabilize one or more body segments is essential if

predictable joint motion and normal function are to be maintained.

Kinematic Chains

Kinematic chains, in the engineering sense, are composed of a series of rigid links that are interconnected by a series of pin-centered joints. The system of joints and links is constructed so that motion of one link at one joint will produce motion at all of the other joints in the system in a predictable manner. The kinematic chain can be open or closed. In an **open kinematic chain,** one joint can move independently of others in the chain. When one end of the chain remains fixed, it creates a closed system or **closed kinematic chain.** Under these conditions, movement at one joint automatically creates movement in other joints in the chain.

These engineering terms have been applied to human movements primarily to describe movements that take place under weight-bearing and NWB conditions, when the distal segment of a limb is not free to move in space. Because the joints of the human body are linked together, motion at one of the joints in the series is, under weight-bearing conditions, accompanied by motion at one or more other joints. For instance, when a person in the erect standing position bends both knees, simultaneous motion must occur at the ankle and hip joints if the person is to remain upright (Fig. 2-25A). The motions of hip flexion and ankle dorsiflexion predictably accompany knee flexion. Under open-chain conditions, the foot is not fixed, and knee flexion can occur independently (see Fig. 2-25B). In the human system of joints and links, the joints of the lower limbs and the pelvis function as a closed kinematic chain when a person is in the erect weight-bearing position, because the feet are fixed on the ground. Most functional activities involving the lower extremities involve closed-chain motion.

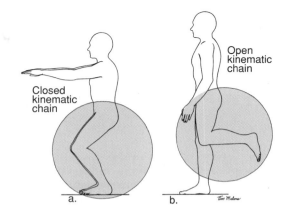

▲ **Figure 2-25** ■ Closed and open kinematic chains. **A.** In a closed kinematic chain, knee flexion is accompanied by hip flexion and ankle dorsiflexion. **B.** Knee motion in an open kinematic chain may occur with or without motion at the hip and ankle. In the diagram, knee flexion is shown without simultaneous motion at the hip and the ankle.

The ends of human limbs, especially the upper extremities, frequently are not fixed but are free to move. In these open kinematic chain motions, joint motion is much more varied. The motion of waving the hand may occur at the wrist without causing motion of the more distal finger joints distally or the more proximal elbow or shoulder. The same motion may also occur through medial and lateral rotation at the shoulder. In an open kinematic chain, motion does not occur in a predictable manner because joints may function either independently or in unison.

Example 2-16

A person may wave the whole upper limb by moving the arm at the glenohumeral joint at the shoulder or may move only at the wrist. In the first instance, all of the degrees of freedom of all of the joints from the shoulder to the wrist are available to the distal segment (hand). If the person is waving from the wrist, only the degrees of freedom at the wrist would be available to the hand, and motion of the hand in space would be more limited than in the first situation.

The concept of kinematic chains, which is useful for analyzing human motion, therapeutic exercise, and the effects of injury and disease on the joints of the body, will be used throughout this text. Although the joints in the human body do not always behave in an entirely predictable manner in either a closed or an open chain, the joints are interdependent. A change in the function or structure of one joint in the system will usually cause a change in the function of a joint either immediately adjacent to the affected joint or at a distal joint. For example, if the ROM at the knee were limited, the hip and/or ankle joints would have to compensate in order that the foot could clear the floor when the person was walking, so that he or she could avoid stumbling.

Joint Motion

■ Range of Motion

The normal ROM of a joint is sometimes called the anatomic or physiologic ROM, because it refers to the amount of motion available to a joint within the anatomic limits of the joint structure.[25] The extent of the anatomic range is determined by a number of factors, including the shape of the joint surfaces, the joint capsule, ligaments, muscle bulk, and surrounding musculotendinous and bony structures. In some joints there are no bony limitations to motion, and the ROM is limited only by soft tissue structures. For example, the knee joint has no bony limitations to motion. Other joints have definite bony restrictions to motion in addition to soft tissue limitations. The humeroulnar joint at the elbow is limited in extension by bony contact of the

ulna on the olecranon fossa of the humerus. The sensation experienced by the examiner performing passive physiologic movements at each joint is referred to as the **end-feel.**

A ROM is considered to be pathologic when motion at a joint either exceeds or fails to reach the normal anatomic limits of motion. When a ROM exceeds the normal limits, the joint is hypermobile. When the ROM is less than what would normally be permitted by the structure, the joint is hypomobile. **Hypermobility** may be caused by a failure to limit motion by either the bony or soft tissues and may lead to instability. **Hypomobility** may be caused by bony or cartilaginous blocks to motion or by the inability of the capsule, ligaments, or muscles to elongate sufficiently to allow a normal ROM. A **contracture,** which is the shortening of soft tissue structures around a joint, is one cause of hypomobility. Either hypermobility or hypomobility of a joint may have undesirable effects, not only at the affected joint but also on adjacent joint structures.

Example 2-17

Limitation of hip extension as a consequence of osteoarthritis may lead to excessive lumbar spine movement to achieve adequate movement of the lower extremity during gait.

■ Osteokinematics

Osteokinematics refers to the movement of the bones in space during physiologic joint motion.[25] These are the movements in the sagittal, frontal, and transverse planes that occur at joints. The movements are typically described by the plane in which they occur, the axis about which they occur, and the direction of movement.

Example 2-18

Osteokinematic movements at the ulnohumeral joint include flexion or extension (direction) of the ulna on the humerus (or humerus on the ulna) in the sagittal plane about a frontal axis. Note that movements are always described as if they are occurring from the anatomical position. Sometimes the direction of the movement is described by the direction of the bone in space: that is, anterior movement ulna on the humerus (flexion) or posterior movement of the humerus on the ulna (extension).

■ Arthrokinematics

Physiologic joint motion involves motion of bony segments (osteokinematics) as well as motion of the joint surfaces in relation to another.[25,27] These movements accompany voluntary movement but cannot be independently produced voluntarily under normal conditions. The term **arthrokinematics** is used to refer to these movements of joint surfaces on one another. Usually one of the joint surfaces is relatively stable and serves as a base for the motion, whereas the other surface moves on this relatively fixed base. The terms roll, slide, and spin (Fig. 2-26) are used to describe the type of motion that the moving part performs.[2,25-27,92] A **roll** refers to the rolling of one joint surface on another, as in a tire rolling on the road. In the knee, the femoral condyles roll on the fixed tibial surface during knee flexion or extension in standing. The direction of rolling is described by the direction of movement of the bone; thus, the femur rolls forward during knee extension in standing. During a pure rolling motion, a progression of points of contact between the surfaces occurs.

Sliding, which is a pure translatory motion, refers to the gliding of one component over another, as when a braked wheel skids. The point of contact changes in the fixed component as the sliding component moves over it. In the hand, the proximal phalanx slides over the fixed end of the metacarpal during flexion and extension. The term **spin** refers to a rotation of the movable component, as when a top spins. Spin is a pure rotatory motion. The same points remain in contact on both the moving and stationary components. At the

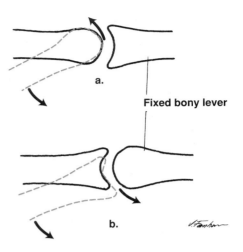

▲ **Figure 2-27** ■ Motion at ovoid joints. **A.** When a convex surface is moving on a fixed concave surface, the convex articulating surface moves in a direction opposite to the direction traveled by the shaft of the bony lever. **B.** When a concave surface is moving on a fixed convex surface, the concave articulating surface moves in the same direction as the remaining portion of the bony lever (proximal phalanx moving on fixed metacarpal).

elbow, the head of the radius spins on the capitulum of the humerus during supination and pronation of the forearm.

During human joint motion, combinations of rolling and sliding arthrokinematic movements usually occur in order to maintain joint integrity. The types of arthrokinematic motion that occur at a particular joint depend on the shape of the articulating surfaces. When a concave articulating surface is moving on a stable convex surface, sliding occurs in the *same direction* as motion of the bony lever (Fig. 2-27). Because the motion of the bony lever is the direction of the roll of the bone, the roll and slide are in the same direction. This allows the joint surfaces to stay in optimum contact with each other. When a convex joint surface moves on a concave surface, the bone must roll in one direction and glide in the opposite direction in order to maintain optimum contact. This is known as the convex-concave rule.

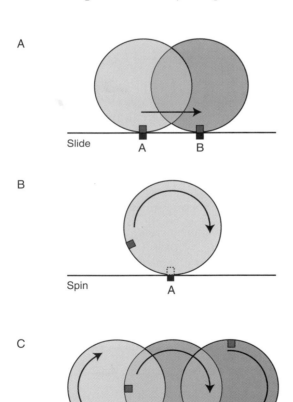

A

Slide
    A   B

B

Spin
    A

C

Roll
   A   B

▲ **Figure 2-26** ■ Arthrokinematic joint motions include sliding (**A**), spinning (**B**), and rolling (**C**).

CONCEPT CORNERSTONE 2-9: *Convex-Concave Joint Surface Motion*

Convex-concave rule: Convex joint surfaces roll and glide in *opposite* directions, whereas concave joint surfaces roll and slide in the *same* direction.

Most joints fit into either an ovoid or a sellar category. In an **ovoid** joint, one surface is convex and the other surface is concave (Fig. 2-28A). In a **sellar** joint, *each* joint surface is *both* convex and concave (see Fig. 2-28B). The arthrokinematic motion of the moving segment is described in relation to the nonmoving segment. Thus, knowledge of the structure of the moving segment and the movement that is occurring allows

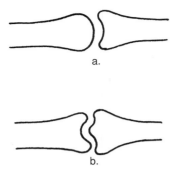

▲ **Figure 2-28** ■ Ovoid and sellar joints. **A.** In an ovoid joint, one articulating surface is convex and the other articulating surface is concave. **B.** In a sellar joint, each articulating surface is concave and convex.

prediction of the arthrokinematics that accompany the movement. The sliding that occurs between articular surfaces is an essential component of joint motion and must occur for normal functioning of the joint. If the articular end of the bone is not free to move (slide) in the appropriate direction, then when the distal end of the bone moves, abnormal forces will be created in the joint.

Example 2-19

Abduction of the distal end of the humerus must be accompanied by downward sliding (inferior movement) of the proximal convex head of the humerus on the concave surface of the glenoid fossa for the distal end to elevate without damage to the joint (Fig. 2-29A). Superior gliding of the humeral head must occur for the distal end of the humerus to be brought back downward into adduction (see Fig. 2-29B). If downward gliding is restricted, abduction of the humerus may cause impingement of anterior soft tissue structures between the humerus and the acromion.

For articular surfaces to be free to slide in the appropriate direction as the bony lever moves, the joint must have a certain amount of **"joint play."** This move-

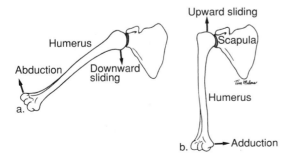

▲ **Figure 2-29** ■ Sliding of joint surfaces. **A.** Abduction of the humerus must be accompanied by inferior sliding of the head of the humerus in the glenoid fossa. **B.** Adduction of the humerus is accompanied by superior sliding of the head of the humerus.

ment of one articular surface on another is not usually under voluntary control and must be tested by the application of an external force. In an optimal situation, a joint has a sufficient amount of play to allow normal motion at the joint's articulating surfaces. If the supporting joint structures are lax, the joint may have too much play and become unstable. If the joint structures are tight, the joint will have too little movement between the articular surfaces, and the amount of motion of the bony lever will be restricted because the appropriate slide will not accompany the physiologic movement.

Case Application 2-10: **Effects of Limited Range of Motion**

> When the cast is removed from George's leg and foot, he has 10° dorsiflexion and 20° plantar flexion, and his subtalar motion is restricted. This will affect the lower kinetic chain during squatting, walking, and other activities. His ability to adapt to uneven surfaces will be compromised by ankle discomfort and by restriction of subtalar joint motion. The latter usually can be readily restored through joint mobilization and will result in much more comfortable walking and standing. Gliding motions of the posterior calcaneus on the talus in a medial or lateral direction will increase eversion or inversion, respectively.

Joint motions commonly include a combination of sliding, spinning, and rolling. Although we typically describe the axis of rotation for various joints in the body and use anatomical landmarks to represent these axes, the combination of sliding and spinning or rolling produces curvilinear motion and a moving axis of motion. An axis that moves during rolling or sliding motions forms a series of successive points. The axis of rotation at any particular point in the motion is called the **instantaneous axis of rotation** (IAR). IARs occur most notably when opposing articular surfaces are of unequal size. In some joints, such as the shoulder, the articulating surface of the moving bone (humerus) is larger than the surface of the stabilized component (glenoid). In other joints, such as the metacarpophalangeal and interphalangeal joints of the fingers, the articulating surface of the moving bone is smaller than the surface of the stabilized component. When the articulating surface of a moving component is larger than the stabilized component, a pure motion such as rolling will result in the larger moving component's rolling off the smaller articulating surface before the motion is completed. Therefore, combination motions, wherein a moving component rolls in one direction and slides in the opposite direction, help to increase the ROM available to the joint and keep opposing joint surfaces in contact with each other. Another method of increasing the range of available motion is by permitting both components to move at the same time. The rolling and sliding arthrokinematic movements of the articular surfaces are not usually visible and thus have not been described in the traditional classification system of joint movement. However, these motions are considered in the six degrees of freedom model described by White and Panjabi.[27] These authors have suggested that motion at the intervertebral symphysis joints between the bodies of the vertebrae in the vertebral column occurs in six planes, around three axes. The implication is that motion at the joints of the body might be more thoroughly described by using a six degrees of freedom model.

All synovial joints have a **close-packed** position in which the joint surfaces are maximally congruent and the ligaments and capsule are maximally taut. The close-packed position is usually at the extreme end of a ROM. In the close-packed position, a joint possesses its greatest stability and is resistant to tensile forces that tend to cause distraction (separation) of the joint surfaces. Little or no joint play is possible. The position of extension is the close-packed position for the humeroulnar, knee, and interphalangeal joints.[2,25] In the **loose-packed** position of a joint, the articular surfaces are relatively free to move in relation to one another. The loose-packed position of a joint is any position other than the close-packed position, although the term is most commonly used to refer to the position at which the joint structures are more lax and the joint cavity has a greater volume than in other positions. In the loose-packed position, the joint has a maximum amount of joint play. An externally applied force, such as that applied by a therapist or physician, can produce movement of one articular surface on another and enable the examiner to assess the amount of joint play that is present. Movement in and out of the close-packed position is likely to have a beneficial effect on joint nutrition because of the squeezing out of the fluid during each compression and imbibing of fluid when the compression is removed.[25]

◆ General Changes with Disease, Injury, Immobilization, Exercise, and Overuse

Each part of a joint has one or more specific functions that are essential for the overall performance of the joint. Therefore, any process that disrupts any one of the parts of a joint will disrupt the total function of the joint. Likewise, anything that affects joint motion will affect all the structures that constitute that joint. This is essential for therapists to remember during rehabilitation after injury. For example, when a bone is broken, the fracture may be the main injury that dictates subsequent treatment, but lack of motion and decreased loading will affect cartilage, ligaments, joint capsule, tendons, and so forth. The ideal rehabilitation protocol will consider the behavior of all the affected structures and design interventions that are tailored to induce adaptations in each structure. This means understanding the time course and nature of the adaptation of each tissue to altered loading conditions.

The complex joints are more likely to be affected by injury, disease, or aging than are the simple joints. The complex joints have more parts and are subject to more wear and tear than are stability joints. Also, the function of the complex joints depends on a number of interrelated factors. For example, the capsule must produce synovial fluid. The fluid must be of the appropriate composition and of sufficient quantity that it can lubricate and provide nourishment for the joint. The hyaline cartilage must be smooth enough so that the joint surfaces can move easily and yet must be permeable so that it can receive some of its nourishment from the joint fluid. The cartilage also must undergo periodic compressive loading and unloading to facilitate movement of the fluid, and the collagen network must be intact to contain the fluid attracted to the PGs. The ligaments and capsules must be strong enough to provide sufficient support for stability and yet be flexible enough to permit normal joint motion. Tendons must be able to withstand the forces generated by muscles as they produce movement.

Disease

The general effects of disease, injury, immobilization, and overuse may be illustrated by using the normal function of a joint structure as a basis for analysis. For example, if the synovial membrane of a joint is affected by a collagen disease such as rheumatoid arthritis, it may be assumed that because the normal function of the synovial membrane is to produce synovial fluid, the production and perhaps the composition of the synovial fluid will be altered in this disease. It could also be postulated that because fluid is altered, the lubrication of the joint also would be altered. The disease process and the changes in joint structure that occur in rheumatoid arthritis involve far more than synovial fluid alteration, but the disease does change the composition and the quantity of the synovial fluid. In another type of arthritis, osteoarthritis, which may be genetic and/or mechanical in origin, the cartilage is the focus of the disease process. On the basis of normal cartilage function, it can be assumed that the cartilage in osteoarthritic joints will not be able to withstand normal stress. Actually, erosion and splitting of the cartilage occur under stress. As a result, friction is increased between the joint surfaces, thus further increasing the erosion process.

Injury

If an injury has occurred, such as the tearing of a ligament, it may be assumed that there will be a lack of support for the joint. In the example of the table with an unstable joint between the leg and the table top, damage and disruption of function may occur as a result of instability. If a heavy load is placed on the damaged table joint, the joint surfaces will separate under the compressive load and the leg may be angled. The once-stable joint now allows mobility, and the leg may wobble back and forth. This motion may cause the screws to loosen or the nails to bend and ultimately to be torn out of one of the wooden components.

Complete failure of the joint may result in splintering of the wooden components, especially when the already weakened joint is subjected to excessive, sudden, or prolonged loads. The effects of a lack of support in a human joint are similar to that in the table joint. Separation of the bony surfaces occurs and may result in wobbling or a deviation from the normal alignment of one of the bony components. These changes in alignment create an abnormal joint distraction on the side where a ligament is torn. As a result, the other ligaments, the tendons, and the joint capsule may become excessively stretched and consequently be unable to provide protection. The supported side of the joint may also be affected and subjected to abnormal compression during weight-bearing or motion. In canine experiments in which an unstable knee joint is produced as a result of transection of the ACL of the knee, morphologic, biochemical, biomechanical, and metabolic changes occur in the articular cartilage shortly after the transection.[12,13] Later, articular cartilage becomes thicker and shows fibrillation, and osteophytes are present. The cartilage also shows much higher water content than in the opposite knee, and the synovial fluid content of the knee is increased. In addition, a sharp increase in bone turnover occurs, as does a thickening of the subchondral bone.[87] According to Van Osch et al., joint instability is a well-known cause of secondary osteoarthritis involving the knee joint.[94]

Immobilization (Stress Deprivation)

In general, any process or event that disturbs the normal function of a specific joint structure will set up a chain of events that eventually affects every part of a joint and its surrounding structures. Immobilization is particularly detrimental to joint structure and function. Immobilization may be externally imposed by a cast, bed rest, weightlessness, or denervation or may be self-imposed as a reaction to pain and inflammation. An injured joint or joint subjected to inflammation and swelling will assume a loose-packed position to accommodate the increased volume of fluid within the joint space. This position may be referred to as the position of comfort because pain is decreased in this position. Each joint has a position of minimum pressure. For the knee and hip joints, the position of comfort is between 30° and 45° of flexion, and for the ankle joint, the position is at 15° of plantar flexion.[55] If the joint is immobilized for a few weeks in the position of comfort, the joint capsule will adapt (shorten), and contractures[95] will develop in the surrounding soft tissues. Consequently, resumption of a normal range of joint motion will be difficult.

■ Effects on Ligament and Tendon

Ligaments and tendons adapt to decreased load by decreasing their collagen content and crosslinking, although their sizes remain the same. The tissue thus weakens, and the resumption of normal loading may cause increased stress and strain.[12,13] The MTJ of tendons loses its interdigitating structure, which makes it weaker.[81] The time course of these adaptations is fairly rapid. Ligaments and tendons have been shown to decrease their tensile strength and stiffness up to 50% after 8 weeks of immobilization.[12,13] It is assumed that ligaments and tendons eventually recover their mechanical properties, but the time course of this recovery appears to be slow, and the total time for recovery is unknown. In general, the time course for the loss of mechanical properties occurs over weeks, whereas recovery can take 12 to 18 months or more.[17] Graded reloading is necessary to restore tendon and ligament strength.

■ Effects on Articular Surfaces and Bone

The effects of immobilization are not confined to the surrounding soft tissues but also may affect the articular surfaces of the joint and the underlying bone. Biochemical and morphologic changes that have been attributed to the effects of immobilization include proliferation of fibrofatty connective tissue within the joint space, adhesions between the folds of the synovium, atrophy of cartilage, regional osteoporosis, weakening of ligaments at their insertion sites as a result of osteoclastic resorption of bone and Sharpey fibers, a decrease in the PG content, and increase in the water content of articular cartilage.[28,94-97] For example, the menisci at the knee are adversely affected by immobilization. In an experiment in which the hindlegs of canines were casted for 4 weeks in a position of 90° flexion, the aggrecan gene expression and PG content in the menisci were reduced and the water content of the tissue increased.[98] Gross atrophy of the menisci was noted. Thinning and softening of the articular cartilage occur, and deformation under compressive test load increases up to 42%. As a result of changes in joint structures brought about by immobilization, decreases may be evident in the ROM available to the joint, the time between loading and failure, and the energy-absorbing capacity of the bone-ligament complex. Swelling or immobilization of a joint also inhibits and weakens the muscles surrounding the joint.[99-102] Therefore, the joint is unable to function normally and is at high risk of additional injury. A summary of the possible effects of prolonged immobilization is presented in Table 2-8.

Case Application 2-11: **Deleterious Effects of Immobilization**

Mr. Chen's joint and surrounding structures, including the following, will undergo striking changes during immobilization:

- bone: weakened, decreased collagen and mineral
- capsule: shrinking, increased resistance to movement
- ligament: decreased crosslinks, decreased tensile strength

Table 2-8	Effects of Increased and Decreased Load on Connective Tissues	
Tissue	Decreased Load	Increased Load
Tendon and ligament	Decreased collagen concentration Decreased crosslinking Decreased tensile strength	Increased cross-sectional area Increased collagen concentration Increased crosslinking Increased tensile strength Increased stiffness
Menisci	Decreased PGs	Increased PGs
Bone	Decreased collagen synthesis Decreased bone formation Increased bone resorption	Denser bone Increased synthesis of collagen and bone
Cartilage	Thinning of cartilage Advancing of subchondral bone Decreased PG synthesis Fewer PG aggregates	Increased PG synthesis Increased volume?
Joint capsule	Disordered collagen fibrils Abnormal crosslinking	Not specifically examined
Synovium	Adhesion formation Fibrofatty tissue proliferation into joint space	Not specifically examined

PG, proteoglycan.

- tendon: decreased crosslinks, disorganization of collagen fibrils, decreased tensile strength
- muscle: loss of sarcomeres in series, decreased contractile proteins
- cartilage: swelling, decreased PG concentration

These changes occur within 8 weeks, but recovery may take 18 months or longer.

 CONCEPT CORNERSTONE 2-10: *Effects of Loading on Connective Tissue*

- Connective tissues become weaker and lose their normal structure if they are not loaded.
- Changes with decreased load occur rapidly.
- Recovery of normal structure and function requires gradual progressive loading.
- Loads should be tailored to the connective tissue.

Recognition of the adverse effects of immobilization has led to the development of the following strategies to help minimize the consequences of immobilization: (1) use of continuous passive motion (CPM) devices after joint surgery, (2) reduction in the duration of casting periods after fractures and sprains, (3) development of dynamic splinting devices to allow joint motion while preventing unwanted motion that may damage healing structures, (4) use of graded loading after immobilization, and (5) extension of the recovery period to months, rather than days or weeks.. The CPM is a mechanical device that is capable of moving joints passively and repeatedly through a specified portion of the physiologic ROM. The speed of the movement and the ROM can be controlled. The CPM devices are able to produce joint motion under low loading conditions, in turn producing medium-frequency alternating compression, which may stimulate cartilage formation. It is easier to control loading with these devices than with active movements, thus avoiding the potentially deleterious compressive-tensile stresses and strains produced by active muscle contractions. Use of CPM was shown to prevent some of the weakening of tendon that occurs during immobilization, although normal tissue strength was not maintained.[103]

Exercise

All tissues appear to respond favorably to gradual progressive loading by adapting to meet the increased mechanical demands. On the local level, exercise influences cell shape and physiologic functions and can have a direct mechanical effect on matrix alignment. The response to exercise varies among tissues and depends on the nature of the stimulus, including the amount, type, and frequency of loading. The local mechanism of connective tissue response to exercise appears to involve cells' detecting tissue strain and modifying the type and amount of tissue synthesized. The volume, nature, and frequency of deformation are important. Low-frequency compressive loading will increase cartilage formation, whereas higher frequencies can enhance bone synthesis. Higher magnitude or sustained loading will induce fibrocartilage formation, whereas tensile loads induce tissue formation resembling that found in tendon or ligament. Maintenance of the normal mechanical state of connective tissues appears to require repetitive loading beyond a threshold level. Below this threshold, the immobilization changes previously described rapidly occur.[69]

■ Bone Response to Exercise

Numerous studies have shown that bone deposition is increased with weight-bearing exercise and in areas of increased muscle force.[104,105] This response of bone form to function, Wolff's law, has been known for over 100 years. Exercise is now used as a therapeutic intervention to prevent bone loss.[106] A systematic review showed that in 11 of 16 studies, postmenopausal women showed improvements in bone density with either exercise or exercise plus calcium or estrogen.[105] The use of interventions to prevent bone loss during space flight and resulting from osteoporosis is an area of active research. Bone formation appears very sensitive to strains, as well as (or instead of) the magnitude of the applied load. Very low magnitude high-frequency vibration has been shown to increase trabecular bone formation by 34%.[107] This suggests that even very low loads, well below the threshold for potential injury, may increase bone density. Rubin et al. have proposed that it is the far lower magnitude, high-frequency (10- to 30-Hz) mechanical signals that continually barrage the skeleton during longer term activities such as standing, which regulate skeletal architecture.[107-109] Only short durations of loading are necessary, and just 10 minutes of low-load, high-frequency stimulation has been shown to prevent bone loss induced by disuse.[107] Lanyon[110] suggested that the asymmetries of strain that occur during normal load-bearing activities create an ever-changing strain distribution, that it is the novelty of the strain that induces bone adaptation, and that the osteogenic response saturates rapidly. He further suggested that exercise regimens designed to control bone architecture can usefully capitalize on this feature of the adaptive (re-)modeling response. Each exercise session need not be prolonged but should include as many novel strain distributions as possible, preferably involving high peak strains and strain rates.

■ Cartilage Response to Exercise

The response of cartilage to immobilization has been described,[111] but the response to increased physiologic loading is largely unknown. It is clear that the health of articular cartilage depends on the application and removal of compressive loads. Chondrocytes are directly connected to their microenvironment, and mechanical forces are transduced into intracellular synthetic activity. The mechanisms of this transduction and the magnitude and frequency of the loading that will optimize cartilage structure are not yet known. This is an area of active research, as cartilage injuries heal very poorly, and the use of transplanted material to repair cartilage defects is being explored. Since Salter's work,[112] it has been well known that motion enhances tissue formation in cartilage defects, but this is fibrocartilage, not hyaline articular cartilage. Unlike fibroblasts in bone, ligament, and tendon, chondrocytes do not migrate and repair areas that have been injured. Defects that extend to subchondral bone are thought to have better healing potential because of the presence of pluri-

potential mesenchymal cells (from bone marrow) that can differentiate into chondroblasts, hence the use of drilling to treat osteochondral defects.[111] There are no quantitative data available about changes in human articular cartilage after immobilization or exercise, although MRI shows promise in this regard. It appears that cyclic low-magnitude, low-frequency ($<$1-Hz) compressive loads may induce or maintain cartilage structure.

■ Tendon Response to Exercise

Tendons respond to increased tensile loads by increasing their collagen concentration, collagen crosslinking, tensile strength, and stiffness. Woo et al. showed that after 12 months of physical training, the extensor digitorum tendons of swine increased their weight, strength, collagen content and stiffness to match the normally stronger flexor digitorum longus, which did not alter in response to the same program.[87] Biochemical changes occured in chicken Achilles tendons after strenuous running, with increased collagen synthesis, crosslinking, tensile strength, and stiffness, although tendon size and weight did not change.[113,114] Chronic increased loading causes tendon hypertrophy and increased crosslinking.[114-116] In other words, both structural and material changes take place. Interestingly, exercise appears to offset some of the changes that occur in connective tissue with age.[117] Progressive tensile loading has been used successfully to treat chronic tendon disorders, under the assumption that the tendon will adapt to the increased loads.[70,118] Despite the facts that symptoms decrease and function improves after such intervention, there is no direct evidence that tendon adaptation has actually occurred as a result of this progressive loading program.

■ Ligament Response to Exercise

The effects of exercise in preventing negative ligament changes with immobilization and the positive effects of activity on ligament healing have been well demonstrated, but the effects of exercise on normal ligament are less clear.[119-122] Recovery of normal ligament structure and mechanics after immobilization, under normal loading conditions, is a slow process that can take months. It appears that exercise may speed this process, but the volume of loading and the time course of the adaptations are not known.[123]

 CONCEPT CORNERSTONE 2-11: *Connective Tissue Adaptation*

All connective tissues will adapt to increased load through changes in structural and/or material properties (form follows function).

The load must be gradual and progressive; as the tissue adapts to the new loading conditions, the load must change to induce further adaptation.

The type of connective tissue formed will match the type and volume of the load:

■ compression: cartilage or bone
■ tension: ligament or tendon

Optimization of load volume and frequency, and the nature of human tissue adaptation, remain largely unknown as yet.

Case Application 2-12: **Facilitation of Tissue Recovery**

The types of exercise that may facilitate tissue recovery in George's case might include:

■ bone: walking, standing with weight shifts, bouncing, on/off pressure
■ cartilage: moderate loads through available ROM
■ ligament: gentle, progressive tensile stress
■ tendon: progressive tensile loading
■ muscle: progressive tensile loading at various speeds (recruit different motor units) and lower load exercise to fatigue (induce metabolic adaptation)
■ capsule: repeated exercise throughout physiological ROM

In general, loads should be kept light for the first 2 to 3 weeks, with the emphasis on repeated motion through the ROM and passive joint mobilization to nontraumatized joints (such as the subtalar joint). When the talocrural joint has adequate dorsiflexion, closed kinetic chain exercises can begin. Although setting exercises (no joint motion) can be used at any point, it is recommended that large loads be avoided while the joint is immobilized.

Overuse

Although immobilization is detrimental, and exercise beyond a threshold level is necessary to maintain connective tissue structure and function, either constant or repetitive loading of articular structures also may have adverse effects. Damage can occur in one of two ways: (1) sudden application of large loads and (2) repeated or sustained application of low loads. The former are nonphysiologic loads that create large stresses and strains, thus creating rupture of the tissue on a microscopic or macroscopic scale (e.g., tendon ruptures, bone fractures). The latter are physiologic loads that are sustained or repeated while creep occurs. Recovery of normal tissue structure takes an as yet unknown time after the load is removed. When a structure that is undergoing creep is subjected to continual loading on the already deformed tissue, the tissues may enter the plastic range and undergo microfailure. This may account for some cases of chronic back pain or tendon injuries. Ligaments subjected to constant tensile loads will lengthen and may undergo permanent change in length if further loading occurs. For example, after loss of the ACL, increased load on the posterior knee joint capsule may cause plastic deformation, leading to increasing knee hypermobility. Cartilage subjected to constant compressive loading will creep and may expe-

rience permanent deformation. Cell death may occur with rigid sustained pressure at focal points on the cartilage, and permeability will be decreased.[7]

Joints and their supporting structures subjected to repetitive loading thus may be injured and fail because they do not have time to recover their original dimensions before they are subjected to another loading cycle, even though the load magnitude is within the normal loading range. Structures are subjected to repeated loading before they have recovered their normal structure. An injury resulting from repetitive strain loading of connective tissues may be called **overuse injury** or **syndrome, repetitive motion disorder,** or **repetitive strain injury.**[9] These disorders have been identified in athletes, dancers, farmers, musicians, and factory and office workers and appear to affect a greater proportion of women than men.[21] However, the reason why women have a greater incidence of these injuries than do men is still under investigation. Hart et al. hypothesized that intrinsic gender differences may exist in the regulation of connective tissue structures.[21] It is well known that hormonal levels fluctuate in women during pregnancy and the menstrual cycle. Investigations of tendons in female rabbits demonstrated that type I collagen significantly decreased and collagenase significantly increased in a number of selected tendons in these rabbits during pregnancy. It appears that the sex hormonal receptors in the tendons responded to the changed levels of hormones in the rabbits.[21] Biopsy material from tendons from human subjects undergoing surgery for repetitive motion disorders shows an inflammatory process in some tendons and a degenerative process in others.[114] In view of the findings to date, it appears that simple tissue fatigue is not a sufficient explanation for the cause of repetitive motion disorders and that additional research is needed to determine all of the factors involved in the cause, effect, prevention, and treatment of repetitive motion disorders. The threshold between loading-induced adaptation and overuse may be a fine one (Fig. 2-30).

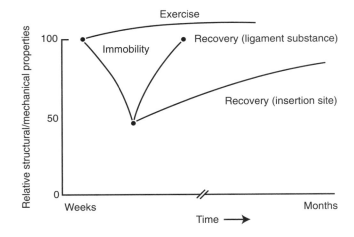

▲ **Figure 2-30** ■ Effects of load alteration of normal and immobilized tissues. Adaptation to decreased load is rapid, whereas recovery is slower. The response of normal tissues to increased load remains uncertain.

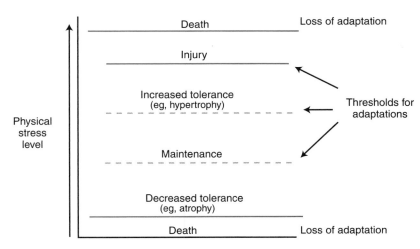

Effect of Physical Stress on Tissue Adaptation

◀ **Figure 2-31** ■ The range of adaptations possible in joint structures in response to different levels of loading. (From Mueller MJ, Maluf KS: Tissue adaptation for physical stress: A proposed "physical stress theory" to guide physical therapist practice, education and research. Phys Ther 82:383-403, 2002, with permission of the American Physical Therapy Association.)

 CONCEPT CORNERSTONE 2-12: *Chronic Overuse Injuries*

■ Chronic overuse injuries may involve repeated or sustained loads while the tissue is still in a deformed state. Time, not load alteration, may be the critical variable.
■ The role of systemic influences (e.g., hormones, nutrition) and neurophysiologic influences (referred pain, focal dystonia) in repetitive injuries remains to be explored.

Summary

This chapter has presented the elementary principles of joint design, a classification system for human joints, and an introduction to the materials found in human joints and the properties of these materials, as well as the effects of disease, immobilization, and overuse on joint structures. The health and strength of joint structures and hence their function depend on a threshold amount of stress and strain; this threshold can move up or down, depending on the mechanical environment. Cartilage and bone nutrition and growth depend on joint movement and muscle contraction. Cartilage nutrition depends on joint movement through a full ROM to ensure that all of the articular cartilage receives the nutrients necessary for survival. Ligaments and tendons depend on a normal amount of stress and strain to maintain and increase strength. Controlled loading and motion applied early in the rehabilitation process stimulate collagen synthesis and help align collagen fibrils. Bone density and strength increase following the stress and strain created by muscle and joint activity. In contrast, bone density and strength decrease when stress and strain are absent. Therefore, micromotion and compression are recommended to promote bony union and healing of fractures. Controlled mobilization, rather than complete immobilization, is preferred. There is still a great deal left to learn about adaptation in connective tissues, especially in humans. It appears that tissues have a movable threshold, below which they atrophy and above which they become injured (Fig. 2-31). Progressive loading involves gradually moving this threshold so that the tissue can withstand the forces accompanying functional activities.

The inadequacy of cartilage repair mechanisms and the slow recovery of bones, ligaments, and tendons suggest that the prevention of injury to joint structures through the avoidance of excessive loading is crucial. Gradual, progressive loading is the ideal. The therapist must skillfully load the tissues with the appropriate direction, magnitude, and frequency of loading to prevent weakening or to induce adaptation. In subsequent chapters, the specific structure and function of each of the major joints in the body will be explored. Knowledge of the basic elements of normal joint structure and function and understanding the changes that function can induce in structure, and vice versa, will help the reader recognize abnormal joint function; analyze the effects of injury, disease, or aging on joint structure and function; and appreciate the complex nature of human joints.

Study Questions

1. Describe the structure of a typical diarthrodial joint.
2. Describe the type of motion that is available at a pivot joint, and give at least two examples of pivot joints.

(Continued on following page)

3. Describe the composition of the interfibrillar component of the extracellular matrix in connective tissue.
4. Describe how diarthrodial joints are lubricated.
5. Describe the movements of the bony lever during motion at an ovoid joint.
6. Describe what is meant by the term "toe region."
7. Explain creep and how it affects joint structure and function.
8. Explain how immobilization affects joint structures.
9. Explain what happens to a material when hysteresis occurs.
10. Explain how an overuse injury may occur.
11. Compare the structure and function of synarthroses with that of diarthroses.
12. Compare a closed chain with an open chain and give examples of each.
13. Compare the composition, properties, and function of ligaments with those of tendons, cartilage, and bone.
14. Compare stress and strain. Give at least one example using a load-deformation curve.

◆ References

1. Michl J: Form follows WHAT? The modernist notion of function as a carte blanche. MagFaculty Architecture Town Planning 1(10):2031, 1995.
2. Williams PL (ed): Gray's Anatomy, 38th ed. New York, Churchill Livingstone, 1995.
3. Culav EM, Clark CH, Merilee MJ: Connective tissues: Matrix composition and its relevance to physical therapy. Phys Ther 79:308, 1999.
4. Ralphs JR, Benjamin M: The joint capsule: Structure, composition, ageing and disease. J Anat 184:503, 1994.
5. Rodeo SA, Suzuki K, Yamauchi M, et al.: Analysis of collagen and elastic fibers in shoulder capsule in patients with shoulder instability. Am J Sports Med 26:634, 1998.
6. Lewis AR, Ralphs JR, Kneafsey B, et al.: Distribution of collagens and glycosaminoglycans in the joint capsule of the proximal interphalangeal joint of the human finger. Anat Rec 250:281, 1998.
7. Walker JM: Cartilage of human joints and related structures. In Zachazewski JE, Magee DJ, Quillen WS (eds): Athletic Injuries and Rehabilitation. Philadelphia, WB Saunders, 1996.
8. Grigg P: Articular neurophysiology. In Zachazewski JE, Magee DJ, Quillen, WS (eds): Athletic Injuries and Rehabilitation. Philadelphia, WB Saunders, 1996.
9. Allan DA: Structure and physiology of joints and their relationship to repetitive strain injuries. Clin Orthop 352:32, 1998.
10. English T, Wheeler ME, Hettinga DL: Inflammatory response of synovial joint structures. In Malone TR, McPoil T, Nitz AJ (eds): Orthopedic and Sports Physical Therapy. St. Louis, Mosby-Year Book, 1997.
11. Hogorvost T, Brand, RA: Mechanoreceptors in joint function. J Bone Joint Surg Am 80:1365, 1998.
12. Noyes FR, DeLucas JL, Torvik PJ: Biomechanics of anterior cruciate ligament failure: An analysis of strain-rate sensitivity and mechanisms of failure in primates. J Bone Joint Surg Am 56:2, 1974.
13. Noyes FR, Torvik PJ, Hyde WB, et al.: Biomechanics of ligament failure II: An analysis of immobilization, exercise, and reconditioning effects in primates. J Bone Joint Surg Am 56:1406–1418, 1974.
14. Decraemer WF, Maes MA, Vanhuyse VJ, et al.: A non-linear viscoelastic constitutive equation for soft biological tissues based upon a structural model. J Biomech 13:559, 1980.
15. Goldstein SA, Armstrong TJ, Chaffin DB, et al.: Analysis of cumulative strain in tendons and tendon sheaths. J Biomech 20:1, 1987.
16. To SYC, Kwan MK, Woo, SL-Y: Simultaneous measurements of strains on two surfaces of tendons and ligaments. J Biomech 21:511, 1988.
17. Woo SL-Y, Gomez MA, Woo YK, et al.: Mechanical properties of tendons and ligaments. II. The relationships of immobilization and exercise on tissue remodeling. Biorheology 19:397, 1982.
18. Akeson WH, Amiel D, Abel MF, et al.: Effects of immobilization on joints. Clin Orthop 219:28–37, 1987.
19. Rong G, Wang Y: The role of the cruciate ligaments in maintaining knee joint stability. Clin Orthop 215:65, 1987.
20. Djurasovic M, Aldridge JW, Grumbles R, et al.: Knee joint immobilization decreases aggrecan gene expression in the meniscus. Am J Sports Med 26:460, 1998.
21. Hart DA, Archambault JM, Kydd A, et al.: Gender and neurogenic variables in tendon biology and repetitive motion disorders. Clin Orthop 351:44, 1998.
22. Simkin PA: In Schumacher HR, Klippel JH, Robinson DR (eds): Primer on the Rheumatic Diseases, 9th ed. Atlanta, Arthritis Foundation, 1988.
23. Hettinga DL: II Normal joint structures and their reaction to injury. J Orthop Sports Phys Ther 1:2, 1979.
24. Radin EL, Paul IL: A consolidated concept of joint lubrication. J Bone Joint Surg Am 54:607.
25. Lehmkuhl D, Smith L: Brunnstrom's Clinical Kinesiology, 4th ed. Philadelphia, FA Davis, 1984.
26. Gowitzke BA, Milner M: Understanding the Scientific Basis of Human Movement, 3rd ed. Baltimore, Williams & Wilkins, 1988.

27. White AA, Panjabi MM: Clinical Biomechanics of the Spine, 2nd ed. Philadelphia, JB Lippincott, 1990.

28. Cohen NP, Foster RJ, Mow VC: Composition and dynamics of articular cartilage: Structure, function and maintaining healthy state. J Orthop Sports Phys Ther 28:203,1998.

29. Bosman FT, Stamenkovic I: Functional structure and composition of the extracellular matrix. J Pathol 200:423–428, 2003.

30. Heinegard D, Paulsson M: Structure and metabolism of proteoglycans. In Piez KA, Reddi AH (eds): Extracellular Matrix Biochemistry, pp 277–328. New York, Elsevier, 1984.

31. Poole AR, Kojima T, Yasuda T, et al.: Composition and structure of articular cartilage: A template for tissue repair. Clin Orthop (391 Suppl):S26-S33, 2001.

32. Covizi DZ, Felisbino SL, Gomes L, et al.: Regional adaptations in three rat tendons. Tissue Cell 33: 483–490, 2001.

33. Vogel KG, Ordog A, Pogany G, et al.: Proteoglycans in the compressed region of human tibialis posterior tendon and in ligaments. J Orthop Res 11: 68–77, 1993.

34. Vogel KG, Thonar EJ: Keratan sulfate is a component of proteoglycans in the compressed region of adult bovine flexor tendon. J Orthop Res 6: 434–442, 1988.

35. Hae Yoon J, Brooks R, Hwan Kim Y, et al.: Proteoglycans in chicken gastrocnemius tendons change with exercise. Arch Biochem Biophys 412:279–286, 2003.

36. Eyre DR: Collagen: Molecular diversity in the body's protein scaffold. Science 207:1315–1322, 1980.

37. Eyre DR: The collagens of articular cartilage. Semin Arthritis Rheum 21(3, Suppl 2):2–11, 1991.

38. Burgeson RE, Nimni ME : Collagen types. Molecular structure and tissue distribution. Clin Orthop 282: 250–272, 1992.

39. Kuivaniemi H, Tromp G, Prockop DJ: Mutations in fibrillar collagens (types I, II, III, and XI), fibril-associated collagen (type IX), and network-forming collagen (type X) cause a spectrum of diseases of bone, cartilage, and blood vessels. Hum Mutat 9:300–315, 1997.

40. Myllyharju J, Kivirikko KI: Collagens and collagen-related diseases. Ann Med 33:7–21, 2001.

41. Kannus P: Structure of the tendon connective tissue. Scand J Med Sci Sports 10:312–320, 2000.

42. Eriksen HA, Pajala A, Leppilahti J, et al.: Increased content of type III collagen at the rupture site of human Achilles tendon. J Orthop Res 20: 1352–1357, 2002.

43. Liu SH, Yang RS, al-Shaikh R, et al.: Collagen in tendon, ligament, and bone healing. A current review. Clin Orthop 318:265–278, 1995.

44. Kastelic J, Galeski A, Baer E: The multicomposite structure of tendon. Connect Tissue Res 6:11–23, 1978.

45. Enoka RM: Neuromechanical Basis of Kinesiology, 2nd ed. Champaign, IL, Human Kinetics, 1994.

46. Bailey AJ, Robins SP, Balian G: Biological significance of the intermolecular crosslinks of collagen. Nature 251:105–109, 1974.

47. Butler DL, Grood ES, Noyes FR, et al.: Biomechanics of ligaments and tendons. Exerc Sport Sci Rev 6:125–181, 1978.

48. Oakes BW: Tendon/ligament basic science. In Harries M, Williams C, Stanish WD, et al. (eds): Oxford Textbook of Sports Medicine. New York, Oxford University Press, 1998.

49. Benjamin M, Kumai T, Milz S, Boszczyk et al.: The skeletal attachment of tendons-tendon "entheses." Comp Biochem Physiol A Mol Integr Physiol 133:931–45, 2002.

50. Benjamin M, Ralphs JR: Tendons and ligaments—An overview. Histol Histopathol 12:1135, 1997.

51. Curwin SL: Tendon injuries: Pathophysiology and treatment. In Zachazewski JE, Magee DJ, Quillen WS (eds): Athletic Injuries and Rehabilitation. Philadelphia, WB Saunders, 1996.

52. Tidball JG, Chan M: Adhesive strength of single muscle cells to basement membrane at myotendinous junctions. J Appl Physiol 67:1063–1069, 1989.

53. Trotter JA: Structure-function considerations of muscle-tendon junctions. Comp Biochem Physiol A Mol Integr Physiol 133:1127–1133, 2002.

54. Buckwalter JA: Articular cartilage: Injuries and potential for healing. J Orthop Sports Phys Ther 28:192, 1998.

55. Walker JM: Pathomechanics and classification of cartilage lesions, facilitation of repair. J Orthop Sports Phys Ther 28:216, 1998.

56. Ghadially FH: Structure and function of articular cartilage. Clin Rheum Dis 7:3, 1980.

57. Lane LB, Bullough PG: Age-related changes in the thickness of the calcified zone and the number of tidemarks in adult human articular cartilage. J Bone Joint Surg Br 62:3, 1980.

58. Bullough PG, Jagannath A: The morphology of the calcification front in articular cartilage. Its significance in joint function. J Bone Joint Surg Br 65:72, 1983.

59. O'Driscoll SW: The healing and regeneration of articular cartilage. J Bone Joint Surg Am 80: 1795–1812, 1998.

60. Mow VC, Holmes MH, Lai WM: Fluid transport and mechanical properties of articular cartilage: A review. J Biomech 17:377–394, 1984.

61. Bachrach NM, Mow VC, Guilak F: Incompressibility of the solid matrix of articular cartilage under high hydrostatic pressures. J Biomech 31:445–451, 1998.

62. Mansour JM, Mow VC: The permeability of articular cartilage under compressive strain and at high pressures. J Bone Joint Surg Am 58:4, 1976.

63. McDonough AL: Effects of immobilization and exercise on articular cartilage—A review of literature. J Orthop Sports Phys Ther 2:5, 1981.

64. Athanasiou KA, Shah AR, Hernandez RJ, et al.: Basic science of articular cartilage repair. Clin Sports Med 20:223–247, 2001.

65. Poole AR: An introduction to the pathophysiology of osteoarthritis. Front Biosci 15:D662-D670, 1999.

66. Mankin HJ, Mankin CJ: Metabolic bone disease: An update. Instr Course Lect 52:769–784, 2003.

67. Carter DR, Orr TE, Fyhrie DP: Relationship between loading history and femoral cancellous bone architecture. J Biomech 22:231, 1989.

68. Gambert SR, Schultz BM, Hamdy RC: Osteoporosis. Clinical features, prevention, and treatment. Endocrinol Metab Clin North Am 24: 317–371, 1995.

69. Stanish WD, Rubinovich RM, Curwin S: Eccentric exercise in chronic tendinitis. Clin Orthop 208: 65–68, 1986.

70. Stanish WD, Curwin S, Mandell S: Tendinitis. Its Etiology and Treatment. New York, Oxford University Press, 2001.

71. Chetlin RD: Contemporary issues in resistance training: What works? ACSM Fit Society Page (Fall): 1, 12–13, 2002.

72. Mueller MJ, Maluf KS: Tissue adaptation to physical stress: A proposed "physical stress theory" to guide physical therapist practice, education, and research. Phys Ther 82:383–403, 2002.

73. van der Meulen MC, Huiskes R: Why mechanobiology? A survey article. J Biomech 35:401–414, 2002.

74. Brand RA: Biomechanics or necromechanics? Or how to interpret biomechanical studies. Iowa Orthop J 22:110–115, 2002.

75. Nordin M, Frankel VH: Basic Biomechanics of the Musculoskeletal System. Philadelphia, Lippincott Williams & Wilkins, 2001.

76. Ozkaya N, Nordin M: Fundamentals of Biomechanics, Equilibrium, Motion and Deformation, 2nd ed. New York, Springer-Verlag, 1999.

77. Alexander RM: Tendon elasticity and muscle function. Comp Biochem Physiol A Mol Integr Physiol 133:1001–1011, 2002.

78. Alexander RM: Springs for wings. Science 268: 50–51, 1995.

79. Finni T, Ikegawa S, Komi PV: Concentric force enhancement during human movement. Acta Physiol Scand 173:369–377, 2001.

80. Birch HL, McLaughlin L, Smith RK, et al.: Treadmill exercise-induced tendon hypertrophy: Assessment of tendons with different mechanical functions. Equine Vet J Suppl 30:222–226, 1999.

81. Tidball JG, Salem G, Zernicke R: Site and mechanical conditions for failure of skeletal muscle in experimental strain injuries. J Appl Physiol 74:1280–1286, 1993.

82. Barfred T: Kinesiological comments on subcutaneous ruptures of the Achilles tendon. Acta Orthop Scand 42:397–405, 1971.

83. Matsumoto F, Trudel G, Uhthoff K, et al.: Mechanical effects of immobilization on the Achilles tendon. Arch Phys Med Rehabil 84: 662–667, 2003.

84. Benjamin M, Ralphs JR: Fibrocartilage in tendons and ligaments—An adaptation to compressive load. J Anat 193:481–494, 1998.

85. Viidik A: Tensile strength properties of Achilles tendon systems in trained and untrained rabbits. Acta Orthop Scand 40:261–272, 1969.

86. Kasashima Y, Smith RK, Birch HL, et al.: Exercise-induced tendon hypertrophy: Cross-sectional area changes during growth are influenced by exercise. Equine Vet J Suppl 34:264–268, 2002.

87. Woo SL, Ritter MA, Amiel D, et al.: The biomechanical and biochemical properties of swine tendons—Long term effects of exercise on the digital extensors. Connect Tissue Res 7:177–183, 1980.

88. Benjamin M, Ralphs JR: Tendons and ligaments—An overview. Histol Histopathol 12:1135, 1997.

89. Frank CB: Ligament injuries: Pathophysiology and healing. In Zachazewski JE, Magee DJ, Quillen WS (eds): Athletic Injuries and Rehabilitation. Philadelphia, WB Saunders, 1996.

90. Eckstein F, Tieschky M, Faber SC, et al.: Effect of physical exercise on cartilage volume and thickness in vivo: MR imaging study. Radiology 207: 243–248, 1998.

91. Armstrong CG, Mow VC: Friction, lubrication and wear of synovial joints. In Owen R, Goodfellow J, Bullough P (eds): Scientific Foundations of Orthopaedics and Traumatology. Philadelphia, WB Saunders, 1980.

92. Goodfellow JW, O'Connor JJ: The design of synovial joints. In Owen R, Goodfellow J, Bullough P (eds): Scientific Foundations of Orthopaedics and Traumatology. Philadelphia, WB Saunders, 1980.

93. Brandt KD, Schauwecker DS, Dansereau S, et al.: Bone scintography in the canine cruciate deficiency model of osteoarthritis. Comparison of the unstable and contralateral knee. J Rheumatol 24: 140, 1997.

94. Van Osch GJVM, van der Kraan PM, Blankevoort L, et al.: Relation of ligament damage with site specific cartilage loss and osteophyte formation in collaginase induced osteoarthritis in mice. J Rheumatol 23:1227, 1996.

95. Perry J: Contractures: A historical perspective. Clin Orthop 219:8, 1987.

96. Akeson WH, Amiel D, Abel MF, et al.: Effects of immobilization on joints. Clin Orthop 219:28–37, 1987.

97. Enneking WF, Horowitz M: The intra-articular effects of immobilization on the human knee. J Bone Joint Surg Am 54:973, 1972.

98. Djurasovic M, Aldridge JW, Grumbles R, et al.: Knee joint immobilization decreases aggrecan gene expression in the meniscus. Am J Sports Med 26:460–466, 1998.

99. de Andrade JR, Grant C, Dixon St J: Joint distension and reflex muscle inhibition in the knee. J Bone Joint Surg 47A:313, 1965.

100. Young A, Stokes M, Iles JF: Effects of joint pathology on muscle. Clin Orthop 219:21, 1987.

101. Spencer JD, Hayes KC, Alexander IJ: Knee joint effusion and quadriceps reflex inhibition in man. Arch Phys Med Rehabil 65:171, 1984.

102. Stokes M, Young A: The contribution of reflex inhibition to arthrogenous muscle weakness. Clin Sci 67:7, 1984.

103. Loitz BJ, Zernicke RF, Vailas AC, et al.: Effects of short-term immobilization versus continuous passive motion on the biomechanical and biochemical properties of the rabbit tendon. Clin Orthop 244:265–271, 1989.

104. Turner CH: Three rules for bone adaptation to mechanical stimuli. Bone 23:399–407, 1998.

105. Wolff I, van Croonenborg JJ, Kemper HC, et al.: The effect of exercise training programs on bone mass: A meta-analysis of published controlled trials in pre- and postmenopausal women. Osteoporos Int 9:1–12, 1999.

106. Todd JA, Robinson RJ: Osteoporosis and exercise. Postgrad Med J 79:320–323, 2003.

107. Rubin C, Turner AS, Bain S, et al.: Anabolism. Low mechanical signals strengthen long bones. Nature 412:603–604, 2001

108. Rubin C, Turner AS, Mallinckrodt C, et al.: Mechanical strain, induced noninvasively in the high-frequency domain, is anabolic to cancellous bone, but not cortical bone. Bone 30:445–452, 2002.

109. Rubin C, Xu G, Judex S: The anabolic activity of bone tissue, suppressed by disuse, is normalized by brief exposure to extremely low-magnitude mechanical stimuli. FASEB J 15:2225–2229, 2001.

110. Lanyon LE: Using functional loading to influence bone mass and architecture: Objectives, mechanisms, and relationship with estrogen of the mechanically adaptive process in bone. Bone 18(Suppl 1):37S-43S, 1996.

111. Vanwanseele B, Lucchinetti E, Stussi E: The effects of immobilization in the characteristics of articular cartilage: Current concepts and future directions. Osteoarthritis Cartilage 10:408–419, 2002.

112. Salter RB: History of rest and motion and the scientific basis for early continuous passive motion. Hand Clin 12:1–11, 1996.

113. Curwin SL, Vailas AC, Wood J: Immature tendon adaptation to strenuous exercise. J Appl Physiol 65:2297–2301, 1988.

114. Gerriets JE, Curwin SL, Last JA: Tendon hypertrophy is associated with increased hydroxylation of nonhelical lysine residues at two specific cross-linking sites in type I collagen. J Biol Chem 268:25553–25560, 1993.

115. Hitchcock TF, Light TR, Bunch WH, et al.: The effect of immediate constrained digital motion on the strength of flexor tendon repairs in chickens. J Hand Surg [Am] 12:590–595, 1987.

116. Buchanan CI, Marsh RL: Effects of exercise on the biomechanical, biochemical and structural properties of tendons. Comp Biochem Physiol A Mol Integr Physiol 133:1101–1107, 2002.

117. Nielsen HM, Skalicky M, Viidik A: Influence of physical exercise on aging rats. III. Life-long exercise modifies the aging changes of the mechanical properties of limb muscle tendons. Mech Ageing Dev 100:243–260, 1998.

118. Silbernagel KG, Thomee R, Thomee P, et al.: Eccentric overload training for patients with chronic Achilles tendon pain—A randomised controlled study with reliability testing of the evaluation methods. Scand J Med Sci Sports 11: 197–206, 2001.

119. Vailas AC, Tipton CM, Matthes RD, et al.: Physical activity and its influence on the repair process of medial collateral ligaments. Connect Tissue Res 9:25–31, 1981.

120. Zuckerman J, Stull GA: Ligamentous separation force in rats by training, detraining and cage restriction. Med Sci Sports 5:44–49, 1973.

121. Gomez MA, Woo SL, Amiel D, et al. The effects of increased tension on healing medial collateral ligaments. Am J Sports Med 19:347–354, 1991.

122. Curwin SL: The aetiology and treatment of tendonitis. In Harries M, Williams C, Stanish WD, et al. (eds.): Oxford Textbook of Sports Medicine, pp 610–630. New York, Oxford University Press, 1998.

123. Józsa L, Kannus P: Human Tendons: Anatomy, Physiology, and Pathology. Champaign, IL, Human Kinetics, 1997.

3

Muscle Structure and Function

Gary Chleboun, PT, PhD

◆ Introduction

The skeletal muscles, like the joints, are designed to contribute to the body's needs for mobility and stability. Muscles serve a mobility function by producing or controlling the movement of a bony lever around a joint axis; they serve a stability function by resisting extraneous movement of joint surfaces and through approximation of joint surfaces. The body is incapable of either supporting itself against gravity or of producing motion without muscle function.

Human movement is a complex interaction of the muscle function and joint lever systems under the control of the nervous system. Daily, clinicians evaluate the muscle function of patients and clients in order to determine extent of the loss of muscle function and to formulate appropriate interventions to regain muscle function. Understanding muscle function begins with a clear picture of the structure of the muscle. It is the structure of the muscle from the various proteins that account for the contractile ability of the muscle to its overall size, length, and fiber type—that ultimately determines the muscle function. The interaction of muscles working over the joints of the body produces the movements we use for daily activities, work, play, and sport. Unfortunately, some of the movements may cause injury to the muscles and tendons. The following case identifies a common muscle injury. Throughout this chapter, you will see how the structure and function of the muscles can be applied to this clinical situation.

3-1   Patient Case

Vik Patel, a 50-year-old man, was playing softball one summer evening. He was trying to catch a fly ball when he stepped back with his right foot and slipped slightly. As his foot slipped, the motion at the ankle was dorsiflexion and the ankle plantar flexor muscles were contracting as he tried to push off so that he could run forward. At the moment of trying to push off, he felt a twinge of pain in the right calf muscle. Vik states that he has pain in the calf muscle and along the Achilles tendon when he tries to stand on his toes and when he does calf-stretching exercises. After evaluation of Vik, it appears that he might have strained the calf muscle or caused some tendinitis.

◈ Elements of Muscle Structure

Skeletal muscles are composed of muscle tissue (contractile) and connective tissue (noncontractile). The muscle tissue has the ability to develop tension in response to chemical, electrical, or mechanical stimuli. The connective tissue, on the other hand, develops tension in response to passive loading.[1] The properties of these tissues and the way in which they are interrelated give muscles their unique characteristics.

Composition of a Muscle Fiber

■ Contractile Proteins

A skeletal muscle is composed of many thousands of muscle fibers. A single muscle contains many **fascicles,** a group of muscle fibers (cells) surrounded by connective tissue (Fig. 3-1A). The arrangement, number, size, and type of these fibers may vary from muscle to muscle,[2,3] but each fiber is a single muscle cell that is enclosed in a cell membrane called the **sarcolemma** (see Fig. 3-1B). Like other cells in the body, the muscle fiber is composed of cytoplasm, which in a muscle is called **sarcoplasm.** The sarcoplasm contains **myofibrils** (see Fig. 3-1C), which are the contractile structures of a muscle fiber and nonmyofibrillar structures such as ribosomes, glycogen, and mitochondria, which are required for cell metabolism.

The myofibril is composed of thick **myofilaments** composed of the protein **myosin** and thin filaments composed of the protein **actin** (see Fig. 3-1D). The interaction of these two myofilaments is essential for a muscle contraction to occur. The thin myofilaments are formed by two chainlike strings of actin molecules wound around each other. Molecules of the globular

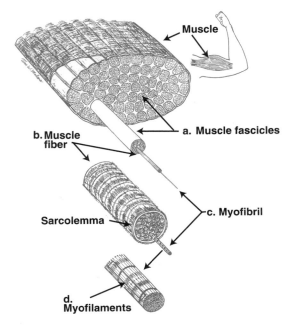

▲ **Figure 3-1** ■ Composition of a muscle fiber. **A.** Groups of muscle fibers form bundles called **fascicles. B.** The muscle fiber is enclosed in a cell membrane called the **sarcolemma. C.** The muscle fiber contains myofibrillar structures called **myofibrils. D.** The myofibril is composed of thick myosin and thin actin **myofilaments.**

protein **troponin** are found in notches between the two actin strings and the protein **tropomyosin** is attached to each troponin molecule (Fig. 3-2A). The troponin and tropomyosin molecules control the binding of actin and myosin myofilaments.

Each of the myosin molecules has globular enlargements called **head groups** (see Fig. 3-2B).[4] The head groups, which are able to swivel and are the binding sites for attachment to the actin, play a critical role in muscle contraction and relaxation. When the entire myofibril is viewed through a microscope, the alternation of thick (myosin) and thin (actin) myofilaments forms a distinctive striped pattern, as seen in Figure 3-1D. Therefore, skeletal muscle is often called **striated muscle.** A schematic representation of the ordering of the myofilaments in a myofibril is presented in Figure 3-3.

■ Structural Proteins

The muscle fiber also consists of several structural proteins (see Patel and Lieber[5] for a review of these proteins). Some of these proteins (**intermediate filaments**) provide a structural scaffold for the muscle fiber, whereas others (e.g., **desmin**) may be involved in the transmission of force along the fiber and to adjoining fibers. One protein, **titin,** has a particularly important role maintaining the position of the thick filament during a muscle contraction and in the development of passive tension.[6,7] Titin is a large protein that is attached along the thick filament and spans the gap from the thick filament to the Z lines (Fig. 3-4). More

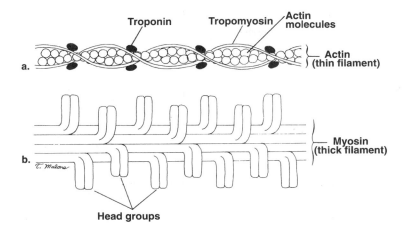

◀ **Figure 3-2** ■ Myofilaments. **A.** The actin molecules are shown as circles. The troponin molecules are globular and are shown located in notches between the two strands of actin molecules. The tropomyosin molecules are thin and are shown lying along grooves in the actin strands. **B.** A myosin myofilament showing head groups or globular enlargements.

will be said about titin in the discussion on the passive length-tension relationship.

The Contractile Unit

■ Organization of the Contractile Unit

The portion of the myofibril that is located between two Z disks is called the **sarcomere** (see Fig. 3-3). The Z disks, which are located at regular intervals throughout the myofibril, not only serve as boundaries for the sarcomere but also link the thin filaments together. Areas of the sarcomere called **bands** or **zones** help to identify the arrangement of the thick and thin filaments. The portion of the sarcomere that extends over both the length of the thick filaments and a small portion of the thin filaments is called the **anisotropic** or **A band.** Areas that include only actin filaments are called **isotropic** or **I bands.**[4] The terms anisotropic and isotropic refer to the behavior of these portions of the fibers when light shines on them. The central portion of the thick filament (A band area) in which there is no overlap with the thin filaments is called the **H zone.** The central portion of the H zone, which consists of the

wide middle portion of the thick filament, is called the **M band.**

■ Cross-Bridge Interaction

Interaction between the thick and thin filaments of the sarcomere leading to muscle contraction is initiated by the arrival of a nerve impulse at the motor end plate, which evokes an electric impulse, or **action potential,** that travels along the muscle fiber.[8] The action potential initiates the release of calcium ions,[9] and the calcium ions cause troponin to reposition the tropomyosin molecules so that receptor sites on the actin are free and the head groups of the myosin can bind with actin. This bonding of filaments is called a **cross-bridge.** Tension is generated with the inclusion of the hydrolysis of adenosine triphosphate (ATP) and the release of adenosine diphosphate (ADP) from the myosin head[1,10,11] (Fig. 3-5).

■ Types of Muscle Contraction

The sliding of the thin filaments toward and past the thick filaments, accompanied by the formation and re-formation of cross-bridges in each sarcomere, will result in shortening of the muscle fiber and the generation of

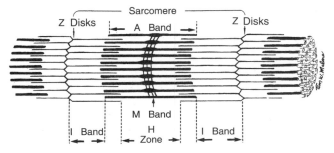

▲ **Figure 3-3** ■ Ordering of myofibrils in a muscle at rest. The sarcomere is the portion of the myofibril that is located between the Z disks. The A band portion of the sarcomere contains an overlap of the myosin and actin filaments. The portion of the A band that contains only myosin filaments without overlap is called the H zone. The M band, located in the central portion of the H zone, contains transversely oriented myosin filaments that connect one myosin filament with another. The I band portion contains only actin fibers.

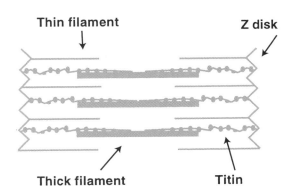

▲ **Figure 3-4** ■ Sarcomere depicting the relationship between titin and the thick and thin filaments.

tension. The muscle fiber will shorten (contract) if a sufficient number of sarcomeres actively shorten and if either one or both ends of the muscle fiber are free to move. The active shortening of a muscle is called a **concentric contraction,** or shortening contraction (Fig. 3-6). In contrast to a shortening contraction, in which the thin filaments are being pulled toward the thick filaments, the muscle may undergo an **eccentric contraction,** or lengthening contraction. In a lengthening contraction, the thin filaments are pulled away from the thick filaments, and cross-bridges are broken and re-formed as the muscle lengthens. Tension is generated by the muscle as cross-bridges are re-formed. Eccentric contractions occur whenever a muscle actively resists motion created by an external force (such as gravity). The muscle fiber will not change length if the force created by the cross-bridge cycling is matched by the external force. The contraction of a muscle fiber without changing length is called an **isometric contraction.**

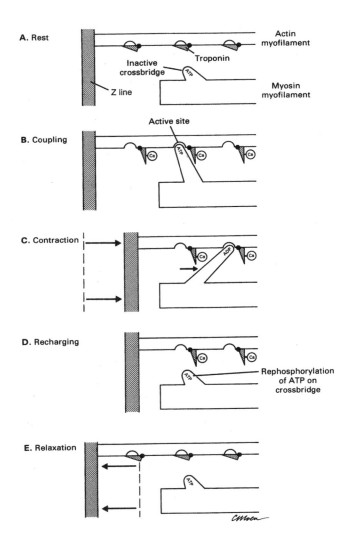

▲ **Figure 3-5** ■ Cross-bridge cycle. **A.** Rest. Cross-bridges project from a myosin myofilament but are not coupled with an actin myofilament. Adenosine triphosphate (ATP) is attached near the head of the cross-bridge; troponin covers the active sites on the actin myofilament; and calcium ions are stored in the sarcoplasmic reticulum. **B.** Coupling. Arrival of the muscle action potential depolarizes the sarcolemma and T tubules; calcium ions are released and react with troponin; and change in the shape of the troponin-calcium complex uncovers active sites on actin; a cross-bridge couples with an adjacent active site, thereby linking myosin and actin myofilaments. **C.** Contraction. Linkage of a cross-bridge and an active site triggers adenosine triphospatase (ATPase) activity of myosin; ATP splits into adenosine diphosphate (ADP) + PO_4 + energy; the reaction produces a transient flexion of the cross-bridge; the actin myofilament is pulled a short distance past the myosin myofilament; and Z disks are moved closer together. **D.** Recharging. The cross-bridge uncouples from the active site and retracts; ATP is replaced on the cross-bridge. The recoupling, flexion, uncoupling, retraction, and recharging processes are repeated hundreds of times per second. **E.** Relaxation. Cessation of excitation occurs; calcium ions are removed from the vicinity of the actin myofilament and are returned to storage sites in the sarcoplasmic reticulum; troponin returns to its original shape, covering active sites on the actin myofilament; and actin and myosin myofilaments return to the rest state. (From Smith LK, Weiss EL, Lemkuhl LD [eds]: Brunnstrom's Clinical Kinesiology, 5th ed. Philadelphia, FA Davis, 1996, p 83, with permission.)

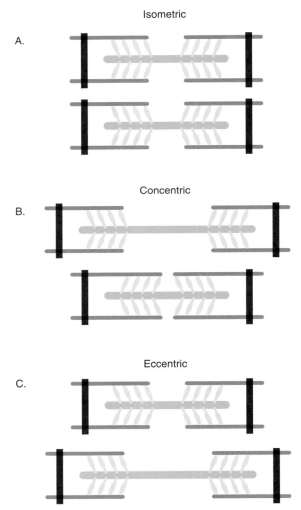

▲ **Figure 3-6** ■ Types of muscle contraction from the perspective of change (or lack of change) in sarcomere length during the contraction. **A.** Isometric contraction with no change in length. **B.** Concentric or shortening muscle contraction. **C.** Eccentric or lengthening muscle contraction. The top illustration in each type of contraction represents the beginning of the contraction, and the bottom illustration represents the end of the contraction.

Continuing Exploration: **Terminology: Muscle Action versus Muscle Contraction**

A potentially more accurate way to describe the types of muscle "contraction" is to use the term "action." Because the word contract means to draw together or shorten, it is an oxymoron to refer to an "eccentric contraction" or "lengthening contraction." However, during the eccentric contraction, the contractile units (cross-bridges) are attempting to contract and pull the thin filaments toward the thick filaments, but the external forces are greater than the internal forces, which results in lengthening. Therefore, the term "contraction" implies the attempt to shorten and the term "eccentric" describes the lengthening. We have chosen to use the more common term "contraction" in this text, but we realize that muscle "action" is a synonymous term.

Case Application 3-1: **Possible Mechanism of Injury**

In the case study at the beginning of the chapter, our patient, Vik, stepped back with his right foot, causing the foot to go into dorsiflexion. The external force was greater than the muscle force; therefore, the muscle was lengthened as it tried to resist the external force (an example of an eccentric contraction). This situation is a common mechanism of injury to the muscle and/or tendon that will result in pain localized to the muscle or tendon.

 CONCEPT CORNERSTONE 3-1: *Muscle Contraction Facts*

The following is a summary of the important facts about muscle contraction at the sarcomere level:

- Tension is generated whenever cross-bridges are formed.
- Calcium influx initiates the muscle contraction.
- ATP hydrolysis fuels the cross-bridge cycle.
- In a concentric contraction, the thin myofilaments are pulled toward the thick myofilaments, and cross-bridges are formed, broken, and re-formed.
- In an eccentric contraction, the thin myofilaments are pulled away from the thick myofilaments, and cross-bridges are broken, re-formed, and broken.
- In an isometric contraction, the length of the muscle fiber is constant.

The Motor Unit

■ Organization of the Motor Unit

Although the sarcomere is the basic unit of tension in a muscle, it is actually part of a larger complex called the motor unit. The **motor unit** consists of the alpha motor neuron and all of the muscle fibers it innervates. The stimulus that the muscle fiber receives initiating the contractile process is transmitted through an **alpha**

motor neuron (Fig. 3-7). The cell body of the neuron is located in the anterior horn of the spinal cord. The nerve cell **axon** extends from the cell body to the muscle, where it divides into either a few or as many as thousands of smaller branches. Each of the smaller branches terminates in a motor end plate that lies in close approximation to the sarcolemma of a single muscle fiber. All of the muscle fibers on which a branch of the axon terminates are part of one motor unit, along with the cell body and the axon.

The contraction of the entire muscle is the result of many motor units firing *asynchronously* and *repeatedly*. The magnitude of the contraction of the entire muscle may be altered by changing the number of motor units that are activated or the frequency at which they are activated. The number of motor units in a muscle, as well as the structure of these units, varies from muscle to muscle.

Motor units vary according to the size of the neuron cell body, diameter of the axon, number of muscle fibers, and type of muscle fibers. Each of these variations in structure affects the function of the motor unit. Some motor units have small cell bodies, and others have large cell bodies. Units that have small cell bodies have small-diameter axons (see Fig. 3-7). Nerve impulses take longer to travel through small-diameter axons than they do through large-diameter axons. Therefore, in the small-diameter units, a stimulus will take longer to reach the muscle fibers than it will in a unit with a large-diameter axon.

The size of the motor unit is determined by the number of muscle fibers that it contains and the size of the motor nerve axon (see Fig. 3-7). The number of fibers may vary from two or three to a few thousand. Muscles that either control fine movements or are used to make small adjustments have small-size motor units. Such motor units generally have small cell bodies and small-diameter axons. Muscles that are used to produce large increments in force and large movements usually have a predominance of large-size motor units, large cell bodies, and large-diameter axons. The motor units of the small muscles that control eye motions may contain as few as six muscle fibers, whereas the gastrocnemius muscles have motor units that contain about 2000 muscle fibers.[4] Muscles with a predominantly large number of fibers per motor unit usually have a relatively smaller total number of motor units than do muscles that have few fibers per motor unit. The platysma muscle in the neck has relatively small motor units consisting of approximately 25 muscle fibers each, but the muscle has a total of 1000 of these motor units. The gastrocnemius, on the other hand, has relatively large motor units consisting of about 2000 muscle fibers per unit, but the muscle has a relatively small number (600) of such units. In most instances, a muscle has at least some mix of small and large motor units.

■ Recruitment of Motor Units

Usually, when an isometric muscle action is desired, the motor units with the small cell bodies and few motor

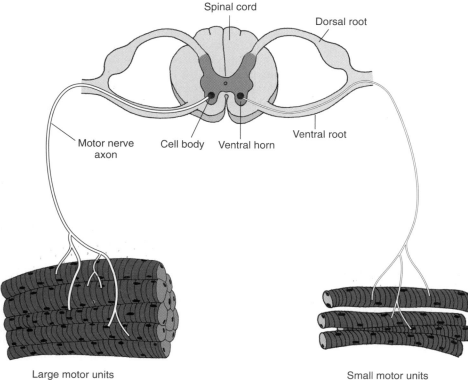

Spinal cord

Dorsal root

Ventral root

Motor nerve axon   Cell body   Ventral horn

Large motor units
- Large axon
- Many fibers, primarily Type II fibers
- Recruited in forceful contractions

Small motor units
- Small axon
- Fewer fibers, primarily Type I fibers
- Recruited first in most activities

◄ **Figure 3-7** ■ An alpha motor neuron. The cell body is in the ventral horn with the motor axon leaving the ventral root. As can be seen in the diagram, the muscle fibers innervated by a single axon are not necessarily located next to one another. The size of the motor unit is determined by the number of muscle fibers that it contains and by the size of the motor nerve axon. Large units may contain as many as a few thousand muscle fibers, whereas small units may contain as few as three.

fibers are recruited first by the nervous system and then, as force is increased, larger motor units are recruited.[12,13] This recruitment strategy is referred to as the size principle of motor unit recruitment.[12] Small motor units generate less tension than do large motor units and require less energy expenditure, and therefore this recruitment strategy is thought to be energy conserving. If a few small motor units are capable of accomplishing the task, the recruitment of large motor units is unnecessary. If the task demands are such that the small motor units are unable to complete the task, larger motor units can be recruited. However, the recruitment strategy may be based not only on energy conservation but also on previous experience; the nature of the task[14] (how rapidly the muscle must respond or the anticipated magnitude of the required force); type of muscle action[13,15] (concentric, eccentric, or isometric); and a mechanism that takes into account the actions of all muscles around a joint, including such considerations as the muscle's mechanical advantage at a particular point in the range of motion (ROM). The recruitment strategy also may involve the selection of motor units from not just one but a variety of muscles surrounding a joint to accomplish a particular task.[16] The frequency of firing of a motor unit also affects the force modulation. The contribution of recruitment or firing frequency to the development of muscle force

may be different, depending on the muscle. Small, distal muscles tend to rely more on increased frequency of firing, and larger, proximal muscles rely more on recruitment of additional motor units.[17]

Case Application 3-2: **Possible Role of High-Velocity Eccentric Contraction in Injury**

Vik was most likely performing a high-velocity eccentric contraction of the plantar flexor muscles, and he may have been selectively recruiting fast motor units rather than relying on the sequential recruitment of slow motor units and then fast motor units. This may have contributed to the high forces he experienced and increased chance of injury.

CONCEPT CORNERSTONE 3-2: *Summary of Factors Affecting Active Muscle Tension*

To review: tension of the whole muscle may be affected by

- the number of muscle fibers (which affects the magnitude of the response to a stimulus).
- the diameter of the axon (which determines the conduction velocity of the impulse).

- the number of motor units that are firing at any one time (which affects the total response of the muscle).
- the frequency of motor unit firing (which affects the total response of the muscle).

In addition, the type of muscle fibers contained within a motor unit will affect the response of a muscle. All of the muscle fibers contained in a single motor unit are of one type, but the type of muscle fibers within a muscle may vary from one motor unit to another motor unit.

Muscle Structure

■ Fiber Types

Three principal types of muscle fibers are found in varying proportions in human skeletal muscles. These fiber types may be distinguished from one another histochemically, metabolically, morphologically, and mechanically. Although there are different systems of nomenclature used in different texts,[18] in this text the three primary muscle fiber types will be referred to as type I (slow), type IIA (intermediate), and type IIB (fast) (Table 3-1).[19] In this classification system, which is the most common system for human skeletal muscle fiber typing, the myofibrillar ATPase activity under varying acidic and alkaline conditions is used to delineate fiber types. In fact, several intermediate fiber types have been identified through this scheme.

Continuing Exploration: **Another Muscle Fiber Classification Scheme**

Another scheme uses the response of the muscle to metabolic enzymes. This scheme identifies three main fiber types as fast-twitch glycolytic (FG), fast-twitch oxidative glycolytic (FOG), and slow-twitch oxidative (SO).[20] This nomenclature is based on the combination of reactions of cellular enzymes with substrates to identify myofibrillar ATPase activity (fast versus slow), succinate dehydrogenase activity (oxidative potential), and α-glycerophosphate dehydrogenase activity (glycolytic potential). It is often assumed that the two schemes are interchangeable; however, this may not be the case. There appears to be much overlap of metabolic enzyme activity between type IIA and type IIB. The fact that meta-

bolic enzyme activity levels depend on the degree of training of the muscle suggests that these two schemes may not be the same. Another scheme, using immunohistochemical analysis (identification of portions of the myosin molecule with antibodies), has found that the type I, IIA, and IIB fibers correspond to specifically different types of myosin molecules (myosin heavy chain [MHC] I, MHC IIA, and MHC IIB).[19] The combination of this scheme and the myosin ATPase system provides an estimate of the contractile properties of the muscle. Whichever classification scheme is used, it should be remembered that there is actually a continuum of fiber types without exact distinctions between types.

Each skeletal muscle in the body is composed of a combination of each of the three types of fibers, but variations exist among individuals in the percentage of each fiber type in similar muscles. The variations in fiber types among individuals are believed to be genetically determined. In postmortem studies, the vastus lateralis, rectus femoris, deltoid, and gastrocnemius muscles have been found to be similar among individuals in that they contain about 50% type II and 50% type I fibers,[2] and the hamstrings contain about 50% to 55% type II and 45% to 50% type I fibers.[21,22] In studies using muscle biopsy samples from younger subjects, the vastus lateralis tends to be about 54% type II fibers and 46% type I fibers.[23] Although the differences may be subtle, fiber type changes with age so that there is a decrease in the number and size of the type II fibers. This may account for the differences seen in many of the studies documenting fiber type percentages.

The soleus muscle, on the other hand, contains up to 80% type I fibers.[24] Muscles that have a relatively high proportion of type I fibers in relation to type II fibers, such as the soleus muscle, are able to carry on sustained activity because the type I fibers do not fatigue rapidly. These muscles are often called **stability** or **postural** muscles. The relatively small, slow motor units of the soleus muscle (with small cell bodies, small-diameter axons, and a small number of muscle fibers per motor unit) are almost continually active during erect standing so as to make the small adjustments in muscle tension that are required to maintain body balance and counteract the effects of gravity. Muscles that have a higher proportion of the type II fibers, such as the hamstring muscles, are sometimes designated as **mobility** or **nonpostural** muscles. These muscles are involved in producing a large ROM of the bony components.[21,22] The type II fibers respond more rapidly to a stimulus but also fatigue more rapidly than do type I fibers. After intermittent bouts of high-intensity exercise, muscles with a high proportion of type II fibers, which involve a large initial response, show greater fatigue and recover more slowly than do muscles with a high proportion of type I fibers.[25] Although muscle fiber type is important in determining the function of a muscle, there are other aspects of muscle structure that also play an important role in determining function.

Table 3-1	Characteristics of Skeletal Muscle Fibers		
	Type I (Slow Oxidative)	Type IIA (Fast Oxidative Glycolytic)	Type IIB (Fast Glycolytic)
Diameter	Small	Intermediate	Large
Muscle color	Red	Red	White
Capillarity	Dense	Dense	Sparse
Myoglobin content	High	Intermediate	Low
Speed of contraction	Slow	Fast	Fast
Rate of fatigue	Slow	Intermediate	Fast

Case Application 3-3: **Muscle Fiber Type Identification of Injured Muscle**

Vik injured his plantar flexor muscles, which include the gastrocnemius and soleus muscles. However, because fiber type is related to muscle function, it is reasonable to make assumptions as to which muscle may have been preferentially injured. Because the soleus muscle is composed primarily of type I fibers (postural control) and the gastrocnemius is composed primarily of type II fibers (power and mobility), the gastrocnemius was likely selectively recruited and therefore more likely injured.

■ Muscle Architecture: Size, Arrangement, and Length

Many human muscles have an approximately equal proportion of fast and slow fiber types. Therefore, the determination of muscle function should not be based solely on this single characteristic. In fact, the architecture of the whole muscle may be more important in determining muscle function than the fiber type.[26] The description of skeletal muscle architecture includes the arrangement of the fibers in relation to the axis of force (amount of pennation), muscle fiber length, muscle length, muscle mass, and the **physiologic cross-sectional area** (**PCSA**). These structural variations affect not only the overall shape and size of the muscles but also the function of the skeletal muscles.

The two most important architectural characteristics that affect muscle function are the muscle fiber length and the PCSA. The fiber length (or the number of sarcomeres along the fiber) directly determines the amount of shortening or lengthening of the fiber. Consequently, a long muscle fiber, with more sarcomeres in series, is capable of shortening over a greater distance than a short muscle fiber. For example, if muscle fibers are capable of shortening to about 50% of resting length, a muscle fiber that is 6 cm long is able to shorten 3 cm, whereas a fiber that is 4 cm long is able to shorten only 2 cm. The significance of the preceding example is that a hypothetical muscle with long fibers is able to move the bony lever to which it is attached through a greater distance than is a muscle with short fibers. However, the relationship between the muscle fiber length and the distance that it is able to move a bony lever is not always a direct relationship. The arrangement of the muscle fibers and the length of the moment arm (MA) of the muscle affect the length-shortening relationship, and, therefore, both fiber length and MA must be considered.

The PCSA is a measure of the cross-sectional area of the muscle perpendicular to the orientation of the muscle fibers. The amount of force that a muscle produces is directly proportional to the number of sarcomeres aligned side by side (or in parallel). Therefore, if there are a large number of fibers packed into a muscle (as in a pennate muscle) or if the fiber increases in size (addition of myofibrils), the ability to produce

force will be increased.[27] A good example of the relationship between muscle architecture and function is the comparison between the quadriceps and hamstring muscles. The quadriceps muscles have a larger PSCA, and the hamstring muscles have longer fibers. This architectural arrangement suggests that the quadriceps muscles are designed for force production and the hamstring muscles are designed for movements requiring a larger ROM. Because most of the hamstring muscles cross two joints (hip and knee), it would be expected that the muscle would need longer fibers for the greater excursion during movements of both the hip and the knee.

Arrangement of fascicles (muscle fiber groups) varies among muscles. The fasciculi may be parallel to the long axis of the muscle (Fig. 3-8A), may spiral around the long axis (see Fig. 3-8B), or may be at an angle to the long axis (see Fig. 3-8C). Muscles that have a parallel fiber arrangement (parallel to the long axis and to each other) are designated as **strap** or **fusiform** muscles. In strap muscles, such as the sternocleidomastoid, the fascicles are long and extend throughout the length of the muscle. However, in the rectus abdominis, which also is considered to be a strap muscle, the fascicles are divided into short segments by fibrous intersections. In fusiform muscles, most but not all of the muscle fibers extend throughout the length of the muscle. In general, muscles with a parallel fiber arrangement will produce a greater ROM of a bony lever than will muscles with a pennate fiber arrangement. This is again related to muscle fiber length, as discussed previously. Fusiform muscles tend to have longer fiber length than do pennated muscles.

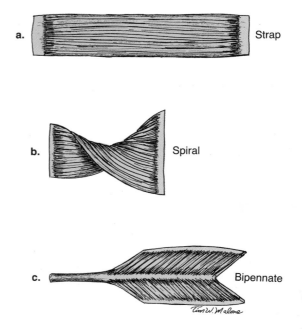

▲ **Figure 3-8** ■ Arrangement of fasciculi in a muscle. **A.** Parallel arrangement. **B.** Spiral arrangement. **C.** Bipennate arrangement.

Muscles that have a fiber arrangement oblique to the muscle's long axis are called pennate muscles because the fiber arrangement resembles that found in a feather. The fibers that make up the fascicles in pennate muscles are usually shorter and more numerous than the fibers in many of the strap muscles. In **unipennate** muscles, such as the flexor pollicis longus, the obliquely set fascicles fan out on only one side of a central muscle tendon. In a **bipennate** muscle, such as the gastrocnemius, the fascicles are obliquely set on both sides of a central tendon. In a **multipennate** muscle, such as the soleus or subscapularis, the oblique fascicles converge on several tendons.

The oblique angle of the muscle fibers in a pennate muscle disrupts the direct relationship between the length of the muscle fiber and the distance that the total muscle can move a bony part and decreases the amount of force that is directed along the long axis of the muscle. Only a portion of the force of the pennate muscles goes toward producing motion of the bony lever. In fact, the more oblique a fiber lies to the long axis of the muscle, the less force the muscle is able to exert at the tendon. This decrease in muscle force is a function of the cosine of the pennation angle. Many human muscles have a pennation angle that is less than 30° at rest. Therefore, the muscle force at the tendon will be decreased by a maximum of 13% (cos 30° = 0.87).[28] When muscle shortens during muscle contraction and joint movement, the pennation angle becomes much more oblique, thus potentially affecting the tendon force to an even greater degree.[29,30] This potential decreased force at the tendon, however, is offset because pennate muscles usually have a large number of muscle fibers as a result of increased fiber packing, thus increasing PCSA. Therefore, despite the loss of force as a result of pennation, a pennated muscle, such as the soleus, is still able to transmit a large amount of force to the tendon to which it attaches.

Muscular Connective Tissue

■ **Organization of Connective Tissue in Muscle**

Muscles and muscle fibers, like other soft tissues in the body, are surrounded and supported by connective tissue. The sarcolemma of individual muscle fibers is surrounded by connective tissue called the **endomysium,** and groups of muscle fibers are covered by connective tissue called the **perimysium.** The myofibril is connected to the endomysium via specialized proteins. The endomysium and perimysium are continuous with the outer connective tissue sheath called the **epimysium,** which envelops the entire muscle (Fig. 3-9). The myotendinous junction is an intricate connection between muscle fibers and the connective tissue of the tendon. Many special proteins are arranged to make this junction strong. Tendons are attached to bones by **Sharpey fibers,** which become continuous with the periosteum.

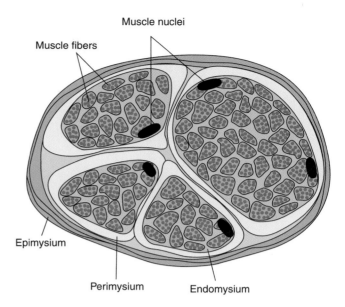

▲ **Figure 3-9** ■ Muscular connective tissue. A schematic cross-sectional view of the connective tissue in a muscle shows how the perimysium is continuous with the outer layer of epimysium and the endomysium surrounds each muscle fiber.

Case Application 3-4: **Myotendinous Junction as a Possible Site of Injury**

Although the myotendinous junction is designed to be strong and able to transmit the larger forces from the muscle to the tendon, the myotendinous junction is often the site of muscle strain injuries. This could be one explanation for the location of the injury in the case of our softball player patient.

Other connective tissues associated with muscles are in the form of fasciae, aponeuroses, and sheaths. Fasciae can be divided into two zones: superficial and deep. The zone of **superficial fasciae,** composed of loose tissue, is located directly under the dermis. This zone contributes to the mobility of the skin, acts as an insulator, and may contain skin muscles such as the platysma in the neck. The zone of **deep fasciae** is composed of compacted and regularly arranged collagenous fibers. The deep fasciae attach to muscles and bones and may form tracts or bands and retinacula. For example, the deep femoral fasciae in the lower extremity forms a tract known as the **iliotibial tract** or **band.** This tract transmits the pull of two of the lower-extremity muscles to the bones of the leg (Fig. 3-10). **Retinacula** are formed by localized transverse thickenings of the fasciae, which form a loop that is attached at both ends to bone (Fig. 3-11A). The tunnels formed by retinacula retain or prevent tendons from bowing out of position during muscle action (see Fig. 3-11B). Sometimes deep fasciae are indistinguishable from aponeuroses, which are sheets of dense white

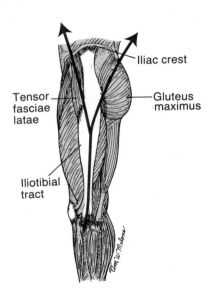

▲ **Figure 3-10** ■ Iliotibial tract. A lateral view of the left lower limb showing the deep fascial iliotibial tract extending from the tubercle of the iliac crest to the lateral aspect of the knee. The right arrow represents the pull of the gluteus maximus. The left arrow represents the pull of the tensor fasciae latae.

compacted collagen fibers that attach directly or indirectly to muscles, fasciae, bones, cartilage, and other muscles. Aponeuroses distribute forces generated by the muscle to the structures to which they are attached.[1]

■ **Parallel and Series Elastic Components of Muscle**

All of the connective tissue in a muscle is interconnected and constitutes the **passive elastic component** of a muscle. The connective tissues that surround the muscle, plus the sarcolemma, the elastic protein titin, and other structures (i.e., nerves and blood vessels), form the **parallel elastic component** of a muscle. When a muscle lengthens or shortens, these tissues also lengthen or shorten, because they function in parallel to the muscle

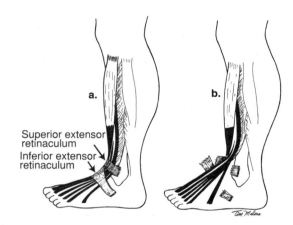

▲ **Figure 3-11** ■ Retinacula. **A.** The superior and inferior retinacula are shown in their normal position, in which they form a tunnel for the tendons from the extensor muscles of the lower leg. **B.** When the retinacula are torn or removed, the tendons move anteriorly.

contractile unit. For example, the collagen fibers in the perimysium of fusiform muscles are slack when the sarcomeres are at rest but straighten out and become taut as sarcomere lengths increase. As the perimysium is lengthened, it also becomes **stiffer** (resistance to further elongation increases). The increased resistance of perimysium to elongation may prevent overstretching of the muscle fiber bundles and may contribute to the tension at the tendon.[31] When sarcomeres shorten from their resting position, the slack collagen fibers within the parallel elastic component buckle (crimp) even further. Whatever tension might have existed in the collagen at rest is diminished by the shortening of the sarcomere. Because of the many parallel elastic components of a muscle, the increase or decrease in passive tension can substantially affect the total tension output of a muscle. This relationship between length and tension will be addressed in the next section.

The tendon of the muscle is considered to function in **series** with the contractile elements. This means that the tendon will be under tension when the muscle actively produces tension. When the contractile elements in a muscle actively shorten, they exert a pull on the tendon. The pull must be of sufficient magnitude to take up the slack (compliance) in the tendon so that the muscle pull can be transmitted through the tendon to the bony lever (Fig. 3-12). Fortunately, the **compliance** (or **extensibility**) of the tendon is relatively small (about 3% to 10% in human muscles). Thus, most of the muscle force can be used for moving the bony lever and is not dissipated stretching the tendon. The tendon is also under tension when a muscle is controlling or braking the motion of the lever in an eccentric contraction. A tendon is under reduced tension only when a muscle is completely relaxed and in a relatively shortened position.

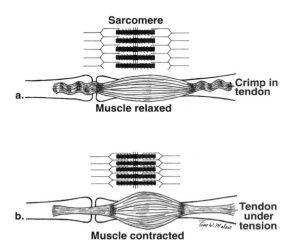

▲ **Figure 3-12** ■ Series elastic component. **A.** The muscle is shown in a relaxed state with the tendon slack (crimping or buckling of collagen fibers has occurred). The sarcomere depicted above the muscle shows minimal overlap of thick and thin filaments and little cross-bridge formation. **B.** The muscle in an actively shortened position shows that the tendons are under tension and no crimp can be observed. The sarcomere depicted above the muscle shows extensive overlap of filaments and cross-bridge formation.

Muscle Function

Muscle Tension

The most important characteristic of a muscle is its ability to develop tension and to exert a force on the bony lever. Tension can be either active or passive, and the total tension that a muscle can develop includes both active and passive components. Total tension, which was identified in Chapter 1 as Fms, is a vector quantity that has (1) magnitude, (2) two points of application (at the proximal and distal muscle attachments), (3) an action line, and (4) direction of pull. The point of application, action line, and direction of pull were the major part of the discussion of muscle force in Chapter 1, but we now need to turn our attention to the determinants of the component called magnitude of the muscle force, or the total muscle tension.

■ Passive Tension

Passive tension refers to tension developed in the parallel elastic component of the muscle. Passive tension in the parallel elastic component is created by lengthening the muscle beyond the slack length of the tissues. The parallel elastic component may add to the active tension produced by the muscle when the muscle is lengthened, or it may become slack and not contribute to the total tension when the muscle is shortened. The total tension that develops during an active contraction of a muscle is a combination of the passive (noncontractile) tension added to the active (contractile) tension (Fig. 3-13) .

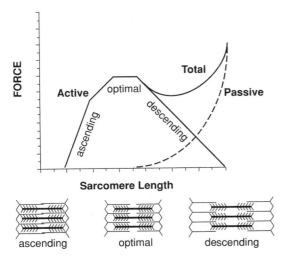

▲ **Figure 3-13** ■ The skeletal muscle sarcomere length-tension relationship. Active, passive, and the total curves are shown. The plateau of the active curve signifies optimal sarcomere length where maximum active tension is developed. Isometric tension decreases as the muscle is lengthened because fewer cross-bridges are able to be formed. Tension decreases as the muscle is shortened because of interdigitation of the thin filaments. The increase in passive tension with elongation of the muscle is shown by the dashed line. Passive plus active tension results in the total amount of tension developed by the muscle fiber.

Continuing Exploration: **Passive Muscle Stiffness**

Passive muscle stiffness is an important property of skeletal muscle. The passive stiffness of an isolated muscle (not connected to bones and joints) is the slope of the passive length-tension relationship. The steeper the slope is, the greater is the stiffness in the muscle. The passive stiffness of a muscle attached to bone and crossing a joint is the slope of the torque-angle relationship (Fig. 3-14). **Titin** is the primary structure of the muscle that accounts for the stiffness of the muscle (see Lieber[28] for a review of the role of titin). On the other hand, the connective tissues in and around the muscle (perimysium and endomysium) are responsible for the extent to which the muscle can be elongated.[31] This is often referred to as the muscle extensibility or flexibility.

■ Active Tension

Active tension refers to tension developed by the contractile elements of the muscle. Active tension in a muscle is initiated by cross-bridge formation and movement of the thick and thin filaments. The amount of active tension that a muscle can generate depends on neural factors and mechanical properties of the muscle fibers. The neural factors that can modulate the amount of active tension include the frequency, number, and size of motor units that are firing. The mechanical properties of muscle that determine the active tension are the isometric length-tension relationship and the force-velocity relationship.

■ Isometric Length-Tension Relationship

One of the most fundamental concepts in muscle physiology is the direct relationship between isometric tension development in a muscle fiber and the length of the sarcomeres in a muscle fiber.[32] The identification of this relationship was, and continues to be, the primary evidence supporting the sliding filament theory of muscle contraction. The isometric sarcomere length-tension relationship was experimentally determined with isolated single muscle fibers under very controlled circumstances. There is an optimal sarcomere length at which a muscle fiber is capable of developing maximal isometric tension (see Fig. 3-13). Muscle fibers develop maximal isometric tension at optimal sarcomere length because the thick and thin filaments are positioned so that the maximum number of cross-bridges within the sarcomere can be formed. If the muscle fiber is lengthened or shortened beyond optimal length, the amount of active tension that the muscle fiber is able to generate when stimulated decreases (see Fig. 3-13). When a muscle fiber is lengthened beyond optimal length, there is less overlap between the thick and thin filaments and consequently fewer possibilities for cross-bridge formation. However, the passive elastic tension in the parallel component may be increased when the muscle is elongated. This passive tension is added to the active tension, resulting in the total tension (see Fig. 3-13).

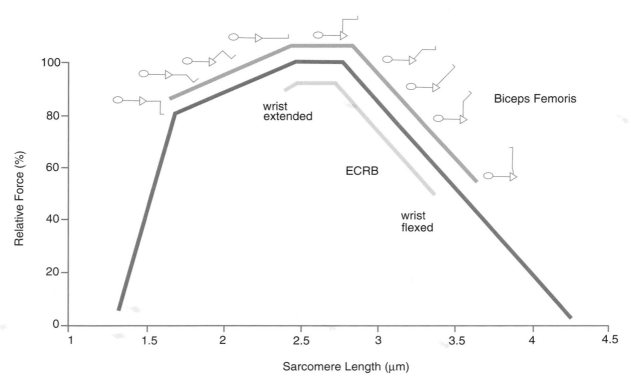

▲ **Figure 3-14** ■ The sarcomere length-tension relationship for the human extensor carpi radialis brevis (ECRB) and the biceps femoris, long head. The data for the ECRB were determined from intraoperative laser diffraction measurement of the sarcomere length, and the data from the biceps femoris were calculated on the basis of ultrasound measurements of the change in fascicle length with joint position.[35] The black line is the presumed length-tension relationship of human muscle, based on the known lengths of human thin and thick filaments. (Adapted from Chleboun GS, France AR, Crill MT, et al.: *In vivo* measurement of fascicle length and pennation angle of the human biceps femoris muscle. Cells Tissues Organs 169:401–409, 2001 with permission.)

A similar loss of isometric tension or diminished capacity for developing tension occurs when a muscle fiber is shortened from its optimal sarcomere length. When the sarcomere is at shorter lengths, the distance between the Z disks decreases and there is interdigitation of the filaments. The interdigitation of the thick and thin filaments may interfere with the formation of cross-bridges from the myosin molecules, thus decreasing the active force.

It must be remembered that the sarcomere length-tension relationship was determined with isometric contractions and therefore should apply, in the strict sense, only to isometric muscle contraction. In addition, as we will see in the following section, the full range of sarcomere lengthening and shortening may be possible only in experiments with isolated muscle. Sarcomere length obviously changes during dynamic contractions (concentric and eccentric contractions) that affect the tension that can be developed in the muscle. However, during dynamic contractions, the length-tension relationship must be combined with the force-velocity relationship to determine the effect that both length and velocity have on the muscle tension.

Application of the Length-Tension Relationship

In applying the length-tension relationship to whole muscle and ultimately to muscle-joint systems is not a simple matter. For example, sarcomere length is not homogeneous throughout the muscle, let alone between muscles with similar functions. This means that for any particular whole muscle length at a particular joint position, there may be sarcomeres at many different lengths corresponding to different points on the length-tension relationship. Also, when the muscle is acting at a joint, the torque produced is not only a function of the muscle force (which depends on muscle length) but also a function of the MA of the muscle. This means that at a certain joint angle, the muscle length may be short (which suggests that force will be low), but the MA may be relatively long, thus maintaining a higher joint torque. From these examples it is clear that the sarcomere length-tension relationship is important in our understanding of muscle physiology, but there are other important factors when whole muscle and joint systems are considered.

Only a few experiments have attempted to determine the isometric sarcomere length-tension relationship in intact human muscle.[33–37] In these experiments on human wrist muscles and thigh muscles, the range of sarcomere length change that is seen with normal joint motion is quite small and is located around optimal length. This design appears to be quite beneficial in that the muscle is not disadvantaged by being too long or too short. Figure 3-14 shows the estimated length-tension relationship for the extensor carpi radialis brevis and the biceps femoris, long head.[35,36]

One empirical application of the sarcomere length-tension relationship is the observation that a muscle has the diminished ability to produce or maintain isometric tension at the extremes of joint motion. This probably occurs only in muscles that cross more than one joint (two-joint or multijoint muscles), in which muscle length excursion is greater than in single-joint muscles. A decrease in the torque produced by the muscle may be encountered when the full ROM is attempted simultaneously at all joints crossed by a multijoint muscle. This decrease in torque is often referred to as "active insufficiency." Although the decrease in isometric torque can be conveniently explained by the length changes in the muscle that result in decreased muscle force, other factors such as the change in MA and the passive restraint of the lengthened antagonists also play a substantial role. Sarcomere length appears to stay close to the optimal length during joint movements; therefore, influence of the MA and passive restraint of the antagonists may be more important than once thought.[33,35–38] Therefore, the term active insufficiency refers to a concept that is much broader than just the active length-tension properties of the muscle.

Example 3-1

The finger flexors cross the wrist, carpometacarpal, metacarpophalangeal, and interphalangeal joints (Fig. 3-15A). When the finger flexors shorten, they will cause simultaneous flexion at all joints crossed. If all of the joints are allowed to flex simultaneously, the finger flexors will probably be shorter and, as a result, may develop less tension. In addition, the finger extensors (antagonists) may be restricting motion and limiting force production. Normally, when the finger flexors contract, the wrist is maintained in slight extension by the wrist extensor muscles (see Fig. 3-15B). The wrist extensors prevent the finger flexors from flexing the wrist, and therefore an optimal length of the flexors is maintained.

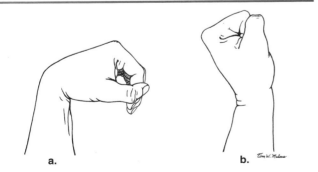

▲ **Figure 3-15** ■ Decrease in active tension with muscle shortening. **A.** The individual is attempting to make a tight fist but is unable to do so because the finger flexors are shortened over both the flexed wrist and fingers. In addition, the finger extensors have become lengthened, potentially restricting motion. **B.** The length-tension relationship of both flexors and extensors has been improved by stabilization of the wrist in a position of slight extension. The individual, therefore, is able to form a tight fist.

■ Force-Velocity Relationship

Another factor that affects the development of tension within a muscle is the speed of shortening of the myofilaments. The speed of shortening is the rate at which the myofilaments are able to slide past one another and form and re-form cross-bridges. Remember that the speed of shortening is related to muscle fiber type as well as muscle fiber length. The force-velocity relationship describes the relationship between the velocity of the muscle contraction and the force produced, therefore providing an explanation for what happens during concentric and eccentric muscle contractions. From the experiments on isolated muscles, the force-velocity relationship states that the velocity of muscle contraction is a function of the load being lifted,[39] but, from a clinical perspective, it may also be stated with the variables reversed (the force generated is a function of the velocity of the muscle contraction) (Fig. 3-16). The maximum shortening speed occurs when there is no resistance to the shortening. However, in this situation, no tension is developed in the muscle because there is no resistance. Conversely, tension may be developed when the resistance to movement of the bony lever prevents visible shortening of the muscle, such as occurs in an isometric contraction. In a concentric muscle contraction, as the shortening speed decreases, the tension in the muscle increases. In an isometric contraction, the speed of shortening is zero, and tension is greater than in a concentric contraction. In an eccentric contraction, as the speed of lengthening increases, the tension in the muscle increases. Not only is this relationship seen in experimental conditions with isolated muscles lifting a load, but it is also seen, to some degree, in intact muscle moving bony levers.[40,41]

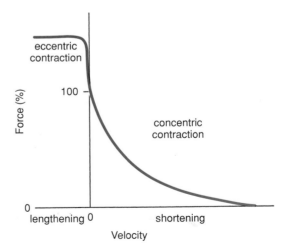

▲ **Figure 3-16** ■ The skeletal muscle force-velocity curve. At maximum velocity of shortening, no force is produced (in other words, maximum velocity of shortening can be attained only with no load on the muscle). As shortening velocity decreases, the force that the muscle can develop increases. At zero velocity, the muscle contracts isometrically. Force increases dramatically and then plateaus when the muscle is lengthened actively.

Case Application 3-5: **Force-Velocity Curve Prediction**

> Vik's plantar flexor muscles were most likely contracting eccentrically as he was planting his foot. Therefore, the force-velocity curve would predict that the muscles were producing high forces, which potentially led to injury of Vik's's muscle or tendon.

Previously, it was mentioned that during dynamic contractions, the length-tension relationship must be combined with the force-velocity relationship because both sarcomere length and velocity of contraction affect the development of muscle tension. It cannot be assumed simply that as the muscle shortens, the tension developed in the muscle follows the isometric length-tension relationship. For example, at high shortening velocities, the muscle tension will be low, regardless of sarcomere length. The fact that most human movements do not occur at a constant velocity of contraction complicates the situation further because the force will vary with changing velocity and changing length.

 CONCEPT CORNERSTONE 3-3: *Factors Affecting Active Muscle Tension*

In summary, active tension in the muscle can be modulated by several factors:

- Tension may be increased by increasing the frequency of firing of a motor unit or by increasing the number of motor units that are firing.
- Tension may be increased by recruiting motor units with a larger number of fibers.
- The greater the number of cross-bridges that are formed, the greater the tension. .
- Muscles that have large physiologic cross-sections are capable of producing more tension than are muscles that have small cross-sections.
- Tension increases as the velocity of active shortening decreases and as the velocity of active lengthening increases.

This basic understanding of the two most important mechanical properties of muscle, the length-tension relationship and the force-velocity relationship, can now be applied to clinical situations.

■ **Types of Muscle Action**

Muscle actions (or contractions) are described as **isometric contraction** (constant length) or dynamic contractions consisting of **concentric contraction** (shortening of the muscle under load) and **eccentric contraction** (lengthening of the muscle under load). The term *isotonic contraction* is not used here because it refers to equal or constant tension, which is unphysiological. The tension generated in a muscle cannot be controlled or kept constant. Therefore, the types of muscle actions that will be considered in the following section are isometric, concentric, and eccentric. Two types of exercise, isokinetic and isoinertial, which are sometimes referred to as types of muscle contraction, will be considered in a later section of this chapter.[42]

Previously, isometric, concentric, and eccentric muscle contractions were introduced in relation to the movement occurring at the sarcomere level. To review: when a muscle fiber is activated so that cross-bridges form, the sarcomeres in the fiber will either stay at constant length, shorten, or lengthen, depending on the load that is applied. An isometric contraction occurs when the muscle is activated and the sarcomere does not change length; a concentric contraction occurs when the sarcomere shortens; and an eccentric contraction occurs when the sarcomere lengthens (the load is greater than the force of the sarcomere).

We can apply this same idea to whole muscle that is attached to bone. When the whole muscle is activated and the bones that it is attached to do not move, it is called an **isometric contraction** (Fig. 3-17). Holding the weight without changing the joint angle means that the muscle is contracting isometrically. During an isometric contraction, no work is being done because the joint is not moving. The formula for work is $W = F \times d$, where W is work, F is the force created by the muscle, and d is the distance that the object, in this case the joint, is moved.

During a **concentric contraction,** the bones move closer together as the whole muscle shortens (Fig. 3-18). **Positive work** is being done by the muscle because the joint moves through a ROM. During an **eccentric contraction,** the bones move away from each other as the muscle tries to control the descent of the weight (Fig. 3-19). The muscle lengthens as the joint moves through the ROM. The work that is being done during an eccentric contraction is called **negative work** because the work is done *on* the muscle rather than *by* the muscle.

The amount of tension that can be developed in a muscle varies according to the type of contraction as was seen in the force-velocity relationship. A greater amount of tension can be developed in an isometric contraction than in a concentric contraction.[43] In general, the tension developed in an eccentric contraction is greater than what can be developed in an isometric

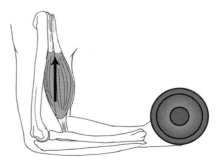

▲ **Figure 3-17** ■ An isometric contraction. Both the distal and proximal bony levers are fixed, and no visible motion occurs when the muscle develops active tension.

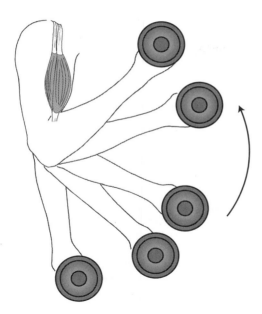

▲ **Figure 3-18** ■ A concentric muscle contraction. When a muscle develops tension, it exerts a pull on both its bony attachments.

contraction. However, this relationship may not hold true for all muscles at all points in a joint's ROM.[44] The reasons for greater tension development in a muscle during an eccentric contraction than in a concentric contraction may be due, in part, to either mechanical factors in the attachment and detachment of cross-bridges or to alterations in the neural activation of the muscle.[45]

■ Production of Torque

As clinicians, we often assess the patient's muscle strength. Whether we assess the strength by using an instrument (such as an isokinetic device) or by simple manual pressure, we are actually determining the amount of joint torque that the muscle can produce. In many physiological experiments on muscle, the muscle is isolated from the bone and the actual muscle force is measured as the muscle is activated. When the muscle is attached to bones in the body, the muscle still produces a force, but it now acts over a MA at the joint to produce a torque.

The MA of the muscle can change with joint position, thus affecting the torque being produced. For example, if the biceps brachii is activated to produce 10 pounds of force with a small MA at one joint position, the torque (muscle strength measured) will be less than if the MA of the muscle were larger at a different joint position (Fig. 3-20). Remember that as the joint moves, the muscle length changes also. From the discussion of the length-tension relationship of the muscle, we know that the muscle force will vary as the muscle is lengthened or shortened. Therefore, at different joint positions, both the MA of the muscle and the length of the muscle will affect the amount of joint torque that can be produced. In addition, during dynamic movements, the velocity of the shortening or lengthening will affect the amount of force that the muscle produces, thus affecting the torque production.

■ Interaction of Muscle and Tendon

The interaction between muscle and tendon (including the aponeurosis) during muscle contraction and

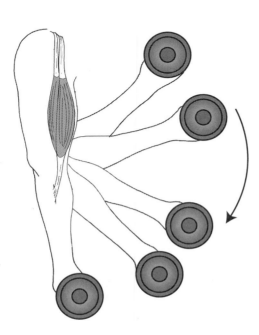

▲ **Figure 3-19** ■ An eccentric contraction. The muscle elongates while continuing to produce active tension.

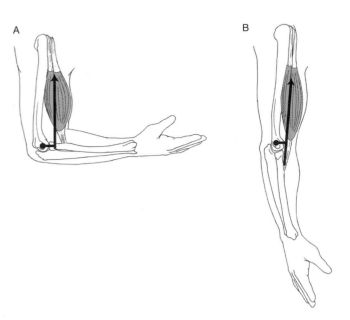

▲ **Figure 3-20** ■ The torque generated by the muscle changes as the moment arm of the muscle changes during joint motion. In position (A) the torque is less than in position (B) because the moment arm is greater (assuming that the force is the same in each position).

movement has some important functional implications. Let us begin with a simple example. During an isometric contraction (as shown in Fig. 3-17), the muscle actually shortens slightly and the tendon lengthens slightly. In many muscles, the fibers may shorten and the tendon may lengthen by as much as 10% of their resting length during an isometric contraction.[46] The compliance of the tendon (or ability to lengthen under load) is important in augmenting the torque production of the muscle. This is the basis for **plyometric exercises,** in which the muscle/tendon complex is stretched before a forceful concentric contraction. The stretch immediately before the concentric contraction helps produce a much greater torque during the concentric contraction. Although the exact mechanism for the increase in torque is debated, evidence shows that the muscle fibers tend to stay at constant length (isometric) while the tendon lengthens, storing energy to be used during the concentric contraction.[47–49]

Case Application 3-6: **Achilles Tendon Involvement?**

Because the Achilles tendon is one of the most compliant tendons in the human body, the patient may have caused undue stretching of the tendon when he stepped back. The high force of the eccentric contraction, coupled with the stretch of the tendon, could have easily caused a strain in the muscle and/or the tendon.

■ **Muscle Action under Controlled Conditions**

Isokinetic Exercise and Testing

Advances in technology have led to the development of testing and exercising equipment that provide for manipulation and control of some of the variables that affect muscle function. In **isokinetic exercise and testing**[50] or **isokinetic muscle contraction,**[43] the angular velocity of the bony component is preset and kept constant by a mechanical device throughout a joint ROM. The concept of an "isokinetic contraction" may not be so much a type of muscle action as it is a description of joint motion. To maintain a constant velocity, the resistance produced by the isokinetic device is *directly proportional* to the torque produced by a muscle at all points in the ROM. Therefore, as the torque produced by a muscle increases, the magnitude of the torque of the resistance increases proportionately. Control of the resistance may be accomplished mechanically by using isokinetic devices such as a Biodex, Cybex, Kin Com, or IsoMed.

Experienced evaluators of human function may attempt to control manually the angular velocity of a bony component by applying resistance that is proportional to the torque produced by a muscle throughout the ROM. In manual muscle testing, the evaluator may apply manual resistance throughout the ROM to a concentric muscle contraction produced by the subject being tested. The evaluator's resistance must adjust constantly so that it is proportional to the torque produced by the muscle being tested at each point in the

ROM. If the evaluator successfully balances the torque output of the subject, a constant angular velocity is achieved. However, manually controlled angular velocity and the manually adjusted resistance required to produce it cannot be given with the same measure of precision or consistency that can be given by a mechanical device. Furthermore, manual resistance cannot be quantified as accurately as mechanical resistance.

The proposed advantage of isokinetic exercise over free weight lifting through a ROM is that isokinetic exercise theoretically accommodates for the changing torques created by a muscle throughout the ROM. As long as the preset speed is achieved, the isokinetic device provides resistance that is proportional to the torque produced by a muscle at all points in the ROM. For example, the least amount of resistance is provided by an isokinetic device at the point in the ROM at which the muscle has the least torque-producing capability. The resistance provided is greatest at the point in the ROM at which the muscle has the largest torque-producing capability.[50]

The maximum isokinetic torques for concentric contractions obtained at high-angular velocities are less than at low-angular velocities. This decline in torque with increasing contraction velocity is expected on the basis of the force-velocity relationship of muscle. In fact, isometric torque values at any point in the ROM are higher than isokinetic concentric torque values at any velocity for the particular point in the joint ROM. Therefore, the closer the angular velocity of a concentric isokinetic contraction approaches zero, the greater is the isokinetic torque.[51,52]

Isokinetic equipment is used extensively for determining the amount of joint torque that a muscle can develop at different velocities, for strength training, and for comparing the relative strength of one muscle group with another. Most isokinetic devices also permit quantification for testing eccentric muscle torque. Isokinetic evaluation of muscle strength has provided much important information about muscle function, and isokinetic exercise is effective for gaining strength. However, there are some limitations to isokinetic evaluation and exercise. For example, at higher speeds, the amount of ROM in which movement is at constant velocity is decreased, and functional movements are rarely performed at constant velocity. Some research shows that isokinetic testing or exercising may differentiate performance in functional tasks or may enhance the training effect for functional activities, and some research shows that it does not.[53–55]

Isoinertial Exercise and Testing

Isoinertial testing and exercising have been developed to quantify dynamic muscle work. Isoinertial exercise is defined as a type of exercise in which muscles act against a constant load or resistance and the measured torque is determined while the constant load is accelerating or decelerating.[42] It is thought to more closely mimic the functional performance of the muscle-joint system than does isokinetic testing and exercising. If the torque produced by the muscle is equal to the torque of the resistance, the muscle contracts isometrically. If the torque produced by the muscle is greater than the resistance, the muscle shortens and the muscle contracts concentrically. Conversely, if the torque produced by the muscle is less than the resistance, the muscle will contract eccentrically. Isoinertial exercise is similar to normal muscle activity in which isometric and either accelerating or decelerating muscle contractions are used in response to a constant load.

Example 3-2

When a person begins to lift a constant external load, the inertia of the load must be overcome by the lifting muscles. At the initial moment of lifting, the muscles contract isometrically as they attempt to develop the torque necessary to match inertial resistance. Once the inertial resistance is exceeded, the muscles contract concentrically as the muscle torque increases and the load begins to move (accelerate).[40] Once in motion, antagonists to the "lifting" muscle may need to contract eccentrically to decelerate the load.

The advantage of both isokinetic and isoinertial devices is that they are capable of quantifying muscle activity. To what degree either testing method can determine accurately the performance level of the person being tested is the primary question. At this point, the answer to this question appears to be that both are able to determine the difference between persons who can perform a functional task well and those who cannot, given that the testing is done in a way that is task specific.[56]

■ Summary of Factors Affecting Active Muscle Tension

Active muscle tension is affected by many factors. Some, such as the size and number of fibers, are intrinsic to the muscle, whereas other factors, such as the influence of the nervous system recruitment patterns, are extrinsic to the muscle.

 CONCEPT CORNERSTONE 3-4: *Summary of Intrinsic and Extrinsic Factors Involving Active Muscle Tension*

The velocity of muscle contraction is affected by:

■ *recruitment order of the motor units:* Units with slow conduction velocities are generally recruited first.
■ *type of muscle fibers in the motor units:* Units with type II muscle fibers can develop maximum tension more rapidly than units with type I muscle fibers; rate of cross-bridge formation, breaking, and re-formation may vary.
■ *the length of the muscle fibers:* Long fibers have a higher shortening velocity than do shorter fibers.

The magnitude of the active tension is affected by:

■ *size of motor units:* Larger units produce greater tension.

■ *number and size of the muscle fibers in a cross-section of the muscle:* The larger the cross-section is, the greater the amount of tension that a muscle may produce.
■ *number of motor units firing:* The greater the number of motor units firing in a muscle, the greater the tension is.
■ *frequency of firing of motor units:* The higher the frequency of firing of motor units, the greater the tension is.
■ *sarcomere length:* The closer the length is to optimal length, the greater the amount of isometric tension that can be generated.
■ *fiber arrangement:* A pennate fiber arrangement gives a greater number of muscle fibers and potentially a larger PCSA, and therefore a greater amount of tension may be generated in a pennate muscle than in a parallel muscle.
■ *type of muscle contraction:* An isometric contraction can develop greater tension than a concentric contraction; an eccentric contraction can develop greater tension than an isometric contraction.
■ *speed:* As the speed of shortening increases, tension decreases in a concentric contraction. As speed of active lengthening increases, tension increases in an eccentric contraction.

Classification of Muscles

Individual muscles may be named in many different ways, such as according to shape (rhomboids, deltoid), number of heads (biceps, triceps, quadriceps), location (biceps femoris, tibialis anterior), or a combination of location and function (extensor digitorum longus, flexor pollicis brevis). Groups of muscles are categorized on the basis of either the actions they perform or the particular role they serve during specific actions. When muscles are categorized on the basis of action, muscles that cause flexion at a joint are categorized as **flexors.** Muscles that cause either extension or rotation are referred to as **extensors** or **rotators,** respectively. When muscles are categorized according to role, individual muscles or groups of muscles are described in terms that demonstrate the specific role that the muscle plays during action. When using this type of role designation, it matters not what action is being performed (flexion, extension) but only what role the muscle plays.

■ Based on Role of the Muscle in Movement

The term **prime mover** (**agonist**) is used to designate a muscle whose role is to produce a desired motion at a joint. If flexion is the desired action, the flexor muscles are the prime movers and the muscles (extensors) that are directly opposite to the desired motion are called the **antagonists.** The desired motion is not opposed by the antagonists, but these muscles have the potential to oppose the action.

Ordinarily, when an agonist (for example, the biceps brachii) is called on to perform a desired motion (elbow flexion), the antagonist muscle (the triceps brachii) is inhibited. If, however, the agonist and the potential antagonist contract simultaneously, then **co-contraction** occurs (Fig. 3-21). Co-contraction of muscles around a joint can help to provide stability for the

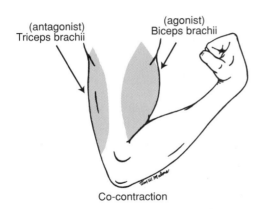

▲ **Figure 3-21** ■ Co-contraction of an agonist and antagonist.

joint and represents a form of synergy that may be necessary in certain situations. Co-contraction of muscles with opposing functions can be undesirable when a desired motion is prevented by involuntary co-contraction, such as occurs in disorders affecting the control of muscle function (e.g., cerebral palsy).

Muscles that help the agonist to perform a desired action are called **synergists.**

Example 3-3

If flexion of the wrist is the desired action, the flexor carpi radialis and the flexor carpi ulnaris are referred to as the "agonists" or "prime movers" because these muscles produce flexion. The finger flexors are the synergists that might directly help the wrist flexors. The wrist extensors are the potential antagonists.

Synergists may assist the agonist directly by helping to perform the desired action, such as in the wrist flexion example, or the synergists may assist the agonist indirectly either by stabilizing a part or by preventing an undesired action.

Example 3-4

If the desired action is finger flexion, such as in clenching of the fist, the finger flexors, which cross both the wrist and the fingers, cannot function effectively (a tight fist cannot be achieved) if they flex the wrist and fingers simultaneously. Therefore, the wrist extensors are used synergistically to stabilize the wrist and to prevent the undesired motion of wrist flexion. By preventing wrist flexion, the synergists are able to maintain the joint in a position that allows the finger flexors to develop greater torque, a combination of optimizing sarcomere length and MA.

Sometimes the synergistic action of two muscles is necessary to produce a pure motion such as radial devi-ation (abduction) of the wrist. The radial flexor, flexor carpi radialis, of the wrist acting alone produces wrist flexion and radial deviation. The radial extensor, extensor carpi radialis brevis and longus, acting alone produces wrist extension and radial deviation. When the wrist extensor and the wrist flexor work together as prime movers to produce radial deviation of the wrist, the unwanted motions are canceled, and the pure motion of radial deviation results (Fig. 3-22). In this example, the muscles that are the potential antagonists of the desired motion are the wrist extensor and flexor on the ulnar side of the wrist (extensor carpi ulnaris and flexor carpi ulnaris, respectively).

■ Based on Muscle Architecture

Placing muscles into functional categories such as flexor and extensor or agonists and antagonists helps to simplify the task of describing the many different muscles and of explaining their actions. However, muscles can change roles. A potential antagonist in one instance may be a synergist in another situation. An example of this can be found in the preceding discussion. The extensors and flexors on the ulnar side of the wrist are antagonists during the motion of radial deviation, but during ulnar deviation, these same muscles are synergists. Despite this apparent change in role, muscles that have similar functions also have similar architectural characteristics. This may seem obvious, because muscle architecture plays such an important role in determining the potential force and velocity of muscle contraction. However, it was not until recently that several studies confirmed that the functional groups of muscles have similar architecture. Examples of this may be seen in experiments with both animals and humans.[26,57,58] In the lower extremity, the knee extensors have a short fiber length and large PCSA, as opposed to the knee flexors, which have a longer fiber

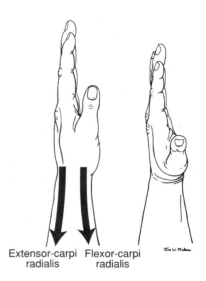

Extensor-carpi   Flexor-carpi
radialis   radialis

▲ **Figure 3-22** ■ Synergistic muscle activity. When the flexor carpi radialis and the extensor carpi radialis work synergistically, they produce radial deviation of the wrist.

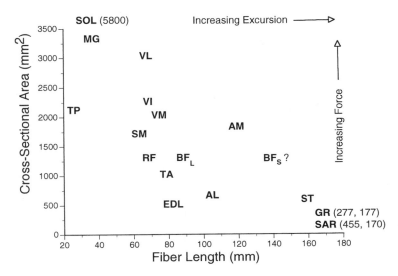

◀ **Figure 3-23** ■ The relationship between PCSA and fiber length of selected muscles of the lower extremity. Note the general grouping of muscles with similar function for example, the soleus (SOL) and medial gastrocnemius (MG); the tibialis anterior (TA) and extensor digitorum longus (EDL); and the vastus lateralis, vastus medialis, and vastus intermedius (VL,VM, VI); gracilis (GR); and sartorius (SAR) (Note: Data are only for fiber length of the biceps femoris short head [BFs].) (Adapted from Lieber RL: Skeletal Muscle Structure and Function: Implications for Rehabilitation and Sports Medicine. Baltimore, Williams & Wilkins, 1992, with permission.)

length and smaller PCSA. The ankle plantar flexors typically have short fiber lengths and large PCSA, thus setting them apart from the ankle dorsiflexors that have longer fiber lengths and smaller PCSA. In the upper extremity, the finger flexors have longer fiber lengths and greater PCSA, as opposed to the shorter and smaller finger extensors (Figs. 3-23 and 3-24).

■ **Based on Length of the Moment Arm**

The orientation of the muscle to the joint has also been used to classify muscles into groups. The length of the muscle MA is an important component of determining the joint torque and, in combination with the fiber length, the ROM through which the muscle can move the joint.[28] The ratio of the fiber length to the MA provides a way of identifying which factor plays a greater role in the production of the joint torque and in deter-

mining the resulting ROM at the joint. For example, the ratio of fiber length to MA is much higher in the wrist extensor muscles than in the wrist flexor muscles, which suggests that fiber length plays a greater role than does MA in the wrist extensors than in the wrist flexors.[33]

Although all skeletal muscles adhere to a general basic structural design, a considerable amount of variability exists among muscles in regard to the number, size, arrangement, and type of muscle fibers. Therefore, attempts to classify muscles into only a few groups may be inappropriate. According to the evidence that subpopulations of motor units from muscles rather than groups of muscles appear to work together for a particular motor task, a more appropriate way of describing muscle action might be in terms of motor units.[17] However, more research needs to be performed in this area before a motor unit classification system can be widely used and accepted.

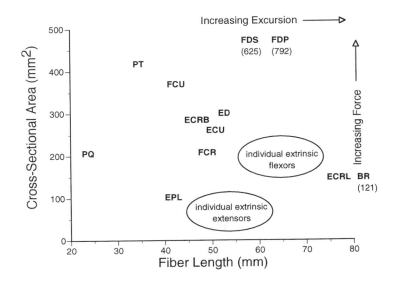

◀ **Figure 3-24** ■ The relationship between PCSA and fiber length of selected muscles of the upper extremity. Note the general grouping of muscles with similar function—for example, the flexor digitorum superficialis (FDS) and profundus (FDP); the extensor carpi radialis brevis (ECRB), extensor carpi ulnaris (ECU), and extensor digitorum (ED); and the individual finger flexors and extensors. (Adapted from Lieber RL: Skeletal Muscle Structure and Function: Implications for Rehabilitation and Sports Medicine. Baltimore, Williams & Wilkins, 1992, with permission.)

Factors Affecting Muscle Function

In addition to the large number of factors that affect muscle function presented previously, a few other factors need to be considered:

- types of joints and location of muscle attachments
- number of joints crossed by the muscle
- passive insufficiency
- sensory receptors

■ Types of Joints and Location of Muscle Attachments

The type of joint affects the function of a muscle in that the structure of the joint determines the type of motion that will occur (flexion and extension) and the ROM. The muscle's location or line of action relative to the joint determines which motion the muscle will perform. In general, muscles that cross the anterior aspect of the joints of the upper extremities, trunk, and hip are flexors, whereas the muscles located on the posterior aspect of these joints are extensors. Muscles located laterally and medially serve as abductors and adductors, respectively, and may also serve as rotators. Muscles whose distal attachments are close to a joint axis are usually able to produce a wide ROM of the bony lever to which they are attached. Muscles whose distal attachments are at a distance from the joint axis, such as the brachioradialis, are designed to provide stability for the joint, because a large majority of their force is directed toward the joint that compresses the joint surfaces. A muscle's relative contribution to stability will change throughout a motion as the rotatory and compressive components of the muscle's force vary indirectly with each other. A muscle provides maximum joint stabilization at the point at which its compressive component is greatest.

Usually one group of muscles acting at a joint is able to produce more torque than another group of muscles acting at the same joint. Disturbances of the normal ratio of agonist-antagonist pairs may create a muscle imbalance at the joint and may place the joint at risk for injury. Agonist-antagonist strength ratios for normal joints are often used as a basis for establishing treatment goals after an injury to a joint. For example, if the shoulder joint were to be injured, the goal of treatment might be to strengthen the flexors and extensors at the injured joint so that they have the same strength ratio as at the uninjured joint.

■ Number of Joints

Many functional movements require the coordinated movement of several joints controlled by a combination of muscles that cross one or many of the joints. To produce a purposeful movement pattern, many authorities believe that the control of the movement is designed to minimize necessary muscle force to accomplish the task (least motor unit activity) and thus minimize muscle fatigue. These strategies of motor control attempt to ensure that movement is done efficiently.

One way of providing an efficient movement pattern is through the coordinated efforts of single-joint and multijoint muscles. In many ways, the number of joints that the muscle crosses determines the muscle function. Single-joint muscles tend to be recruited to produce force and work, primarily in concentric and isometric contractions. This recruitment strategy occurs primarily when a simple movement is performed at one joint, but it may also be used during movements involving multiple joints. Multijoint muscles, in contrast, tend to be recruited to control the fine regulation of torque during dynamic movements involving eccentric more than concentric muscle actions.[59,60] Multijoint muscles tend to be recruited during more complex motions requiring movement around multiple axes. For example, the movement of elbow flexion with concurrent supination uses the biceps brachii (a multijoint muscle) with added contribution of the brachialis (a single-joint muscle). This may seem obvious because of the attachment of the biceps brachii to the radius, which allows supination, whereas the brachialis attaches to the ulna and allows only flexion of the elbow.[61] If a single-joint motion is desired, a single-joint muscle is recruited because recruitment of a multijoint muscle may require the use of additional muscles to prevent motion from occurring at the other joint or joints crossed by the multijoint muscles. For example, elbow flexion with the forearm in pronation is accomplished primarily with the brachialis and not the biceps brachii.

Single-joint and multijoint muscles may also work together in such a way that the single-joint muscle can assist in the movement of joints that it does not cross. For example, the simple movement of standing from a chair requires knee and hip extension. The hip extension is accomplished by activation of the single-joint hip extensor muscles (gluteus maximus) and the multijoint hip extensors (hamstrings). The concomitant knee extension is accomplished by activation of the single-joint knee extensor muscles (vastus muscles) and the multijoint knee extensors (rectus femoris). An interesting corollary is that the single-joint knee extensors may actually assist in hip extension in this movement of standing from a chair. If the hamstrings are active, the knee extension (produced by the vastus muscles) will pull on the active hamstring muscles (which act as a tie-rod), which results in hip extension.

■ Passive Insufficiency

If a person's elbow is placed on the table with the forearm in a vertical position and the hand is allowed to drop forward into wrist flexion, the fingers tend to extend (Fig. 3-25A). Extension of the fingers is a result of the insufficient length of the finger extensors that are being stretched over the flexed wrist. The insufficient length is termed **passive insufficiency.** If the person moves his or her wrist backward into wrist extension, the fingers will tend to flex (see Fig. 3-25B).

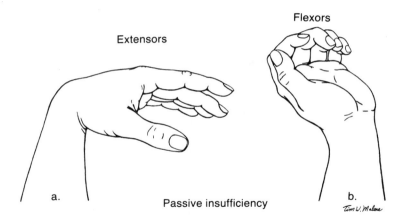

Extensors

Flexors

a.

b.

Passive insufficiency

◀ **Figure 3-25** ■ Passive insufficiency. **A.** The finger extensors become passively insufficient as they are lengthened over the wrist and fingers during wrist flexion. The passive tension that is developed causes extension of the fingers (tenodesis). **B.** The finger flexors become passively insufficient as they are lengthened over the wrist and fingers during wrist extension. The passive tension developed in the finger flexors causes the fingers to flex.

Flexion of the fingers is a result of insufficient length of the finger flexors as they are stretched over the extended wrist.

Under normal conditions, one-joint muscles rarely, if ever, are of insufficient length to allow full ROM at the joint. Two-joint or multijoint muscles, however, frequently are of insufficient length or extensibility to permit a full ROM to be produced simultaneously at all joints crossed by these muscles. The passive tension developed in these stretched muscles is sufficient to either check further motion of the bony lever (passive resistance torque = torque of the effort force) or, if one segment of the joint is not fixed, may actually pull the bony lever in the direction of the passive muscle pull. If the bone is not free to move in the direction of passive muscle pull, damage to the muscle being stretched may occur. Usually, pain will signal a danger point in stretching, and active contraction of the muscle will be initiated to protect the muscle.

When a multijoint muscle on one side of a joint becomes excessively shortened, a multijoint muscle on the opposite side of the joint often becomes excessively lengthened.

Example 3-5

The finger flexors and extensors are an excellent example of this principle. When the finger flexors actively flex the wrist and fingers, the finger extensors are being lengthened over the wrist and finger joints, thereby limiting the amount of finger and wrist flexion.

In this example, at the same time that the finger flexors are shortened, the inactive finger extensors are being passively stretched over all of the joints that they cross. The extensors are providing a passive resistance to wrist and finger flexion at the same time that the finger flexors are having difficulty performing the movement (Fig. 3-26). Insufficient length of the extensors is responsible for pulling the fingers into slight extension when the wrist is flexed before finger flexion

is attempted. The combination of excessive lengthening of passive muscle and attempted shortening of active muscle is threatening to the integrity of the muscle, and such positions are not usually encountered in normal activities of daily living, but they may be encountered in sports activities.

■ Sensory Receptors

Two important sensory receptors, the **Golgi tendon organ** and the **muscle spindle,** affect muscle function. The Golgi tendon organs, which are located in the tendon at the myotendinous junction, are sensitive to tension and may be activated either by an active muscle contraction or by an excessive passive stretch of the muscle. When the Golgi tendon organs are excited, they send a message to the nervous system to inhibit the muscle in whose tendon the receptor lies.

The **muscle spindles,** which consist of 2 to 10 specialized muscle fibers (**intrafusal fibers**) enclosed in a connective tissue sheath, are interspersed throughout

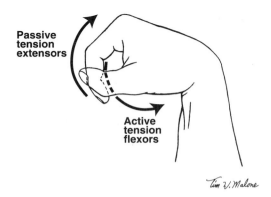

Passive tension extensors

Active tension flexors

▲ **Figure 3-26** ■ Increase in passive tension with passive muscle lengthening. When a person attempts to make a tight fist with the wrist fully flexed, the active shortening of the finger and wrist flexors results in passive lengthening of the finger extensors. The length of the finger extensors is insufficient to allow full range of motion at both the wrist and the fingers and therefore passively limits the ability of the finger flexors to make a tight fist.

the muscle. These spindle fibers are sensitive to the length and the velocity of lengthening of the muscle fibers (**extrafusal fibers**). They send messages to the brain (cerebellum) about the state of stretch of the muscle. When the muscle fiber shortens, the spindles stop sending messages because they are no longer stretched. When the signal decreases, the higher centers send a message to the intrafusal muscle fibers in the spindle to shorten so that they once again are able to respond to the length change in the muscle.

The muscle spindle is responsible for sending the message to the muscle in which it lies to contract when the tendon of a muscle is tapped with a hammer (Fig. 3-27). The quick stretch of the muscle caused by tapping the tendon activates the muscle spindles, and the muscle responds to the unexpected spindle message by a brief contraction. This response is called by various names: for example, **deep tendon reflex (DTR)**, **muscle spindle reflex (MSR)**, or, simply, **stretch reflex.** Both the Golgi tendon organs and the muscle spindles provide constant feedback to the central nervous system during movement so that appropriate adjustments can be made, and they help protect the muscle from injury by monitoring changes in muscle length.

The presence of the stretch reflex is beneficial for preventing muscle injury but presents a problem in treatment programs or fitness programs, in which stretching of a muscle is desirable for improving flexibility and restoring a full range of joint motion. Muscle contraction or reflex activation of motor units during intentional stretching of a muscle may create a resistance to the stretching procedure and makes stretching more difficult and possibly ineffective. Methods of stretching that may prevent reflex activity and motor unit activation during stretching have been investigated.[62,63] The noncontractile components of a muscle also provide resistance to stretching and need to be considered when a muscle-stretching program is implemented.

Receptors that lie in joint capsules and ligaments may have an influence on muscle activity through their signals to the central nervous system. Swelling of the joint capsule and noxious stimuli such as pinching of the capsule will cause reflex inhibition of muscles.

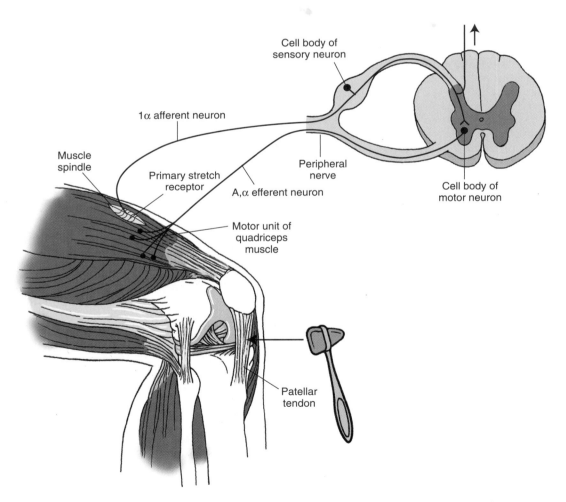

▲ **Figure 3–27** ■ The stretch reflex. When the muscle spindle is stretched by the tap of the hammer, the 1α afferent neuron sends a message to the alpha motor neuron, which results in contraction of the stretched muscle. (Adapted from Smith LK, Weiss EL, Lehmkuhl LD [eds]: Brunnstrom's Clinical Kinesiology, 5th ed. Philadelphia, FA Davis, 1996, p 100, with permission.)

Nociceptors and other receptors in and around the knee joint can have flexor excitatory and extensor inhibitory action. Even a small joint effusion that is undetectable by the naked eye can cause inhibition.[64–66]

The effects of the sensory receptors on muscle activity add an aspect of involuntary control of muscle function to the factors previously discussed. A review of the recent literature related to motor control or "movement science" is beyond the scope of this text, but some aspects of motor control will be presented in Chapter 13.

◆ Effects of Immobilization, Injury, and Aging

Immobilization

Immobilization affects both muscle structure and function. The effects of immobilization depend on immobilization position (shortened or lengthened), percentage of fiber types within the muscle, and length of the immobilization period.

■ **In Shortened Position**

Studies focusing on single muscle fibers and on whole muscles have found that immobilization in a shortened position produces the following structural changes:

- decrease in the number of sarcomeres[67,68]
- increase in sarcomere length[67,69,70]
- increase in the amount of perimysium[70]
- thickening of endomysium[70]
- increase in the amount of collagen
- increase in ratio of connective tissue to muscle fiber tissue
- loss of weight and muscle atrophy[69,71,72]

Changes in function that result from immobilization in the shortened position reflect the structural changes. The decrease in the number of sarcomeres, coupled with an increase in the length of sarcomeres, brings muscle to a length at which it is capable of developing maximal tension in the immobilized position. The loss of sarcomeres displaces the length-tension relationship of the muscle so that the maximum tension generated corresponds to the immobilized position. Therefore, the muscle is able to generate maximal tension in the shortened position. Although this altered capacity for developing tension may be beneficial while the muscle is immobilized in the shortened position, the muscle will not be able to function effectively at the joint it crosses immediately after cessation of the immobilization. The muscle that has adapted to its shortened state will resist lengthening passively, thus checking joint motion. Furthermore, the overall tension-generat-

ing capacity of the muscle is decreased and the increase in connective tissue in relation to muscle fiber tissue results in increase in stiffness to passive stretch.

■ **In Lengthened Position**

Muscles immobilized in the lengthened position exhibit fewer structural and functional changes than do muscles immobilized in the shortened position. The primary structural changes are an increase in the number of sarcomeres, a decrease in their length, and muscle hypertrophy that may be followed by atrophy.[67,70,73] The primary functional changes in muscles immobilized in a lengthened rather than in a shortened position are an increase in maximum tension-generating capacity and displacement of the length-tension curve close to the longer immobilized position. Passive tension in the muscle approximates that of the muscle before immobilization.[69]

Prevention of the effects of immobilization in the shortened position may require only short periods of daily movement. With only 30 minutes of daily ROM activities out of the cast, the negative effects of immobilization in a shortened position were eliminated in animal models.[73] In summary, a word of caution concerning the interpretation of the response of muscle to immobilization: the studies on sarcomere adaptation to immobilization have all been done with specific muscles in animals. It is not clear whether these changes are apparent in all muscles and in humans.

Injury

■ **Overuse**

Overuse may cause injury to tendons, ligaments, bursae, nerves, cartilage, and muscle. The common etiology of these injuries is repetitive trauma that does not allow time for complete repair of the tissue. The additive effects of repetitive forces lead to microtrauma, which in turn triggers the inflammatory process and results in swelling. The tissue most commonly affected by overuse injuries is the musculotendinous unit. Tendons can fatigue with repetitive submaximal loading and are most likely to be injured when tension is applied rapidly and obliquely and when the muscle group is stretched by external stimuli. Bursae may become inflamed with resultant effusion and thickening of the bursal wall as a result of repetitive trauma. Nerves can be subjected to compression injuries by muscle hypertrophy, decreased flexibility, and altered joint mechanics.[74]

■ **Muscle Strain**

Muscle strain injuries can occur from a single high-force contraction of the muscle while the muscle is lengthened by external forces (such as body weight). The muscle usually fails at the junction between the muscle and tendon.[21,75] Subsequently, there is localized bleeding and a significant acute inflammatory response, resulting in swelling, redness, and pain.

Case Application 3-7: **Tissue Healing**

> Because it is possible that the patient strained the plantar flexor muscles, there are probably some swelling and pain in the calf muscles. It would be best for Vik to rest the limb by decreasing his activities to allow the tissues to heal. As the tissues heal, he will need to begin a rehabilitation program to regain mobility and strength. He may not be able to return to strenuous activities until 4 to 8 weeks after the initial injury.

■ **Eccentric Exercise-Induced Muscle Injury**

Injuries to muscles may occur as a result of even a single bout of eccentric exercise. After 30 to 40 minutes of eccentric exercise (walking downhill) or as few as 15 to 20 repetitions of high-load eccentric contractions, significant and sustained reductions in maximal voluntary contractions occur. Also, a loss of coordination, **delayed-onset muscle soreness** (**DOMS**), swelling, and a dramatic increase in muscle stiffness have been reported. The DOMS reaches a peak 2 to 4 days after exercise.[76–78] DOMS occurs in muscles performing eccentric exercise but not in muscles performing concentric exercise.[76] The search for a cause of DOMS is still under investigation. It is known to be related to the forces experienced by muscles and may be a result of mechanical strain in the muscle fibers or in their associated connective tissues.[79,80] Morphologic evidence shows deformation of the Z disk (Z-disk streaming) and other focal lesions after eccentric activity that induces soreness. Biomechanical and histochemical studies have demonstrated evidence for collagen breakdown and for other connective tissue changes.[76]

Aging

■ **Fiber Number and Fiber Type Changes**

As a person ages, skeletal muscle strength decreases as a result of changes in fiber type and motor unit distribution. After the sixth decade of life, there is a loss of muscle fibers; some muscles (vastus lateralis) show a 25% to 50% loss of fibers in persons in their 70s and 80s.[81] In addition, there is a gradual decrease in the number and size of type II fibers, and then the muscle is left with a relative increase in type I fibers.[82] There is also a decrease in the number of motor units, with the remaining motor units increased in the number of fibers per motor unit.[82,83]

■ **Connective Tissue Changes**

Aging will also increase the amount of connective tissue within the endomysium and perimysium of the skeletal muscle. It is generally assumed that the increased connective tissue results in decreased ROM and increased muscle stiffness,[84,85] although there have been reports that muscle stiffness may not change or may decrease with aging.[86,87] All of these changes in the muscle result in decreased muscle strength and, more important, a loss in muscle power. This loss of muscle power, or the ability to contract the muscle with high force and high velocity, may be a potential cause of falls in the elderly.[88] Resistance exercise training in the elderly appears to have positive effects on aging muscles, causing an increase in the size of muscle fibers and an increase in strength and functional performance.[89] However, the response to resistance training is more limited in the elderly than in the young.[90]

Summary

There are many factors that affect the function of the muscles. From the individual proteins and the whole muscle architecture that determine the structure of the muscle to the neural and biomechanical relationships that determine performance of the muscle, the interrelationships between structure and function in muscles are complex and often indistinguishable. Muscles are more adaptable and, in many ways, more complex than the joints that they serve. Artificial joints have been designed and used to replace human joints, but it is as yet impossible to design a structure that can be used to replace a human muscle.

All skeletal muscles adhere to the general principles of structure and function that have been presented in this chapter. Muscles produce the forces that power an incredible array of movements. During human movements, muscles not only provide the force to move the limbs but also provide the force for stabilization. In the following chapters, the structure and function of specific muscles and the relationship of the muscles to specific joints will be explored. The way in which muscles support the body in the erect standing posture and provide movement during walking will be examined in the last two chapters of this book.

 Study Questions

1. Describe the contractile and noncontractile elements of muscle.
2. Explain what happens at the sarcomere level when a muscle contracts.
3. Identify the antagonists in each of the following motions: abduction at the shoulder, flexion at the shoulder, and abduction at the hip.

(Continued on following page)

4. Describe action in the following muscles when the distal bony segment is fixed and the proximal bony segment moves: triceps, biceps, gluteus medius, iliopsoas, and hamstrings. Give examples of activities in which this type of action of these muscles would occur.

5. Compare the function of the quadriceps and hamstrings muscles on the basis of the architectural characteristics of each muscle group.

6. Diagram the changes in the MA of the biceps brachii muscle from full elbow extension to full flexion. Explain how these changes will affect the function of the muscle.

7. Identify the muscles that are involved in lowering oneself into an armchair by using one's arms. Is the muscle contraction eccentric or concentric? Please explain your answer.

8. Describe the factors that could affect the development of active tension in a muscle. Suggest positions of the upper extremity in which each of the following muscles would not be able to develop maximal tension: biceps brachii, triceps brachii, and flexor digitorum profundus. Describe the position in which the same muscles would passively limit motion (be passively insufficient).

9. Explain how a motor unit composed of type I fibers differs from a motor unit composed of type II fibers.

10. List the factors that affect muscle function and explain how each factor affects muscle function.

11. Explain how isokinetic exercise differs from other types of exercise such as weight lifting and isometrics.

12. Explain isoinertial exercise.

13. Describe the effects of immobilization on muscles.

14. Describe the adaptations that occur in skeletal muscle to aging.

References

1. Williams PL, Warwick R, Dyson M, et al. (eds): Gray's Anatomy, 37th ed. London, Churchill Livingstone, 1995.

2. Johnson MA, Pogar J, Weightman D, et al.: Data on the distribution of fibre types in thirty-six human muscles: An autopsy study. J Neurol Sci 18:111, 1973.

3. Gans C: Fiber architecture and muscle function. Exerc Sports Sci Rev 10:160–207, 1982.

4. Netter FH: The Ciba Collection of Medical Illustrations, vol 8. Summit, NJ, Ciba-Geigy Corporation, 1987.

5. Patel TJ, Lieber RL: Force transmission in skeletal muscle: From actomyosin to external tendons. Exerc Sport Sci Rev 25:321–363, 1997.

6. Horowits R, Kempner ES, Bisher ME, et al.: A physiological role for titin and nebulin in skeletal muscle. Nature 323:160–164, 1986.

7. Wang K, McCarter R, Wright J, et al.: Viscoelasticity of the sarcomere matrix of skeletal muscles: The titin-myosin composite filament is a dual-stage molecular spring. Biophys J 64:1161–1177, 1993.

8. Peachey LD, Franzini-Armstrong C: Structure and function of membrane systems of skeletal muscle cells. In Peachey LD (ed): Handbook of Physiology, pp 23–73. Bethesda, MD, American Physiological Society, 1983.

9. Entman ML, Van Winkle WB (eds): Sarcoplasmic Reticulum in Muscle Physiology, vol 1. Boca Raton, FL, CRC Press, 1986.

10. Huxley AF: Muscle structure and theories of contractions. Prog Biophys Biophys Chem 7:225–318, 1957.

11. Huxley AF, Simmons RM: Proposed mechanism of force generation in striated muscle. Nature 233:533–538, 1971.

12. Henneman E, Somjen G, Carpenter DO: Functional significance of cell size in spinal motoneurons. J Neurophysiol 28:560–580, 1965.

13. Linnamo V, Moritani T, Nicol C, et al.: Motor unit activation patterns during isometric, concentric and eccentric actions at different force levels. J Electromyogr Kinesiol 13:93–101, 2003.

14. Gielen CCAM, Denier van der Gon JJ: The activation of motor units in coordinated arm movements in humans. News Physiol Sci 5:159–163, 1990.

15. Howell JN, Fuglevand AJ, Walsh ML, et al.: Motor unit activity during isometric and concentric-eccentric contractions of the human first dorsal interosseus muscle. J Neurophysiol 74:901–904, 1995.

16. Van Zuylen EJ, Gielen AM, Denier van der Gon JJ: Coordination and inhomogeneous activation of human arm muscles during isometric torques. J Neurophys 60:1523–1548, 1988.

17. Conwit RA, Stashuk D, Tracy B, et al.: The relationship of motor unit size, firing rate and force. Clin Neurophysiol 110:1270–1275, 1999.

18. Rosse C, Clawson DK: The Musculoskeletal System in Health and Disease. Hagerstown, MD, Harper & Row, 1980.

19. Peter JB, Barnard RJ, Edgerton VR, et al.: Metabolic profiles on three fiber types of skeletal muscle in guinea pigs and rabbits. Biochemistry 11: 2627–2633, 1972.

20. Staron RS: Human skeletal muscle fiber types: Delineation, development, and distribution. Can J Appl Physiol 22:307–327, 1997.

21. Garrett, WE, Califf, JC, and Bassett, FH: Histochemical correlates of hamstring injuries. Am J Sports Med 12:98–103, 1984.

22. Eriksson K, Hamberg P, Jansson E, et al.: Semiten-

dinosus muscle in anterior cruciate ligament surgery: Morphology and function. Arthroscopy 17: 808–817, 2001.

23. Staron RS, Leonardi MJ, Karapondo DL, et al.: Strength and skeletal muscle adaptations in heavy-resistance-trained women after detraining and retraining. J Appl Physiol 70:631–640, 1991.

24. Saltin B, Henriksson J, Nygaard E, et al.: Fiber types and metabolic potentials of skeletal muscles in sedentary man and endurance runners. Ann N Y Acad Sci 301:3–29, 1977.

25. Colliander EB, Dudley GA, Tesch PA: Skeletal muscle fiber type composition and performance during repeated bouts of maximal concentric contractions. Eur J Appl Physiol 58:81–86, 1988.

26. Lieber RL, Jacobson MD, Fazeli BM, et al.: Architecture of selected muscles of the arm and forearm: Anatomy and implications for tendon transfer. J Hand Surg [Am] 17:787–798, 1992.

27. Sacks RD, Roy RR: Architecture of the hind limb muscle of cats: Functional significance. J Morphol 173:185–195, 1982.

28. Lieber RL: Skeletal Muscle Structure and Function, and Plasticity: The Physiological Basis for Rehabilitation, 2nd ed. Baltimore, Lippincott Williams & Wilkins, 2002.

29. Maganaris CN, Baltzopoulos V, Sargeant AJ: *In vivo* measurements of the triceps surae complex architecture in man: Implications for muscle function. J Physiol 512:603–614, 1998.

30. Kawakami Y, Ichinose Y, Fukunaga T: Architectural and functional features of human triceps surae muscles during contraction. J Appl Physiol 85: 398–404, 1998.

31. Purslow PP: Strain-induced reorientation of an intramuscular connective tissue network: Implications for passive muscle elasticity. J Biomech 22:21–31, 1989.

32. Gordon AM, Huxley AF, Julian FJ: The variation in isometric tension with sarcomere length in vertebrate muscle fibers. J Physiol 184:170–192, 1966.

33. Lieber RL, Ljung B, Friden J: Intraoperative sarcomere length measurements reveal differential design of human wrist extensor muscles. J Exp Biol 200:19–25, 1997.

34. Ichinose Y, Kawakami Y, Ito M, et al.: Estimation of active force-length characteristics of human vastus lateralis muscle. Acta Anat (Basel) 159:78–83, 1997.

35. Lieber RL, Loren GJ, Friden J: *In vivo* measurement of human wrist extensor muscle sarcomere length changes. J Neurophysiol 71:874–881, 1994.

36. Cheboun GS, France AR, Crill MT, et al.: *In vivo* measurement of fascicle length and pennation angle of the human biceps femoris muscle. Cells Tissues Organs 169:401–409, 2001.

37. Maganaris CN: Force-length characteristics of *in vivo* human skeletal muscle. Acta Physiol Scand 172:279–285, 2001.

38. Lutz GJ, Rome LC: Built for jumping: The design of the frog muscular system. Science 263:370–372, 1994.

39. Hill AV: First and Last Experiments in Muscle Mechanics. Cambridge, UK, Cambridge University Press, 1970.

40. Griffin JW: Differences in elbow flexion torque measured concentrically, eccentrically, and isometrically. Phys Ther 67:1205–1208, 1987.

41. Perrine JJ, Edgerton VR: Muscle force-velocity and power-velocity relationships under isokinetic loading. Med Sci Sports 10:159–166, 1978.

42. Parnianpour M, Nordin M, Kahanovitz N, et al.: The triaxial coupling of torque generation of trunk muscles during isometric exertions and the effect of fatiguing isoinertial moments on the motor output and movement patterns. Spine 13:982–990, 1988.

43. Knapik JJ, Wright JE, Mawdsley RH, et al.: Muscle groups through a range of joint motion. Phys Ther 63:938–947, 1983.

44. Singh M, Karpovich PV: Isotonic and isometric forces of forearm flexors and extensors. J Appl Physiol 21:1435–1437, 1966.

45. Enoka RM: Eccentric contractions require unique activation strategies by the nervous system. J Appl Physiol 81:2339–2346, 1996.

46. Maganaris CN, Paul JP: Load-elongation characteristics of *in vivo* human tendon and aponeurosis. J Exp Biol 203:751–756, 2000.

47. Fukunaga T, Kawakami Y, Kubo K, et al.: Muscle and tendon interaction during human movements. Exerc Sport Sci Rev 30:106–110, 2002.

48. Ishikawa M, Finni T, Komi PV: Behaviour of vastus lateralis muscle-tendon during high intensity SSC exercises *in vivo*. Acta Physiol Scand 178:205–213, 2003.

49. Kurokawa S, Fukunaga T, Fukashiro S: Behavior of fascicles and tendinous structures of human gastrocnemius during vertical jumping. J Appl Physiol 90:1349–1358, 2001.

50. Hislop H, Perrine JJ: The isokinetic exercise concept. Phys Ther 47:114–117, 1967.

51. Murray P, Gardner GM, Mollinger LA, et al.: Strength of isometric and isokinetic contractions: Knee muscles of men aged 20 to 86. Phys Ther 60: 412–419, 1980.

52. Knapik JL, Ramos ML: Isokinetic and isometric torque relationships in the human body. Arch Phys Med Rehabil 61:64, 1980.

53. Moffroid MT, Whipple R, Hofkosh J, et al.: A study of isokinetic exercise. Phys Ther 49:735–747, 1969

54. Kovaleski JE, Heitman RH, Trundle TL, et al.: Isotonic preload versus isokinetic knee extension resistance training. Med Sci Sports Exerc 27: 895–899, 1995.

55. Cordova ML, Ingersoll CD, Kovaleski JE, et al.: A comparison of isokinetic and isotonic predictions of a functional task. J Athl Train 30:319–322, 1995.

56. Murphy AJ, Wilson GJ: The assessment of human dynamic muscular function: A comparison of isoinertial and isokinetic tests. J Sports Med Phys Fitness 36:169–177, 1996.

57. Burkholder T, Fingado B, Baron S, et al.: Relationship between muscle fiber types and sizes and muscle architectural properties in the mouse hindlimb. J Morphol 221:177–190, 1994.

58. Wickiewicz TL, Roy RR, Powell PL, et al.: Muscle architecture of the human lower limb. Clin Orthop 179:275–283, 1983.

59. van Ingen Schenau GJ, Dorssers WM, Welter TG, et al.: The control of mono-articular muscles in multijoint leg extensions in man. J Physiol 484: 247–254, 1995.

60. Sergio LE, Ostry DJ: Coordination of mono- and bi-articular muscles in multi-degree of freedom elbow movements. Exp Brain Res 97:551–555, 1994.

61. van Groeningen CJJE, Erkelens CJ: Task-dependent differences between mono- and bi-articular heads of the triceps brachii muscle. Exp Brain Res 100:345–352, 1994.

62. Guissard N, Duchateau J, Hainaut K: Muscle stretching and motoneuron excitability. Eur J Appl Physiol 58:47–52, 1988.

63. Entyre BR, Abraham LD: Antagonist muscle activity during stretching: A paradox revisited. Med Sci Sports Exerc 20:285–289, 1988.

64. Young A, Stokes M, Iles JF, et al.: Effects of joint pathology on muscle. Clin Orthop 219:21–26, 1987.

65. Spencer J, Hayes KC, Alexander IJ: Knee joint effusion and quadriceps reflex inhibition in man. Arch Phys Med Rehabil 65:171–177, 1984.

66. Stokes M, Young A: The contribution of reflex inhibition to arthrogenous muscle weakness. Clin Sci 67:7–14, 1984.

67. Tabary JC, Tabary C, Tardieu C, et al.: Physiological and structural changes in the cat's soleus muscle due to immobilization at different lengths by plaster casts. J Physiol 224:231–244, 1987.

68. Wills, et al.: Effects of immobilization on human skeletal muscle. Orthop Rev 11(11):57–64, 1982.

69. Williams PE, Goldspink G: Changes in sarcomere length and physiological properties in immobilized muscle. J Anat 127:459–468, 1978.

70. Williams PE, Goldspink G: Connective tissue changes in immobilized muscle. J Anat 138: 343–350, 1984.

71. Witzman FA: Soleus muscle atrophy induced by cast immobilization: Lack of effect by anabolic steroids. Arch Phys Med Rehabil 69:81–85, 1988.

72. Booth F: Physiologic and biomechanical effects of immobilization on muscle. Clin Orthop 219:15–20, 1986.

73. Williams PE: Use of intermittent stretch in the prevention of serial sarcomere loss in immobilized muscle. Ann Rheum Dis 49:316–317, 1990.

74. Herring SA, Nilson KL: Introduction to overuse injuries. Clin Sports Med 6:225–239, 1987.

75. Garrett WE: Muscle strain injuries. Am J Sports Med 24(6 Suppl):S2–S8, 1996.

76. Clarkson PM, Hubal MJ: Exercise-induced muscle damage in humans. Am J Phys Med Rehabil 81(11 Suppl):S52–S69, 2002.

77. Howell JN, Chleboun GS, Conatser RR: Muscle stiffness, strength loss, swelling and soreness following exercise-induced injury in humans. J Physiol 464:183–196, 1993.

78. Chleboun GS, Howell JN, Conatser RR, et al.: Relationship between muscle swelling and stiffness after eccentric exercise. Med Sci Sports Exerc 30: 529–535, 1998.

79. Lieber RL, Friden J: Muscle damage is not a function of muscle force but active muscle strain. J Appl Physiol 74:520–526, 1993.

80. Warren GL, Hayes DA, Lowe DA, et al.: Mechanical factors in the initiation of eccentric contraction-induced injury in rat soleus muscle. J Physiol 464:457–475, 1993.

81. Lexell J, Henriksson-Larsen K, Winblad B, et al.: Distribution of different fiber types in human skeletal muscle: Effects of aging studied in whole muscle cross sections. Muscle Nerve 6:588–595, 1983.

82. Lexell J, Taylor CC, Sjostrom M: What is the cause of the ageing atrophy? Total number, size and proportion of different fiber types studied in whole vastus lateralis muscle from 15 to 83-year old men. J Neurol Sci 84:275–294, 1988.

83. Doherty TJ, Vandervoort AA, Brown WF: Effects of aging on the motor unit: A brief review. Can J Appl Physiol 18:331–358, 1993.

84. Alnaqeeb MA, Alzaid NS, Goldspink G: Connective tissue changes and physical properties of developing and aging skeletal muscle. J Anat 139:677–689, 1984.

85. Gajdosik R, Vander Linden DW, Williams AK: Influence of age on concentric isokinetic torque and passive extensibility variables of the calf muscles of women. Eur J Appl Physiol 74:279–286, 1996.

86. Winegard KJ, Hicks AL, Vandervoort AA: An evaluation of the length-tension relationship in elderly human plantarflexor muscles. J Gerontol A Biol Sci Med Sci 52:B337–B343, 1997.

87. Oatis CA: The use of a mechanical model to describe the stiffness and damping characteristics of the knee joint in healthy adults. Phys Ther 73:740–749, 1993.

88. Skelton DA, Beyer N: Exercise and injury prevention in older people. Scand J Med Sci Sports 13:77–85, 2003.

89. Grimby G, Aniansson A, Hedberg M, et al.: Training can improve muscle strength and endurance in 78- to 84-yr-old men. J Appl Physiol 73:2517–2523, 1992.

90. Brown M: Resistance exercise effects on aging skeletal muscle in rats. Phys Ther 69:46–53, 1989.

Axial Skeletal Joint Complexes

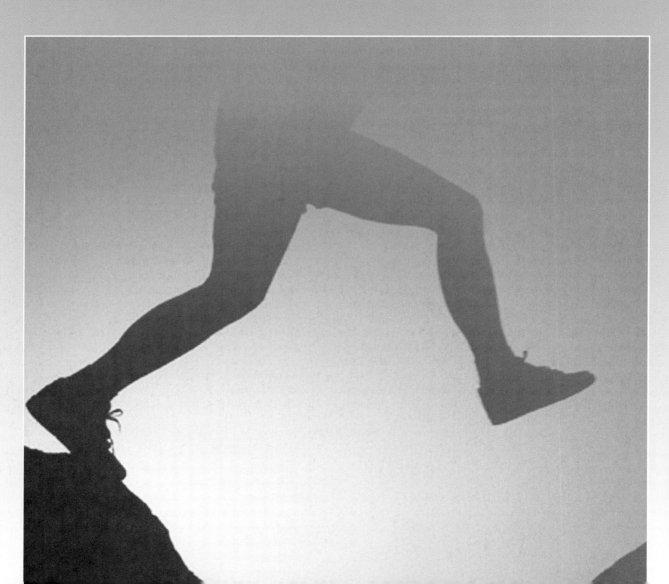

Chapter 4

The Vertebral Column

Diane Dalton, PT, MS, OCS

◆ Introduction

The vertebral column is an amazingly complex structure that must meet the seemingly contradictory demands of mobility and stability of the trunk and the extremities and of providing protection for the spinal cord. Although the pelvis is not considered to be part of the vertebral column, the pelvic attachment to the vertebral column through the sacroiliac joints (SIJs) will be included in this chapter because of the interrelationship of these joints to those of the lumbar region.

4-1	**Patient Case**

Our patient, Malik Johnson, is a 33-year-old male construction worker who for several months has been experiencing moderate to severe low back pain which radiates into his right buttock. He has pain with sitting, carrying, and all lifting activities, especially activities involving lifting from a stooped position. He also has pain with upper extremity tasks such as hammering and using power tools. The pain is particularly severe when he first gets to work in the morning and when he performs any of these activities. He can relieve the pain somewhat if he lies down but has been able to tolerate work for only approximately 4 hours at a time. His history includes several episodes of low back pain that were severe but much shorter in duration, inasmuch as they lasted for only a few days, and resolved on their own.

◆ General Structure and Function

Structure

The vertebral column resembles a curved rod, composed of 33 vertebrae and 23 intervertebral disks. The vertebral column is divided into the following five regions: cervical, thoracic, lumbar, sacral, and coccygeal (Fig. 4-1). The vertebrae adhere to a common basic structural design but show regional variations in size and configuration that reflect the functional demands of a particular region. The vertebrae increase in size from the cervical to the lumbar regions and then

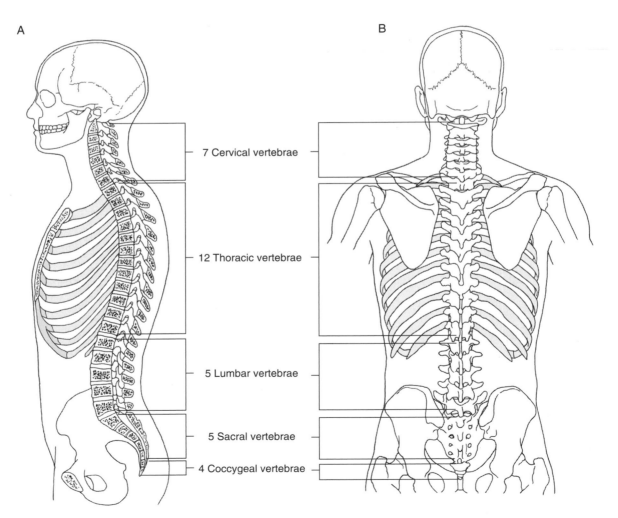

A

B

7 Cervical vertebrae

12 Thoracic vertebrae

5 Lumbar vertebrae

5 Sacral vertebrae

4 Coccygeal vertebrae

▲ **Figure 4-1** ■ Five distinct regions of the vertebral column.

decrease in size from the sacral to coccygeal regions. Twenty-four of the vertebrae in the adult are distinct entities. Seven vertebrae are located in the cervical region, 12 in the thoracic region, and 5 in the lumbar region. Five of the remaining nine vertebrae are fused to form the sacrum, and the remaining four constitute the coccygeal vertebrae.

In the frontal plane, the vertebral column bisects the trunk when viewed from the posterior aspect. When viewed from the sagittal plane, the curves are evident (see Fig. 4-1). The curve of the vertebral column of a baby in fetal life exhibits one long curve that is convex posteriorly, whereas secondary curves develop in infancy. However, in the column of an adult, four distinct anteroposterior curves are evident (Fig. 4-2). The two curves (thoracic and sacral) that retain the original posterior convexity throughout life are called **primary curves,** whereas the two curves (cervical and lumbar) that show a reversal of the original posterior convexity are called **secondary curves.** Curves that have a posterior convexity (anterior concavity) are referred to as **kyphotic curves;** curves that have an anterior convexity (posterior concavity) are called **lordotic curves.** The secondary or lordotic curves develop as a result of the accommodation of the skeleton to the upright posture.

A curved vertebral column provides significant advantage over a straight rod in that it is able to resist much higher compressive loads. According to Kapandji, a spinal column with the normal lumbar, thoracic, and cervical curves has a 10-fold ability to resist axial compression in comparison with a straight rod.[1]

The vertebral column functions as a closed chain with both the head and the ground. We can easily see how this occurs through contact of the feet to the ground, but we often forget the need for the head to remain in a somewhat stable position as we move to allow the sensory organs, particularly the eyes and ears, to be optimally positioned for function. Each of the many separate but interdependent components of the vertebral column is designed to contribute to the overall function of the total unit, as well as to perform specific tasks.

The first section of this chapter will cover the general components of the mobile segment, followed by regional variations and the SIJs. The second section of the chapter will cover the muscles of the vertebral column and pelvis.

■ The Mobile Segment

It is generally held that the smallest functional unit in the spine is the mobile segment; that is, any two adjacent vertebrae, the intervening intervertebral disk (if there is one), and all the soft tissues that secure them together.

■ A Typical Vertebra

The structure of a typical vertebra consists of two major parts: an anterior, cylindrically shaped vertebral body and a posterior, irregularly shaped vertebral or neural arch (Fig. 4-3). The vertebral body is designed to be the weight-bearing structure of the spinal column. It is suitably designed for this task, given its blocklike shape with generally flat superior and inferior surfaces. In order to minimize the weight of the vertebrae and allow dynamic load-bearing, the vertebral body is not a solid block of bone but a shell of cortical bone surrounding a cancellous cavity.[2] The cortical shell is reinforced by trabeculae in the cancellous bone, which provide resistance to compressive forces.

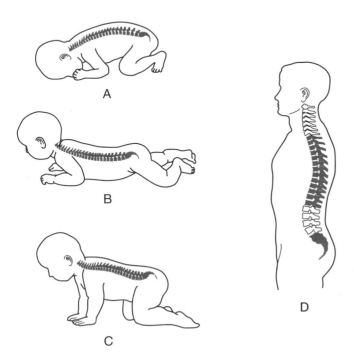

▲ **Figure 4-2** ■ Primary and secondary curves. *The colored areas represent the two primary curves.* (From McKinnis, LN: Fundamentals of Orthopedic Radiology, 1997, with permission from F.A. Davis Company).

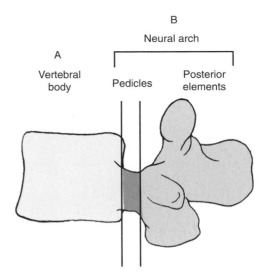

▲ **Figure 4-3** ■ A. The anterior portion of a vertebra is called the **vertebral body. B.** The posterior portion of a vertebra is called the **vertebral** or **neural arch.** The neural arch is further divided into the **pedicles** and the **posterior elements.**

The **neural arch** can be further divided into the pedicles and the posterior elements. The **pedicles** are the portion of the neural arch that lie anterior to the articular processes on either side and serve as the connection between the posterior elements and the vertebral bodies. Their function is to transmit tension and bending forces from the posterior elements to the vertebral bodies. They are well designed for this function, inasmuch as they are short, stout pillars with thick walls. In general, the pedicles increase in size from the cervical to lumbar regions, which makes sense inasmuch as greater forces are transmitted through the pedicles in the lumbar region.

The remaining posterior elements are the laminae, the articular processes, the spinous process, and the transverse processes (Fig. 4-4). The laminae are centrally placed and serve as origination points for the rest of the posterior elements. The **laminae** are thin, vertically oriented pieces of bone that serve as the "roof" to the neural arch, which protects the spinal cord. In addition, the laminae transmit forces from the posterior elements to the pedicles and, through them, onto the vertebral body. This force transfer occurs through a region of the laminae called the pars interarticularis. The **pars interarticularis,** as its name suggests, is the portion of the laminae that is between the superior and inferior articular processes (Fig. 4-5). The pars interarticularis is subjected to bending forces as forces are transmitted from the vertically oriented lamina to the more horizontally oriented pedicles. The pars interarticularis is most developed in the lumbar spine, where the forces are the greatest in magnitude. Typically, an increase in cortical bone occurs to accommodate the increased forces in this region. However, in some individuals, the cortical bone is insufficient, making them susceptible to stress fractures.[2]

■ CONCEPT CORNERSTONE 4-1: *Spondylolisthesis*

When stress fractures of the pars interarticularis occur bilaterally, the result is **spondylolisthesis**.[1,2] The posterior elements are completely separated from the remainder of the neural arch and

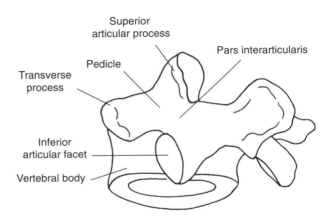

▲ **Figure 4-5** ■ The **pars interarticularis** is the portion of the laminae between the articular processes.

the vertebral body. The vertebral body, then, will begin to slip forward on the vertebra below. Although this can occur in any segment, it frequently occurs at the L5/S1 segment because of the angulation of the segment and the anterior shear forces that exist there (Fig. 4-6).

The altered location of the slipped vertebra changes its relationship to adjacent structures and creates excessive stress on associated supporting ligaments and joints. Overstretched ligaments may lead to the lack of stability or hypermobility of the segment. Narrowing of the posterior joint space, which occurs with forward slippage of a vertebra, may cause stress to spinal nerves, the spinal cord, or the cauda equina. Pain in spondylolisthesis may arise from excessive stress on any of the following pain-sensitive structures: anterior and posterior longitudinal ligaments (PLL), interspinous ligament, spinal nerves, dura mater, vertebral bodies, zygapophyseal joint capsules, synovial linings, or the muscles.

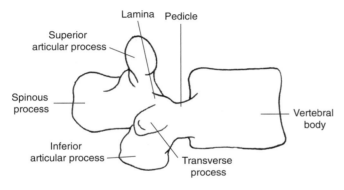

▲ **Figure 4-4** ■ The posterior elements are the **laminae,** the **articular processes,** the **spinous process,** and the **transverse processes.**

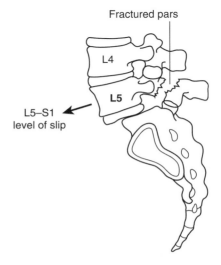

▲ **Figure 4-6** ■ Spondylolisthesis. (From McKinnis, LN: Fundamentals of Orthopedic Radiology, 1997, with permission from F.A. Davis Company).

Case Application 4-1: Spondylolisthesis as a Possible Cause of Pain

Spondylolisthesis could be a possible source of Malik's back pain, inasmuch as it can create excessive stress on the pain-sensitive structures listed previously. In particular for Malik's pain, the posterior ligaments, lumbar spinal nerves and dura mater, lumbar zygapophyseal joints, or the lumbar muscles that control anterior shear could all be producing his symptoms. The primary symptom of Malik's that is atypical of someone with spondylolisthesis, however, is pain in the sitting position. Flexion-based activities such as sitting are usually pain free or much less painful with patients who have spondylolisthesis. This is due to the decreased anterior shear forces on the lumbar spine in the sitting position. Extension-based activities are most painful.

The **spinous processes** and two **transverse processes** are sites for muscle attachments and serve to increase the lever arm for the muscles of the vertebral column. The **articular processes** consist of two superior and two inferior facets for articulation with facets from the cranial and caudal vertebrae, respectively. In the sagittal plane, these articular processes form a supportive column, frequently referred to as the **articular pillar**.[2] Table 4-1 summarizes the components of a typical vertebra.

The vertebrae are subjected to a wide variety of forces; however, they have a typical bony architecture that suggests a typical loading pattern.[3] Vertebral bone trabecular systems that develop in response to the stresses placed on the vertebral bodies and the neural arch are found within the spongy bone[4] (Fig. 4-7). The vertebrae have vertically oriented trabeculae with horizontal connections near the end plate and with denser bone areas near the pedicle bases.[3,5] The vertical systems within the body help to sustain the body weight and resist compression forces (Fig. 4-8). There are also

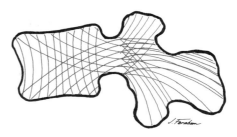

▲ **Figure 4-7** ■ Schematic representation of the internal architecture of a vertebra. The various trabeculae are arranged along the lines of force transmission.

fan-shaped trabeculae introduced into the vertebral body at the area of the pedicle in response to bending and shearing forces transmitted through this region.[3]

■ **The Intervertebral Disk**

The intervertebral disk has two principle functions: to separate two vertebral bodies, thereby increasing available motion, and to transmit load from one vertebral

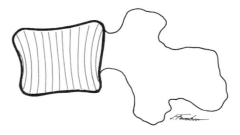

▲ **Figure 4-8** ■ The vertical trabeculae of the vertebral bodies are arranged to resist compressive loading.

Table 4-1	Components of a Typical Vertebra	
	Description	Function
Body	Block of trabecular bone covered by a layer of cortical bone	To resist compressive loads
Pedicle	Short, stout pillars with thick walls that connect the vertebral body to the posterior elements	To transmit the bending forces from the posterior elements to the vertebral body
Lamina	The vertical plate that constitutes the central portion of the arch posterior to the pedicles	To transmit the forces from the articular, transverse, and spinous processes to the pedicles
Transverse processes	Lateral projections of bone that originate from the laminae	Serve as muscle attachments and provide mechanical lever
Spinous process	Posterior projection of bone that originates from the central portion of the lamina, dividing it into two	Serves as muscle attachment and provides mechanical lever; may also serve as a bony block to motion
Vertebral foramen	Opening bordered by the posterior vertebral body and the neural arch	Combined with all segments, forms a passage and protection for the spinal cord

body to the next. Therefore, the size of the intervertebral disk is related to both the amount of motion and the magnitude of the loads that must be transmitted. The intervertebral disks, which make up about 20% to 33% of the length of the vertebral column, increase in size from the cervical to the lumbar regions.[6] The disk thickness varies from approximately 3 mm in the cervical region, where the weight-bearing loads are the lowest, to about 9 mm in the lumbar region, where the weight-bearing loads are the greatest.[1] Although the disks are smallest in the cervical region and largest in the lumbar region, it is the ratio between disk thickness and vertebral body height that determines the available motion.[1] The greater the ratio, the greater the mobility. The ratio is greatest in the cervical region, followed by the lumbar region, and the ratio is smallest in the thoracic region. This reflects the greater functional needs for mobility found in the cervical and lumbar regions and for stability in the thoracic region.

The majority of the information regarding structure and function of the intervertebral disks has been gleaned from studies of the lumbar region. It was long thought that the disks of the cervical and thoracic regions had a structure similar to those of the lumbar region. It appears that this is not the case, particularly with regard to the intervertebral disks of the cervical region.[7–9] This section will describe the general structure and function of the intervertebral disk. Specific variations will be described with the regional structure.

The intervertebral disks are composed of three parts: (1) the **nucleus pulposus,** (2) the **anulus fibrosus,** and (3) the **vertebral end plate** (Fig. 4-9). The nucleus pulposus is the gelatinous mass found in the center, the anulus fibrosus is the fibrous outer ring, and the vertebral end plate is the cartilaginous layer covering the superior and inferior surfaces of the disk, separating it from the cancellous bone of the vertebral bodies above and below. All three structures are composed of water, collagen, and proteoglycans (PGs); however, the relative proportions of each vary. Fluid and PG concentrations are highest in the nucleus and lowest in the outer anulus fibrosus and the outer vertebral end plate (closest to the vertebral body). Conversely, collagen concentrations are highest in the vertebral end plate and outer anulus and lowest in the nucleus pulposus. Although the nucleus pulposus is clearly distinct from the anulus fibrosus in the center and the anulus fibrosus is clearly distinct from the nucleus in the outer rings, there is no clear boundary separating the two structures where they merge. They are distinct structures only where they are furthest apart.

Nucleus Pulposus

The nucleus pulposus is 70% to 90% water, depending on age and time of day.[2] PGs make up approximately 65% of the dry weight, which, as you recall, have an ability to attract water molecules because of the presence of glycosaminoglycans, hence the high water content.[2] Collagen fibers contribute 15% to 20% of the dry weight, and the remainder of the dry weight contains many cells, including elastin, proteins, proteolytic enzymes, chondrocytes, and other types of collagen.[2]

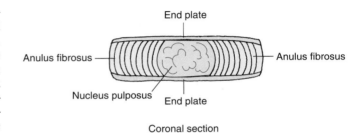

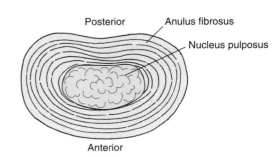

Coronal section

Transverse section

▲ **Figure 4-9** ■ A schematic representation of a lumbar intervertebral disk showing the **nucleus pulposus,** the **anulus fibrosus,** and the **vertebral end plate.**

The nucleus pulposus has both type I and type II collagen; however, type II predominates because of its ability to resist compressive loads. In fact, very little if any type I collagen is present in the center portion of the nucleus pulposus.[2,10] The nucleus pulposus has been frequently likened to a water balloon. When compressed, it deforms, and the increased pressure stretches the walls of the balloon in all directions (Fig. 4-10).

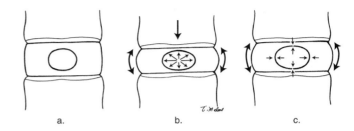

▲ **Figure 4-10** ■ Compression of an intervertebral disk. **A.** In this schematic representation of a disk, the nucleus pulposus is shown as a round ball in the middle of the anulus fibrosus. **B.** Under compressive loading, the pressure is exerted in all directions as the nucleus pulposis attempts to expand. Tension in the anulus fibrosus rises as a result of the nuclear pressure. **C.** A force equal in magnitude but opposite in direction is exerted by the anulus fibrosus on the nucleus pulposus, which restrains radial expansion of the nucleus pulposus and establishes equilibrium. The nuclear pressure is transmitted by the anulus fibrosus to the end plates.

Anulus Fibrosus

In general, the anulus fibrosus is 60% to 70% water, also depending on age and time of day. Collagen fibers make up 50% to 60% of the dry weight, with proteoglycans contributing only 20% of the dry weight.[2] Clearly, the relative proportions of these components are different from the nucleus pulposus, reflecting the difference in structure. The remainder of the dry weight is made up of approximately 10% elastin and other cells such as fibroblasts, and chondrocytes.[2] Again, type I and type II collagen are present; however, type I collagen predominates in the anulus fibrosus, particularly in the outer portions.[2,10] This makeup reflects the need for the anulus fibrosus rather than the nucleus pulposus to resist greater proportions of tensile forces. The anulus fibers are attached to the cartilaginous end plates on the inferior and superior vertebral plateaus of adjacent vertebrae and to the epiphyseal ring region by Sharpey fibers.

Vertebral End Plates

The vertebral end plates are layers of cartilage 0.6 to 1mm thick that cover the region of the vertebral bodies encircled by the ring apophysis on both the superior and inferior surfaces.[2] They cover the entire nucleus pulposus but not the entire anulus fibrosus. The vertebral end plate is strongly attached to the anulus fibrosus and only weakly attached to the vertebral body, which is why it is considered to be a component of the disk rather than the vertebral body.[2,10] The vertebral end plates consist of proteoglycans, collagen, and water, as in the rest of the disk. In addition, there are cartilage cells aligned along the collagen. As in the other regions of the disk, there is a higher proportion of water and proteoglycans closest to the nucleus pulposus and a higher proportion of collagen closest to the anulus fibrosus and the subchondral bone of the vertebral body. The cartilage of the vertebral end plates is both hyaline cartilage and fibrocartilage. Hyaline cartilage is present closest to the vertebral body and is found mainly in young disks. Fibrocartilage is present closest to the nucleus pulposus and, with increasing age, becomes the major component of the vertebral end plate, with little or no hyaline cartilage remaining, reflecting the need to tolerate high compressive forces.

Innervation and Nutrition

The intervertebral disks are innervated in the outer one third to one half of the fibers of the anulus fibrosus.[2] In the cervical and lumbar regions, the innervation has been demonstrated to be by branches from the vertebral and sinuvertebral nerves. The sinuvertebral nerve also innervates the peridiskal connective tissue and specific ligaments associated with the vertebral column.[2]

The intervertebral disks do not receive blood supply from any major arterial branches. The metaphyseal arteries form a dense capillary plexus in the base of the end plate cartilage and the subchondral bone deep to the end plate, and small branches from these metaphyseal arteries do supply the outer surface of the anulus fibrosus.[2,11] The remainder of the disk receives its nutrition via diffusion through these sources.

■ **Articulations**

Two main types of articulations are found in the vertebral column: **cartilaginous** joints of the **symphysis** type between the vertebral bodies, including the interposed disks, and **diarthrodial,** or **synovial,** joints between the zygapophyseal facets located on the superior articular processes of one vertebra and the zygapophyseal facets on the inferior articular processes of an adjacent vertebra above. The joints between the vertebral bodies are referred to as the **interbody joints.** The joints between the zygapophyseal facets are called the **zygapophyseal** (**apophyseal** or **facet**) joints (Fig. 4-11). Synovial joints also are present where the vertebral column articulates with the ribs (see Chapter 5), with the skull, and with the pelvis at the **SIJs.**

Interbody Joints

Available movements at the interbody joints include **gliding, distraction and compression,** and **rotation** (also

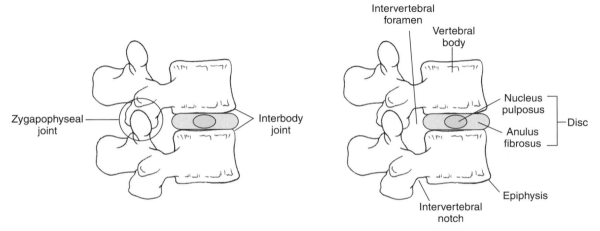

▲ **Figure 4-11** ■ Interbody and zygapophyseal joints.

called tilt or rocking in the spine) (Fig. 4-12). Gliding motions can occur in the following directions: anterior to posterior, medial to lateral, and torsional. Tilt motions can occur in anterior to posterior and in lateral directions. These motions, together with the distraction and compression, constitute six degrees of freedom.[6] The amounts of each of these motions are small and vary by region according to structural differences in the disks and the vertebral bodies, as well as in the ligamentous supports. In addition, the zygapophyseal joints influence the total available motion of the interbody joints.

Zygapophyseal Articulations

The zygapophyseal joints are composed of the articulations between the right and left superior articulating facets of a vertebra and the right and left inferior facets of the adjacent cranial vertebra. The zygapophyseal joints are diarthrodial joints and have regional variations in structure. Intra-articular accessory joint structures have been identified in the zygapophyseal joints.[2,12–14] These accessory structures appear to be of several types, but most are classified as either adipose tissue pads or fibroadipose meniscoids.[2] The structures are most likely involved in protecting articular surfaces that are exposed during flexion and extension of the vertebral column.

■ Ligaments and Joint Capsules

The ligamentous system of the vertebral column is extensive and exhibits considerable regional variability. Six main ligaments are associated with the intervertebral and zygapophyseal joints. They are the **anterior and posterior longitudinal ligaments** and **PLL**; the **ligamentum flavum**; and the **interspinous, supraspinous,** and **intertransverse ligaments** (Figs. 4-13 and 4-14).

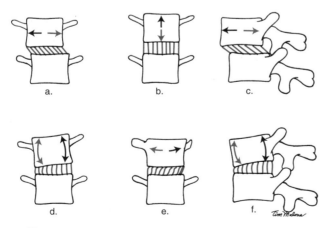

▲ **Figure 4-12** ■ Translations and rotations of one vertebra in relation to an adjacent vertebra. **A.** Side-to-side translation (gliding) occurs in the frontal plane. **B.** Superior and inferior translation (axial distraction and compression) occur vertically. **C.** Anteroposterior translation occurs in the sagittal plane. **D.** Side-to-side rotation (tilting) in a frontal plane occurs around an anteroposterior axis. **E.** Rotation occurs in the transverse plane around a vertical axis. **F.** Anteroposterior rotation (tilting) occurs in the sagittal plane around a frontal axis.

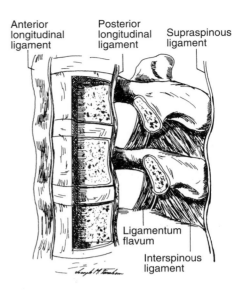

▲ **Figure 4-13** ■ The anterior and posterior longitudinal ligaments are located on the anterior and posterior aspects of the vertebral body, respectively. The ligament flavum runs from lamina to lamina on the posterior aspect of the vertebral canal. Portions of the lamellae have been removed to show the orientation of the collagen fibers.

Anterior and Posterior Longitudinal Ligaments

The anterior longitudinal ligament (ALL) and posterior longitudinal Ligament (PLL) are associated with the interbody joints. The anterior longitudinal ligament runs along the anterior and lateral surfaces of the vertebral bodies from the sacrum to the second cervical vertebra. Extensions of the ligament from C2 to the occiput are called the anterior atlanto-occipital and anterior atlantoaxial ligaments. The anterior longitudinal ligament has at least two layers that are made up of thick bundles of collagen fibers.[15,16] The fibers in the superficial layer are long and bridge several vertebrae, whereas the deep fibers are short and run between single pairs of vertebrae. The deep fibers blend with the fibers of the anulus fibrosus and reinforce the anterolateral portion of the intervertebral disks and the anterior interbody joints. The ligament is well developed in the lordotic sections (cervical and lumbar) of the vertebral column but has little substance in the region of thoracic kyphosis. The anterior longitudinal ligament increases in thickness and width from the lower thoracic vertebrae to L5/S1.[15] The tensile strength of the ligament is greatest at the high cervical, lower thoracic, and lumbar regions, with the greatest strength being in the lumbar region.[17] The ligament is compressed in flexion (Fig. 4-15A) and stretched in extension (see Fig. 4-15B). It may become slack in the neutral position of the spine when the normal height of the disks is reduced, such as might occur when the nucleus pulposus is destroyed or degenerated.[18] The anterior longitudinal ligament is reported to be twice as strong as the PLL.[17]

The PLL runs on the posterior aspect of the vertebral bodies from C2 to the sacrum and forms the

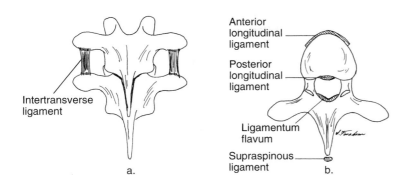

Intertransverse ligament

Anterior longitudinal ligament

Posterior longitudinal ligament

Ligamentum flavum

Supraspinous ligament

a.   b.

◀ **Figure 4-14** ■ **A.** The intertransverse ligament connects the transverse processes. **B.** The relative positions of the other ligaments are shown in a superior view of the vertebra.

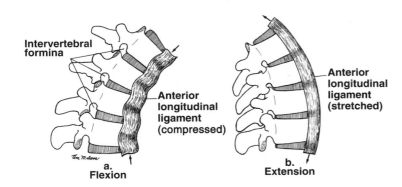

Intervertebral formina

Anterior longitudinal ligament (compressed)

Anterior longitudinal ligament (stretched)

a. **Flexion**   b. **Extension**

◀ **Figure 4-15** ■ Anterior longitudinal ligament (ALL). **A.** The ALL is slack and may be compressed in forward flexion of the vertebral column. **B.** The ALL is stretched in extension of the vertebral column.

ventral surface of the vertebral canal. It also consists of at least two layers: a superficial and a deep layer. In the superficial layer, the fibers span several levels. In the deep layer, the fibers extend only to adjacent vertebrae, interlacing with the outer layer of the anulus fibrosus and attaching to the margins of the vertebral end plates in a manner that varies from segment to segment.[15] Superiorly, the ligament becomes the tectorial membrane from C2 to the occiput. In the lumbar region, the ligament narrows to a thin ribbon that provides little support for the interbody joints. The PLL's resistance to axial tension in the lumbar area is only one sixth of that of the anterior longitudinal ligament.[17] The PLL is stretched in flexion (Fig. 4-16A) and is slack in extension (see Fig. 4-16B).

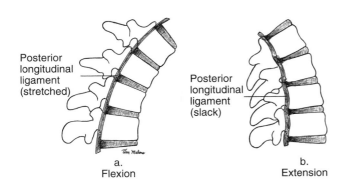

Posterior longitudinal ligament (stretched)

Posterior longitudinal ligament (slack)

a. Flexion   b. Extension

▲ **Figure 4-16** ■ Posterior longitudinal ligament (PLL). **A.** The PLL is stretched during forward flexion of the vertebral column. **B.** The ligament is slack and may be compressed during extension.

Case Application 4-2: **Potential Role of the PLL in Low Back Injury**

The narrow PLL in the lumbar region does not provide much support to the intervertebral disks, which is one of the factors contributing to the increased incidence of disk herniations in a posterolateral direction in the lumbar spine. A posterior disk herniation could be one of the causes of Malik's pain, especially as he has increased pain in a flexed position, which produces a large amount of stress on this area of the PLL.

Ligamentum Flavum

The ligamentum flavum is a thick, elastic ligament that connects lamina to lamina from C2 to the sacrum and forms the smooth posterior surface of the vertebral canal.[19] Some fibers extend laterally to cover the articular capsules of the zygapophyseal joints.[16] From C2 to the occiput, this ligament continues as the posterior atlanto-occipital and atlantoaxial membranes. The ligamentum flavum is strongest in the lower thoracic region and weakest in the midcervical region.[17] Although the highest strain in this ligament occurs during flexion when the ligament is stretched,[2,17] this ligament is under constant tension even when the spine is in a neutral position, because of its elastic nature.[16,20] This highly elastic nature serves two purposes. First, it creates a continuous compressive force on the disks, which causes the intradiskal pressure to remain high. The raised pressure in the disks makes the disks stiffer and thus more able to provide support for the spine in the neutral position.[21] Second, a highly elastic ligament in this location is advantageous because the ligament will not buckle on itself during movement. If the ligament did buckle on itself, it would compress the spinal cord in the vertebral canal, especially with any movement into flexion.

Interspinous Ligaments

The interspinous ligament connects spinous processes of adjacent vertebra. It is described as a fibrous sheet consisting of type I collagen, proteoglycans, and profuse elastin fibers.[22] The interspinous ligament, along with the supraspinous ligament, is the first to be damaged with excessive flexion.[23] The interspinous ligament is innervated by medial branches of the dorsal rami and thought to be a possible source of low back pain.[24] The interspinous ligament has been found to contribute to lumbar spine stability and to degenerate with aging.[24]

Continuing Exploration: **Interspinous Ligament**

The orientation of the fibers of the interspinous ligament has been subject to debate. Some authors have described the fibers as running predominantly parallel to the spinous processes, whereas others describe oblique fiber orientation as well. Of those that describe oblique orientation, the direction varies from anterior to posterior and from posterior to anterior.[22,24,25] The function of the ligament is also subject of debate; however, most authors agree that it resists flexion. It may also resist end-range extension and posterior shear of the superior vertebra on the inferior one.[22,24,26] McGill suggested that the ligament also produces anterior shear during full flexion and that this should be considered in exercise prescription.[26] For example, individuals with shear pathologies such as spondylolisthesis are often prescribed full flexion exercises, which, McGill suggested, may in fact be contraindicated because of the increased anterior shear forces.[26]

Supraspinous Ligament

The supraspinous ligament is a strong cordlike structure that connects the tips of the spinous processes from the seventh cervical vertebra to L3 or L4.[2,27] The fibers of the ligament become indistinct in the lumbar area, where they merge with the thoracolumbar fascia and insertions of the lumbar muscles. In the cervical region, the ligament becomes the **ligamentum nuchae.** The supraspinous ligament, like the interspinous ligament, is stretched in flexion, and its fibers resist separation of the spinous processes during forward flexion. During hyperflexion, the supraspinous ligament, along with the interspinous ligament, is the first to fail.[28] The supraspinous ligament contains mechanoreceptors, and deformation of the ligament appears to play a role in the recruitment of spinal stabilizers such as the multifidus muscles.[29]

Intertransverse Ligaments

The structure of the paired intertransverse ligaments is extremely variable. In general, the ligaments pass between the transverse processes and attach to the deep muscles of the back. In the cervical region, only a few fibers of the ligaments are found. In the thoracic region, the ligaments consist of a few barely discernible fibers that blend with adjacent muscles. In the lumbar region, the ligaments consist of broad sheets of connective tissue that resembles a membrane. The membranous fibers of the ligament form part of the thoracolumbar fascia. The ligaments are alternately stretched and compressed during lateral bending. The ligaments on the right side are stretched and offer resistance during lateral bending to the left, whereas the ligaments on the left side are slack and compressed during this motion. Conversely, the ligaments on the left side are stretched during lateral bending to the right and offer resistance to this motion.

Zygapophyseal Joint Capsules

The zygapophyseal joint capsules assist the ligaments in providing limitation to motion and stability for the vertebral column. The roles of the joint capsules also vary by region. In the cervical spine, the facet joint capsules, although lax, provide the primary soft tissue restraint to axial rotation and lateral bending, but they provide little restraint to flexion and extension.[30] The zygapophyseal joint capsules of the lumbar spine, in addition to the anular fibers, also provide primary restraint to axial rotation,[31,32] however those of the thoracic spine do not provide primary restraint to axial rotation.

The capsules are strongest in the thoracolumbar region and at the cervicothoracic junction[17] sites where the spinal configuration changes from a kyphotic to lordotic curve and from a lordotic to kyphotic curve, respectively, and the potential exists for excessive stress in these areas. The joint capsules, like the supraspinous and interspinous ligaments, are vulnerable to hyperflexion, especially in the lumbar region. It has been suggested that the joint capsules in the lumbar region provide more restraint to forward flexion than any of the posterior ligaments because they fail after the supraspinous and interspinous ligaments when the spine is hyperflexed.[33] Table 4-2 provides a summary of the ligaments and their functions.

Function

■ Kinematics

The motions available to the column as a whole are flexion and extension, lateral flexion, and rotation. These motions appear to occur independently of each other; however, at the level of the individual motion segment, these motions are often coupled motions. **Coupling** is defined as the consistent association of one motion about an axis with another motion around a different axis. The most predominant motions that exhibit coupled behaviors are lateral flexion and rotation. Pure lateral flexion and pure rotation do not occur in any region of the spine. In order for either motion to occur, at least some of the other must occur as well.[6,34]

Table 4-2	Major Ligaments of the Vertebral Column	
Ligaments	Function	Region
Anulus fibrosus (outer fibers)	Resists distraction, translation, and rotation of vertebral bodies.	Cervical, thoracic, and lumbar.
Anterior longitudinal ligament	Limits extension and reinforces anterolateral portion of anulus fibrosus and anterior aspect of intervertebral joints.	C2 to sacrum but well developed in cervical, lower thoracic, and lumbar regions.
Anterior atlantoaxial (continuation of the anterior longitudinal, ligament)	Limits extension.	C2 to the occipital bone.
Posterior longitudinal ligament	Limits forward flexion and reinforces posterior portion of the anulus fibrosus.	Axis (C2) to sacrum. Broad in the cervical and thoracic regions and narrow in the lumbar region.
Tectorial membrane (continuation of the posterior longitudinal ligament)	Limits forward flexion.	Axis (C2) to occipital bone.
Ligamentum flavum	Limits forward flexion, particularly in the lumbar area, where it resists separation of the laminae.	Axis (C2) to sacrum. Thin, broad, and long in cervical and thoracic regions and thickest in lumbar region.
Posterior atlantoaxial (continuation of the ligamentum flavum)	Limits flexion.	Atlas (C1) and axis (C2)
Supraspinous ligaments	Limit forward flexion.	Thoracic and lumbar (C7–L3 or L4). Weak in lumbar region.
Ligamentum nuchae	Limits forward flexion.	Cervical region (occipital protuberance to C7)
Interspinous ligaments	Limit forward flexion.	Primarily in lumbar region, where they are well developed.
Intertransverse ligaments	Limit contralateral lateral flexion.	Primarily in lumbar region.
Alar ligaments	Limit rotation of head to same side and lateral flexion to the opposite side.	Atlas (C1 and C2)
Iliolumbar ligament	Resists anterior sliding of L5 and S1.	Lower lumbar region.
Zygapophyseal joint capsules	Resist forward flexion and axial rotation.	Strongest at cervicothoracic junction and in the thoracolumbar region.

Coupling patterns, as well as the types and amounts of motion that are available, are complex, differ from region to region, and depend on the spinal posture, curves, orientation of the articulating facets, fluidity, elasticity, and thickness of the intervertebral disks and extensibility of the muscles, ligaments, and joint capsules.[34,35]

Motions at the interbody and zygapophyseal joints are interdependent. The *amount* of motion available is determined primarily by the size of the disks, whereas the *direction* of the motion is determined primarily by the orientation of the facets.

The intervertebral disks increase movement between two adjacent vertebrae. If the vertebrae lay flat against each other, the movement between them would be limited to translation alone.[2] The vertebrae are also allowed to rock or tilt on each other because the soft, deformable disk is between them. This arrangement adds tremendous range of motion (ROM) (Fig. 4-17). The fibers of the anulus fibrosus behave as a ligamentous structure and act as restraints to motion.

The motions of flexion and extension occur as a result of the tilting and gliding of a superior vertebra over the inferior vertebra. As the superior vertebra moves through a ROM, it follows a series of different arcs, each of which has a different instantaneous axis of rotation.[36,37] The nucleus pulposus acts like a pivot but, unlike a ball, is able to undergo greater distortion because it behaves as a fluid.

Regardless of the magnitude of motion created by the ratio of disk height to width, a gliding motion occurs at the interbody and zygapophyseal joints as the vertebral body tilts (rotates) over the disk at the interbody joint. The orientation of the zygapophyseal facet surfaces, which varies from region to region, determines the direction of the tilting and gliding within a particular region. If the superior and inferior zygapophyseal facet surfaces of three adjacent vertebrae lie in the sagittal plane, the motions of flexion and extension are facilitated (Fig. 4-18A). On the other hand, if the zygapophyseal facet surfaces are placed in the frontal plane, the predominant motion that is allowed is lateral flexion (Fig. 4-18B).

Flexion

In vertebral flexion, antrior tilting and gliding of the superior vertebra occur and cause widening of the intervertebral foramen and separation of the spin-

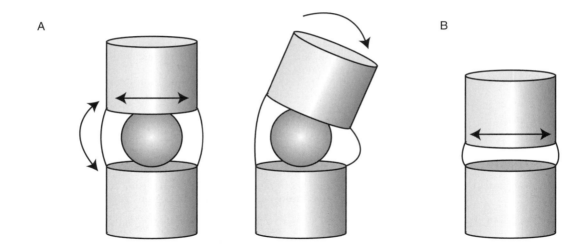

▲ **Figure 4-17** ■ **A.** The addition of an intervertebral disk allows the vertebra to tilt, which dramatically increases ROM at the interbody joint. **B.** Without an intervertebral disk, only translatory motions could occur.

ous processes (Fig. 4-19A). Although the amount of tilting is dependent partly on the size of the disks, tension in the supraspinous and interspinous ligaments resists separation of the spinous processes and thus limits the extent of flexion. Passive tension in the zygapophyseal joint capsules, ligamentum flavum, PLL, posterior anulus fibrosus, and the back extensors also imposes controls on excessive flexion. With movement into flexion, the anterior portion of the anulus fibrosus is compressed and bulges anteriorly, whereas the posterior portion is stretched and resists separation of the vertebral bodies.

Extension

In extension, posterior tilting and gliding of the superior vertebra occur and cause narrowing of the intervertebral foramen, and the spinous processes move closer together (see Fig. 4-19B). The amount of motion available in extension, in addition to being limited by the size of the disks, is limited by bony contact of the spinous processes and passive tension in the zygapophyseal joint capsules, anterior fibers of the anulus fibrosus, anterior trunk muscles, and the anterior longitudinal ligament. In general, there are many more ligaments that limit flexion than there are ligaments that limit extension. The only ligament that limits extension is the anterior longitudinal ligament. This is likely the reason that this ligament is so strong in comparison with the posterior ligaments. The numerous checks to flexion follow the pattern of ligamentous checks to motion where bony limits are minimal. Fewer

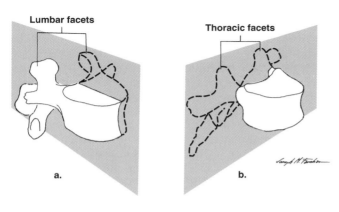

▲ **Figure 4-18** ■ **A.** Sagittal plane orientation of the lumbar zygapophyseal facets favors the motions of flexion and extension. **B.** Frontal plane orientation of the thoracic zygapophyseal facets favors lateral flexion.

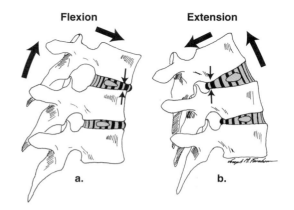

▲ **Figure 4-19** ■ **A.** The superior vertebra tilts and glides anteriorly over the adjacent vertebra below during flexion. The anterior tilting and gliding cause compression and bulging of the anterior anulus fibrosus and stretching of the posterior anulus fibrosus. **B.** In extension, the superior vertebra tilts and glides posteriorly over the vertebra below. The anterior anulus fibers are stretched, and the posterior portion of the disk bulges posteriorly.

ligamentous checks to extension are necessary, given the presence of numerous bony checks.

Lateral Flexion

In lateral flexion, the superior vertebra laterally tilts, rotates, and translates over the adjacent vertebra below (Fig. 4-20). The anulus fibrosus is compressed on the concavity of the curve and stretched on the convexity of the curve. Passive tension in the anulus fibers, intertransverse ligaments, and anterior and posterior trunk muscles on the convexity of the curve limits lateral flexion. The direction of rotation that accompanies lateral flexion differs slightly from region to region because of the orientation of the facets.

All interbody and zygapophyseal joint motion that occurs between the vertebrae from L5 to S1 adheres to the general descriptions that have been presented. Regional variations in the structure, function, and musculature of the column are covered in the following sections. Table 4-3 summarizes the regional variations in the structure of the vertebrae.

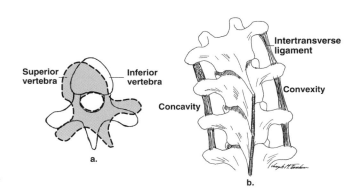

▲ **Figure 4-20** ■ **A.** The superior vertebra tilts laterally and rotates over the adjacent vertebra below during lateral flexion. **B.** Lateral flexion and rotation of the vertebra are limited by tension in the intertransverse ligament on the convexity of the curve.

Table 4-3	Regional Variations in Vertebral Structure		
Part	Cervical Vertebrae	Thoracic Vertebrae	Lumbar Vertebrae
Body	The body is small with a transverse diameter greater than anterior-posterior diameter. Anterior surface of the body is convex; posterior surface is flat. The superior surface of the body is saddle-shaped because of the presence of uncinate processes on the lateral aspects of the superior surfaces.	The transverse and anterior-posterior diameters of the bodies are equal. Anterior height is greater than posterior height. Two demifacets for articulation with the ribs are located on the posterolateral corners of the vertebral plateaus.	The body is massive, with a transverse diameter greater than the anterior-posterior diameter and height.
Arches	Cervical Vertebrae	Thoracic Vertebrae	Lumbar Vertebrae
Pedicles	Project posterolaterally.	Variable in shape and orientation.	Short and thick.
Laminae	Project posteromedially and are thin and slightly curved.	Short, thick, and broad.	Short and broad.
Superior zygapophyseal facets	Face superiorly and medially.	Thin and flat and face posteriorly, superiorly, and laterally.	Vertical and concave and face postero-medially. Support mamillary processes on posterior borders.
Inferior zygapophyseal facets	Face anteriorly and laterally.	Face anteriorly, superiorly, and medially.	Vertical, convex, and face anterolaterally.
Transverse processes	Possess foramina for vertebral artery, vein, and venous plexus. Also have a gutter for spinal nerve.	Processes are large with thickened ends. Possess paired oval facets for articulation with the ribs. Show a caudal decrease in length.	Processes are long and slender and extend horizontally. They support accessory processes on the posterior inferior surfaces of the root.
Spinous processes	Short, slender, and extend horizontally. Have bifid tips.	T1–T10 slope inferiorly. T11 and T12 have a triangular shape.	Broad, thick, and extend horizontally.
Vertebral foramen	Large and roughly triangular.	Small and circular.	Triangular. Larger than the thoracic but smaller than the cervical.

■ **Kinetics**

The vertebral column is subjected to axial compression, tension, bending, torsion, and shear stress not only during normal functional activities but also at rest.[38] The column's ability to resist these loads varies among spinal regions and depends on the type, duration, and rate of loading; the person's age and posture; the condition and properties of the various structural elements (vertebral bodies, joints, disks, muscles, joint capsules, and ligaments); and the integrity of the nervous system.[39]

Axial Compression

Axial compression (force acting through the long axis of the spine at right angles to the disks) occurs as a result of the force of gravity, ground reaction forces, and forces produced by the ligaments and muscular contractions. The disks and vertebral bodies resist most of the compressive force, but the neural arches and zygapophyseal joints share some of the load in certain postures and during specific motions. The compressive load is transmitted from the superior end plate to the inferior end plate through the trabecular bone of the vertebral body and the cortical shell. The cancellous body contributes 25% to 55% of the strength of a lumbar vertebra before the age of 40 years, and the cortical bone carries the remainder. After age 40, the cortical bone carries a greater proportion of the load as the trabecular bone's compressive strength and stiffness decrease with decreasing bone density.[40] Depending on the posture and region of the spine, the zygapophyseal joints carry from 0% to 33% of the compression load. The spinous processes also may share some of the load when the spine is in hyperextension.

The nucleus pulposus acts as a ball of fluid that can be deformed by a compression force. The pressure created in the nucleus pulposus actually is greater than the force of the applied load.[41] When a weight is applied to the nucleus pulposus from above, the nucleus pulposus exhibits a swelling pressure and tries to expand outward toward the anulus fibrosus and the end plates (see Fig. 4-10). As the nucleus attempts to distribute the pressure in all directions, stress is created in the anulus fibrosus, and central compressive loading occurs on the vertebral end plates. The forces of the nucleus pulposus on the anulus fibrosus and of the anulus fibrosus on the nucleus pulposus form an interaction pair. Normally, the anulus fibrosus and the end plates are able to provide sufficient resistance to the swelling pressure in the nucleus pulposus to reach and maintain a state of equilibrium. The pressure exerted on the end plates is transmitted to the superior and inferior vertebral bodies. The disks and trabecular bone are able to undergo a greater amount of deformation without failure than are the cartilaginous end plates or cortical bone when subjected to axial compression. The end plates are able to undergo the least deformation and therefore will be the first to fail (fracture) under high compressive loading. The disks will be the last to fail (rupture).

The intervertebral disks, like all viscoelastic materials, exhibit **creep.** This phenomenon produces typical diurnal changes in disk composition and function. When the intervertebral disks are subjected to a constant load, they exhibit creep. Under sustained compressive loading such as that incurred in the upright posture, the rise in the swelling pressure causes fluid to be expressed from the nucleus pulposus and the anulus fibrosus. The amount of fluid expressed from the disk depends both on the size of the load and the duration of its application. The expressed fluid is absorbed through microscopic pores in the cartilaginous end plate. When the compressive forces on the disks are decreased, the disk imbibes fluid back from the vertebral body.[42] The recovery of fluid that returns the disk to its original state explains why a person getting up from bed is taller in the morning than in the evening. The average variation in height during the day has been demonstrated to be 19 mm with a loss of approximately 1.5 mm (almost 20%) in height from each of the lumbar intervertebral disks.[43–45] Running is a form of dynamic loading that decreases disk height more rapidly than static loading. The height of the vertebral column is a widely used indicator of cumulative compression. In a study involving 31 men, Ahrens found that the men had a mean loss of 0.89 cm and 0.72 cm after a 6-mile run.[46]

Continuing Exploration: **Effects of Creep Loading on the Intervertebral Disks**

Adams and colleagues reported mechanical changes in the disk with creep loading as loss of intervertebral disk height, increased bulging of the disk, increased stiffness in compression, and more flexibility in bending.[43] The result of these changes is that the neural arch and the ligaments, especially the zygapophyseal joints, are subjected to large compressive and bending forces. The authors stated that these normal changes cause different spinal structures to be more heavily loaded at different times of the day. In addition, Adams and colleagues reported that with prolonged compressive forces, there will be a shift in load from the nucleus pulposus to the anulus fibrosus, especially the posterior aspects.[43] This increased load can cause buckling or prolapse of the anulus fibrosus. Also, the decreased exchange of fluid causes decrease in metabolism, thereby decreasing nutrition and healing.[43–45]

Bending

Bending causes both compression and tension on the structures of the spine. In forward flexion, the anterior structures (anterior portion of the disk, anterior ligaments, and muscles) are subjected to compression; the posterior structures are subjected to tension. The resistance offered to the tensile forces by collagen fibers in the posterior outer anulus fibrosus, zygapophyseal joint capsules, and posterior ligaments help to limit extremes of motion and hence provide stability in flexion. Creep occurs when the vertebral column is subjected to sustained loading, such as might occur in either the fully flexed postures commonly assumed in gardening or in the fully extended postures assumed in painting the ceiling. The resulting deformation (elongation or compression) of supporting structures such as ligaments, joint capsules, and intervertebral disks leads to an increase in the ROM beyond normal limits and places the vertebral structures at risk of injury. If the creep deformation of tissues occurs within the toe region of the stress-strain curve, the structures will return to their original dimensions in either minutes or hours after a cessation of the gardening or painting activity.

In extension, the posterior structures generally are either unloaded or subjected to compression, whereas the anterior structures are subjected to tension.[47] In general, resistance to extension is provided by the anterior outer fibers of the anulus fibrosus, zygapophyseal joint capsules, passive tension in the anterior longitudinal ligament, and possibly by contact of the spinous processes. In lateral bending, the ipsilateral side of the disk is compressed; that is, in right lateral bending, the right side of the disk is compressed, whereas the outer fibers of the left side of the disk are stretched. Therefore, the contralateral fibers of the outer anulus fibrosus and the contralateral intertransverse ligament help to provide stability during lateral bending by resisting extremes of motion.

Torsion

Torsional forces are created during axial rotation that occurs as a part of the coupled motions that take place in the spine. The torsional stiffnesses in flexion and lateral bending of the upper thoracic region from T1 to T6 are similar, but torsional stiffness increases from T7/T8 to L3/L4. Torsional stiffness is provided by the outer layers of both the vertebral bodies and intervertebral disks and by the orientation of the facets.[48] The outer shell of cortical bone reinforces the trabecular bone and provides resistance to torsion.[48] When the disk is subjected to torsion, half of the anulus fibrosus fibers resist clockwise rotations, whereas fibers oriented in the opposite direction resist counterclockwise rotations. It has been suggested that the anulus fibrosus may be the most effective structure in the lumbar region for resisting torsion[49]; however, the risk of rupture of the disk fibers is increased when torsion, heavy axial compression, and bending are combined.[50]

Shear

Shear forces act on the midplane of the disk and tend to cause each vertebra to undergo translation (move anteriorly, posteriorly, or from side to side in relation to the inferior vertebra). In the lumbar spine, the zygapophyseal joints resist some of the shear force, and the disks resist the remainder. When the load is sustained, the disks exhibit creep, and the zygapophyseal joints may have to resist all of the shear force. Table 4-4 summarizes vertebral function.

Table 4-4	Summary: Vertebral Function
Structure	**Function**
Body	Resists compressive forces. Transmits compressive forces to vertebral end plates.
Pedicles	Transmit bending forces (exerted by muscles attached to the spinous and transverse processes) to the vertebral bodies.
Laminae	Resist and transmit forces (that are transmitted from spinous and zygapophyseal articular processes) to pedicles. Serve as attachment sites for muscles and ligaments.
Transverse processes	Serve as attachment sites for muscles and ligaments.
Spinous processes	Resist compression and transmit forces to laminae. Serve as attachment sites for ligaments and muscles.
Zygapophyseal facets	Resist shear, compression, tensile and torsional forces. Transmit forces to laminae.
Nucleus pulposus	Resists compression forces to vertebral end plates and translates vertical compression forces into circumferential tensile forces in anulus fibrosus
Anulus fibrosus	Resists tensile, torsional, and shear forces.

Case Application 4-3: **Effects of Creep Loading on Low Back Structures**

Malik has a job that involves lifting and carrying heavy loads in a repetitive manner. Therefore, the intervertebral disks in his lumbar region will have experienced creep loading as a result of these loads. These repetitive loads, combined with the flexed postures that he sustains daily, may have caused damage to the posterior aspects of the anulus fibrosus and decreased fluid exchange to the disk. As a result, the neural arch, particularly the zygapophyseal joints, could be overloaded. In addition, with fluid loss, the capsuloligamentous support could be compromised as a result of the loss in disk height. (Recall too, that the anular fibers in this region of the spine do not have as much support from the PLL.) Also, Malik may have increased mobility at one or more segments and decreased abililty to resist bending and shear forces. Another possibility is that the pain Malik is feeling may be a result of tears in the anulus fibrosus, damage to posterior ligaments (such as the PLL or the interspinous ligament), or damage to the capsules or joint surfaces of the lumbar zygapophyseal joints, all of which are innervated and potential sources of pain.

◈ Regional Structure and Function

The complexity of a structure that must fulfill many functions is reflected in the design of its component parts. Regional structures are varied to meet different but equally complex functional requirements. Structural variations evident in the first cervical and thoracic vertebrae, fifth lumbar vertebra, and sacral vertebrae represent adaptations necessary for joining the vertebral column to adjacent structures. Differences in vertebral structure are also apparent at the cervicothoracic, thoracolumbar, and lumbosacral junctions, at which a transition must be made between one type of vertebral structure and another. The vertebrae located at regional junctions are called **transitional vertebrae** and they usually possess characteristics common to two regions. The cephalocaudal increase in the size of the vertebral bodies reflects the increased proportion of body weight that must be supported by the lower thoracic and lumbar vertebral bodies. Fusion of the sacral vertebrae into a rigid segment reflects the need for a firm base of support for the column. In addition to these variations, a large number of minor alterations in structure occur throughout the column. However, only the major variations are discussed here.

Structure of the Cervical Region

The cervical vertebral column consists of seven vertebrae in total. Morphologically and functionally, the cervical column is divided into two distinct regions: the upper cervical spine, or craniovertebral region, and the lower cervical spine (Fig. 4-21). The **craniovertebral region** includes the **occipital condyles** and the first two cervical vertebrae, **C1** and **C2**, or, respectively, the **atlas** and **axis.** The **lower cervical spine** includes the vertebrae of **C3 to C7.** The vertebrae from C3 to C6 display similar characteristics and are therefore considered to be the typical cervical vertebrae. The atlas, axis, and C7 exhibit unique characteristics and are considered the atypical cervical vertebrae. All of the cervical vertebrae have the unique feature of a foramen (transverse foramen) on the transverse process, which serves as passage for the vertebral artery.

■ Craniovertebral Region

Atlas

The atlas (C1) is frequently described to be like a washer sitting between the occipital condyles and the axis. The functions of the atlas are to cradle the occiput and to transmit forces from the occiput to the lower cervical vertebrae. These functions are reflected in the bony structure. The atlas is different from other vertebrae in that it has no vertebral body or spinous process and is shaped like a ring (Fig. 4-22). There are two large lateral masses that have a vertical alignment under each occipital condyle that reflect the function of transmitting forces. The lateral masses are connected by an anterior and posterior arch that form the ring structure and also create large transverse processes for muscle attachments.[8] The lateral masses include four articulating facets: two superior and two inferior. The superior zygapophyseal facets are large, typically kidney-shaped, and deeply concave to accommodate the large, convex articular surfaces of the occipital condyles. There is, however, large variation in the size and shape of these facets. The inferior zygapophyseal facets are slightly convex and directed inferiorly for articulation with the superior zygapophyseal facets of the axis (C2). The atlas also possesses a facet on the internal surface of the

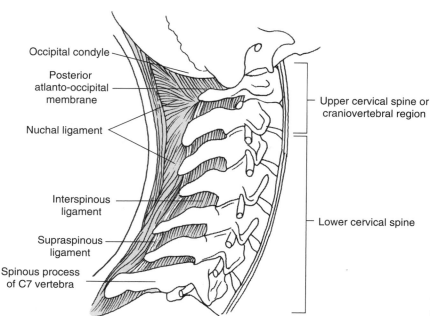

Occipital condyle

Posterior atlanto-occipital membrane

Nuchal ligament

Interspinous ligament

Supraspinous ligament

Spinous process of C7 vertebra

Upper cervical spine or craniovertebral region

Lower cervical spine

◀ **Figure 4-21** ■ The cervical region consists of the upper cervical spine, or craniovertebral region, and the lower cervical spine.

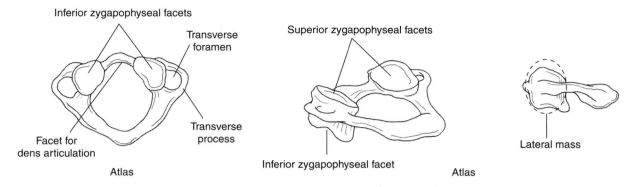

Inferior zygapophyseal facets

Transverse foramen

Superior zygapophyseal facets

Facet for dens articulation

Transverse process

Inferior zygapophyseal facet

Lateral mass

Atlas

Atlas

Atlas

▲ **Figure 4-22** ■ The atlas is a markedly atypical vertebra. It lacks a body and a spinous process.

anterior arch for articulation with the dens (**odontoid process**) of the axis.

Axis

The primary functions of the axis are to transmit the combined load of the head and atlas to the remainder of the cervical spine and to provide motion into axial rotation of the head and atlas.[8] The axis is atypical in that the anterior portion of the body extends inferiorly and a vertical projection called the dens arises from the superior surface of the body (Fig. 4-23). The dens has an anterior facet for articulation with the anterior arch of the atlas and a posterior groove for articulation with the transverse ligament. The arch of the axis has inferior and superior zygapophyseal facets for articulation with the adjacent inferior vertebra and the atlas, respectively. The spinous process of the axis is large and elongated with a bifid (split into two portions) tip. The superior zygapophyseal facets of the axis face upward and laterally. The inferior zygapophyseal facets face anteriorly.[51]

■ **Articulations**

The two **atlanto-occipital joints** consist of the two concave superior zygapophyseal facets of the atlas articulat-

ing with the two convex occipital condyles of the skull. These joints are true synovial joints with intra-articular fibroadipose meniscoids and lie nearly in the horizontal plane.

There are three synovial joints that compose the **atlantoaxial joints**: the median atlantoaxial joint between the dens and the atlas and two lateral joints between the superior zygapophyseal facets of the axis and the inferior zygapophyseal facets of the atlas (Fig. 4-24). The median joint is a synovial trochoid (pivot) joint in which the dens of the axis rotates in an osteoligamentous ring formed by the anterior arch of the atlas and the **transverse ligament.** The two lateral joints appear, on the basis of bony structure, to be plane synovial joints; however, the articular cartilages of both the atlantal and axial facets are convex, rendering the zygapophyseal facet joints biconvex.[52] The joint spaces that occur as a result of the incongruence of the biconvex structure are filled with meniscoids.

■ **Craniovertebral Ligaments**

Besides the longitudinal ligaments mentioned earlier in the chapter, a number of other ligaments are specific to the cervical region. Many of these ligaments attach to

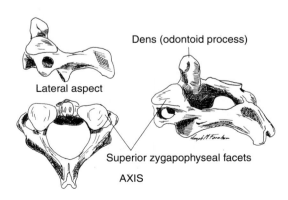

Dens (odontoid process)

Lateral aspect

Superior zygapophyseal facets

AXIS

▲ **Figure 4-23** ■ The dens (odontoid process) arises from the anterior portion of the body of the axis. The superior zygapophyseal facets are located on either side of the dens.

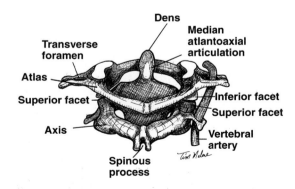

Dens

Median atlantoaxial articulation

Transverse foramen

Atlas

Superior facet

Axis

Inferior facet

Superior facet

Vertebral artery

Spinous process

▲ **Figure 4-24** ■ Atlantoaxial articulation. The median atlantoaxial articulation is seen, with the posterior portion (transverse ligament) removed to show the dens and the anterior arch of the atlas. The two lateral atlantoaxial joints between the superior zygapophyseal facets of the axis and the inferior facets of the atlas can be seen on either side of the median atlantoaxial joint.

the axis, atlas, or skull and reinforce the articulations of the upper two vertebrae. Four of the ligaments are continuations of the longitudinal tract system; the four remaining ligaments are specific to the cervical area.

The **posterior atlanto-occipital** and **atlantoaxial** membranes are the continuations of the ligamentum flavum (Fig. 4-25A). Their structure, however, varies from the ligamentum flavum in that they are less elastic and therefore permit a greater ROM, especially into rotation.[53] The **anterior atlanto-occipital** and **atlantoaxial** membranes are the continuations of the anterior longitudinal ligament (see Fig. 4-25B). The **tectorial membrane** is the continuation of the PLL in the upper two segments and is a broad, strong membrane that originates from the posterior vertebral body of axis, covers the dens and its cruciate ligament, and inserts at the anterior rim of the foramen magnum[53] (Fig. 4-26). The thick **ligamentum nuchae,** which extends from the spinous process of C7 to the external occipital protuberance, is an evolution of the supraspinous ligaments (see Fig. 4-13). The ligamentum nuchae serves as a site for muscle attachment and likely helps to resist the flexion moment of the head.

Transverse Ligament

The **transverse ligament** stretches across the ring of the atlas and divides the ring into a large posterior section for the spinal cord and a small anterior space for the dens. The transverse length of the ligament is about 21.9 mm.[54] The transverse ligament has a thin layer of articular cartilage on its anterior surface for articulation with the dens. Longitudinal fibers of the transverse ligament extend superiorly to attach to the occipital bone, and inferior fibers descend to the posterior portion of the axis. The transverse ligament and its longitudinal bands are sometimes referred to as the **atlantal cruciform ligament** (Fig. 4-27). The transverse portion of the ligament holds the dens in close approximation against the anterior ring of the atlas and serves as an articular surface. Its primary role, however, is to prevent anterior displacement of C1 on C2. This ligament is critical in maintaining stability at the C1/C2 segment. Its superior and inferior longitudinal bands provide some assistance in this role. The transverse atlantal ligament is very strong, and the dens will fracture before the ligament will tear.[27] Integrity of the transverse

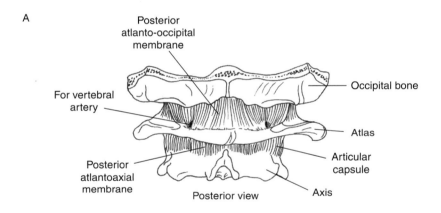

A

Posterior atlanto-occipital membrane

For vertebral artery

Occipital bone

Atlas

Posterior atlantoaxial membrane

Articular capsule

Axis

Posterior view

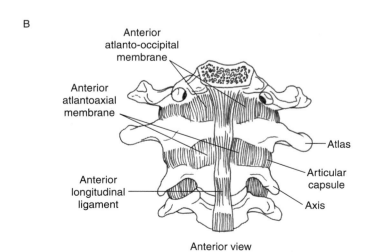

B

Anterior atlanto-occipital membrane

Anterior atlantoaxial membrane

Atlas

Articular capsule

Anterior longitudinal ligament

Axis

Anterior view

▲ **Figure 4-25** ■ A. Posterior atlanto-occipital and atlantoaxial membranes. B. Anterior atlanto-occipital and atlantoaxial membranes.

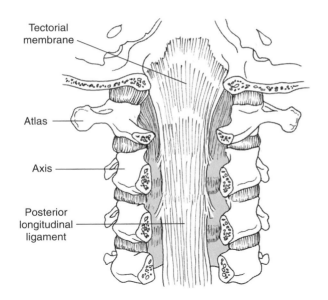

▲ **Figure 4-26** ■ The **tectorial membrane** is a continuation of the posterior longitudinal ligament in the craniovertebral region.

ligament can be compromised, however, particularly with such diseases as rheumatoid arthritis and with other conditions such as Down syndrome.

Alar Ligaments

The two **alar ligaments** are also specific to the cervical region (see Fig. 4-27). These paired ligaments arise from the axis on either side of the dens and extend laterally and superiorly to attach to roughened areas on the medial sides of the occipital condyles[55] and to the lateral masses of the atlas.[54] The ligaments are approximately 1 cm in length and about a pencil width in diameter and consist mainly of collagen fibers arranged in parallel.[55] These ligaments are relaxed with the head in midposition and taut in flexion.[55] Axial rotation of the head and neck tightens both alar ligaments.[55] The right upper and left lower portions of the alar ligaments limit left lateral flexion of the head and neck.[6] These ligaments also help to prevent distraction of C1 on C2. The

alar ligaments are weaker than the transverse atlantal ligament. The **apical ligament** of the dens connects the axis and the occipital bone of the skull. It runs in a fan-shaped arrangement from the apex of the dens to the anterior margin of the foramen magnum of the skull.[27]

■ The Lower Cervical Region

Typical Cervical Vertebrae

Body

The body (Fig. 4-28) of the cervical vertebra is small, with a transverse diameter greater than anteroposterior diameter and height. The upper and lower end plates from C2 to C7 also have transverse diameters (widths) that are greater than the corresponding anteroposterior diameters. The transverse and anteroposterior diameters increase from C2 to C7 with a significant increase in both diameters in the upper end plate of C7.[56] The posterolateral margins of the upper surfaces of the vertebral bodies from C3 to C7 support **uncinate processes** that give the upper surfaces of these vertebrae a concave shape in the frontal plane. The uncinate processes are present prenatally and after birth gradually enlarge from 9 to 14 years of age.[57] The anterior inferior border of the vertebral body forms a lip that hangs down toward the vertebral body below, which produces a concave shape of the inferior surface of the superior vertebra in the sagittal plane.

Arches

Pedicles. The pedicles project posterolaterally and are located halfway between the superior and inferior surfaces of the vertebral body.

Laminae. The laminae are thin and slightly curved. They project posteromedially.

Zygapophyseal Articular Processes (Superior and Inferior). The processes support paired superior facets that are flat and oval and face superoposteriorly. The width and height of the superior zygapophyseal facets gradually increase from C3 to C7. The paired inferior facets face anteriorly and lie closer to the frontal plane

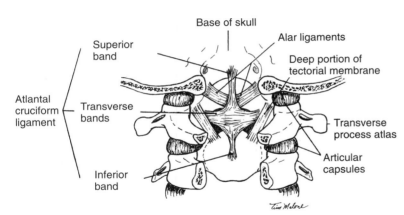

◀ **Figure 4-27** ■ The transverse atlantal ligament. This is a posterior view of the vertebral column in which the posterior portion of the vertebrae (spinous processes and portion of the arches) has been removed to show the atlantal cruciform and alar ligaments.

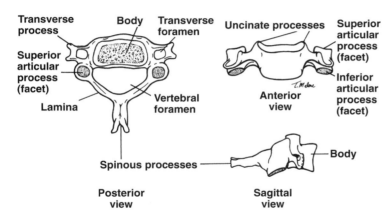

Transverse process
Body
Transverse foramen
Uncinate processes
Superior articular process (facet)

Superior articular process (facet)
Inferior articular process (facet)

Lamina
Vertebral foramen
Anterior view

Spinous processes
Body

Posterior view
Sagittal view

◀ **Figure 4-28** ■ The body of a typical cervical vertebra is small and supports uncinate processes on the posterolateral superior and inferior surfaces.

than do the superior facets.[27] The superior facets of C3 and C7 are more steeply oriented than the others.

Transverse Processes. A foramen is located in the transverse processes bilaterally for the vertebral artery, vein, and venous plexus. Also, there is a groove for the spinal nerves.

Spinous Processes. The cervical spinous processes are short, slender, and extend horizontally. The tip of the spinous process is bifid. The length of the spinous processes decreases slightly from C2 to C3, remains constant from C3 to C5, and undergoes a significant increase at C7.[56]

Vertebral Foramen. The vertebral foramen is relatively large and triangular.

■ **Intervertebral Disk**

The structure of the intervertebral disk in the cervical region is distinctly different from that in the lumbar region (Fig. 4-29). Mercer and Bogduk, in several works, contributed most of the information known about the structure of the cervical disks.[7,8,52] They

reported that instead of a fibrous ring completely surrounding a gelatinous center, there is a discontinuous ring surrounding a fibrocartilaginous core.

The fibers of the anulus fibrosus are not arranged in alternating lamellar layers as in the lumbar region. In addition, they do not surround the entire perimeter of the nucleus pulposus. Instead, the anular fibers in this region have a crescent shape when viewed from above, being thick anteriorly and tapering laterally as they approach the uncinate processes[7,52] (see Fig. 4-29A). Anteriorly, the anulus fibrosus is thick with oblique fibers in the form of an inverted "V" whose apex points to the location of the axis of rotation on the anterior end of the upper vertebra.[7,52] Laterally, there is no substantive anulus fibrosus, and posteriorly, it is only a thin layer of vertically oriented fibers. Posterolaterally, the nucleus is contained only by the PLL.

Fissures in the disk develop along with the uncinate processes and become clefts by approximately 9 years of age (see Fig. 4-29B). These clefts become the joint cavity of what has been known as the uncovertebral joints or "joints of Luschka."[7,52]

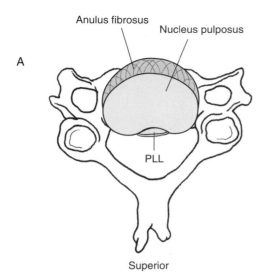

Anulus fibrosus
Nucleus pulposus

A

PLL

Superior

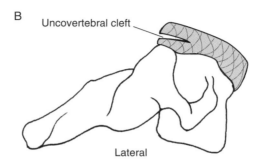

B
Uncovertebral cleft

Lateral

◀ **Figure 4-29** ■ Cervical intervertebral disk. **A.** Superior view shows crescent-shaped anulus fibrosus. **B.** Lateral view shows uncovertebral cleft.

Differences between Cervical and Lumbar Disks

Damage to and pain from the cervical disks are unlikely to be similar in mechanism or pathoanatomy to disks of the lumbar region, because of differences in structure and function of the disks between the two regions. Combined flexion and rotation movements will not damage the posterolateral fibers of the anulus fibrosus in the cervical region as they do in the lumbar region, because there are no posterolateral anular fibers. Disk herniations in the cervical region that cause spinal nerve compression will most likely also involve strain of the PLL.[9]

■ Interbody Joints of the Lower Cervical Region (C3 to C7)

The interbody joints of the lower cervical region are saddle joints, and motion therefore occurs in only two planes (Fig. 4-30). In the frontal plane, the inferior surface of the cranial vertebra is convex and sits in the concave surface of the caudal vertebra created by the uncinate processes. In the sagittal plane, the inferior surface of the cranial vertebra is concave and the superior surface of the caudal vertebra is convex because of the uncinate processes.[9] The motions that occur are predominantly rocking motions with few translatory motions available.[9,52]

■ Zygapophyseal Joints

The zygapophyseal joints in the cervical spine, as in other regions, are true synovial joints and contain fibroadipose meniscoids.[8,9,52] The joint capsules are lax to allow a large ROM; however, they do restrict motion

at the end of the available ranges. The joints that are oriented approximately 45° from the frontal and horizontal planes lie midway between the two planes.

Function of the Cervical Region

Although the cervical region demonstrates the most flexibility of any of the regions of the vertebral column, stability of the cervical region, especially of the atlanto-occipital and atlantoaxial joints, is essential for support of the head and protection of the spinal cord and vertebral arteries. The design of the atlas is such that it provides more free space for the spinal cord than does any other vertebra. The extra space helps to ensure that the spinal cord is not impinged on during the large amount of motion that occurs here. The bony configuration of the atlanto-occipital articulation confers some stability, but the application of small loads produces large rotations across the occipitoatlantoaxial complex[58,59] and also across the lower cervical spine.[58]

■ Kinematics

The cervical spine is designed for a relatively large amount of mobility. Normally, the neck moves 600 times every hour whether we are awake or asleep.[57] The motions of flexion and extension, lateral flexion, and rotation are permitted in the cervical region. These motions are accompanied by translations that increase in magnitude from C2 to C7.[60] However, the predominant translation occurs in the sagittal plane during flexion and extension.[61,62] Excessive anteroposterior translation is associated with damage to the spinal cord.[61]

The atlanto-occipital joints allow for only nodding movements between the head and the atlas[63–65] (Fig. 4-31). In all other respects, the head and atlas move

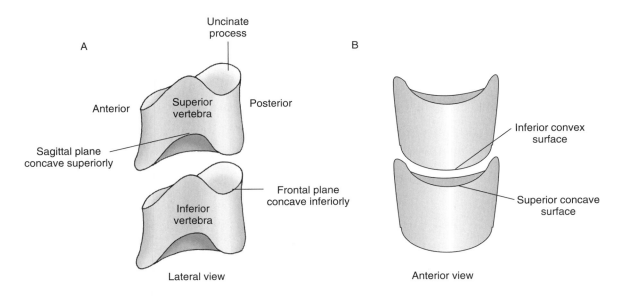

Interbody joints of lower cervical spine

▲ **Figure 4-30** ■ **A.** Lateral view of an interbody saddle joint of the lower cervical spine. **B.** Anterior view showing how the convex inferior surface of the superior vertebra fits into the concave superior surface of the inferior vertebra.

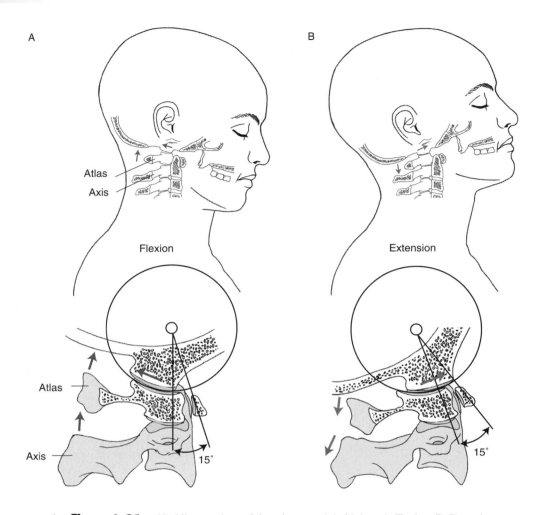

▲ **Figure 4-31** ■ Nodding motions of the atlanto-occipital joints. **A.** Flexion. **B.** Extension.

together and function as one unit.[52] The deep walls of the atlantal sockets prevent translations, but the concave shape does allow rotation to occur.[8] In flexion, the occipital condyles roll forward and slide backward. In extension, the occipital condyles roll backward and slide forward. Axial rotation and lateral flexion are not physiological motions at these joints, inasmuch as they cannot be produced by muscle action.

There is little agreement about the extent of the range of motion (ROM) available at the atlanto-occipital joints. The combined ROM for flexion-extension reportedly ranges from 10° to 30°.[58,63–65] The total ROM available in both axial rotation and lateral flexion is extremely limited by tension in the joint capsules that occurs as the occipital condyles rise up the walls of the atlantal sockets on the contralateral side of either the rotation or lateral flexion.[55,66]

Motions at the atlantoaxial joint include rotation, lateral flexion, flexion, and extension. Approximately 55% to 58% of the total rotation of the cervical region

occurs at the atlantoaxial joints[55,66] (Fig. 4-32). The atlas pivots about 45° to either side, or a total of about 90°. The alar ligaments limit rotation at the atlantoaxial joints. The remaining 40% of total rotation available to the cervical spine is distributed evenly in the lower joints.[66]

The shape of the zygapophyseal joints and the interbody joints dictates the motion at the lower cervical segments. Pure anterior translation does not occur, because it would cause the zygapophyseal joints to abut one another. Flexion of these segments must include anterior tilt of the cranial vertebral body coupled with anterior translation. Given the 45° slope, tilt of the vertebral body, in addition to anterior translation, is necessary to get full motion from these joints (Fig. 4-33). Extension includes posterior tilt of the cranial vertebral body, coupled with posterior translation. Lateral flexion and rotation are also coupled motions, because movement of either alone would cause the zygapophyseal joints to abut one another and prevent motion.

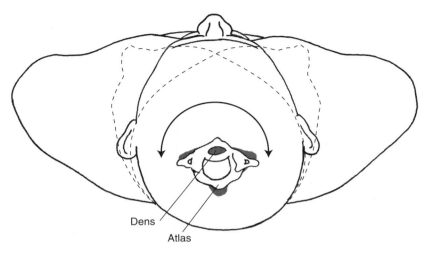

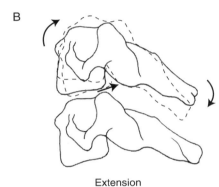

◄ **Figure 4-32** ■ Superior view of rotation at the atlantoaxial joints: The occiput and atlas pivot as one unit around the dens of axis.

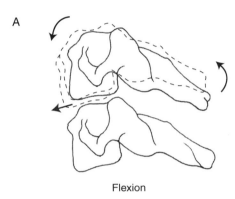

A

B

Flexion

Extension

◄ **Figure 4-33** ■ **A.** Flexion of the lower cervical spine combines anterior translation and sagittal plane rotation of the superior vertebra. **B.** Extension combines posterior translation with sagittal plane rotation.

Lateral flexion is coupled with ipsilateral rotation, and rotation is coupled with ipsilateral lateral flexion. These motions are also a combination of vertebral tilt to the ipsilateral side and translations at the zygapophyseal joints.[35,52]

Mercer and Bogduk[8,9,52] suggested that the notion of lateral flexion and horizontal rotation are an artificial construct. In their view, movement should be viewed as gliding that occurs in the plane of the zygapophyseal joints (Fig. 4-34). In this plane, the coupled motions are evident. Lower cervical segments generally favor flexion and extension ROM; however, there is great variability in reported ranges of motion in the individual cervical segments. In general, the range for flexion and extension increases from the C2/C3 segment to the C5/C6 segment, and decreases again at the C6/C7 segment.[9] The zygapophyseal joint capsules and the ligaments, in addition to the shape of the joints, dictate motions at all of the cervical segments. The zygapophyseal joint capsules are generally lax in the cervical region, which contributes to the large amount of motion available here. The height in relation to the diameter of the disks also plays an important role in determining the amount of motion available in the cervical spine. The height is large in comparison with the

anteroposterior and transverse diameters of the cervical disks. Therefore, a large amount of flexion, extension, and lateral flexion may occur at each segment, especially in young persons, when there is a large amount of water in the disks.

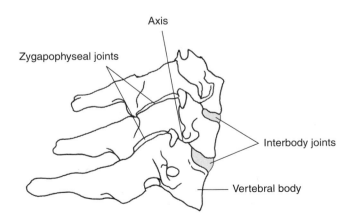

▲ **Figure 4-34** ■ Motion at the lower cervical interbody joints occurs in the plane of the zygapophyseal joints about an axis perpendicular to the plane.

The disk at C5/C6 is subject to a greater amount of stress than other disks because C5/C6 has the greatest range of flexion-extension and is the area where the mechanical strain is greatest.[60]

■ Kinetics

Although the cervical region is subjected to axial compression, tension, bending, torsion, and shear stresses as in the remainder of the spinal column, there are some regional differences. The cervical region differs from the thoracic and lumbar regions in that the cervical region bears less weight and is generally more mobile.

No disks are present at either the atlanto-occipital or atlantoaxial articulations; therefore, the weight of the head (compressive load) must be transferred directly through the atlanto-occipital joint to the articular facets of the axis. These forces are then transferred through the pedicles and laminae of the axis to the inferior surface of the body and to the two inferior zygapophyseal articular processes. Subsequently, the forces are transferred to the adjacent inferior disk. The laminae of the axis are large, which reflects the adaptation in structure that is necessary to transmit these compressive loads. The trabeculae show that the laminae of both the axis and C7 are heavily loaded, whereas the intervening ones are not. Loads diffuse into the lamina as they are transferred from superior to inferior articular facets.[67]

The loads imposed on the cervical region vary with the position of the head and body and are minimal in a well-supported reclining body posture. In the cervical region from C3 to C7 compressive forces are transmitted by three parallel columns: a single anterocentral column formed by the vertebral bodies and disks and two rodlike posterolateral columns composed of the left and right zygapophyseal joints. The compressive forces are transmitted mainly by the bodies and disks, with a little over one third transmitted by the two posterolateral columns.[59,67,68] Compressive loads are relatively low during erect stance and sitting postures and high during the end ranges of flexion and extension.[21] Cervical motion segments tested in bending and axial torsion exhibit less stiffness than do lumbar motion segments but exhibit similar stiffness in compression.[69] In an experiment with cadaver specimens, combinations of sagittal loads *in vitro* demonstrated that the midcervical region from C2 to C5 is significantly stiffer in compression and extension from C5 to T1.[70] Specimens that were axially rotated before being tested in flexion and compression failed at a lower flexion angle (17°) than at the mean angle (25°) of nonaxially rotated specimens. The implication is that the head should be held in a nonrotated position during flexion/extension activities to reduce the risk of injury.[70]

Structure of the Thoracic Region

The majority of the thoracic vertebrae adhere to the basic structural design of all vertebrae except for some minor variations. The 1st and 12th thoracic vertebrae are **transitional vertebrae** and therefore possess characteristics of the cervical and lumbar vertebrae, respectively. The **first thoracic vertebra** has a typical cervical shaped body with a transverse diameter practically twice the anteroposterior diameter. The spinous process of T1 is particularly long and prominent. The **12th thoracic vertebra** has thoracic-like superior zygapophyseal articular facets that face posterolaterally. The inferior zygapophyseal facets, however, are more lumbar-like and have convex surfaces that face anterolaterally to articulate with the vertical, concave, posteromedially facing superior zygapophyseal facets of the first lumbar vertebra. Additional differences in T1, T11, and T12 include the presence of full costal facets rather than demifacets, inasmuch as ribs 1, 11, and 12 articulate only with their corresponding vertebral bodies. The pedicles in the thoracic region are generally directed more posteriorly and less laterally than any other region, which creates a smaller vertebral canal in the thoracic region than in the cervical or lumbar regions. The laminae are short, thick, and broad. The end plates show a gradual increase in transverse and anteroposterior diameters from T1 to T12. The inferior end plate width increases by 55%, and the superior end plate anteroposterior diameter increases by 75%. Increase in width for both superior and inferior end plates is greatest at T11/T12.[71]

■ Typical Thoracic Vertebrae

Body

The body of a typical thoracic vertebra has equal transverse and anteroposterior diameters (Fig. 4-35), which lends to greater stability. The vertebral bodies are wedge shaped with posterior height greater than anterior height, which produces the normal kyphotic posture of the thoracic spine. In a study of 144 vertebrae, Panjabi and coworkers found that the posterior height of each vertebra increased from approximately 14.3 mm at T1 to 22.7 mm at T12, representing an increase of 60%, or a 0.8-mm increase per vertebral level.[71] **Demifacets** (or half facets) for articulation with the heads of the ribs are located on the posterolateral corners of the vertebral plateaus.

Arches

Pedicles. These generally face posteriorly with little to no lateral projection, creating a small vertebral canal.

Laminae. The laminae are short, thick, and broad.

Zygapophyseal Articular Processes. The superior zygapophyseal facets are thin and almost flat and face posteriorly and slightly superolaterally. The inferior zygapophyseal facets face anteriorly and slightly superomedially. The facets lie nearly in the frontal plane. The orientation of the facets changes at either T10 or T11 so that the superior facets face posterolaterally and the inferior facets face anterolaterally, and they lie closer to the sagittal plane.

Transverse Processes. The transverse processes have thickened ends that support paired large oval

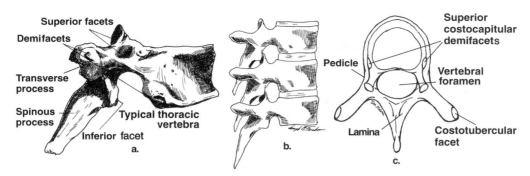

▲ **Figure 4-35** ■ **A.** Lateral view of the thoracic vertebra shows the superior and inferior facets of the zygapophyseal joints and the demifacets for articulation with the ribs. **B.** Overlapping of spinous processes in thoracic region. **C.** Superior view of a thoracic vertebra, showing the small, circular shape of the vertebral foramen, the costotubercular facets for articulation with the tubercles of the ribs, and the superior costocapitular facets for articulation with the heads of the ribs.

facets (**costotubercular facets**) for articulation with the tubercles of the ribs.

Spinous Processes. The spinous processes slope inferiorly and, from T5 to T8, overlap the spinous process of the adjacent inferior vertebra. The spinous processes of T11 and T12 are triangular and project horizontally. For most of the thoracic spine, the tip of the spinous process lies at the level of the caudal vertebral body.

Vertebral Foramen. The vertebral foramen is small and circular.

■ **Intervertebral Disks**

There has been little study of the structure of the thoracic intervertebral disks; however, the structure is generally held to be similar to disks in the lumbar region, with differences only in size and shape. Thoracic intervertebral disks are thinner than those of other regions, especially in the upper thoracic segments. Also, the ratio of disk size to vertebral body size is smallest in the thoracic region, which results in greater stability and less mobility for this region. The intervertebral disks are also somewhat wedge shaped, with the posterior height greater than the anterior height, which contributes to the thoracic kyphosis.[72] The thoracic intervertebral disks are primary restraints to movement and are considered the primary stabilizer of the mobile segment.[73]

■ **Articulations**

Interbody Joints

The interbody joints of the thoracic spine involve flat vertebral surfaces that allow for all translations to occur. The intervertebral disk allows for tipping of the vertebral bodies; however, the relatively small size limits the available motion.

Zygapophyseal Joints

The zygapophyseal joints are plane synovial joints with fibroadipose meniscoids present. These joints lay approximately 20° off the frontal plane, which allows greater ROM into lateral flexion and rotation and less

ROM into flexion and extension (see Fig. 4-18B). The joint capsules are more taut than those of the cervical and lumbar regions, which also contributes to less available ROM.

■ **Ligaments**

The ligaments associated with the thoracic region are the same as ligaments described at the beginning of the chapter except that the ligamentum flavum and anterior longitudinal ligaments are thicker in the thoracic region than in the cervical region.

Function of the Thoracic Region

The thoracic region is less flexible and more stable than the cervical region because of the limitations imposed by structural elements such as the rib cage, spinous processes, taut zygapophyseal joint capsules, the ligamentum flavum, and the dimensions of the disks and the vertebral bodies. Each thoracic vertebra articulates with a set of paired ribs by way of two joints: the **costovertebral** and the **costotransverse** joints. The vertebral components of the costovertebral joints are the demifacets located on the vertebral bodies. The vertebral components of the costotransverse joints are the oval facets on the transverse processes. These joints are discussed in detail in Chapter 5.

■ **Kinematics**

All motions are possible in the thoracic region, but the range of flexion and extension is extremely limited in the upper thoracic region (T1 to T6), because of the rigidity of the rib cage and because of the zygapophyseal facet orientation in the frontal plane. In the lower part of the thoracic region (T9 to T12), the zygapophyseal facets lie more in the sagittal plane, allowing an increased amount of flexion and extension. Lateral flexion and rotation are free in the upper thoracic region. The ROM in lateral flexion is always coupled with some axial rotation. The amount of accompanying axial rotation decreases in the lower part of the region because of the change in orientation of the zygapophyseal facets at T10 or T11. In the upper part of the thoracic region, lateral flexion and rotation are coupled in the same direction, whereas rotation in the lower region may be accompanied by lateral flexion in the opposite direction.[16] In this region, however, the direction of coupled rotation may vary widely among individuals.[6]

Flexion in the thoracic region is limited by tension in the PLL, the ligamentum flavum, the interspinous ligaments, and the capsules of the zygapophyseal joints. Extension of the thoracic region is limited by contact of the spinous processes, laminae, and zygapophyseal facets and by tension in the anterior longitudinal ligament, zygapophyseal joint capsules, and abdominal muscles. Lateral flexion is restricted by impact of the zygapophyseal facets on the concavity of the lateral-flexion curve and by limitations imposed by the rib cage.[61] Rotation in the thoracic region also is limited by the rib cage. When a thoracic vertebra rotates, the motion is accompanied by distortion of the associated rib pair (Fig. 4-36). The posterior portion of the rib on the side to which the vertebral body rotates becomes more convex as the anterior portion of the rib becomes flattened. The amount of rotation that is possible depends on the ability of the ribs to undergo distortion and the amount of motion available in the costovertebral and costotransverse joints. As a person ages, the costal cartilages ossify and allow less distortion. This results in a reduction in the amount of rotation available with aging.

■ Kinetics

The thoracic region is subjected to increased compression forces in comparison with the cervical region, because of the greater amount of body weight that needs to be supported and the region's kyphotic shape. The line of gravity falls anterior to the thoracic spine. This produces a flexion moment on the thoracic spine that is counteracted by the posterior ligaments and the spinal extensors. The greatest flexion moment is at the peak of the kyphosis as a result of the increased moment arm of the line of gravity.[6]

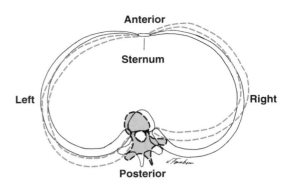

▲ **Figure 4-36** ■ Rotation of a thoracic vertebral body to the left produces a distortion of the associated rib pair that is convex posteriorly on the left and convex anteriorly on the right.

Structure of the Lumbar Region

The first four lumbar vertebrae are similar in structure. The fifth lumbar vertebra has structural adaptations for articulation with the sacrum.

■ Typical Lumbar Vertebrae

Body

The body (Fig. 4-37A) of the typical lumbar vertebra is massive, with a transverse diameter that is greater than the anterior diameter and height. The size and shape reflect the need to support great compressive loads caused by body weight, ground reaction forces, and muscle contraction.

Arches

Pedicles. The pedicles are short and thick and project posterolaterally.
Laminae. The laminae are short and broad.
Zygapophyseal Articular Processes (facets). According to Bogduk, both the superior and inferior zygapophyseal facets vary considerably in shape and orientation (see Fig. 4-37A).[74] **Mamillary processes,** which appear as small bumps, are located on the posterior

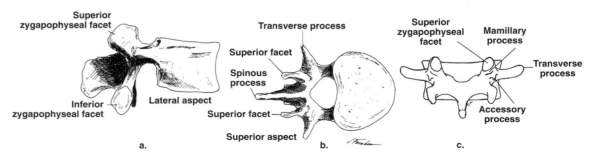

▲ **Figure 4-37** ■ **A.** Lateral view of a typical lumbar vertebra shows the large body and zygapophyseal facets. **B.** Superior view of a typical lumbar vertebra shows transverse and spinous processes and superior zygapophyseal facets. **C.** Posterior view of a lumbar vertebra shows the location of the mamillary and accessory processes. The mamillary processes appear as small, smooth bumps on the posterior edges of each zygapophyseal facet. The accessory processes are easily recognizable as the bony prominences on the posterior surfaces of the transverse processes close to the attachment of the transverse processes to the pedicles.

edge of each superior zygapophyseal facet[74] (see Fig. 4-37C). The mamillary processes serve as attachment sites for the multifidus and medial intertransverse muscles.[27] The inferior zygapophyseal facets are vertical and convex and face slightly anteriorly and laterally.[27]

Transverse Process. The transverse process is long and slender and extends horizontally. **Accessory processes,** which are small and irregular bony prominences, are located on the posterior surface of the transverse process near its attachment to the pedicle[74] (see Fig. 4-37C). The accessory processes serve as attachment sites for the multifidus and medial intertransverse muscles.

Spinous Process. The spinous process is broad and thick and extends horizontally.

Vertebral Foramen. The vertebral foramen is triangular and larger than the thoracic vertebral foramen but smaller than the cervical vertebral foramen.

The fifth lumbar vertebra is a transitional vertebra and differs from the rest of the lumbar vertebrae in that it has a wedge-shaped body wherein the anterior portion of the body is of greater height than the posterior portion. The L5/S1 lumbosacral disk also is wedge shaped. The superior diskal surface area of L5 is about 5% greater than the areas of disks at L3 and L4. The inferior diskal surface area of L5 is smaller than the diskal surface area at other lumbar levels. Also, the spinous process is smaller than other lumbar spinous processes, and the transverse processes are large and directed superiorly and posteriorly.

The **lumbosacral articulation** is formed by the fifth lumbar vertebra and first sacral segment. The first sacral segment, which is inclined slightly anteriorly and

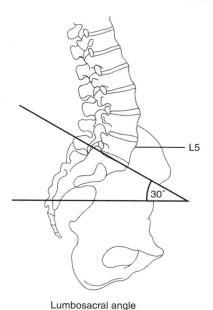

Lumbosacral angle

▲ **Figure 4-38** ■ The lumbosacral angle is determined by measuring the angle formed by a line drawn parallel to the superior aspect of the sacrum and a horizontal line.

inferiorly, forms an angle with the horizontal called the **lumbosacral angle**[75] (Fig. 4-38). The size of the angle varies with the position of the pelvis and affects the superimposed lumbar curvature. An increase in this angle will result in an increase in lordosis of the lumbar curve and will increase the amount of shearing stress at the lumbosacral joint (Fig. 4-39).

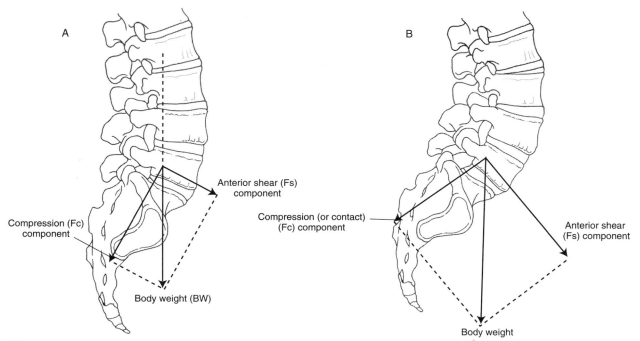

▲ **Figure 4-39** ■ Shear stresses at the lumbosacral joint. **A.** Anterior shear with typical lumbosacral angle of 30°. Body weight acting on L5 results in L5's having both a compressive force (Fc) and an anterior shear force (Fs) in relation to the inclined surface of S1. **B.** With an increased lumbosacral angle of 45°, the force of the body weight acting on L5 results in a shear force (Fs) that is equal to or greater than the compressive force (Fc) in relation to the inclined surface of S1.

■ Intervertebral Disks

Specific regional variations occur in the intervertebral disks of the lumbar region, which differ from the disks of the cervical region in that the collagen fibers of the anulus fibrosus are arranged in sheets called **lamellae** (Fig. 4-40). The lamellae are arranged in concentric rings that surround the nucleus. Collagen fibers in adjacent rings are oriented in opposite directions at 120° to each other.[6,10] The advantage of the varying fiber orientation by layer is that the anulus fibrosus is able to resist tensile forces in nearly all directions. The lumbar intervertebral disks are the largest in the body (as are the vertebral bodies). The shape of each disk is not purely elliptical but concave posteriorly. This provides a greater cross-sectional area of anulus fibrosus posteriorly and hence increased ability to resist the tension that occurs here with forward bending[2] (Fig. 4-41).

■ Articulations

Interbody Joints

The interbody joints of the lumbar region are capable of translations and tilts in all directions.

Zygapophyseal Joints

The zygapophyseal joints of the lumbar region, like all others, are true synovial joints and contain fibroadipose meniscoid structures. The joint capsules are more lax than in the thoracic region but more taut than those of the cervical region. The dorsal capsule has been demonstrated to be fibrocartilaginous in nature, which suggests that this portion of the capsule is subject to compressive as well as tensile forces.[32]

In a newborn, the zygapophyseal joints in the lumbar region lie predominantly in the frontal plane in the presence of lumbar kyphosis. As the child develops and assumes an upright posture, the curve of the lumbar region changes to lordosis, and the orientation of the zygapophyseal joints change as well. The orientations of the adult lumbar zygapophyseal joints display great variability both between individuals and within individuals; however, the majority of them have a curved structure that is biplanar in orientation. The anterior aspect of each joint remains in the frontal plane, and the poste-

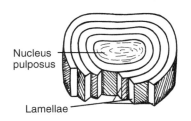

▲ **Figure 4-40** ■ Schematic representation of an intervertebral disk, showing arrangement of lamellae in anulus fibrosus. The collagen fibers in any two adjacent concentric bands or sheets (lamellae) are oriented in opposite directions.

rior aspect lies close to or in the sagittal plane (Fig. 4-42). The degrees to which this happens vary. The frontal plane orientation provides resistance to the anterior shear that naturally is present in the lordotic lumbar region. The sagittal plane orientation allows the great range of flexion and extension ROM and provides resistance to rotation.

Case Application 4-4: **Variations in Zygapophyseal Joints**

The shape of an individual's lumbar zygapophyseal joints may be a factor that predisposes some people to injury and protects others. For example, it may be that Malik has lumbar zygapophyseal joints at the L5/S1 segment that are oriented entirely in the frontal plane, and they therefore offer little bony resistance to anterior shear forces.

■ Ligaments and Fascia

The majority of the ligaments associated with the lumbar region are the same ligaments described previously (ligamentum flavum, PLL, anterior longitudinal ligament, interspinous and supraspinous ligaments, and joint capsules). However, a few of these ligaments have variations specific to the lumbar region and need to be mentioned here before the iliolumbar ligaments and the thoracolumbar fascia are introduced.

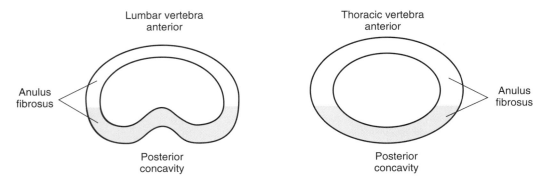

◀ **Figure 4-41** ■ Lumbar intervertebral disks are concave posteriorly, which provides a greater portion of anulus fibrosus located posteriorly. This provides more anulus fibrosus available to resist the posterior stretch that occurs in flexion. (From Bogduk, N: Clinical Anatomy of the Lumbar Spine and Sacrum, (3rd ed.), 1997, with permission from Elsevier).

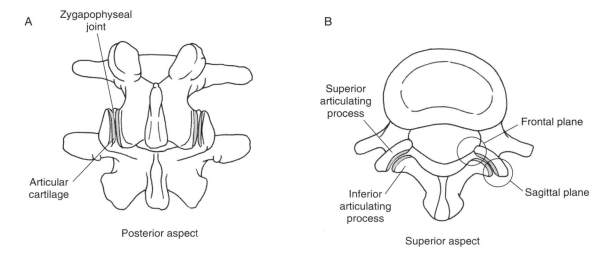

Figure 4-42 ■ The biplanar orientation of the lumbar zygapophyseal joints. The posterior view (**A**) demonstrates the predominant sagittal plane orientation; however, a superior view (**B**) with the vertebral body of the cranial vertebra removed demonstrates the biplanar orientation. (From Bogduk, N: Clinical Anatomy of the Lumbar Spine and Sacrum, (3rd ed.), 1997, with permission from Elsevier).

The supraspinous ligament is well developed only in the upper lumbar region and may terminate at L3, although the most common termination site appears to be at L4. The ligament is almost always absent at L5/S1. The deep layer of the supraspinous ligament is reinforced by tendinous fibers of the multifidus muscle. The middle fibers of the supraspinous ligament blend with the dorsal layer of the thoracolumbar fascia. The intertransverse ligaments are not true ligaments in the lumbar area and are replaced by the iliolumbar ligament at L4.[74] The PLL is only a thin ribbon in the lumbar region, whereas the ligamentum flavum is thickened here.[76] In a study of 132 lumbar spine ligaments, Pintar and associates found that the interspinous ligament had the least overall stiffness and the joint capsules the highest. The anterior longitudinal ligament is strong and well developed in this region.[76]

Iliolumbar Ligaments

The iliolumbar ligaments consist of a series of bands that extend from the tips and borders of the transverse processes of L4 and L5 to attach bilaterally on the iliac crests of the pelvis (Fig. 4-43). There are three primary bands: the ventral (or anterior) band, which runs from the ventral caudal aspect of the transverse process of L5 to the ventral surface of the iliac crest at the iliac tuberosity; the dorsal (or posterior) band, which runs from the tip of the transverse process of L5 to the cranial part of the iliac crest at the iliac tuberosity; and the sacral band (sometimes called the lumbosacral ligament), which runs from the ventral aspect of the transverse process of L5 and the ala of the sacrum to the sacral surface of the iliac tuberosity of the iliac crest.[77] The iliolumbar ligaments as a whole are very strong and play a significant role in stabilizing the fifth lumbar vertebra (preventing the vertebra from anterior displacement) and in resisting flexion, extension, axial rotation, and lateral bending of L5 on S1.[74,78–80]

Thoracolumbar Fascia

The thoracolumbar fascia (also called the lumbodorsal fascia) consists of three layers: the posterior, middle, and anterior (Fig. 4-44). The posterior layer is large, thick, and fibrous and arises from the spinous processes and supraspinous ligaments of the thoracic, lumbar, and sacral spines. The posterior layer gives rise to the latissimus dorsi cranially, travels caudally to the sacrum and ilium, and blends with the fascia of the contralateral gluteus maximus. Deep fibers are continuous with the sacrotuberous ligament and connected to the

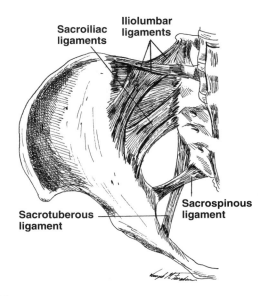

Figure 4-43 ■ The sacroiliac and iliolumbar ligaments reinforce the sacroiliac and lumbosacral articulations, respectively. The sacrospinous ligament forms the inferior border of the greater sciatic notch, and the sacrotuberous ligament forms the interior border of the lesser sciatic notch.

posterior superior iliac spines, iliac crests, and PLL.[81] The posterior layer also travels laterally over the erector spinae muscles and forms the lateral raphe at the lateral aspect of the erector spinae. The internal abdominal oblique and the transversus abdominal muscles arise from the lateral raphe. The posterior layer becomes the middle layer and travels medially again along the anterior surface of the erector spinae and attaches back to the transverse processes and intertransverse ligaments of the lumbar spine. These two layers completely surround the lumbar extensor muscle group. The anterior layer of the thoracolumbar fascia is derived from the fascia of the quadratus lumborum muscle, where it joins the middle layer, inserts into the transverse processes of the lumbar spine, and blends with the intertransverse ligaments.[74]

McGill described the fascia as a stabilizing corset that forms a "hoop" around the abdomen along the abdominal muscles and their fascia[26] (see Fig. 4-44). Gracovetsky designated the anterior layer of the thoracolumbar fascia as the "passive part" and the posterior layer as the "active part."[82] According to Gracovetsky, the passive part serves to transmit tension produced by a contraction of the hip extensors to the spinous processes. The active portion is activated by a contraction of the transversus abdominis muscle, which tightens the fascia. The fascia transmits tension longitudinally to the tips of the spinous processes of L1/L4 and may help the spinal extensor muscles to resist an applied load.[82] Vleeming found that both the gluteus maximus and contralateral latissimus dorsi tensed the superficial layer and provided a pathway for the mechanical transmission of forces between the pelvis and the trunk.[81]

Case Application 4-5: **Soft Tissue Structures as Possible Source of Pain**

> Given the tasks that Malik performs daily, he is continually experiencing large anterior shear forces. The iliolumbar ligaments, the posterior anulus fibrosus, the PLL, and the joint capsules are being subjected to stresses, which could lead to failure of some or all of these structures. Each of these structures is innervated and may be a source of his pain.

Function of the Lumbar Region

■ Kinematics

The lumbar region is capable of movement in flexion, extension, lateral flexion, and rotation. The lumbar zygapophyseal facets favor flexion and extension, because of the predominant sagittal plane orientation (see Fig. 4-18A). Flexion of the lumbar spine is more limited than extension and, normally, it is not possible to flex the lumbar region to form a kyphotic curve. The amount of flexion varies at each interspace of the lumbar vertebrae, but most of the flexion takes place at the

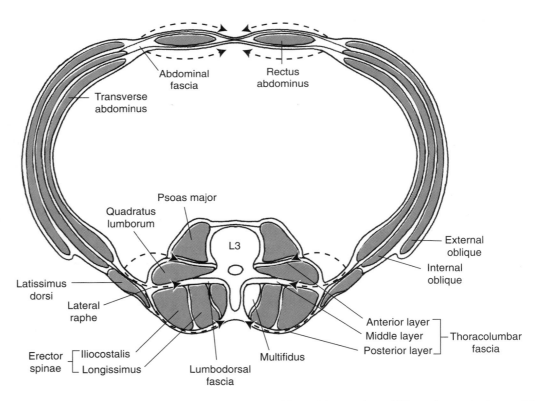

▲ **Figure 4-44** ■ A superior view of a cross-section to identify the abdominal hoop. The anterior, middle, and posterior layers of the thoracolumbar fascia, along with the abdominal fascia, are the passive parts. The muscles are the active parts, which pull (dashed arrows) on the fascia to tighten the hoop.

lumbosacral joint.[83,84] During flexion and extension, the greatest mobility of the spine occurs between L4 and S1, which is also the area that must support the most weight.

Rotation in this region, however, is more limited because of the shape of the zygapophyseal joints (Fig. 4-45). The effectiveness of the zygapophyseal joints in resisting axial rotation depends on the extent that the superior facets face medially (in the sagittal plane). The greater the medial orientation of the joint surfaces, the greater the resistance to axial rotation.

In the lumbar region, pure flexion and extension can occur,[34] but coupled motions always occur with lateral flexion and axial rotation. With lateral flexion, pronounced flexion and slight ipsilateral rotation occurs. With axial rotation, however, substantial lateral flexion in a contralateral direction occurs, but only a slight amount of flexion occurs.[34] Lateral flexion and rotation are most free in the upper lumbar region and progressively diminish in the lower region. The largest lateral flexion ROM and axial rotation occurs between L2 and L3.[84] Little or no lateral flexion or rotation is possible at the lumbosacral joint because of the most common orientation of the zygapophyseal joints, at 45° to the sagittal plane.[74] There is, however, a considerable amount of variation in the degree of axial rotation of lumbar vertebrae. In addition to being affected by facet orientation, the amount of rotation available at each vertebral level appears to be affected by the position of the lumbar spine. When the lumbar spine is flexed, the ROM in rotation is less than when the lumbar spine is in the neutral position. The posterior anulus fibrosus and the PLL seem to play an important role in limiting axial rotation when the spine is flexed. The zygapophyseal joint capsules limit rotation in both the neutral and extended positions of the spine.[85]

Continuing Exploration: **Lumbar-Pelvic Rhythm**

Cailliet described a specific instance of coordinated, simultaneous activity of lumbar flexion and anterior tilting of the pelvis in the sagittal plane during trunk flexion and extension. He called the combined lumbar and pelvic motion **lumbar-pelvic rhythm.** The activity of bending over to touch one's toes with knees straight depends on lumbar-pelvic rhythm.[86] According to Cailliet, the first part of bending forward consists of lumbar flexion, followed next by anterior tilting of the pelvis at the hip joints (Fig. 4-46). A return to the erect posture is initiated by posterior tilting of the pelvis at the hips, followed by extension of the lumbar spine. The initial pelvic motion delays lumbar extension until the trunk is raised far enough to shorten the moment arm of the external load, thus reducing the load on the erector spinae.

Nelson and coworkers studied lumbar-pelvic motion in 30 healthy women, age 19 to 35 years, who lifted and replaced a 9.5-kg weight on the floor. They found that lumbar and pelvic motion were variable among these individuals and tended to occur simultaneously during trunk flexion and more sequentially during trunk extension.[87] The use of a weight may have affected the lumbar-pelvic rhythm, but this study raises questions about exactly when and how trunk and pelvic motion occurs. McGill reported that he and his colleagues had never seen this strict sequence described by Cailliet in any of the vast number of studies that they had done.[26]

There is no argument, however, that the integration of motion of the pelvis about the hip joints with motion of the vertebral column not only increases the ROM available to the total column but also reduces the amount of flexibility required of the lumbar region. Hip motion may even, as McGill suggested, eliminate the need for full lumbar flexion, which would serve a protective function by protecting the anulus fibrosus and posterior ligaments from being fully lengthened.[26]

The contribution to motion from multiple areas to produce a larger ROM than could be accomplished by a single area is similar to what is found at the shoulder in scapulohumeral rhythm. A restriction of motion at either the lumbar spine or at the hip joints may disturb the rhythm and prevent a person from reaching the toes. Restriction of motion at one segment also may result in hypermobility of the unrestricted segment.

Rotation in the lumbar spine

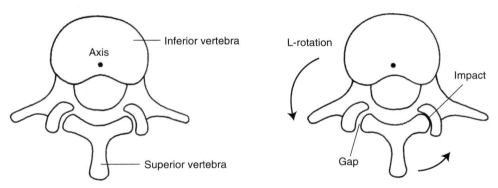

▲ **Figure 4-45** ■ Zygapophyseal mechanics in rotation of the lumbar vertebra. The sagittal plane orientation provides resistance to rotation. With left rotation, the right zygapophyseal joint will abut, limiting the ROM, and the left zygapophyseal joint will gap.

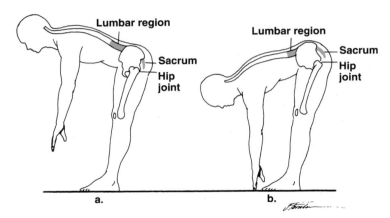

◀ **Figure 4–46** ■ Lumbar-pelvic rhythm. The lumbar spine flexes (**A**) and the pelvis rotates anteriorly (**B**) in the sagittal plane.

■ Kinetics

Compression

One of the primary functions of the lumbar region is to provide support for the weight of the upper part of the body in static as well as in dynamic situations. The increased size of the lumbar vertebral bodies and disks in comparison with their counterparts in the other regions helps the lumbar structures support the additional weight. The lumbar region must also withstand the tremendous compressive loads produced by muscle contraction. Experimental testing of 10 cadaver spines subjected to 1000-N compressive loading demonstrated that the lumbar interbody joints shared 80% of the load, and the zygapophyseal facet joints in axial compression shared 20% of the total load.[88] This percentage can change with altered mechanics: with increased extension or lordosis, the zygapophyseal joints will assume more of the compressive load. Also, with degeneration of the intervertebral disk, the zygapophyseal joints will assume increased compressive load.

Khoo and colleagues compared lumbosacral loads (ground reaction forces and accelerations plus forces generated by erector spinae and rectus abdominis muscle groups) at the center of the L5/S1 joint in static versus dynamic situations in 10 men. Lumbosacral loads in the erect standing posture were in the range of 0.82 to 1.18 times body weight, whereas lumbosacral loads during level walking were in the range of 1.41 to 2.07 times body weight (an increase of 56.3%).[89] Changes in position of the body will change the location of the body's line of gravity and thus change the forces acting on the lumbar spine. See Chapter 13 for a discussion of compressive loads on the lumbar spine with different positions.

Shear

In the upright standing position, the lumbar segments are subjected to anterior shear forces cause by the lordotic position, the body weight, and ground reaction forces (see Fig. 4-39). This anterior shear or translation of the vertebra is resisted by direct impaction of the inferior zygapophyseal facets of the superior vertebra against the superior zygapophyseal facets of the adjacent vertebra below. The effectiveness of the zygapophyseal joint in providing resistance to anterior translation during flexion depends on the extent to which the inferior vertebra's superior facets lie in the frontal plane and face posteriorly. The more that the superior zygapophyseal facets of an adjacent inferior vertebra face posteriorly, the greater the resistance they are able to provide to forward displacement because the posteriorly facing facets lock against the inferior facets of the adjacent superior vertebra.

CONCEPT CORNERSTONE 4-3: *Variations in Zygapophyseal Joints*

The shape of the zygapophyseal joints, the zygapophyseal joint capsules, the fibers of the anulus fibrosus, and the iliolumbar ligaments in the lower segments provide structural resistance to anterior shear forces in the lumbar segments. Individual variation in joint structure, therefore, can be a contributing factor to pain in this region. If an individual has zygapophyseal joints oriented totally in the sagittal plane, the capsuloligamentous structures will be taxed, and eventually they may become lengthened and be a source of pain, because they are innervated structures. Even if an individual has zygapophyseal joints with a biplanar orientation, excessive anterior shear forces can cause damage. In this case, in addition to the lengthened capsuloligamentous structures, the zygapophyseal joints themselves can experience excessive compression in the anterior regions and produce pain. Fortunately, there is a dynamic restraint to anterior shear, the deep erector spinae muscles, which will be discussed later in the chapter.

Case Application 4-6: **Excessive Anterior Shear Forces**

The shape of Malik's zygapophyseal joints may or may not be known from diagnostic tests. Regardless, it is likely that these joints have been under repetitive stress because of his job tasks. The excessive anterior shear forces may be a likely source of pain from microtrauma to the joint capsules and ligaments, fibroadipose meniscoids, and/or degenerative changes to the joint surfaces themselves. In any case, including exercises to maximize the ability of the deep erector spinae to control the excessive anterior shear forces will be important to Malik's rehabilitation. In the meantime, changing Malik's activity to minimize the anterior shear forces that he encounters will likely decrease his symptoms. If his activity cannot be changed sufficiently a lumbosacral brace or corset may be considered to provide proprioceptive input for positioning and possibly to protect him from further injury.

Structure of the Sacral Region

Five sacral vertebrae are fused to form the triangular or wedge-shaped structure that is called the sacrum. The base of the triangle, which is formed by the first sacral vertebra, supports two articular facets that face posteriorly for articulation with the inferior facets of the fifth lumbar vertebra. The apex of the triangle, formed by the fifth sacral vertebra, articulates with the coccyx.

■ Sacroiliac Articulations

The two **SIJs** consist of the articulations between the left and right articular surfaces on the sacrum (which are formed by fused portions of the first, second, and third sacral segments) and the left and right iliac bones (Fig. 4-47). The SIJs are unique in that both the structure and function of these joints change significantly from birth through adulthood.

Articulating Surfaces on the Sacrum

The articulating surfaces on the sacrum are auricular (C)-shaped[90] and are located on the sides of the fused sacral vertebrae lateral to the sacral foramina. The fetal and prepubertal surfaces are flat and smooth, whereas the postpubertal surfaces are marked by a central groove or surface depression that extends the length of the articulating surfaces.[90,91] The articular surfaces are covered with hyaline cartilage. The overall mean thickness of the sacral cartilage is greater than that of the iliac cartilage.[92–95]

Articulating Surfaces on the Ilia

The articular surfaces on the ilia are also C-shaped. In the first decade of life, the iliac joint surfaces are smooth and flat and covered with fibrocartilage. The type of cartilage covering the iliac articular surfaces in the adult continues to be a matter of debate. The cartilage is different in gross appearance and is thinner than the sacral articular cartilage. It was usually described as fibrocartilage.[90,96] However, type II collagen, which is typical of hyaline cartilage, has been identified in the iliac cartilage,[97] and the iliac cartilage is described in the 38th edition of *Gray's Anatomy* as being hyaline cartilage.[27] After puberty, the joint surfaces develop a central ridge that extends the length of the articulating surface and corresponds to the grooves on the sacral articulating surfaces.[92,98]

■ Ligaments

The **anterior, interosseous,** and **posterior sacroiliac ligaments** are directly associated with the SIJs. A separate portion of the posterior sacroiliac ligament is called either the **long posterior sacroiliac ligament**[27] or the **long dorsal sacroiliac ligament.**[99] The **iliolumbar ligaments,** which connect the fifth lumbar vertebra to the sacrum and the **sacrospinous ligaments,** and the **sacrotuberous ligaments,** which connect the sacrum to the ischium, are indirectly associated with the SIJs (Fig. 4-48). The iliolumbar ligaments were described previously in the lumbar region.

Sacroiliac Ligaments

The sacroiliac ligaments as a whole extend from the iliac crests to attach to the tubercles of the first four sacral vertebrae. The sacroiliac ligaments, which are reinforced by fibrous expansions from the quadratus lumborum, erector spinae, gluteus maximus, gluteus minimus, piriformis, and iliacus muscles, contribute to the joint's stability. The fascial support is greater posteriorly than anteriorly because more muscles are located

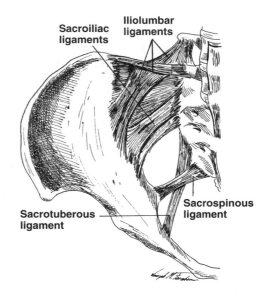

▲ **Figure 4-48** ■ The sacroiliac and iliolumbar ligaments reinforce the sacroiliac and lumbosacral articulations, respectively. The sacrospinous ligament forms the inferior border of the greater sciatic notch, and the sacrotuberous ligament forms the interior border of the lesser sciatic notch.

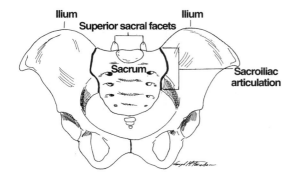

▲ **Figure 4-47** ■ The sacroiliac joints consist of the articulations between the first three sacral segments and the two ilia of the pelvis.

posteriorly.[91] The anterior sacroiliac ligaments are considered by *Gray's Anatomy* to be capsular ligaments because of the ligaments' intimate connections to the anteroinferior margins of the joint capsules.[27] According to Bogduk, the anterior sacroiliac ligaments cover the anterior aspects of the SIJs and join the ilia to the sacrum.[74]

The interosseous sacroiliac ligaments, which constitute the major bonds between the sacrum and the ilia, are considered to be the most important ligaments directly associated with the SIJs.[27,74] The ligaments are composed of superficial and deep portions, which are divided into superior and inferior bands. The superficial bands unite the superior articular processes and lateral crests of the first two sacral segments to the ilia. This portion of the interosseous ligament is referred to as the **short posterior sacroiliac ligament**.[27,74] The deeper portions of the interosseous sacroiliac ligament extend from depressions posterior to the sacral articular surface to depressions on the iliac tuberosities. The posterior sacroiliac ligaments connect the lateral sacral crests to the posterior superior iliac spines and iliac crests.

The paired long dorsal sacroiliac ligaments have superior attachments to the posterior superior sacroiliac spines (PSISs) and adjacent parts of the ilium. Inferiorly, the ligaments are attached to the lateral crest of the third and fourth sacral segments. The medial fibers are connected to the deep lamina of the posterior layer of the thoracolumbar fascia and the aponeurosis of the erector spinae (ESA).[99] The **sacrospinous** ligaments connect the ischial spines to the lateral borders of the sacrum and coccyx. The **sacrotuberous** ligaments connect the ischial tuberosities to the posterior spines at the ilia and the lateral sacrum and coccyx. The sacrospinous ligament forms the inferior border of the greater sciatic notch; the sacrotuberous ligament forms the inferior border of the lesser sciatic notch.[100,101]

■ Symphysis Pubis Articulation

The symphysis pubis is a cartilaginous joint located between the two ends of the pubic bones. The end of each pubic bone is covered with a layer of articular cartilage and the joint is formed by a fibrocartilaginous disk that joins the hyaline cartilage-covered ends of the bones. The disk has a thin central cleft,[1] which in women may extend throughout the length of the disk.[102] The three ligaments that are associated with the joint are the **superior pubic ligament,** the **inferior pubic ligament,** and the **posterior ligament**.[1] The superior ligament is a thick and dense fibrous band that attaches to the pubic crests and tubercles and helps support the superior aspect of the joint. The inferior ligament arches from the inferior rami on one side of the joint to the inferior portion of the rami on the other side and thus reinforces the inferior aspect of the joint. The posterior ligament consists of a fibrous membrane that is continuous with the periosteum of the pubic bones.[1] The anterior portion of the joint is reinforced by aponeurotic expansions from a number of muscles that cross the joint (Fig. 4-49). Kapandji described the muscle expansions as forming an anterior ligament consist-

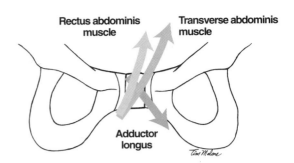

▲ **Figure 4-49** ■ The aponeurotic extensions of the muscles crossing the anterior aspect of the symphysis pubis.

ing of expansions of the transversus abdominis, rectus abdominis, internal obliquus abdominis, and adductor longus.[1]

Function of the Sacral Region

■ Kinematics

The SIJs permit a small amount of motion that varies among individuals. Both the amount and type of motion available at these joints has been and continues to be a matter of controversy. At most, it appears as if the motion available is very slight and not easily defined. The SIJs are linked to the symphysis pubis in a closed kinematic chain, and therefore any motion occurring at the symphysis pubis is accompanied by motion at the SIJs and vice versa.

The smooth SIJ surfaces in early childhood permit gliding motions in all directions, which is typical of a synovial plane joint.[90] However, after puberty, the joint surfaces change their configuration and, according to Walker, motion in the adult is restricted to a very few millimeters of translation and or rotation.[92] However, a considerable amount of controversy exists with regard to both the type and amount of motion available at the SIJs.

Nutation is the term commonly used to refer to movement of the sacral promontory of the sacrum anteriorly and inferiorly while the coccyx moves posteriorly in relation to the ilium (Fig. 4-50A). **Counternutation** refers to the opposite movement, in which the anterior tip of the sacral promontory moves posteriorly and superiorly while the coccyx moves anteriorly in relation to the ilium (see Fig. 4-50B). The change in position of the sacrum during nutation and counternutation affects the diameter of the pelvic brim and pelvic outlet. During nutation, the anteroposterior diameter of the pelvic brim is reduced and the anteroposterior diameter of the pelvic outlet is increased. During counternutation, the reverse situation occurs. The anteroposterior diameter of the pelvic brim is increased, and the diameter of the pelvic outlet is decreased.[1] These changes in diameter are of particular importance during pregnancy and childbirth, and it is possible that the most motion that occurs at the SIJs may occur in pregnancy and childbirth, when the joint structures are

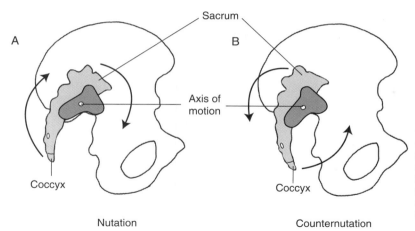

Sacrum

A

B

Axis of motion

Coccyx

Coccyx

Nutation

Counternutation

◀ **Figure 4-50** ■ **A.** Nutation. The arrow at the top of the sacrum indicates the anterior-inferior motion of the anterior tip of the sacral promontory during nutation. The arrow arising from the coccyx indicates the posterior-superior movement of the coccyx. **B.** Counternutation. The sacral promontory moves posteriorly and superiorly in counternutation, and the coccyx moves anteriorly and inferiorly.

under hormonal influence and ligamentous structures are softened. Accurate descriptions of the SIJs and the motions that occur at these joints have been difficult to obtain because the planes of the joint surfaces are oblique to the angle of an x-ray beam used to make a standard anteroposterior radiograph of the pelvis.[97]

During pregnancy, **relaxin,** a polypeptide hormone is produced by the corpus luteum and decidua. This hormone is thought to activate the collagenolytic system, which regulates new collagen formation and alters the ground substance by decreasing the viscosity and increasing the water content. The action of relaxin is to decrease the intrinsic strength and rigidity of collagen and is thought to be responsible for the softening of the ligaments supporting the SIJs and the symphysis pubis. Consequently, the joints become more mobile and less stable, and the likelihood of injury to these joints is increased. The combination of loosened posterior ligaments and an anterior weight shift caused by a heavy uterus may allow excessive movement of the ilia on the sacrum and result in stretching of the SIJ capsules.

The SIJs and symphysis pubis are closely linked functionally to the hip and joints and therefore affect and are affected by movements of the trunk and lower extremities. For example, weight shifting from one leg to another is accompanied by motion at the SIJs. Fusions of the lower lumbar vertebrae have been found to cause compensatory increases in motion at the SIJs.[103]

The joints of the pelvis are linked to the hip and vertebral column in non–weight-bearing as well as in weight-bearing postures. Hip flexion in a supine position tilts the ilia posteriorly in relation to sacrum. This pelvic motion causes nutation at the SIJs, which increases the diameter of the pelvic outlet. During the process of birth, the increase in the diameter of the pelvic outlet facilitates delivery of the fetal head. Counternutation is brought about by hip extension in the supine position and enlarges the pelvic brim. Therefore, a hip-extended position is favored early in the birthing process to facilitate the descent of the fetal head into the pelvis, whereas the hip-flexed position is used during delivery.[104]

■ **Kinetics**

Stability of the SIJs is extremely important because these joints must support a large portion of the body weight. In normal erect posture, the weight of head, arms, and trunk (HAT) is transmitted through the fifth lumbar vertebra and lumbosacral disk to the first sacral segment. The force of the body weight creates a nutation torque on the sacrum. Concomitantly, the ground reaction force creates a posterior torsion on the ilia. The countertorques of nutation and counternutation of the sacrum and posterior torsion of the ilia are prevented by the ligamentous tension and fibrous expansions from adjacent muscles that reinforce the joint capsules and blend with the ligaments.[92]

In one study, Pool-Goudzwaard and colleagues investigated the role that the iliolumbar ligaments played in stabilizing the SIJs.[77] These authors demonstrated that the iliolumbar ligaments have a significant role in stabilizing the SIJ as well as the lumbosacral junction. The ventral band of the iliolumbar ligament is of particular importance in restricting sagittal plane SIJ mobility.

Also, tension developed in the sacrotuberous, sacrospinous, and anterior sacroiliac ligaments counteracts the nutation of the sacrum, although the sacrotuberous and sacrospinous ligaments have not been found to play a major role in pelvic stability.[105] However, the sacrotuberous and interosseous ligaments compress the SIJ during nutation.[99] The long dorsal sacroiliac ligament is under tension in counternutation and relaxed in nutation.[106] The interosseous sacroiliac ligament binds the ilia to the sacrum.[74]

Surface irregularities and texture of the SIJs also contribute to stability of the joint in the adult. In a study of SIJs, the highest coefficients of friction were found in sample joints with ridges, depressions, and coarse-textured cartilage. Sample joints with ridges, depressions, and smooth cartilage showed higher coefficients of friction than did samples without ridges and depressions. These findings suggest that the complementary ridges and depressions as well as the coarse surface textures found in the adult reflect a dynamic, normal development of the SIJs. Vertical load-bearing is facilitated by these changes, but motion is limited by the changes.[92,101,107,108]

Shearing forces are created at the symphysis pubis during the single-leg-support phase of walking, as a result of lateral pelvic tilting. In a normal situation, the joint is capable of resisting the shearing forces, and no appreciable motion occurs. If, however, the joint is dislocated, the pelvis becomes unstable during gait, with increased stress on the sacroiliac and hip joints as well as the vertebral column.

◆ Muscles of the Vertebral Column

The Craniocervical/Upper Thoracic Regions

The muscles of the craniocervical region serve two primary roles: to hold the head upright against gravity and to infinitely position the head in space in order to optimally position the sensory organs. The muscles of the cervicothoracic region also serve two primary roles: again, to position the head and neck in space and to stabilize the head and neck to allow and produce movement of the scapula. The line of gravity in an upright standing position passes anteriorly to the axis of rotation in the cervical region, producing a flexion moment (Fig. 4-51). The posterior muscles, along with the ligamentous structures previously discussed,

counter this flexion moment. The need to position the head for the special sensory organs often includes rapid, coordinated movements, such as when a loud noise is heard and there is rapid turning of the head to locate the source of the sound. The muscular structure and function are complex in order to serve the demands for such great amounts of motion and yet provide sufficient stability to protect the spinal cord and allow for use of the upper extremities.

■ Posterior Muscles

We will examine the muscles from superficial to deep and begin with the posterior muscles (Figs. 4-52 and 4-53). The trapezius muscle is the most superficial of the posterior muscles. The trapezius spans from the occiput to the lower thoracic spine and contains a prominent tendinous region over the cervicothoracic junction.[53] The trapezius belongs predominantly to the shoulder region; however, when the upper extremities are fixated, the trapezius can produce extension of the head and neck. Acting unilaterally, the upper trapezius can produce ipsilateral lateral flexion and contralateral rotation of the head and neck.

The levator scapula is deep to the trapezius. It runs from the root of the spine of the scapula and courses superiorly, medially, and anteriorly to insert on the cervical transverse processes. This muscle has a large cross-sectional area. The levator scapula is a scapular elevator and downward rotator when the neck is stable, but if the upper extremity is stabilized, it will produce ipsilateral lateral flexion and rotation of the cervical spine. In addition, the anterior inclination plays an important role in the mechanics of the cervical spine. The levator scapula is optimally aligned to produce a posterior shear force on the cervical spine.[53] Porterfield and DeRosa[53] likened the levator scapulae to the deep erector spinae of the lumbopelvic area, which will be

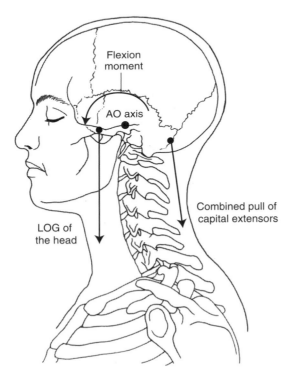

▲ **Figure 4-51** ■ The line of gravity in the cervical region passes anteriorly to the axis of rotation, producing a flexion moment. The extensor muscles must contract to counter this moment.

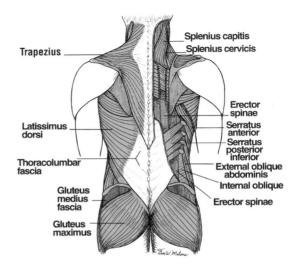

▲ **Figure 4-52** ■ Posterior back muscles. The superficial muscles have been removed on the right side to show the erector spinae. The anterior layer of the thoracolumbar fascia is intact on the left side of the back.

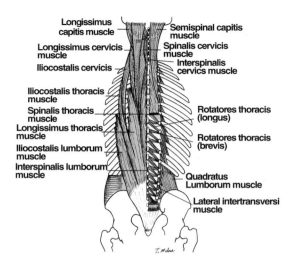

▲ **Figure 4-53** ▪ Erector spinae and deep back muscles. The erector spinae muscle has been removed from the right side of the neck to show the deep back muscles.

discussed later. The cervical spine is subjected to constant anterior shear forces caused by gravity and the lordotic position of the spine in this region. The levator scapulae help resist these forces (Fig. 4-54). An increase in the cervical lordosis, as is often seen in excessive forward head posture, will further increase the anterior shear forces on the cervical vertebrae and may cause overactivity of the levator scapula to resist these excessive anterior shear forces.

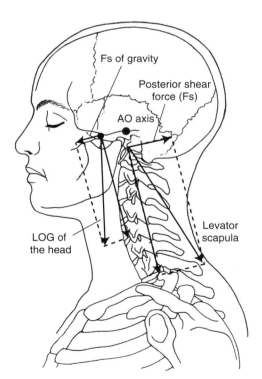

▲ **Figure 4-54** ▪ The cervical spine is subjected to anterior shear forces as a result of the lordosis and anterior line of gravity. The levator scapulae help resist the anterior shear forces by producing posterior shear.

Continuing Exploration: **Treatment for Overactivity of Levator-Scapula Muscle**

Porterfield and DeRosa[53] suggested that overactivity in the presence of a forward head posture may be the reason that so many people have pain and tenderness to palpation in the levator scapulae. Conventional treatment will often involve stretching this strained muscle. Porterfield and DeRosa[53] cautioned that stretching this muscle may actually worsen the situation and cause further irritation, because it will decrease the muscle's ability to control the anterior shear if it is overly lengthened. Rather, removal of the excessive anterior shear forces is necessary. In addition, the levator scapulae may need endurance and strength training.

The splenius capitis and splenius cervicis muscles are deep to the levator scapulae. The splenius muscles are large, flat muscles running from the spinous processes of the cervical and thoracic spine and the ligamentum nuchae to the superior nuchal line, the mastoid process, and the cervical transverse processes (see Fig. 4-52). These muscles serve as prime movers of the head and neck as a result of their large cross-sectional area and the large moment arm. They produce extension when working bilaterally and ipsilateral rotation when working unilaterally. However, these muscles show little electromyographic activity in normal stance.

The semispinalis capitis and semispinalis cervicis muscles are deep to the splenius group. These muscles have the most optimal line of pull and a large moment arm to produce extension of the head and neck and an increase in the cervical lordosis. They run from the occiput to the cervical spinous processes (semispinalis capitis) and the thoracic transverse processes to the cervical spinous processes (semispinalis cervicis) (see Fig. 4-53). These muscles together form the cordlike bundle of muscles palpated laterally to the cervical spinous processes.[53] Porterfield and DeRosa[53] likened the function of the semispinalis group to that of the multifidus muscles in the lumbar region in that they have optimal alignment and moment arm for increasing the lordosis of the cervical and lumbar regions, respectively (Fig. 4-55). It is important to note that the greater occipital nerve pierces the semispinalis capitis muscle on its way to innervate the skull. This can be a site of nerve irritation and entrapment when the semispinalis capitis is overactive or shortened as in a forward head posture. Occipital region headaches can result.

The longissimus capitis and longissimus cervicis are deep and lateral to the semispinalis group (see Fig. 4-53). Their deep position places them close to the axis of rotation for flexion and extension, rendering them ineffective extensors because of the small moment arm. They do, however, produce compression of the cervical segments. The lateral position allows them to produce ipsilateral lateral flexion when working unilaterally, and when working bilaterally, they serve as frontal plane stabilizers of the cervical spine.[53]

The suboccipital muscles are the deepest posterior muscles and consist of the rectus capitus posterior

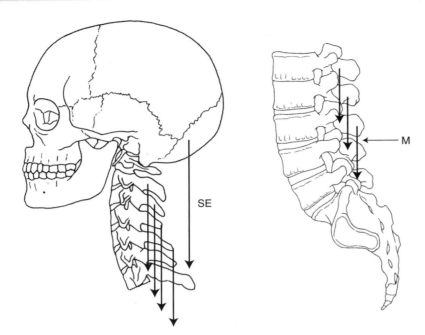

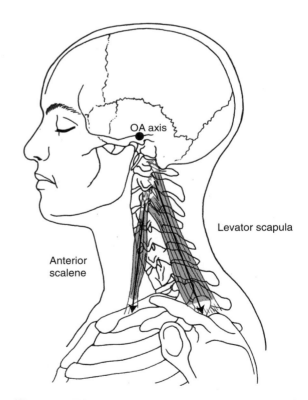

◄ **Figure 4-55** ■ Function of the semispinalis capitis in comparison with the lumbar multifidus muscle. The semispinalis capitis has an optimal lever arm for cervical extension. M, multifidus muscle; SE, semispinalis capitis muscle. (From Porter, JA, and DeRosa, C; Mechanical Neck Pain. Saunders/Elsevier, 1995, with permission.)

minor and major, inferior oblique, and superior oblique muscles. As a group, they run between the occiput and C2, allowing independent movement of the craniovertebral region on the lower cervical spine. Together, they produce occipital extension. Unilaterally, they produce ipsilateral rotation and lateral flexion. Given the small cross-sectional area of these muscles, some authors have questioned their ability to generate force and produce movement; rather, they may serve primarily a proprioceptive role and produce small movements in order to fine-tune motion.[109]

■ Lateral Muscles

The scalene muscles are located on the lateral aspect of the cervical spine and serve as frontal plane stabilizers along with the longissimus muscles posteriorly when they are acting as a group. In the sagittal plane, the anterior scalene muscles, which run from the first rib to the anterior tubercles of the transverse processes of C3 to C6, work with the levator scapulae to provide stability (Fig. 4-56). The anterior scalene muscles, when working bilaterally, will flex the cervical spine and produce an anterior shear. Unilaterally, the anterior scalene muscles will produce ipsilateral lateral flexion and contralateral rotation to the cervical spine. The middle scalene muscles run from the first rib to the anterior tubercles of the transverse processes of C3 to C7. The middle scalene muscles are more laterally placed than are the anterior scalene muscles, and their line of pull makes them excellent frontal plane stabilizers.[53] The posterior scalene muscles run from the second rib to the posterior tubercles of the transverse processes of C3 to C7. The posterior scalene muscles predominantly laterally flex the neck. The role of the scalene muscles in breathing will be discussed in Chapter 5. The anterior and middle scalene muscles form a triangle through which the brachial plexus and the subclavian artery and vein pass (Fig. 4-57). This can be a site for compression on the neurovascular structures by the anterior scalene muscle: scalenus anticus syndrome, described by Cailliet. This can produce pain, numbness, and tingling to the arm.[65]

The sternocleidomastoid muscle runs from the

▲ **Figure 4-56** ■ In the sagittal plane, the anterior scalene muscles work in synergy with the levator scapulae to provide stability for the cervical spine.

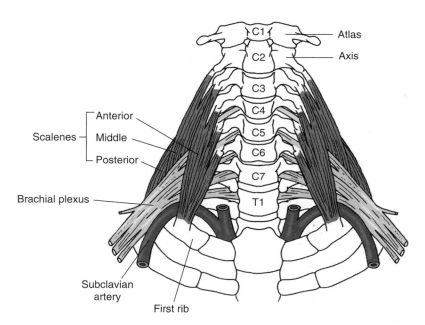

◀ **Figure 4-57** ■ The brachial plexus and the subclavian artery and vein pass between the anterior and middle scalene muscles.

sternum, distal clavicle, and acromion to the mastoid process. The angle of inclination is posterior, medial, and superior. It is unique in that, because of this orientation, it lies anterior to the axis of rotation in the lower cervical spine, producing flexion when acting bilaterally but posterior to the axis at the skull, producing extension of the head on the neck. Acting unilaterally, the sternocleidomastoid muscle will produce ipsilateral lateral flexion and contralateral rotation of the head and neck.

■ **Anterior Muscles**

The longus capitis run from the anterior tubercles of the cervical transverse processes to the occiput. The longus colli run from the thoracic vertebral bodies to the anterior tubercles of the cervical transverse processes and cranially from the anterior tubercles of the transverse processes to the atlas. These two muscles lie close to the vertebral bodies and therefore are relatively close to the axis of rotation. Although they do have sufficient moment arm to produce flexion, they also produce a fair amount of compression. The longus capitis and longus colli work in synergy with the trapezius to stabilize the head and neck to allow the trapezius to upwardly rotate the scapula[53] (Fig. 4-58). Given that muscles always contract from both ends, were it not for the longus capitis and longus colli, the trapezius would extend the head and neck rather than upwardly rotate the scapula, in view of the vastly greater weight and moment arm of the upper extremity in comparison with the head.

 CONCEPT CORNERSTONE 4-4: *Cervical Motion*

Porterfield and DeRosa[53] suggested that this synergy between the longus capitis and longus colli muscles and the trapezius muscle helps explain why hyperextension injuries to the neck (whiplash)

can result in pain and inability to raise the arm overhead. If damage has occurred to the longus capitis and longus colli, these muscles will be unable to stabilize the head and neck in order for the trapezius to successfully upwardly rotate the scapula.

The rectus capitis anterior and rectus capitis lateralis are able to produce flexion as a result of their line of pull; however, as with the suboccipital muscles, the

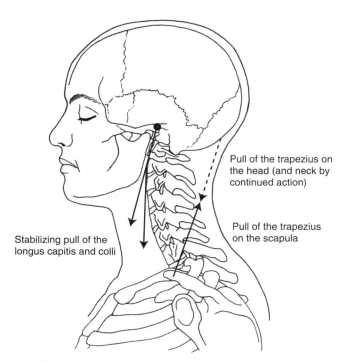

▲ **Figure 4-58** ■ In the sagittal plane, the trapezius, longus capitis, and longus colli work in synergy to elevate the scapula.

small cross-sectional area and moment arms probably render them capable of serving a greater proprioceptive function rather than prime mover.

Lower Thoracic/Lumbopelvic Regions

Muscles of the lower spine regions serve the roles of producing and controlling movement of the trunk and stabilizing the trunk for motion of the lower extremities. The muscles also assist in attenuating the extensive forces that affect this area.

■ Posterior Muscles

Again, we will examine the muscles from superficial to deep and begin with the posterior muscles. The thoracolumbar fascia is the most superficial structure. As discussed previously, several major muscle groups of this region are associated with the thoracolumbar fascia. The fascia gives rise to the latissimus dorsi, the gluteus maximus, the internal and external abdominal oblique, and the transversus abdominis. In addition, the fascia surrounds the erector spinae and the multifidus muscles of the lumbar region. These attachments are significant in that tensile forces can be exerted on the thoracolumbar fascia through muscle contraction of these muscles. Tension on the thoracolumbar fascia will

produce a force that exerts compression of the abdominal contents. Along with contraction of the abdominal muscles, this compression is similar to that of an external corset. The coupled action of the latissimus dorsi, contralateral gluteus maximus, and tension through the thoracolumbar fascia will compress the lumbosacral region and impart stability[26,110] (Fig. 4-59).

The erector spinae consist of the longissimus and iliocostalis muscle groups. In general, these muscles are identified as extensors of the trunk. Bogduk[2] examined the function of the longissimus thoracis and the iliocostalis lumborum and further described these muscles as each having a lumbar portion (pars lumborum) and a thoracic portion (pars thoracis). The longissimus thoracis pars thoracis and the iliocostalis lumborum pars thoracis form the more superficial layer and the longissimus thoracis pars lumborum and the iliocostalis lumborum pars lumborum form a deeper layer.

Anatomically and functionally, therefore, it is easier to group the muscles together as the superficial layer and the deep layer. The **superficial layer** runs from the ribs and thoracic transverse processes to form muscle bellies that are laterally located in the thoracic region. The muscles have long tendons that join together to form the ESA, which inserts into the spinous processes of the lower lumbar spine, sacrum, and iliac crest (Fig. 4-60). This superficial layer, with its long moment arm and excellent line of pull, produces extension of the

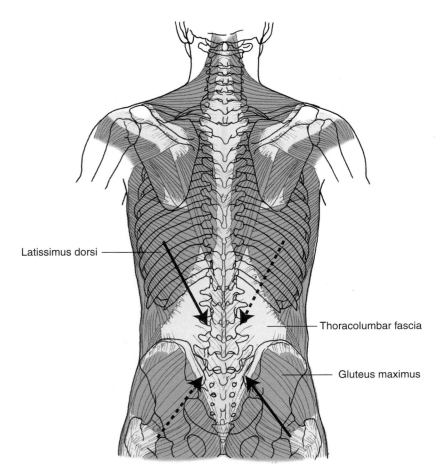

Latissimus dorsi

Thoracolumbar fascia

Gluteus maximus

◀ **Figure 4-59** ■ Coupled action of the latissimus dorsi, contralateral gluteus maximus, and tension through the thoracolumbar fascia will compress and stabilize the lumbosacral region.

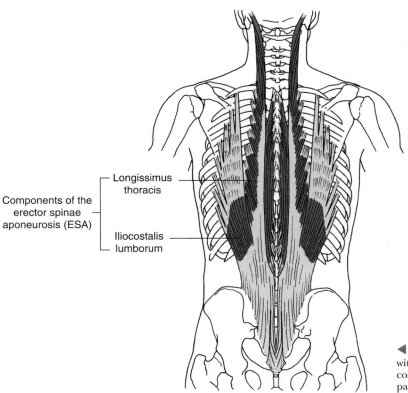

Components of the erector spinae aponeurosis (ESA)
⎧
⎨
⎩
Longissimus thoracis

Iliocostalis lumborum

◀ **Figure 4-60** ■ The superficial erector spinae with the erector spinae aponeurosis (ESA). IL, iliocostalis lumborum pars thoracis; LT, longissimus thoracis pars thoracis.

thoracic and lumbar regions when acting bilaterally. These muscles are considered to be the primary extensors of the trunk (Fig. 4-61). Acting unilaterally, they are able to laterally flex the trunk and contribute to rotation. During trunk flexion from a standing position, the erector spinae are responsible for contracting eccentrically to control the motion. The gravitational moment will produce forward flexion, but the extent and rate of flexion are controlled partially by eccentric contractions of the extensors with the ESA and partially by the thoracolumbar fascia and posterior ligamentous system. The erector spinae act eccentrically until approximately two thirds of maximal flexion has been attained, at which point they become electrically silent.[74,80,82] This is called the **flexion-relaxation phenomenon,** which is thought to occur at the point when stretched and deformed passive tissues are able to generate the required moment. However, the extensor muscles may be relaxed only in the electrical sense because they may be generating force elastically through passive stretching.[106] According to Gracovetsky,[82] control of flexion becomes the responsibility of the passive elastic response of the ESA, the thoracolumbar fascia, and the posterior ligamentous system. The posterior ligaments (supraspinous and interspinous ligaments) have longer moment arms than do the extensor muscles and thus have a mechanical advantage over the extensors.

Bogduk and others[2,111,112] identified the **deep layer** of the erector spinae as being entirely separate from the superficial layer and consisting of individual fascicles with common tendinous insertions. Bogduk[2] reported that the fascicles arise from the ilium at the

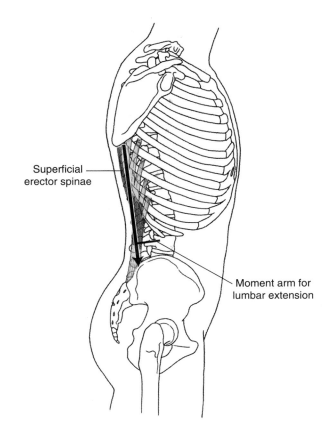

Superficial erector spinae

Moment arm for lumbar extension

▲ **Figure 4-61** ■ Sagittal view of the force vectors of the superficial erector spinae, demonstrating the excellent line of pull and large moment arm for extension.

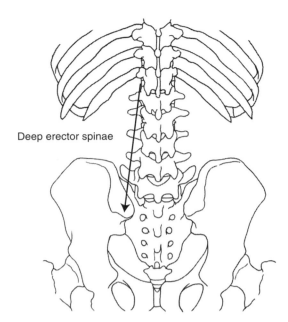

Deep erector spinae

▲ **Figure 4-62** ■ The fascicles of the deep erector spinae.

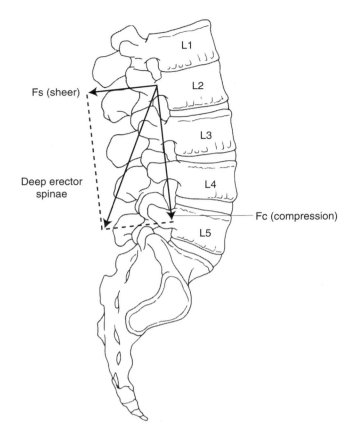

Fs (sheer)

Deep erector spinae

Fc (compression)

L1
L2
L3
L4
L5

▲ **Figure 4-63** ■ Sagittal view of the force vectors of the deep erector spinae, demonstrating the compression and posterior shear components.

PSIS and just lateral on the iliac crest and course superiorly, medially, and anteriorly to insert on the lumbar transverse processes (Fig. 4-62). Some debate remains, however, inasmuch as Daggfeldt et al.[111] reported some attachment to the ESA (and therefore not independent function) of the upper lumbar fascicles. Porterfield and DeRosa[110] described these deep erector spinae as similar in orientation and function to the levator scapulae in the cervical region. These muscles lie close to the axis of rotation and therefore do not have sufficient moment arm to be the prime movers into extension. Their oblique orientation, however, allows the muscles to exert a posterior shear force to the vertebrae. In addition to posterior shear, they also exert compressive forces (Fig. 4-63). Because of their oblique line of action and ability to produce posterior shear, these muscles provide an extremely important dynamic resistance to the constant anterior shear forces of the lumbar region caused by the lordotic position and the forces of gravity and ground reaction forces combined. These muscles, then, have great clinical significance. McGill[26] reported, however, that with lumbar spine flexion, these muscles lose their oblique orientation and therefore lose their ability to resist anterior shear forces. A flexed spine, therefore, is unable to dynamically resist anterior shear forces, which can cause damage.

Continuing Exploration: **Negative Effects of Overstretching the Deep Erector Spinae**

Like the levator scapulae in the cervical region, the deep erector spinae will become overworked and may be painful when subjected to excessive anterior shear forces. These muscles can become painful as a result of the excessive strain. Caution should be taken, however, in regard to stretching these mus-

cles. Overstretching of these muscles can remove the only dynamic restraint to the excessive anterior shear forces and either further load the noncontractile structures or, if they have already been damaged, remove the only remaining restraint. In either case, it is likely to worsen the symptoms. It is more likely that these muscles need greater endurance and strength training.

Case Application 4-7: **Deep Erector Spinae Muscle Sprain**

In addition to the noncontractile tissues previously discussed, Malik could also be experiencing pain arising directly from the deep erector spinae muscles, which became strained as a result of continual attempts to control for excessive anterior shear forces. If this were the case, gaining stretch and relaxation of the deep erector spinae would be an inappropriate goal of rehabilitation for Malik, because this would cause only further stress to the noncontractile tissues. Rather, it would be important to gain greater endurance for these muscles and decrease the external anterior shear forces until such time as the muscles could provide the support. This may be an appropriate time to use a lumbar corset, for example.

CONCEPT CORNERSTONE 4-5: *Location and Function of the Erector Spine*

Name	Location	Function
Deep Erector Spinae		
Longissimus thoracis pars lumborum (5 fascicles)	One from each lumbar TP to the PSIS	Ipsilateral lateral flexion Posterior shear: greatest at lower lumbar levels Assist with extension but close to axis of rotation; better MA at upper levels
Iliocostalis lumborum pars lumborum (4 fascicles)	One from each tip of the lumbar TP to the iliac crest	Ipsilateral lateral flexion Better rotators, due to greater MA Posterior shear, especially at lower levels Assist with extension but close to axis
Superficial Erector Spinae		
Longissimus thoracis pars thoracis (12 fascicles)	One from each thoracic TP and ribs via the ESA to L3-S3 SP	Extension of thoracic spine Extension of lumbar spine via increasing lordosis Assist with ipsilateral lateral flexion
Iliocostalis lumborum pars thoracis (7 or 8 fascicles)	One from each of the lower 7-8 ribs to PSIS and sacrum with contribution to the ESA	Extension of lumbar spine via increasing lordosis Assist with ipsilateral lateral flexion

ESA, erector spinae aponeurosis; MA, moment arm; PSIS, posterior superior sacroiliac spine; SP, posterior superior iliac spine; TP, transverse process.

The multifidus muscles of the spine are complex and demonstrate segmental and regional differences. In the lumbar region, the multifidus muscles are not truly transversospinales, as most anatomy texts depict. They run generally from the dorsal sacrum and the ilium in the region of the PSIS to the spinous processes of the lumbar vertebrae. They also have separate fascicles that run from the mamillary processes to the spinous process of the cranial vertebrae. The line of pull in the lumbar region is more vertically oriented. In the thoracic region, the multifidus muscles are transversospinales, inasmuch as they are more laterally oriented with an oblique line of pull. They run from the transverse process of the vertebra to the spinous processes of the more cranial vertebrae covering one to three segments. The lumbar multifidus muscles are deep to the ESA only below L3. They are a thick mass that fills the area of the sacral sulcus and are easily palpable here.[110,113]

As the multifidus muscles in the lumbar region have a greater cross-sectional area and more vertically oriented fibers than those of the thoracic region, it appears that they are better suited to produce extension. The thoracic multifidus muscles are better suited to produce rotation.[113] The lumbar multifidus muscles are arranged in segmental fascicles, which suggests that their principle action is on focal lumbar segments.[2,114]

The fibers of the lumbar multifidus muscles become increasingly more vertical in a caudal direction. The line of action will produce extension by increasing the lumbar lordosis (see Fig 4-55). In so doing, the fibers will add compressive loads to the posterior aspect of the interbody joints. The role of the lumbar multifidus muscles in rotation is to work in synergy with the abdominal muscles by opposing the flexion moment that the abdominal muscles produce.[2] McGill[114] suggested that the role of the lumbar multifidus muscles is to produce extensor torque to allow correction of individual segments that are the foci of stress.

Rotatores and intertransversarii muscles are frequently described as producing lateral flexion and rotation, respectively. Because of small cross-sectional areas and small moment arms, however, it appears likely that these muscles serve more of a proprioceptive role.[26]

■ **Lateral Muscles**

The quadratus lumborum is deep to the erector spinae and multifidus muscles. The quadratus lumborum, when acting bilaterally, serves as an important frontal plane stabilizer (Fig. 4-64A). Porterfield and DeRosa[110] also described the quadratus lumborum as serving an important role in stabilization in the horizontal plane as well. When acting unilaterally, the quadratus lumborum can laterally flex the spine and attachments to the lumbar transverse processes, allowing it to control rotational motion as well (see Fig. 4-64C). If lateral flexion occurs from erect standing, the force of gravity will continue the motion, and the contralateral quadratus lumborum will control the movement by contracting eccentrically. If the pelvis is free to move, the quadratus lumborum will "hike the hip" or laterally tilt the pelvis in the frontal plane (see Fig. 4-64B).

■ **Anterior Muscles**

The rectus abdominis is the prime flexor of the trunk. It is contained within the abdominal fascia, which separates the rectus abdominis into sections and attaches the rectus abdominis to the aponeurosis of the abdominal wall. The abdominal fascia also has attachment to the aponeurosis of the pectoralis major. McGill[114] and Porterfield and DeRosa[110] discussed the importance of these fascial connections as they transmit forces across midline and around the trunk. Tension on this fascial

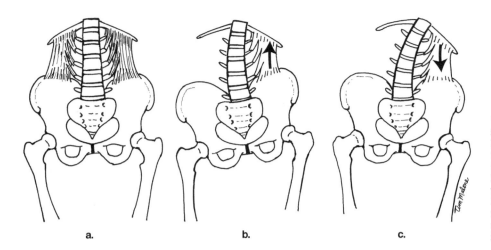

a.   b.   c.

◄ **Figure 4-64** ■ **A.** The illustration shows the attachments of the right and left quadratus lumborum muscles. **B.** A unilateral contraction of the left quadratus lumborum muscle will lift and tilt the left side of the pelvis and hike the hip when the trunk is fixed and the pelvis and leg are free to move. **C.** A unilateral contraction of the left quadratus lumborum muscle when the pelvis and left leg are fixed will cause ipsilateral trunk flexion.

system will provide stability in a corset type of manner around the trunk.

The abdominal wall consists of the external oblique, the internal oblique, and the transversus abdominis muscles. These muscles together form what McGill[114] called the "hoop" around the entire abdomen with the abdominal wall as the anterior aspect and the thoracolumbar fascia and its muscle attachments as the posterior aspect (see Fig. 4-44). This hoop plays an important role in stability of the lumbopelvic region. The transversus abdominis has been shown to mechanically control the SIJ through significant compressive forces due to the transverse (perpendicular) orientation of the muscle to the SIJ.[115] Richardson et al.[115] demonstrated that contraction of the transversus abdominis decreased laxity at the SIJ. Cholewicki et al.[116] demonstrated that in a neutral spine posture in standing, there is trunk flexor-extensor muscle coactivation at a low level. Furthermore, they measured this activation level to increase with an external load and with decreased spinal stiffness, which supports the hypothesis that this "hoop" can provide stability to the lumbopelvic region and that increased muscle activity can compensate for loss of stiffness in the spinal column caused by injury.

Case Application 4-8: **Exercises to Stabilize Trunk**

Knowledge of the function of the trunk musculature needs to be applied to the development of exercises for trunk stabilization for patients like Malik. The fascial connection to the pectoralis major is important in that exercises that use the upper extremity in a functional manner can be used to target trunk stability, because they will produce tension on this fascia. In this way, the exercises can be functional and, in addition, they will not need to produce trunk movement and therefore will be less likely to produce pain, particularly in the early stages of rehabilitation. Exercises that activate this "hoop" both statically and dynamically will be critical for achieving spinal stabilization in states of pathology to the lumbopelvic region.

The psoas major runs from the lumbar transverse processes, the anterolateral vertebral bodies of T12 to L4, and the lumbar intervertebral disks to the lesser trochanter of the femur. It courses inferiorly and laterally, and the distal tendon merges with that of the iliacus. The primary role of the psoas major is flexion of the hip. McGill[114] reported that it is active only when there is active hip flexion. The iliacus runs from the iliac crest over the pubic ramus to the lesser trochanter with the tendon of the psoas major. The primary role of the iliacus is also hip flexion. The role of the psoas major at the lumbar spine appears to be to buttress the forces of the iliacus, which, when activated, cause anterior ilial rotation and thus lumbar spine extension.[114] The psoas major also provides stability to the lumbar spine during hip flexion activities by providing great amounts of lumbar compression during activation. Some anterior shear is also produced when it is activated.

Continuing Exploration: **Exercises for Low Back Pain**

When developing therapeutic exercises for people with low back disorders, it is important to choose exercises that, while taking advantage of training these muscle groups that we have discussed, also impose the lowest possible loads through this region, especially early in the healing stages. Traditionally, this reasoning has not often been applied in rehabilitation programs.

Exercises to increase the strength of the back extensors are often performed in the prone position to take advantage of the resistance provided by gravity to back, leg, and arm extension. Callaghan and colleagues[117] assessed loading of the L4/L5 segment in 13 male volunteers during commonly prescribed exercises. The authors found that the lowest compression forces at the L4/L5 segment were found in single-leg extension in the quadriped position (on hands and knees) (Fig. 4-65A). Raising an arm and leg simultaneously (right arm and left leg) increased compression forces by 1000 N and upper erector spinae muscle activity levels by 30% in comparison with single-leg extension in the hands and knees position (see Fig. 4-65B). The right erector spinae and contralateral abdominal muscles were activated during single right-leg extension to maintain a neutral pelvis and spine posture and to balance internal moments and lateral shear forces.

The authors recommended that only single-leg extension exercises be performed because the lumbar posture is more neutral and the compression forces are relatively low (approximately 2500 N). They further recommended that the exercise in which the subject raises the upper body and legs from a prone lying position never be prescribed for anyone at risk for low back injury or reinjury to the lumbar spine, because during this exercise, lumbar compression forces of up to 6000 N are incurred. The extremely high compression forces are a result of bilateral muscle activity when the spine is hyperextended. In this posture, the facets are subjected to high loads, and the interspinous ligament is in danger of being crushed.[117]

Trunk sit-ups and curl-ups are often performed as a method of abdominal strengthening. McGill measured compression forces during these tasks, with both bent knees and straight knees. He found the compression forces to be approximately 3300 N, without much variation between the types.[118] McGill suggested that. given these large compressive loads, most people, let alone those who have sustained injury to this area, should not perform sit-ups of any type.[26]

■ **Injury Prevention with Lifting Tasks:
Squat Lift versus Stoop Lift**

The prevalence of back problems in the general population and the difficulties of resolving these problems has generated a great deal of research both to explain

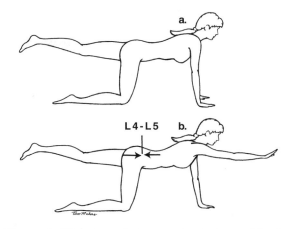

▲ **Figure 4-65** ■ **A.** Single-leg extension in the quadriped position creates low compression forces at the L4/L5 segment. **B.** Raising the opposite leg and arm simultaneously increases compression forces at the L4/L5 segment by 1000 N and upper erector spinae muscle activity by 30% in comparison with single-leg raising.

the mechanisms involved in lifting and to determine the best method of lifting so that back injuries can be prevented. A great deal of focus has been on the squat versus stoop lift (Fig. 4-66). During a stoop lift, trunk flexion is achieved primarily by thoracolumbar flexion, and there is little to no knee flexion. During a squat lift, the spine remains as erect as possible and trunk flexion is achieved primarily by hip and knee flexion.

Continuing Exploration: **Squat Lifting versus Stoop Lifting**

Controversy persists in the literature as to whether there is biomechanical evidence in support of advocating the squat lifting technique over the stoop lifting technique to prevent low back pain. A review by

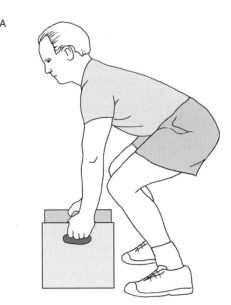

Squat lift

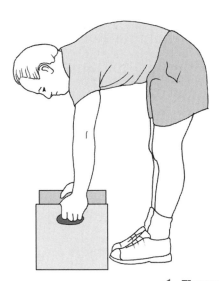

Stoop lift

◀ **Figure 4-66** ■ Squat (**A**) versus stoop (**B**) lift.

van Dieen and coworkers in 1999 concluded that the literature does not support advocating squat lifting over stoop lifting.[119] However, The National Health Service Centre for Reviews and Dissemination cautioned that the review by van Dieen and coworkers contained methodological flaws that affected the authors' conclusions.[120] The points that follow appear to support the use of the squat lift.

The extensor muscles are at a disadvantage in the fully flexed position of the spine because of shortened moment arms in this position, a change in the line of pull, and the possibility of passive insufficiency resulting from the elongated state of the muscles. In a neutral lumbar spine posture, the deep layer of the erector spinae is capable of producing posterior shear, which will help to offset the tremendous amounts of anterior shear that occur with trunk flexion, particularly if the person is carrying an additional load.[26,114] The diminished capacity of the extensors to generate torque and to counteract the anterior shear forces in the forward flexed position are important reasons why stoop lifting is discouraged.[26,114]

Another factor involved is intradiskal pressures. Wilke and colleagues updated the classic works of Nachemson, studying *in vivo* measurements of intervertebral disk pressure.[121] Both Wilke and Nachemson found that intervertebral disk pressures were substantially higher when a load was held in a stooped position than in a squat position.[121,122]

In contrast, there is some evidence that squat lifting results in higher compression forces than does stoop lifting. However, damaging shear forces were two to four times higher for the stoop lift than for the squat lift.[119,123] Although excessive compressive loads can and will produce damage, the spine is better designed to tolerate compressive loads in comparison with shear forces. Preventing these excessive shear forces, therefore, is critical in preventing injury.[114]

Other, less controversial critical factors in lifting in any posture appear to be the distance from the body to the object to be lifted,[74] the velocity of the lift, and the degree of lumbar flexion.[124] The farther away the load is from the body, the greater is the gravitational moment acting on the vertebral column. Greater muscle activity is required to perform the lift, and consequently greater pressure is created in the disk. The higher the velocity of the lift is, the greater is the amount of weight that can be lifted, but the higher is the load on the lumbar disks. The relative spinal load and applied erector spinae force increase significantly with the velocity of trunk extension.[125]

■ **Continuing Exploration: Role of Intra-abdominal Pressure (IAP) in Lifting**

An increase in IAP is frequently demonstrated during lifting tasks. What role the increase in IAP plays as a mechanism of support to the lumbopelvic region during lifting tasks has been the subject of

much debate. Bartelink suggested that an increased IAP decreases spinal compressive loads by pushing up on the rib cage. The author reasoned that closing the glottis and bearing down exerts a force downward on the pelvic floor and upward on the diaphragm, which puts tension through the lumbar region and decreases some compression by producing an extensor moment.[126]

McGill and Norman[127] challenged this theory by arguing that the large compressive loads caused by contraction of the abdominal muscles negate any potential unloading affect and that a net increase in compression through the lumbar spine would result from increased IAP. Cholewicki and colleagues[128] suggested that the increase in IAP has more to do with providing stability to the lumbar region and less to do with generating extensor torque. McGill and Norman agreed with Cholewicki and coworkers that the role of the increased IAP is to stiffen the trunk and prevent tissue strain or failure from buckling of the spine.[127,128]

Hodges and colleagues[129] provided some recent evidence to support the theory that an increased IAP produces an extensor torque; however, they created the increase in IAP without abdominal contraction by stimulating the phrenic nerve. It appears that further studies are needed to delineate the role of the increase in IAP during lifting tasks.

Case Application 4-9: Instruction for Proper Lifting Techniques

An important aspect of rehabilitation for Malik will be to teach him appropriate bending and lifting mechanics. One of his primary complaints is pain with lifting from a stooped position. This position will cause greater anterior shear forces through the lumbar region and may be responsible for his pain. In treatment, therefore, he should be taught how to bend and lift in the squat position, keeping a neutral lumbar spine position. This will remove some strain from the deep erector spinae and allow them to participate in control of the anterior shear forces. In addition, it may be necessary in the early stages of rehabilitation to keep Malik from using increased IAP when he lifts, because the added compressive forces may be further irritating the intervertebral disks, which could be producing pain.

Muscles of the Pelvic Floor

■ **Structure**

Although the **levator ani** and **coccygeus** muscles neither play a major supporting role for the vertebral column nor produce movement of the column, these muscles are mentioned here because of their proximity to the column and possible influence on the linkages that form the pelvis. The levator ani muscles comprise two distinct parts, the iliococcygeus and the pubococcygeus, which help to form the floor of the pelvis and separate the pelvic cavity from the perineum. The left and right broad muscle sheets of the levator ani form the major portion of the floor of the pelvis. The medial borders of the right and left muscles are separated by the visceral outlet, through which pass the urethra, vagina (in the female), and anorectum. The pubococcygeal part of the muscle arises from the posterior aspect of the pubis and has attachments to the sphincter, urethra, walls of the vagina (in the female), and the pineal body and rectum (in both genders). The iliococcygeal portion, which arises from the obturator fascia, is thin. Its fibers blend with the fibers of the anococcygeal ligament, form a raphe, and attach to the last two coccygeal segments. The coccygeus muscle arises from the spine of the ischium and attaches to the coccyx and lower portion of the sacrum. The gluteal surface of the muscle blends with the sacrospinous ligament (Fig. 4-67).

■ **Function**

Voluntary contractions of the levator ani muscles help constrict the openings in the pelvic floor (urethra and anus) and prevent unwanted micturition and defecation (stress incontinence). Involuntary contractions of these muscles occur during coughing or holding one's breath when the IAP is raised. In women, these muscles surround the vagina and help to support the uterus. During pregnancy the muscles can be stretched or traumatized, which can result in stress incontinence whenever the IAP is raised. In men, damage to these muscles may occur after prostate surgery. The coccygeus muscle assists the levator ani in supporting the pelvic viscera and maintaining IAP.

◆ Effects of Aging

Age-Related Changes

Over the life span, the vertebral column is exposed to recurrent loads that change the morphology of the column. However, normal age-related changes also occur in the structures of the vertebral column.

The vertebral bone undergoes changes in the

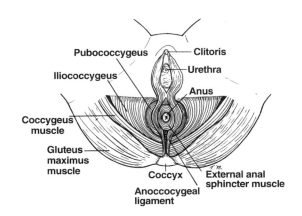

▲ **Figure 4-67** ■ Muscles of the pelvic floor.

amount and form of the trabeculae. The numbers of both horizontal and vertical trabeculae decrease with age, and the horizontal trabeculae become significantly thinner.[130] This loss can decrease the loads that the vertebrae are able to withstand before failure.

Each of the structures of the intervertebral disk undergo changes that include loss of the amount of proteoglycans and change in the specific type of proteoglycan, with resultant loss of water content. In addition, there is an increase of collagen in these structures and loss of elastin. This results in a loss of the ability for the disk to transfer loads from one vertebra to another as the swelling ability of the nucleus decreases. The overall disk height will also decrease somewhat.

The vascularization of the disk also changes. *In utero*, blood vessels can be demonstrated within the fibers of the anulus fibrosus.[131] By the end of the second year of life, these have predominantly degenerated. Thus, the disk relies on the diffusion of nutrients through the vertebral end plate. The vertebral end plate, with aging, gradually becomes more collagenous, and the process of diffusion is hindered. The fibers of the anulus fibrosus in the cervical spine of adults normally demonstrate lateral fissures that subdivide the disk into two halves at the uncovertebral joints. These fissures can first be observed in children at approximately 9 years of age.[131] After formation of these fissures, joint pseudocapsules develop with vascularized synovial folds. The formation of these fissures appears to be load-related and is located predominantly in the regions of C3 to C5.

With large and/or repetitive loads, further changes occur in the disks. The disks demonstrate a dramatic decrease in their elasticity and proteoglycans.[131,132] Eventually, the intervertebral disk will become so dry that it begins to crumble. In the lumbar region, the inner layers of the anulus fibrosus begin to buckle outward, and the lamellae separate. Fissures and tears can occur within the anular fibers, which can decrease the ability of the disk to provide stiffness during movement.[132] The vertebral end plates may become ossified. The adjacent spongy bone of the vertebral body can begin to sclerose. On occasion, blood vessels grow into the disks and trigger ossification.[131] The disk can prolapse or protrude as a result of the pressure of the nucleus and the lack of ability of the anulus fibrosus to sustain it. Schmorl's nodes are formed when the nuclear material prolapses through the vertebral end plate and into the cancellous bone of the vertebra. This material may cause an autoimmune response when it comes in contact with the blood supply in the cancellous bone.[110] This is typically labeled degenerative disk disease.

In this case of degenerative disk disease, there is a more substantial loss of disk height, which causes all ligaments to be placed on slack. The ligamentous prestress normally provided by the ligamentum flavum will decrease, which in turn will impair spinal stiffness. This can also allow the ligament to buckle on itself with movement, potentially compressing the spinal cord. In addition, the ligamentum flavum begins to calcify with age, and this occasionally leads to ossification, which can also potentially cause compression of the spinal nerve in the vicinity of the zygapophyseal joints or the spinal cord within the canal.[133,134]

The zygapophyseal joints can also demonstrate age-related changes and eventual degeneration. Some authors have argued that these changes in the zygapophyseal joints must be secondary to disk degeneration, as a substantial amount of weight-bearing through these joints must occur to cause deterioration. This increase in weight-bearing may be due to the loss of disk height. However, this is not always the case.[131] There have been descriptions of degenerative zygapophyseal joints without disk degeneration. The mechanism of this is not as well understood. If, however, the disks degenerate and a substantive decrease in height occurs, what follows is hypermobility as a result of slackened capsules and longitudinal ligaments. The vertebra may also slip forward or backward on the vertebra below (listhesis or retrolisthesis). There will be excessive shear forces generated, and the zygapophyseal joints will also become subject to more load-bearing.

The result of these changes becomes the same as with what happens to the larger joints of the extremities: damage of the cartilage, including fissures and cysts, and osteophyte formation. These changes can lead to localized pain or pressure on spinal nerves or the central canal or, in the cervical region, compression of the vertebral artery in the transverse foramen.[131]

The joints of Luschka, or uncovertebral joints, are frequent sites for age-related and degenerative changes. Osteophytes on the uncinate processes occur predominantly in the lower segments C5/C6 or C6/C7. The motion of lateral bending becomes extremely limited when these osteophytes occur.

 CONCEPT CORNERSTONE 4-6: *Osteophyte Formation*

Clinicians should remember the frequency of osteophyte formation at the uncinate processes and subsequent lateral bending limitations when examining cervical ROM. Restoration of lateral bending motion is often not a realistic expectation.

Summary

In summary, it is extremely important to understand the normal structure and function, including normal variability, of the vertebral column in order to understand the structures at risk for injury and the best ways to treat people with dysfunction. Injury or failure occurs when the applied load exceeds the strength of a particular tissue. Repetitive strain causes injury by either the repeated application of a relatively low load or by application of a sustained load for a long duration (prolonged sitting or stooped posture).

The effects of an injury, aging, disease, or development deficit on the vertebral column may be analyzed by taking the following points into consideration:

1. the normal function that the affected structure is designed to serve
2. the stresses that are present during normal situations
3. the anatomic relationship of the structure to adjacent structures
4. the functional relationship of the structure to other structures

Study Questions

1. Which region of the vertebral column is most flexible? Explain why this region has greater flexibility.
2. Describe the relationship between the zygapophyseal joints and the interbody joints.
3. What is the zygapophyseal facet orientation in the lumbar region? How does this orientation differ from that of other regions? How does the orientation in the lumbar region affect motion in that region?
4. Describe the relative strength of the longitudinal ligaments in the lumbar region. How does this differ from the other regions? Are some structures more susceptible to injury in this region on the basis of this variation?
5. Which structures would be affected if a person has an increased anterior convexity in the lumbar area? Describe the type of stress that would occur, where it would occur, and how it would affect different structures.
6. Describe the function of the intervertebral disk during motion and in weight-bearing.
7. Describe the differences in structure between the cervical and lumbar intervertebral disks.
8. Identify the factors that limit rotation in the lumbar spine. Explain how the limitations occur.
9. Which muscles cause extension of the lumbar spine? In which position of the spine are they most effective?
10. Describe the forces that act on the spine during motion and at rest.
11. Explain how "creep" may adversely affect the stability of the vertebral column.
12. Describe how muscles and ligaments interact to provide stability for the vertebral column.
13. What role has been attributed to the thoracolumbar fascia in stability of the lumbopelvic region?
14. Describe the dynamic and static restraints to anterior shear in the lumbar region.
15. Describe the dynamic restraints to anterior shear in the cervical region.

◆ References

1. Kapandji IA: The Physiology of the Joints 3, 2nd ed. Edinburgh, Churchill Livingstone, 1974.
2. Bogduk N: Clinical Anatomy of the Lumbar Spine and Sacrum, 3rd ed. New York, Churchill Livingstone, 1997.
3. Huiskes R, Ruimerman R, van Lenthe GH, et al.: Effects of mechanical forces on maintenance and adaptation of form in trabecular bone. Nature 405:704, 2000.
4. Smit T, Odgaard A, Schneider E: Structure and function of vertebral trabecular bone. Spine 22:2823, 1997.
5. Banse X, Devogelaer JP, Munting E, et al.: Inhomogeneity of human vertebral cancellous bone: Systematic density and structure patterns inside the vertebral body. Bone 28:563, 2001.
6. White AA, Panjabi MM: Clinical Biomechanics of the Spine, 2nd ed. Philadephia, JB Lippincott, 1990.
7. Mercer S, Bogduk N: The ligaments and annulus fibrosus of human adult cervical intervertebral discs. Spine 24:619, 1999.
8. Mercer S, Bogduk N: Joints of the cervical vertebral column. J Orthop Sports Phys Ther 31(4): 174, 2001.
9. Mercer S: Structure and function of the bones and joints of the cervical spine. In Oatis C (ed): Kinesiology: The Mechanics & Pathomechanics of Human Movement. Philadelphia, Lippincott Williams & Wilkins, 2004.
10. Lundon K, Bolton K: Structure and function of the lumbar intervertebral disk in health, aging, and pathologic conditions. J Orthop Sports Phys Ther 31:291, 2001.
11. Rudert M, Tillmann B: Lymph and blood supply of the human intervertebral disc. Cadaver study of correlations to discitis. Acta Orthop Scand 64:37, 1993.
12. Mercer S, Bogduk N: Intra-articular inclusions of the cervical synovial joints. Br J Rheum 32:705, 1993.
13. Yoganandan N, Kumaresan S, Pintar FA: Biomechanics of the cervical spine, part 2. Cervical spine soft tissue responses and biomechanical modeling. Clin Biomech (Bristol, Avon) 16:1, 2001.
14. Inami S, Kaneoka K, Hayashi K, et al.: Types of synovial fold in the cervical facet joint. J Orthop Sci 5:475, 2000.
15. Putz R: The detailed functional anatomy of the ligaments of the vertebral column. Anat Anz 174: 40, 1992.
16. Maiman DJ, Pintar FA: Anatomy and clinical biomechanics of the thoracic spine. Clin Neurosurg 38:296, 1992.
17. Myklebust JB, Pintar F, Yoganandan N, et al.: Tensile strength of spinal ligaments. Spine 13:526, 1988.
18. Hedtmann A, Steffen R, Methfessel J, et al.: Measurements of human spine ligaments during loaded and unloaded motion. Spine 14:175, 1989.
19. Olszewski AD, Yaszemski MJ, White A: The anatomy of the human lumbar ligamentum flavum. Spine 21:2307, 1996.
20. Crisco JJ 3rd, Panjabi MM, Dvorak J: A model of the alar ligaments of the upper cervical spine in axial rotation. J Biomech 24:607, 1991.
21. Nordin M, Frankel VH: Basic Biomechanics of the Musculoskeletal System, 2nd ed. Philadelphia, Lea & Febiger, 1989.
22. Dickey J, Bednar DA, Dumas GA: New insight into the mechanics of the lumbar interspinous ligament. Spine 21:2720, 1996.
23. Adams MA, Hutton WC, Stott JRR: The resistance to flexion of the lumbar intervertebral joint. Spine 5:245, 1980.
24. Fujiwara A, Tamai K, An HS, et al.: The interspinous ligament of the lumbar spine: Magnetic resonance images and their clinical significance. Spine 25:358, 2000.
25. Moore K, Dalley A: Clinically Oriented Anatomy, 4th ed. Philadelphia, Lippincott Williams & Wilkins, 1999.
26. McGill S: Low Back Disorders: Evidence-Based Prevention and Rehabilitation. Champaign, IL, Human Kinetics, 2002.
27. Williams PL (ed): Gray's Anatomy, 38th ed. New York, Churchill Livingstone, 1995.
28. Adams MA, Hutton WC: The mechanical function of the lumbar apophyseal joints. Spine 8:327, 1983.
29. Solomonow M, Zhou BH, Harris M, et al.: The ligamento-muscular stabilizing system of the spine. Spine 23:2552, 1998.
30. Onan O, Heggeness MH, Hipp JA: A motion analysis of the cervical facet joint. Spine 23:430, 1998.
31. Krismer M, Haid C, Rabl W: The contribution of anulus fibers to torque resistance. Spine 21:2551, 1996.
32. Boszczyk BM, Boxczyk AA, Putz R, et al.: An immunohistochemical study of the dorsal capsule of the lumbar and thoracic facet joints. Spine 26:E338, 2001.
33. Twomey LT, Taylor JR: Sagittal movements of the human vertebral column: A qualitative study of the role of the posterior vertebral elements. Arch Phys Med Rehabil 64:322, 1983.
34. Cholewicki J, Crisco JJ 3rd, Oxland TR, et al.: Effects of posture and structure on three-dimensional coupled rotations in the lumbar spine: A biomechanical analysis. Spine 21:2421, 1996.
35. Panjabi M, Crisco JJ, Vasavada A, et al.: Mechanical properties of the human cervical spine as shown by three-dimensional load-displacement curves. Spine 26:2692, 2001.
36. Bogduk N, Amevo B, Pearcy M: A biological basis for instantaneous centers of rotation of the verte-

bral column. Proc Inst Mech Eng [H] 209:177, 1995.

37. Haher TR, O'Brien M, Felmly WT, et al.: Instantaneous axis of rotation as a function of three columns of the spine. Spine 17(6 Suppl):S149, 1992.

38. Gracovetsky SA: The resting spine: A conceptual approach to the avoidance of spinal reinjury during rest. Phys Ther 67:549, 1987.

39. Parnianpour M, Nordin M, Frankel VH, et al.: The effect of fatigue on the motor output and pattern of isodynamic trunk movement. Isotechnol Res Abstr April 1988.

40. Keller TS, Hansson TH, Abram AC, et al.: Regional variations in the compressive properties of lumbar vertebral trabeculae: Effects of disc degeneration. Spine 14:1012, 1989.

41. Nachemson AL: The lumbar spine: An orthopedic challenge. Spine 1:1, 1976.

42. Twomey LT, Taylor JR, Oliver MJ: Sustained flexion loading, rapid extension loading of the lumbar spine, and the physical therapy of related injuries. Physiother Pract 4:129, 1988.

43. Adams MA, Dolan P, Hutton WC, et al.: Diurnal changes in spinal mechanics and their clinical significance. J Bone Joint Surg Br 72:266, 1990.

44. McMillan DW, Garbutt G, Adams MA: Effect of sustained loading on the water content of intervertebral discs: Implications for disc metabolism. Ann Rheum Dis 55:880,1996.

45. Keller TS, Nathan M: Height change caused by creep in intervertebral discs: A sagittal plane model. J Spinal Disord 12:313, 1999.

46. Ahrens SF: The effect of age on intervertebral disc compression during running. J Orthop Sports Phys Ther 20:17, 1994.

47. Klein JA, Hukins DWL: Relocation of the bending axis during flexion-extension of lumbar intervertebral discs and its implications for prolapse. Spine 8:1776, 1983.

48. Klein JA, Hukins DWL: Functional differentiation in the spinal column. Eng Med 12:83, 1983.

49. Haher TR, Felmy W, Baruch H, et al.: The contribution of the three columns of the spine to rotational stability: A biomechanical model. Spine 14:663, 1989.

50. Shirazi-Adl A: Strain in fibers of a lumbar disc. Spine 14:98, 1989.

51. Panjabi MM, Oxland T, Takata K, et al.: Articular facets of the human spine. Spine 18:1298, 1993.

52. Bogduk N, Mercer S: Biomechanics of the cervical spine. I: Normal kinematics. Clin Biomech 15:633, 2000.

53. Porterfield J, DeRosa C: Mechanical Neck Pain: Perspectives in Functional Anatomy. Philadelphia, WB Saunders, 1995.

54. Panjabi MM, Oxland TR, Parks H: Quantitative anatomy of the cervical spine ligaments. J Spinal Disord 4:270, 1991.

55. Crisco JJ, Panjabi MM, Dvorak, J: A model of the alar ligaments of the upper cervical spine in axial rotation. J Biomech 24:607, 1991.

56. Panjabi MM, Duranceau J, Goel V, et al.: Cervical human vertebrae: Quantitative three-dimensional anatomy of the middle and lower regions. Spine 16:861,1991.

57. Bland JH, Boushey DR: Anatomy and physiology of the cervical spine. Semin Arthritis Rheum 20:1, 1990.

58. Goel VK, Clark CR, Gallaes K, et al.: Momentrotation relationships of the ligamentousoccipitoatlanto-axial complex. J Biomech 21:673, 1988.

59. Panjabi M, Dvorak J, Duranceau J, et al.: Three-dimensional movements of the upper cervical spine. Spine 13:726, 1988.

60. Dvorak J, Panjabi MM, Novotny JE, et al.: *In vivo* flexion/extension of the normal cervical spine. J Orthop Res 9:828, 1991.

61. Oda I, Abumi K, Lu D, et al.: Biomechanical role of the posterior elements, costovertebral joints, and ribcage in the stability of the thoracic spine. Spine 21:1423, 1996.

62. Milne N: The role of the zygapophysial joint orientation and uncinate processes in controlling motion in the cervical spine. J Anat 178:189, 1991.

63. Kent BA: Anatomy of the trunk: A review. Part 1. Phys Ther 54:7, 1974.

64. Basmajian JV: Primary Anatomy, 7th ed. Baltimore, Williams & Wilkins, 1976.

65. Cailliet R: Neck and Arm Pain, 3rd ed. Philadelphia, FA Davis, 1991.

66. Dumas JL, Sainte Rose M, Dreyfus P, et al.: Rotation of the cervical spinal column. A computed tomography *in vivo* study. Surg Radiol Anat 15:333, 1993.

67. Pal GP, Routal RV: The role of the vertebral laminae in the stability of the cervical spine. J Anat 188:485, 1996.

68. Pal GP, Sherk HH: The vertical stability of the cervical spine. Spine 13:447, 1988.

69. Maroney SP, Schultz AB, Miller JAA, et al.: Load-displacement properties of lower cervical spine motion segments. J Biomech 21:769, 1988.

70. Shea M, Edwards WT, White AA, et al.: Variations in stiffness and strength along the cervical spine. J Biomech 24:95, 1991.

71. Panjabi MM, Takata K, Goel V, et al.: Thoracic human vertebrae: Quantitative three-dimensional anatomy. Spine 16:888, 1991.

72. Goh S, Price RI, Leedman PJ, et al.: The relative influence of vertebral body and intervertebral disc shape on thoracic kyphosis. Clin Biomech (Bristol, Avon) 14:439, 1999.

73. Oda I, Abumi K, Cunningham BW, et al.: An *in vitro* human cadaveric study investigating the biomechanical properties of the thoracic spine. Spine 27(3):E64, 2002.

74. Winkel D: Diagnosis and Treatment of the Spine: Nonoperative Orthopaedic Medicine and Manual Therapy. Rockville, MD, Aspen, 1996.

75. Cailliet R: Low Back Pain Syndrome, 5th ed. Philadelphia, FA Davis, 1995.

76. Pintar FA, Yoganandan N, Myers T, et al.: Biomechanical properties of human lumbar spine ligaments. J Biomech 25:1351, 1992.

77. Pool-Goudzwaard A, Hoek van Dijke G, Mulder P, et al.: The iliolumbar ligament: Its influence on stability of the sacroiliac joint. Clin Biomech 18:99, 2003.

78. Basadonna P-T, Gasparini D, Rucco V: Iliolumbar ligament insertions. Spine 21:2313, 1996.

79. Rucco V, Basadonna P-T, Gasparini D: Anatomy of the iliolumbar ligament: A review of its anatomy and a magnetic resonance study. Am J Phys Med Rehabil 75:451, 1996.

80. Macintosh JE, Bogduk N: The morphology of the lumbar erector spinae. Spine 12:658, 1987.

81. Vleeming A, Pool-Goudzwaard AL, Stoeckart R, et al.: The posterior layer of the thoracolumbar fascia: Its function in load transfer from spine to legs. Spine 20:753, 1995.

82. Gracovetsky S: The Spinal Engine. New York, Springer-Verlag, 1988.

83. Goel VK, Kong W, Han JS, et al.: A combined finite element and optimization investigation of lumbar spine mechanics with and without muscles. Spine 18:1531, 1993.

84. Panjabi MM, Oxland TR, Yamamoto I, et al.: Mechanical behavior of the human lumbar and lumbosacral spine as shown by three-dimensional load-displacement curves. J Bone Joint Surg Am 76:413, 1994.

85. Gunzburg R, Hutton WC, Crane G, et al.: Role of the capsulo-ligamentous structures in rotation and combined flexion-rotation of the lumbar spine. J Spinal Disord 5:1, 1992.

86. Cailliet R: Soft Tissue Pain and Disability, 3rd ed. Philadelphia, FA Davis, 1996.

87. Nelson JM, Walmsley RPO, Stevenson JM: Relative lumbar and pelvic motion during loaded spinal flexion/extension. Spine 20:199,1995.

88. Haher TR, O'Brien M, Dryer JW, et al.: The role of the lumbar facet joints in spinal stability: Identification of alternative paths of loading. Spine 19:2667, 1994.

89. Khoo BCC, Goh JC, Lee JM, et al.: A comparison of lumbosacral loads during static and dynamic activities. Australas Phys Eng Sci Med 17:55, 1994.

90. Bowen V, Cassidy JD: Macroscopic and microscopic anatomy of the sacroiliac joint from embryonic life until the eighth decade. Spine 6:620, 1981.

91. Mierau DR, Cassidy JD, Hamin T, et al.: Sacroiliac joint dysfunction and low back pain in school aged children. J Manipulative Physiol Ther 7:81, 1994.

92. Walker JM: The sacroiliac joint: A critical review. Phys Ther 72:903, 1992.

93. Salsabili N, Valojerdy MR, Hogg DA: Variations in thickness of articular cartilage in the human sacroiliac joint. Clin Anat 8:388,1995.

94. Cassidy JD: The pathoanatomy and clinical significance of the sacroiliac joints. J Manipulative Physiol Ther 15:41, 1992.

95. McLauchlan GJ, Gardner DL: Sacral and iliac articular cartilage thickness and cellularity: Relationship to subchondral bone end-plate thickness and cancellous bone density. Rheumatology 41:375, 2002.

96. DonTigny, RL: Function and pathomechanics of the sacroiliac joint: A review. Phys Ther 65:35, 1985.

97. Reilly JP, Gross RH, Emans JB, et al.: Disorders of the sacro-iliac joint in children. J Bone Joint Surg Am 70:31, 1988.

98. Bernard TN, Cassidy JD: The sacroiliac joint syndrome. Pathophysiology, diagnosis, and management. In Vleeming, A et al. (eds): First Interdisciplinary World Congress on Low Back Pain and Its Relation to the Sacroiliac Joint. San Diego, University of California, 1992.

99. Vleeming A, Pool-Goudzwaard AL, Hammudoghlu D, et al.: The function of the long dorsal sacroiliac ligament: its implication for understanding low back pain. Spine 21:556, 1996.

100. Gould JA, Davies GJ (eds): Orthopaedics and Sports Physical Therapy. St. Louis, CV Mosby, 1985.

101. Freeman MD, Fox D, Richards T: The superior intracapsular ligament of the sacroiliac joint: Presumptive evidence for confirmation of Illi's ligament. J Manipulative Physiol Ther 13:384, 1990.

102. Palastanga N, Field D, Soames R: Anatomy and Human Movement: Structure and Function, 3rd ed. Oxford, UK, Butterworth Heinemann, 2000.

103. Grieve GP: The sacro-iliac joint. Physiotherapy 62:8, 1979.

104. MacLaughlin SM, Oldale KNM: Vertebral body diameters and sex prediction. Ann Hum Biol 19:285, 1992.

105. Vrahas M, Hern TC, Diangelo D, et al.: Ligamentous contributions to pelvic stability. Orthopedics 18:271, 1995.

106. McGill SM, Kippers V: Transfer of loads between lumbar tissues during flexion-relaxation phenomenon. Spine 19:2190, 1994.

107. Vleeming A, Stoeckart R, Volkers AC, et al.: Relation between form and function in the sacroiliac joint. Part I: Clinical anatomical aspects. Spine 15:130, 1990.

108. Vleeming A, Volkers AC, Snijders CJ, et al.: Relation between form and function in the sacroiliac joint. Part II: Biomechanical aspects. Spine 15:11, 1990.

109. Pidcoe P, Mayhew T: Mechanics and pathomechanics of the cervical musculature. In Oatis C (ed): Kinesiology: The Mechanics & Pathomechanics of Human Movement. Philadelphia, Lippincott Williams & Wilkins, 2004.

110. Porterfield J, DeRosa C: Mechanical Low Back Pain: Perspectives in Functional Anatomy, 2nd ed. Philadelphia, WB Saunders, 1998.

111. Daggfeldt K, Huang QM, Thorstensson A: The visible human anatomy of the lumbar erector spinae. Spine 25:2719, 2000.

112. Bustami FM: A new description of the lumbar erector spinae muscle in man. J Anat 144:81, 1986.

113. Bojadsen TWA, Silva ES, Rodrigues AJ, et al.: Comparative study of Mm. Multifidi in lumbar and thoracic spine. J Electromyogr Kinesiol 10:143, 2000.

114. McGill S: Mechanics and pathomechanics of muscles acting on the lumbar spine. In Oatis C (ed): Kinesiology: The Mechanics & Pathomechanics of Human Movement. Philadelphia, Lippincott Williams & Wilkins, 2004.

115. Richardson CA, Snijders CJ, Hides JA, et al.: The relation between the transversus abdominis muscles, sacroiliac joint mechanics, and low back pain. Spine 27:399, 2002.

116. Cholewicki J, Panjabi MM, Khachatryan A: Stabilizing function of trunk flexor-extensor muscles around a neutral spine posture. Spine 22:2207, 1997.

117. Callaghan JP, Gunning JL, McGill SM: The relationship between lumbar spine load and muscle activity during extensor exercises. Phys Ther 78:8, 1998.

118. McGill SM: Low back exercises: Evidence for improving exercise regimens. Phys Ther 78:754, 1998.

119. van Dieen J, Hoozemans MJ, Toussaint HM: Stoop or squat: A review of biomechanical studies on lifting technique. Clin Biomech (Bristol, Avon) 14:685, 1999.

120. National Health Service Centre for Reviews and Dissemination: Stoop or squat. Database of Abstracts of Reviews of Effectiveness, Issue 3, 2003.

121. Wilke HJ, Neef P, Caimi M, et al.: New *in vivo* measurements of pressures in the intervertebral disc in daily life. Spine 24(8):755, 1999.

122. Nachemson A: The load on lumbar discs in different positions of the body. Clin Orthop 45:107, 1966.

123. Potvin JR, McGill SM, Norman RW: Trunk muscle and lumbar ligament contributions to dynamic lifts with varying degrees of trunk flexion. Spine 16:1099, 1991.

124. Dolan P, Mannion AF, Adams MA: Passive tissues help the muscles to generate extensor moments during lifting. J Biomech 27:1077, 1994.

125. Granata KP, Marras WS: The influence of trunk muscle coactivity on dynamic spinal loads. Spine 20:913,1995.

126. Bartelink DL: The role of abdominal pressure in relieving the pressure on the lumbar intervertebral disc. J Bone Joint Surg Br 39:718.

127. McGill S, Norman R: Reassessment of the role of intra-abdominal pressure in spinal compression. Ergonomics 30:1565, 1987.

128. Cholewicki J, Juluru K, McGill SM, et al.: Intra-abdominal pressure mechanism for stabilizing the lumbar spine. J Biomech 32:13, 1999.

129. Hodges P, Cresswell AG, Daggfeldt K, et al.: *In vivo* measurement of the effect of intra-abdominal pressure on the human spine. J Biomech 34:347, 2001.

130. Thomsen JS, Ebbesen EN, Mosekilde LI: Age-related differences between thinning of horizontal and vertical trabeculae in human lumbar bone as assessed by a new computerized method. Bone 31:136, 2002.

131. Prescher A: Anatomy and pathology of the aging spine. Eur J Radiol 27:181, 1998.

132. Thompson R, Pearcy MJ, Downing KJ, et al.: Disc lesions and the mechanics of the intervertebral joint complex. Spine 25:3026, 2000.

133. Maigne JY, Ayral X, Guerin-Surville H: Frequency and size of ossifications in the caudal attachments of the ligamentum flavum of the thoracic spine. Role of rotatory strains in their development. An anatomic study of 121 spines. Surg Radiol Anat 14:119, 1992.

134. Mak K, Mak KL, Gwi-Mak E: Ossification of the ligamentum flavum in the cervicothoracic junction: case report on ossification found on both sides of the lamina. Spine 27:E11, 2002.

Chapter 5

The Thorax and Chest Wall

Julie Starr, PT, MS, CCS, Diane Dalton, PT, MS, OCS

◆ Introduction

The thorax, consisting of the thoracic vertebrae, the ribs, and the sternum (Fig. 5-1A and B), has several important functions. The thorax provides a base for the attachment of muscles of the upper extremities, the head and neck, the vertebral column, and the pelvis. The thorax also forms protection for the heart, lungs, and viscera. Therefore, there needs to be a certain amount of inherent stability to the thorax. Probably the most important function of the chest wall is its role in ventilation. The process of ventilation depends on the mobility of the bony rib thorax and the ability of the muscles of ventilation to move it.[1,2]

    Function, especially ventilatory function, can be affected when pathology interferes with the structure of the bony thorax. For example, scoliosis is a pathologic lateral curvature of the spine, frequently associated with rotation of the vertebrae.[3] A right thoracic scoliosis (named by the side of the convexity of the curve) results in left lateral flexion of the thoracic spine (Fig. 5-2A). The coupled rotation in a typical right thoracic scoliosis causes the bodies of the vertebrae to rotate to the right and the spinous processes to rotate left. The right transverse processes of the vertebrae rotate posteriorly, carrying the ribs with them (see Fig. 5-2B). This is the mechanism causing the classic posterior rib hump of scoliosis. On the concave side of the scoliotic curve, the effects are just the opposite. The transverse processes of the vertebrae move anteriorly, bringing the articulated ribs forward. The rib distortion that results from the vertebral rotation is evident bilaterally in Figure 5-2A. These musculoskeletal abnormalities limit range of motion of the chest cage and the spine and, therefore, decrease ventilation abilities.[4] The coupling and interaction of the bony thorax and the ventilatory muscles and their relationship to ventilation will be the focus of this chapter.

5-1   Patient Case

Mary Nasser is a 12-year-old who is trying out for her town's tennis team. This is the first time she has ever really played tennis beyond lessons in childhood. She began to have complaints of shortness of breath with portions of practice that involved a high level of exertion. She saw her primary care physician, who picked up evidence of a scoliosis (curvature of the spine) in her initial screening. Spine radiographs were done, and Mary was diagnosed with an idiopathic right thoracic scoliosis, with a 40° curve. A medical workup was negative for an acute pulmonary process. Mary was referred to an orthopedic surgeon and to physical therapy for management of the scoliosis and shortness of breath.

◆ General Structure and Function

Rib Cage

The rib cage is a closed chain that involves many joints and muscles. The anterior border of the rib cage is the sternum, the lateral borders are the ribs, and the posterior border is formed by the thoracic vertebrae. The superior border of the rib cage is formed by the jugular

A

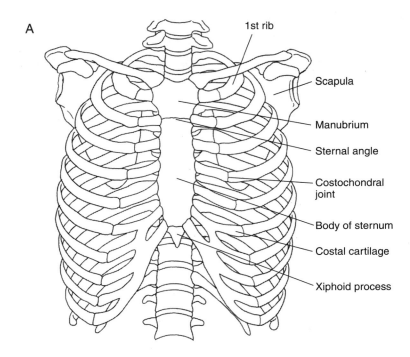

1st rib

Scapula

Manubrium

Sternal angle

Costochondral joint

Body of sternum

Costal cartilage

Xiphoid process

B

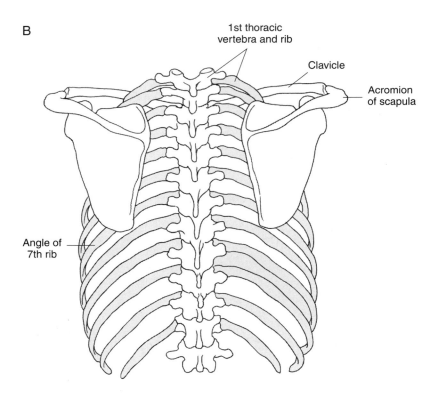

1st thoracic vertebra and rib

Clavicle

Acromion of scapula

Angle of 7th rib

▲ **Figure 5-1** ■ Anterior (**A**) and posterior (**B**) views of the thorax are shown, including its component parts: the sternum, 12 pairs of ribs and their costocartilages, and the thoracic vertebrae.

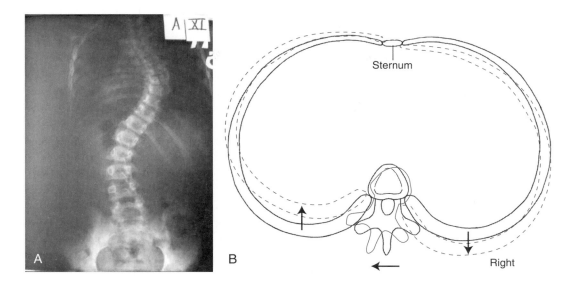

▲ **Figure 5-2** ■ **A.** A right thoracic scoliosis (named by the side of the convexity) of 52° shows the evident rib distortion that results from accompanying rotation of the involved vertebrae. There is also a lumbar curve of 32°. **B.** The bodies of the thoracic vertebrae in scoliosis typically rotate to the right, resulting in posterior displacement of the right transverse process and the attached right rib, as well as anterior displacement of the opposite transverse process and left rib.

notch of the sternum, by the superior borders of the first costocartilages, and by the first ribs and their contiguous first thoracic vertebra. The inferior border of the rib cage is formed by the xiphoid process, the shared costocartilage of ribs 6 through 10, the inferior portions of the 11th and 12th ribs, and the 12th thoracic vertebra (see Fig. 5-1).

The sternum is an osseous protective plate for the heart and is composed of the **manubrium, body,** and **xiphoid process** (Fig. 5-3). The manubrium and the body form a dorsally concave angle of approximately 160°. The xiphoid process often angles dorsally from the body of the sternum and may be difficult to palpate.

There are 12 thoracic vertebrae that make up the posterior aspect of the rib cage. One of the unique aspects of the typical thoracic vertebra is that the vertebral body and transverse processes have six costal articulating surfaces, four on the body (a superior and an inferior costal facet, or demifacet, on each side) and one costal facet on each transverse process (Fig. 5-4). The rib cage also includes 12 pairs of ribs. The ribs are curved flat bones that gradually increase in length from rib 1 to rib 7 and then decrease in length again from rib 8 to rib 12.[5] The posteriorly located head of each rib

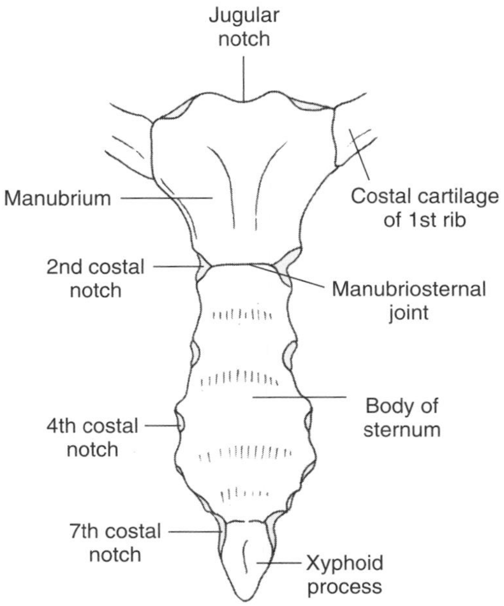

▲ **Figure 5-3** ■ The sternum is composed of the manubrium, the body of the sternum, and the xiphoid process. The costal notches for the chondrosternal joints are also evident in this anterior view.

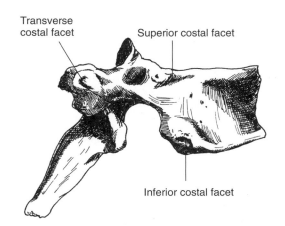

▲ **Figure 5-4** ■ The costal facets on the typical thoracic vertebrae are found on the superior and inferior aspects of the posterior body and the anterior transverse processes.

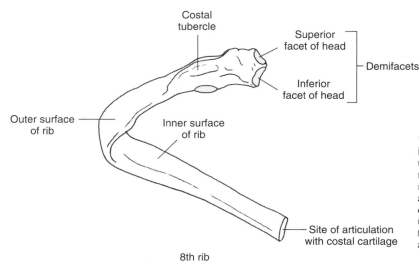

Costal
tubercle

Superior
facet of head

Inferior
facet of head

Demifacets

Outer surface
of rib

Inner surface
of rib

Site of articulation
with costal cartilage

8th rib

◀ **Figure 5-5** ■ The typical rib (ribs 2 through 9) is a curved flat bone. The posteriorly located head of the rib has superior and inferior facets that are separated by a ridge called the crest of the head. The superior and inferior facets (also known as demifacets) articulate, respectively, with the superior and inferior costal facets on the body of the vertebrae; the facet on the costal tubercle articulates with the transverse costal facet on the transverse process of the vertebra; the rib articulates anteriorly with costal cartilages.

articulates with thoracic vertebral bodies; and the costal tubercles of ribs 1 to 10 also articulate with the transverse processes of a thoracic vertebra (Fig. 5-5). Anteriorly, ribs 1 to 10 have a costocartilage that join them either directly or indirectly to the sternum through the costal cartilages (Fig. 5-6). The first through the seventh ribs are classified as **vertebrosternal** (or **"true"**) **ribs** because each rib, through its costocartilage, attaches directly to the sternum. The costocartilage of the 8th through 10th ribs articulates with the costocartilages of the superior rib, indirectly articulating with the sternum through rib 7. These ribs are classified as **vertebrochondral** (or **"false"**) **ribs.** The 11th and 12th ribs are called **vertebral** (or **"floating"**) **ribs**

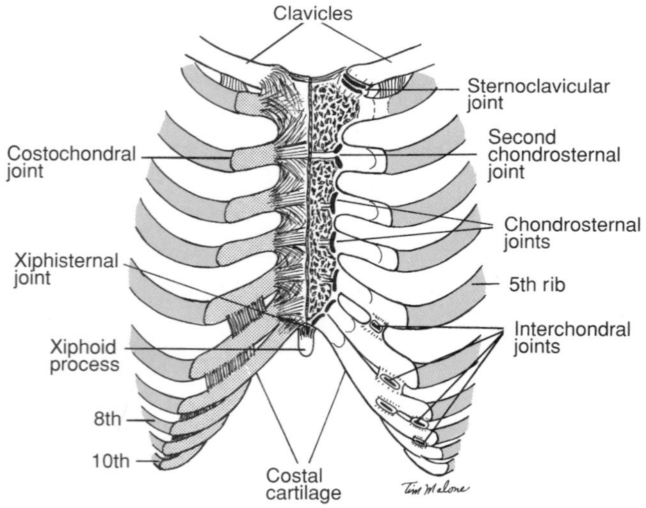

Clavicles

Sternoclavicular
joint

Costochondral
joint

Second
chondrosternal
joint

Chondrosternal
joints

Xiphisternal
joint

5th rib

Interchondral
joints

Xiphoid
process

8th

10th

Costal
cartilage

Tim Malone

▲ **Figure 5-6** ■ In this anterior view of the rib cage, the ribs articulate with the costal cartilages. The ribs join the costal cartilages at the costochondral joints. The costal cartilages of the first through the seventh ribs articulate directly with the sternum through the chondrosternal joints. The costal cartilages of the 8th through the 10th ribs articulate indirectly with the sternum through the costal cartilages of the adjacent superior rib at the interchondral joints.

because they have no anterior attachment to the sternum.[5]

■ **Articulations of the Rib Cage**

The articulations that join the bones of the rib cage include the **manubriosternal (MS)**, **xiphisternal (XS)**, **costovertebral (CV)**, **costotransverse (CT)**, **costochondral (CC)**, **chondrosternal (CS)**, and the **interchondral** joints.

Manubriosternal and Xiphisternal Joints

The manubrium and the body of the sternum articulate at the MS joint (see Fig. 5–3). This joint is also known as the sternal angle or the angle of Louis and is readily palpable.[1,6] The MS joint is a synchondrosis. The MS joint has a fibrocartilaginous disk between the hyaline cartilage–covered articulating ends of the manubrium and sternum—structurally similar to the symphysis pubis of the pelvis. Ossification of the MS joint occurs in elderly persons.[6,7] The xiphoid process joins the inferior aspect of the sternal body at the XS joint. The XS joint is also a synchondrosis that tends to ossify by 40 to 50 years of age.[8]

Costovertebral Joints

The typical CV joint is a synovial joint formed by the head of the rib, two adjacent vertebral bodies, and the interposed intervertebral disk. Ribs 2 to 9 have typical CV joints, inasmuch as the heads of these ribs each have two articular facets, or so-called **demifacets**[6,9] (see Fig. 5-5). The demifacets are separated by a ridge called the crest of the head of the rib. The small, oval, and slightly convex demifacets of the ribs are called the **superior** and **inferior costovertebral facets.** Adjacent thoracic vertebrae have facets corresponding to those of the 9 ribs that articulates with them. The head of each of the second through ninth ribs articulates with an **inferior** facet on the superior of the two adjacent vertebrae and with a superior facet on the inferior of the two

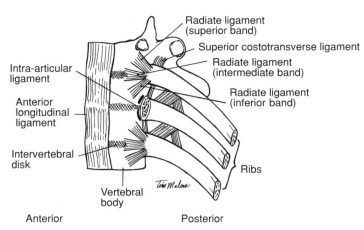

Anterior   Posterior

◀ **Figure 5-7** ■ A lateral view of the CV joints and ligaments. The three bands of the radiate ligament reinforce the CV joints. The superior and inferior bands of the radiate ligament attach to the joint capsule (removed) and to the superior and inferior vertebral bodies, respectively. The intermediate band attaches to the intervertebral disk. The middle CV joint is shown with the radiate ligament bands removed to demonstrate the intra-articular ligament that attaches the head of the rib to the anulus.

adjacent vertebrae (Fig. 5-7). The inferior and superior facets on the adjacent vertebrae articulate, respectively, with the superior and inferior facets on the head of the rib. The heads of the second through ninth ribs fit snugly into the "angle" formed by the adjacent vertebral demifacets and the intervening disk and are numbered by the inferior vertebra with which a rib articulates. The 1st, 10th 11th, and 12th ribs are atypical ribs because they articulate with only one vertebral body and are numbered by that body.[5,8,9] The CV facets of T10 to T12 are located more posteriorly on the pedicle of the vertebra.[6]

The typical CV joint is divided into two cavities by the **interosseous** or **intra-articular ligament.**[8,9] This ligament extends from the crest of the head of the rib to attach to the anulus fibrosus of the intervertebral disk.[6,9] The **radiate ligament** is located within the capsule, with firm attachments to the anterolateral portion of the capsule. The radiate ligament has three bands: the superior band, which attaches to the superior vertebra; the intermediate band, which attaches to the intervertebral disk; and the inferior band, which attaches to the inferior vertebra[5,6,8] (see Fig. 5-7). A fibrous capsule surrounds the entire articulation of each CV joint.

The atypical CV joints of ribs 1 and 10 through 12 are more mobile than the typical CV joints because the rib head articulates with only one vertebra. The interosseous ligament is absent in these joints; therefore, they each have only one cavity.[9] The radiate ligament is present in these joints, with the superior band still attaching to the superior vertebra. Both rotation and gliding motions occur at all of the CV joints.[10]

Costotransverse Joints

The CT joint is a synovial joint formed by the articulation of the costal tubercle of the rib with a costal facet on the transverse process of the corresponding vertebra[9] (Fig. 5-8). There are 10 pairs of CT joints articulating vertebrae T1 through T10 with the rib of the same number. The CT joints on T1 through approximately T6 have slightly concave costal facets on the transverse processes of the vertebrae and slightly con-

vex costal tubercles on the corresponding ribs. This allows slight rotation movements between these segments. At the CT joints of approximately T7 through T10, both articular surfaces are flat and gliding motions predominate. Ribs 11 and 12 do not articulate with their respective transverse processes of T11 or T12.

The CT joint is surrounded by a thin, fibrous capsule. Three major ligaments support the CT joint capsule. These are the **lateral costotransverse ligament,** the **costotransverse ligament,** and the **superior costotransverse ligament** (Fig. 5-9). The lateral costotransverse ligament is a short, stout band located between the lateral portion of the costal tubercle and the tip of the corresponding transverse process.[9,10] The costotransverse ligament is composed of short fibers that run within the costotransverse foramen between the neck of the rib posteriorly and the transverse process at the same level.[6,9] The superior costotransverse ligament runs from the crest of the neck of the rib to the inferior border of the cranial transverse process.

Costochondral and Chondrosternal Joints

The CC joints are formed by the articulation of the 1st through 10th ribs anterolaterally with the costal cartilages (see Fig. 5-6). The CC joints are synchondroses.[6] The periosteum and the perichondrium are continu-

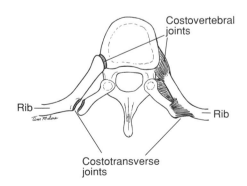

▲ **Figure 5-8** ■ A superior view of the costovertebral and costotransverse joints shows the capsuloligamentous structures on the right. The joint capsules and ligaments are removed on the left to show the articulating surfaces.

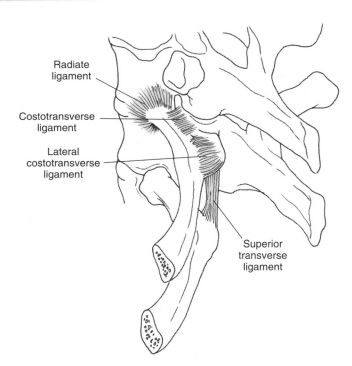

▲ **Figure 5-9** ■ Ligaments supporting the costotransverse joint, including (1) the costotransverse ligament, (2) the lateral costotransverse ligament, and (3) the superior costotransverse ligament.

ous, giving support to the union. The CC joints have no ligamentous support.

The CS joints are formed by the articulation of the costal cartilages of ribs 1 to 7 anteriorly with the sternum (see Fig. 5-6). Rib 1 attaches to the lateral facet of the manubrium, rib 2 is attached via two demifacets at the manubriosternal junction, and ribs 3 through 7 articulate with the lateral facets of the sternal body. The CS joints of the first, sixth, and seventh ribs are synchondroses. The CS joints of ribs 2 to 5 are synovial joints.

The CS joints of the first through seventh ribs have capsules that are continuous with the periosteum and support the connection of the cartilage as a whole.[9] Ligamentous support for the capsule includes **anterior** and **posterior radiate costosternal ligaments**. The **sternocostal ligament** is an intra-articular ligament, similar to the intra-articular ligament of the CV joint, that divides the two demifacets of the second CS joint.[5,8,9] The CS joints may ossify with aging.[5] The **costoxiphoid ligament** connects the anterior and posterior surfaces of the seventh costal cartilage to the front and back of the xiphoid process.

Interchondral Joints

The 7th through the 10th costal cartilages each articulate with the cartilage immediately above them. For the 8th through 10th ribs, this articulation forms the only connection to the sternum, albeit indirect (see Fig. 5-6). The interchondral joints are synovial joints and are supported by a capsule and interchondral ligaments. The interchondral articulations, like the CS joints, tend to become fibrous and fuse with age.

 CONCEPT CORNERSTONE 5-1: *Rib Cage Summary*

In summary, the 1st to 10th ribs articulate posteriorly with the vertebral column by two synovial joints (the CV and CT joints) and anteriorly through the costocartilages to the manubriosternum, either directly or indirectly. These joints form a closed kinematic chain in which the segments are interdependent and motion is restricted. These articulations with their associated ligamentous support give the thoracic cage the stability necessary to protect the organs and yet enough flexibility to maximize function.[9] The 11th and 12th ribs have a single CV joint, no CT joint, and no attachment anteriorly to the sternum. These ribs form an open kinematic chain, and the motion of these ribs is less restricted.

■ **Kinematics of the Ribs and Manubriosternum**

The movement of the rib cage is an amazing combination of complex geometrics governed by the types and angles of the articulations, the movement of the manubriosternum, and the contribution of the elasticity of the costal cartilages.

Controversy exists in the literature regarding the mechanisms and types of motions that are actually occurring for each rib. The major controversy regarding rib motion centers on the types of motion at the CV articulations and whether the ribs can be deformed during inspiration and expiration. Kapandji and others believed the CV and CT joints are mechanically linked, with a single axis passing through the center of both joints.[2,8–10] Saumarez argued that the rib is rigid and, therefore, cannot rotate about a single fixed axis but rather moves as successive rotations about a shifting axis.[11]

Investigators are generally in agreement regarding the structure and motion of the first rib. The anterior articulation of rib 1 is larger and thicker than that of any other rib.[5] The first costal cartilage is stiffer than the other costocartilages. Also, the first CS joint is cartilaginous (synchondrosis), not synovial, and therefore is firmly attached to the manubrium. Finally, the first CS joint is just inferior and posterior to the sternoclavicular joint. For these reasons, there is very little movement of the first rib at the anterior CS joint. Posteriorly, the CV joint of the first rib has a single facet, which increases the mobility at that joint. During inspiration, the CV joint moves superiorly and posteriorly, elevating the first rib.

According to what appears to be the more commonly accepted theory, there is a single axis of motion for the 1st to 10th ribs through the center of the CV and CT joints. This axis for the upper ribs lies close to the frontal plane, allowing thoracic motion predominantly in the sagittal plane. The axis of motion for the lower ribs is nearly in the sagittal plane, allowing for thoracic motion predominantly in the frontal plane (Fig. 5-10). The axis of motion for the 11th and 12th ribs passes through the CV joint only, because there is no CT joint present. The axis of motion for these last two ribs also lies close to the frontal plane.

During inspiration, the ribs elevate. In the upper ribs, most of the movement occurs at the anterior

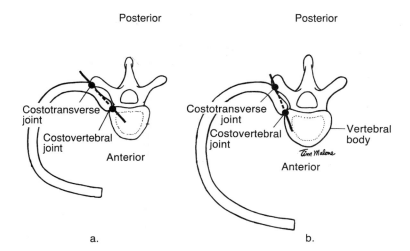

Posterior   Posterior

Costotransverse joint
Costovertebral joint
Anterior
a.

Costotransverse joint
Costovertebral joint
Vertebral body
Anterior
b.

◀ **Figure 5-10** ■ **A.** The common axis of motion for the upper ribs passes through the centers of the CV and CT joints and lies nearly in the frontal plane. **B.** The axis through the CV and CT joints for the lower ribs lies closer to the sagittal plane.

aspect of the rib, given the nearly coronal axis at the vertebrae. The costocartilage become more horizontal.[9] The movement of the ribs pushes the sternum ventrally and superiorly. The excursion of the manubrium is less than that of the body of the sternum because the first rib is the shortest, with the caudal ribs increasing in length until rib 7. The discrepancy in length causes movement at the MS joint.[6] The motion of the upper ribs and sternum has its greatest effect by increasing the anteroposterior (A-P) diameter of the thorax. This combined rib and sternal motion that occurs in a predominantly sagittal plane has been termed the "pump-handle" motion of the thorax (Fig. 5-11).

Elevation of the lower ribs occurs about the axis of motion lying nearly in the sagittal plane. The lower ribs have a more angled shape (obliquity increases from rib

1 to rib 10) and an indirect attachment anteriorly to the sternum. These factors allow the lower ribs more motion at the lateral aspect of the rib cage. The elevation of the lower ribs has its greatest effect by increasing the transverse diameter of the lower thorax. This motion that occurs in a nearly frontal plane has been termed the "bucket-handle" motion of the thorax (Fig. 5-12).

There is a gradual shift in the orientation of the axes of motion from cephalad to caudal; therefore, the intermediate ribs demonstrate qualities of both types of motion.[5,8–10,12] The 11th and 12th ribs each have only one posterior articulation with a single vertebra and no anterior articulation to the sternum; therefore, they do not participate in the closed-chain motion of the thorax.

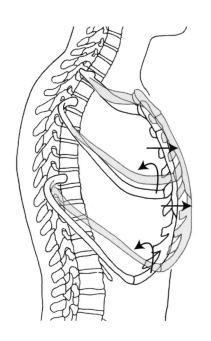

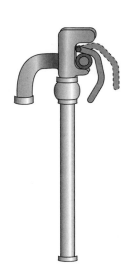

◀ **Figure 5-11** ■ Elevation of the upper ribs at the CV and CT joints results in anterior and superior movement of the sternum (and accompanying torsion of the costal cartilages), referred to as the "pump-handle" motion of the thorax.

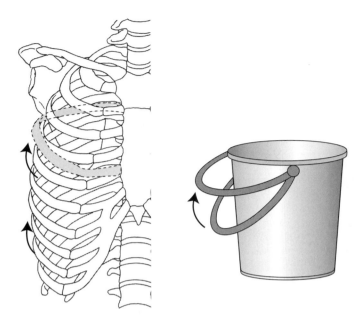

▲ **Figure 5-12** ■ Elevation of the lower ribs at the CV and CT joints results in a lateral motion of the rib cage, referred to as "bucket-handle" motion of the thorax.

Continuing Exploration: **Effects of Scoliosis on the Rib Cage**

The single axis of motion of the ribs is through the CV and CT joints. Therefore, changes in the alignment of these joints will change the mobility of the thorax. In scoliosis, the thoracic vertebrae not only laterally deviate but also rotate, altering the alignment of the costovertebral and costotransverse articulating surfaces (see Fig. 5-2A and B). Although the rib cage volume changes only slightly in scoliosis, it is asymmetrically distributed with the concave side of the thorax (with anterior rib distortion) increasing in volume and the convex side (with posterior rib distortion) decreasing in volume.[13] Figure 5-13A is a view of a normal thorax in a 4-year-old. Figure 5-13B is a view of the thorax of a 4-year-old with a congenital right thoracic scoliosis, showing the rib distortion that occurs with extreme vertebral rotation. The ventilatory abilities in patients with scoliosis are affected by the angle of the deformity, the length of the deformity, the region of the deformity, the amount of rotation of the deformity, and the age at onset.[14,15]

Case Application 5-1: **Rib Distortion in Scoliosis**

Mary is seen by an orthopedic physician, who confirms measurement of her midthoracic scoliotic curve at 40°. This degree of scoliotic angulation in the midthoracic region is likely to be accompanied by rotation of the involved vertebrae and a possible decrease in her pulmonary reserve. This may be a contributing factor in Mary's shortness of breath during tennis play. In addition to the high ventilatory demands of competitive ten-

A

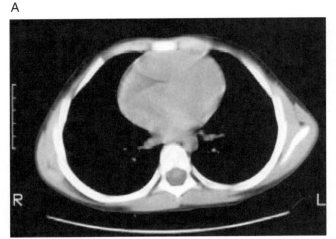

B

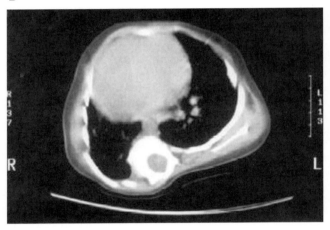

▲ **Figure 5-13** ■ Although the rib cage volume changes only slightly in scoliosis, it is asymmetrically distributed, with the concave side of the thorax increasing in volume and the convex side decreasing in volume.[17]

nis, the task is also an asymmetrical one that may be further compromising Mary's ability to meet the ventilatory demands of her sport.

Muscles Associated with the Rib Cage

The muscles that act on the rib cage are generally referred to as the **ventilatory muscles.** The ventilatory muscles are striated skeletal muscles that differ from other skeletal muscles in a number of ways: (1) the muscles of ventilation have increased fatigue resistance and greater oxidative capacity; (2) these muscles contract rhythmically throughout life rather than episodically; (3) the ventilatory muscles work primarily against the elastic properties of the lungs and airway resistance rather than against gravitational forces; (4) neurologic control of these muscles is both voluntary and involuntary; and (5) the actions of these muscles are life sustaining.

Any muscle that attaches to the chest wall has the potential to contribute to ventilation. The recruitment of muscles for ventilation is related to the type of breathing being performed.[16] In quiet breathing that occurs at rest, only the primary inspiratory muscles are needed for ventilation. During active or forced breathing that occurs with increased activity or with pulmonary pathologies, accessory muscles of both inspiration and expiration are recruited to perform the increased demand for ventilation.

The ventilatory muscles are most accurately classified as either **primary** or **accessory muscles of ventilation.** A muscle's action during the ventilatory cycle, especially the action of an accessory muscle, is neither simple nor absolute, which makes the categorizing of ventilatory muscles as either inspiratory muscles or expiratory muscles inaccurate and misleading.

■ **Primary Muscles of Ventilation**

The primary muscles are those recruited for quiet ventilation. These include the **diaphragm,** the **intercostal muscles** (particularly the **parasternal muscles**), and the **scalene muscles.**[17,18] These muscles all act on the rib cage to promote inspiration. There are no primary muscles for expiration, inasmuch as expiration at rest is passive.

Continuing Exploration: **Measures of Lung Volume and Capacity**

Vital capacity (VC) is a combination of inspiratory reserve volume (IRV), tidal volume (TV), and expiratory reserve volume (ERV). Vital capacity is the volume of air that can be blown out of the lungs from a full inspiration to a full exhalation. Inspiratory capacity (IC) is a combination of IRV and TV; it is the volume of air that can be breathed in from resting exhalation.

Functional residual capacity (FRC) is a combination of expiratory reserve volume and reserve volume (RV); it is the volume of air that remains in the lungs after a quiet exhalation.

Total lung capacity (TLC) is a combination of all four lung volumes: IRV, TV, ERV, and RV. Tidal volume is the portion of the total lung capacity that is used during quiet breathing. Table 5-1 summarizes the definitions graphically. With increased ventilatory demands, the volume of each breath needs to increase, moving that breath into both the inspira-

tory reserve volume and the expiratory reserve volume. With increased ventilatory demands, the rate of breathing (breaths/minute) will also increase.

Diaphragm

The diaphragm is the primary muscle of ventilation, accounting for approximately 70% to 80% of inspiration force during quiet breathing.[17] The diaphragm is a circular set of muscle fibers that arise from the sternum, costocartilages, ribs, and vertebral bodies. The fibers travel cephalad (superiorly) to insert into a **central tendon.**[19,20] The **lateral leaflets** of the boomerang-shaped central tendon form the tops of the domes of the right and left hemidiaphragms. Functionally, the muscular portion of the diaphragm is divided into the **costal portion,** which arises from the sternum, costocartilage and ribs, and the **crural portion,** which arises from the vertebral bodies[21] (Fig. 5-14).

The costal portion of the diaphragm attaches by muscular slips to the posterior aspect of the xiphoid process and inner surfaces of the lower six ribs and their costal cartilages.[19,20] The costal fibers of the diaphragm run vertically from their origin, in close apposition to the rib cage, and then curve to become more horizontal before inserting into the central tendon. The vertical fibers of the diaphragm, which lie close to the inner wall of the lower rib cage, are termed the **zone of apposition**[2] (see Fig. 5-14A).

The crural portion of the diaphragm arises from the anterolateral surfaces of the bodies and disks of L1 to L3 and from the **aponeurotic arcuate ligaments.** The **medial arcuate ligament** arches over the upper anterior part of the psoas muscles and extends from the L1 or L2 vertebral body to the transverse process of L1, L2, or L3. The **lateral arcuate ligament** covers the quadratus lumborum muscles and extends from the transverse process of L1, L2, or L3 to the 12th rib[19,22] (see Fig. 5-14B).

During **tidal breathing,** the fibers of the zone of apposition of the diaphragm contract, causing a descent of the diaphragm but only a slight change in the contour of the dome. As the dome descends, the abdominal contents compress, increasing intra-abdominal pressure.[22] With a deeper breath, the abdomen, now compressed, acts to stabilize the central tendon of the diaphragm (Fig. 5-15A), With a continued contraction of the costal fibers of the diaphragm against the central tendon that is stabilized by abdominal pressure, the lower ribs are now lifted and rotated outwardly in

Table 5-1	Lung Volumes and Lung Capacities		

Lung Volumes	Lung Capacities		
Inspiratory reserve volume (IRV)	Vital Capacity (VC)	Inspiratory Capacity (IC)	Total Lung Capacity (TLC)
Tidal volume (TV)			
Expiratory reserve volume (ERV)		Functional Residual Capacity (FRC)	
Residual volume (RV)	Reserve Capacity (RV)		

A

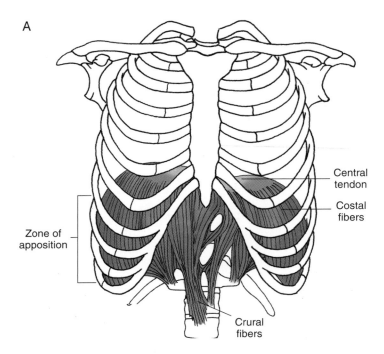

B

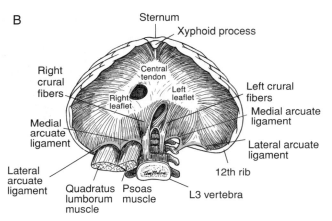

▲ **Figure 5-14** ■ **A.** In an anterior view, the fibers of the diaphragm can be seen to arise from the sternum, costocartilages, and ribs (costal fibers) and from the vertebral bodies (crural fibers). The costal fibers run vertically upward from their origin in close apposition to the rib cage and then curve and become more horizontal before inserting into the central tendon. **B.** An inferior view of the diaphragm shows the leaflets of the central tendon, as well as the medial and lateral arcuate ligaments bilaterally.

the bucket-handle motion[23–25] (see Fig. 5-15B). As the diaphragm reaches the end of its contraction, the fibers become more horizontally aligned, and further contraction no longer lifts the lower rib cage.[26]

The crural portion of the diaphragm has a less direct inspiratory effect on the lower rib cage than does the costal portion.[2,21] Indirectly, the action of the crural portion results in a descending of the central tendon, increasing intra-abdominal pressure. This increased pressure is transmitted across the apposed diaphragm to help expand the lower rib cage.[2,21]

The thoracoabdominal movement during quiet inspiration is a result of the pressures that are generated by the contraction of the diaphragm. When the diaphragm contracts and the central tendon descends, the increase in abdominal pressure causes the abdomi-

nal contents to be displaced anteriorly and laterally. The resultant increase in thoracic size with descent of the diaphragm results in the decreased intrapulmonary pressure that is responsible for inspiration (Fig. 5-16). Exhalation shows a decrease in thoracic size. As the diaphragm returns to its domed shape, the abdominal contents return to their starting position. In persons with chronic obstructive pulmonary disease (COPD), chronic hyperinflation of the lungs results in a resting position of the diaphragm that is lower (more flattened) than normal. Consequently, with more severe disease, an active contraction of the diaphragm pulls the lower ribs inwardly more than pulling the diaphragm down (Fig. 5-17). With an active contraction of the diaphragm in severe COPD, there is less of a reduction in thoracic size and a decreased inspiration.

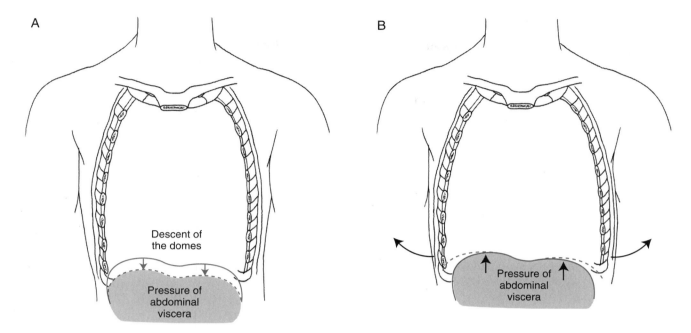

A

Descent of
the domes

Pressure of
abdominal
viscera

B

Pressure of
abdominal
viscera

▲ **Figure 5-15** ■ **A.** During tidal breathing, the diaphragm contracts, causing a descent of the dome of the diaphragm and an increase in intra-abdominal pressure. The increase in intra-abdominal pressure eventually prevents further descent of (stabilizes) the central tendon of the diaphragm. **B.** Continued contraction of the costal fibers of the diaphragm on the stabilized central tendon results in expansion (bucket-handle motion) of the lower ribs.

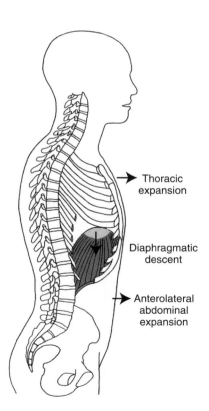

Thoracic
expansion

Diaphragmatic
descent

Anterolateral
abdominal
expansion

▲ **Figure 5-16** ■ With quiet inspiration, the normal thoracoabdominal movement is caused by contraction of the diaphragm. The diaphragm descends, increasing thoracic size and displacing the abdominal viscera anteriorly and laterally. With passive exhalation, the thorax decreases in size, and the abdominal viscera return to their resting position.

Continuing Exploration: **Compliance**

Compliance is a measurement of the distensibility of a structure or system. During diaphragm contraction, the abdomen becomes the fulcrum for lateral expansion of the rib cage. Therefore, compliance of the abdomen is a factor in the inspiratory movement of the thorax.

$$\text{Compliance} = \triangle\text{volume}/\triangle\text{pressure}$$

$$\text{Compliance} = \text{change in volume per unit of pressure}$$

Increased compliance of the abdomen, as in spinal cord injury in which the abdominal musculature may not be innervated, decreases lateral rib cage expansion as a result of the inability to stabilize the central tendon. Without stabilization of the central tendon, the costal fibers of the diaphragm cannot lift the lower ribs. Decreased compliance of the abdomen, as in pregnancy, limits caudal diaphragmatic excursion and causes lateral and upward motion of the rib cage to occur earlier in the ventilatory cycle.

Intercostal Muscles

The **external** and **internal intercostal muscles** are categorized as ventilatory muscles. However, only the **parasternal muscles** (or portions of the internal intercostals adjacent to the sternum) are considered primary muscles of ventilation. To provide a coordinated discussion of ventilatory musculature, the entire group

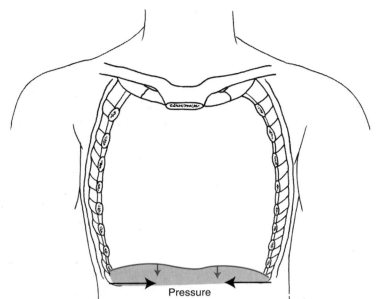

Pressure

◀　**Figure 5-17**　■　Patients with chronic obstructive pulmonary disease (COPD) have a resting position of the diaphragm that is flattened by hyperinflation. In severe disease, contraction of the diaphragm pulls the lower rib cage inward.

of intercostal muscles will be described together in this section.

The internal and external intercostal and the **subcostales** muscles (Fig. 5-18) connect adjacent ribs to one another and are named according to their anatomic orientation and location. The internal intercostal muscles arise from a ridge on the inner surfaces of the 1st through 11th ribs, and each inserts into the superior border of the rib below. The fibers of the internal intercostal muscles lie deep to the external intercostal muscles and run caudally and posteriorly. The internal intercostals begin anteriorly at the chondrosternal junctions and continue posteriorly to the angles of the ribs, where they become an aponeurotic layer called the **posterior intercostal membrane.** The external intercostal fibers run caudally and anteriorly, at an oblique angle to the internal intercostal muscles.[2] The external intercostal muscles begin posteriorly at the tubercles of the ribs and extend anteriorly to the costochondral junctions, where they form the **anterior intercostal membrane.** Given these attachments, only the internal intercostal muscles are present anteriorly from the chondrosternal junctions to the costochondral joints. These are the segments of the internal intercostal muscles that are referred to as the parasternal muscles. There are only external intercostal muscles present posteriorly from the tubercle of the ribs to the angle of the ribs (see Fig. 5-18). Laterally, both internal intercostal and external intercostal muscle layers are present and may be referred to in this location as the **interosseous** or **lateral intercostal muscles.**

The subcostal muscles (see Fig. 5-18) are also intercostal muscles but are generally found only in the lower rib cage. The subcostal muscles are found at the rib angles and may span more than one intercostal space before inserting into the inner surface of a caudal rib. Their fiber direction and action are similar to those of the internal intercostal muscles. The external inter-

costal muscles originate on the inferior borders of the 1st through 11th ribs, and each inserts into the superior border of the rib below.

The functions of the intercostal muscles during ventilation are intricate and controversial. In 1749, Hamberger proposed the simplistic theory that the external intercostal muscles tend to raise the lower rib up to the higher rib, which is an inspiratory motion, and the internal intercostal muscles tend to lower the higher rib onto the lower rib, which is an expiratory

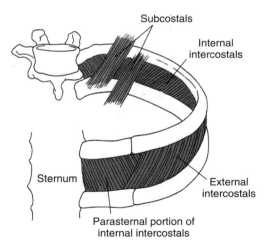

Subcostals

Internal intercostals

Sternum

External intercostals

Parasternal portion of internal intercostals

▲　**Figure 5-18**　■　Intercostal muscles. The internal intercostal muscles originate anteriorly at the chondrosternal junction and continue posteriorly to the angle of the rib, where they become an aponeurotic layer. The anteriorly located fibers of the internal intercostals are referred to as the parasternal fibers. The external intercostal muscles begin at the tubercle of the rib and continue anteriorly to the costochondral junction. The subcostal fibers run parallel to the internal intercostal muscles but are generally found only in the lower rib cage at the rib angle, and they may span more than one intercostal space.

motion.[5] Electromyographic (EMG) studies have shown that, although the external intercostal muscles are active during inspiration and the internal intercostal muscles are active during exhalation,[27] both sets of intercostal muscles may be active during both phases of respiration as minute ventilation increases[28] (see Continuing Exploration: Minute Ventilation). Either set of intercostal muscles can raise the rib cage from a low lung volume or lower the rib cage from a high lung volume.[29] The activation of the intercostal muscles during the ventilatory cycle is from cranial to caudal, meaning that the recruitment of fibers begins in the higher intercostal spaces early in inspiration and moves downward as inspiration progresses. Activation of the lower intercostal muscles appears to occur only during deep inhalation.[30]

Continuing Exploration: **Minute Ventilation**

Minute ventilation is the amount of air that is breathed in (or out) in one minute:

$$\text{Minute ventilation } (V_E) = [TV] \times [\text{respiratory rate (RR)}]$$

The parasternal muscles, the most anterior portion of the internal intercostal muscles, are considered primary inspiratory muscles during quiet breathing.[2,31] The action of the parasternal muscles appears to be a rotation of the CS junctions, resulting in elevation of the ribs and anterior movement of the sternum. The primary function of the parasternal muscles, however, appears to be stabilization of the rib cage.[32–34] This stabilizing action of the parasternal muscles opposes the decreased intrapulmonary pressure generated during diaphragmatic contraction, preventing a paradoxical, or inward, movement of the upper chest wall during inspiration.[34]

The function of the lateral (internal and external) intercostal muscles involves both ventilation and trunk rotation.[2,35,36] The lateral intercostal muscles, although active during the respiratory cycle, have a relatively small amount of activity in comparison with the parasternal muscles and the diaphragm.[37] The major role of the lateral intercostal muscles is in axial rotation of the thorax, with the contralateral internal and external intercostal muscles working synergistically to produce trunk rotation (e.g., right external and left internal intercostal muscles are active during trunk rotation to the left).[37]

Scalene Muscles

The scalene muscles are also primary muscles of quiet ventilation.[18] The scalene muscles attach on the transverse processes of C3 to C7 and descend to the upper borders of the first rib (scalenus anterior and scalenus medius) and second rib (scalenus posterior) (Fig. 5-19). Their action lifts the sternum and the first two ribs in the pump-handle motion of the upper rib cage.[18,23,31] Activity of the scalene muscles begins at the onset of inspiration and increases as inspiration gets closer to total lung capacity. The length-tension relationship of the scalene muscles allows them to generate a greater force late into the respiratory cycle, when the force from the diaphragm is decreasing. The scalene muscles also function as stabilizers of the rib cage. The scalene muscles, along with the parasternal muscles, counteract the paradoxical movement of the upper chest caused by the decreased intrapulmonary pressure created by the diaphragm's contraction.

■ Accessory Muscles of Ventilation

The muscles that attach the rib cage to the shoulder girdle, head, vertebral column, or pelvis may be classified as **accessory muscles** of ventilation. These muscles assist with inspiration or expiration in situations of stress, such as increased activity or disease.

When the trunk is stabilized, the accessory muscles

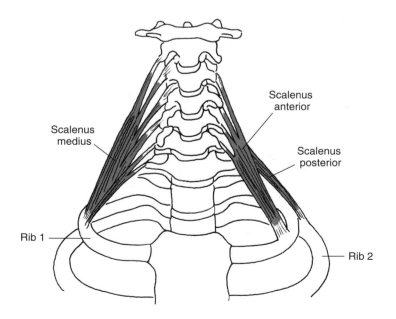

▶ **Figure 5-19** ■ The scalenus anterior, scalenus medius, and scalenus posterior. Their action lifts the sternum and the first two ribs in the pump-handle motion.

of ventilation move the vertebral column, arm, head, or pelvis on the trunk. During times of increased ventilatory demand, the rib cage can become the mobile segment. The accessory muscles of inspiration, therefore, increase the thoracic diameter by moving the rib cage upward and outward.[23] The accessory muscles of expiration move the diaphragm upward and the thorax downward and inward. The most commonly described accessory muscles are shown in Figure 5-20A and B and discussed in the following paragraphs.

The **sternocleidomastoid** runs from the manubrium and superior medial aspect of the clavicle to the mastoid process of the temporal bone. The usual bilateral action of the sternocleidomastoid is flexion of the cervical vertebrae. With the help of the **trapezius** muscle stabilizing the head, the bilateral action of the sternocleidomastoid muscles moves the rib cage superiorly, which expands the upper rib cage in the pump-handle motion. The recruitment of this muscle seems to occur toward the end of a maximal inspiration.[38]

The sternocostal portion of the **pectoralis major** muscle can elevate the upper rib cage when the shoulders and the humerus are stabilized. The clavicular head of the pectoralis major can be either inspiratory or expiratory in action, depending on the position of the upper extremity. When the arm is positioned so that the humeral attachment of the pectoralis major is below the level of the clavicle, the clavicular portion acts as an expiratory muscle by pulling the manubrium and upper ribs down. With the humeral attachment of the pectoralis major above the level of the clavicle, such as when the arm is raised, the muscle becomes an inspiratory muscle, pulling the manubrium and upper ribs up and out. The **pectoralis minor** can help elevate the third, fourth, and fifth ribs during a forced inspiration. The **subclavius,** a muscle between the clavicle and the first rib, can also assist in raising the upper chest for inspiration.

Posteriorly, the fibers of the **levatores costarum** run from the transverse processes of vertebrae C7 through T11 to the posterior external surface of the next lower rib between the tubercle and the angle and can assist with elevation of the upper ribs.[9,39] The **serratus posterior superior** (**SPS**) has its superior attachment at the spinous processes of the lower cervical and upper thoracic vertebrae, and attaches caudally via four thin bands just lateral to the angles of the second through fifth ribs. The SPS and the **serratus posterior inferior** (**SPI**) (see Fig. 5-20B) have been assumed to be accessory muscles of respiration based in large part on their anatomical origins and insertions. The presumed actions would be elevation the ribs by the SPS, and lowering of the ribs and stabilizing the diaphragm by the SPI. In an article by Vilensky et al., this function was questioned.[40] Because there is no EMG evidence to support a ventilatory role of these muscles, the authors concluded that no respiratory function should be attributed to either muscle.[40]

The abdominal muscles (**transversus abdominis, internal oblique abdominis, external oblique abdominis,** and **rectus abdominis)** are expiratory muscles, as well as trunk flexors and rotators. The major function of the abdominal muscles with regard to ventilation is to assist with forced expiration. The muscle fibers pull the ribs and costocartilage caudally, into a motion of exhalation. By increasing intra-abdominal pressure, the abdominal muscles can push the diaphragm upward into the thoracic cage, increasing both the volume and speed of exhalation.

Although considered accessory muscles of exhalation, the abdominal muscles play two significant roles during inspiration. First, the increased intra-abdominal pressure created by the active abdominal muscles during forced exhalation pushes the diaphragm cranially and exerts a passive stretch on the costal fibers of the diaphragm.[2] These changes prepare the respiratory system for the next inspiration by optimizing the length-tension relationship of the muscle fibers of the diaphragm. Second, the increased abdominal pressure created by lowering of the diaphragm in inspiration must be countered by tension in the abdominal musculature. Without sufficient compliance in the abdominal muscles, the central tendon of the diaphragm cannot be effectively stabilized so that lateral chest wall expansion occurs. During periods of increased ventilatory needs, the increased muscular activity of the abdominal muscles assists in both exhalation and inhalation.[2,20]

The **transversus thoracis** (triangularis sterni) muscles are a flat layer of muscle that runs deep to the parasternal muscles. The transversus thoracis muscles originate from the posterior surface of the caudal half of the sternum and run cranially and laterally, inserting into the inner surface of the costal cartilages of the third through seventh ribs.[2] These muscles are recruited for ventilation along with the abdominal muscles to pull the rib cage caudally. Studies have shown that these muscles are primarily expiratory muscles, especially when expiration is active, as in talking, coughing, or laughing, or in exhalation into functional residual capacity.[41,42]

Gravity acts as an accessory to ventilation in the supine position. Gravity, acting on the abdominal viscera, performs the same function as the abdominal musculature in stabilizing the central tendon of the diaphragm. In fact, in the supine position, the abdominal muscles and the trangularis sterni are silent on the EMG monitoring during quiet breathing.

Continuing Exploration: **Respiratory Changes in Scoliosis**

Not only do the anatomical changes that occur in scoliosis alter the alignment and motion of the thorax, but also there is a consequence to the length-tension relationship and the angle of pull of the muscles of ventilation. On the side of the convexity, with sufficient curvature, the intercostal space is widened and the intercostal muscles are elongated. On the side of the concavity, the ribs are approximated and the intercostal muscles are adaptively

A

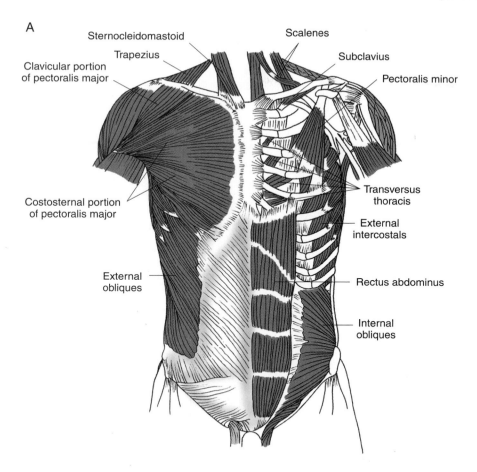

Sternocleidomastoid

Scalenes

Trapezius

Subclavius

Clavicular portion
of pectoralis major

Pectoralis minor

Costosternal portion
of pectoralis major

Transversus
thoracis

External
intercostals

External
obliques

Rectus abdominus

Internal
obliques

B

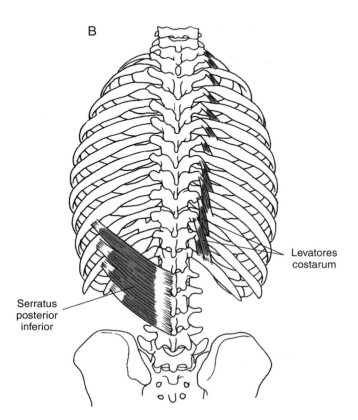

Levatores
costarum

Serratus
posterior
inferior

▲ **Figure 5-20** ■ Accessory muscles of ventilation are those
used during times of increased ventilatory demand. **A.** The right side
of the figure shows some of the anterior superficial muscles of the
thorax that can be accessory muscles of ventilation, whereas the left
side of the thorax shows the deeper accessory muscles of ventilation.
B. The serratus posterior inferior and the levatores costarum are
deep posterior muscles that may also assist with ventilation.

shortened (see Fig. 5-2A). Lung volumes and capacities are reduced from those in someone without thoracic deformity, as a result of the altered biomechanics of the scoliotic thorax[43] (Fig. 5-21).

Case Application 5-2: **Treatment for Scoliosis**

Bracing has been shown to be an effective treatment approach for limiting progression of curves and possibly decreasing severity of curves in some patients.[44] The Boston Scoliosis Brace (Fig. 5-22) is one option for Mary at this time. The Boston Scoliosis Brace places direct pressure on the rib cage in order to treat the scoliosis, but it also decreases thoracic mobility necessary for ventilation. The brace also has a tight-fitting abdominal pad that increases intra-abdominal pressure, restricting the descent of the diaphragm. Lung volumes and capacities are reduced by approximately 15% to 20% while the brace is worn.[45,46] This impairment, although significant, is reversible when the brace is removed.[47] Bracing is likely a good option for Mary, because her curve measures 40°. If there is improvement in the curve, it may improve her ability to tolerate high-level activities such as tennis.

Mary is still skeletally immature, and her 40° curve may increase with continued growth. If bracing is not successful in limiting progression, surgical correction may be considered at some point. Surgical treatment of scoliosis generally substantially reduces or corrects the lateral curvature of the spine. Pulmonary function tests show that any accompanying restrictions to ventilation are improved with surgical intervention, although they are not fully normalized.[48,49] Failure to normalize pulmonary mechanics may result from incomplete correction of the lateral and spinal deviations, irreversible pulmonary parenchymal changes, continued rotation of the vertebrae, and decreased flexibility of the thoracic spine.[48]

Coordination and Integration of Ventilatory Motions

The coordination and integration of the skeletal and muscular chest wall components during breathing are complex and difficult to measure. Investigators have used EMG techniques, electrical stimulation, ultrasound, computed tomography (CT) scans, and computerized motion analysis techniques to analyze and describe chest wall motion and muscular actions.[27,35–37,39] Studies have served to confirm the complexity of the coordinated actions of the many muscle groups involved even in quiet breathing. The recruitment of ventilatory muscles is dependent on the activities in which a person is participating, including not only sports, household, and job activities but also maintenance of posture, locomotion, speech, and defecation. A high and complex level of coordination is necessary for the primary and accessory muscles of ventilation to contribute to additional tasks while they continue to perform the necessary function of ventilation.

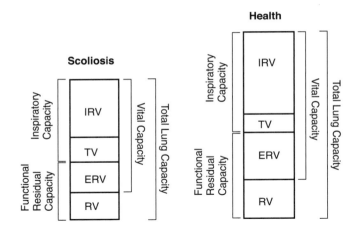

IRV = Inspiratory reserve volume; TV = Tidal volume;
ERV = Expiratory reserve volume; RV = Residual volume

▲ **Figure 5-21** ■ Lung volumes and capacities in health and in a patient with scoliosis.

 CONCEPT CORNERSTONE 5-2: *Summary of the Ventilatory Sequence During Breathing*

Although the coordinated function and sequence of breathing are complex when activities are combined, the following sequence of motions and muscle actions is typical of a healthy person at rest during quiet breathing. The diaphragm contracts, and the central tendon moves caudally. The parasternal and scalene muscles stabilize the anterior upper chest wall to prevent a paradoxical inward movement caused by the decreasing intrapulmonary pressure. As intra-abdominal pressure increases, the abdominal contents are displaced in such a way that the anterior epigastric abdominal wall

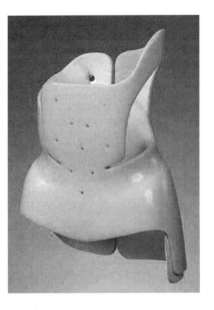

▲ **Figure 5-22** ■ The Boston Scoliosis Brace consists of a firmly fitting pelvic girdle that extends upward to apply forces (as appropriate to the individual) to the ribs in a way that reverses (or limits exacerbation of) the scoliotic curvature.

is pushed ventrally. Further outward motion of the abdominal wall is countered by the abdominal musculature, which allows the central tendon to stabilize on the abdominal viscera. The appositional (costal) fibers of the diaphragm now pull the lower ribs cephalad and laterally, which results in the bucket-handle movement of the lower ribs. With continued inspiration, the parasternal, scalene, and levatores costarum muscles actively rotate the upper ribs and elevate the manubriosternum, which results in an anterior motion of the upper ribs and sternum. The lateral motion of the lower ribs and anterior motion of the upper ribs and sternum can occur simultaneously. Expiration during quiet breathing is passive, involving the use of the recoil of the elastic components of the lungs and chest wall.

✦ Developmental Aspects of Structure and Function

Differences Associated with the Neonate

The compliance, configuration, and muscle action of the chest wall changes significantly from the infant to the elderly person. The newborn has a cartilaginous, and therefore extremely compliant, chest wall that allows the distortion necessary for the infant's thorax to travel through the birth canal. The increased compliance of the rib cage is at the expense of thoracic stability. The infant's chest wall muscles must act as stabilizers, rather than mobilizers, of the thorax to counteract the reduced intrapulmonary pressure created by the lowered diaphragm during inspiration. Complete ossification of the ribs does not occur for several months after birth.

Whereas the ribs in the adult thorax slope downward and the diaphragm is elliptically shaped (Fig. 5-23A), the rib cage of an infant shows a more horizontal alignment of the ribs, with the angle of insertion of the costal fibers of the diaphragm also more horizontal than those of the adult (see Fig. 5-23B). There is an increased tendency for these fibers to pull the lower ribs inward, thereby decreasing efficiency of ventilation and increasing distortion of the chest wall.[50,51] There is very little motion of the rib cage during tidal breathing of an infant.

Only 20% of the muscle fibers of the diaphragm are fatigue-resistant fibers in the healthy newborn, in comparison with 50% in the adult. This discrepancy predisposes infants to earlier diaphragmatic fatigue.[51] Accessory muscles of ventilation are also at a disadvantage in the infant. Until infants can stabilize their upper extremities, head, and spine, it is difficult for the accessory muscles of ventilation to produce the action needed to be helpful during increased ventilatory demands.

As the infant ages and the rib cage ossifies, muscles can begin to mobilize rather than stabilize the thorax. As the infant gains head control, he is also gaining accessory muscle use for increased ventilation. As the toddler assumes the upright position of sitting and standing, gravitation forces and postural changes allow

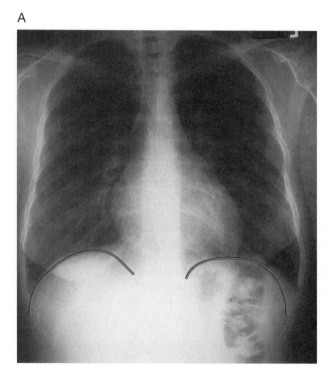

▲ **Figure 5-23** ■ **A.** In the adult, the ribs slope downward, and the diaphragm has an elliptical shape. **B.** The rib cage of an infant shows a nearly horizontal alignment of the ribs, and the angle of insertion of the costal fibers of the diaphragm is also more horizontal.

for the anterior rib cage to angle obliquely downward. This elliptical thorax allows for a greater bucket-handle motion of the rib cage. The attachments for the muscles of ventilation move with the increasingly angled ribs, improving their action on the thorax. Throughout childhood, the numbers of alveoli and airways continue to increase. [52] In early adolescence, the sizes of the alveoli and airways continue to expand, as demonstrated by increases in pulmonary function test results.

Differences Associated with the Elderly

Skeletal changes that occur with aging affect pulmonary function. Many of the articulations of the chest wall undergo fibrosis with advancing age.[53,54] The interchondral and costochondral joints can fibrose, and the chondrosternal joints may be obliterated. The xiphosternal junction usually ossifies after age 40. The chest wall articulations that are true synovial joints may undergo morphologic changes associated with aging, which results in reduced mobility. The costal cartilages ossify, which interferes with their axial rotation.[10] Overall, chest wall compliance is significantly reduced with age. Reduction in diaphragm-abdomen compliance has also been reported and is at least partially related to the decreased rib cage compliance, especially in the lower ribs that are part of the zone of apposition.[55]

Aging also brings anatomical changes to the lung tissue that affect the function of the lungs. The airways narrow, the alveolar duct diameters increase, and there are shallower alveolar sacs. There is a reorientation and decrease of the elastic fibers. Overall, there is a decrease in the elastic recoil and an increase in pulmonary compliance.[54] Because the resting position of the thorax depends on the balance between the elastic recoil properties of the lungs pulling the ribs inwardly and the outward pull of the bones, cartilage, and muscles, the reduced recoil property of the lung tissue allows the thorax to rest with an increased A-P diameter (a relatively increased inspiratory position). An increased kyphosis is often observed in older individuals, which decreases the mobility not only of the thoracic spine but also of the rib cage.

The result of these skeletal and tissue changes is an increase in the amount of air remaining in the lungs after a normal exhalation (i.e., an increase in functional residual capacity). If the lungs retain more air at the end of exhalation, there will be a decrease in inspiratory capacity of the thorax. Functionally, the changes result in a decrease in the ventilatory reserve available during times of need, such as during an illness or increased activity.

Skeletal muscles of ventilation of the elderly person have a documented loss of strength, fewer muscle fibers, a lower oxidative capacity, a decrease in the number or the size of fast-twitch type II fibers, and a lengthening of the time to peak tension.[54,56] The resting position of the diaphragm becomes less domed, with a decrease in abdominal tone in aging.[10] There is an early

recruitment pattern for accessory muscles of ventilation. For example, the transverse thoracic muscles are active during quiet expiration in older subjects in the standing position.[41]

CONCEPT CORNERSTONE 5-3: *Summary of Rib Cage Changes with Aging*

In elderly persons, there is likely to be a decreased compliance of the bony rib cage, an increased compliance of the lung tissue, and an overall decreased compliance of the respiratory system as a result of the effects of aging. There is a decrease effectiveness of the ventilatory muscles, and ventilation becomes more energy expensive with age. There is a decreased ventilatory reserve available during times of increased ventilatory need, such as increased activity or illness.

◆ Pathological Changes in Structure and Function

In this chapter, the effects of the musculoskeletal system on ventilation have been discussed. In scoliosis, a change in the musculoskeletal structure renders a change to ventilation. It is interesting to note that the opposite can also be true; changes in the pulmonary system can affect the biomechanics of the thorax. A brief discussion of this relation is presented, with COPD as the framework.

Chronic Obstructive Pulmonary Disease

The major manifestation of COPD is damage to the airways and destruction of the alveolar walls. As tissue destruction occurs with disease, the elastic recoil property of the lung tissue is diminished. Passive exhalation that depends upon this elastic recoil property becomes ineffective in removing air from the thorax. Air trapping and hyperinflation occur. The static position of the thorax changes as more air is now housed within the lungs at the end of exhalation. This affects the lung volume and ventilatory capacities (Fig. 5-24).

The static resting position of the thorax is a function of the balance between the elastic recoil properties of the lungs pulling inward and the normal outward spring of the rib cage. In COPD, there is an imbalance in these two opposing forces. As elasticity decreases, an increase in the A-P diameter (more of a barrel shape) of the hyperinflated thorax is apparent, along with flattening of the diaphragm at rest (Fig. 5-25). The range of motion, or excursion, of the thorax is limited. Although the basic problem in COPD is an inability to exhale, it is clear that inspiratory reserve is compromised.

Hyperinflation affects not only the bony components of the chest wall but also the muscles of the thorax. The fibers of the diaphragm are shortened, decreasing the available range of contraction. The angle of pull of the flattened diaphragm fibers becomes

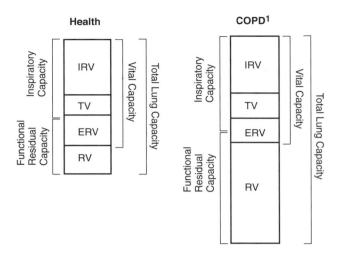

Health				COPD[1]			
	IRV				IRV		
	TV				TV		
	ERV				ERV		
	RV				RV		

IRV = Inspiratory reserve volume; TV = Tidal volume;
ERV = Expiratory reserve volume; RV = Residual volume

[1]COPD = Chronic obstructive pulmonary disease

▲ **Figure 5-24** ■ Lung volumes and capacities in health and in a patient with COPD.

more horizontal with a decreased zone of apposition. In severe cases of hyperinflation, the fibers of the diaphragm will be aligned horizontally. Contraction of this very flattened diaphragm will pull the lower rib cage inward, actually working against lung inflation[57] (see Fig. 5-17).

With compromise of the diaphragm in COPD, the majority of inspiration is now performed by other inspiratory muscles that are not as efficient as the diaphragm. The barrel-shaped and elevated thorax puts the sternocleidomastoid muscles in a shortened position, making them much less efficient. The parasternal and scalene muscles are able to generate a greater force as the lungs approach total lung capacity; consequently, hyperinflation has a less dramatic effect on them.[58] The diaphragm has a limited ability to laterally expand the rib cage, and so inspiratory motion must occur within the upper rib cage. In a forceful contraction of the functioning inspiratory muscles of the upper rib cage, the diaphragm and the abdominal contents actually may be pulled upward.[59] This is a paradoxical thorocoabdominal breathing pattern because the abdomen is pulled inward and upward during inspiration (Fig. 5-26), and is pushed back out and down during exhala-

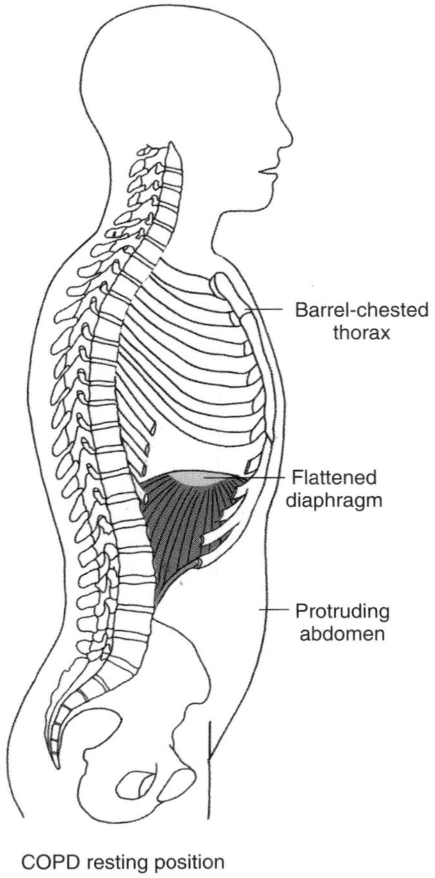

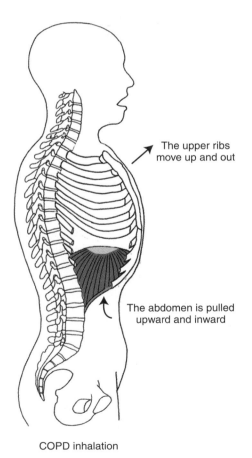

Barrel-chested thorax

Flattened diaphragm

Protruding abdomen

COPD resting position

▲ **Figure 5-25** ■ Resting position of a person with COPD. The thorax is barrel-shaped, and the diaphragm flattened from hyperinflation, and the abdomen protrudes as a result of increased intra-abdominal pressure.

The upper ribs move up and out

The abdomen is pulled upward and inward

COPD inhalation

▲ **Figure 5-26** ■ Paradoxical thorocoabdominal movement in COPD. With a strong pull of the accessory muscles of inspiration, there is an increase in the motion of the upper chest. Because the diaphragm is ineffective in descending, the abdominal viscera are pulled in and up. With exhalation, the thorax decreases in size, and the abdominal viscera return to their resting position.

tion. The paradoxical pattern is a reflection of the maintained effectiveness of the upper inspiratory rib cage musculature and the reduced effectiveness of the diaphragm.[60] The disadvantages of these biomechanical alterations of hyperinflation are compounded by the increased demand for ventilation in COPD. More work is required of a less effective system. The energy cost of ventilation, or the work of breathing, in COPD is markedly increased.

Summary

In this chapter, comprehensive coverage of the structure and function of the bony thorax and the ventilatory muscles has been provided. Additional information on the structure and function of accessory muscles of ventilation as these muscle may affect the shoulder complex will be presented in Chapter 7.

Study Questions

1. Describe the articulations of the chest wall and thorax, including the CV, CT, CC, CS, interchondral, and MS joints.
2. What is the normal sequence of chest wall motions during breathing? Explain why these motions occur.
3. What is the role of the diaphragm, the intercostal muscles, and the abdominal muscles during breathing?
4. Describe the "accessory" muscles and explain their functions.
5. Compare the action of the abdominal muscles with that of the scalene muscles.
6. What effect does COPD have on the inspiratory muscles?
7. How does the aging process affect the structure and function of the thorax?

References

1. Brannon F, Foley M, Starr J, et al.: Cardiopulmonary Rehabilitation: Basic Theory and Practice, 3rd ed. Philadelphia, FA Davis, 1998.
2. De Troyer A, Estenne M: Functional anatomy of the respiratory muscles. Clin Chest Med 9:175–193, 1988.
3. Stehbens W: Pathogenesis of idiopathic scoliosis revisited. Exp Mol Pathol 74:49–60, 2003.
4. Leong JCY, Lu, WW, Karlberg EM: Kinematics of the chest cage and spine during breathing in healthy individuals and in patients with adolescent idiopathic scoliosis. Spine 24:1310–1323, 1999.
5. Williams PL: Gray's Anatomy, 38th ed. St. Louis, Elsevier, 1995.
6. Moore KL, Dalley AF: Clinically Oriented Anatomy, pp 60 -173. Baltimore, Lippincott Williams & Wilkins, 1999.
7. Palastanga N, Field D, Soames R: Anatomy and Human Movement: Structure and Function, 4th ed. Boston, Butterworth Heinemann, 2002.
8. Grieve GP: Common Vertebral Joint Problems, 2nd ed, pp 32–39, 110–129. New York, Churchill Livingstone, 1988.
9. Winkel D: Diagnosis and Treatment of the Spine, pp 393–401. Gaithersburg, MD, Aspen, 1996.
10. Kapandji IA: The Physiology of the Joints: The Trunk and Vertebral Column, 3rd ed. New York, Churchill Livingstone, 1990.
11. Saumarez RC: An analysis of possible movements of human upper rib cage. J Appl Physiol 60:678–689, 1986.
12. Wilson TA, Rehder K, Krayer S, et al.: Geometry and respiratory displacement of human ribs. J Appl Physiol 62:1872–1877, 1987.
13. Closkey R, Schultz A, Luchies C: A model for studies of the deformable rib cage. J Biomechanics 25:529–539, 1992.
14. Brainthwaite MA: Cardiorespiratory consequences of unfused idiopathic scoliosis patients. Br J Dis Chest 80:360–369, 1986.
15. Campbell RM, Smith MD, Thomas C, et al.: The characteristics of thoracic insufficiency syndrome associated with fused ribs and congenital scoliosis. J Bone Joint Surg Am 85:399–408, 2003.
16. Estenne M, Derom E, De Troyer A: Neck and abdominal muscle activity in patients with severe thoracic scoliosis. Am J Respir Crit Care Med 158:452–457, 1998.
17. Tobin MI: Respiratory muscles in disease. Clin Chest Med 9:263–286, 1988.
18. De Troyer A, Estenne M: Coordination between rib cage muscles and diaphragm during quiet breathing in humans. J Appl Physiol 57:899–906, 1984.
19. Panicek DM, Benson CB, Gottlieb RH, et al.: The diaphragm: Anatomic, pathologic and radiographic considerations. Radiographics 8:385–425, 1988.

20. Celli BR: Clinical and physiologic evaluation of respiratory muscle function. Clin Chest Med 10:199–214, 1989.

21. De Troyer A, Sampson M, Sigrist S, et al.: The diaphragm: Two muscles. Science 213:237–238, 1981.

22. Deviri, E, Nathan, H, Luchansky, E: Medial and lateral arcuate ligaments of the diaphragm: Attachment to the transverse process. Anat Anz 166:63–67, 1988.

23. Celli BR: Respiratory muscle function. Clin Chest Med 7:567–584, 1986.

24. Epstein S: An overview of respiratory muscle function. Clin Chest Med 15:619–638, 1994.

25. De Troyer A, Sampson M, Sigrist S, et al.: Action of costal and crural parts of the diaphragm on the rib cage in dog. J Appl Physiol 53:30–39, 1982.

26. Reid WD, Dechman G: Considerations when testing and training the respiratory muscles. Phys Ther 75:971–982, 1995.

27. De Troyer A, Kelly S, Zin WA: Mechanical action of the intercostal muscles on the ribs. Science 220:87–88, 1983.

28. LeBars P, Duron B: Are the external and internal intercostal muscles synergistic or antagonistic in the cat? Neurosci Lett 51:383–386, 1984.

29. Van Luneren E: Respiratory muscle coordination. J Lab Clin Med 112:285–300, 1988.

30. Koepke GH, Smith EM, Murphy AJ, et al.: Sequence of action of the diaphragm and intercostal muscles during respiration. I. Inspiration. Arch Phys Med Rehabil 39:426–430, 1958.

31. De Troyer A: Actions of the respiratory muscles or how the chest wall moves in upright man. Bull Eur Physiopathol Respir 20:409–413, 1984.

32. De Troyer A, Heilporn A: Respiratory mechanics in quadriplegia. The respiratory function of the intercostal muscles. Am Rev Respir Dis 122:591–600, 1980.

33. Macklem PT, Macklem DM, De Troyer A: A model of inspiratory muscle mechanics. J Appl Physiol 55:547–557, 1983.

34. Cala SJ, Kenyon CM, Lee A, et al.: Respiratory ultrasonography of human parasternal intercostal muscles *in vivo*. Ultrasound Med Biol 24:313–326, 1998.

35. De Troyer A, Kelly S, Macklem PT, et al.: Mechanics of intercostal space and actions of external and internal intercostal muscles. J Clin Invest 75:850–857, 1985.

36. Rimmer KP, Ford GT, Whitelaw WA: Interaction between postural and respiratory control of human intercostal muscles. J Appl Physiol 79:1556–1561, 1995.

37. Whitelaw WA, Ford GT, Rimmer KP, et al.: Intercostal muscles are used during rotation of the thorax in humans. J Appl Physiol 72:1940–1944, 1992.

38. Raper AJ, Thompson WT, Shapiro W, et al.: Scalene and sternomastoid muscle function. J Appl Physiol 21:497–502, 1966.

39. Goldman MD, Loh L, Sears TA: The respiratory activity of human levator costal muscle and its modification by posture. J Physiol 362:189–204, 1985.

40. Vilensky J, Baltes M, Weikel L, et al.: Serratus posterior muscles: Anatomy, clinical relevance and function. Clin Anat 14:237–241, 2001.

41. De Troyer A, Ninane V, Gilmartin JJ, et al.: Triangularis sterni muscle use in supine humans. J Appl Physiol 62:919–925, 1987.

42. Estenne M, Ninane V, De Troyer A: Triangularis sterni muscle use during eupnea in humans: Effect of posture. Respir Physiol 74:151–162, 1988.

43. Upadhyay S, Mullaji A, Luk K, et al.: Relation of spinal and thoracic cage deformities and their flexibilities with altered pulmonary functions in adolescent idiopathic scoliosis. Spine 20:2415–2420, 1995.

44. Rowe DE, Bernstein SM, Riddick MF, et al.: A meta-analysis of the efficacy of non-operative treatment for idiopathic scoliosis. J Bone Joint Surg Am 79:664–674, 1997.

45. Lisboa C, Moreno R, Fava M, et al.: Inspiratory muscle function in patients with severe kyphoscoliosis. Am Rev Respir Dis 46:53–62, 1985.

46. Refsum HE, Naess-Andersen CF, Lange EJ: Pulmonary function and gas exchange at rest and exercise in adolescent girls with mild idiopathic scoliosis during treatment with Boston thoracic brace. Spine 15:420-3, 1990.

47. Korovessis P, Filos K, Feorgopoulos D: Long term alterations of respiratory function in adolescents wearing a brace for idiopathic scoliosis. Spine 21:1979–1984, 1996.

48. Gagnon S, Jodoin A, Martin R: Pulmonary function test study and after spinal fusion in young idiopathic scoliosis. Spine 14:486–490. 1989.

49. Upadhyay SS, Ho EKW, Gunawardene WMS, et al.: Changes in residual volume relative to vital capacity and total lung capacity after arthrodesis of the spine in patients who have adolescent idiopathic scoliosis. J Bone Joint Surg Am 75:46–52, 1993.

50. Crane, LD: Physical therapy for the neonate with respiratory dysfunction. In Irwin S, Tecklin JS (eds): Cardiopulmonary Physical Therapy, 3rd ed, pp 486–515. St. Louis, CV Mosby, 1995.

51. Davis GM, Bureau MA: Pulmonary and chest wall mechanics in the control of respiration in the newborn. Clin Perinatol 14:551–579, 1987.

52. Reid L: Lung growth. In Zorab PA (ed): Scoliosis and Growth: Proceedings of a Third Symposium, pp 117–121. Edinburgh, Churchill Livingstone, 1971.

53. Krumpe PE, Knudson RJ, Parsons G, et al.: The aging respiratory system. Clin Geriatr Med 1:143–175, 1985.

54. Chan ED, Welsh CH: Geriatric respiratory medicine. Chest 114:1704–1733, 1998.

55. Estenne M, Yernault JC, De Troyer A: Rib cage and diaphragm-abdomen compliance in humans: Effects of age and posture. J Appl Physiol 59:1842–1848, 1985.

56. Makrides L, Heigenhauser GJ, McCartney N, et al.: Maximal short-term exercise capacity in healthy subjects aged 15–70 years. Clin Sci (Lond) 69:197–205, 1985.

57. De Troyer A: Effect of hyperinflation on the diaphragm. Eur Respir J 10:703–713, 1997.

58. Decramer M: Hyperinflation and respiratory muscle interaction. Eur Respir J 10:934–941, 1997.

59. Camus P, Desmeules M: Chest wall movements and breathing pattern at different lung volumes [abstract]. Chest 82:243, 1982.

60. De Troyer A: Respiratory muscle function in chronic obstructive pulmonary disease. In Cassabury R, Petty T (eds): Principles and Practice of Pulmonary Rehabilitation. Philadelphia, WB Saunders, 1995.

Chapter 6

The Temporomandibular Joint

Don Hoover, PT, PhD, Pamela Ritzline, PT, EdD

6-1   Patient Case

Wendy Doe is a 31-year-old housewife with three children younger than 6 years. Her visit to the clinic is prompted by frequent headaches and intermittent aching pain in the right jaw area. Wendy is right-handed, and her history is unremarkable except for a reported history of allergies and a period of physical abuse that occurred over a period of months when she was 23 years old. She reports that the headaches started intermittently after she was first struck in the face by her boyfriend. Over the years, the headaches have gotten progressively more intense and frequent. The symptoms in the area of her right jaw are reportedly triggered when she tries to eat an apple or a large sandwich. She also reports an occasional "popping" noise that accompanies opening her mouth but states that the noise is not associated with pain.

    Wendy's physical examination reveals a forward head posture, rounded shoulders, and increased thoracic kyphosis. Her right shoulder is slightly elevated. She demonstrates limitations in active movement when performing mouth opening, mandibular protrusion, and left lateral excursion of the mandible. Restricted movement of the mandibular condyle on the right side during mouth opening is noted. Active range of motion of the cervical spine is limited, especially the upper segmental levels. Passive range of motion of the cervical spine is also limited. Palpation of the right temporomandibular (TM) joint is painful. Wendy also reports tenderness with palpation of the muscles at the back of her head, the sides of her face, and under her chin bilaterally. Wendy's strength and reflexes appear to be within normal limits.

Screening of body systems beyond the musculoskeletal system is negative.

◆ Introduction

The **TM joint** is unique within the body both structurally and functionally. Structurally, the mandible is a horseshoe-shaped bone (Fig. 6-1) that articulates with the temporal bone at each end; thus, the mandible has two different but connected articulations. Each TM joint also has a disk that separates the articulation into discrete upper and lower joints that each function slightly differently. Therefore, mandibular movement affects four distinct joints simultaneously. In all, the TM joint is a complex joint that moves in all planes of motion.

    Each TM joint is formed by the **condyle** (or **head**) **of the mandible** inferiorly and the **articular eminence** of the temporal bone superiorly (Fig. 6-2), with an interposed **articular disk** (Fig. 6-3). The lower joint formed by the mandibular condyle and the inferior surface of the disk is a simple hinge joint. The upper joint formed by the articular eminence and the superior surface of the disk is a plane or gliding joint. Classic work by Sicher[1] described the TM joint as a hinge joint with movable sockets, and later authors supported this description.[2,3] The TM joint is classified as a synovial joint, although no hyaline cartilage covers the articular

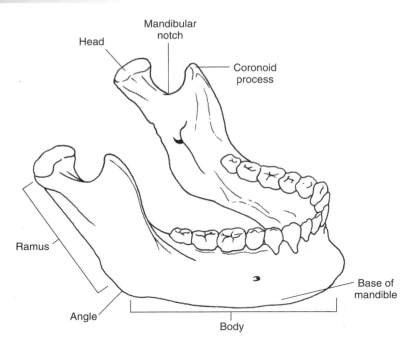

Head

Mandibular
notch

Coronoid
process

Ramus

Angle

Body

Base of
mandible

◄ **Figure 6-1** ■ The mandible.

surfaces. The surfaces are instead covered by dense collagenous tissue described as fibrocartilage, with a great
capacity to remodel in response to physical load.[4] Both
the articular eminence of the temporal bone and the
condyle of the mandible are convex structures, resulting in an incongruent joint. The disk increases stability
while minimizing loss of mobility. The articular disk is
necessary to reduce friction and avoid biomechanical
stress on the joint.[4-6] Functionally, few other joints are
moved as often as the TM joint. Mandibular motion
plays a role in phonation, facial expression, mastica-
tion, and swallowing. The muscles surrounding the TM
joint create great forces during biting or chewing, and
yet they generate finely controlled motion that requires
little force during speaking and swallowing. These activities have obvious importance in the lives of all individuals. The TM joint exhibits a combination of complexity,
almost continuous use, and capacity for force and
finesse that is remarkable.

◆ Structure

Articular Surfaces

The proximal or stationary segment of the TM joint is
the temporal bone. The condyles of the mandible sit
in the **glenoid fossa** of the temporal bone (see Fig. 6-3).
The glenoid fossa is located between the **posterior glenoid spine** and the articular eminence of the temporal
bone. The glenoid fossa, on superficial inspection,
looks like the articular surface for the TM joint.
However, the bone in that area is thin and translucent
and not at all appropriate for an articular surface.[1-3,7-9]
The articular eminence, however, has a major area of
trabecular bone and serves as the primary articular surface for the mandibular condyle.[10,11]

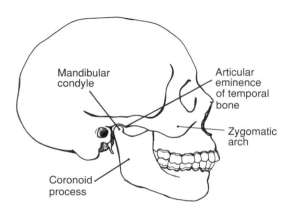

Mandibular
condyle

Articular
eminence
of temporal
bone

Zygomatic
arch

Coronoid
process

▲ **Figure 6-2** ■ Lateral view of the articulation of the mandible
with the articular eminence of the temporal bone.

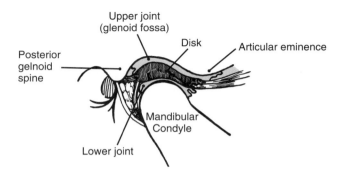

Upper joint
(glenoid fossa)

Disk

Articular eminence

Posterior
gelnoid
spine

Mandibular
Condyle

Lower joint

▲ **Figure 6-3** ■ A cross-sectional lateral view of the TM joint
shows the fibrocartilage-covered load-bearing surfaces on the condyle
of the mandible and the articular eminence. The TM disk divides the
articulation into an upper joint and a lower joint, each with its own
synovial lining. The anterior and posterior attachments of the joint
capsule (squiggly lines) to the disk are shown.

The mandible is the distal or moving segment of the TM joint. The mandible is divided into a body and two rami, with each ramus having a **coronoid process** and a mandibular condyle (see Fig. 6-1). In the closed-mouth position, the coronoid process sits under the zygomatic arch, but it can be palpated below the arch when the mouth is open. The coronoid process serves as an attachment for the muscle.

The mandibular condyles are located at the end of the ramus at its most posterosuperior aspect, with each having a medial and a lateral pole (Fig. 6-4). Each condyle protrudes medially 15 to 20 mm from the ramus.[1,2,7,12] The portion of the condyle that can be readily palpated is the lateral pole. This bony landmark lies just in front of the external auditory meatus of the ear. The medial pole is deep and cannot be palpated. However, the posterior aspect of the condyle can be palpated if a fingertip is placed into the external auditory meatus and the pad of the finger is pushed anteriorly (Fig. 6-5).[8] As the jaw is opened and closed, the movement under the fingertip is that of the mandibular condyle. Lines following the axis of mediolateral poles of each condyle will intersect just anterior to the foramen magnum (see Fig. 6-4).[1,3,4] The anterior portion of the mandibular condyle is the articular portion and is composed of trabecular bone.[10,11]

The articular surfaces of the articular eminence of the temporal bone and the mandibular condyle are covered with dense, avascular collagenous tissue that contains some cartilaginous cells.[13] Because some of the cells are cartilaginous, the covering is often referred to as fibrocartilage.[7,9] The articular collagen fibers are aligned perpendicular to the bony surface in the deeper layers to withstand stresses. The fibers near the surface of the articular covering are aligned in a parallel arrangement to facilitate gliding of the joint surfaces.[7,9] The presence of fibrocartilage rather than hyaline cartilage is significant because fibrocartilage can repair and remodel.[7,9] Typically, fibrocartilage is present in areas that are intended to withstand repeated and high-level stress. The TM joints are subjected not only to the repetitive stress of jaw motions

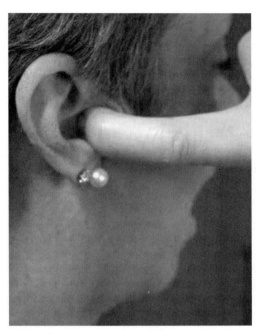

▲ **Figure 6-5** ■ Palpation of the posterior mandibular condyle through the external auditory meatus.

but also to tremendous bite forces that have been measured at 597 N for women and 847 N for men.[14] The TM joint surfaces are amenable to some degree of adaptation, but there is no clear-cut point between adaptive and maladaptive changes.[15] Unlike the fibrocartilage on the mandibular condyles and articular eminences, the articular disk of the TM joint does not have the ability to repair and remodel.[16]

Articular Disk

The articular disk of the TM joint is biconcave; that is, both its superior and inferior surfaces are concave (Fig. 6-6). Styles and Whyte described the disk as having a "bowtie" appearance on magnetic resonance imaging (MRI) film, with the "knot" lying at the thinnest portion.[17] The articular disk varies in thickness, from 2 mm anteriorly to 3 mm posteriorly and to 1 mm in the middle.[12] The disk of the TM joint allows the convex surface of the articular eminence and the convex surface of the condyle to remain congruent throughout the range of TM motion.[9,12] The anterior and posterior portions of the disk are vascular and innervated; the middle segment, however, is avascular and not innervated.[9,12,18] The lack of vascularity and innervation is consistent with the fact that the middle portion of the disk is the force-accepting segment.

The disk has a complex set of attachments. The disk appears to be firmly attached to the medial and lateral poles of the condyle of the mandible but not to the TM joint capsule medially or laterally.[3] These attachments allow the condyle to rotate freely on the disk in an anteroposterior direction. Although the medial and lateral attachments of the disk cannot be

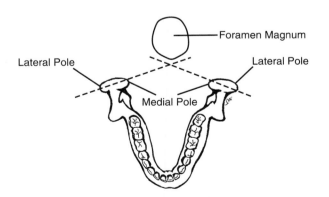

▲ **Figure 6-4** ■ A superior view of the mandible (removed from the skull) shows the medial and lateral poles of the mandibular condyles. Mandibular rotation occurs around axes that pass through the medial and lateral poles of the right and left condyles, with the lines intersecting anterior to the foramen magnum of the skull.

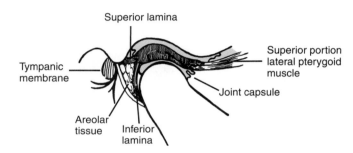

▲ **Figure 6-6** ■ The TM disk attaches posteriorly to the joint capsule and to the superior and inferior laminae (segments of the bilaminar retrodiskal pad). The disk attaches anteriorly to the joint capsule and to the lateral pterygoid muscle.

readily shown, Figure 6-6 shows the anterior and posterior attachments of the disk. The disk is attached to the joint capsule anteriorly, as well as to the tendon of the **lateral pterygoid muscle.** The anterior attachments restrict posterior translation of the disk. Posteriorly, the disk is attached to a complex structure, the components of which are collectively called the **bilaminar retrodiskal pad.** The two bands (or laminae) of the bilaminar retrodiskal pad are each attached to the disk. The superior lamina is attached posteriorly to the tympanic plate (at the posterior glenoid fossa).[12,19] The superior lamina is made of elastic fibers that allow the superior band to stretch. The superior lamina allows the disk to translate anteriorly along the articular eminence during mouth opening (Fig. 6-7); its elastic properties assist in repositioning the disk posteriorly during mouth closing. The inferior lamina is attached to the neck of the condyle and is inelastic. The inferior lamina simply serves as a tether on the disk, limiting forward translation, but does not assist with repositioning the disk during mouth closing.[12,16,17] Neither of the laminae of the retrodiskal pad is under tension when the TM joint is at rest. Between the two laminae is loose areolar connective tissue rich in arterial and neural supply.[6,12,16]

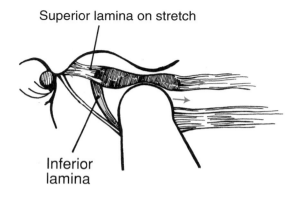

▲ **Figure 6-7** ■ With full mouth opening, the disk and the condyle together translate anteriorly. The inferior lamina limits translation, and the elastic properties of the superior lamina both control anterior translation and assist with posterior translation during mouth closing.

A healthy TM disk is viscoelastic and well suited to the distribution of force, showing only minor changes in connective tissue fiber waviness even under significant stress.[18] The disk consists primarily of collagen, glycosaminoglycans (GAGs), and elastin. Collagen is largely responsible for the disk's maintaining its shape. Elastin contributes to the disk's regaining its form during unloading. GAG composition maintains disk resiliency and resists mechanical compressive force. The biomechanical behavior of the disk may change according to changes in its composition.[18] Such changes in composition may occur as a result of aging, mechanical stress, or both.[14]

Capsule and Ligaments

The TM joint capsule is not as well defined as many joint capsules. According to *Gray's Anatomy*, the joint is supported by short capsular fibers running from the temporal bone to the disk and from the disk to the neck of the condyle.[13] The portion of the capsule above the disk is quite loose, whereas the portion of the capsule below the disk is tight.[3,13] Consequently, the disk is more firmly attached to the condyle below and freer to move on the articular eminence above. The capsule is quite thin and loose in its anterior, medial, and posterior aspects, but the lateral aspect (Fig. 6-8) is stronger and is reinforced with long fibers (temporal bone to condyle).[3,13] The lack of strength of the capsule anteriorly and the incongruence of the bony articular surfaces predisposes the joint to anterior dislocation of the mandibular condyle.[1] The capsule is highly vascularized and innervated, which allows it to provide a great deal of information about position and movement.

The primary ligaments of the TM joint are the **temporomandibular (TM) ligament,** the **stylomandibular ligament,** and the **sphenomandibular ligament** (see Fig. 6-8). The TM ligament is a strong ligament that is composed of two parts. The outer oblique portion (shown in Fig. 6-8) attaches to the neck of the condyle and the articular eminence. It serves as a suspensory ligament and limits downward and posterior motion of the mandible, as well as limiting rotation of the condyle during mouth opening.[3,9,12] The inner portion of the ligament is attached to the lateral pole of the condyle and posterior portion of the disk and to the articular eminence. Its fibers are almost horizontal and resist posterior motion of the condyle. Limitation of posterior translation of the condyle protects the retrodiskal pad.[12] Neither of the bands of the TM ligament limits forward translation of the condyle or disk, but they do limit lateral displacement.[19]

The stylomandibular ligament is a band of deep cervical fascia that runs from the styloid process of the temporal bone to the posterior border of the ramus of the mandible. Some authors have identified its function as limitation to protrusion of the jaw,[2,9,12] whereas others have stated that it has no known function.[1,20,21]

The sphenomandibular ligament attaches to the spine of the sphenoid bone and to the middle surface

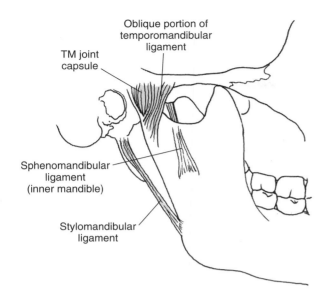

▲ **Figure 6-8** ■ A lateral view of the TM joint capsule and ligaments.

of the ramus of the mandible. Abe and colleagues[22] stated that the sphenomandibular ligament also has continuity with the disk medially. Some authors have stated that it serves to suspend the mandible[5] and to check the mandible from excessive forward translation.[2,9,16] Other authors, however, have stated that this ligament also has no function.[13,20,21]

Upper and Lower Temporomandibular Joints

The TM disk divides the TM joint into two separate joint spaces, each with its own synovial lining. Synovial fluid supplies the nutritional demands of the fibrocartilage covering the joint surfaces and the avascular middle portion of the disk. Intermittent pressure on these collagenous structures during joint motion causes the synovial fluid to be pumped in and out of them, providing their nutrition.

The lower joint of the TM articulation functions effectively as a hinge joint. The firm attachments of the disk to the medial and lateral poles of the condyle allow free rotation of the condyle under the disk around an axis through both poles of the condyle, with little translatory motion occurring. The upper joint of the TM articulation functions as a plane joint, with the loose attachment of the disk to the temporal bone allowing translatory movement between the disk and articular eminence. The attachments between the disk and condylar poles that permit rotation between these structures in the lower joint cause the condyle and disk to translate forward (glide) together as a unit with upper joint motion.

The biconcave shape of the disk provides unique advantages to the TM articulation's dual joint surfaces. The disk's shape provides increased congruence through

a wide range of positions, allowing greater flexibility of the disk as the condyle first rotates beneath it and then translates with it over the articular eminence.[3,12,16,17] The thick-thin-thick arrangement of the disk also provides a self-centering mechanism for the disk on the condyle.[3,12,16,17] As pressure between the condyle and the articular eminence increases, the disk rotates on the condyle so that the thinnest portion of the disk is between the articulating surfaces. Like other connective tissues in the body, the function of the disk may be disrupted by physical stress over time or profound trauma.[14] As we examine the motions of the jaw (mandible), the role of and potential for problems with the disk will become more evident.

◆ Function

The TM joint is one of the most frequently used joints in the body. It is involved in talking, chewing, and swallowing. Most TM joint movements are empty-mouth movements[16] (e.g., talking); that is, they occur with no resistance from food or contact between the upper and lower teeth. The joint is well designed for this intensive use. The cartilage covering the articular surfaces is designed to tolerate repeated and high-level stress. In addition to a joint structure that supports the high level of usage, the musculature is designed to provide both power and intricate control.[16] Speech requires fine control of the jaw, and the ability to chew requires great strength.

Mandibular Motions

The motions of the TM joint are mouth opening (**mandibular depression**), mouth closing (**mandibular elevation**), jutting the chin forward (**mandibular protrusion**), sliding the teeth backward (**mandibular retrusion**), and sliding the teeth to either side (**lateral deviation** of the mandible). These motions are created by various combinations of rotation and gliding in the upper and lower joints. The motions involved in chewing, talking, and swallowing become quite complex. For purposes of this chapter, we will describe only the movements of the mandible that occur without resistance (empty-mouth movements).

■ Mandibular Elevation and Depression

In normally functioning TM joints, mandibular elevation and depression are relatively symmetrical motions. The motion at each TM joint follows a similar pattern. Two distinct and somewhat conflicting descriptions of the movement of mouth opening can be found in the literature. One conceptual framework describes two sequential phases: rotation and glide.[2,4,21] In the rotation phase of mouth opening, there is pure anterior rotation (spin) of the condyle on the disk in the lower joint (Fig. 6-9A). This has also been described as posterior rotation of the disk on the condyle. The second

A

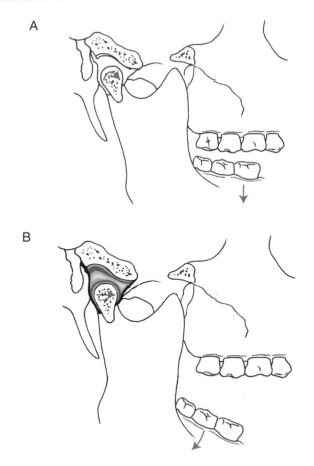

B

▲ **Figure 6-9** ■ **A.** During initial mouth opening, the motion at the TM joint may be limited to anterior rotation of the condyle on the disk. **B.** Anterior translation of the condyle and disk together on the articular eminence may occur in the latter stages of mouth opening.

phase involves translation of the disk-condyle unit anteriorly and inferiorly along the articular eminence (see Figs. 6-9B and 6-7). This motion occurs in the upper joint between the disk and the articular eminence and accounts for the remainder of the opening. Normal mouth opening is considered to be 40 to 50 mm.[5,8] Of that motion, between 11 mm[13,23] and 25 mm[12] is gained from rotation of the condyle in the disk, whereas the remainder is from translation of the disk and condyle along the articular eminence.

The second model, based on more recent research, argues that the components of rotation and gliding are present but occur concomitantly rather than sequentially (Fig. 6-10).[23–25] That is, both rotation and gliding are present throughout the range of mandibular depression and elevation, starting at the initiation of mouth opening. Isberg and Westesson also noted that the amount of rotation has a positive correlation with the steepness of the articular eminence.[23]

For a quick and rough, but useful, estimate of function, the clinician may use the proximal interphalangeal (PIP) joints to assess opening. If two PIP joints can be placed between the upper and lower central

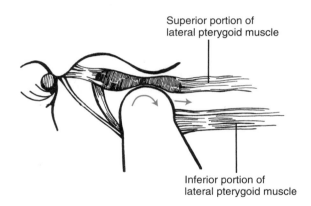

Superior portion of lateral pterygoid muscle

Inferior portion of lateral pterygoid muscle

▲ **Figure 6-10** ■ Another conceptual framework holds that condylar rotation on the disk and anterior translation of the disk and condyle on the articular eminence occur concomitantly during mouth opening.

front incisors, the amount of opening is functional, although a fit of three PIP joints is considered normal (Fig. 6-11).[4] Dijkstra and associates demonstrated a positive correlation between the amount of mouth opening and the length of the mandible. This should be considered in determining what is normal for each patient.[26]

Mandibular elevation (mouth closing) is the reverse of depression. It consists of translation of the disk-condyle unit posteriorly and superiorly and of posterior rotation of the condyle on the disk.

Control of the Disk during Mandibular Elevation and Depression

The articular disk is controlled both actively and passively during mouth opening and closing. The passive control is exerted by the capsuloligamentous attachments of the disk to the condyle. Active control of the disk may be exerted through the disk's attachment

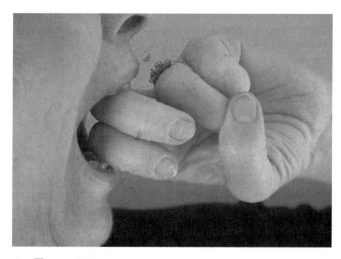

▲ **Figure 6-11** ■ Mandibular depression (mouth opening) is considered within normal limits if the proximal interphalangeal joints of two fingers can be inserted between the teeth.

anteriorly to the superior portion of the lateral ptery-goid muscle (see Fig. 6-6 and Fig. 6-10), although evi-dence suggests that these attachments may not be consistently present.[22,27] Bell also proposed two other muscles that may assist with maintaining the disk posi-tion.[16] These two muscles are derived from the masseter muscle and are attached to the anterolateral portion of the disk. They help overcome the medial pull of the anteromedially directed lateral pterygoid.

During mouth opening, the medial and lateral at-tachments of the disk to the condyle limit the motion between the disk and condyle to rotation. During trans-lation of the condyle, the biconcave shape of the disk causes it to follow the condyle without any additional active or passive assistance. The inferior retrodiskal lam-ina limits forward excursion of the disk. The superior portion of the lateral pterygoid muscle appears to be positioned to assist with anterior translation of the disk but does *not* show activity during mouth opening.[8,16]

During mouth closing, the elastic character of the superior retrodiskal lamina applies a posterior distrac-tive force on the disk. In addition, the superior portion of the lateral pterygoid now demonstrates activity that is assumed to eccentrically control the posterior movement of the disk. The activity of the superior lateral pterygoid allows the disk-condyle complex to translate upward and posteriorly during mouth closing and then main-tains the disk in a forward position until the condyle has completed its posterior rotation on the disk or until the disk has rotated anteriorly on the condyle.[28-30]

Abe and colleagues suggested that the spheno-mandibular ligament also assists this action. Again, the medial and lateral attachments of the disk to the con-dyle limit the motion to rotation of the disk around the condyle.[22]

■ Mandibular Protrusion and Retrusion

This motion occurs when all points of the mandible move forward the same amount. The condyle and disk together translate anteriorly and inferiorly along the articular eminence. No rotation occurs in the TM joint during protrusion. The motion is all translation and occurs in the upper joint alone. The teeth are separated when protrusion occurs (Fig. 6-12). During protrusion, the posterior attachments of the disk (the bilaminar retrodiskal tissue) stretch 6 to 9 mm to allow the motion to occur.[12] Protrusion should be adequate to allow the upper and lower teeth to touch edge to edge.[8]

Retrusion occurs when all points of the mandible move posteriorly the same amount. Tension in the tem-poromandibular ligament limits this motion, as does compression of the soft tissue in the retrodiskal area between the condyle and the posterior glenoid spine. Although rarely measured, retrusion is limited to an estimated 3 mm of translation.[12]

■ Mandibular Lateral Deviation

In lateral deviation of the mandible (chin) to one side, one condyle spins around a vertical axis and the other

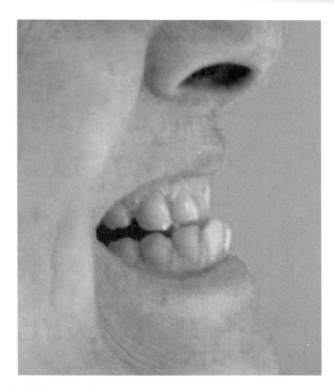

▲ **Figure 6-12** ■ With maximum mandibular protrusion, the lower teeth should be in front of the upper teeth.

condyle translates forward.[12,13] For example, deviation to the right would involve the right condyle spin-ning and the left condyle translating or gliding forward (Fig. 6-13). The result is movement of the chin to the right. Normally, the amount of lateral excursion of the joint is about 8 mm.[8] A functional measurement of lateral motion of the mandible involves the use of the

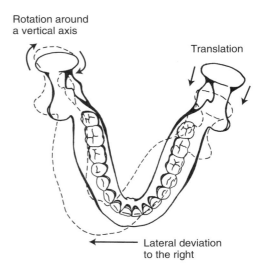

Rotation around a vertical axis

Translation

Lateral deviation to the right

▲ **Figure 6-13** ■ In this superior view of the mandible, lateral deviation of the mandible (chin) to the right occurs effectively as a rotation (spin) of the right condyle around a vertical axis, and the left condyle translates anteriorly.

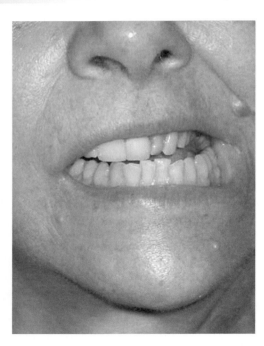

▲ **Figure 6-14** ■ With normal lateral deviation of the mandible to the right, the midline of the lower teeth should move the full width of the right upper central incisor.

width of the two upper central incisors. If the mandible can move the full width of one of the central incisors in each direction, motion is considered normal (Fig. 6-14).[8]

Lateral deviation of the mandible can be considered a normal asymmetrical movement of the jaw. Another normal asymmetrical movement involves rotation of one condyle around an anteroposterior axis while the other condyle depresses.[12] This results in a frontal plane motion of the mandible in which the chin moves downward and deviates from the midline slightly toward the condyle that is spinning. This motion typically occurs during biting on one side of the jaw. Although these motions were just described separately, they are commonly combined into one complex motion used in chewing and grinding food.

Case Application 6-1: **Palpation and Asymmetry of Motion**

Wendy Doe demonstrates decreased active range of motion with mouth opening, with mandibular protrusion and left lateral deviation. When palpating fingers are placed in her ears, the mandibular condyles moved with marked asymmetry during mouth opening. The left condyle appears to move considerably more than the right. This may indicate that the condyles are not rotating or that the condyles and disk are not translating either with the same magnitude or in the same sequence on the right and the left. This may indicate either hypomobility on the right, or hypermobility on the left.

Muscular Control of the Temporomandibular Joint

The primary muscle responsible for mandibular depression is the **digastric** muscle (Fig. 6-15).[16] The posterior portion of the digastric muscle arises from the mastoid notch, whereas the anterior portion arises from the inferior mandible. The tendon that joins the anterior and posterior portions is connected by a fibrous loop to the hyoid bone in the neck. The hyoid bone must be stabilized for the digastric muscle to act as a depressor of the mandible. The lateral pterygoid muscles are considered to be mandibular depressors,[3,10,13,29] but Bell considered this limited to the inferior portion alone (with the superior portion silent during mouth opening).[16] Gravity is also a mandibular depressor. The contribution of the mandibular elevators to eccentric control of mandibular depression is unclear.[3]

Mandibular elevation is accomplished primarily by several muscles. The **temporalis muscle** attaches to the inside of the coronoid process (Fig. 6-16). The **masseter muscle** is attached to the outer surface of the angle and ramus of the mandible (Fig. 6-17). The **medial pterygoid muscle** is attached to the inner surface of the angle and ramus of the mandible (Fig. 6-18).[13,28] As we have already seen, the superior portion of the lateral pterygoid is also active during mouth closing in what is assumed to be eccentric control of the disk as the disk-condyle complex translates upward and posteriorly and then in maintaining the disk in a forward

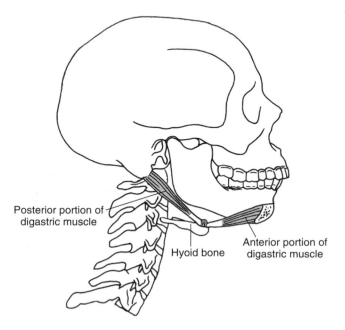

▲ **Figure 6-15** ■ The posterior portion of the digastric muscle arises from the mastoid notch, and the anterior portion arises from the inferior mandible. The tendon that joins the anterior and posterior portions is connected by a fibrous loop to the hyoid bone in the neck.

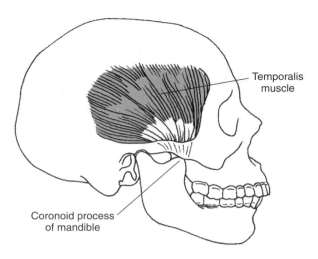

▲ **Figure 6-16** ■ The temporalis muscle, with its attachment to the medial aspect of the coronoid process.

Temporalis muscle

Coronoid process of mandible

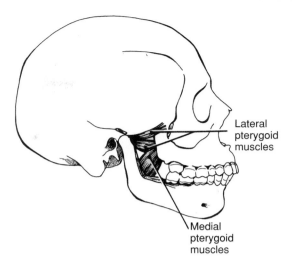

▲ **Figure 6-18** ■ The medial and lateral pterygoid muscles.

Lateral pterygoid muscles

Medial pterygoid muscles

position until the condyle has completed its posterior rotation as the condyle returns to its normal rest position.

 CONCEPT CORNERSTONE 6-1: *Summary: Mandibular Elevation and Depression*

Mouth opening (mandibular depression) is initiated by concentric action of the digastric muscles bilaterally, and by the inferior portion of the lateral pterygoid muscles. Mouth closing (mandibular elevation) is produced by the collective concentric action of the masseter, temporalis, and medial pterygoid muscles, with eccentric control of the TM disks by the superior lateral pterygoid muscles.

The other simple mandibular motions of protrusion, retrusion, and lateral deviation are produced by the same muscles that elevate and depress the

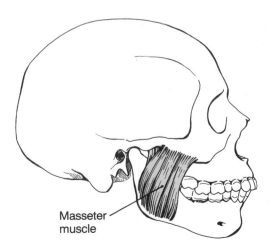

Masseter muscle

▲ **Figure 6-17** ■ The masseter muscle.

mandible but in different sequences. Mandibular protrusion is produced by bilateral action of the masseter, medial pterygoid,[4,21] and lateral pterygoid muscles.[12,31] Retrusion is produced through the bilateral action of the posterior fibers of the temporalis muscles with assistance from the anterior portion of the digastric muscle.[13] Lateral deviation of the mandible is caused by unilateral action of a selected set of these muscles. The medial and lateral pterygoid muscles each deviate the mandible to the opposite side.[12,13] The temporalis muscle can deviate the mandible to the same side. Although the temporalis and lateral pterygoid muscles on the left, for example, appear to create opposite motions of the mandible, concomitant contractions of the right lateral pterygoid and right temporalis muscles function as a force couple. The lateral pterygoid muscle is attached to the medial pole of the condyle and pulls the condyle forward. The temporalis muscle on the same side is attached to the coronoid process and pulls it posteriorly. Together they effectively spin the condyle to create deviation of the mandible to the left. Because the temporalis muscle is also an elevator of the mandible, this combination of muscular activity is particularly useful in chewing.

Relationship with the Cervical Spine

The cervical spine and the TM joint are intimately connected. Many of the muscles that attach to the mandible also have attachments to the head (cranium), to the hyoid bone, and to the clavicle. Consequently, muscles may act not only on the mandible but also on the atlanto-occipital joint and cervical spine. Head and neck position, too, may affect the tension in cervical muscles that, in turn, may affect the position or function of the mandible. Proper posture minimizes the force produced by the cervical extensors and other cervical muscles necessary to support the weight of the head. Poor cervical posture over time may lead to adaptive shortening or lengthening in muscles around the head and cervical spine, affecting range of motion, muscular force production capacity, and joint morphology in the involved region. Many of the symptoms reported by a person with TM joint dysfunction are similar to the symptoms reported by a person with primary cervical spine problems. With the intimate relationship of these two areas, any client being seen for complaints in one area should have the other examined as well.[11,32–34]

Continuing Exploration: **TM/Cervical Joint Interrelationships**

A forward head posture frequently involves extension of the occiput and the upper cervical spine, leading to compensatory flattening of the lower cervical spine and upper thoracic spine to achieve a level head position[35] (Fig. 6-19A). With the occiput extended on the atlas (C1), the suboccipital tissues adapt and shorten. The suboccipital tissues include the anterior atlantoaxial and atlanto-occipital ligaments (cephalad continuations of the ligamentum flavum), the posterior belly of the digastric muscles, the stylohyoid muscles, and the upper fibers of the upper trapezius, semispinalis capitis, and splenius capitis muscles.[36] The forces necessary to maintain the head against gravity with a poor cervical posture and forward head result in muscle imbalance and altered movement patterns. Such alterations typi-

cally lessen the capacity of particular structures to meet the thresholds for adaptive responses to physical stresses. Increased tension from shortening of the suboccipital tissues may lead to headaches that originate in the suboccipital area, limitation in active range of motion of the upper cervical spine, and TM joint dysfunction. Furthermore, pain in the TM region may be referred from the cervical region.[34,37] Thus, it is proposed that cervical posture should be normalized to successfully treat dysfunction in the TM joint complex[32,34,37] (Fig. 6-19B).

Continuing Exploration: **TM/Respiratory/ Cervical Dysfunction**

TM joint disorders may develop as a result of dysfunctional growth and developmental patterns that may accompany conditions such as chronic sinus allergies.[38] To illustrate, a child with allergies who has difficulty breathing through the nose will often hyperextend the upper cervical spine to more fully open the upper respiratory tract. Such a cervical posture places the upper and lower teeth in contact with each other and may affect the resting position of the TM joint. In turn, the muscles surrounding the TM joint complex expend greater energy to maintain this posture and have more difficulty resting and repair. Resistance to inspiration may also lead to use of accessory muscles of respiration (scalene and sternocleidomastoid muscles) to assist with breathing. Use of these accessory muscles may lead to a forward

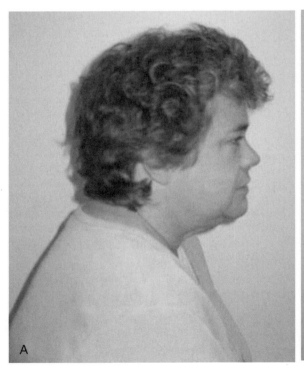 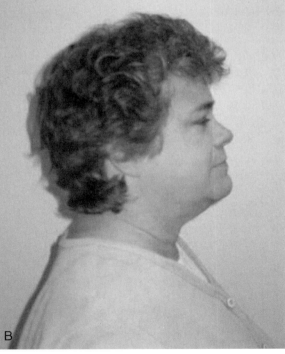

▲ **Figure 6-19** ■ **A.** Poor cervical posture increases the physical demands on the suboccipital structures, contributing to TM joint dysfunction. **B.** Corrected cervical posture restores the muscles of the cervical spine and TM joint to a more balanced length-tension relationship.

head posture.[38] Such a posture contributes over time to a cycle of increasing musculoskeletal dysfunction, including repeated episodes of TM inflammation that can result in fibrosis of the TM joint capsule.

Case Application 6-2: **Posture and TM Joint Relations**

Wendy Doe's complaints of frequent headaches and intermittent aching pain in the right jaw area may be associated with her posture. Wendy's physical examination reveals a forward head, rounded shoulders, and an increased thoracic kyphosis (see Fig. 6-19A). The observed elevation of Wendy's right shoulder may indicate tightness of the suboccipital tissues, consistent with her demonstrated limitation in active movement when performing mandibular depression (mouth opening), mandibular protrusion, and left lateral excursion of the mandible. Wendy also reports tenderness with palpation of the muscles at the back of her head, the sides of her face, and under her chin bilaterally. Tenderness and muscle guarding may be related to the stresses placed on the tissues from improper positioning.[35]

Dentition

Occlusion, or contact of the teeth, is intimately involved in the function of the TM joint. Although the teeth are only together approximately 15 minutes of each day, the presence and position of the teeth are critical to normal TM joint function. Chewing is one of the functions of the TM joint, and contact of the upper and lower teeth limits motion of the TM joint during empty-mouth movements. The complexities of the TM joint and the interrelated issues with the teeth underscore the necessity of the comprehensive management of TM joint disorders.

Normal adult dentition includes 32 teeth divided into four quadrants. The only teeth we will refer to by name are the upper and lower central incisors. These are the two central teeth of the maxilla and the two central teeth of the mandible.[39] When the central incisors are in firm approximation, the position is called **maximal intercuspation**[7] or the **occlusal position**.[13] This is not, however, the normal resting position of the mandible. Rather, 1.5 to 5.0 mm of **"freeway" space** between the upper and lower incisors is normally maintained.[12,16] This freeway space is particularly important. By maintaining this space, the intra-articular pressure within the TM joint is decreased, the stress on the articular structures is reduced, and the tissues of the area are able to rest and repair.[12]

Age-Related Changes in the Temporomandibular Joint

The TM joint is affected by the aging process. However, as is the case when age-related changes in other joints in the musculoskeletal system are considered, we must understand that normal aging is not necessarily synonymous with degenerative changes, nor are all degenerative changes synonymous with disability. Rowe and Kahn[40] described successful aging as "multidimensional, encompassing the avoidance of disease and disability, the maintenance of high physical and cognitive function, and sustained engagement in social and productive activities." We know that tissues are likely to become less supple, less elastic, and less able to withstand maximal forces with aging, leading to biomechanical changes in musculoskeletal tissues as one progresses through the life span. However, these changes will not necessarily become pathologic or lead to biomechanical dysfunction. Conversely, degenerative changes may be a result of preexisting dysfunction and not a result of aging alone.

In a study at autopsy of 37 TM joints of persons age 55 to 99 years, Nannmark et al. reported structural changes in 38% of the examined mandibular condyles.[41] The authors found no signs of inflammatory cell infiltration in any TM joint specimens, which suggested that observed changes were secondary to biomechanical stresses rather than to inflammatory processes. Twenty-two (59%) of the TM disks had perforations, roughness, or were thinned. However, only 3 (8%) of the disks were in an anterior position, and each of these was perforated. The authors concluded that osteoarthritis may be expected in 14% to 40% of adults, with increased frequency with age in both men and women.[41]

De Leeuw and colleagues conducted radiography and MRI of 46 former patients 30 years after diagnosis of osteoarthrosis and **internal derangement** of the TM joint.[42] Internal derangement of the TM joint is an abnormal positional and functional relationship between the disk and articulating surfaces.[3] De Leeuw and colleagues' patients were between the ages of 50 and 70 years at the time of the follow-up study. The investigators also performed similar imaging on 22 age-matched controls without known TM joint dysfunction.[42] Radiographic signs were more common and severe in the former patients. A higher percentage of osteoarthrosis and internal derangement of the disk was noted on MRI not only on the side of TM joint problems but also in the contralateral joints. However, the contralateral joints appeared to have developed these degenerative changes largely asymptomatically (with only 25% reporting any symptoms and none having sought treatment). Control subjects only infrequently showed MRI evidence of osteoarthrosis or internal derangement.

The work done by Nannmark et al. and by de Leeuw and colleagues appears to indicate that TM degeneration is not an expected part of aging and that degenerative changes evident on radiograph or MRI are not necessarily associated with symptoms or dysfunction.

Tanaka and coworkers found that disks from patients with severe internal derangement demonstrated more extensive degenerative changes than those from controls.[18] The authors described patterns of collagen fiber running more irregularly in deranged disks than in the disks of the control group. The authors related the structural changes in the disks with internal derangement to the diminished capacity of these tissues to withstand mechanical stress. Tanaka and coworkers found a cause-effect relationship, with internal derangement leading to disk damage.[18]

Dysfunctions

Although many dysfunctions may impact the TM joint, mechanical stress is the most critical factor in the multifactorial etiology.[10,18,43] Some dysfunctions are caused by direct trauma such as motor vehicle accidents or falls. Others are the result of years of poor postural or oral habits such as forward head posture or **bruxism** (grinding of the teeth). Most clients with temporomandibular dysfunction (TMD) will not fit neatly into a specific category or dysfunction classification, which makes evaluation and treatment of TMD a particularly challenging clinical endeavor. Furthermore, only 20% to 30% of individuals affected with internal derangement of the TM joint develop symptomatic TM joints,[3] with symptoms that may progress or may resolve spontaneously.[17] Because of the complex interrelationships associated with various types of TMD, practitioners interested in diagnosis and treatment of this clinical population should seek advanced education in this area. Here, we will present a small group of problems that were chosen to represent the most common forms of TM joint complex dysfunction: inflammatory conditions, capsular fibrosis, osseous mobility conditions, articular disk displacement, and degenerative conditions.

Inflammatory Conditions

Inflammatory conditions of the TM joint include capsulitis and synovitis. Capsulitis involves inflammation of the joint capsule, and synovitis is characterized by a fluctuating swelling caused by effusion within the synovial membrane of the joint. Rheumatoid arthritis is the most common cause of such inflammatory conditions, but gout, psoriatic arthritis, ankylosing spondylitis, systemic lupus erythematosus, juvenile chronic arthritis, and calcium pyrophosphate dehydrate deposition may also contribute to inflammation of the synovia.[3] Individuals with inflammatory conditions may experience diminished mandibular depression as a result of pain and inflammation within the joint complex.[4]

Rheumatoid arthritis is a chronic systemic condition with articular and extra-articular involvement. The primary symptoms of rheumatoid arthritis include pain, stiffness, edema, and warmth. This autoimmune disorder targets the capsule, ligamentous structures, and synovial lining of the joint complex, resulting in joint instability, joint deformity, or ankylosis.[44] Multiple bilateral joints are typically involved with this disease. Clients with rheumatoid arthritis should be managed medically by a rheumatologist, particularly during the acute stage of the disease. Detailed discussion of rheumatoid arthritis is beyond the scope of this text;

however, clinicians should be aware that rheumatoid arthritis often involves the temporomandibular joint.[44]

Capsular Fibrosis

Inflammation can lead to adhesions that restrict the movement of the disk and limit the function of the TM joint.[17] Capsular fibrosis in the TM joint complex may arise from unresolved or chronic inflammation of the joint capsule, which results in the overproduction of fibrous connective tissue.[4,44] The resultant fibrosis causes progressive damage and loss of tissue function.[4,44] A client history suggesting repeated episodes of capsulitis is key in identifying this condition. Circumstances leading to chronic capsulitis and, in turn, capsular fibrosis may include prolonged periods of immobilization, trauma, or arthritis.[4] Active motion of the TM joint capsule will typically elicit pain. Physical examination will reveal limited or altered osteokinematic motions, suggestive of a decrease in translatory motion in the involved side.[4]

Case Application 6-3: **Trauma and TM Dysfunction**

Ms. Doe's musculoskeletal complaints may be attributable to capsular fibrosis, as well as to her poor posture. It is likely that she had an acute episode of capsulitis in response to first to being hit in the face by her boyfriend. A common mechanism would be that the trauma to the face caused a stretching force on the ipsilateral TM joint and a compression force on the contralateral TM joint, resulting in an inflammatory process with edema and pain in both TM areas. Repeated assaults may have exacerbated the inflammation without the opportunity for resolution, leading to a chronic and progressive capsular fibrosis.[4]

Osseous Mobility Conditions

Osseous mobility disorders of the TM joint complex include joint hypermobility and dislocation. Many similarities exist in the history and clinical findings for these two conditions. Excessive motion, or hypermobility, of the TM joint is a common phenomenon found in both symptomatic and nonsymptomatic populations.[4] Joint hypermobility may be a generalized connective tissue disorder that involves all joints of the body, including the TM joints.[28,38,45–47] The hypermobility is a result of laxity of the joint capsules, tendons, and ligaments. Individuals seen clinically for this condition typically report the jaw "going out of place," producing noises, or "catching" when the mouth is in the fully opened position. Physical examination of patients with TM joint hypermobility reveals an increased indentation posterior to the lateral pole. Joint noises occur at the end of mandibular depression and at the beginning of mandibular closing. These noises may be heard by the patients but are more often palpable only by the clinician. Hypermobility of one TM joint results in deflection of the mandible toward the contralateral side with mouth opening. In addition, mandibular depression will exceed 40 mm.[4] Yang et al. examined the MRIs of 98 patients diagnosed with TM joint hypermobility, or overmovement of the condyle during jaw opening.[28] They found pathological changes (hypertrophy, atrophy, or contracture) in 77% of the lateral pterygoid muscles, with changes more common in the superior portion of the muscle. The authors often found anterior disk displacement with reduction in the patients who reported more symptoms than in persons with normal mobility or with disk displacement without reduction.[28]

Many aspects of the history and physical examination of an individual with dislocation of the TM joint are similar to those in an individual with hypermobility. However, with TM joint dislocation, full mouth opening results in deflection (lateral deviation) of the jaw to the contralateral side of the involved TM joint, and the inability to close the mouth. The individual may or may not experience pain with this condition. With dislocation, both the mandibular condyle and the disk have translated anteriorly well beyond the articular crest of the tubercle of the temporal bone, thus "sticking" in the extreme end-range position.[4,17] This condition is usually temporary and resolves with joint mobilization; however, intervention is beyond the scope of this text and therefore will not be discussed.

Articular Disk Displacement

The articular disk of the TM joint may sublux, contributing to dysfunction in this joint.[17,29] Articular disk displacement conditions include disk displacement with reduction and disk displacement without reduction.[4,28,29] Without intervention, disk displacement with reduction often evolves to disk displacement without reduction.[4,17,28,29] Disk displacement (internal derangement) may be identified through diagnostic imaging or through physical examination.[17] MRI is the imaging modality of choice for identifying disk displacement.[3]

Individuals exhibiting disk displacement with reduction experience "joint noise" at two intervals: during mandibular opening and mandibular closing. This joint noise is known as a **reciprocal click**[4,17] and is a key sign in diagnosing disk displacement with reduction. In this situation, the mandibular condyle is in contact with the retrodiskal tissue at rest, rather than with the disk. On mouth opening, the condyle slips forward and under the disk to obtain a normal relationship with the disk. When the condyle slips under the disk, an audible click is often present. Once the condyle is in the proper relationship with the disk, motion continues normally through opening and closing until the condyle again slips out from under the disk, when another click is heard. A click would be expected to signify that the condyle and disk have lost a normal relationship. In the case of an anteriorly dislocated disk, however, the initial click signifies regaining a normal relationship. When the click occurs early in opening and late in closing, the amount of anterior displacement of the disk is rela-

tively limited. The later the click occurs in the opening phase, the more severe the disk dislocation is.[4] Some evidence exists that the timing of the clicks during opening and closing can determine treatment prognosis.[48]

Individuals with disk displacement with reduction may remain in this state or progress rapidly, within months, to an acute condition of disk displacement without reduction. The posterior attachments to the disk become overstretched and unable to relocate the disk during mandibular depression, which results in the loss of the reciprocal clicks.[17] Yang et al. discovered on MRI a highly significant correlation between abnormalities of the lateral pterygoid muscles and TM joints with disk displacements both with and without reduction of the disk.[28] The abnormalities of the lateral pterygoid muscle noted included hypertrophy, contracture, and atrophy of the superior and inferior bellies of the lateral pterygoid muscles of the involved TM joint. Recall that the lateral pterygoid muscle attaches to the anterior portion of the disk and is normally active with mouth closing, presumed to be eccentrically controlling the return to resting position. Hypertrophy of this muscle indicates overactivity, which thus possibly leads to the excessive anterior translation of the articular disk.[28]

Whether acute or chronic, disk displacement without reduction indicates that the disk does not relocate onto the mandibular condyle. Thus, clients with acute disk displacement without reduction demonstrate limited mandibular motion as a result of the disk's creating a mechanical obstruction to condylar motion, rather than facilitating condylar translation. Individuals with disk displacement without reduction typically describe an inability to fully depress the mandible, as well as difficulty performing functional movements involving the jaw such as chewing, talking, or yawning.

Degenerative Conditions

Primarily two conditions affect the TM joint: osteoarthritis and rheumatoid arthritis. Rheumatoid arthritis is discussed previously under inflammatory conditions. Kessler and Hertling[5] stated that 80% to 90% of the population older than 60 years have some symptoms of osteoarthritis in the TM joint. Yang et al. concurred with MRI evidence to substantiate their findings.[28] According to Mahan,[19] osteoarthritis usually occurs unilaterally (unlike rheumatoid arthritis, which is usually bilateral in presentation). The primary cause of osteoarthritis is repeated minor trauma to the joint, particularly trauma that creates an impact between the articular surfaces.[17,19] Styles and Whyte[17] suggested that the radiographic features of degenerative changes in the TM joint, including joint space narrowing, erosions, osteophyte formation, sclerosis, and remodeling, are similar to those seen elsewhere in the body. Loss of posterior teeth may also contribute to degenerative changes because simple occlusion of the remaining teeth alters the forces that occur between the TM joint forces.[4,19]

CONCEPT CORNERSTONE 6-2: *Signs and Symptoms of TM Joint Dysfunction*

Clinical signs and symptoms of TM joint dysfunction vary widely, depending on the extent of the condition and the presence of complicating factors. Signs and symptoms may include

- pain in the area of the jaw
- increased or decreased active or passive range of motion
- popping or clicking noises
- difficulty with functional activities (e.g., eating, talking) or parafunctional activities (e.g., clenching, nail biting, pencil chewing) of the mandible
- catching or locking of the jaw
- forward head posture

Case Application 6-4: **Patient Summary**

Wendy Doe sought physical therapy because of frequent headaches and intermittent aching in the right jaw area. Her symptoms may be attributable to a number of potential sources in isolation—trauma to the TM joint, poor cervical posture, forward head position—or in some combination of these sources. Factors such as stress of work and family life or bruxism may also play a role in her clinical presentation. Although the research literature does not explicitly draw a direct link between these variables, it does suggest that these biomechanical variables may play a role in a patient's pain presentation. In turn, clinical interventions aimed at improving structural balance of the head, neck, and thorax are important augmentations to any direct intervention at the TM joint. Task modification in her work environment and stress management may also be therapeutic adjuncts.

Summary

The TM joints are unique both structurally and functionally. The magnitude and frequency of jaw movement, the daily resistance encountered during chewing, the physical stress imposed by sustained sitting and standing postures, and the chronic adaptation of muscles around the TM joint complex make it particularly vulnerable to problems. The influence of the cervical spine upon the TM joint must always be recognized. Intervention for clients with temporomandibular disorders presents many clinical challenges, and practitioners with interest in this population should seek advanced education beyond the entry level in this specialty area. As we proceed in subsequent chapters to examine the joint complexes of the appendicular skeleton, it will be seen that each complex has its own unique features. We will not see again, however, the complexity of intra-articular and diskal motions seen at the TM joints.

 Study Questions

1. Describe the articulating surface of the TM joint.
2. What is the significance of the differing thicknesses and the differing vascularity of the disk?
3. How do the superior and inferior laminae of the retrodiskal area differ?
4. Describe the motions in the upper and lower joints during mouth opening and closing.
5. What limits posterior motion of the condyle? How is the motion limited?
6. What would be the consequences of having a left TM joint that could not translate?
7. What would be the consequences of having a right disk that could not rotate freely over the condyle?
8. Describe the control of the disk in moving from an open-mouth to a closed-mouth position.
9. What is the potential impact of the posture of the cervical spine on the function of the TM joint complex?
10. Compare and contrast the functional presentation of a hypomobile versus hypermobile TM joint complex.

 References

1. Sicher H: Functional anatomy of the temporomandibular joint. In Sarnat B (ed): The Temporomandibular Joint, 2nd ed. Springfield, IL, Charles C Thomas, 1964.
2. Hylander W: Functional anatomy. In Sarnat BG, Laskin DM (eds): The Temporomandibular Joint: A Biological Basis for Clinical Practice. Philadelphia, WB Saunders, 1992.
3. Sommer O, Aigner F, Rudisch A, et al.: Cross-sectional and functional imaging of the temporomandibular joint: Radiology, pathology, and basic biomechanics of the jaw. In Radiographics 23:e14, 2003.
4. Kraus S: Temporomandibular joint. In Saunders H, Saunders R (eds): Evaluation, Treatment, and Prevention of Musculoskeletal Disorders, 3rd

ed. Bloomington, MN, Educational Opportunities, 1993.

5. Kessler R, Hertling D: Management of Common Musculoskeletal Disorders: Physical Therapy Principles and Methods, 3rd ed. Philadelphia, Lippincott-Raven, 1996.

6. Magee D: Orthopedic Physical Assessment, 4th ed. Philadelphia, WB Saunders, 2002.

7. Ermshar C: Anatomy and neuroanatomy. In Morgan D, House L, Wall W, et al. (eds): Diseases of the Temporomandibular Apparatus: A Multidisciplinary Approach, 2nd ed. St. Louis, CV Mosby, 1982.

8. Kraus S: Temporomandibular joint. In Saunders H, Saunders R (eds): Evaluation, Treatment, and Prevention of Musculoskeletal Disorders, 2nd ed. New York, Viking Press, 1985.

9. Eggleton TL, Langton DM: Clinical anatomy of the TMJ complex. In Krauss SL (ed): Temporomandibular Disorders, 2nd ed. New York, Churchill Livingstone, 1994.

10. Matsumoto M, Matsumoto W, Bolognese A: Study of the signs and symptoms of temporomandibular dysfunction in individuals with normal occlusion and malocclusion. Cranio 20:274–281, 2002.

11. Moya H, Miralles R, Zuniga C, et al.: Influence of stabilization occlusal splint on craniocervical relationships. Part I: Cephametric analysis. Cranio 12:47–51, 1994.

12. Bourbon B: Anatomy and biomechanics of the TMJ. In Kraus S (ed): TMJ Disorders: Management of the Craniomandibular Complex. New York, Churchill Livingstone, 1988.

13. Williams P: Gray's Anatomy, 38th ed. New York, Churchill Livingstone, 1999.

14. Waltimo A, Kononen M: A novel bite force recorder and maximal isometric bite force values for healthy young adults. Scand J Dent Res 101:171–175, 1993.

15. Mueller M, Maluf K: Tissue adaptation to physical stress: A proposed "physical stress theory" to guide physical therapist practice, education, and research. Phys Ther 2:383–403, 2002.

16. Bell W: Temporomandibular Disorders: Classification, Diagnosis, Management, 3rd ed. Chicago, Year Book Medical, 1990.

17. Styles C, Whyte A: MRI in the assessment of internal derangement and pain within the temporomandibular joint: A pictorial essay. Br J Oral Maxillofac Surg 40:220–228, 2002.

18. Tanaka E, Shibaguchi T, Tanaka M, et al.: Viscoelastic properties of the human temporomandibular joint disc in patients with internal derangement. J Oral Maxillofac Surg 58:997–1002, 2000.

19. Mahan P: The temporomandibular joint in function and pathofunction. In Solberg W, Clark GT (eds): Temporomandibular Joint Problems: Biologic Diagnosis and Treatment. Chicago, Quintessence, 1980.

20. Loughner B, Gremillion HA, Mahan PE, et al.: The medial capsule of the human temporomandibular joint. J Oral Maxillofac Surg 55:363–369, 1997.

21. Helland M: Anatomy and function of the temporomandibular joint. J Orthop Sports Phys Ther 1:145–152, 1980.

22. Abe S, Ouchi Y, Ide Y, et al.: Perspectives on the role of the lateral pterygoid muscle and the sphenomandibular ligament in temporomandibular joint functions. Cranio 15:203–207, 1997.

23. Isberg A, Westesson P: Steepness of articular eminence and movement of the condyle and disk in asymptomatic temporomandibular joints. Oral Surg Oral Med Oral Pathol Oral Radiol Endod 86:152–157, 1998.

24. Lindauer SJ, Sabol G, Isaacson RJ, et al.: Condylar movement and mandibular rotation during jaw opening. Am J Orthod Dentofacial Orthop 107:573–577, 1995.

25. Ferrario VF, Sforza C, Miani A Jr, et al.: Open-close movements in the human temporomandibular joint: Does a pure rotation around the intercondylar hinge axis exist? J Oral Rehabil 23:401–408, 1996.

26. Dijkstra PU, Hof AL, Stegenga B, et al.: Influence of mandibular length on mouth opening. J Oral Rehabil 26:117–122, 1999.

27. Naidoo L: Lateral pterygoid muscle and its relationship to the meniscus of the temporomandibular joint. Oral Sur Oral Med Oral Pathol Oral Radiol Endod 82:4–9, 1996.

28. Yang X, Pernu H, Pyhtinen J, et al.: MRI findings concerning the lateral pterygoid muscle in patients with symptomatic TMJ hypermobility. Cranio 19:260–268, 2001.

29. Yang X, Pernu H, Pyhtinen J, et al.: MR abnormalities of the lateral pterygoid muscle in patients with nonreducing disk displacement of the TMJ. Cranio 20:209–221, 2002.

30. Bade H, Schenck C, Koebke J: The function of discomuscular relationships in the human temporomandibular joint. Acta Anat (Basel) 151:258–267, 1994.

31. Murray GM, Orfanos T, Chan JY, et al.: Electromyographic activity of the human lateral pterygoid muscle during contralateral and protrusive jaw movements. Arch Oral Biol 44:269–285, 1999.

32. Hellsing E: Changes in the pharyngeal airway in relation to extension of the head. Eur J Orthod 11:359–365, 1989.

33. Evcik D, Aksoy O: Correlation of temporomandibular joint pathologies, neck pain and postural differences. J Phys Ther Sci 12:97–100, 2000.

34. Ciancaglini R, Testa M, Radaelli G: Association of neck pain with symptoms of temporomandibular dysfunction in the general adult population. Scand J Rehab Med 31:17–22, 1999.

35. Saunders H, Saunders R: Evaluation, Treatment and Prevention of Musculoskeletal Disorders, 3rd ed. Chaska, MN, The Saunders Group, 1993.

36. Netter F: Atlas of Human Anatomy, 3rd ed. Teterboro, NJ, Icon Learning Systems, 2003.

37. Ali H: Diagnostic criteria for temporomandibular joint disorders: A physiotherapist's perspective. Physiotherapy 88:421–426, 2002.

38. Antoniott T, Rocabado M: Exercise and Total Well-Being for Vertebral and Craniomandibular Disorders. Santiago, Chile, Alfabeta Impresories, 1990.

39. Brand R, Isselhard D: Anatomy of Orofacial Structures, 2nd ed. St. Louis, CV Mosby, 1982.

40. Rowe J, Kahn R: Successful aging and disease prevention. Adv Ren Replace Ther 7:70–77, 2000.

41. Nannmark U, Sennerby L, Haraldson T: Macroscopic, microscopic and radiologic assessment of the condylar part of the TMJ in elderly subjects. An autopsy study. Swed Dent J 14:163–169, 1990.

42. de Leeuw R, Boering G, van der Kuijl B, et al.: Hard and soft tissue imaging of the temporomandibular joint 30 years after diagnosis of osteoarthrosis and internal derangement. J Oral Maxiofac Surg 54: 1270–1280, 1996.

43. Arnett GW, Milam SB, Gottesman L: Progressive mandibular retrusion–idiopathic condylar resorption. Part II. Am J Orthod Dentofac Orthop 110: 117–127, 1996.

44. Goodman C, Boissanault W: Pathology: Implications for the Physical Therapist, 2nd ed. Philadelphia, WB Saunders, 2003.

45. Winocur E, Gavish A, Halachmi M, et al.: Generalized joint laxity and its relation with oral habits and temporomandibular disorders in adolescent girls. J Oral Rehabil 27:614–622, 2000.

46. Buckingham R, Braun T, Harinstein D, et al.: Temporomandibular joint dysfunction syndrome: A close association with systemic joint laxity. Oral Surg Oral Med Oral Pathol 72:514–519, 1991.

47. Westling L, Carlsson G, Helkimo M: Background factors in craniomandibular disorders with special reference to general joint hypermobility, parafunction, and trauma. J Craniomandib Disord 4:89–98, 1990.

48. Kirk W, Calabrese D: Clinical evaluation of physical therapy in the management of internal derangement of the temporomandibular joint. J Oral Maxillofac Surg 47:113–119, 1989.

Upper Extremity Joint Complexes

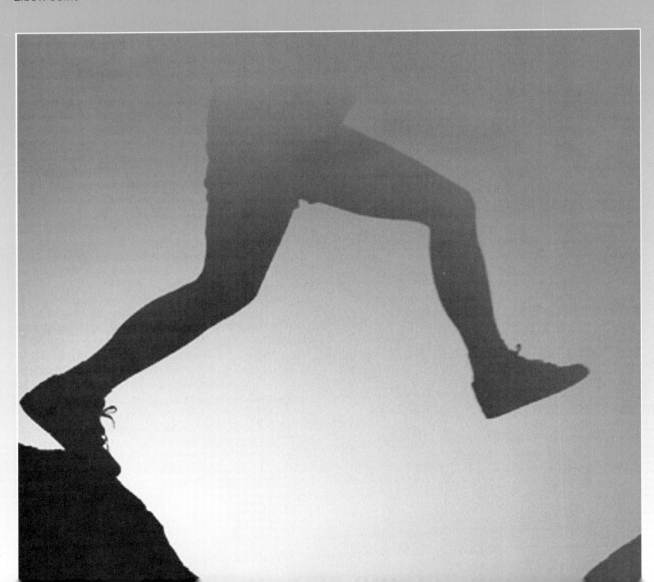

Chapter 7

The Shoulder Complex

Paula M. Ludewig, PT, PhD, John D. Borstead, PT, PhD

Introduction

The shoulder complex, composed of the clavicle, scapula, and humerus, is an intricately designed combination of three joints linking the upper extremity to the thorax. The articular structures of the shoulder complex are designed primarily for mobility, allowing us to move and position the hand through a wide range of space. The **glenohumeral (GH) joint,** linking the humerus and scapula, has greater mobility than any other joint in the body. Although the components of the shoulder complex constitute half of the mass of the entire upper limb,[1] the components are connected to the axial skeleton by a single joint (the **sternoclavicular [SC] joint**). As a result, muscle forces serve as a primary

mechanism for securing the shoulder girdle to the thorax and providing a stable base of support for upper extremity movements.

The contradictory requirements on the shoulder complex for both mobility and stability are met through active forces, or **dynamic stabilization,** a concept for which the shoulder complex is considered a classic example. In essence, dynamic stability exists when a moving segment or set of segments is limited very little by passive forces such as articular surface configuration, capsule, or ligaments and instead relies heavily on active forces or dynamic muscular control. Dynamic stabilization results in a wide range of mobility for the complex and provides adequate stability when the complex is functioning normally. However, the competing mobility and stability demands on the shoulder girdle and the intricate structural and functional design result in the shoulder complex being highly susceptible to dysfunction and instability.

Susan Sorenson is a 42-year-old dental hygienist who presents to the clinic with a chief complaint of right shoulder pain. She localizes the pain primarily to the lateral proximal humerus (C5 dermatome region) but also reports pain in the upper trapezius. Symptoms include pain and fatigue with elevating her arm and the inability to sleep on her right shoulder. Her medical history includes a diagnosis of early-stage breast cancer in the right breast 6 months ago. She had a lumpectomy with sentinel node biopsy, followed by radiation treatments for 5 weeks. She finished treatment almost 6 months ago. She reports feelings of tightness over the anterior chest region when she raises her right arm. Her history also includes a right acromioclavicular joint separation many years ago for which she was immobilized in a sling for several weeks and never underwent any further treatment.

◆ Components of the Shoulder Complex

The osseous segments of the shoulder complex are the clavicle, scapula, and humerus (Fig. 7-1). These three segments are joined by three interdependent linkages: the **SC joint,** the **acromioclavicular (AC) joint,** and the **GH joint.** The articulation between the scapula and the thorax is often described as the **scapulothoracic (ST) "joint,"** although it does not have the characteristics of a fibrous, cartilaginous, or synovial union. Instead, scapular motion on the thorax is directly a function of SC, AC, or combined SC and AC joint motion. The ST joint is frequently described in the literature as a "functional" joint. An additional functional articulation that is, at times, considered to be part of the shoulder complex is the **subacromial (or suprahumeral) "joint."** This functional joint is formed by movement of the head of the humerus below the coracoacromial arch. Although the movement between these two components plays an important role in shoulder function and dysfunction, we will refer to it as the **suprahumeral space** and consider it a component of the GH joint rather than a separate linkage.

The joints that compose the shoulder complex in combination with trunk motion can contribute as much as 180° of elevation to the upper extremity. **Elevation** of the upper extremity refers to the combination of scapular, clavicular, and humeral motion that occurs when the arm is raised either *forward* or *to the side* (including sagittal plane flexion, frontal plane abduction, and all the motions in between). Motion of the scapula on the thorax normally contributes about one third of the total motion necessary for elevation of the arm through the linked SC and AC joint motions, whereas the GH joint contributes about two thirds of the total motion. Although integrated function of all three joints is of primary interest, each of the articulations and compo-

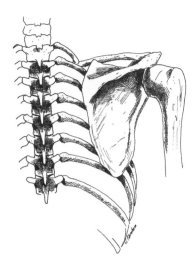

▲ **Figure 7-1** ■ A posterior view of the three components of the shoulder complex: the humerus, the scapula, and the clavicle.

nents of the shoulder complex must be examined individually before integrated dynamic function can be appreciated.

Sternoclavicular Joint

The SC joint serves as the only structural attachment of the clavicle, scapula, and upper extremity to the axial skeleton. Movement of the clavicle at the SC joint inevitably produces movement of the scapula under conditions of normal function, because the scapula is attached to the lateral end of the clavicle. In order for the scapula to not move with the clavicle during SC motion, equal and opposite motions would have to occur at the AC joint; this is not typical with an intact claviculoscapular linkage. Similarly, any motions of the scapula must result in motion at the SC joint (unless scapular motions are isolated to the AC joint—which is, again, unlikely under normal circumstances). The SC joint is a plane synovial joint with three rotatory and three translatory degrees of freedom. This joint has a synovial capsule, a joint disk, and three major ligaments.

■ Sternoclavicular Articulating Surfaces

The SC articulation consists of two saddle-shaped surfaces, one at the sternal or medial end of the clavicle and one at the notch formed by the manubrium of the sternum and first costal cartilage (Fig. 7-2). Because tremendous individual differences exist across people and the saddle shape of these surfaces is very subtle, the SC joint is often classified as a plane synovial joint. The sternal end of the clavicle and the manubrium are incongruent; that is, there is little contact between their articular surfaces. The superior portion of the medial clavicle does not contact the manubrium at all; instead it serves as the attachment for the **SC joint disk** and the **interclavicular ligament.** At rest, the SC joint space is

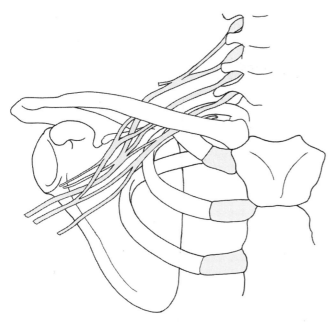

▲ **Figure 7-2** ■ The sternoclavicular joint is the articulation of the medial clavicle with the manubrium and first costal cartilage.

wedge-shaped and open superiorly.[2] Movements of the clavicle in relation to the manubrium result in changes to the areas of contact between the clavicle, the SC joint disk, and the manubriocostal cartilage.

■ **Sternoclavicular Disk**

As is generally true at an incongruent joint, the SC joint has a fibrocartilage joint disk, or meniscus, that increases congruence between joint surfaces. The upper portion of the SC disk is attached to the postero-superior clavicle. The lower portion is attached to the manubrium and first costal cartilage, as well as to the anterior and posterior aspects to the fibrous capsule.[3] The disk diagonally transects the SC joint space (Fig. 7-3) and divides the joint into two separate cavi-

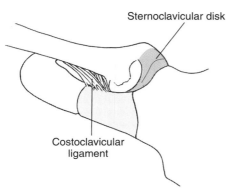

Sternoclavicular disk

Costoclavicular
ligament

▲ **Figure 7-3** ■ The sternoclavicular disk transects the joint into two separate joint cavities. The axes for motion appear to occur at the location of the costoclavicular ligament.

ties.[1] Given its attachments, the disk acts like a hinge or pivot point during clavicle motion.

In elevation and depression of the clavicle, the medial end of the clavicle rolls and slides on the relatively stationary disk, with the upper attachment of the disk serving as a pivot point. In protraction/retraction of the clavicle, the SC disk and medial clavicle roll and slide together on the manubrial facet, with the lower attachment of the disk serving as a pivot point.[1] The disk, therefore, is considered part of the manubrium in elevation/depression and part of the clavicle in pro-traction/retraction. As the disk switches its participation from one articular segment to the other during clavicular motions, mobility between the segments is maintained and stability is enhanced. The resultant movement of the clavicle in both elevation/depression and protraction/retraction is a fairly complex set of motions, with the mechanical axis for these two movements located not at the SC joint itself but at the more laterally located **costoclavicular ligament** (see Fig. 7-3).

The SC disk serves an important stability function by increasing joint congruence and absorbing forces that may be transmitted along the clavicle from its lateral end. In Figure 7-3, it can be seen that the unique diagonal attachment of the SC disk will check medial movement of the clavicle that might otherwise cause the large medial articular surface of the clavicle to override the shallow manubrial facet. The disk also has substantial contact with the medial clavicle, permitting the disk to dissipate the medially directed forces that would otherwise cause high pressure at the small manubrial facet. Although one might think that medially directed forces on the clavicle are rare, we shall see that this is not the case when we examine the function of the AC joint, the **upper trapezius muscle,** and the **coracoclavicular ligament.**

Continuing Exploration: **Three-Compartment SC Joint**

Anatomic examination of the SC articulation has led to the proposal that there are three, rather than two, functional units of the SC joint: a lateral compartment between the disk and clavicle for elevation and depression; a medial compartment between the disk and manubrium for protraction and retraction; and a costoclavicular joint for anterior and posterior long axis rotation. Anterior and posterior rotation are thought to occur between a portion of the disk over the first rib and a "conus" on the anteroinferior edge of the articular surface of the medial clavicle.[4]

■ **Sternoclavicular Joint Capsule and Ligaments**

The SC joint is surrounded by a fairly strong fibrous capsule but must depend on three ligaments for the majority of its support. These are the **sternoclavicular ligaments,** the costoclavicular ligament, and the interclavicular ligament (Fig. 7-4). The anterior and posterior SC ligaments reinforce the capsule and function primarily to check anterior and posterior translatory movement of the medial end of the clavicle. The costoclavicular ligament is a very strong ligament found between the clavicle and the first rib. The costoclavicular ligament has two segments or laminae. The anterior lamina has fibers directed laterally from the first rib to the clavicle, whereas the fibers of the posterior lamina are directed medially from the rib to the clavicle.[3,5] Both segments check elevation of the lateral end of the clavicle and, when the limits of the ligament are reached, may contribute to the inferior gliding of the medial clavicle that occurs with clavicular elevation.[6] The costoclavicular ligament is also positioned to counter the superiorly directed forces applied to the clavicle by the sternocleidomastoid and sternohyoid muscles. The medially directed fibers of the posterior lamina will resist medial movement of the clavicle,[7] absorbing some of the force that would otherwise be imposed on the SC disk. The interclavicular ligament resists excessive depression of the distal clavicle and superior glide of the medial end of the clavicle. The limitation to clavicular depression is critical to protecting structures such as the brachial plexus and subclavian artery that pass under the clavicle and over the first rib. In fact, when the clavicle is depressed and the interclavicular ligament and superior capsule are taut, the tension in the interclavicular ligament can support the weight of the upper extremity.[8]

■ Sternoclavicular Motions

The three rotatory degrees of freedom at the SC joint are most commonly described as elevation/depression, protraction/retraction, and anterior/posterior rotation of the clavicle. Motions of any joint are typically described by identifying the direction of movement of the portion of the lever that is farthest from the joint. The horizontal alignment of the clavicle (rather than the vertical alignment of most of the appendicular levers of the skeleton) can sometimes create confusion and impair visualization of the clavicular motions. The motions of elevation/depression (Fig. 7-5) and protraction/retraction (Fig. 7-6) should be visualized by referencing movement of the lateral end of the clavicle. Clavicular anterior/posterior rotation are long axis rolling motions of the entire clavicle (Fig. 7-7). Three degrees of translatory motion at the SC joint can also

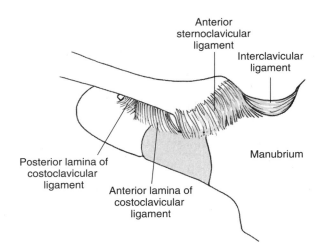

▲ **Figure 7-4** ■ The sternoclavicular joint ligaments.

occur, although they are very small in magnitude. Translations of the medial clavicle on the manubrium are usually defined as occurring in anterior/posterior, medial/lateral, and superior/inferior directions (see Figs. 7-5 and 7-6).

Elevation and Depression of the Clavicle

The motions of elevation and depression occur around an approximately anteroposterior (A-P) axis (see Fig. 7-5) between a convex clavicular surface and a concave surface formed by the manubrium and the first costal cartilage. With elevation, the lateral clavicle rotates upward, and with depression, the lateral clavicle rotates downward. The cephalocaudal shape of the articular surfaces and the location of the axis indicate that the convex surface of the clavicle must slide inferiorly on the concave manubrium and first costal cartilage, in a direction opposite to movement of the lateral end of the clavicle. The SC joint axis is described as lying lateral to the joint at the costoclavicular ligament. The location of this functional (rather than anatomic) axis relatively far from the joint reflects a large intra-articular motion of the medial clavicle. The range of available clavicular elevation has been described as up

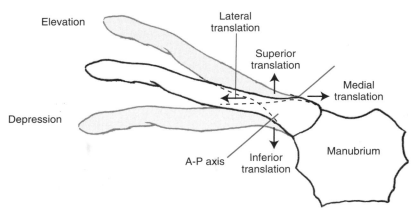

◀ **Figure 7-5** ■ Clavicular elevation/depression at the SC joint occurs as movement of the lateral clavicle about an A-P axis. The medial clavicle also has small magnitudes of medial/lateral translation and superior/inferior translation at the SC joint.

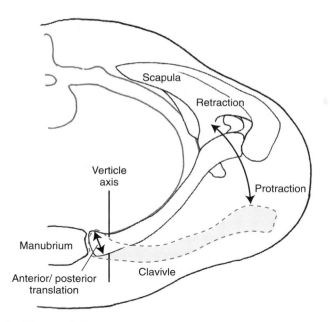

▲ Figure 7-6 ■ Shown in a superior view, clavicular protraction/retraction at the SC joint occurs as movement of the lateral clavicle (and attached scapula) around a vertical axis. The medial clavicle also has a small magnitude of anterior/posterior translation at the SC joint.

to 48°, whereas passive depression is limited, on average, to less than 15°.[9] The full magnitude of the available range of elevation is generally not utilized during functional ranges of arm elevation.[10,11]

Protraction and Retraction of the Clavicle

Protraction and retraction of the clavicle occur at the SC joint around an approximately vertical (superoinferior) axis that also appears to lie at the costoclavicular ligament (see Fig. 7-6). With protraction, the lateral clavicle rotates anteriorly, and with retraction, the lateral clavicle rotates posteriorly. The configuration of joint surfaces in this plane is the opposite of that for elevation/depression; the medial end of the clavicle is concave, and the manubrial side of the joint is convex. During protraction, the medial clavicle is expected to slide anteriorly on the manubrium and first costal cartilage. There is about 15° to 20° protraction and 20° to 30° retraction of the clavicle available.[9,11,12]

Anterior and Posterior Rotation of the Clavicle

Anterior/posterior, or long axis, rotation of the clavicle (see Fig. 7-7) occurs as a spin between the saddle-shaped surfaces of the medial clavicle and manubriocostal facet. Unlike many joints that can rotate in either direction from resting position of the joint, the clavicle rotates primarily in only one direction from its resting position. The clavicle rotates posteriorly from neutral, bringing the inferior surface of the clavicle to face anteriorly. This has also been referred to as backward or upward rotation rather than posterior rotation.[1] From its fully rotated position, the clavicle can rotate anteriorly again to return to neutral. Available anterior rotation past neutral is very limited, generally described as less than 10°.[1] The range of available clavicular posterior rotation is cited to be as much as 50°.[10] The axis of rotation runs longitudinally through the clavicle, intersecting the SC and AC joints.

■ Sternoclavicular Stress Tolerance

The bony segments of the SC joint, its capsuloligamentous structure, and the SC disk combine to produce a joint that meets its dual functions of mobility and stability well. The SC joint serves its purposes of joining the upper limb to the axial skeleton, contributing to upper limb mobility, and withstanding imposed stresses. Although the SC joint is considered incongruent, the joint does not undergo the degree of degenerative change common to the other joints of the shoulder complex.[13,14] Strong force-dissipating structures such as the SC disk and the costoclavicular ligament minimize articular stresses and also prevent excessive intra-articular motion that might lead to subluxation or dislocation. Dislocations of the SC joint represent only 1% of joint dislocations in the body.[15]

Acromioclavicular Joint

The AC joint attaches the scapula to the clavicle. It is generally described as a plane synovial joint with three

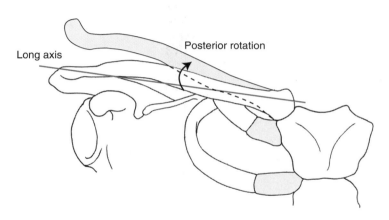

◀ Figure 7-7 ■ Clavicular rotation at the SC joint occurs as a spin of the entire clavicle around a long axis that has a medial/lateral orientation. As the clavicle posteriorly rotates, the lateral end flips up; anterior rotation is a return to resting position.

rotational and three translational degrees of freedom. It has a joint capsule and two major ligaments; a joint disk may or may not be present. The primary function of the AC joint is to allow the scapula additional range of rotation on the thorax and allow for adjustments of the scapula (tipping and internal/external rotation) outside the initial plane of the scapula in order to follow the changing shape of the thorax as arm movement occurs. In addition, the joint allows transmission of forces from the upper extremity to the clavicle.

■ Acromioclavicular Articulating Surfaces

The AC joint consists of the articulation between the lateral end of the clavicle and a small facet on the acromion of the scapula (Fig. 7-8). The articular facets, considered to be incongruent, vary in configuration. They may be flat, reciprocally concave-convex, or reversed (reciprocally convex-concave).[5] The inclination of the articulating surfaces varies from individual to individual. Depalma[13] described three joint types in which the angle of inclination of the contacting surfaces varied from 16° to 36° from vertical. The closer the surfaces were to the vertical, the more prone the joint was to the wearing effects of shear forces. Given the variable articular configuration, intra-articular movements for this joint are not predictable.

■ Acromioclavicular Joint Disk

The disk of the AC joint (see Fig. 7-8 inset) is variable in size between individuals, at various ages within an individual, and between sides of the same individual. Through 2 years of age, the joint is actually a fibrocartilaginous union. With use of the upper extremity, a joint space develops at each articulating surface that may leave a "meniscoid" fibrocartilage remnant within the joint.[14]

■ Acromioclavicular Capsule and Ligaments

The capsule of the AC joint is weak and cannot maintain integrity of the joint without reinforcement of the **superior** and **inferior acromioclavicular** and the **coracoclavicular ligaments** (Fig. 7-9). The superior acromioclavicular ligament assists the capsule in apposing articular surfaces and in controlling A-P joint stability. The fibers of the superior AC ligament are reinforced by aponeurotic fibers of the trapezius and **deltoid** muscles, which makes the superior joint support stronger than the inferior.[7]

The coracoclavicular ligament, although not belonging directly to the anatomic structure of the AC joint, firmly unites the clavicle and scapula and provides much of the joint's stability. This ligament is divided into a lateral portion, the **trapezoid ligament,** and a medial portion, the **conoid ligament.** The trapezoid ligament is quadrilateral in shape and is nearly horizontal in orientation. The conoid ligament, medial and slightly posterior to the trapezoid, is more triangular and vertically oriented.[5] The two portions are separated by adipose tissue and a large bursa.[8] Both these ligaments attach to the undersurface of the clavicle, the conoid ligament very posteriorly, influencing their function in a way that will be described later. Although the AC capsule and ligament can resist small rotary and translatory forces at the AC joint, restraint of larger displacements is credited to the coracoclavicular ligament.

The conoid portion of the coracoclavicular ligament provides the primary restraint for the AC joint in the superior and inferior directions, whereas the trape-

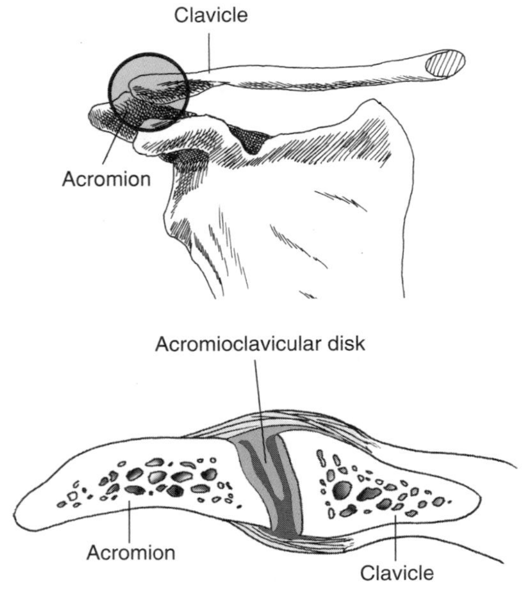

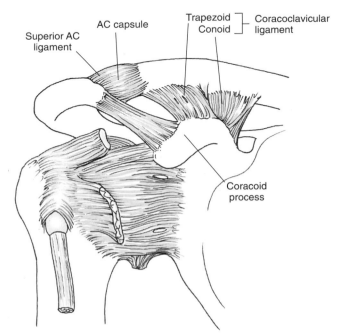

▲ **Figure 7-8 ■** The acromioclavicular joint. **Inset.** A cross-section of the AC joint shows the disk and the angulation of the articular surfaces.

▲ **Figure 7-9 ■** The AC joint capsule and ligaments, including the coracoclavicular ligament with its conoid and trapezoid portions.

zoid portion provides the majority of resistance to posterior translatory forces applied to the distal clavicle.[16,17] In addition, both portions of the coracoclavicular ligament limit upward rotation of the scapula at the AC joint. When medially directed forces on the humerus (such as those produced with leaning on the arm) are transferred to the glenoid fossa of the scapula, medial displacement of the scapula's acromion on the clavicle is prevented by tension in and the strength of the coracoclavicular ligament (especially the horizontal trapezoid portion) that transfer the force to the clavicle, and then on to the very strong SC joint (Fig. 7-10). One of the most critical roles played by the coracoclavicular ligament, as shall be seen later, is in coupling the posterior rotation of the clavicle to scapula rotation during elevation of the upper extremity.

■ **Acromioclavicular Motions**

The articular facets of the AC joint are small, afford limited motion, and have a wide range of individual differences. For these reasons, studies are inconsistent in identifying the movement and axes of motion for this joint. The primary rotatory motions that take place at the AC joint are **internal/external rotation, anterior/posterior tipping or tilting,** and **upward/downward rotation**. These motions occur around axes that are oriented to the plane of the scapula rather than to the cardinal planes. Although internal/external rotation occurs around an essentially vertical axis, anterior/posterior tipping occurs around an oblique "coronal" axis, and anterior/posterior tipping around an oblique "A-P" axis (Fig. 7-11). Terminology for the AC motions, as well as for motions of the scapula on the thorax, varies widely. The AC joint also influences and is influenced by rotation of the clavicle around its long axis. In

addition, translatory motions at the AC joint can occur, although, as in the case of the SC joint, these motions are typically small in magnitude. These translations are usually defined as anterior/posterior, medial/lateral, and superior/inferior.

Internal and External Rotation

Internal/external rotation of the scapula in relation to the clavicle occurs around an approximately vertical axis through the AC joint. Internal and external rotation at the AC joint can best be visualized as bringing the glenoid fossa of the scapula anteromedially and posterolaterally, respectively (Fig. 7-12). These motions occur to maintain contact of the scapula with the horizontal curvature of the thorax as the clavicle protracts and retracts, sliding the scapula around the thorax in scapular protraction and retraction, and to "aim" the glenoid fossa toward the plane of humeral elevation (see Fig. 7-12 inset). The orientation of the glenoid fossa is important to maintain congruency with the humeral head; maximize the function of GH muscles, capsule, and ligaments; maximize stability of the GH joint; and maximize available motion of the arm. The available range of motion (ROM) at the AC joint is difficult to measure. Dempster provided a range of 30° for combined internal and external ROM in cadaveric AC joints separated from the thorax.[1] Smaller values (20° to 35°) have been reported *in vivo* during arm motions, although up to 40° to 60° may be possible with full-range motions reaching forward and across the body.[9,11,12]

Anterior and Posterior Tipping

The second AC motion is anterior/posterior tipping or tilting of the scapula in relation to the clavicle around an oblique "coronal" axis through the joint. Anterior

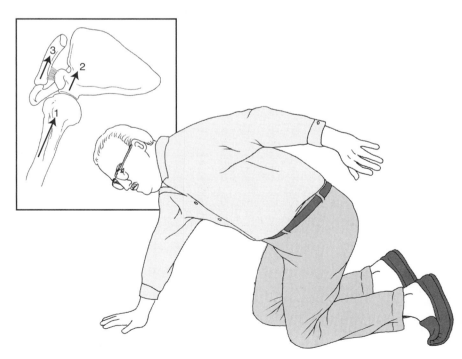

◀ **Figure 7-10** ■ When a person bears weight on the arm, a medially directed force up the humerus (1) is transferred to the scapula (2) through the glenoid fossa and then to the clavicle (3) through the coracoclavicular ligament.

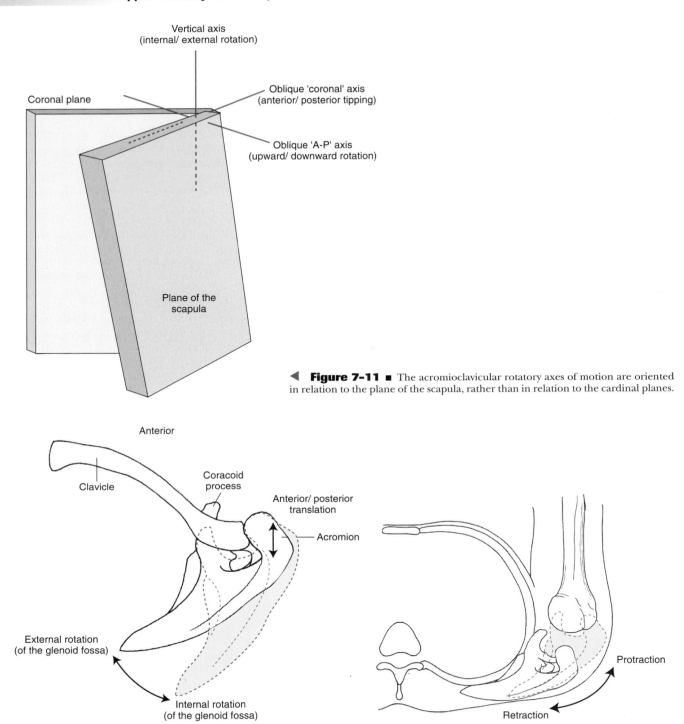

◀ **Figure 7-11** ■ The acromioclavicular rotatory axes of motion are oriented in relation to the plane of the scapula, rather than in relation to the cardinal planes.

▲ **Figure 7-12** ■ A superior view of scapular internal and external rotation at the AC joint. Although the directional arrows are drawn at the vertebral border, the motions are named with the glenoid fossa of the scapula as the reference. The acromion also has small amounts of anterior and posterior translatory motions that can occur. **Inset.** Protraction and retraction of the scapula require internal and external rotation, respectively, for the scapula to follow the convex thorax and orient the glenoid fossa with the plane of elevation.

tipping will result in the acromion tipping forward and the inferior angle tipping backward (Fig. 7-13). Posterior tipping will rotate the acromion backward and the inferior angle forward. Scapular tipping, like internal/external rotation of the scapula, occurs to maintain the contact of the scapula with the contour of the rib cage and orient the glenoid fossa. As the scapula moves upward or downward on the rib cage in elevation or depression, the scapula must adjust its position to maintain full contact with the vertical curvature of the ribs (see Fig. 7-13 inset). Elevation of the scapula on the thorax, such as occurs with a shoulder shrug, can result

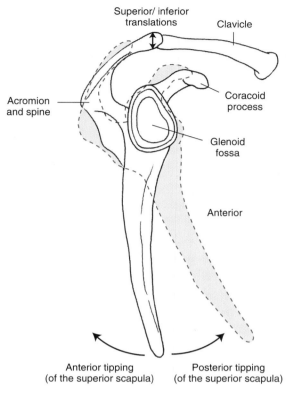

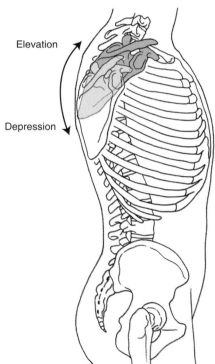

▲ **Figure 7-13** ■ A lateral view of scapular anterior and posterior tipping at the AC joint. Although the directional arrows are drawn at the inferior angle, the motions are named with the superior aspect of the scapula as the reference. The acromion also has small amounts of anterior and posterior translatory motions that can occur. **Inset.** Elevation and depression of the scapula require anterior and posterior tipping, respectively, for the scapula to follow the convex thorax.

in anterior tipping. The scapula does not always follow the curvature of the thorax precisely. During normal flexion or abduction of the arm, the scapula posteriorly tips on the thorax as the scapula is upwardly rotating. Available passive motion into anterior/posterior tipping at the AC joint is 60° in cadaveric AC joint specimens separated from the thorax.[1] The magnitude of anterior/posterior tipping during *in vivo* arm elevation has been quantified as approximately 30°, although up to 40° or more may be possible in the full range from maximum flexion to extension.[11]

Upward/Downward Rotation

The third AC joint motion is upward/downward rotation of the scapula in relation to the clavicle about an oblique "A-P" axis approximately perpendicular to the plane of the scapula, passing midway between the joint surfaces of the AC joint. Upward rotation tilts the glenoid fossa upward (Fig. 7-14), and downward rotation is the opposite motion. The amount of available passive motion into upward/downward rotation specifically at the AC joint is limited by the attachment of the coracoclavicular ligament. In order for upward rotation to occur at the AC joint, the coracoid process and superior border of the scapula need to move inferiorly away from the clavicle, a motion restricted by tension in the coracoclavicular ligaments. However, Dempster described

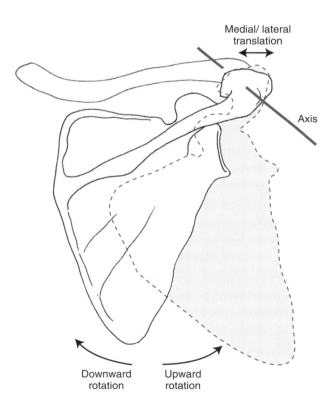

▲ **Figure 7-14** ■ Upward/downward rotation of the scapula at the AC joint occurs around an approximately A-P (perpendicular to the plane of the scapula) axis. Although the directional arrows are drawn at the inferior angle, the motions are named with the glenoid fossa of the scapula as the reference. The acromion also has a small magnitude of medial and lateral translatory motions that can occur.

30° of available passive ROM into upward/downward rotation.[1] The amount of available upward rotation is dependent in part on clavicular long axis rotation. Because of the attachment of the coracoclavicular ligaments to the undersurface and posterior edge of the clavicle, posterior rotation at the SC joint releases tension on the coracoclavicular ligaments and "opens up" the AC joint, allowing upward rotation to occur.[10] Conway described 30° of upward rotation and 17° of downward rotation actively at the AC joint *in vivo*.[9]

■ Acromioclavicular Stress Tolerance

Unlike the stronger SC joint, the AC joint is extremely susceptible to both trauma and degenerative change. This is likely to be due to its small and incongruent surfaces that result in large forces per unit area. Degenerative change is common from the second decade on,[14] with the joint space itself commonly narrowed by the sixth decade.[18] Treatment of sprains, subluxations, and dislocations of this joint occupies a large amount of the literature on the shoulder complex. Controversy exists on description and classification of AC subluxations and dislocations, as well as on nonsurgical and surgical management.[19] An increased understanding of the mechanics of this joint supports the importance of normal AC motions in healthy functioning of the shoulder complex.[20]

> #### *Continuing Exploration:* **Classifying Acromioclavicular Dislocations**
>
> The AC joint is susceptible to traumatic injury through accidents or contact sports. These AC separations are graded on the basis of the direction and amount of displacement. Various classification schemes exist; most commonly, **type I** injuries consist of a sprain to the AC ligaments, **type II** injuries typically have ruptured AC ligaments and sprained coracoclavicular ligaments, and **type III** injuries result in rupture of both sets of ligaments, with a result of 25% to 100% greater coracoclavicular space than normal. Types I, II, and III AC separations all involve inferior displacement of the acromion in relation to the clavicle caused by the loss of support from the coracoclavicular ligaments. **Type IV** injuries have a posteriorly displaced lateral clavicle, often pressing into the trapezius posteriorly, with complete rupture of both the AC and coracoclavicular ligaments. **Type V** injuries also involve an inferior displacement of the acromion and complete rupture of both sets of ligaments and are distinguished from type III by a severity of between three and five times greater coracoclavicular space than normal. **Type VI** injuries have an inferiorly displaced clavicle in relation to the acromion, with complete ligament rupture and displacement of the distal clavicle into a subacromial or subcoracoid position. Types IV, V, and VI are much rarer injuries, and each necessitates surgical management.[21]

> **Case Application 7-1:** **AC Joint Injury**
>
> Our patient, Ms. Sorenson, reports a past AC joint separation treated by immobilization with the arm at the side in a sling. This treatment is consistent with an injury ranging from type I to a type III in severity, which are frequently not surgically stabilized. With a type I injury, she may have healed well and may have normal AC joint function. If the past injury was a type III injury, she may still have a substantial instability or disruption of the claviculoscapular linkage. The position and prominence of the distal clavicle on the right in comparison with her left noninvolved side can provide some insight into her past injury. A prominent distal clavicle with a step down to the acromion (step sign) would be consistent with inferior scapular (or superior clavicle) positioning related to a past type II or III injury. Although this injury is commonly not surgically stabilized because many surgeons believe it unnecessary, follow-up studies indicate high rates of residual symptoms in persons with past AC joint injuries. These rates of residual symptoms range from 36% in type I injuries to 69% in type III injuries, which suggests that more aggressive treatment and rehabilitation may be warranted with AC injuries.[20]

Scapulothoracic Joint

The ST "joint" is formed by the articulation of the scapula with the thorax. It is not a true anatomic joint because it has none of the usual joint characteristics (union by fibrous, cartilaginous, or synovial tissues). In fact, the articulation of the scapula with the thorax depends on the integrity of the anatomic AC and SC joints. The SC and AC joints are interdependent with the ST joint because the scapula is attached by its acromion process to the lateral end of the clavicle through the AC joint; the clavicle, in turn, is attached to the axial skeleton at the manubrium of the sternum through the SC joint. Any movement of the scapula on the thorax *must* result in movement at either the AC joint, the SC joint, or both; that is, the functional ST joint is part of a true closed chain with the AC and SC joints and the thorax. Observation and measurement of individual SC and AC joint motions are more difficult than observing or measuring motions of the scapula on the thorax. Consequently, ST position and motions are described and measured far more frequently than are the SC and AC joint motions upon which ST motions are dependent.

■ Resting Position of the Scapula

Normally, the scapula rests at a position on the posterior thorax approximately 2 inches from the midline, between the second through seventh ribs (see Fig. 7-1). The scapula also is internally rotated 30° to 45° from the coronal plane (Fig. 7-15A), is tipped anteriorly approximately 10° to 20° from vertical (Fig. 7-15B), and is upwardly rotated 10° to 20° from vertical.[22] The magnitude of upward rotation has as its reference a "longitudinal" axis perpendicular to the axis running from the root of the scapular spine to the AC joint (Fig. 7-15C). If the vertebral or medial border of the scapula is used as the reference axis, the magnitude of upward rotation at rest is usually described as 2° to 3° from vertical.[23] Although these "normal" values for the resting scapula are cited, substantial individual variability exists in scapular rest position, even among healthy subjects.[23]

The motions of the scapula from this resting or reference position include three rotations that were already described because they occur at the AC joint. These are upward/downward rotation, internal/external rotation, and anterior/posterior tipping. Of these three AC joint rotations, only upward/downward rotation is readily observable at the ST, and it is therefore considered for our purposes to be a "primary" scapular motion. Internal/external rotation and anterior/posterior tipping are *normally* difficult to observe and are therefore considered for our purposes to be "secondary" scapular motions. The scapula presumably also has

available the translatory motions of scapular **elevation/depression** and **protraction/retraction.** These "primary" (readily observable) scapular motions are typically described as if they occur independently of each other. The linkage of the scapula to the AC and SC joints, however, actually prevents scapular motions both from occurring in isolation and from occurring as true translatory motions. Instead, scapular motions on the thorax must occur in combinations, such as the simultaneous upward rotation, external rotation, and posterior tipping that occur when the arm is abducted.

■ Motions of the Scapula

Upward/Downward Rotation

Upward rotation of the scapula on the thorax (Fig. 7-16) is the principal motion of the scapula observed during active elevation of the arm and plays a significant role in increasing the range of elevation of the arm

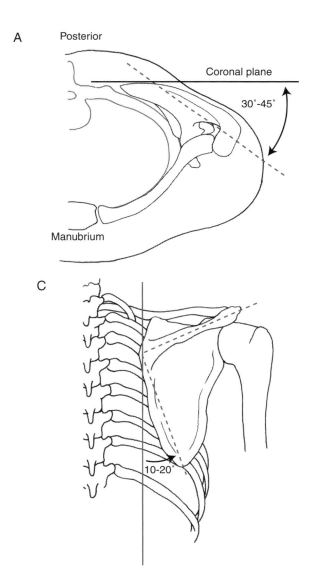

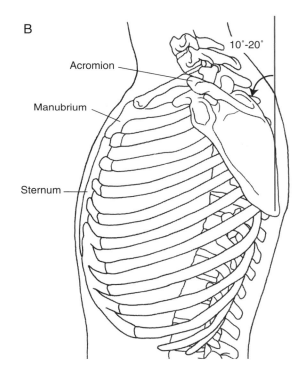

◀ **Figure 7-15** ■ The resting position of the scapula on the thorax. **A.** In this superior view, it can be seen that the scapula rests in an internally rotated position 30° to 45° anterior to the coronal plane. **B.** In this side view, it can be seen that the scapula at rest is tipped anteriorly approximately 10° to 20° to the vertical plane. **C.** In this posterior view, the "longitudinal" axis of the scapula (90° to an axis through the spine) is upwardly rotated 10° to 20° from vertical.

overhead. Approximately 60° of upward rotation of the scapula on the thorax is typically available. Given the closed-chain relationship between the SC, AC, and ST joints, differing proportions of upward/downward rotation of the scapula are contributed by SC joint elevation/depression, by SC joint posterior/anterior rotation, and by AC joint upward/downward rotation. Most often, scapular upward/downward rotation results from a combination of these SC and AC motions.

 CONCEPT CORNERSTONE 7-1: *Terminology*

In describing upward and downward rotation of the scapula, we define upward and downward motion by the upward and downward movement of the glenoid fossa, respectively. Other authors use the inferior angle of the scapula as the referent, with upward and downward rotation then described as movement of the inferior angle away from the vertebral column (upward rotation) or movement of the inferior angle toward the vertebral column (downward rotation). Some authors also refer to upward/downward rotation of the scapula (regardless of reference point on the scapula) by the names abduction/adduction or lateral/medial rotation, respectively.[1,24]

Elevation/Depression

Scapular elevation and depression can be isolated (relatively speaking) by shrugging the shoulder up and depressing the shoulder downward. Elevation and depression of the scapula on the thorax are commonly described as translatory motions in which the scapula moves upward (cephalad) or downward (caudally) along the rib cage from its resting position. Scapular elevation, however, occurs through elevation of the clavicle at the SC joint and requires subtle adjustments in anterior/posterior tipping and internal/external

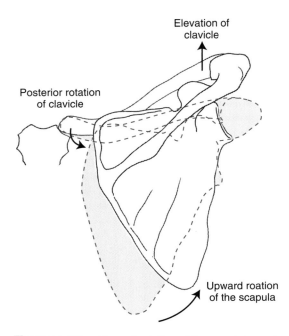

▲ **Figure 7-16** ■ Upward rotation of the scapula is produced by clavicular elevation and posterior rotation at the SC joint and by rotations at the AC joint.

rotation at the AC joint to maintain the scapula in contact with the thorax (Fig. 7-17).

Protraction/Retraction

Protraction and retraction of the scapula on the thorax are often described as translatory motions of the scapula away from or toward the vertebral column, respectively. However, if protraction of the ST joint occurred as a pure translatory movement, the scapula would move directly away from the vertebral column,

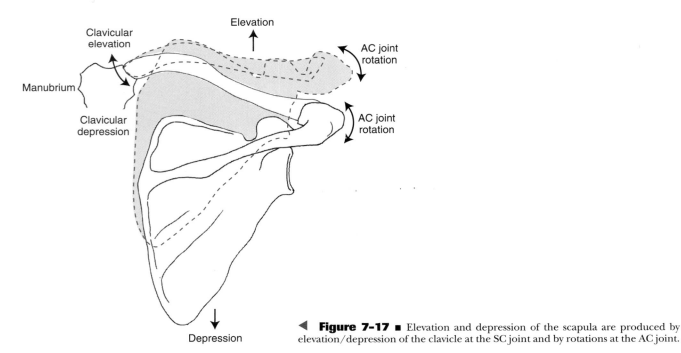

◄ **Figure 7-17** ■ Elevation and depression of the scapula are produced by elevation/depression of the clavicle at the SC joint and by rotations at the AC joint.

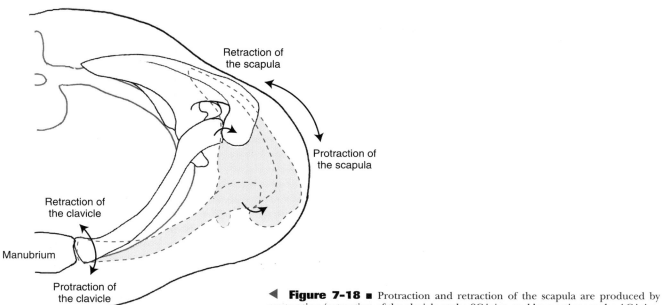

Retraction of
the scapula

Protraction of
the scapula

Retraction of
the clavicle

Manubrium

Protraction of
the clavicle

◀ **Figure 7-18** ■ Protraction and retraction of the scapula are produced by protraction/retraction of the clavicle at the SC joint, and by rotations at the AC joint.

and the glenoid fossa would face laterally. Only the vertebral border of the scapula would remain in contact with the rib cage. In reality, full scapular protraction results in the glenoid fossa facing anteriorly with the full scapula in contact with the rib cage. The scapula follows the contour of the ribs by rotating internally and externally at the AC joint in combination with clavicular protraction and retraction at the SC joint (Fig. 7-18).

Internal/External Rotation

The scapular motions of internal and external rotation are normally not overtly identifiable on physical observation but are critical to its movement along the curved rib cage. Internal/external rotation of the scapula on the thorax should normally accompany protraction/retraction of the clavicle at the SC joint. Internal rotation of the scapula on the thorax that is isolated to (or occurs excessively at) the AC joint results in prominence of the vertebral border of the scapula as a result of loss of contact with the thorax. This is often referred to clinically as scapular "winging" (Fig. 7-19). Excessive internal rotation may be indicative of pathology or poor neuromuscular control of the ST muscles.

Anterior/Posterior Tipping

As is true for internal/external rotation, anterior/posterior tipping is normally not overtly obvious on clinical observation and yet is critical to maintaining contact of the scapula against the curvature of the rib cage. Anterior/posterior tipping of the scapula on the thorax occurs at the AC joint and normally will accompany anterior/posterior rotation of the clavicle at the SC joint. Anterior tipping that is isolated to or occurs excessively at the AC joint will result in prominence of the inferior angle of the scapula (Fig. 7-20). An anteriorly tipped scapula may occur in pathologic situations (poor neuromuscular control) or in abnormal posture.

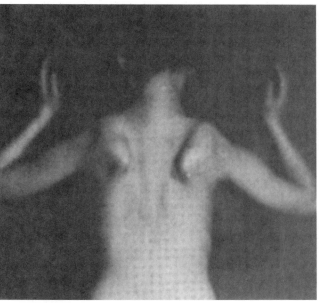

▲ **Figure 7-19** ■ These scapulae are "winged" bilaterally. Excessive internal rotation of the scapulae at the AC joint causes prominence of the medial borders of the scapulae with attempted elevation of the arms.

■ Scapulothoracic Stability

Stability of the scapula on the thorax is provided by the structures that maintain integrity of the linked AC and SC joints. The muscles that attach to both the thorax and scapula maintain contact between these surfaces while producing the movements of the scapula. In addition, stabilization is provided through the ST musculature by pulling or compressing the scapula to the thorax.[24]

The ultimate functions of scapular motion are to orient the glenoid fossa for optimal contact with the

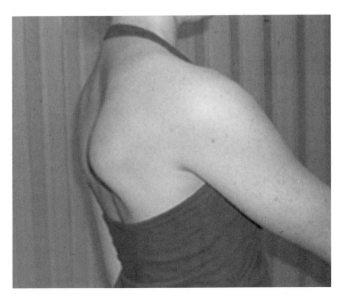

▲ **Figure 7-20** ■ This scapula is anteriorly tipped with attempted elevation of the arm, causing the inferior angle of the scapula to lift off the thorax and become visually prominent.

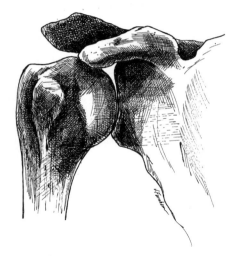

▲ **Figure 7-21** ■ The glenohumeral joint.

maneuvering arm, to add range to elevation of the arm, and to provide a stable base for the controlled motions between the humeral head and glenoid fossa. The scapula, with its associated muscles and linkages, performs these mobility and stability functions so well that it serves as a premier example of dynamic stabilization in the human body.

Glenohumeral Joint

The GH joint is a ball-and-socket synovial joint with three rotational and three translational degrees of freedom. It has a capsule and several associated ligaments and bursae. The articulation is composed of the large head of the humerus and the smaller glenoid fossa (Fig. 7-21). Because the glenoid fossa of the scapula is the proximal segment of the GH joint, any motions of the scapula (and its interdependent SC and AC linkages) may influence GH joint function. The GH joint has sacrificed articular congruency to serve the mobility needs of the hand and is subsequently susceptible to degenerative changes, instability, and derangement.

■ Glenohumeral Articulating Surfaces

The glenoid fossa of the scapula serves as the proximal articular surface for this joint. The orientation of the shallow concavity of the glenoid fossa in relation to the thorax varies, as we have already seen, with the resting position of the scapula on the thorax and with motion at the SC and AC joints. However, the orientation of the glenoid fossa may vary with the form of the scapula itself. The glenoid fossa may be tilted slightly upward or downward when the arm is at the side,[25-27] although representations most commonly show a slight upward tilt.

The fossa also does not always lie in a plane perpendicular to the plane of the scapula; it may be anteverted or retroverted up to 10°, with 6° to 7° of retroversion most typical.[26] With anteversion, the glenoid fossa faces slightly anterior in relation to the plane or body of the scapula and, with retroversion, slightly posterior. The curvature of the surface of the glenoid fossa is greater in length than in width, with substantial variability between subjects.[28] The radius of curvature of the fossa is increased by articular cartilage that is thinner in the middle and thicker on the periphery, which improves congruence with the much larger radius of curvature of the humeral head [29]

The humerus is the distal segment of the GH joint. The humeral head has an articular surface that is larger than that of the proximal glenoid articular surface, forming one third to one half of a sphere.[2] As a general rule, the head faces medially, superiorly, and posteriorly with regard to the shaft of the humerus and the humeral condyles. An axis through the humeral head and neck in relation to a longitudinal axis through the shaft of the humerus forms an angle of 130° to 150° in the frontal plane (Fig. 7-22A).[2] This is commonly known as the **angle of inclination** of the humerus. In the transverse plane, the axis through the humeral head and neck in relation to the axis through the humeral condyles forms an angle that varies far more than other parameters but is usually described as approximately 30° posteriorly (Fig. 7-22B). This angle is known as the **angle of torsion.** The normal posterior position of the humeral head with regard to the humeral condyles may be termed **posterior torsion, retrotorsion,** or **retroversion** of the humerus.

Because of the internally rotated resting position of the scapula on the thorax, retroversion of the humeral head *increases* congruence of the GH joint by "turning" the humeral head back toward the glenoid fossa of the scapula (Fig. 7-23). Reduced retroversion (or anteversion) results in a more anterior position of the humeral head on the glenoid surface when the arm is in an anatomically neutral position (Fig. 7-24). Humeral

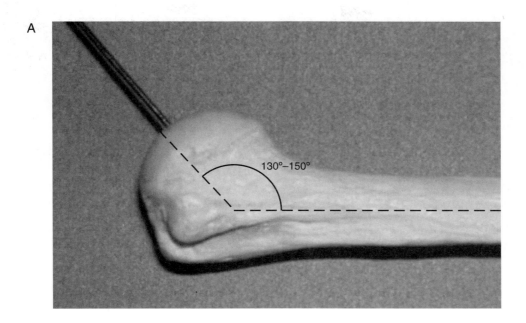

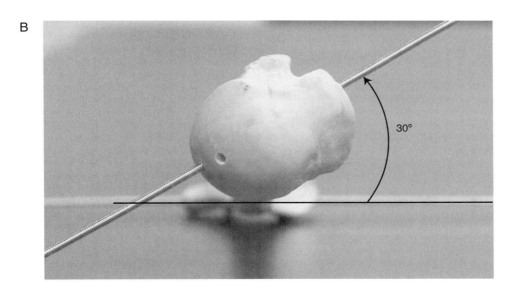

▲ **Figure 7-22** ■ **A.** The normal angle of inclination (the angle between the humeral head and the shaft) varies between 130° and 150°. **B.** The humeral head is normally angled posteriorly approximately 30° (angle of torsion) with regard to an axis through the humeral condyles.

anteversion can result in an increased range of medial rotation of the humerus and a reduced range of external rotation that places the humeral head at risk for anterior subluxation at the end range. Increased retroversion results in a more posterior position of the humeral head on the glenoid surface when the arm is in an anatomically neutral position (Fig. 7-25). Humeral retroversion can result in increased range of external rotation of the humerus and a reduced range of medial rotation that puts the humeral head at risk for posterior subluxation at end range. Increased GH external rotation and decreased GH medial rotation have been demonstrated in the dominant arm of throwing athletes, and evidence suggests that an increase in humeral retroversion may be one contributing mechanism for this ROM adaptation.[30,31]

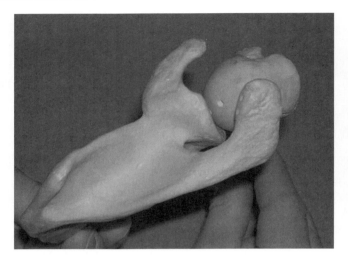

▲ **Figure 7-23** ■ The slightly retroverted angle of torsion turns and effectively centers the humeral head on the glenoid fossa of the scapula when the scapula is in its internally rotated resting position on the thorax and the humerus is in neutral rotation.

■ Glenoid Labrum

When the arms hang dependently at the side, the two articular surfaces of the GH joint have little contact. The majority of the time, the inferior surface of the humeral head rests on only a small inferior portion of the fossa [2,32,33] (see Fig. 7-21). The total available articular surface of the glenoid fossa is enhanced by an accessory structure, the **glenoid labrum.** This structure surrounds and is attached to the periphery of the glenoid fossa (Fig. 7-26), enhancing the depth or curvature of the fossa by approximately 50%.[34,35] Although the labrum was traditionally thought to be synovium-lined fibrocartilage, more recently it has been proposed that it is actually a redundant fold of dense fibrous connective tissue with little fibrocartilage other than at the attachment of the labrum to the periphery of the fossa.[36] The labrum superiorly is loosely attached,

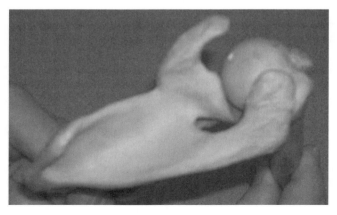

▲ **Figure 7-24** ■ Reduced retroversion or anteversion of the humerus places the humeral head anteriorly with regard to the glenoid fossa of the scapula when the scapula is in its internally rotated resting position on the thorax and the humerus is in neutral rotation.

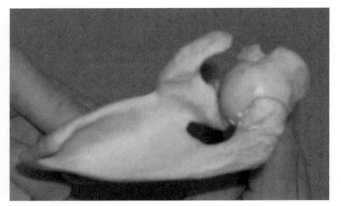

▲ **Figure 7-25** ■ Retroversion of the humerus places the humeral head posteriorly with regard to the glenoid fossa of the scapula when the scapula is in its internally rotated resting position on the thorax and the humerus is in neutral rotation.

whereas the inferior portion is firmly attached and relatively immobile.[37] The glenoid labrum also serves as the attachment site for the glenohumeral ligaments and the tendon of the **long head of the biceps brachii.**[38]

■ Glenohumeral Capsule and Ligaments

The entire GH joint is surrounded by a large, loose capsule that is taut superiorly and slack anteriorly and inferiorly in the resting position (arm dependent at the side) (Fig. 7-27). The capsular surface area is twice that of the humeral head.[39] More than 2.5 cm of distraction of the head from the glenoid fossa is allowed in the loose-packed position.[5] The relative laxity of the GH capsule is necessary for the large excursion of joint surfaces but provides little stability without the reinforcement of ligaments and muscles. When the humerus is abducted and laterally rotated on the glenoid fossa, the capsule twists on itself and tightens, making abduction and lateral rotation the close-packed position for the GH joint.[40] The capsule is reinforced by the **superior, middle,** and **inferior GH ligaments,** as well as by the **coracohumeral ligament** (Fig. 7-28). However, a thin area of capsule between the superior and the middle GH ligaments (known as the **foramen of Weitbrecht**) is a particular point of weakness in the capsule. Although the capsule is reinforced anteriorly by the **subscapularis** tendon(see Fig. 7-26), the foramen of Weitbrecht is a common site of extrusion of the humeral head with anterior dislocation of the joint.

The three GH ligaments (superior, middle, and inferior) vary considerably in size and extent and may change with age. Figure 7-26 shows the three ligaments as they appear on the interior surface of the joint capsule. Externally, the superior GH ligament passes from the superior glenoid labrum to the upper neck of the humerus deep to the coracohumeral ligament. Harryman and colleagues described the superior GH ligament, the superior capsule, and the coracohumeral ligament as interconnected structures that bridge the space between the **supraspinatus** and **subscapularis**

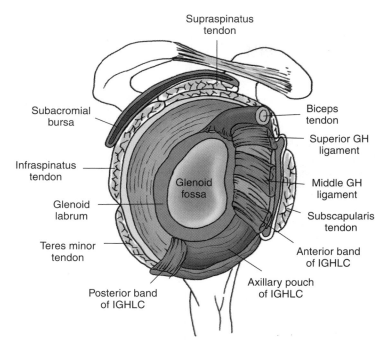

Supraspinatus tendon

Subacromial bursa

Infraspinatus tendon

Glenoid labrum

Teres minor tendon

Posterior band of IGHLC

Glenoid fossa

Axillary pouch of IGHLC

Biceps tendon

Superior GH ligament

Middle GH ligament

Subscapularis tendon

Anterior band of IGHLC

◄ **Figure 7-26** ■ In a direct view into the glenoid fossa (humerus removed), it can be seen that the glenoid labrum increases the articular area of the glenoid fossa and serves as the attachment for the GH capsule and capsular ligaments.

muscle tendons, forming what they described as the **rotator interval capsule**[41] (Fig. 7-29).

The middle GH ligament runs obliquely from the superior anterior labrum to the anterior aspect of the proximal humerus below the superior GH ligament attachment (see Figs. 7-26 and 7-28). This ligament blends with the anterior capsule but has also been found to be absent in up to 30% of subjects in several anatomic studies. The inferior GH ligament has been described as having at least three portions and thus has been termed the **inferior GH ligament complex (IGHLC)**.[42] The three components of the complex are the anterior and posterior bands and the axillary pouch in between (see Fig. 7-26). The IGHLC shows position-dependent variability in function,[43] as well as variations in viscoelastic behavior.[35]

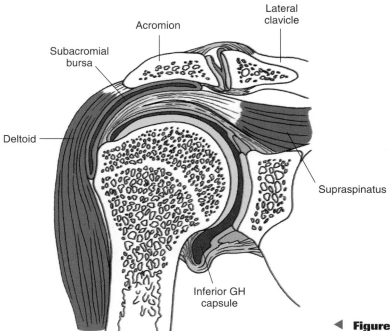

Acromion

Lateral clavicle

Subacromial bursa

Deltoid

Supraspinatus

Inferior GH capsule

◄ **Figure 7-27** ■ When the arm is at rest at the side, the superior capsule is taut, whereas the inferior capsule is slack.

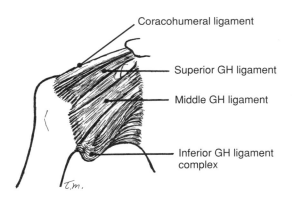

▲ **Figure 7-28** ■ The ligamentous reinforcements to the GH capsule: the superior, middle, and inferior GH ligaments, along with the coracohumeral ligament.

Numerous studies of the restraints provided by the GH ligaments indicate different contributions to GH stability. There appears to be reasonable consensus, however, that the superior GH ligament (and its associated rotator interval capsule structures) contribute most to anterior and inferior stability by limiting anterior and inferior translations of the humeral head when the arm is at the side (0° abduction) (Fig. 7-30A). The middle GH ligament contributes primarily to anterior stability by limiting anterior humeral translation with the arm at the side and up to 45° of abduction (see Fig. 7-30B). With abduction beyond 45° or with combined abduc-

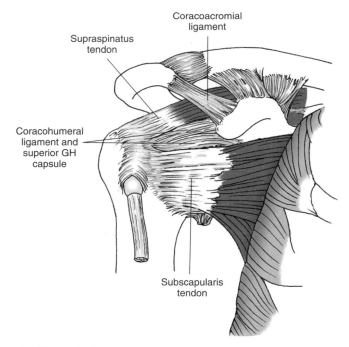

▲ **Figure 7-29** ■ The rotator interval capsule is made up of the superior GH capsule, superior GH ligament, and coracohumeral ligament. Together, these structures bridge the gap between the supraspinatus and subscapularis muscle tendons.

tion and rotation (see Fig. 7-30C), the IGHLC plays the major role of stabilization.[35,42-45] With abduction, the axillary redundancy or slack is taken up, and the IGHLC resists inferior humeral head translations. With subsequent humeral external rotation from an abducted position (see Fig. 7-30D), the anterior band of the IGHLC fans out to provide anterior stability and resistance to anterior humeral translation. With humeral abduction and medial rotation (see Fig. 7-30E), the posterior band of the IGHLC fans out and provides posterior stability and resistance to posterior humeral translation.[46] In all positions of humeral abduction, the capsule and GH ligaments tighten with rotation of the humerus, producing tension and consequently increasing GH stabilization.[47]

The coracohumeral ligament (see Fig. 7-29) originates from the base of the coracoid process and may be defined as having two bands. The first inserts into the edge of the supraspinatus and onto the greater tubercle, where it joins the superior GH ligament; the other band inserts into the subscapularis and lesser tubercle.[41,48] The two bands form a tunnel through which the tendon of the long head of the biceps brachii passes.[49] The location and interconnections of the ligament imply a fairly complex function. As part of the rotator interval capsule, it appears to be most important in limiting inferior translation of the humeral head in the dependent arm. However, there is some indication that it may also assist in preventing superior translation, especially when the dynamic stabilizing force of the rotator cuff muscles is impaired.[48] In addition, the coracohumeral ligament is usually reported as resisting humeral external rotation with the arm adducted.[2]

■ **Coracoacromial Arch**

The **coracoacromial** (or **suprahumeral**) **arch** is formed by the coracoid process, the acromion, and the coracoacromial ligament that spans the two bony projections (Fig. 7-31). Often the inferior surface of the AC joint is included as well. The coracoacromial arch forms an osteoligamentous vault that covers the humeral head and forms a space within which the subacromial bursa, the rotator cuff tendons, and a portion of the tendon of the long head of the biceps brachii lie. The coracoacromial arch protects the structures beneath it from direct trauma from above. Such trauma is relatively common and can occur through such simple daily tasks as carrying a heavy bag over the shoulder. The arch also prevents the head of the humerus from dislocating superiorly, because an unopposed upward translatory force on the humerus would cause the head of the humerus to hit the coracoacromial arch. As a consequence, however, the contact of the humeral head with the undersurface of the arch (while beneficially preventing dislocation) can simultaneously cause painful impingement or mechanical abrasion of the structures lying in the subacromial space. The supraspinatus is particularly vulnerable because of its passage beneath all of the potentially impinging superior structures except the coracoid (see Fig. 7-31).

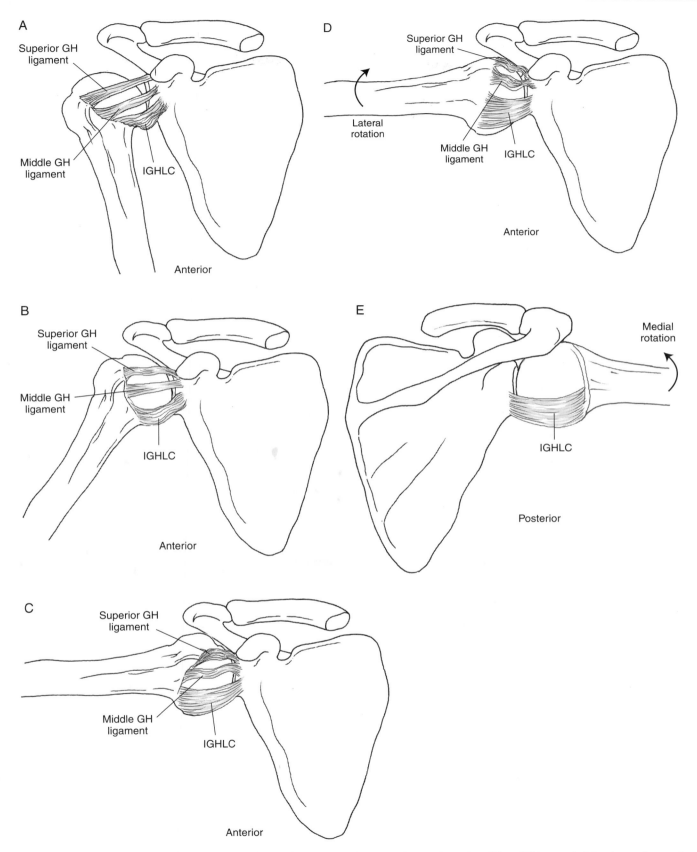

▲ **Figure 7-30** ■ The GH ligaments at rest (**A**); at 45° humeral abduction and neutral rotation (**B**); at 90° humeral abduction and neutral rotation (**C**); at 90° humeral abduction and external rotation (**D**); and at 90° humeral abduction and medial rotation (**E**).

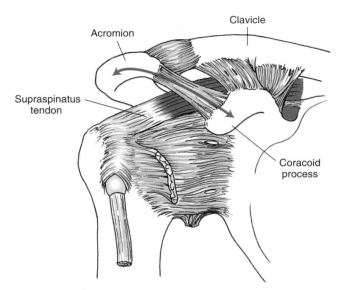

▲ **Figure 7-31** ■ The coracoacromial arch is formed by the coracoid process anteriorly, the acromion posteriorly, and the coracoacromial ligament superiorly. Together, these structures form an osteoligamentous arch over the humeral head.

The subacromial space, or area between the humeral head and coracoacromial arch, is also referred to as the suprahumeral space or supraspinatus outlet. Radiographically, this space has been quantified by measuring a superior-to-inferior acromiohumeral interval. This interval averages 10 mm in healthy subjects with the arm adducted at the side.[50] During elevation of the arm, this space decreases to about 5 mm.[51] The subacromial space must accommodate the soft tissue structures identified previously, as well as the articular cartilage and the capsuloligamentous structures. For this reason, Flatow et al. suggested that even during normal motion into humeral elevation, there is some contact of the rotator cuff structures beneath the anterior acromion.[51]

When the subacromial space is narrowed, the likelihood of impingement of the rotator cuff tendons and subacromial bursa during elevation of the arm increases. Narrowing of the space can be caused by anatomic factors such as changes in the shape of the acromion inferiorly, changes in the slope of the acromion, acromial bone spurs, AC joint osteophytes, a large coracoacromial ligament, or a size mismatch between the humeral head and area beneath the coracoacromial arch.[52,53] Abnormal scapular or humeral motions can also functionally reduce the size of the suprahumeral space. Inadequate posterior tipping or upward rotation of the scapula during arm elevation or abnormal superior or anterior translation of the humeral head on the glenoid fossa brings the humeral head and rotator cuff tendons in closer proximity to the humerus and increases the risk of impingement.[22,54,55] Finally, inflammation, fibrosis and thickening of the soft tissues can occur with repetitive impingement, further reducing the available subacromial space for clearance of the soft tissues during arm elevation. Abnormal anatomic factors and motion abnormalities have been identified in persons with impingement,[22,53–55] as well as a reduction in the available subacromial space during arm elevation.[56]

Continuing Exploration: **Symptoms of Impingement**

Ms. Sorenson reports shoulder pain localized to the proximal lateral humerus. This localization of pain is consistent with pain originating from the rotator cuff tendons, the long head of the biceps tendon, or the subacromial bursa. Her pain may be related to a rotator cuff or biceps tendonitis and possible shoulder impingement. Repetitive impingement can create tendonitis and progress to partial- and full-thickness rotator cuff tears.[53] In addition, she reports pain when sleeping on the right shoulder. This is a common complaint of persons with pain originating from the subacromial space. Additional compression of the humeral head into the subacromial space is experienced with lying on the affected side.

■ **Bursae**

In part because of the confined nature and proximity of structures in the subacromial space, several bursae are associated with the shoulder complex in general and with the GH joint specifically. The presence of bursae are indicative of the potential for frictional forces between structures. Although all bursae contribute to function, the most important are the **subacromial** and **subdeltoid** bursae (see Fig. 7-27). These bursae separate the supraspinatus tendon and head of the humerus from the acromion, coracoid process, coracoacromial ligament, and deltoid muscle. The bursae may be separate but are commonly continuous with each other. Collectively, the two are known as the subacromial bursa. The subacromial bursa permits smooth gliding between the humerus and supraspinatus tendon and surrounding structures. Interruption or failure of this gliding mechanism is a common cause of pain and limitation of GH motion, although it rarely occurs as a primary problem. The inferior wall of the subacromial bursa is also the superior portion of the supraspinatus tendon sheath. Subacromial bursitis is most commonly secondary to inflammation or degeneration of the supraspinatus tendon.[14] It is important to identify that, in the absence of inflammation, the bursa are merely layers of synovial tissue in contact with each other with a very thin layer of fluid between. When inflamed, the space occupied by the bursa increases. With an intact rotator cuff, the subacromial bursa does not communicate with the GH joint space.

■ **Glenohumeral Motions**

The GH joint is usually described as having three rotational degrees of freedom: flexion/extension, abduction/adduction, and medial/lateral rotation. The range of each of these motions occurring solely at the GH joint varies considerably. Flexion and extension occur about a coronal axis passing through the center of the humeral head. The GH joint is often considered to have 120° of flexion and about 50° of extension.[57] However, more recent work measuring three-dimensional GH motion reported peak humeral flexion of only 97° in relation to the scapula in a small sample of subjects averaging 50 years of age.[58] The higher values classically attributed to GH flexion may not have fully isolated GH motion from trunk and scapular motion.

Medial and lateral rotation occur about a long axis parallel to the shaft of the humerus and passing though the center of the humeral head. The range of medial/lateral rotation of the humerus varies with position. With the arm at the side, medial and lateral rotation may be limited to as little as 60° of combined motion.[58] Abducting the humerus to 90° frees the arc of rotation, with GH values reported to 120°.[2] The restricted arc of medial/lateral rotation when the arm is at the side may be related to different alignment of the greater and lesser tubercles, which creates a mechanical block, or to different areas of capsular or muscular tightness when the arm is adducted versus abducted.

Abduction/adduction of the GH joint occur around an A-P axis passing through the humeral head center. The maximum range of abduction at the GH joint is the topic of much disagreement. There is general consensus, however, that the range of abduction of the humerus in the frontal plane (whether done actively or passively) will be diminished if the humerus is maintained in neutral or medial rotation. The restriction to abduction in medial or neutral rotation is commonly attributed to impingement of the greater tubercle on the coracoacromial arch. When the humerus is laterally rotated 35° to 40°,[59,60] the greater tubercle will pass under or behind the arch so that abduction can continue.

The ROMs for abduction of the GH joint (if impact of the greater tubercle is avoided) are reported to be anywhere from 90° to 120°.[1,2,14,58,61,62] Inman and coworkers[10] found active abduction to be limited to 90° when the scapula did not participate in the motion but claimed that 120° of motion was available passively. Further increasing the variability between investigations, some studies examined the range of abduction in the traditional frontal plane, whereas others have investigated elevation in the plane of the scapula (30° to 45° anterior to the frontal plane). The available passive range for abduction in the scapular plane may be slightly greater than for abduction in the frontal plane.[60] When the humerus is elevated in the plane of the scapula (referred to as abduction in the plane of the scapula, scapular abduction, or **scaption** in clinical jargon), there is presumably less restriction to motion because the capsule is less twisted than when the humerus is brought further back into the frontal plane. An,[59] however, found maximum elevation not in the plane of the scapula but 10° to 37° anterior to that plane. Although it has been proposed that abduction in the scapular plane does not require concomitant lateral rotation to achieve maximal range, this premise has also been disputed.[59,60]

Intra-articular Contribution to Glenohumeral Motions

Full ROM of the GH joint is, to a reasonable degree, a function of the intra-articular movement of the incongruent articular surfaces. The convex humeral head is a substantially larger surface and may have a different radius of curvature than the shallow concave fossa. Given this incongruence, rotations of the joint around its three axes do not occur as pure spins but have changing centers of rotation and shifting contact patterns within the joint. There is a somewhat surprising lack of consensus on the extent and direction of movement of the humeral head on the fossa.[35] However, elevation of the humerus requires that the articular surface of the humeral head slide inferiorly (caudally) in a direction opposite to movement of the shaft of the humerus. Failure of the humeral articular surface to slide downwardly in abduction of the humerus would cause superior (cephalad) rolling of the humeral head surface on the fossa. The large humeral head would soon run out of glenoid surface, and the head of the humerus would impinge upon the overhanging coracoacromial arch (Fig. 7-32A). If, as it should, the articular surface of the head of the humerus slides inferiorly while the head rolls up the fossa, full ROM can be achieved (see Fig. 7-32B).

There is consensus that inferior sliding of the humeral head's articular surface is necessary to minimize upward rolling of the humeral head. However, it appears that the humeral head as a whole (its center of rotation) still moves somewhat superiorly (translates upwardly) on the glenoid fossa in spite of the downward sliding (Fig. 7-33), although the magnitude of reported upward shift differs among investigators.[35,54,60,63,64] The humeral articular surface may also slide anteriorly or posteriorly and medially or laterally on the glenoid fossa. The humeral head's center is believed to move slightly superior (1 to 2 mm of translation) until about 60° of active elevation motion.[27,54,63,64] With further elevation, the humeral head's center is believed to remain relatively stable and centered on the glenoid fossa. Less agreement exists with regard to anterior and posterior translations of the humeral head's center. Slight anterior positioning and translation (1 to 2 mm) has been reported during active elevation.[63] Other authors have

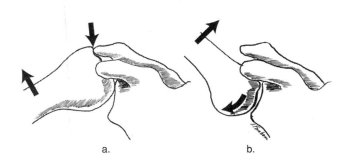

▲ **Figure 7-32** ■ **A.** Without downward sliding of the articular surface of the humeral head, the humeral head will roll up the glenoid fossa and impinge upon the coracoacromial arch. **B.** With downward sliding of the humeral head's articular surface as the humeral abducts, a full range of motion can occur without impingement.

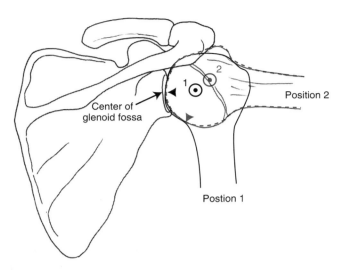

▲ **Figure 7-33** ■ Slight superior translation of the center of the humeral head can still occur during humeral abduction despite inferior sliding of the head's articular surface.

reported slight posterior translations early in the range or slight anterior translations early in the range and posterior translations from 60° to 120° of active elevation.[54,64] All studies of active translations show smaller magnitudes of motion (<5 mm) during active motions than is available in a passive laxity examination, in which translations up to 20 mm have been reported.[65] These data support the premise that rotator cuff forces help to stabilize and center the humeral head on the glenoid fossa. Most investigators also agree that many variables determine the patterns of movement of the humeral head on the glenoid fossa, including articular geometry, capsuloligamentous influences, influences of arm position, and muscle forces.

Much of the confusion surrounding reported motions of the humeral head on the glenoid fossa may be attributed to the differences in the point on the humerus that is being followed (combinations of rolling and sliding versus translations), as well as to the small magnitudes of these motions and the limitations of currently available measurement systems.

Continuing Exploration: **The Role of the Capsule**

The GH capsule and its associated GH ligaments provide stability to the GH joint by limiting anterior, inferior, or posterior humeral head translation on the glenoid fossa. The stabilizing function of these structures is minimal at less than 90° of humeral motion when only the superior segment of the capsule is under any significant tension. The blending of the rotator cuff tendons into the capsule and ligaments results in some ability to actively influence tension of the capsule and ligaments through muscle contraction. Toward the end range of humeral motion, however, the capsule becomes passively tight and has been demonstrated to actually produce rather than restrict humeral head center translations.[66] With asymmetrical tightening of the capsule,

this obligate translation occurs in a direction away from the tight and toward the loose capsular tissue.[66] For example, with increasing medial rotation, the posterior capsule becomes tight and produces anterior translation of the humeral head center that is not restricted by the relatively slack anterior capsule. A tight posterior capsule is, therefore, one potential mechanism for shoulder impingement, inasmuch as it may produce increased anterior humeral head translation and minimize the subacromial space.[54]

■ Static Stabilization of the Glenohumeral Joint in the Dependent Arm

Given the incongruence of the GH articular surfaces, the bony surfaces alone cannot maintain joint contact in the dependent position (arm hanging at the side). As the humeral head rests on the fossa, gravity acts on the humerus parallel to the shaft in a downward direction (caudally directed translatory force). This appears to require a vertical upward pull to maintain equilibrium. Such a vertical force could be supplied by muscles such as the deltoid, supraspinatus, or the long heads of the biceps brachii and triceps brachii. Basmajian and Bazant[25] and MacConaill and Basmajian[40] reported that all muscles of the shoulder complex are electrically silent in the relaxed, unloaded limb and even when the limb is tugged vigorously downward. The mechanism of joint stabilization, therefore, appears to be passive. The line of gravity (LoG) acting on the upper extremity (and extended through the humerus) creates a downward force on the humerus (and an inferiorly directed force on the humeral head). Given the magnitude of passive tension in the structures of the rotator interval capsule (superior capsule, superior GH ligament, and coracohumeral ligament) that are taut when the arm is at the side,[41,43,44] the resultant pull of both the LoG and the rotator interval capsule creates a line of force that compresses the humeral head into the lower portion of the glenoid fossa (Fig. 7-34), where the humeral head commonly sits when the arm is at the side.

In addition to the passive tension in the rotator interval capsule, two other mechanisms help provide static stability of the dependent arm. In a healthy GH joint, the capsule has an airtight seal, which produces negative intra-articular pressure. This pressure creates a relative vacuum that resists inferior humeral translation caused by the force of gravity.[43] Loss of intra-articular pressure, produced by venting the capsule or tears in the glenoid labrum, results in large increases in inferior humeral translations.[67,68] It has also been demonstrated that the degree of glenoid inclination influences the stability of the GH joint with the arm in the dependent position.[45] If there is a slight upward tilt of the glenoid fossa either anatomically in the structure of the scapula or through scapular upward rotation, the tilt of the fossa will produce a partial bony block against humeral inferior translation.

When the available passive forces are inadequate for static stabilization, as may occur in the heavily loaded arm, activity of the supraspinatus is recruited.[25] This is not surprising, given that the supraspinatus ten-

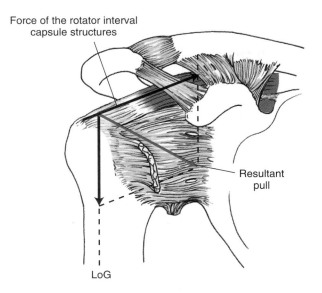

Force of the rotator interval capsule structures

Resultant pull

LoG

▲ **Figure 7-34** ■ Mechanism for stabilization of the dependent arm. With the arm relaxed at the side, the downward pull of gravity on the arm (vector extended from the center of gravity of the upper extremity) is opposed by the passive tension in the rotator interval capsule. The resultant of these opposing forces stabilizes the humeral head on the glenoid fossa.

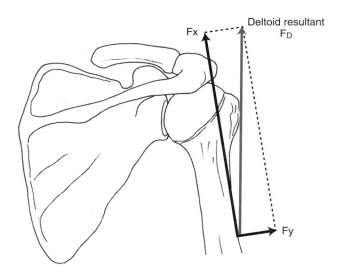

Fx

Deltoid resultant F_D

Fy

▲ **Figure 7-35** ■ The action line of all three segments of the deltoid follows the line of pull of the middle deltoid. The resultant (F_D) resolves into a very large translatory component (Fx) and a small rotatory component (Fy) so that an isolated contraction of the deltoid would cause the deltoid to produce more superior translation than does rotation of the humerus.

don has attachments to the rotator interval capsule.[48] In fact, the role of the supraspinatus may be more critical than its electromyographic (EMG) activity indicates. Although the supraspinatus may not be active when the arm is hanging at the side, paralysis or dysfunction in the supraspinatus may lead to gradual inferior subluxation of the GH joint. Without the reinforcing passive tension of the intact supraspinatus muscle, the sustained load on the structures of the rotator interval capsule apparently causes these structures to gradually stretch (become plastic), which results in a loss of joint stability. Although the subscapularis does not show activity in the loaded dependent arm, resting tension in this muscle may also, through its connections to the rotator interval, provide some support to those structures. Inferior GH subluxation is commonly encountered in patients with diminished rotator cuff function caused by stroke or other brain injury.

■ Dynamic Stabilization of the Glenohumeral Joint

The Deltoid and Glenohumeral Stabilization

It is generally accepted that the deltoid muscle is a prime mover (along with the supraspinatus) for GH abduction. The anterior deltoid is also considered the prime mover in GH flexion. Both abduction and flexion are elevation activities with many biomechanical similarities. The segment or segments of the deltoid that participate in elevation will vary with role and function.[69,70] However, examination of the resultant action line of the deltoid muscle in abduction can be used to highlight the stabilization needs of the GH joint in elevation activities. Figure 7-35 shows the action line of the deltoid muscle with the arm at the side. The action lines of the three segments of the deltoid acting together

coincide with the fibers of the middle deltoid. When the muscle action line (F_D) is resolved into its parallel (Fx) and perpendicular (Fy) components in relation to the long axis of the humerus, the parallel component directly cephalad (superiorly) is by far the larger of the two components. That is, the majority of the force of contraction of the deltoid causes the humerus and humeral head to translate superiorly; only a small proportion of force is applied perpendicular to the humerus and directly contributes to rotation (abduction) of the humerus.

At many other joints, a force component parallel to the long bone has a stabilizing effect because the parallel component contributes to joint compression. However, the articular surface of the humerus is not in line with the shaft of the humerus. Consequently, the force (Fx) applied parallel to the long axis of the bone creates a shear force (approximately parallel to the contacting articular surfaces) rather than a stabilizing (compressive) effect. The large superiorly directed force of the deltoid, if unopposed, would cause the humeral head to impact the coracoacromial arch before much abduction had occurred. The rotatory torque produced by the relatively small perpendicular component of the deltoid (Fy) will not be particularly effective until the translatory forces are in equilibrium. If the humeral head migrated upward into the coracoacromial arch, the inferiorly directed contact force of the arch would offset the Fx component of the deltoid, theoretically permitting rotation of the humeral head to continue. However, pain from impinged structures in the subacromial space is likely to prevent much motion. The inferior pull of gravity cannot offset the Fx component of the deltoid, because the resultant force of the deltoid must exceed that of gravity before any rotation can occur. That is, the deltoid cannot independently abduct (elevate) the arm. Another force or set of forces must be introduced to work synergistically with the deltoid for the deltoid to work effectively. This is the role of the muscles of the rotator, or musculo-tendinous, cuff.

The Rotator Cuff and Glenohumeral Stabilization

The supraspinatus, **infraspinatus, teres minor,** and sub-scapularis muscles compose the **rotator** or **musculo-tendinous cuff** (also referred to by the acronym **SITS** muscles). These muscles are considered to be part of a "cuff" because the inserting tendons of each muscle of the cuff blend with and reinforce the GH capsule. Of more importance, all have action lines that significantly contribute to the dynamic stabilization of the GH joint. The action lines of the four segments of the rotator cuff (the superiorly located supraspinatus, posteriorly located infraspinatus and teres minor, and the more anteriorly located subscapularis muscles) are shown in Figure 7-36. If any one or all three of the vector pulls of the infraspinatus, teres minor, or subscapularis muscles is resolved into its components (Fig. 7-37), it can be seen that the rotatory force component (Fy) not only tends to cause at least some rotation of the humerus, given its orientation to the long axis of the bone, but Fy also compresses the head into the glenoid fossa. This is an example of a rotatory component (rather than a translatory component) creating joint stabilization. This is due to the fact that the articular surface of the humerus lies nearly perpendicular to the shaft and provides a clear illustration of how a rotatory component may do more than "rotate" a bone around a joint axis.

Although the infraspinatus, teres minor, and sub-scapularis muscles of the rotator cuff are important GH joint compressors, equally (or perhaps more) critical to the stabilizing function of these particular muscles is the inferior (caudal) translatory pull (Fx) of the muscles. The sum of the three negative (inferior) transla-

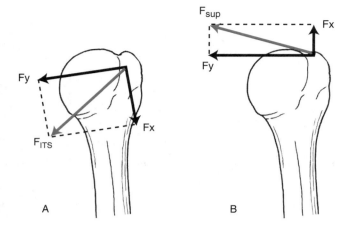

▲ **Figure 7-37** ■ **A.** The infraspinatus, teres minor, and sub-scapularis muscles individually or together have a similar line of pull. The rotatory component (Fy) compresses as well as rotates, and the translatory component (Fx) helps offset the superior translatory pull of the deltoid. **B.** The supraspinatus has a superiorly directed transla-tory component (Fx) and a rotatory component (Fy) that is more compressive than that of the other rotator cuff muscles and can independently abduct the humerus.

tory components of these three muscles of the rotator cuff nearly offsets the superior translatory force of the deltoid muscle. Sharkey and Marder[71] showed that abduction without the infraspinatus, teres minor, and subscapularis muscles resulted in substantial superiorly directed shifts in humeral position in cadaver models.

The teres minor and infraspinatus muscles, in addition to their stabilizing role, contribute to abduction of the arm by providing the external rotation that typically occurs with elevation of the humerus to help clear the greater tubercle from beneath the acromion. Although the weak adduction force of the teres minor muscle and the medial rotary force of the subscapularis muscle appear to contradict their role in elevation of the arm, Otis and colleagues[72] found the effectiveness of these muscles in their contradictory functions to be dimin-ished during abduction of the arm. That is, the infra-spinatus and subscapularis muscles added to the abduction torque, whereas the teres minor muscle added to the lateral rotatory torque. The medial and lateral rotatory forces also help center the humeral head in an anterior/posterior direction, with increased anterior and posterior displacements evident when rotator cuff forces are reduced.[73] Saha[28] referred to these cuff muscles as "steerers."

The action of the deltoid and the combined actions of the infraspinatus, teres minor, and subscapularis muscles approximate a force couple. The nearly equal and opposite forces for the deltoid and these three rotator cuff muscles acting on the humerus approxi-mate an *almost* perfect spinning of the humeral head around a relatively stable axis of rotation.

The Supraspinatus and Glenohumeral Stabilization

Although the supraspinatus muscle is part of the rota-tor cuff, the action line of the supraspinatus muscle,

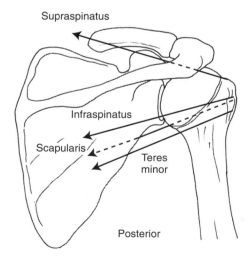

▲ **Figure 7-36** ■ The action line of the four segments of the rotator cuff: the supraspinatus, infraspinatus, teres minor, and sub-scapularis muscles.

unlike the action lines of the other three rotator cuff muscles, has a superior (cephalad) translatory component, rather than the inferior (caudal) component found in the other muscles of the cuff (see Fig. 7-37B). Given its line of pull, the supraspinatus is not able to offset the upward dislocating action of the deltoid.[74] The supraspinatus is still an effective stabilizer of the GH joint, however, because its rotatory component is proportionally larger than that of the other rotator cuff muscles. The more superior location of the supraspinatus results in an action line that lies farther from the GH joint axis than the action lines of the cuff muscles. The supraspinatus has a large enough moment arm (MA) that it is capable of independently producing a full or nearly full range of GH joint abduction while simultaneously stabilizing the joint.[40] Gravity acts as a stabilizing synergist to the supraspinatus by offsetting the small upward translatory pull of the muscle.

Continuing Exploration: **The Supraspinatus as an Independent Abductor**

The supraspinatus can, at least theoretically, independently produce abduction of the arm through most or all of its range, whereas the deltoid cannot. The resultant of the forces of a supraspinatus contraction and gravity is essentially identical to that which we saw in Figure 7-34. The action line of the supraspinatus is the same as that of the rotator interval capsule with which it blends (and to which it contributes passive tension at rest). With a concentric contraction of the supraspinatus, the proportionally small superiorly directly translatory force is offset by the inferiorly directed force of gravity, which results in linear equilibrium but effective rotation. The resultant of the gravitational and supraspinatus forces contributes to an inferior gliding of the humeral head surface during abduction of the arm, allowing full articulation of the joint surfaces and preventing abnormal superior displacement. The supraspinatus can also contribute small amounts of either medial or lateral rotation torque, depending on the position of the arm, although the MA for long axis rotation is very small.[75]

The Long Head of the Biceps Brachii and Glenohumeral Stabilization

The long head of the biceps brachii runs superiorly from the anterior shaft of the humerus through the bicipital groove between the greater and lesser tubercles to attach to the supraglenoid tubercle and superior labrum. It enters the GH joint capsule through an opening between the supraspinatus and subscapularis muscles, where it penetrates the capsule but not the synovium (Fig. 7-38). Within the bicipital groove, the biceps tendon is enveloped by a tendon sheath and tethered there by the **transverse humeral ligament** that runs between the greater and lesser tubercles. The long head of the biceps brachii, because of its position at the superior capsule and its connections to structures of the rotator interval capsule,[48] is sometimes considered

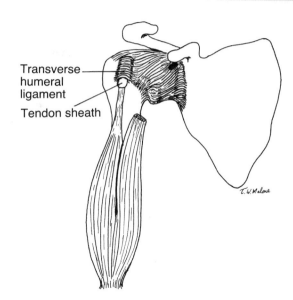

Transverse humeral ligament

Tendon sheath

▲ **Figure 7-38** ■ The long head of the biceps brachii passes through a fibro-osseous tunnel formed by the bicipital groove and the transverse humeral ligament. It is protected within the tunnel by a tendon sheath.

to be part of the reinforcing cuff of the GH joint. The biceps muscle is capable of contributing to the force of flexion and can, if the humerus is laterally rotated, contribute to the force of abduction and anterior stabilization.[10] Although elbow and shoulder position may influence its function, the long head appears to contribute to GH stabilization by centering the head in the fossa and by reducing vertical (superior and inferior) and anterior translations.[76–79] Pagnani and colleagues hypothesized that the long head may produce its effect by tightening the relatively loose superior labrum and transmitting increased tension to the superior and middle GH ligaments.[79] This concept follows from their observation that lesions of the anterosuperior labrum did not affect stability of the GH joint unless the attachment of the long head of the biceps brachii was also disrupted.[80] The overall contribution of the long head to GH stabilization is supported by the observation that the tendon hypertrophies with rotator cuff tears.[79]

 CONCEPT CORNERSTONE 7-2: *Dynamic Stabilization*

Given what we know about the GH joint thus far, we can summarize that dynamic stabilization at any point in the range is a function of (1) the force of the prime mover or movers, (2) the force of gravity, (3) the force of the muscle stabilizers, (4) articular surface geometry, and (5) passive capsuloligamentous forces. Inman and coworkers[10] appropriately added the factors of (6) the force of friction and (7) the joint reaction force, because any shear force within the GH joint creates some friction across its joint surfaces and because all forces that compress the head into the glenoid fossa must be opposed by an equal force from the glenoid fossa in the opposite direction (joint reaction force). Joint reaction forces can reach magnitudes of 9 to 10 times the weight of the upper extremity as the arm is elevated through muscular compression alone.[10,34] When the medially directed forces have slightly superior or inferior components, sheer forces are the result. The greatest sheer forces during humeral elevation typically occur between 30° and 60° of elevation.[34]

Costs of Dynamic Stabilization of the Glenohumeral Joint

When all stabilization factors are intact, the head of the humerus rotates into flexion or abduction around a relatively stable axis with minimal translation. Over time, however, even normal stresses resulting from the complex dynamic stabilization process may lead to degenerative changes or dysfunction at the GH joint. Any disruption in the synergistic action of the dynamic stabilization factors may accelerate degenerative changes in or around the joint.

The supraspinatus muscle is a particularly key structure in dynamic stabilization. The supraspinatus is either passively stretched or actively contracting when the arm is at the side (depending on load); it also participates in humeral elevation throughout the ROM. Consequently, the tendon is under tension most of a person's waking hours and is vulnerable to tensile overload and chronic overuse.[7] Mechanical compression and impingement of the stressed supraspinatus tendon can occur when the subacromial space is reduced by osteoligamentous factors, when there is increased superior or anterior translation of the humeral head center with less favorable GH mechanics, when the scapula does not posteriorly tip or upwardly rotate adequately during humeral elevation, or when occupational factors require heavy lifting or sustained overhead arm postures. The supraspinatus tendon is the most vulnerable of the cuff muscles. However, the overuse and potential impingement issues also apply to the other cuff muscles. Symptomatic and asymptomatic rotator cuff tears are seen in almost all people over the age of 70, with the supraspinatus likely to show lesions before the other tendons of the cuff.[81] Rotator cuff tendinitis or tears typically produce pain between 60° and 120° of humeral elevation in relation to the trunk. This range constitutes what is known as the **painful arc.** It is within this ROM that the tendons of the rotator cuff are passing beneath the coracoacromial arch. Beyond 120°, the tendons have rotated past the overlying arch structures.[82]

Case Application 7-2: **Supraspinatus Tendon Tears**

We have already noted that Susan Sorenson's symptoms are consistent with and may be related to subacromial impingement. She reports pain with elevation of the arm. Her job as a dental hygienist requires sustained elevation of her arms in the lower range of the painful arc (60° to 80°). Rates of shoulder pain consistent with rotator cuff involvement are higher than the norm for occupational groups that need to sustain such shoulder postures. Ms. Sorenson's past breast cancer treatment may also have altered the position of the scapula and the dynamic stabilization of the GH joint. Even a small amount of superior translation of the humeral head

may contribute to changes that occur in the pressure within the subacromial bursa as the humerus elevates, especially if the subacromial space is reduced by other factors. The increased subacromial bursa pressures are related to both arm position and load, with greater pressures in the bursa evident as the arms are loaded and maintained in an elevated position.[83] The increased pressure of the subacromial bursa, especially with a concomitant supraspinatus contraction as the arm elevates, may produce further narrowing of the subacromial space and may decrease blood supply to the supraspinatus tendon, where small anastomosing vessels are responsible for tendon nutrition.[14] Such restriction of blood supply may be one factor contributing to an increasing incidence of supraspinatus tendon tears from minor trauma with increasing age.[84] Supraspinatus tendon tears, however, are not attributable to the aging process alone but are considered multifactorial.

Degenerative changes in the AC joint may result in pain in the same area of the shoulder as pain from supraspinatus or rotator cuff lesions. Pain due to AC degeneration is more typically found when the arm is raised beyond the painful arc or when the arm is adducted across the body, compressing the AC joint surfaces.[85] The long head of the biceps brachii similarly can produce pain in the anterosuperior shoulder. Because the long head of the biceps tendon also passes directly beneath the impinging structures of the coracoacromial arch, it is subject to some of the same degenerative changes and the same trauma seen in the tendons of the rotator cuff. Whether the biceps is actively contributing to elevation of the arm or to joint stabilization or is passive, the tendon of the biceps must slide within the bicipital groove and under the transverse humeral ligament as the humerus moves around any of its three rotatory axes. If the bicipital tendon sheath is worn or inflamed, or if the tendon is hypertrophied (as often seen with rotator cuff tears), the gliding mechanism may be interrupted and pain produced. A tear in the transverse humeral ligament may result in the tendon of the long head popping in and out of the bicipital groove with rotation of the humerus, a potentially wearing and painful microtrauma.

Case Application 7-3: **AC Joint Degenerative Changes**

In addition to or instead of rotator cuff or biceps tendonitis or a partial rotator cuff tear, Ms. Sorenson's shoulder pain may be related to AC joint degeneration. Because of her history of an AC joint separation, she is more likely to have secondary AC joint degeneration.[20] If she has a painful arc of motion between 60° and 120° of elevation, this is more indicative of a rotator cuff or biceps primary source of pain, whereas pain later in the motion may be indicative of the AC degeneration as the primary source of pain.

Mechanical deviations in GH stabilization factors may result in injury to other structures of the joint besides the rotator cuff (e.g., the glenoid labrum) and to subluxation of the GH joint. Dislocation of the GH joint can also occur and is, in fact, the most frequently dislocated of all joints in the body. Capsuloligamentous and muscle reinforcement to the GH joint is weakest inferiorly, but it is most common for the GH joint to dislocate anteriorly because of the type of forces to which it is exposed. Although the subscapularis and the GH ligaments reinforce the capsule anteriorly, a force applied to an abducted, laterally rotated arm can force the humeral head through the foramen of Weitbrecht. A predisposition to GH subluxation or dislocation is multifactorial. Saha suggested that greatest susceptibility exists when individual structural variations are in the direction of (1) anterior tilt of the glenoid fossa in relation to the scapular plane, resulting in less of a mechanical block of the glenoid fossa to anterior translation; (2) excessive retroversion of the humeral head; or (3) weakened rotator cuff muscles.[28] Alternatively, Weiser suggested that scapular medial rotation results in less anterior humeral head translation and greater tension in the anterior capsule.[86]

Integrated Function of the Shoulder Complex

The shoulder complex acts in a coordinated manner to provide the smoothest and greatest ROM possible to the upper limb. Motion available to the GH joint alone would not account for the full range of elevation (abduction or flexion) available to the humerus. The remainder of the range is contributed by the scapula on the thorax through its SC and AC linkages. Combined scapulohumeral motion (1) distributes the motion between the joints, permitting a large ROM with less compromise of stability than would occur if the same range occurred at one joint; (2) maintains the glenoid fossa in an optimal position in relation to the head of the humerus, increasing joint congruency while decreasing shear forces; and (3) permits muscles acting on the humerus to maintain a good length-tension relation while minimizing or preventing active insufficiency of the GH muscles.

Scapulothoracic and Glenohumeral Contributions

The scapula on the thorax contributes to elevation (flexion and abduction) of the humerus by upwardly rotating the glenoid fossa 50° to 60° from its resting position.[11] If the humerus were fixed to the fossa, this alone would result in up to 60° of elevation of the humerus. The humerus, of course, is not fixed but can move independently on the glenoid fossa. The GH joint contributes 100° to 120° of flexion and 90° to 120° of abduction. The combination of scapular and humeral

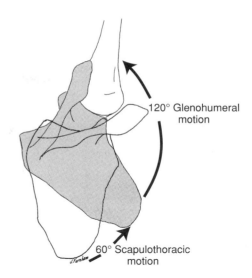

▲ **Figure 7-39** ■ When the total range of elevation is considered to be 180°, it is common to attribute 120° of the ROM to the humerus at the GH joint and 60° to the scapula on the thorax—with the two segments moving concomitantly rather than sequentially.

movement results in a maximum range of elevation of 150° to 180° (Fig. 7-39).[58,87] Some of the variability in ranges reported by investigators is due to individual structural variations (especially for the GH joint); another factor in variability may be the extent to which trunk contributions were isolated from humeral motions during the measurement. The *overall* ratio of 2° of GH to 1° of ST motion during arm elevation is commonly used, and the combination of concomitant GH and ST motion most commonly referred to as **scapulohumeral rhythm**. According to the 2-to-1 ratio framework, flexion or abduction of 90° in relation to the thorax would be accomplished through approximately 60° of GH and 30° of ST motion. It must also be recognized, however, that elevation of the arm is often accompanied not only by elevation of the humerus but also by lateral rotation of the humerus in relation to the scapula. During abduction of the humerus in the plane of the scapula, an average of 43° of lateral rotation from the resting position has been reported, with peak lateral rotation generally occurring between 90 and 120° of humeral elevation.[22]

The 2-to-1 ratio of GH to ST contribution to elevation of the arm is acknowledged to be an oversimplification, with substantial variability in scapular and humeral contributions at different points in the ROMs, and among individuals. The distinction must also be made between elevation of the arm from vertical and elevation of the arm relative to the trunk. The trunk may laterally flex or extend to gain additional range for the arm. However, we will consistently refer to elevation of the arm *in relation to the trunk* unless otherwise stated. As long as the trunk does *not* participate in the motion, the degree of elevation of the arm from vertical and elevation of the arm relative to the trunk will be the same.

CONCEPT CORNERSTONE 7-3: *Variations in Scapulohumeral "Rhythm"*

During the initial 60° of flexion or the initial 30° of abduction of the humerus, Inman and coworkers reported an inconsistent amount and type of scapular motion in relation to GH motion.[10] The scapula has been described as seeking a position of stability in relation to the humerus during this period (setting phase).[10,70] In this early phase, motion occurs primarily at the GH joint, although stressing the arm may increase the scapular contribution.[62] A number of studies have investigated this "rhythm," with ratios reported varying between 1.25:1 and 2.69:1.[27,28,61,62,88] Ratios are often described as nonlinear, indicating changing ratios during different portions of the ROM for elevation of the arm. The rhythm varies among individuals and may vary with external constraints.[88] Synchronous upward rotation of the scapula with GH elevation is certainly an important concept. However, the utility of the term "rhythm" seems limited because there does not appear to be a definitive scapulohumeral "rhythm" and because scapulohumeral "rhythm" provides limited insight into pathologies.

The scapula contributes to elevation of the arm not only by upwardly rotating on the thorax but also through other ST motions. Because of a number of differences between studies, the exact magnitudes of different scapular motions varies across studies. The general patterns of scapular motions, however, are relatively consistent. As the arm is elevated into flexion, scapular plane abduction, or frontal plane abduction, the scapula posteriorly tips on the thorax.[11,22–24] As the arm moves from the side to 150° of elevation, the magnitude of this motion is about 30°.[11] This posterior tipping allows the inferior angle of the scapula to move anteriorly and stay in contact with the thorax as it rotates upward and around the rib cage. Posterior tipping of the scapula also has the effect of bringing the anterior acromion up and back. This may serve to minimize reduction in the subacromial space as the humerus elevates.

During elevation, the scapula is, in general, externally rotating on the thorax.[11,22,24] External rotation of the scapula is important to maintaining the scapula, particularly the medial border, in contact with the thorax as the scapula upwardly rotates during arm elevation. Studies consistently report this motion of the scapula during frontal plane abduction of the humerus. The magnitude of external rotation during scapular plane abduction of the humerus, however, may be less. McClure and colleagues reported about 25° of external rotation of the scapula during abduction of the humerus in the plane of the scapula, most of which occurs at more than 90° of motion.[11] In flexion, the scapula initially protracts and internally rotates to orient the glenoid fossa anteriorly (in the sagittal plane). Studies describe slight internal rotation of the scapula early in the motion and less external rotation during the motion than occurs in other elevation activities.[11,24] Structural limitations or inability of muscles to appropriately stabilize the scapula may result in anterior tipping, internal rotation, and downward rotation of the scapula with attempted flexion of the arm (Fig. 7-40).

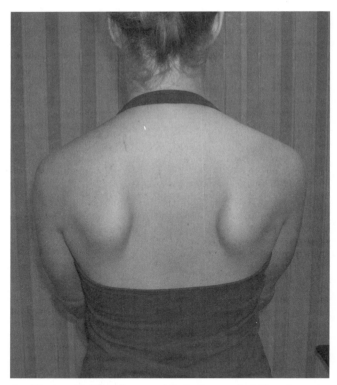

▲ **Figure 7-40** ■ Structural limitations or inability of muscles to appropriately stabilize the scapula may result in anterior tipping, internal rotation, and downward rotation of the scapula during elevation of the arm, lifting the inferior and medial angles of the scapula off the thorax.

Sternoclavicular and Acromioclavicular Contributions

Elevation of the arm in any plane involves motion of the SC and AC joints to produce ST joint motion, because the ST joint is part of a closed chain. Given the complexity of the linkages, there is no consensus on the relative contribution of the SC and AC joints to the 60° arc of upward rotation of the scapula as the scapula moves through its full ROM.

The initial ST upward rotation as the arm is flexed or abducted appears to be caused by clavicular elevation at the SC joint.[70] This scapular upward rotation occurs around an approximately A-P axis, passing through the costoclavicular ligament (SC motion) and projecting backward through the root of the scapular spine (ST motion) (Fig. 7-41). As elevation of the arm progresses, the ST axis of rotation gradually shifts laterally, reaching the AC joint in the final range of scapular upward rotation (Fig. 7-42). This major shift in the axis of rotation happens because the ST joint motion can occur only through a combination of motions at the SC and AC joints. When the axis of scapular upward rotation is near the root of the scapular spine, ST motion is primarily a function of SC joint motion; when the axis of scapular upward rotation is at the AC joint, AC joint motions predominate; and when the axis of scapular upward rotation is in an intermediate position, both the SC and AC joints are contributing to ST motion.

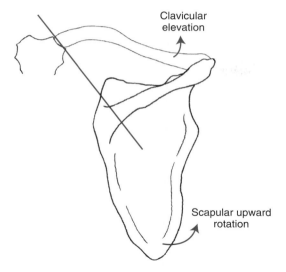

▲ **Figure 7-41** ■ With elevation of the arm, the scapulothoracic upward rotation contribution begins as elevation at the SC joint around an axis that appears to pass posteriorly from the costoclavicular ligament to the root of the spine of the scapula.

Inman and coworkers in 1944 described relative contributions of the SC and AC joint to ST upward rotation during arm elevation to be about 50% from SC elevation and 50% from AC upward rotation (20° to 30° each to obtain 50° to 60° upward rotation).[10] However, current three-dimensional descriptions of clavicular motion show only about 10° of clavicular elevation during arm elevation. If additional upward rotation of the

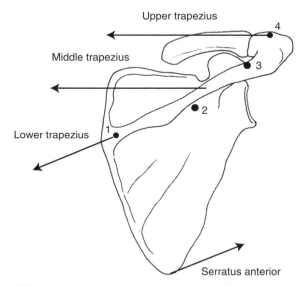

▲ **Figure 7-42** ■ At the initiation of scapular motion during elevation of the arm, the action lines of the upper trapezius, middle trapezius, and serratus anterior muscles combine to produce upward rotation of the scapula. The axis of scapular upward rotation progresses from its initial position (1) near the root of the scapular spine, laterally (2 and 3) to its final location near the AC joint (4) at the end of the motion. At the end of scapular upward rotation, the action lines of the upper trapezius and the extended vector of the lower trapezius pass close to axis 4; consequently, they have a reduced moment arm for contributing to upward rotation.

scapula is to occur at the AC joint, the limitation to AC motion imposed by the coracoclavicular ligament must be overcome. Tension in the coracoclavicular ligament (especially the conoid portion[7]) is produced as the coracoid process of the scapula gets pulled downward, with muscle forces attempting to upwardly rotate the scapula at the AC joint. The tightened conoid ligament pulls its posteroinferior clavicular attachment forward and down as the coracoid process drops, causing the clavicle to posteriorly rotate. Posterior rotation of the clavicle around its longitudinal axis will result in additional ST upward rotation (see Fig. 7-7). The ST upward rotation occurs both as the lateral end of the S-shaped clavicle flips up and as the tension in the coracoclavicular ligament is reduced, to permit upward rotation at the AC joint. The magnitude of posterior rotation of the clavicle may be anywhere from 30° to 55°.[7]

For the clavicle to rotate about its longitudinal axis, it appears to require mobility of both the SC and the AC joints. However, according to some authors, internal fixation of the AC joint does not significantly impair range of elevation, whereas attempted internal fixation of the SC joint most often results in extrusion of the fixating hardware.[7] As the ability to measure three-dimensional clavicular motion improves, our understanding of the contributions of these joints to ST motion will be enhanced.

Throughout elevation of the arm (flexion, scapular plane abduction, or frontal plane abduction), the clavicle also retracts at the SC joint, typically 20° to 25°, contributing to external rotation of the scapula on the thorax.[11] As the scapula adjusts to the differing contour of the rib cage, the AC joint allows varying amounts of anterior/posterior tipping and internal/external rotation, contributing to the overall ST motions previously described. The magnitudes of AC motion can be expected to differ among flexion, scapular plane abduction, and frontal plane abduction of the arm, as well as to differ with variations in scapular resting position, rib cage configuration, and muscle dynamics. Although the range varies somewhat, the component motions of the SC and AC joints are similar regardless of whether the motion is performed in the sagittal, scapular, or frontal planes. The other difference between performance of sagittal plane and frontal plane elevation is that the clavicle and scapula begin the flexion in less retraction and more internal rotation in order to bring the glenoid fossa forward, keeping the fossa in line with the shaft of the elevating humerus.

■ **Upward Rotators of the Scapula**

Although there might not be consensus (or consistency) in the way in which the SC and AC joints contribute to upward rotation of the scapula, there is agreement that the motions of the scapula are primarily produced by a balance of the forces between the **trapezius** and **serratus anterior** muscles through their attachments on the clavicle and the scapula (see Fig. 7-42). The upper portion of the trapezius muscle is attached to the clavicle and positioned to contribute directly to the initial elevation of the clavicle. The serratus anterior muscle makes its contribution to the combined clavicular and scapular motion through its action on the scapula. Given the hypothesized location of the axis for scapular upward rotation at the initiation of the motion (position 1), the middle trapezius may also contribute, although the serratus anterior muscle has a much greater MA. The lower portion of the trapezius muscle is not in a position to produce any upward rotational torque on the scapula during the initial stages of the motion.[89]

There are substantial implications for the large shift in the axis of rotation for scapular upward rotation with regard to muscle function. As the axis of rotation shifts laterally toward the AC joint (toward position 4 in Fig. 7-42), the upper and middle trapezius have progressively smaller MAs for ST upward rotation. Although the lower trapezius is classically described as an upward rotator, its action line appears to lie in line with or below the progressive axes for scapular rotation, which makes this segment of the trapezius either ineffective as an upward rotator or, in the latter stages of motion, a downward rotator of the scapula. The serratus anterior muscle maintains a large MA for ST upward rotation throughout the entire range of elevation.

Despite a line of action that is not contributory to ST upward rotation, the lower trapezius is clearly active during arm elevation and plays a role in the balance of forces to move and control the scapula on the thorax.[10] If the serratus anterior muscle acted in isolation, the lateral line of action would result in substantial lateral translation and less effective upward rotation of the scapula. The medial line of action of the trapezius offsets the lateral translatory action of the serratus and results in more effective upward rotation by the serratus.

Continuing Exploration: **Trapezius Function Reconsidered**

Johnson et al.[89] proposed lines of action for the trapezius muscle that differ from the traditional anatomic descriptions of muscle fiber orientation. Typically, the upper trapezius is shown with a superior and medial line of action on the scapula, and the lower trapezius with an inferior medial line of action (Fig. 7-43). Johnson et al. suggested, on the basis of cadaveric dissection, that the upper trapezius fibers act minimally on the scapula but more through elevation of the clavicle, thus indirectly upwardly rotating the scapula on the thorax. The middle trapezius would be capable of upwardly rotating the scapula with a small MA; this role would decrease as the axis of rotation approaches the AC joint later in elevation (see Fig. 7-42). Johnson et al. also suggested, on the basis of actual fiber orientation and cross-sectional area, that the lower trapezius action line should be directed more medially and less inferiorly. Subsequently, this muscle, as previously discussed, would have minimal if any MA to contribute to scapular upward rotation (see Fig. 7-42). These descriptions are consistent with Dvir and Berme's[70] model of shoulder function, which identifies the serratus ante-

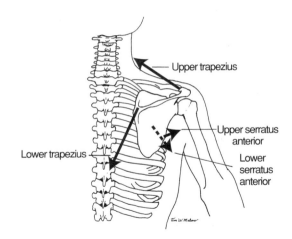

▲ **Figure 7-43** ■ Classically described action lines for the upward rotators of the scapula.

rior muscle as the prime mover of the scapula and the trapezius as the prime stabilizer.

The contribution of ST muscles to producing and controlling other ST motions (anterior/posterior tipping and internal/external rotation) is not well described. The serratus anterior muscle, with its insertions into the inferior angle and medial border of the scapula, plays a primary role in stabilizing the scapula to the thorax. Although the function of the serratus anterior muscle is classically considered to be production of scapular protraction, its line of action is capable of producing AC joint external rotation as it pulls the scapula laterally on the thorax. In fact, paralysis of the serratus anterior muscle is classically characterized by scapular "winging." The scapular winging is internal rotation of the scapula, produced by the remaining muscles without the stabilizing external rotation influence of the serratus. The serratus anterior muscle also has a large MA to produce posterior tipping of the scapula. The trapezius may have some ability to contribute to tipping or internal/external rotation torques in some positions of the arm; however, it would have relatively small MAs for these motions.

Structural Dysfunction

Completion of the range of elevation of the arm depends on the ability of GH, SC, and AC joints each to make the needed contribution. Disruption of movement in any of the participating joints will result in a loss of ROM. Once restrictions to function are introduced, the concept of scapulohumeral rhythm is altered; that is, a reduction in GH joint range will *not* result in a proportional decrease in ST range. The ratio of movement is no longer consistent because the body will likely recruit remaining motion at other joints. Although it is not necessarily predictable, restriction to motion at any one joint in the shoulder complex may result in the development of some hypermobility (and reduced stability) in remaining articulations.

Example 7-1

Glenohumeral Joint Hypomobility

If motion at the GH joint is restricted by pain or disease, the total range available to the humerus will be reduced. Whatever portion of the motion remains at the GH joint will still be accompanied by full ST motion. A restriction of the humerus, limiting GH joint abduction to approximately 60°, can combine with up to 60° of ST motion to provide a total available range of 120° as the arm is raised from the side.

Example 7-2

Sternoclavicular Joint Hypomobility

Hypothetical fusion of the SC joint would substantially minimize ST movement. Because both clavicular elevation and rotation occur through the SC joint, SC fusion would eliminate both contributors of scapular upward rotation. The arm would elevate only at the GH joint with limited contribution of AC joint upward rotation, because the clavicle could not posteriorly rotate to reduce coracoclavicular ligament tightness. It should be noted, however, that fixation of the very stable SC joint rarely occurs. In such an unusual instance, one would expect over time to develop hypermobility and increased instability of the AC joint.

Example 7-3

Acromioclavicular Joint Hypomobility

Although hypermobility and instability of the AC joint are more common, fusion of the joint generally occurs only through surgical fixation. With limited or no AC joint mobility within the closed chain of the AC, SC, and ST joint, motions of the clavicle at the SC joint (and therefore motions of the scapula on the thorax) would be limited. If the clavicle attempted to posteriorly rotate with a fused AC joint (and a fixed scapuloclavicular relationship), the clavicular rotation would force the inferior angle of the scapula into the thorax, and further motion would be checked. Mobility of the AC joint (relative anterior tipping) seems to be necessary to allow the clavicle to posteriorly rotate. Normal clavicular (and scapular) protraction at the initiation of flexion of the arm is also dependent on the ability of the AC joint to allow the scapula to internally rotate to orient the glenoid fossa anteriorly and to accommodate to the curvature of the thorax. If the scapula could not internally rotate at the AC joint as the clavicle and scapula protract, the glenoid fossa and lateral border of the scapula would press against the thorax and limit further protraction.

◆ Muscles of Elevation

Perry described elevation and depression as the two primary patterns of shoulder complex function.[90] Elevation activities are described as those requiring muscles to overcome or control the weight of the limb and its load. The completion of normal elevation depends not only on freedom of movement and integrity of the SC, AC, and ST joints but also on the appropriate strength and function of the muscles producing and controlling movement. A closer look at the activity of these muscles should enhance an understanding of normal function, as well as contribute to an understanding of the deficits seen in pathologic situations.

Deltoid Muscle Function

The deltoid is at resting length (optimal lengthtension) when the arm is at the side. When at resting length, the deltoid's angle of pull will result in a predominance of superior translatory pull on the humerus with an active contraction (see Fig. 7-35). With an appropriate synergistic inferior pull from the infraspinatus, teres minor, and subscapularis muscles, the rotatory components of the deltoid muscle are an effective primary mover for flexion and abduction. While the anterior deltoid is the prime mover for flexion, the anterior deltoid can assist with abduction after 15° of GH motion.[72] During abduction in the plane of the scapula, the anterior and middle deltoid segments are optimally aligned to produce elevation of the humerus.[31] The action line of the posterior deltoid has too small a MA (and too small a rotatory component) to contribute effectively to frontal plane abduction; it serves primarily as a joint compressor[32,69] and in functions such as horizontal abduction.

As the humerus elevates, the translatory component of the deltoid diminishes its superior dislocating influence as the action line shifts increasingly toward the glenoid fossa. At the same time, the rotatory component of the deltoid must counteract the increasing torque of gravity as the arm moves toward horizontal. Analysis by EMG shows gradually increasing activity in the deltoid, peaking at 90° of humeral abduction with a plateau for the remainder of the motion (Saha[28] found a peak at 120° with a drop-off to moderate activity at 180°). The peak activity in flexion does not occur until the end of the range and there is less total activity.[10,28] Although the MA of the deltoid gets larger as the humerus elevates[33] and the torque of gravity diminishes once the arm is above the horizontal, the high activity level of the deltoid continues. The shortening deltoid is not able to produce as much active tension and passive tension is diminished. As a result, a greater number of motor units must be recruited to maintain even equivalent force output. The multipennate structure and considerable cross section of the deltoid help compensate for the relatively small MA, low mechanical advantage, and less than optimal length-tension relationship.

Maintenance of an appropriate length-tension relationship of the deltoid is strongly dependent on simultaneous scapular movement or scapular stabilization. When the scapula is restricted and cannot upwardly rotate, the loss of tension in the deltoid with increased shortening results in achievement of only 90° of GH abduction (whether the supraspinatus is available for assistance or not).[2,10] If the scapular upward rotators (trapezius and serratus anterior muscles) are absent, the middle and posterior fibers of the activate deltoid (originating on the acromion and spine of the scapula) will act not on the heavier arm but on the lighter scapula; that is, without the stabilizing tension in the upward rotators, the middle and posterior deltoid will downwardly rotate the scapula (Fig. 7-44). Although the deltoid can still achieve the 90° of GH motion attributed to it when the scapular motion is restricted, the 90° occurs on a downwardly rotated scapula. The net effect of attempted abduction by the deltoid in the presence of trapezius and serratus anterior muscle paralyses is that the arm will rise from the side only about 60° to 75° (see Fig. 7-19).[91]

As we discussed earlier, effective deltoid activity also depends on intact rotator cuff muscles. With complete derangement of the cuff, a contraction of the deltoid results in a shrug of the shoulder (scapular upward rotation and upward translation of the humerus) rather than in abduction of the humerus from the side. Stimulation of the axillary nerve (innervating the deltoid and teres minor muscles alone) produces approximately 40° of abduction.[92] Partial tears in or partial paralysis of the cuff will weaken the rotation produced by the deltoid.

Supraspinatus Muscle Function

The supraspinatus muscle is considered an abductor of the humerus. Like the deltoid muscle, however, it func-

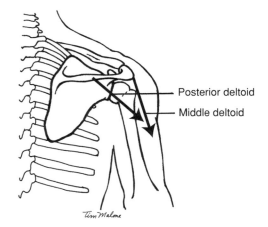

Posterior deltoid
Middle deltoid

Tim Malone

▲ **Figure 7-44** ■ Without the trapezius, the scapula rests in a downwardly rotated position as a result of the unopposed effect of gravity on the scapula. When abduction of the arm is attempted, the middle and posterior fibers of the activated deltoid—unopposed by the trapezius—will act on the lighter scapula to increase the downward rotatory pull on the scapula.

tions in all planes of elevation of the humerus. Its role, according to MacConaill and Basmajian,[40] is quantitative rather than specialized. The pattern of activity of the supraspinatus is essentially the same as that found in the deltoid.[10] The MA of the supraspinatus is fairly constant throughout the ROM and is larger than that of the deltoid for the first 60° of shoulder abduction.[32] When the deltoid is paralyzed, the supraspinatus alone can bring the arm through most if not all of the GH range, but the motion will be weaker. With a suprascapular nerve block that paralyzes the supraspinatus and the infraspinatus, the strength of elevation in the plane of the scapula is reduced by 35% at 0° and by 60% to 80% at 150°.[93] The secondary functions of the supraspinatus are to compress the GH joint, to act as a "steerer" for the humeral head, and to assist in maintaining the stability of the dependent arm. With isolated and complete paralysis of the supraspinatus muscle, or an isolated supraspinatus tear, some loss of abduction force is evident, but most of its functions can be performed by remaining musculature. Isolated paralysis of the supraspinatus is unusual, however, because its innervation is the same as the infraspinatus and related to that of the teres minor muscle. Most commonly, tears of the rotator cuff muscles do not remain isolated to the supraspinatus but extend to the infraspinatus or subscapularis, producing a more extensive deficit than seen with paralysis of the supraspinatus alone.

Infraspinatus, Teres Minor, and Subscapularis Muscle Function

When Inman and coworkers[10] assessed the combined actions of the infraspinatus, teres minor, and subscapularis muscles, EMG activity indicated a nearly linear rise in action potentials from 0° to 115° elevation. Activity dropped slightly between 115° and 180°. Total activity in flexion was slightly greater than that in abduction. In abduction, an early peak in activity of these muscles appeared at 70° of elevation. Steindler[2] hypothesized that the early peak was a response to the need for downward sliding of the humeral head, whereas the latter peak at 115° was a result of increased activity of these muscles in producing lateral rotation of the humerus. As noted earlier, the medial rotatory function of the subscapularis muscle diminishes with abduction,[72] serving instead to steer the head of the humerus horizontally while continuing to work with the other cuff muscles to compress and stabilize the joint.[28]

Upper and Lower Trapezius and Serratus Anterior Muscle Function

The upper trapezius and upper serratus anterior muscles form one segment of a balance of forces that drives the scapula in elevation of the arm. These two muscle segments, along with the levator scapula muscle, also support the shoulder girdle against the downward pull of gravity. Although support of the scapula in the pendant limb in many individuals is passive, loading the limb will produce activity in these muscles.[10,40] The second segment of the balance of forces is formed by the lower trapezius and lower serratus anterior muscles. When activity of the upper and lower trapezius and serratus anterior muscles was monitored by EMG during humeral elevation, the curves were similar and complementary. Activity in the trapezius rises linearly to 180° in abduction, with more undulating activity in flexion. The serratus anterior muscle shows a linear increase in action potentials to 180° in flexion, with undulating activity in abduction.[10] Saha found the upper and lower trapezius activity peaked and reached plateau before the end of the range, with some decrease in activity at maximal elevation.[28] The middle trapezius muscle is also active during elevation (especially abduction) and may contribute to upward rotation of the scapula early in the ROM.

Continuing Exploration: **EMG and Muscle Function**

EMG must be interpreted as only an indirect representation of muscle force production. If the length of the muscle is not held constant, an increase in EMG is not necessarily indicative of increased force production but, rather, may be increased activation to compensate for muscle shortening, as is proposed to be the rationale for increased end-range activity of the deltoid. Higher activation levels are commonly seen for muscles at the end ranges of motion, despite the necessity for peak torque production near the midrange of motion, at which gravitational resistance torques are often greatest. In addition, for increased EMG activation to relate to increased muscle force, the velocity of contraction and type of contraction (concentric, eccentric, isometric) must not be changing across comparison conditions.

EMG activity of a muscle during a specific motion does not define the function of the muscle. Often, muscles are active to offset unwanted translatory components of another muscle force, rather than to produce a primary rotational torque. This was seen previously with lower trapezius function and will occur additionally with rhomboid function during arm elevation.

In active abduction of the arm, the force of the trapezius seems more critical than the force of the serratus anterior muscle to ST motion. When the trapezius is intact and the serratus anterior muscle is paralyzed, active abduction of the arm can occur through its *full range,* although it is weakened. When the trapezius is paralyzed (even though the serratus anterior muscle may be intact), active abduction of the arm is both weakened and *limited in range* to 75°, with remaining range occurring exclusively at the GH joint[2] This active range of abduction is only slightly better than the range that can be obtained by the deltoid when neither of the upward rotators of the scapula are present (60° to 75°).[92] Without the trapezius (with or without the serratus anterior muscle), the scapula rests in a down-

wardly rotated position as a result of the unopposed effect of gravity on the scapula.

Case Application 7-4: **Trapezius Overuse**

Excess activation of the trapezius has been identified in some patients with shoulder impingement symptoms.[22] This can result in an imbalance of forces between the trapezius and serratus. The result can be a shoulder shrug type of motion when trying to elevate the arm and less efficient upward rotation of the scapula on the thorax. Prolonged overuse of the upper trapezius can result in muscle fatigue and pain in this muscle. The pain over the upper trapezius region that Ms. Sorenson reports may be related to an upper trapezius overuse pattern with arm elevation.

Although the trapezius seems to be more critical to upward rotation of the scapula in abduction, the serratus anterior muscle seems to be the more critical of the two muscles in producing scapular upward rotation during flexion of the arm. If the serratus anterior muscle is intact, trapezius muscle paralysis results in loss of force of shoulder flexion, but there is *no range deficit.* If the serratus anterior muscle is paralyzed (even in the presence of a functioning trapezius), flexion will be both diminished in strength and *limited in range* to 130° or 140° of flexion. When the scapular retraction component of the trapezius is unopposed by the serratus anterior muscle, the trapezius is unable to upwardly rotate the scapula more than 20° of its potential 60°.[2]

The role of the serratus anterior muscle in normal shoulder function appears to be essential in many aspects. This includes its being the only muscle capable of producing simultaneous scapular upward rotation, posterior tipping, and external rotation, the three component motions of the scapula that have been identified as occurring during elevation of the arm. The serratus also has the largest MAs of any of theST muscles, regardless of the changing ST axis of rotation. The serratus is the primary stabilizer of the inferior angle and medial border of the scapula to the thorax. Finally, reductions of serratus anterior muscle activation have been identified in patients with shoulder impingement,[26] which is further suggestive of the importance of this muscle to normal shoulder function.

The serratus anterior and trapezius muscles are prime movers for upward rotation of the scapula. These two muscles are also synergists for the deltoid during abduction at the GH joint. The trapezius and serratus anterior muscles, as upward scapular rotators, prevent the undesired downward rotatory movement of the scapula by the middle and posterior deltoid segments that are attached to the scapula. The trapezius and serratus anterior muscles maintain an optimal length-tension relationship with the deltoid and permit the deltoid to carry its heavier distal lever through full ROM. Thus, the role of the scapular forces of the trapezius and the serratus anterior muscles is both agonistic to scapular movement and synergistic with GH movement.

Rhomboid Muscle Function

The **rhomboid major** and **minor** muscles are active in elevation of the arm, especially in abduction. These muscles serve a critical function as stabilizing synergists to the muscles that upwardly rotate the scapula. If the rhomboids, downward rotators of the scapula, are active during upward rotation of the scapula, these muscles must be working eccentrically to control the change in position of the scapula produced by the trapezius and the serratus anterior muscles. Paralysis of these muscles causes disruption of the normal scapulohumeral rhythm and may result in diminished ROM.[2] Like the lower trapezius, the rhomboid muscles act primarily to offset the lateral translation component of the serratus anterior muscle.

◆ Muscles of Depression

Depression is the second of the two primary patterns of shoulder complex function.[90] Depression involves the *forceful* downward movement of the arm in relation to the trunk. If the arm is fixed by weight-bearing or by holding on to an object (e.g., a chinning bar), shoulder depression will move the trunk upward in relation to the arm. In depression activities, the scapula tends to rotate downward and adduct during the humeral motion, but there is not a consistent or overall ratio of movement of one segment in comparison with the other.

Latissimus Dorsi and Pectoral Muscle Function

When the upper extremity is free to move in space, the **latissimus dorsi** muscle may produce adduction, extension, or medial rotation of the humerus. Through its attachment to both the scapula and humerus, the latissimus dorsi can also adduct and depress the scapula and shoulder complex. When the hand and/or forearm is fixed in weight-bearing, the latissimus dorsi muscle will pull its caudal attachment on the pelvis toward its cephalad attachment on the scapula and humerus. This results in lifting the body up as in a seated pushup. When the hands are bearing weight on the handles of a pair of crutches, a contraction of the latissimus dorsi will unweight the feet as the trunk rises beneath the fixed scapula, allowing the legs to swing forward through the crutches. Some studies have found the latissimus dorsi muscle to be active in abduction and flexion of the arm.[27,28] Its activity may contribute to GH joint stability because the latissimus dorsi causes compression of the joint when the arm is above the horizontal.

The **clavicular portion** of the **pectoralis major** muscle can assist the deltoid in flexion of the GH joint, but the **sternal** and **abdominal portions** are primary depressors of the shoulder complex. The combined action of the pectoralis major's sternal and abdominal portions parallels that of the latissimus dorsi muscle, although the pectoralis is located anterior to the GH joint rather than posterior. In activities involving weight-bearing on the hands, the pectoralis major and the latissimus dorsi muscles in combination can depress the shoulder complex, while synergistically offsetting anterior/posterior movement of the humerus and protraction/retraction of the scapula. The depressor function of these muscles is further assisted by the **pectoralis minor** muscle, which directly depresses the scapula through its attachment on the coracoid process.

Teres Major and Rhomboid Muscle Function

The **teres major** muscle, like the latissimus dorsi, adducts, medially rotates, and extends the humerus. The teres major muscle is active primarily during resisted activities but may also be active during unresisted extension and adduction activities behind the back.[94] Function of the teres major muscle is strongly dependent on activity of the rhomboid muscles. The teres major muscle originates on the scapula and attaches to the humerus. Consequently, its proximal segment is lighter than the segment to which it attaches distally. The proximal scapular segment must be stabilized to permit the teres major muscle to act effectively as an extensor and adductor of the distal humeral segment. Without stabilization, the teres major muscle would upwardly rotate the lighter scapula rather than move

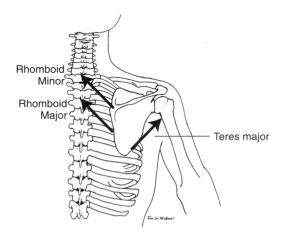

▲ **Figure 7-45** ■ In order for the teres major muscle to extend the heavier humerus rather than upwardly rotate the lighter scapula, the synergy of the rhomboid muscles is necessary to stabilize the scapula.

the heavier humerus (Fig. 7-45). The rhomboid muscles, as downward rotators of the scapula, offset the undesired upward rotatory force of the teres major muscle. By fixing the scapula as the teres major muscle contracts, the rhomboids allow the teres major muscle to move the heavier humerus. The rhomboids are assisted in stabilization of the scapula during humeral extension or adduction by the anteriorly located pectoralis minor muscle.

Continuing Exploration: **Breast Cancer and Radiation**

Standard treatment for breast cancer treated by breast-conserving therapy (lumpectomy) includes using two-field tangential radiation of the whole breast and chest wall.[95,96] Because of the contour of the rib cage, the ipsilateral pectoral muscles are generally included in the field. Radiation may be associated with release of certain cytokines and growth factors in exposed tissue cells that stimulate radiation-induced fibroblast proliferation, collagen deposition, and fibrosis,[97] with the potential to result in secondary muscular and soft tissue fibrosis.[96,98] A clinical consequence of muscular fibrosis may be increased passive resistance to stretch, including the pectoralis major and minor muscles. There is evidence of reduced shoulder ROM and impaired mobility at higher rates in patients after breast cancer treated with radiation than in patients who underwent treatments that did not include radiation.[99,100]

Case Application 7-5: **Patient Summary**

In addition to her contributing history of AC joint separation and her job requirements, Ms. Sorenson's treatment for breast cancer can be a contributing factor. The pectoralis major muscle is capable of producing medial rotation of the humerus and, indirectly, clavicular protraction. The pectoralis minor is capable of producing scapular downward rotation, internal rotation, and anterior tipping on the thorax. These motions are all antagonistic to motions of the scapula and humerus that must occur during normal arm elevation. Because of the attachment of the pectoralis minor muscle to the coracoid process and rib cage (Fig. 7-46), fibrotic changes and decreased extensibility as a result of radiation treatment could cause the muscle to limit scapular upward rotation, posterior tipping and external rotation, as well as clavicular retraction. Decreased extensibility in the pectoralis major could limit her ability to externally rotate the humerus as she elevates her arm. The reduced muscle extensibility may limit ROM. A subtle but potentially important effect may also be to increase the risk for impingement of the rotator cuff tendons and long head of the biceps brachii in elevation

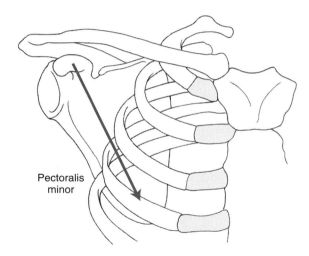

▲ **Figure 7-46** ■ The attachment of the pectoralis minor muscle to both the coracoid process of the scapula and the rib cage may limit the ability of the scapula to upwardly rotate, posteriorly tip, and externally rotate during elevation of the arm.

of the arm. The risk may be increased as a result of a decreased subacromial space because of the inability of the scapula to posteriorly tip and externally rotate to clear the acromion during elevation. The reduction in scapular upward rotation may also result in hypermobility of the GH joint, which increases the likelihood that the humerus will impinge on the coracoacromial arch. Furthermore, a restriction in lateral rotation of the humerus from pectoral major tightness may not allow the greater tubercle to adequately clear the acromion. These risk factors from potential muscle fibrosis, Ms. Sorenson's potential AC joint degenerative changes, and her need to maintain elevation of her arms for sustained periods of time during her workday may be multifactorial contributors to subacromial impingement and potential rotator cuff tearing.

Summary

In this chapter, we laid the foundation for understanding more distal upper extremity joint function by exploring the intricate dynamic stabilization of the shoulder complex. The more distal joints of the upper extremity depend on the dual mobility/stability roles of the shoulder complex. Whereas function in the hand, for instance, can continue on a limited basis with loss of shoulder mobility, loss of shoulder stability can render the remaining function in the hand unusable. In the next chapter, we will explore the elbow as the intermediary between the shoulder and the hand.

Study Questions

1. Identify the intra-articular motions of the SC for elevation/depression, protraction/retraction, and axial rotation.
2. What are the roles of the costoclavicular and interclavicular ligaments at the SC joint?
3. Discuss the relevance of the sternoclavicular disk to SC joint congruency, joint motion, and joint function.
4. Identify the scapular movements that take place at the AC joint.
5. Discuss the relevance of the coracoclavicular ligament to the AC joint function.
6. Discuss the configuration of the humerus and the glenoid fossa as they relate to GH joint stability. What role do the glenoid labrum and joint capsule play in joint stability?
7. What is the most frequent direction of GH dislocation? Why is this true?
8. Compare the relative stability and tendency toward degenerative changes in the GH, AC, and SC joints.
9. What are the advantages of the coracohumeral arch? What are the disadvantages?
10. What intra-articular motions must occur at the GH joint for full abduction to occur? What is the normal range? What range will be available to the joint if the humerus is not able to laterally rotate?
11. What muscle is the prime mover in shoulder GH flexion and abduction? What synergy is necessary for normal function of this muscle? Why?
12. Why is the supraspinatus able to abduct the shoulder without additional muscular synergy?
13. What accounts for the static stabilization of the GH joint when the arm is at the side? What happens if you excessively load the hanging (dependent) limb?
14. Identify five factors that play a role in the dynamic stabilization of the GH joint in either flexion or abduction of that joint.
15. What is the total ROM available to the humerus in elevation? How is this full range achieved?
16. How does the shape of the clavicle contribute to elevation of the arm?
17. What muscles are necessary to produce the normal scapular and humeral movements in elevation of the arm?
18. If the scapulothoracic joint were fused in neutral position, what range of elevation would still be available to the upper extremity actively?
19. What is the most common traumatic problem at the AC joint? What deficits is a person with this disability likely to encounter?
20. What are the consequences of a rupture of the coracoclavicular ligaments?
21. If the GH joint were immobilized by osteoarthritis, what range of elevation would be available to the upper extremity?
22. If isolated paralysis of the supraspinatus were to occur, what would be the likely functional deficit?
23. If the muscles of the rotator cuff were paralyzed, what would be the effect when abduction of the arm was attempted?
24. When there is paralysis of the trapezius and the serratus anterior muscles, what is the functional deficit when abduction of the arm is attempted?
25. If the deltoid alone were paralyzed, what would happen with attempted abduction of the arm? With attempted flexion of the arm?
26. What is the role of the rhomboids in elevation of the arm?
27. What differences would you see in attempted abduction if the trapezius alone were paralyzed, in comparison with paralysis of both the trapezius and the serratus anterior muscles?
28. What muscular synergy does the teres major muscle require to perform its function?
29. Describe why electromyographic activity of the deltoid in normal abduction shows a gradual rise in activity to between 90° and 120°, with a plateau thereafter.
30. Which of the joints of the shoulder complex is most likely to undergo degenerative changes over time? Which is least likely?

References

1. Dempster W: Mechanics of shoulder movement. Arch Phys Med Rehabil 45:49, 1965.
2. Steindler A: Kinesiology of the Human Body. Springfield, IL, Charles C Thomas, 1955.
3. Brossmann J, Stabler A, Preidler KW, et al.: Sternoclavicular joint: MR imaging—Anatomic correlation. Radiology 198:193–198, 1996.
4. Barbaix E, Lapierre M, Van Roy P, et al.: The sternoclavicular joint: Variants of the discus articularis. Clin Biomech (Bristol, Avon) 15(Suppl 1): S3-S7, 2000.
5. Williams P: Gray's Anatomy, 38th ed. New York, Churchill Livingstone, 1995.
6. Pronk G, van der Helm F, Rozendaal L: Interaction between the joints of the shoulder mechanism: The function of the costoclavicular, conoid and trapezoid ligaments. Proc Inst Mech Eng [H] 207:219–229, 1993.
7. Pratt N: Anatomy and biomechanics of the shoulder. J Hand Ther 7:65–76, 1994.
8. Sarrafian S: Gross and functional anatomy of the shoulder. Clin Orthop 173:11–18, 1983.
9. Conway A: Movements at the sternoclavicular and acromioclavicular joints. Phys Ther Rev 41: 421–432, 1961.
10. Inman B, Saunders J, Abbott L: Observations of function of the shoulder joint. J Bone Joint Surg Br 26:1, 1944.
11. McClure P: Direct 3-dimensional measurement of scapular kinematics during dynamic movements *in vivo.* J Shoulder Elbow Surg 10:269–277, 2001.
12. Fung M, Kato S, Barrance PJ, et al.: Scapular and clavicular kinematics during humeral elevation: A study with cadavers. J Shoulder Elbow Surg 10: 278–285, 2001.
13. Depalma A: Degenerative Changes in Sternoclavicular and Acromioclavicular Joints in Various Decades. Springfield, IL, Charles C Thomas, 1957.
14. Cailliet R: Shoulder Pain, 2nd ed. Philadelphia, FA Davis, 1991.
15. Sadr B, Swann M: Spontaneous dislocation of the sterno-clavicular joint. Acta Orthop Scand 50: 269–274, 1979.
16. Lee K-W, Debski RE, Chen CH, et al.: Functional evaluation of the ligaments at the acromioclavicular joint during anteroposterior and superoinferior translation. Am J Sports Med 25:858–862, 1997.
17. Debski R, Parsons IM 4th, Woo SL, et al.: Effect of capsular injury on acromioclavicular joint mechanics. J Bone Joint Surg Am 83:1344–1351, 2001.
18. Petersson C: Degeneration of the acromioclavicular joint. Acta Orthop Scand 54:434, 1983.
19. MacDonald P, Alexander, MJ, Frejuk, J, et al.: Comprehensive functional analysis of shoulders following complete acromioclavicular separation. Am J Sports Med 16:475–480, 1988.
20. Cox J: The fate of the acromioclavicular joint in athletic injuries. Am J Sports Med 9:50–53, 1981.
21. Turnbull J: Acromioclavicular joint disorders. Med Sci Sports Exerc 30:26–32, 1998.
22. Ludewig P, Cook T: Alterations in shoulder kinematics and associated muscle activity in people with symptoms of shoulder impingement. Phys Ther 80:276–291, 2000.
23. Ludewig P, Cook T, Nawoczenski D: Three-dimensional scapular orientation and muscle activity at selected positions of humeral elevation. J Orthop Sports Phys Ther 24:57–65, 1996.
24. van der Helm F, Pronk, G: Three-dimensional recording and description of motions of the shoulder mechanism. J Biomech Eng 117:27–40, 1995.
25. Basmajian J, Bazant F: Factors preventing downward dislocation of the adducted shoulder. J Bone Joint Surg Am 41:1182–1186, 1959.
26. Saha A: Dynamic stability of the glenohumeral joint. Acta Orthop Scand 42:490, 1971.
27. Poppen N, Walker P: Normal and abnormal motion of the shoulder. J Bone Joint Surg Am 58:195, 1976.
28. Saha A: Theory of Shoulder Mechanism: Descriptive and Applied. Springfield, IL, Charles C Thomas, 1961.
29. Soslowsky LJ, Flatow EL, Bigliani LU, et al.: Articular geometry of the glenohumeral joint. Clin Orthop 285:181–190, 1992.
30. Crocket H, Gross LB, Wilk KE, et al.: Osseous adaptation and range of motion at the glenohumeral joint in professional baseball pitchers. Am J Sports Med 30:20–26, 2002.
31. Reagan KM, Meister K, Horodyski MB, et al.: Humeral retroversion and its relationship to glenohumeral rotation in the shoulder of college baseball players. Am J Sports Med 30:354–360, 2002.
32. Poppen N, Walker P: Forces at the glenohumeral joint in abduction. Clin Orthop 135:165, 1978.
33. Walker P, Poppen N: Biomechanics of the shoulder joint during abduction on the plane of the scapula. Bull Hop Joint Dis 38:107, 1977.
34. Howell S, Galinat, B: The glenoid labral socket: A constrained articular surface. Clin Orthop 243:122–125, 1989.
35. Bigliani L, Kelkar R, Flatow E, et al.: Glenohumeral stability. Clin Orthop 330:13–30, 1996.
36. Moseley H, Overgaarde K: The anterior capsule mechanism in recurrent dislocation of the shoulder. Morphological and clinical studies with special references to the glenoid labrum and glenohumeral ligaments. J Bone Joint Surg Br 44:913, 1962.
37. Cooper D, Arnozcky S, O'Brien S: Anatomy, histology and vascularity of the glenoid labrum: An anatomical study. J Bone Joint Surg Am 74:46–52, 1992.
38. Beltran J, Bencardino J, Padron M, et al.: The middle glenohumeral ligament: Normal anatomy, vari-

ants and pathology. Skeletal Radiol 31:253–262, 2002.

39. Rothman R, Marvel J Jr, Heppenstall R: Anatomic considerations in the glenohumeral joint. Orthop Clin North Am 6:341, 1975.

40. MacConaill M, Basmajian J: Muscles and Movement: A Basis for Human Kinesiology. Baltimore, Williams & Wilkins, 1969.

41. Harryman DT, Sidles JA, Harris SL, et al.: The role of the rotator interval capsule in passive motion and stability of the shoulder. J Bone Joint Surg Am 74:53–66, 1992.

42. O'Brien SJ, Neves MC, Arnoczky SP, et al.: The anatomy and histology of the inferior glenohumeral ligament complex of the shoulder. Am J Sports Med 18:449–456, 1990.

43. Warner JJP, Deng X, Warren RF, et al.: Static capsuloligamentous restraints to superior-inferior translation of the glenohumeral joint. Am J Sports Med 20:675–685, 1992.

44. O'Connell PW, Nuber GW, Mileski RA, et al.: The contribution of the glenohumeral ligaments to anterior stability of the shoulder joint. Am J Sports Med 18:579–584, 1990.

45. Itoi E, Motzkin N, Morrey B, et al.: Scapular inclination and inferior stability of the shoulder. J Shoulder Elbow Surg 1:131–139, 1992.

46. Halder A, Itoi E, An KN: Anatomy and biomechanics of the shoulder. Orthop Clin North Am 31:159–176, 2000.

47. Gohlke F, et al.: The pattern of the collagen fiber bundles of the capsule of the glenohumeral joint. J Shoulder Elbow Surg 3:111–128, 1994.

48. Soslowsky L, Carpenter J, Bucchieri J, et al.: Biomechanics of the rotator cuff. Orthop Clin North Am 28:17–30, 1997.

49. Ferrari DA: Capsular ligaments of the shoulder. Am J Sports Med 18:20–24, 1990.

50. Petersson CJ, Redlund-Johnell I: The subacromial space in normal shoulder radiographs. Acta Orthop Scand 55:57–58, 1984.

51. Flatow E, Ateshian G, Soslowsky L, et al.: Computer simulation of glenohumeral and patellofemoral subluxation: Estimating pathological articular contact. Clin Orthop 306:28–33, 1994.

52. Meskers C, van der Helm FC, Rozing PM: The size of the supraspinatus outlet during elevation of the arm in the frontal and sagittal plane: A 3-D model study. Clin Biomech 17:257–266, 2002.

53. Zuckerman JD, Kummer FJ, Cuomo F, et al.: The influence of coracoacromial arch anatomy on rotator cuff tears. J Shoulder Elbow Surg 1:4–14, 1992.

54. Ludewig P, Cook T: Translations of the humerus in persons with shoulder impingement symptoms. J Orthop Sports Phys Ther 32:248–259, 2003.

55. Lukasiewicz A, McClure P, Michener L, et al.: Comparison of 3-dimensional scapular position and orientation between subjects with and without shoulder impingement. J Orthop Sports Phys Ther 29:574–583, 1999.

56. Graichen H, Bonel H, Stammberger T, et al.: Three-dimensional analysis of the width of the sub-acromial space in healthy subjects and patients with impingement syndrome. AJR Am J Roentgenol 172:1081–1086, 1999.

57. Norkin C, White D: Measurement of Joint Motion: A Guide to Goniometry, 2nd ed. Philadelphia, FA Davis, 1995.

58. Rundquist P, Anderson DD, Guanche CA, et al.: Shoulder kinematics in subjects with frozen shoulder. Arch Phys Med Rehabil 84:1473–1479, 2003.

59. An K-N: Three-dimensional kinematics of glenohumeral elevation. J Orthop Res 9:143–149, 1991.

60. Soslowsky L, Flatow E, Bigliani L, et al.: Quantitation of *in situ* contact areas at the glenohumeral joint: A biomechanical study. J Orthop Res 10:524–534, 1992.

61. Freedman L, Monroe R: Abduction of the arm in the scapular plane: Scapular and glenohumeral movements. J Bone Joint Surg Am 48:150, 1966.

62. Doody S, Waterland J: Shoulder movements during abduction in the scapular plane. Arch Phys Med Rehabil 51:595, 1970.

63. Graichen H, Stammberger T, Bonel H, et al.: Glenohumeral translation during active and passive elevation of the shoulder—A 3D open-MRI study. J Biomech 33:609–613, 2000.

64. Kelkar R, et al.: A stereophotogrammetric method to determine the kinematics of the glenohumeral joint. Adv Bioeng 22:143–146, 1992.

65. Harryman DT II, Sidles JA, Harris SL, et al.: Laxity of the normal glenohumeral joint: A quantitative *in-vivo* assessment. J Bone Joint Surg 1:66–76, 1990.

66. Harryman DT II, Sidles JA, Clark JM, et al.: Translation of the humeral head on the glenoid with passive glenohumeral motion. J Bone Joint Surg Am 72:1334–1343, 1990.

67. Gibb T, Sidles JA, Harryman DT II, et al.: The effect of capsular venting on glenohumeral laxity. Clin Orthop 268:120–127, 1991.

68. Habermeyer P, Schuller U, Wiedemann E: The intra-articular pressure of the shoulder: An experimental study on the role of the glenoid labrum in stabilizing the joint. Arthroscopy 8:166–172, 1992.

69. DeLuca C, Forrest W: Force analysis of individual muscles acting simultaneously on the shoulder joint during isometric abduction. J Biomech 6:385, 1973.

70. Dvir Z, Berme N: The shoulder complex in elevation of the arm: A mechanism approach. J Biomech 1:219, 1978.

71. Sharkey N, Marder R: The rotator cuff opposes superior translation of the humeral head. Am J Sports Med 23:270–275, 1995.

72. Otis J, Jiang C, Wickiewicz T, et al.: Changes in the moment arms of the rotator cuff and deltoid muscles with abduction and rotation. J Bone Joint Surg Am 76:667–676, 1994.

73. Wuelker N, Korell M, Thren K: Dynamic glenohumeral joint stability. J Shoulder Elbow Surg 7:43–52, 1998.

74. Wuelker N, Plitz W, Roetman B, et al.: Function of

the supraspinatus muscle. Acta Orthop Scand 65:442–446, 1994.

75. Ihashi K, Matsushita N, Yagi R, et al.: Rotational action of the supraspinatus muscle on the shoulder joint. J Electromyogr Kinesiol 8:337–346, 1998.

76. Itoi E, Kuechle D, Newman S, et al.: Stabilising function of the biceps in stable and unstable shoulders. J Bone Joint Surg Br 75:546–550, 1993.

77. Itoi E, Hsu HC, An KN: Biomechanical investigation of the glenohumeral joint. J Shoulder Elbow Surg 5:407–424, 1996.

78. Malicky D, Soslowsky L, Blasier R, et al.: Anterior glenohumeral stabilization factors: Progressive effects in a biomechanical model. J Orthop Res 14:22–288, 1996.

79. Pagnani M, Deng X, Warren R, et al.: Role of the long head of the biceps brachii in glenohumeral stability: A biomechanical study in cadavera. J Shoulder Elbow Surg 5:255–262, 1996.

80. Pagnani M, Deng X, Warren R, et al.: Effect of lesions of the superior portion of the glenoid labrum on glenohumeral translation. J Bone Joint Surg Am 77:1003–1010, 1995.

81. Gschwend N, Ivosevic-Radovanovic D, Patte D: Rotator cuff tear—Relationship between clinical and anatomopathological findings. Arch Orthop Trauma Surg 107:7–15, 1988.

82. Flatow EL, Soslowsky LJ, Ticker JB, et al.: Excursion of the rotator cuff under the acromion: Patterns of subacromial contact. Am J Sports Med 22:779–788, 1994.

83. Sigholm G, Styf J, Dorner L, et al.: Pressure recording in the subacromial bursa. J Orthop Res 6:123–128, 1988.

84. Ozaki J, Fujimoto S Nakagawa Y, et al.: Tears of the rotator cuff of the shoulder associated with pathological changes in the acromion. J Bone Joint Surg Am 70:1224–1230, 1988.

85. Kessel L, Watson M: The painful arc syndrome. Clinical classification as a guide to management. J Bone Joint Surg Br 59:166–172, 1977.

86. Weiser W, Lee TQ, McMaster WC, et al.: Effects of simulated scapular protraction on anterior glenohumeral stability. Am J Sports Med 27:801–805, 1999.

87. Barnes CJ, Van Steyn SJ, Fischer RA: The effects of age, sex, and shoulder dominance on range of motion of the shoulder. J Shoulder Elbow Surg 10:242–246, 2001.

88. McQuade K, Smidt G: Dynamic scapulohumeral rhythm: The effects of external resistance during elevation of the arm in the scapular plane. J Orthop Sports Phys Ther 27:125–133, 1998.

89. Johnson G, Bogduk N, Nowitzke A, et al.: Anatomy and actions of the trapezius muscle. Clin Biomech 9:44–50, 1994.

90. Perry J: Normal upper extremity kinesiology. Phys Ther 58:265, 1978.

91. Smith L, Weiss E, Lehmkuhl L: Brunnstrom's Clinical Kinesiology, 5th ed. Philadelphia, FA Davis, 1996.

92. Celli L, Balli A, de Luise G, et al.: Some new aspects of the functional anatomy of the shoulder. Ital J Orthop Traumatol 11:83–91, 1985.

93. Colachis S, Strohm B: Effects of suprascapular and axillary nerve block on muscle force in the upper extremity. Arch Phys Med Rehabil 52:22–29, 1971.

94. Basmajian J, DeLuca C: Muscles Alive, 5th ed. Baltimore, Williams & Wilkins, 1985.

95. Breast Cancer (PDQ)®: Treatment. Washington, DC, U.S. Department of Health and Human Service, National Cancer Institute, 2004. Accessed 10/11/04 at: http://cancernet.nci.nih.gov/cancertopics/pdq/treatment/breast/HealthProfessional/page7#Section_108.

96. Borger JH, Kemperman H, Smitt HS, et al.: Dose and volume effects on fibrosis after breast conservation therapy. Int J Radiat Oncol Biol Phys 30:1073–1081, 1994.

97. Basavaraju SR, Easterly CE: Pathophysiological effects of radiation on atherosclerosis development and progression, and the incidence of cardiovascular complications. Med Phys 29:2391–2403, 2002.

98. Lefaix JL, Daburon F, Martin M, et al.: [Gamma irradiation and delayed effects: Muscular fibrosis.] Pathol Biol (Paris) 38:617–625, 1990.

99. Chetty U, Jack W, Prescott RJ, et al.: Management of the axilla in operable breast cancer treated by breast conservation: A randomized clinical trial. Edinburgh Breast Unit. Br J Surg 87:163–169, 2000.

100. Ryttov N, Holm NV, Qvist N, et al.: Influence of adjuvant irradiation on the development of late arm lymphedema and impaired shoulder mobility after mastectomy for carcinoma of the breast. Acta Oncol 27:667–670, 1988.

Chapter 8

The Elbow Complex

Cynthia C. Norkin, PT, EdD

◆ Introduction

The joints and muscles of the elbow complex are designed to serve the hand. They provide mobility for the hand in space by apparent shortening and lengthening of the upper extremity. This function allows the hand to be brought close to the face for eating and grooming or to be placed at a distance from the body equal to the length of the entire upper extremity. Rotation at the elbow complex provides additional mobility for the hand. In conjunction with providing mobility for the hand, the elbow complex structures also provide stability for skilled or forceful movements of the hand when performing activities with tools or implements. Many of the 15 muscles that cross the elbow complex[1] also act at either the wrist or shoulder, and therefore the wrist and shoulder are linked with the elbow in enhancing function of the hand.

The elbow complex includes the elbow joint (humeroulnar and humeroradial joints) and the proxi-mal and distal radioulnar joints. The elbow joint is considered to be a compound joint that functions as a modified or loose hinge joint. One degree of freedom is possible at the elbow, permitting the motions of flex-ion and extension, which occur in the sagittal plane around a coronal axis. A slight bit of axial rotation and side-to-side motion of the ulna occurs during flexion and extension, and that is why the elbow is considered to be a modified or loose hinge joint rather than a pure hinge joint.[2] Two major ligaments and five muscles are directly associated with the elbow joint. Three of the muscles are flexors that cross the anterior aspect of the joint. The other two muscles are extensors that cross the posterior aspect of the joint.

The proximal and distal radioulnar joints are linked and function as one joint. The two joints acting together produce rotation of the forearm and have 1 degree of freedom of motion. The radioulnar joints are diarthrodial uniaxial joints of the pivot (trochoid) type and permit rotation (supination and pronation), which occurs in the transverse plane around a longitudinal axis. Six ligaments and four muscles are associated with these joints. Two muscles are for supination, and two are for pronation. The elbow joint and the proximal radioulnar joint are enclosed in a single joint capsule but constitute distinct articulations.

8-1	**Patient Case**

James Daly, a 40-year-old carpenter, has come into our clinic complaining of pain in his right lateral forearm. He says that he has experienced numerous episodes of pain in the same area over the past few years. Usually the pain has lessened, but not entirely disappeared, after a short rest period of 1 or 2 days. The current episode of pain is more severe than he has experienced in the past; it has continued for a much longer period of time and has not been relieved by a short period of rest. He reports that the pain is worse when he attempts to hammer, saw, or split wood for his wood stove. "Just lifting the chain saw causes pain."

We notice that James is holding his right elbow in considerable flexion. Palpation reveals tenderness in the area over our patient's right lateral epicondyle, common extensor tendon, and muscle belly of the one of the wrist extensors. Some tenderness also appears to be present along the path of the radial nerve. Active wrist and/or finger extension increases the pain in the lateral elbow area. A test of our patient's grip strength was attempted but not completed because of the degree of discomfort that James was experiencing.

Our task is to determine which structures are involved in producing our patient's pain. Once we identify the structure involved and make a diagnosis, we need to select the most appropriate treatment by examining the evidence regarding the effectiveness of various treatment options.

◆ Structure: Elbow Joint (Humeroulnar and Humeroradial Articulations)

Articulating Surfaces on the Humerus

The articulating surfaces on the anterior aspect of the distal humerus are the hourglass-shaped **trochlea** and the spherical **capitulum** (Fig. 8-1). These structures are situated between the medial and lateral humeral epicondyles. The trochlea, which forms part of the **humeroulnar articulation,** is set at an angle on the medial aspect of the distal humerus and lies slightly anterior to the humeral shaft. A groove called the **trochlear groove** spirals obliquely around the trochlea and divides it into medial and lateral portions. The medial portion of the trochlea projects distally more than the lateral portion and results in a valgus angulation of the forearm.

The indentation in the humerus located just above the trochlea is called the **coronoid fossa** and is designed to receive the coronoid process of the ulna at the end of elbow flexion range of motion (ROM). The capitulum, which is part of the humeroradial articulation, is located on the anterior lateral surface of the distal humerus. The capitulum, like the trochlea, lies anterior to the shaft of the humerus. A groove called

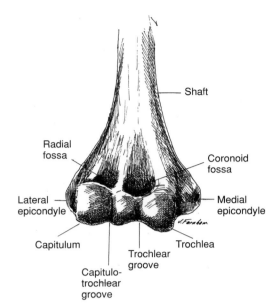

▲ **Figure 8-1** ■ Articulating surfaces on the anterior aspect of the right distal humerus.

the **capitulotrochlear groove** separates the capitulum from the trochlea (see Fig. 8-1). The indentation located on the humerus just above the capitulum is called the **radial fossa** and is designed to receive the head of the radius in elbow flexion. Posteriorly, the distal humerus is indented by a deep fossa called the **olecranon fossa,** which is designed to receive the olecranon process of the ulna at the end of elbow extension ROM (Fig. 8-2).

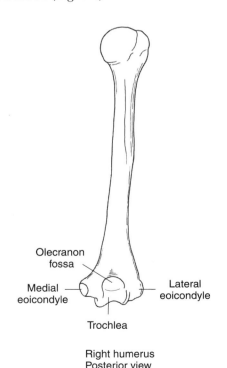

Right humerus
Posterior view

▲ **Figure 8-2** ■ The olecranon fossa on the posterior aspect of the distal humerus.

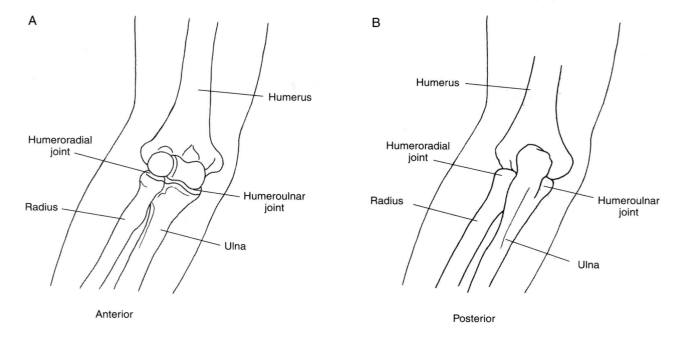

A

Humerus

Humeroradial joint

Radius

Humeroulnar joint

Ulna

Anterior

B

Humerus

Humeroradial joint

Radius

Humeroulnar joint

Ulna

Posterior

▲ **Figure 8-3** ■ **A.** Anterior aspect of the elbow joint. **B.** Posterior aspect of the elbow joint.

Articulating Surfaces on the Radius and Ulna

The articulating surfaces of the ulna and radius correspond to the humeral articulating surfaces (Fig. 8-3A and B). The ulnar articulating surface of the humero-ulnar joint is a deep semicircular concave surface called the **trochlear notch.** [3] The proximal portion of the notch is divided into two unequal parts by the **trochlear ridge,** which corresponds to the **trochlear groove** on the humerus (Fig. 8-4A). The ulnar coronoid process forms the distal end of the notch, whereas the olecranon process projects over the proximal end (see Fig. 8-4B). The radial articulating surface of the humeroradial joint is composed of the proximal end of the radius, known as the **head of the radius** (Fig. 8-5A). The radial head has a slightly cup-shaped concave surface called the **fovea** that is surrounded by a rim (see Fig. 8-5B). The radial head's convex rim fits into the capitulotrochlear groove.

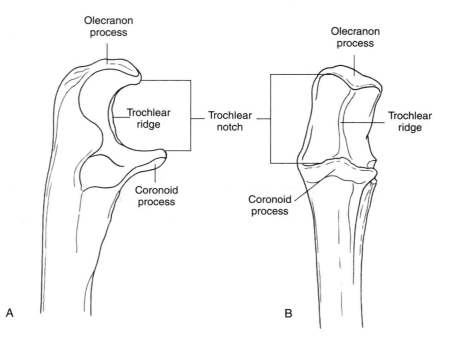

Olecranon process

Trochlear ridge

Trochlear notch

Coronoid process

Olecranon process

Trochlear notch

Trochlear ridge

Coronoid process

A

B

◄ **Figure 8-4** ■ **A.** Lateral view of the trochlear notch and ridge. The coronoid process forms the distal end of the trochlear notch and the olecranon process projects over the proximal end. **B.** Anterior view of the trochlear notch and ridge.

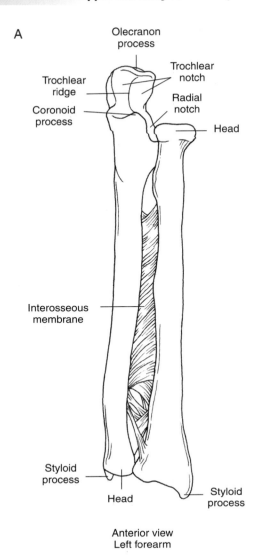

A

Olecranon
process

Trochlear
notch

Trochlear
ridge

Radial
notch

Coronoid
process

Head

Interosseous
membrane

Styloid
process

Head

Styloid
process

Anterior view
Left forearm

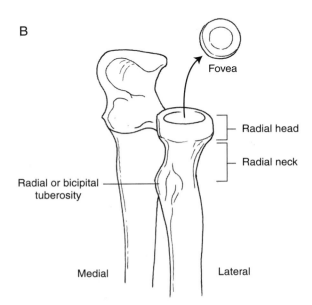

B

Fovea

Radial head

Radial neck

Radial or bicipital
tuberosity

Medial

Lateral

▲ **Figure 8-5** ■ A. Head of the radius. B. Fovea and rim.

Articulation

Articulation between the ulna and humerus at the humeroulnar joint occurs primarily as a sliding motion of the ulnar trochlear ridge on the humeral trochlear groove. In extension, sliding continues until the olecranon process enters the olcranon fossa (Fig. 8-6A). In flexion, the trochlear ridge of the ulna slides along the trochlear groove until the coronoid process reaches the floor of the coronoid fossa in full flexion[3] (see Fig. 8-6B).

Although the opposing articulating surfaces of the trochlear and trochlear notch appear to be completely congruent, experiments with cadaveric specimens have shown that the articulating surface of the trochlea does not contact the articulating surface at the bottom center of the notch unless the joint is heavily loaded.[4–7]

For example, Eckstein and colleagues[4] determined that at loads of 25 N (simulating resisted elbow extension), with the elbow positioned at 30° increments up to 120° of flexion, no surface contact occurred between the trochlea and the depths of the trochlear notch in all six elbow specimens studied (Fig. 8-7A). At a load of 500 N (approximately 112 lb), the articulating surface contact areas expanded from the sides toward the depths of the notch (see Fig. 8-7B).

Articulation between the radial head and the capitulum at the humeroradial joint involves sliding of the shallow concave radial head over the convex surface of the capitulum. The humeral capitulum is slightly smaller than the corresponding radial fovea, and so the joint surfaces are slightly incongruent.[8] In full extension, no contact occurs between the articulating surfaces (Fig. 8-8A). In flexion, the rim of the radial head slides in the capitulotrochlear groove and enters the radial fossa as the end of the flexion range is reached[9] (see Fig. 8-8B).

Joint Capsule

The humeroulnar and humeroradial joints and the superior radioulnar joint are enclosed in a single joint capsule (Fig. 8-9). Anteriorly, the proximal attachment of the capsule is just above the coronoid and radial fossae, and distally it is inserted into the ulna on the margin of the coronoid process. The capsule blends with the proximal border of the annular ligament except posteriorly, where the capsule passes deep below the annular ligament to attach to the posterior and inferior margins of the neck of the radius.[3] Laterally, the capsule's attachment to the radius blends with the fibers of the lateral collateral ligament (LCL). Medially, the capsule blends with fibers of the medial collateral ligament (MCL). Posteriorly, the capsule is attached to the humerus along the upper edge of the olecranon fossa.

The capsule is fairly large, loose, and weak anteriorly and posteriorly, and it contains folds that are able to unfold to allow for a full range of elbow motion. Laterally and medially, the capsule is reinforced by the

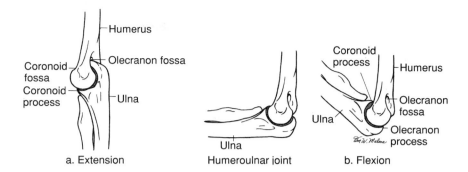

▲ **Figure 8-6** ■ Schematic representation of motions of the ulna on the humerus at the humeroulnar joint. **A.** In extension, the olecranon process enters the olecranon fossa. **B.** In flexion, the coronoid process reaches the coronoid fossa.

collateral ligaments. Fat pads are located between the capsule and the synovial membrane adjacent to the olecranon, coronoid, and radial fossae.[3]

The capsule's synovial membrane lines the coronoid, radial, and olecranon fossae. It also lines the flat medial trochlear surface and the lower part of the annular ligament. A triangular synovial fold inserted between the proximal radius and ulna partly divides the elbow joint into two joints.[3] Duparc et al.[10] found that in the majority of joints examined in 50 adult cadavers, the triangular synovial fold was located at the proximal radioulnar joint near the junction of the annular ligament and the joint capsule. The synovial folds varied from 1 to 4 mm in thickness, from 9 to 51 mm in length, and from 110 mm in width and contained fat pads and nerve fibers.[10]

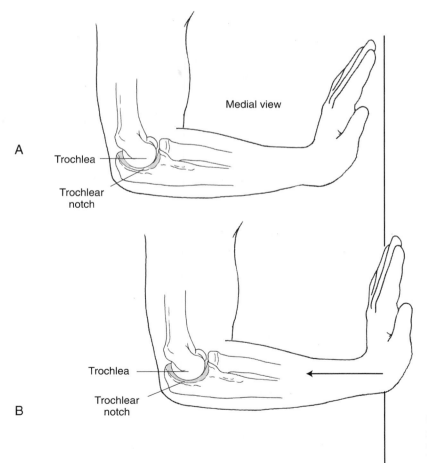

◀ **Figure 8-7** ■ **A.** No surface contact occurs between the trochlea and the center of the troclear notch from 30° to 120° of flexion. Contact is primarily on the sides of the notch under no-load conditions. **B.** Contact areas expand from the sides toward the center when a load is applied.

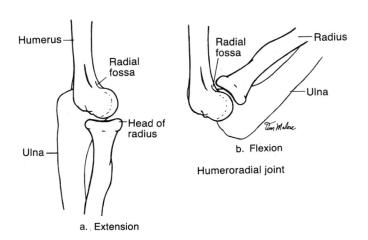

a. Extension

b. Flexion

Humeroradial joint

◀ **Figure 8-8** ■ Schematic representation of motions of the radius at the humeroradial joint. **A.** In full extension, there is no contact between the capitulum and the radial head. **B.** During flexion, the rim of the radius slides in the capitulotrochlear groove, and in full flexion, it reaches the radial fossa on the humerus.

Case Application 8-1: **Hypertrophied Synovial Fold**

Hypertrophied triangular synovial folds have been identified as a source of pain in cases of **lateral epicondylalgia** (pain in the region of the lateral epicondyle).[10] Therefore, it is possible that our patient's lateral elbow pain arises from irritation of the nerve fibers in a hypertophied triangular synovial fold.

Ligaments

Most of our knowledge of ligamentous functioning stems from tests on joint specimens that are subjected to various stresses. Initially, ligaments are intact during these tests, but subsequently they are sectioned or transected to determine the effects of the cutting on joint stability. On the basis of the results of the testing, researchers make judgments about the role or roles that a particular ligament plays at a joint.

Most hinge joints in the body have collateral ligaments, and the elbow is no exception. Collateral ligaments are located on the medial and lateral sides of hinge joints to provide medial/lateral stability to the joint and to keep joint surfaces in apposition. The two main ligaments associated with the elbow joints are the **medial (ulnar)** and **lateral (radial) collateral** ligaments.

■ Medial (Ulnar) Collateral Ligament

The MCL is considered to be the major soft tissue restraint of valgus stress at the medial aspect of the elbow. The elbow joint's normal valgus configuration subjects the medial aspect of the joint to a high degree of valgus stress, especially during throwing and golfing

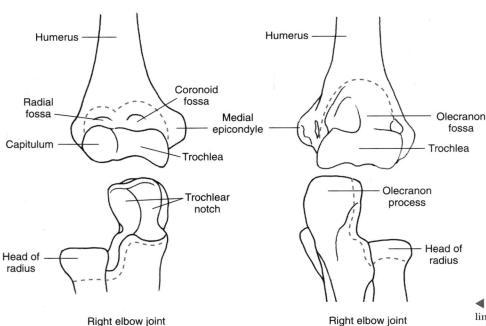

Right elbow joint
Anterior view

Right elbow joint
Posterior view

◀ **Figure 8-9** ■ The red dashed lines show the anterior and posterior attachments of the elbow joint capsule.

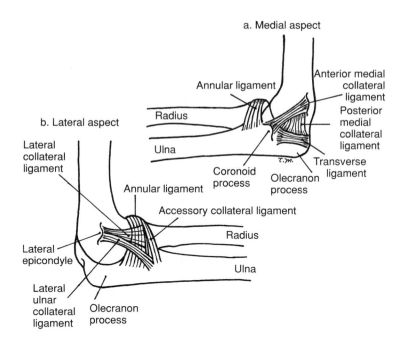

a. Medial aspect

Annular ligament

Anterior medial collateral ligament

Radius

Posterior medial collateral ligament

Ulna

Coronoid process

Olecranon process

Transverse ligament

b. Lateral aspect

Lateral collateral ligament

Annular ligament

Accessory collateral ligament

Radius

Lateral epicondyle

Ulna

Lateral ulnar collateral ligament

Olecranon process

◀ **Figure 8-10** ■ **A.** Three parts of the medial (ulnar) collateral ligament are shown on the medial aspect of the right elbow. The musculature and joint capsule have been removed to show the ligament's attachments. **B.** The lateral collateral ligament complex inlcudes the lateral (radial) collateral ligament, lateral ulnar collateral ligament, and annular ligament. The musculature and the joint capsule have been removed to show the ligaments' attachments.

activities. The MCL is described as consisting of two parts (anterior and posterior)[11-13] or three parts (anterior, oblique or transverse, and posterior)[14-17] (Fig. 8-10A). The anterior part of the MCL extends from the anterior aspect, tip, and medial edge of the medial epicondyle of the humerus to attach on the ulnar coronoid process. Mechanoreceptors (Golgi organs, Ruffini terminals, Pacini corpuscles, and free nerve endings) are densely distributed near the ligament's humeral and ulnar attachments.[18]

The anterior portion of the MCL is considered to be the primary restraint of valgus stress from 20° to 120° of elbow flexion.[19,20] Callaway and colleagues[17] described the composition of the anterior portion of the MCL as having an anterior band and a posterior band that tighten in a reciprocal manner as the elbow flexes and extends. The anterior band of the anterior portion was found by these authors to be the primary restraint of valgus at 30°, 60°, and 90° of flexion and the coprimary restraint up to 120°.[17]

The posterior part of the MCL is not as distinct as the anterior part, and sometimes its fibers blend with the fibers from the medial portion of the joint capsule. The posterior portion of the MCL extends from the posterior aspect of the medial epicondyle of the humerus to attach to the ulnar coronoid and olecranon processes. The posterior MCL limits elbow extension but plays a less significant role than the anterior MCL in providing valgus stability for the elbow.[19,20]

The oblique (transverse) fibers of the MCL extend between the olecranon and ulnar coronoid processes. This portion of the ligament assists in providing valgus stability and helps to keep the joint surfaces in approximation.

CONCEPT CORNERSTONE 8-1: *Functional Summary for Medial Collateral Ligament*

1. stabilizes the elbow against valgus torques[17-20]
2. limits extension at the end of the elbow extension ROM[11,12]
3. guides joint motion throughout flexion ROM[11]
4. provides some resistance to longitudinal distraction of joint surfaces.

■ **Lateral (Radial) Collateral Ligamentous Complex**

The lateral collateral ligamentous complex includes the LCL, the lateral ulnar collateral ligament (LUCL),[12,14,21] and the annular ligament[22] (see Fig. 8-10B). The LCL is a fan-shaped structure that extends from the inferior aspect of the lateral epicondyle of the humerus to attach to the annular ligament (the ligament encircling the head of the radius) and to the olecranon process. Ligamentous tissue extending from the lateral epicondyle to the lateral aspect of the ulnar and the annular ligament is referred to as the LUCL.[12] The LUCL adheres closely to the supinator, extensor, and anconeus muscles and lies just posterior to the LCL.[23]

Certain functions are attributed to individual ligaments in the complex, and other functions are thought to be the result of the entire complex. The LCL provides reinforcement for the humeroradial articulation, offers some protection against varus stress in some positions of the elbow, and assists in providing resistance to longitudinal distraction of the joint surfaces.[24] Some fibers of the LCL remain taut throughout the flexion ROM when either a varus or valgus moment is applied.[12] O'Driscoll[25] described the LCL as a key structure that is always disrupted in elbow dislocations.

Olsen and colleagues[26] concluded that the LCL was the primary soft tissue restraint and the LUCL and the annular ligament were secondary restraints to combined forced varus and supination stresses and forced valgus stress. The authors found that sectioning either the LUCL or annular ligament resulted in either no or minor (2°) laxity during forced varus stress and supination and a 4° laxity in forced valgus stress. However, sectioning of the LCL led to a maximum laxity of 15.4° during forced varus stress and supination and 23° in forced valgus stress.[26]

It appears that the LUCL has the potential for assisting the LCL in resisting varus stress at the elbow and assisting in providing lateral support to the elbow joint.[27] Imatani and colleagues[23] suggested that the LUCL is not a major restraint but contributes to posterolateral stability by securing the ulna to the humerus. Also, it may provide support to the annular ligament. Kim and associates[28] suggested that the LUCL is not a static stabilizer but acts as a dynamic stabilizer together with related muscles.

Continuing Exploration: **Controversy Regarding the Roles of the LCL, the LUCL, and the Annular Ligament**

Dunning and coworkers[29] found that when the annular ligament was intact, either the LCL or the LUCL could be transected without causing posterolateral rotatory instability. In contrast, Hannouche and Begue[30] found that subluxation of the humeroulnar joint occurred either when the anterior and medial bundles of the LCL were sectioned at their humeral attachment or when the medial bundle and annular ligament were sectioned at their ulnar insertion. The authors concluded that posterolateral instability is largely maintained by the anterior and medial bundles of the LCL and the annular ligament.

 Concept Cornerstone 8-2: *Functional Summary for Lateral Collateral Ligamentous Complex*

1. stabilizes elbow against varus torque[21,22,24,26]
2. stabilizes against combined varus and supination torques[21,22,26]
3. reinforces humeroradial joint and assists in providing some resistance to longitudinal distraction of the articulating surfaces[24]
4. stabilizes radial head, thus providing a stable base for rotation[26]
5. maintains posterolateral rotatory stability[22,23,27,29-31]
6. prevents subluxation of humeroulnar joint by securing ulna to humerus
7. prevents forearm from rotating off of the humerus in valgus and supination during flexion from fully extended position

---

Case Application 8-2: **LCL Complex**

It is possible that either the LCL or LUCL has been overstretched and incurred some microtrauma, which could be a source of our patient's pain. Both ligaments are attached to the joint capsule, which has free nerve endings and mechanoreceptors distributed near the humeral and ulnar capsular attachments.[18] Isolated tears of the LCL are uncommon, but chronic insufficiency may lead to symptomatic posterolateral joint subluxation.[31] Complete disruption of the LCL complex is most often seen in fracture dislocations and fractures involving the coronoid or radial head.[32] If our patient James were experiencing painful clicking or locking of the elbow, the clinician might suspect posterolateral instability and conduct the appropriate manual tests, as well as requesting stress x-rays.[25] However, we have no reason to suspect posterolateral instability or a fracture or dislocation, because our patient has not complained of any painful clicking or locking of the elbow. Therefore, we can probably rule out complete disruption of the LCL as a source of his pain. Furthermore, complete disruptions of the lateral ligaments usually occur as a result of a fall in which the radius is fractured, and our patient has no history of a fall. Some amount of stretching and microtrauma involving one of the structures in the LCL complex could still be present and difficult to diagnose because microscopic tears and partial disruption of fibers might not cause observable instability.

Muscles

Nine muscles cross the anterior aspect of the elbow joint, but only three of these muscles (the **brachialis, biceps brachii,** and **brachioradialis**) have primary functions at the elbow joint. The **supinator teres** and **pronator teres** have major functions at the radiolunar joints. The remaining four muscles (**flexor carpi radialis, flexor carpi ulnaris, flexor digitorum superficialis,** and **palmaris longus**), which arise by a common tendon from the medial epicondyle of the humerus, have primary functions at other joints, including the wrist, hand, and fingers, but are considered to be weak flexors of the elbow (Fig. 8-11A).

The major flexors of the elbow are the brachialis, the biceps brachii, and the brachioradialis. The brachialis muscle arises from the anterior surface of the lower portion of the humeral shaft and attaches by a thick, broad tendon to the ulnar tuberosity and coronoid process. The biceps brachii arises from two heads, one short and the other long. The short head arises as a thick, flat tendon from the coracoid process of the scapula, and the long head arises as a long, narrow tendon from the scapula's supraglenoid tubercle. The muscle fibers arising from the two tendons unite in the middle of the upper arm to form the prominent muscle bulk of the upper arm. Muscle fibers from both heads insert by way of the strong flattened tendon on the rough posterior area of the tuberosity of the radius. Other fibers of the biceps brachii insert into the bicipital aponeurosis that extends medially to blend with the

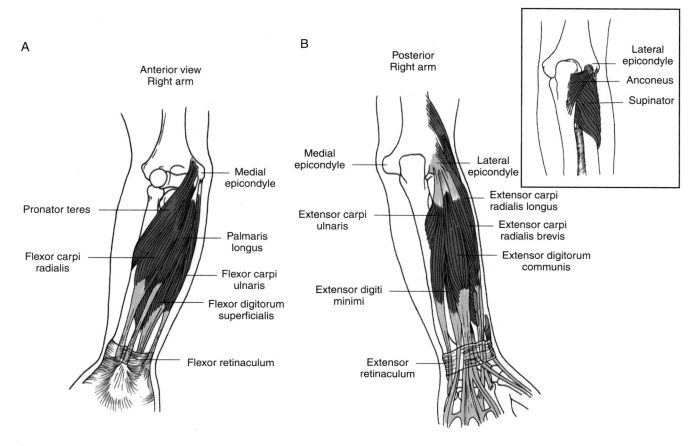

▲ **Figure 8-11** ■ **A.** Insertion of the flexor muscles on the medial epicondyle of the humerus.. **B.** Insertion of the extensor muscles on the lateral epicondyle of the humerus.

fascia that lies over the forearm flexors.[3] The brachioradialis muscle arises from the lateral supracondylar ridge of the humerus and inserts into the distal end of the radius just proximal to the radial styloid process.

The two extensors of the elbow are the **triceps** and the **anconeus.** The triceps has three heads, (long, medial, and lateral). The long head crosses both the glenohumeral joint at the shoulder as well as the elbow joint. The long head arises from the infraglenoid tubercle of the scapula by a flattened tendon that blends with the glenohumeral joint capsule. The medial and lateral heads cross only the elbow joint. The medial head covers an extensive area as it arises from the entire posterior surface of the humerus. In contrast, the lateral head arises from only a narrow ridge on the posterior humeral surface. The three heads insert via a common tendon into the olecranon process. The anconeus is a small triangular muscle that arises from the posterior surface of the lateral epicondyle of the humerus and extends medially to attach to the lateral aspect of the olecranon process and the adjacent proximal quarter of the posterior surface of the ulna[3] (see Fig. 8-11).

In addition to the anconeus muscle, a number of muscles with primary actions at the wrist and fingers insert into the lateral humeral epicondyle by way of a common extensor tendon. These muscles include the **extensor carpi radialis longus (ECRL), extensor carpi radialis brevis (ECRB), extensor digitorum communis (EDC), extensor carpi ulnaris (ECU),** and **extensor digiti minimi (EDM)** (see Fig. 8-11B).

Case Application 8-3: **Muscles and Tendons**

The ECRL, ECRB, and ECU are active in gripping , hammering, and sawing activities. Therefore, the repetitive pull of these muscles during our patient's workday could have injured the common extensor tendon or another tendon either in its substance or at the entheses. The muscles also could have been strained. Therefore, it is possible that James's pain could come from (1) the common extensor tendon, (2) the tendon's attachment site (enthesis on the lateral humeral epicondyle), or (3) one of the muscles. Disorders at the enthesis (enthesopathies) are commonly seen in tennis elbow and jumper's knee.[33] Also, because James has had numerous episodes of similar pain over a number of years, we might suspect that this is a chronic condition and, therefore, there may be degenerative changes affecting the tendon if it is the source of pain.

The types of changes that might be seen in either our patient's tendon or his muscle are presented in Table 8-1. These changes are from examinations of biopsy material from patients with chronic lateral elbow pain diagnosed as **lateral epicondylitis** (inflammation of the lateral epicondyle and surrounding tissues). Many of the changes listed appear to be suggestive more of a degenerative process than of a simple inflammatory process and are similar to changes observed in aged supraspinatus tendons.[34]

Magnetic resonance imaging (MRI) is a less invasive diagnostic method than a biopsy, but it is more expensive. Mackay and colleagues[38] used MRI to identify signs of edema, thickening, and tears in common extensor tendons and peritendon edema in patients with lateral elbow pain. Savnik and associates, also using MRI, found separation of the ECRB tendon from the LCL.[39] Edema is more more suggestive of an inflammatory process than are some of the changes identified in Table 8-1.

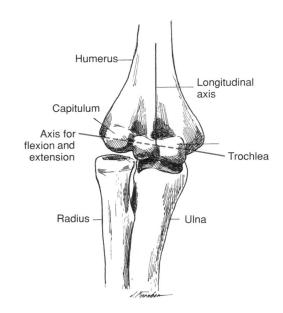

▲ **Figure 8-12** ■ The axis of motion for flexion and extension. The axis of motion is centered in the middle of the trochlea on a line that intersects the longitudinal (anatomic) axis of the humerus.

Function: Elbow Joint (Humeroulnar and Humeroradial Articulations)

Axis of Motion

Traditionally, the axis for flexion and extension has been described as being a relatively fixed axis that passes horizontally through the center of the trochlea and capitulum and bisects the longitudinal axis of the shaft of the humerus[40,41] (Fig. 8-12). However, some studies have found that the axis is not as fixed as previously thought.[42–44]

An exact determination of the axis of motion at the elbow is important because of the need to position elbow prostheses in such a way that they correctly mimic elbow joint motion. In the past, elbow prostheses that were modeled as pure hinge devices often became loose during motion. Screw displacement axes (SDAs) are used to define the elbow axis accurately for proper prosthesis positioning. However, investigations have been complicated because the location of the SDA is

influenced by the type of flexion motion (active or passive) and by forearm position (pronation or supination), which indicates that the elbow behaves like a loose hinge joint rather than like a pure hinge joint.[43] Variations found in the instantaneous axis inclination **support** the hypothesis that activity of the various muscles may influence the pattern of motion during active flexion, and differences in contours of the joint surfaces may explain interindividual differences during passive motion.[42] Intraindividual and interindividual variations in the axes appear to be greater in the frontal plane than in the horizontal plane.[42]

For example, Ericson and coworkers,[42] using a radiostereometric analysis technique and x-rays taken at 30° intervals up to 120° of active elbow flexion, found that the orientation of the instantaneous axes varied (between subjects) within the arc of flexion from 2.1° to 14.3° in the frontal plane and from 1.6° to 9.8° in the horizontal plane. However, the inclination of the mean axis in the horizontal plane differed little from

Table 8-1	Tennis Elbow: Changes in Tendons and Muscle in Patients with Lateral Epicondylitis		
Chard et al.[34]: Biopsies (N = 20 patients, 27–56 yr)	Galliani et al.[35]: Biopsies (N = 11 patients, 38–54 yr)	Steinborn et al.[36]: Biopsies (N = 23 patients, 29–58 yr)	Ljung et al.[37]: Biopsies (N = 20 patients)
Common extensor tendon	**Common extensor tendon insertion**	**Common extensor tendon**	**Extensor carpi radialis brevis muscle**
Loss of tenocytes	Loss of tenocytes	Fatty degeneration	Moth-eaten fibers
Calcification	Calcifying processes	Intratendinous cartilage formation	Fiber necrosis
Glycosaminoglycan infiltration	Biochemical and spatial degeneration of collagen	Fibrosclerotic degeneration	Fiber degeneration
Fibrocartilaginous transformation	Hyaline degeneration	Fibrovascular proliferation	Increased percentage of fast-twitch type 2A fibers
	Fibrocartilage metaplasia		

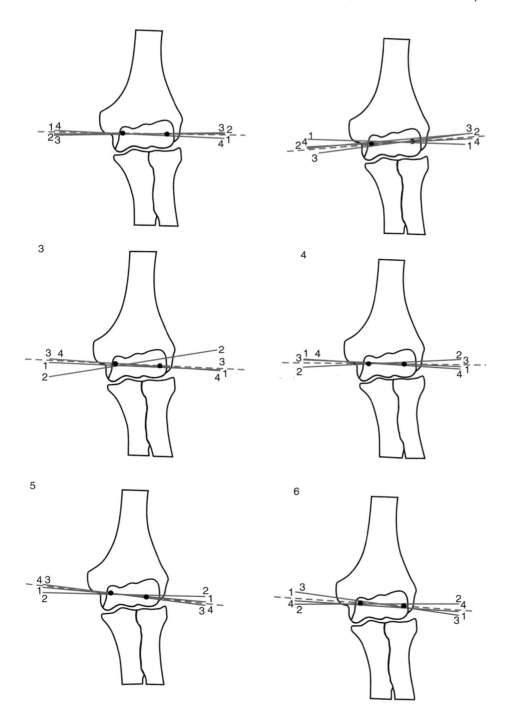

▲ **Figure 8-13** ■ Variations in the instantaneous axis for flexion and extension. (From Ericson A, Arndt A, Stark A, et al.: Variation in the position and orientation of the elbow flexion axis. J Bone Joint Surg Br 85:539, 2003.)

a line through the centers of the trochlea and capitulum (Fig. 8-13).

Bottlang and colleagues[44] found that the envelope for valgus-varus laxity was greatest between 0° and 40° of flexion and decreased considerably when flexion exceeded 100°. Like Ericson and coworkers[42], however, Bottlang and colleagues[44] found that all instantaneous rotation axes nearly intersected on the medial facet of the trochlea.

■ Long Axes of the Humerus and Forearm

When the upper extremity is in the anatomic position , the long axis of the humerus and the long axis of the forearm form an acute angle medially when they meet at the elbow. The angulation in the frontal plane is caused by the configuration of the articulating surfaces at the humeroulnar joint. The medial aspect of the trochlea extends more distally than does the lateral aspect, which shifts the medial aspect of the ulna trochlear notch more distally and results in a lateral deviation (or valgus angulation) of the ulna in relation to the humerus.. This normal valgus angulation is called the **carrying angle** or **cubitus valgus** (Fig 8-14A). The average angle in full elbow extension is about 15° (see Fig. 8-14B). An increase in the carrying angle beyond the average is considered to be abnormal, especially if it occurs unilaterally. A varus angulation at the elbow is referred to as **cubitus varus** and is usually abnormal (see Fig. 8-14C).

Normally, the carrying angle disappears when the forearm is pronated and the elbow is in full extension and when the supinated forearm is flexed against the humerus in full elbow flexion.[9] The configuration of the trochlear groove determines the pathway of the forearm during flexion and extension. In the most common configuration of the groove, the ulna is guided progressively medially from extension to flexion, so that in full flexion, the forearm comes to rest in the same plane as the humerus[9] (Fig. 8-15A). In exten-

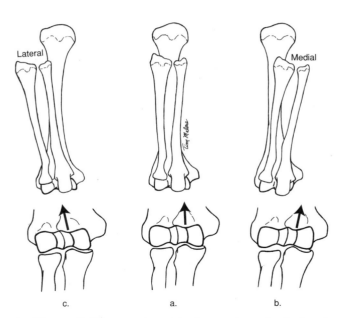

▲ **Figure 8-15** ■ Position of the forearm in passive flexion. **A.** In the most common configuration of the trochlear groove, the ulna is guided progressively medially from extension to flexion so that in full flexion the forearm comes to rest in the same plane as the humerus. **B.** The forearm comes to rest slightly medially to the humerus in passive flexion. **C.** The forearm comes to rest slightly laterally in the least common configuration of the trochlear groove.

sion, the forearm moves laterally until it reaches a position slightly lateral to the axis of the humerus in full extension. Variations in the direction of the groove will alter the pathway of the forearm, so that when the elbow is passively flexed, the forearm will come to rest either medial[9,40] (see Fig. 8-15B) or lateral (see Fig. 8-15C) to the humerus[9] in full flexion.

Range of Motion

A number of factors determine the amount of motion that is available at the elbow joint. These factors include the type of motion (active or passive), the position of the forearm (relative pronation-supination), and the position of the shoulder. The range of active flexion at the elbow is usually less than the range of passive motion, because the bulk of the contracting flexors on the anterior surface of the humerus may interfere with the approximation of the forearm with the humerus. The active ROM for elbow flexion with the forearm supinated is typically considered to be from about 135° to 145°, whereas the range for passive flexion is between 150° and 160°.[9] The position of the forearm also affects the flexion ROM. When the forearm is either in pronation or midway between supination and pronation, the ROM is less than it is when the forearm is supinated. The position of the shoulder may affect the ROM available to the elbow. Two joint muscles, such as the biceps brachii and the triceps, that cross both the shoulder and elbow joints may limit ROM at the elbow if a full ROM is attempted at both joints simultaneously.

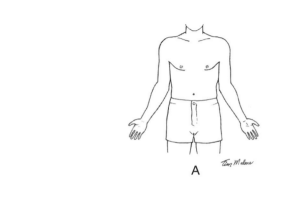

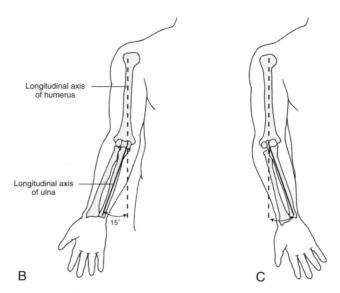

Longitudinal axis of humerus

Longitudinal axis of ulna

15°

B   C

▲ **Figure 8-14** ■ The carrying angle of the elbow. **A.** The forearm lies slightly lateral to the humerus when the elbow is fully extended in the anatomic position. **B.** The long axis of the humerus and the long axis of the forearm form the carrying angle. **C.** Cubitus varus.

Two-Joint Muscle Effects on Elbow ROM

Passive tension in the triceps may limit elbow flexion when the shoulder is simultaneously moved into full flexion (Fig 8-16A). Passive tension created in the long head of the biceps brachii by passive shoulder hyperextension may limit full elbow extension. Torque produced by the long head of the biceps brachii may diminish as the muscle shortens over both joints in full active shoulder and elbow function (see Fig. 8-16B). In simultaneous active shoulder hyperextension and full elbow extension, torque in the long head of the triceps may decrease as the muscle attempts to actively shorten over both the shoulder and the elbow.

Other factors that limit the ROM but help provide stability for the elbow are the configuration of the joint surfaces, the ligaments, and joint capsule. The elbow has inherent articular stability at the extremes of extension and flexion.[20,24] In full extension, the humeroulnar joint is in a **close-packed position.** In this position, bony contact of the olecranon process in the olecranon fossa limits the end of the extension range, and the configuration of the joint structures helps provide valgus and varus stability. The bony components, MCL, and anterior joint capsule contribute equally to resist valgus stress in full extension.[24] The bony components provide half of the resistance to varus stress in full extension, and the lateral collateral complex and joint capsule provide the other half of the resistance.[24] Resistance to joint distraction in the extended position is provided entirely by soft tissue structures. The ante-

rior portion of the joint capsule provides the majority of the resistance to anterior displacement of the distal humerus out of the olecranon fossa, whereas the MCL and LCL contribute only slightly.[20,24]

Approximation of the coronoid process with the coronoid fossa and of the rim of the radial head in the radial fossa limits extremes of flexion. In 90° of flexion, the anterior part of the MCL provides the primary resistance to both distraction and valgus stress. If the anterior portion of the MCL becomes lax through overstretching, medial instability will result when the elbow is in flexed positions. Also, the carrying angle will increase. The majority of the resistance to varus stress when the elbow is flexed to 90° is provided by the osseous structures of the joint, and only a slight amount is provided by the LCL and the joint capsule. The anterior joint capsule contributes only slightly to varus/valgus stability and provides little resistance to distraction when the elbow is flexed.[20,24] Co-contractions of the flexor and extensor muscles of the elbow, wrist, and hand help to provide stability for the elbow during forceful motions of the wrist and fingers and in activities in which the arms are used to support the body weight. During pulling activities, such as when a person grasps and attempts to pull a fixed rod toward the body, the elbow joints are compressed by the contractions of muscles that cross the elbow and act on the wrist and hand.[45]

Swelling and or pain also may limit the range of elbow motion. McGuigan and Bookout[46] investigated the effects of intra-articular fluid on the ROM. They found that the flexion arc of motion decreased 2.1° per millimeter of injected fluid.

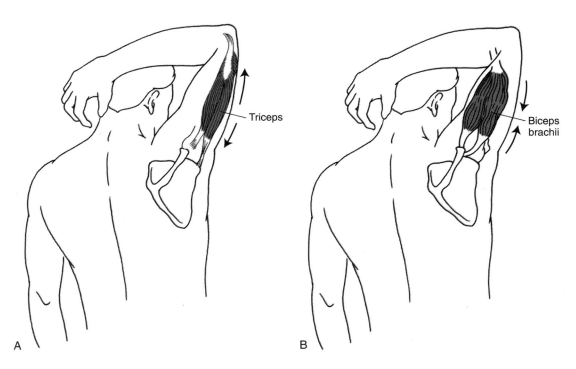

▲ **Figure 8-16** ■ **A.** Passive tension in the long head of the biceps brachii may limit elbow flexion. **B.** Passive tension in the long head of the biceps brachii may limit elbow extension.

Case Application 8-4: **Inflammation and Swelling at the Enthesis**

When we first met James, he was holding his right elbow in a considerable amount of flexion. Inflammation at the enthesis is often accompanied by swelling and might be the cause of our patient's elbow pain. If excess fluid accumulates within the joint, the joint capsule stretches and causes pain. To reduce the pain, patients will often assume a position in which stretching of the joint capsule is at a minimum. Elbow flexion of about 80° is considered to be the elbow position at which the least amount of tension is present in the joint capsule.[47] Therefore, it is a position of relative comfort for patients with interarticular swelling.

Muscle Action

 CONCEPT CORNERSTONE 8-4: *Summary of Factors Affecting Elbow Muscle Activity*

The role that the elbow muscles play in motion at the elbow is determined by a number of factors, including:

■ number of joints crossed by the muscle (one joint or two joint muscles)
■ physiologic cross-sectional area (PCSA)
■ location in relation to joint
■ position of the elbow and adjacent joints
■ position of the forearm
■ magnitude of the applied load
■ type of muscle action (concentric, eccentric, isometric, isokinetic)
■ speed of motion (slow or fast)
■ moment arm (MA) at different joint positions
■ fiber types

A great deal of our information regarding muscle action comes from studies using electromyography (EMG). This technique is used to monitor the electrical activity that is produced by the firing of motor units. With EMG, it is possible to determine the relative proportion of motor units that are firing in a particular muscle during a specific muscle contraction. In addition, the muscle activation patterns of agonists and antagonists, as well as synergistic activity among both agonists and antagonists, may be identified during the performance of different tasks.

■ Flexors

Elbow Flexors

The brachialis is considered to be a **mobility** muscle because its insertion is close to the elbow joint axis. It has a large strength potential in that it has a large PCSA and a large work capacity (volume).[1] Its MA is greatest at slightly more than 100° of elbow flexion,[48] at which its ability to produce torque is greatest (Fig. 8-17).

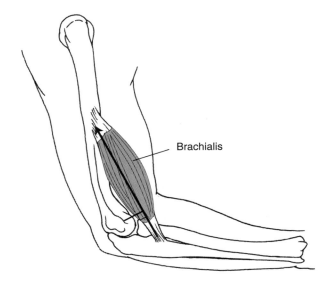

Brachialis

▲ **Figure 8-17** ■ Moment arm of the brachialis at 100° of elbow flexion.

Because the brachialis is inserted on the ulna, it is unaffected by changes in the forearm position brought about by rotation of the radius. Being a one-joint muscle, it is not affected by the position of the shoulder. According to EMG studies, the brachialis muscle works in flexion of the elbow in all positions of the forearm, with and without resistance. It also is active in all types of contractions (isometric, concentric, and eccentric) during slow and fast motions.[49] The fact that the brachialis works in all conditions may be related to the finding that the central nervous system (CNS) appeared to favor using one-joint muscles over two-joint muscles to perform an isometric activity.[50]

The biceps brachii, like the brachialis, is also considered to be a mobility muscle because of its insertion close to the elbow joint axis. The long head of the biceps brachii has the largest volume among the flexors, but the muscle has a relatively small PCSA.[1] The MA of the biceps is largest between 80° and 100° of elbow flexion and, therefore, the biceps is capable of producing its greatest torque in this range[48] (Fig. 8-18A). The MA of the biceps is rather small when the elbow is in full extension, and most of the muscle force is translatory and toward joint compression (see Fig. 8-18B). Therefore, when the elbow is fully extended, the biceps is less effective as an elbow flexor than when the elbow is flexed to 90°. When the elbow is flexed beyond 100°, the translatory component of the muscle force is directed away from the elbow joint and, therefore, acts as a distracting or dislocating force.

The functioning of the biceps is affected by the position of the shoulder, inasmuch as both heads of the muscle cross both the shoulder and the elbow. If full flexion of the elbow is attempted with the shoulder in full flexion, especially when the forearm is supinated, the muscle's ability to generate torque is diminished. Also, the activation of the biceps was found to be significantly affected by elbow joint angle during concen-

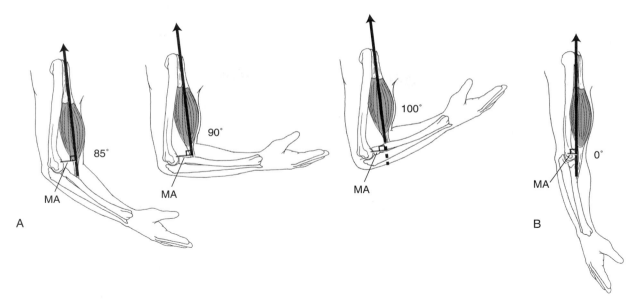

▲ **Figure 8-18** ■ **A.** Moment arm of the biceps at 85° to 100° of elbow flexion. **B.** Moment arm of the biceps at full extension.

tric and isometric contractions but not during isometric or isokinetic contraction.[51] In an EMG study of the flexors and extensors, the biceps brachii was active for supination torques.[52] Subjects in a study by Naito and associates were asked to maintain the elbow in flexion while performing alternating motions of supination and pronation at slow and fast speeds. EMG activity increased in the biceps during slow supination and decreased during pronation.[53]

The biceps brachii is active during unresisted elbow flexion with the forearm supinated and when the forearm is midway between supination and pronation in both concentric and eccentric contractions, but it tends *not* to be active when the forearm is pronated. However, when the magnitude of the resistance increases much beyond limb weight, the biceps is active in all positions of the forearm.[51]

The brachioradialis is inserted at a distance from the joint axis, and therefore the largest component of muscle force goes toward compression of the joint surfaces and hence toward stability. The brachioradialis has a relatively small mean PCSA (1.2 cm) but a relatively large average peak MA (7.7 cm) in comparison with other elbow flexors.[48] The peak MA for the brachioradialis occurs between 100° and 120° of elbow flexion.[48] The brachioradialis does not cross the shoulder and therefore is unaffected by the position of the shoulder. The position of the elbow joint was found to affect brachioradialis muscle activity only during voluntary maximum eccentric contractions. Elbow joint angle had no effect on concentric, isometric, or isokinetic maximum voluntary contractions.[51]

The brachioradialis shows no electrical activity during eccentric flexor activity when the motion is performed slowly with the forearm supinated.[54] Also, the brachioradialis shows no activity during slow, unresisted, concentric elbow flexion. When the speed of the motion is increased, the brachioradialis shows moder-

ate activity if a load is applied and the forearm is either in a position midway between supination and pronation or in full pronation.[49] In an EMG experiment on the effects of forearm motion on muscle activity wherein nine healthy subjects maintained their elbows in 90° flexion while pronating and supinating the forearm, the brachioradialis showed high levels of activity during rapid alternating supination/pronation motions. Higher levels of activity were noted when the forearm was pronated than when it was supinated.[53]

The pronator teres, as well as the palmaris longus, flexor digitorum superficialis, flexor carpi radialis, and flexor carpi ulnaris, is a weak elbow flexor with primary actions at the radioulnar and wrist joints.[3]

■ Extensors

The effectiveness of the triceps as a whole is affected by changes in the position of the elbow but not by changes in position of the forearm, because the triceps attaches to the ulna and not the radius. Activity of the long head of the triceps is affected by changing shoulder joint positions because the long head crosses both the shoulder and the elbow. The long head's ability to produce torque may diminish when full elbow extension is attempted with the shoulder in hyperextension. In this instance, the muscle is shortened over both the elbow and shoulder simultaneously.

The medial and lateral heads of the triceps, being one-joint muscles, are not affected by the position of the shoulder. The medial head is active in unresisted active elbow extension,[49] but all three heads are active when heavy resistance is given to extension or when quick extension of the elbow is attempted in the gravity-assisted position. Maximum isometric torque generation is at a position of 90° of elbow flexion.[55,56] However, the total amount of extensor torque generated at 90° varies with the position of the shoulder and the

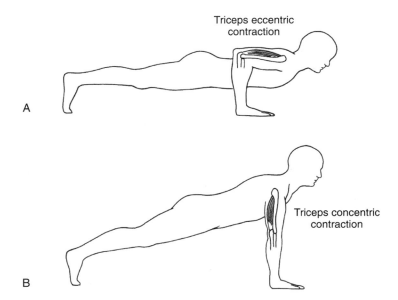

Triceps eccentric contraction

A

Triceps concentric contraction

B

◄ **Figure 8-19** ■ Action of the triceps in a push-up. **A.** The triceps muscle works eccentrically in reverse action to control elbow flexion during the lowering phase of a push-up. **B.** The triceps works concentrically in reverse action to produce the elbow extension that raises the body in a push-up.

body.[57] The triceps is active eccentrically to control elbow flexion as the body is lowered to the ground in a push-up (Fig. 8-19A). The triceps is active concentrically to extend the elbow when the triceps acts in a closed kinematic chain, such as in a push-up (see Fig. 8-19B). The triceps may be active during activities requiring stabilization of the elbow. For example, it acts as a synergist to prevent flexion of the elbow when the biceps is acting as a supinator. The other extensor of the elbow, the anconeus, assists in elbow extension and apparently also acts as a stabilizer during supination and pronation.

Synergistic actions of elbow flexor and extensor muscles have been investigated during isometric contractions in response to a variety of stresses, including varus stress, valgus stress, flexion, and extension.[58] Some flexor muscle pairs, such as the brachialis and brachioradialis, and the extensor pairs of the anconeus and medial head of the triceps brachii are coactivated in a similar manner for all stresses. However, the synergistic patterns of other muscles at the elbow are complex and vary with the joint angle, direction of the stress, and the type of muscle contraction. For example, the brachialis and the long head of the biceps brachii work synergistically during isometric contractions only from 0° to 45° of flexion. In a no-load situation in which subjects held their elbows at 90° of flexion while they supinated and pronated their forearms, reciprocal activity among the elbow flexors permitted the biceps to work to produce supination without increasing the amount of elbow flexion.[53]

In addition to the fact that synergies are affected by the direction and variety of stress, synergistic activity also appears to be affected by the type of muscle contraction being used (isometric, concentric, eccentric).[53] Nakazawa and associates found that activation patterns in the biceps brachii and the brachioradialis varied with the type of muscle contraction during elbow flexion against a load.[54] The synergistic actions of the muscles

of the elbow and their relation to elbow and wrist function are still being investigated. Dounskaia and coworkers, in an EMG study of arm cycling, suggested that a hierarchical organization of control for elbow-wrist coordination was operative in this activity. Muscles of the elbow were responsible for movement of the entire linkage, and the wrist muscles were responsible for making the corrections to the movement that were necessary to complete the task.[59] Zhang and Nuber[50] found that in voluntary isometric extension, the uniarticular lateral and medial heads of the triceps provided 70% to 90% of the total elbow extension moment. The anconeus muscle contributed about 15% of the extension moment. In contrast, the biarticular long head of the triceps contibuted significantly less. Authors concluded that this was an example of the fact that the CNS selectively recruits uniarticular muscles rather than two-joint muscles to complete a task. In another study, Prodoehl and colleagues[60] demonstrated that muscle activation patterns changed with the force requirements of the task and the amount of available muscle force.

 CONCEPT CORNERSTONE 8-5: *Summary of Muscle Activation Patterns*

Muscle activation patterns appear to be affected by

1. number of joints crossed
2. type of muscle action (concentric, eccentric, isometric, isokinetic)
3. speed of motion
4. resistance
5. requirements of the task
6. direction of the stress
7. activity of other muscles

Structure: Superior and Inferior Articulations

Superior Radioulnar Joint

The articulating surfaces of the proximal radioulnar joint include the **ulnar radial notch,** the **annular ligament,** the capitulum of the humerus, and the head of the radius. The radial notch is located on the lateral aspect of the proximal ulna directly below the trochlear notch (Fig. 8-20A). The surface of the radial notch is concave and covered with articular cartilage. A circular ligament called the annular ligament is attached to the anterior and posterior edges of the notch. The ligament is lined with articular cartilage, which is continuous with the cartilage lining of the radial notch. The annular ligament encircles the rim of the radial head, which is also covered with articular cartilage (see Fig. 8-20B). Mechanoreceptors are evenly distributed throughout the ligament.[18] The capitulum and the proximal surface of the head of the radius are actually part of the elbow and have already been discussed in the section on the elbow joint.

Inferior Radioulnar Joint

The articulating surfaces of the distal radioulnar joint include the **ulnar notch,** the **articular disk,** and the **head of the ulna** (Fig. 8-21). The ulnar notch of the radius is located at the distal end of the radius along the interosseous border. The radius of curvature of the concave ulnar notch is 4 to 7 mm larger than that of the ulnar head. The articular disk is sometimes referred to as either the **triangular fibrocartilage (TFC)** because of its triangular shape or as a part of **the triangular fibrocartilage complex (TFCC)** because of its extensive fibrous connections.

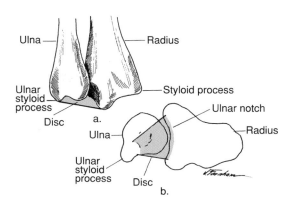

▲ **Figure 8-21** ■ The inferior radioulnar joint of a left forearm. **A.** An anterior view of the inferior radioulnar joint shows the disk in its normal position in a supinated left forearm. **B.** An inferior view of the disk shows how the disk covers the inferior aspect of the distal ulna and separates the ulna from the articulation at the wrist.

The disk has been described as resembling a shelf whose medial border is embedded in a wedge of vascular connective tissue containing fine ligamentous bands that join the disk to the ulna and articular capsule.[61] The base of the articular disk is attached to the distal edge of the ulnar notch of the radius. The apex of the articular disk has two attachments. One attachment is to the fovea on the ulnar head. The other attachment is to the base of the ulnar styloid process.[62,63] Medially, the articular disk is continuous with the fibers of the ulnar collateral ligament, which arises from the sides of the styloid process.[63] The margins of the articular disk are thickened[63,64] and are either formed by or are integral parts of the dorsal and palmar capsular radioulnar ligaments (Fig. 8-22). The ligaments are firmly attached to the radius; the ulnar attachments are some what less firmly attached. The thickness of the dorsal and palmar margins and of the apex of the disk is approximately 3 to 6 mm,[63,64] in contrast to the central area of the articular disk, which is often so thin that it is transparent.[63] Also, the central area may be perforated, and the number of perforations increases with age from 7% in the

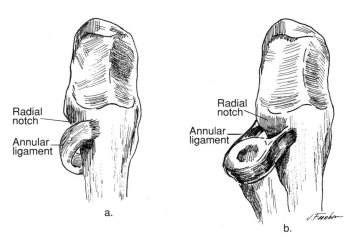

▲ **Figure 8-20** ■ The annular ligament. **A.** Attachments of the annular ligament. **B.** The head of the radius has been pulled away from its normal position adjacent to the radial notch to show how the ligament partially surrounds the radial head.

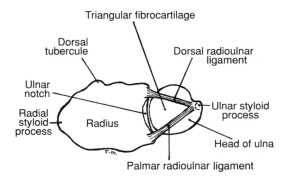

▲ **Figure 8-22** ■ The illustration includes the distal aspects of a left radius and ulna, as well as the articular disk and articulating surfaces of the distal radioulnar joint. The articular disk is shown with radioulnar ligaments bordering the sides of the disk.

third decade to 53.1% for individuals who are in the sixth decade and older.[63] Chidgey and colleagues, in a study of 12 fresh cadaver wrists, found that the articular disks had a high collagen content with sparsely but equally distributed elastin fibers. The same authors found that 80% of the central portion of the articular disk was avascular, in comparison with the peripheral area, which was only 15% to 20% avascular. The radioulnar ligaments were well vascularized.[65] Ohmori and Azuma found free nerve endings in the ulnar side of the articular disk, particularly around the periphery. The authors suggested that, in view of their findings, the disk may be a source of wrist pain.[66]

The articular disk has two articulating surfaces: the proximal (superior) surface and the distal (inferior) surface. The proximal surface of the disk articulates with the ulnar head at the distal radioulnar joint, whereas the distal surface articulates with the carpal bones as part of the radiocarpal joint.[3] Both the proximal and distal surfaces of the articular disk are concave. The superior surface of the articular disk is deepened to accommodate the convexity of the ulnar head; the distal surface is adapted to accommodate the carpal bones.[63] The peripheral parts of both the ulnar and carpal disk surfaces are covered by synovium coming from their respective joint capsules.[63]

The ulnar head is convex and is covered with articular cartilage distally.[67,68] The head has two articular surfaces, the pole and the seat, which articulate with the articular disk and the ulnar notch of the radius, respectively. The convex pole is U-shaped and faces the disk. The convex seat faces the ulnar notch of the radius.[62]

Radioulnar Articulation

The proximal and distal radioulnar joints are mechanically linked; therefore, motion at one joint is always accompanied by motion at the other joint. The distal radioulnar joint is also considered to be functionally linked to the wrist in that compressive loads are transmitted through the distal radioulnar joint from the hand to the radius and ulna.[68]

Pronation of the forearm occurs as a result of the radius's crossing over the ulna at the superior radioulnar joint. During pronation and supination, the rim of the head of the radius spins within the osteoligamentous enclosure formed by the radial notch and the annular ligament. At the same time, the surface of the head spins on the capitulum of the humerus. At the distal radioulnar joint, the concave surface of the ulnar notch of the radius slides around the ulnar head, and the disk follows the radius by twisting at its apex and sweeping along beneath the ulnar head. Joint surface contact is optimal only with the forearm in a neutral position between supination and pronation. In maximal pronation and supination, the articulating surfaces have only minimal contact.[69] In full supination, the seat of the ulnar head rests on the palmar aspect of the ulnar notch, whereas in full pronation, it rests against the dorsal lip of the ulnar notch[62,70] (Fig. 8-23).

Ligaments

The three ligaments associated with the proximal radioulnar joint are the annular and quadrate liga-

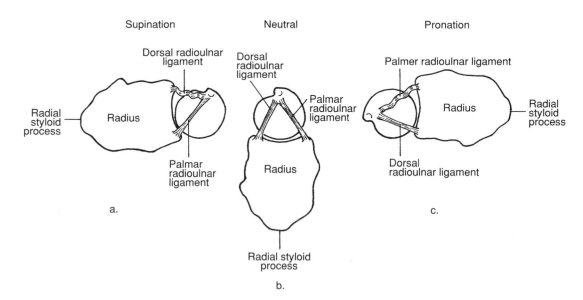

▲ **Figure 8-23** ■ Articulating surfaces and dorsal and palmar radioulnar ligaments at the distal radioulnar joint. **A.** The head of the ulna is shown in contact with the palmar aspect of the ulnar notch in full supination. The palmar radioulnar ligament is taut, and the dorsal ligament is lax. **B.** In the neutral position, the articulating surface of the head of the ulna has maximum contact with the radial articulating surface. **C.** In full pronation, the head of the ulna has contact only with the dorsal lip of the ulnar notch. The dorsal radioulnar ligament is taut, and the palmar ligament is lax.

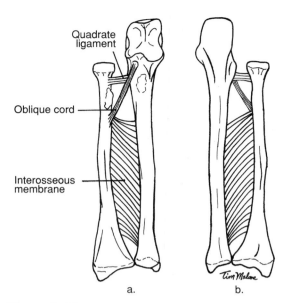

Figure 8-24 ■ Ligamentous structures that provide stability for the proximal and distal radioulnar joints. The head of the radius has been slightly separated from the ulna, and the annular ligament has been removed to show the quadrate ligament. **A.** The anterior aspect of the radius and ulna are shown with the right forearm in a supinated position. The quadrate ligament is shown extending from the inferior edge of the radial notch to attach on the neck of the radius. The ventral oblique cord extends from below the radial notch to attach just below the bicepital tuberosity. **B.** A posterior view of the right radius and ulna in the supinated position. The interosseous membrane is shown extending between the radius and ulna for a considerable portion of their length. The dorsal oblique cord is not shown in this figure.

ments and the oblique cord (Fig. 8-24). The **annular ligament** is a strong band that forms four fifths of a ring that encircles the radial head (see Fig. 8-20B). The inner surface of the ligament is covered with cartilage and serves as a joint surface. The proximal border of the annular ligament blends with the joint capsule, and the lateral aspect is reinforced by fibers from the LCL.[3] The **quadrate ligament** extends from the inferior edge of the ulna's radial notch to insert in the neck of the radius. The quadrate ligament reinforces the inferior aspect of the joint capsule and helps maintain the radial head in apposition to the radial notch. The quadrate ligament also limits the spin of the radial head in supination and pronation. The **oblique cord** is a flat fascial band on the ventral forearm that extends from an attachment just inferior to the radial notch on the ulna to insert just below the bicipital tuberosity on the radius. The fibers of the oblique cord are at right angles to the fibers of the interosseous membrane (IOM).[3] The functional significance of the oblique cord is not clear, but it may assist in preventing separation of the radius and ulna.

The dorsal and palmar radioulnar ligaments, as well as the IOM, which stabilizes both proximal and distal joints, reinforce the distal radioulnar joint. The dorsal and palmar ligaments are formed by longitudinally oriented collagen fiber bundles originating from the dorsal and palmar aspects of the ulnar notch of the

radius.[69] The two ligaments extend along the margins of the articular disk to insert on the ulnar fovea and base of ulnar styloid process[62] (see Fig. 8-23). The palmar radioulnar ligament is at least 2 mm longer than the dorsal radioulnar ligament.[71] According to Linscheid, the dorsal radioulnar ligament averages 18 mm in length, whereas the palmar radioulnar ligament averages 22 mm.[62]

The **interosseous membrane (IOM)**, which is located between the radius and the ulna, is a complex structure consisting of the following three components: a central band, a thin membranous portion, and a dorsal oblique cord (see Fig. 8-5). The **central band** is described as being a strong, thick, ligamentous[72,73] or tendinous structure[74] consisting of bundles of fibers that run obliquely from the radius to the ulna. The central band has a very high collagen content arranged in fibrillar structures surrounded by elastin. The collagen content is more abundant in proximal bundles than it is in distal bundles.[75] When the tensile strength of the central band was compared with that of the patellar tendon, the investigators[73] found that the ultimate tensile strength of the central band was 84% of the strength of the patellar tendon. In contrast to the central band, the **membranous portion** is described as a soft and thin structure that lies adjacent proximally and distally to the central band.[74] The **dorsal oblique cord** is considered to be part of the IOM and should not be confused with the oblique cord located on the ventral aspect of the forearm, which is not considered to be part of the IOM. The dorsal oblique cord extends from the proximal quarter of the ulna to the middle region of the radius.[72,74] Its fibers run counter to the central band.

The IOM maintains space between the radius and ulna during forearm rotation,[76] and according to an MRI study by Nakamura and associates,[77] the central band remains taut throughout forearm rotation, apparently to keep the radius and ulna from splaying apart. In contrast, the membranous portion of the IOM evidenced wavy deformations at maximum supination and in the neutral position. Deformations also occurred around the oblique cord at maximum pronation. The IOM protects the proximal radioulnar joint by transferring some of the compressive loads at the distal radius to the proximal ulna.[78] The IOM maintains transverse stability of forearm during compressive load transfer from the hand to the elbow[79] (see Fig. 8-28).

Maximum strain in the fibers of the central band was found to occur when the forearm was in a neutral position (midway between supination and pronation). Force in the IOM that depends on elbow flexion angle and forearm rotation ranges from a minimum of 8 N in full elbow extension with neutral forearm rotation to a maximum of 43 N at 30° of elbow flexion and with the forearm supinated. The largest of all forces was found in supination in all flexion angles.[80] The average proportion of total load in each bone in supination was 68% in the distal radius, 32% in the distal ulna, 51% in the proximal radius, and 49% in the proximal ulna. The IOM transfers loads from the wrist to the proximal forearm via fibers that run from the proximal radius to the distal ulna. The fibers in the central band are relaxed in both full supination and full pronation.[3,72] The IOM provides stability for both the superior and inferior radioulnar joints.

A tract extends from the interosseus membrane and inserts in the distal radioulnar joint capsule between the tendon sheaths of the EDM and the ECU muscles. The tract's deep fibers insert directly into the articular disk (triangular fibrocartilage). The tract of the interosseus membrane is taut in pronation and loose in supination.[81] The articular disk also provides stability for the inferior radioulnar joint by binding the distal radius and ulna together. The distal radioulnar joint capsule, which is a separate entity from the triangular fibrocartilage, can be a source of limitation of motion when it is invaded by scar tissue after wrist injuries.[82]

Muscles

The primary muscles associated with the radioulnar joints are the **pronator teres, pronator quadratus, biceps brachii,** and **supinator.** The pronator teres has two heads: a humeral head and an ulnar head. The humeral head comes from the common flexor tendon on the medial epicondyle of the humerus. The smaller ulnar head arises from the medial aspect of the coronoid process of the ulna. Both heads attach distally to the surface of the lateral side of the radius at its greatest convexity. The pronator quadratus, which is located at the distal end of the forearm, also has two heads (superficial and deep). Both of these heads arise from the ulna and cross the IOM anteriorly to insert on the radius. The fibers of the superficial head pass transversely across the IOM, whereas the fibers of the deep head extend obliquely across the IOM to insert on the radius.[83] The biceps brachii has been discussed previously. The supinator is a short, broad muscle that arises from the lateral epicondyle of the humerus, the radial collateral ligament, the annular ligament, and the lateral aspect of the ulna. The muscle crosses the posterior aspect of the IOM to insert into the radius just medial and inferior to the bicipital tuberosity.

Another group of muscles that are active during supination and pronation, especially when gripping is involved and during resisted motion, include the flexor carpi ulnaris and ECU, the brachioradialis, and the flexor carpi radialis and ECRB. The anconeus muscle may also play a role in supination and pronation . This muscle arises from the posterior surface of the lateral humeral epicondyle and attaches to the lateral aspect of the olecranon and proximal quarter of the posterior surface of the ulna.

Case Application 8-5: **Role of the Extensor Carpi Radialis**

The ECRB may play a role in our patient James's pain, inasmuch as it exerts a pull on the lateral epicondyle and is active during gripping. Repetitive pulling during hammering and using a screwdriver and the chain saw may have damaged the enthesis of the common extensor tendon or another extensor tendon and caused inflammation at the medial epicondyle and posssibly swelling within the joint capsule.

Two tests that we performed on our patient were indicative of a diagnosis of lateral epicondylitis. A third test that we performed that is used to determine whether pain is coming from the ECRB tendon involves giving resistance to the end of our patient's extended third finger. When this activity causes pain over the lateral epicondyle, it suggests a probable diagnosis of lateral epicondylitis. James had pain over the lateral epicondyle when we performed this test, and so now we had three tests indicating a diagnosis of lateral epicondylitis.

◆ Function: Radioulnar Joints

Axis of Motion

The axis of motion for pronation and supination is a longitudinal axis extending from the center of the radial head to the center of the ulnar head.[9,84] In supination, the radius and ulna lie parallel to one another, whereas in pronation, the radius crosses over the ulna (Fig. 8-25). There is very little motion of the ulna during pronation and supination. Motion of the proximal ulna is negligible. Motion of the distal ulna is of less magnitude than that of the radius and opposite in direction to motion of the radius.[68] The ulnar head moves distally and dorsally in pronation and proximally and medially in supination. Therefore, at the distal radioulnar joint, the ulnar head glides in the ulnar notch of the radius from the dorsal lip of the ulnar

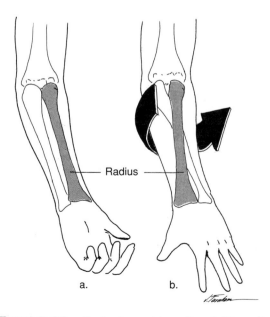

▲ **Figure 8-25 ■** Supination and pronation. **A.** The radius and ulna are parallel to each other in the supinated position of the forearm. **B.** In the pronated position, the radius crosses over the ulna. Drawing shows a left upper extremity.

notch in pronation to a position on the palmar aspect of the ulnar notch in full supination.[62]

Range of Motion

A total ROM of 150° has been ascribed to the radioulnar joints.[3,67,84] The ROM of pronation and supination is assessed with the elbow in 90° of flexion. This position of the elbow stabilizes the humerus so that radioulnar joint rotation may be distinguished from rotation that is occurring at the shoulder joint. When the elbow is fully extended, active supination and pronation occur in conjunction with shoulder rotation. Limitation of pronation when the elbow is extended may be caused by passive tension in the biceps brachii. Pronation in all elbow positions is limited by bony approximation of the radius and ulna and by tension in the dorsal radioulnar ligament and the posterior fibers of the MCL of the elbow.[20] Supination is limited by passive tension in the palmar radioulnar ligament and the oblique cord. The quadrate ligament limits spin of the radial head in both pronation and supination, and the annular ligament helps to maintain stability of the proximal radioulnar joint by holding the radius in close approximation to the radial notch.

Muscle Action

The pronators produce pronation by exerting a pull on the radius, which causes its shaft and distal end to turn over the ulna (Fig. 8-26). The pronator teres has its major action at the radioulnar joints, but the long head, as a two-joint muscle, plays a slight role in elbow flexion. The pronator teres contributes some of its force toward stabilization of the proximal radioulnar

joint, inasmuch as the muscle's translatory component helps maintain contact of the radial head with the capitulum.

The pronator quadratus, a one-joint muscle, is unaffected by changing positions at the elbow. The pronator quadratus is active in unresisted and resisted pronation and in slow or fast pronation. The deep head of the pronator quadratus is active during both resisted supination and resisted pronation and is thought to act as a dynamic stabilizer to maintain compression of the distal radioulnar joint.[83,84]

In a mechanical study on cadavers, the pronators were found to be most efficient around the neutral position of the forearm when the elbow was flexed to 90°.[85] In a different study in which the supinators and pronators were tested in the absence of gripping but against resistance, no significant differences were found between supination and pronation torques with the forearm in a neutral position. However, supination torque generation was greatest with the forearm in pronated positions, and pronation torque generation was greatest with the forearm in supinated positions.[86]

The supinators, like the pronators, act by pulling the shaft and distal end of the radius over the ulna (Fig. 8-27). The supinator muscle may act alone during unresisted slow supination in all positions of the elbow or forearm. The supinator also can act alone during unresisted fast supination when the elbow is extended. However, activity of the biceps is always evident when supination is performed against resistance and during fast supination when the elbow is flexed to 90°. As the forearm moves into pronation, its supination torque increases and reaches a maximum at about 20° of pronation.. The biceps has been found to exert four times as much supination torque with the forearm in the pronated position than in other forearm posi-

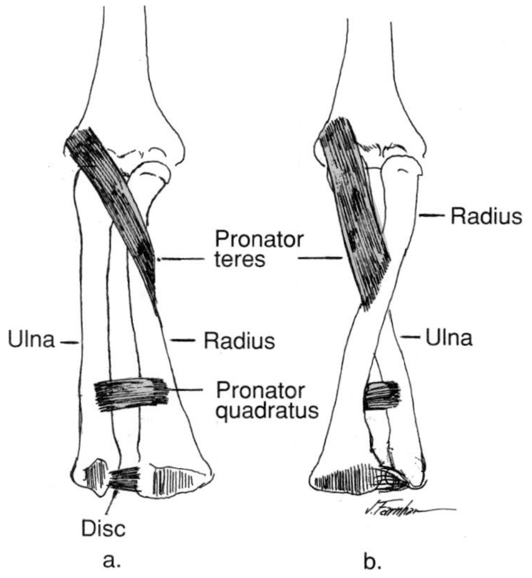

▲ **Figure 8-26** ■ Pronation of the forearm. The pronator teres and pronator quadratus produce pronation by pulling the radius over the ulna. Drawing shows a left forearm in the supinated position (**A**) and in the pronated position (**B**).

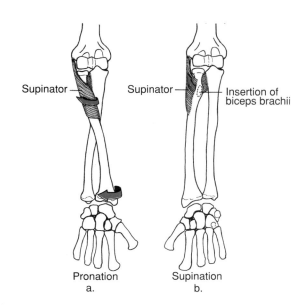

▲ **Figure 8-27** ■ Supination of the right forearm. **A.** In the pronated position, the supinator muscle wraps around the proximal radius. A contraction of the supinator or the biceps or both pulls the radius over the ulna. **B.** The supinator muscle and the insertion site of the biceps are shown in the supinated position.

tions.[85] A mean maximum supination torque of 16 Nm was recorded with the forearm 75% pronated, in comparison with a mean maximum supination torque of 13.1 Nm for the neutral forearm position with the elbow at 45° of flexion.[52] The anconeus muscle is active in supination and pronation, and an elbow stabilization role has been suggested to explain this activity. As determined by isometric testing, the supinators are stronger than the pronators.[87]

Stability

Muscular support of the distal radioulnar joint is attributed to the pronator quadratus[71,83,84,88,89] and the ECU tendon.[62,72,90] Also according to Linscheid, the ulnar head of the pronator teres may help by binding the ulna to the radius while the humeral head depresses the ulna during pronation.[62] The deep head of the pronator quadratus is active throughout supination and pronation and therefore is thought to provide dynamic stabilization for the distal radioulnar joint.[87] Activity in the ECU muscle exerts a depressive force on the dorsal aspect of the ulnar head as the tendon is stretched over the head during supination. Tension in the tendon helps to maintain the position of the ulnar head during both supination and pronation.[90]

The ECRB also provides support for the forearm, as evidenced by the maximum voluntary effort (MVE) in the ECRB that occurs in both supination (26% to 43% MVE) and pronation torques (27% to 55% MVE). The ECRB appears to act both as a stabilizer to the forearm for gripping during pronation torques (depending on forearm angle) and as a prime mover for wrist extension for supination torques.[52]

Case Application 8-6: **Link between Gripping during Forearm Rotations and High Muscle Activity**

The direct link found by O'Sullivan and Gallwey[52] between gripping during forearm rotations and high muscular activity in the ECRB not only helps to explain the mechanism of injury in lateral epicondylitis but also has implications for the prognosis for our patient. A poor prognosis in cases of lateral epicondylitis is associated with manual job employment with a high level of physical strain at work and a high level of pain at baseline.[91]

Ligamentous support of the distal radioulnar joint is provided by the dorsal and palmar radioulnar ligaments and the IOM and its tract, and the articular disk provide ligamentous support of the distal radioulnar joint. The dorsal radioulnar ligament becomes taut in pronation, whereas the palmar radioulnar ligament becomes taut in supination[63,69,71,84,88,92] (see Fig. 8-23). According to Schiend,[70] the radioulnar ligaments have limited cross-sectional areas and low structural stiffness, but they are able to prevent separation of the radius from the ulna during loading and also allow for force transmission from the radius to the ulna through the

distal radioulnar joint.[70] However, these ligaments do not augment longitudinal stability. They allow approximately 5 mm of play between the radius and ulna before providing resistance to further distraction.[62] The radioulnar ligaments, the articular disk, and the pronator quadratus maintain the ulna within the ulnar notch and prevent the ulna from subluxating or dislocating. However, these ligaments allow a high degree of mobility. The IOM provides stability for the distal joint by binding the radius and ulna together. Also, according to Skahen and coworkers, the IOM in combination with the triangular fibrocartilaginous complex provide important longitudinal stabilization.[72,93] Markolf and associates studied radioulnar load sharing at the wrist and elbow with the elbow in varus, valgus, and neutral positions.[94] When the elbow was in the varus position (no contact between the radial head and capitulum), force was transmitted from the distal radius through the IOM to the proximal ulna (Fig. 8-28). When the elbow was in the valgus position (contact between the radial head and the capitulum), the force was transmitted through the radius. When the forearm was in the neutral position, the mean force in the distal end of the ulna averaged 7% of the applied wrist load, whereas

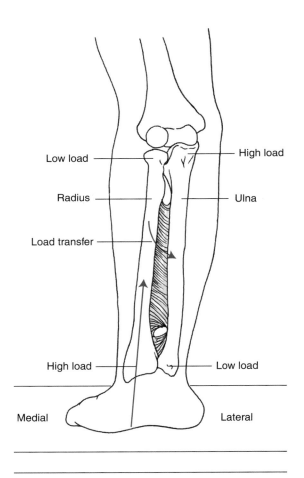

▲ **Figure 8-28 ■** IOM force transmission from radius to the ulna.

the force in the proximal ulna averaged 93% of the load applied to the wrist[94]. The tract associated with the IOM is taut in pronation and loose in supination. During pronation, the tract protects the ulnar head in a sling. It also provides stability for the joint by reinforcing the dorsal aspect of the joint capsule.[81]

The articular disk acts as a cushion in allowing compression force transmission from the carpals to the ulna and acts as a stabilizer of the ulnar side of the carpals.[68] Also, the disk assists in the transmission of compressive forces from the radius to the ulna.[78,94,95] Adams and Holley[92] used a distractive force to simulate the effects of the separation of articulating surfaces that accompanies a power grip. These authors found that strain distribution in the disk was dependent on forearm position.[92] Tension across the entire disk decreased in supination and increased in the radial portion of the disk in pronation.[92] The authors concluded that the articular disk regularly bears both compressive and tensile strains.[92] According to Mikic, compressive forces are transmitted through the central portion of the disk, and some of the load is converted to tensile loading within the peripheral margins.[63] A summary of ligamentous and muscular support for the distal radioulnar joint is presented in Table 8-2.

◆ Mobility and Stability: Elbow Complex

Functional Activities

The joints and muscles of the elbow complex are used in almost all activities of daily living such as dressing, eating, carrying, and lifting. They are also used in tasks such as splitting firewood, hammering nails, and playing tennis. Most of the activities of daily living require a combination of motion at both the elbow and radioulnar joints. Morrey and associates measured elbow and forearm motion in 33 healthy subjects during 15 activities.[96] The authors concluded that a total arc of about

100° of elbow flexion (between 30° and 130°) and about 100° of forearm rotation (50° supination and 50° pronation) is sufficient to accomplish simple tasks such as eating, brushing hair, brushing teeth, and dressing. For example, about 40° of pronation and 20° of supination are necessary to use a telephone.[96] Therefore, mobility of the complex is necessary for normal functioning in most areas of activity. As can be seen in Table 8-3,[97,98] among the 10 activities listed, using the telephone requires the largest arc of motion in both flexion (92.8°) and pronation and supination (63.5°). Cutting with a knife requires the smallest arc of flexion and of pronation/supination.

Relationship to the Hand and Wrist

The design of the radioulnar joints enhances the mobility of the hand. In primitive mammalian species, the ulna was a major weight-bearing structure and was connected directly to the carpals through a dense immobile syndesmosis.[84] The complete separation of the ulna from the carpals by the articular disk and the formation of a true diarthrodial joint lined with articular cartilage are features that permit pronation and supination to occur in every position of the hand to the forearm. Pronation and supination of the forearm, when the elbow is flexed at 90°, rotates the hands so that the palm faces either superiorly or inferiorly. The mobility afforded the hand is achieved at the expense of stability because the movable forearm is unable to provide a stable base for attachment of the wrist and hand muscles. Therefore, many of the muscles that act on the wrist and hand are attached on the distal end of the humerus rather than on the forearm.

The location of the hand and wrist muscles at the elbow and the fact that these muscles cross the elbow create close structural and functional relationships between the elbow and wrist/hand complexes. Anatomically, the hand and wrist muscles help reinforce the elbow joint capsule and contribute to stability of the elbow complex. In a study of 11 cadaveric specimens, Davidson and coworkers[99] found that the

Table 8-2	Ligamentous and Muscular Contributions to Stability at the Proximal and Distal Radioulnar joints	
Joint	Ligamentous	Muscular
Proximal radioulnar joint	Annular and quadrate ligaments[11]	Passive tension in the biceps brachii in the full extended elbow position
	Oblique cord[21] (limits supination)	Pronator teres (helps maintain contact of radial head and capitulum)
	Interosseous membrane	
Distal radioulnar joint	Interosseous membrane[49,50]	Pronator quadratus[39,52,57]
	Dorsal radioulnar ligament (limits pronation)[39,46,56]	Anconeus
	Palmar radioulnar ligament (limits supination)[39,46,56]	Extensor carpi ulnaris[39,48,58]
	Triangular fibrocartilage[39,40,47,59]	Pronator teres
	Joint capsule	

Table 8-3	Elbow and Forearm Motion During Functional Activities: Mean Values in Degrees						
Activity	Flexion			Pronation and Supination			Source
	Min	Max	Arc	Pronation Max	Supination Max	Arc	
Use telephone	42.8	135.6	92.8	40.9	22.6	63.5	Morrey[24]
	75	140	65				Packer[25]
Rise from chair	20.3	94.5	74.2	33.8	−9.5*	24.3	Morrey
	15	100	85				Packer
Open door	24.0	57.4	33.4	35.4	23.4	58.8	Morrey
Read newspaper	77.9	104.3	26.4	48.8	−7.3*	41.5	Morrey
Pour pitcher	35.6	58.3	22.7	42.9	21.9	64.8	Morrey
Put glass to mouth	44.8	130.0	85.2	10.1	13.4	23.5	Morrey
Drink from cup	71.5	129.2	57.7	−3.4†	31.2	27.8	Safaee-Rad[26]
Cut with knife	89.2	106.7	17.5	41.9	−26.9*	15.0	Morrey
Eat with fork	85.1	128.3	43.2	10.4	51.8	62.2	Morrey
	93.8	122.3	28.5	38.2	58.8	97.0	Safaee-Rad
Eat with spoon	101.2	123.2	22.0	22.9	58.7	81.6	Safaee-Rad
	70	115	45				Packer

*The minus sign indicates pronation.
† The minus sign indicates supination.
From Norkin CC, White DJ: Measurement of Joint Motion: A Guide to Goniometry, 3rd ed. Philadelphia, FA Davis, 2003.

humeral head of the flexor carpi ulnaris muscle is the only muscle that lies directly over the anterior portion of the MCL at elbow flexion positions between 90° and 120°. Because the medial elbow is subjected to the largest valgus stress during the cocking and acceleration phases of throwing, which occur between 80° and 120° of elbow flexion, the flexor carpi ulnaris muscle has the potential to provide significant reinforcement for the MCL during throwing activities.[99] During muscular contractions, the wrist muscles may contribute to the torque production of the elbow muscles. However, the muscles may have a more important functional role by producing compression of the articulating surfaces at the elbow. The importance of compression or stabilization of the elbow can be seen in the work of Amis and associates,[45] who investigated the effect of tensile loads on the forearm during a pulling activity. They found that both the humeroradial and humeroulnar articulations are subjected to compressive forces during pulling activities and that the MCL was heavily loaded. Andersson and Schultz found that during a pulling task, the flexors, at an elbow position of 90° of flexion, exerted a flexor force of 6000 N.[100]

◆ Effects of Age and Injury

Like other joints in the body, the joints and muscles of the elbow complex may be subject to the effects of age, injury, and immobilization.

Age

As can be seen in sampling of experimental findings presented in Table 8-4, the decrease in muscle strength that accompanies increasing age appears to be affected by the type of muscle action involved (eccentric/con-

Table 8-4	Effects of Aging on Elbow Muscles		
Frontera et al.[101]	Hughes et al.[102]	Lynch et al.[103]	Gallagher et al.[104]
n=12 men **Age 1st eval, 65 yr** **Age 2nd eval, 77 yr**	**n=68 women** **n=52 men** **Age 1st eval, 47–78 yr** **Age 2nd eval, 56–88 yr**	**n=339 women** **n=364 men** **Age, 19–93 yr**	**n=60 men** **age, 20–60 yr**
Isokinetic strength losses ranged from 20% to 30% at slow and fast velocities over the 12-year period.	Isokinetic strength in the elbow flexors and extensors declined by 2% per decade for women and by 12% per decade for men.	Muscle quality (peak torque per unit of muscle mass) for concentric peak torque showed a 28% decrease in men and a 20% decrease in women. Eccentric peak torque showed a 25% decline in men, but the decline was not significant in women.	Active flexion/extension peak torque, power, and angle of peak torque production measured bilaterally showed highly significant differences between young and old. However, no age-related differences occurred in supination and pronation.

centric), muscle group involved and gender among other factors such as level of physical activity.[102–107]

Continuing Exploration: **Research Findings Related to Aging of the Elbow Muscles**

Significant differences between young and old groups have been found in the location where peak torque is produced in a ROM.[103] Valour and Pousson found that maximal isometric force and series elastic component compliance of the elbow flexors were significantly less in the elderly than in younger groups, but the antagonist coactivation was similar for both groups.[107] Klein and associates found that the area of type I fibers in the biceps brachii muscle and maximum voluntary strength of the elbow flexors was lower in old than in young persons, but the percentages of type II fibers and type I fiber areas were not different between young and old persons.[108]

Injury

Injuries to the elbow are fairly frequent, and in early adolescence the elbow is one of the most common sites for apophysitis or strains at the apophysis.[109] An understanding of the mechanisms of elbow injuries and their relation to elbow joint structures is necessary for determining the effects of the injuries on joint function.

■ **Compression Injuries**

Resistance to longitudinal compression forces at the elbow is provided for mainly by the contact of bony components; therefore, excessive compression forces at the elbow often result in bony failure. Falling on the hand when the elbow is in a close-packed (extended)

position may result in the transmission of forces through the bones of the forearm to the elbow (Fig. 8-29A). If the forces are transmitted through the radius, as may happen with a concomitant valgus stress, a fracture of the radial head may result from impact of the radial head on the capitulum (see Fig. 8-29B). If the force from the fall is transmitted to the ulna, a fracture of either the coronoid or olecranon processes may occur from impact of the ulna on the humerus. If neither the radius nor the ulna absorbs the excessive force by fracturing, then the force may be transmitted to the humerus and may result in a fracture of the supracondylar area.

Muscle contractions also may cause high compression forces at the elbow. For example, during the acceleration and deceleration phases of baseball pitching, the compression forces at the elbow can attain 90% of body weight.[110] Nerve compression, bony fracture, or dislocation may also result from muscle contractions. Repetitive forceful contractions of the flexor carpi ulnaris muscle may compress the ulnar nerve as it passes through the cubital tunnel between the medial epicondyle of the humerus and olecranon process of the ulna[111–113] (Fig. 8–30). According to Chen et al.,[113] the ulnar nerve may be subjected not only to compression but also to traction and friction stresses during flexion and extension. The result of these stresses can cause an injury called cubital tunnel syndrome in which motion of the fourth and fifth fingers is impaired. Even in an MRI examination of 20 normal fresh-frozen elbow specimens, the ulnar nerve changed in area as much as 50% during elbow flexion and extension.[114]

■ **Distraction Injuries**

Ligaments and muscles provide for resistance of the joints of the elbow complex to longitudinal traction. A tensile force of sufficient magnitude exerted on a pronated and extended forearm may cause the radius

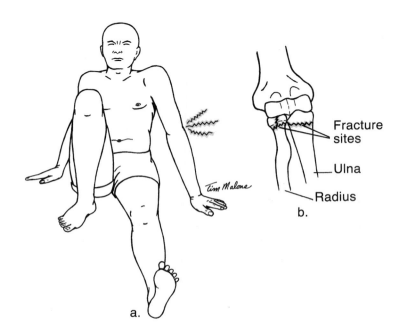

Fracture sites

Ulna

Radius

b.

a.

◄ **Figure 8-29** ■ A fall on the hand with the elbow in a close-packed position may involve transmission of forces through the bones of the forearm to the elbow. **A.** Transmission of forces from the hand to the elbow may occur through either the radius or ulna or through both. **B.** Impact of the radial head on the capitulum may cause either a fracture of the radial head or neck or both. A fracture of the coronoid or olecranon process or both may result from forces transmitted through the ulna.

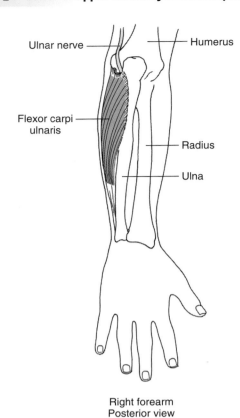

Right forearm
Postrior view

▲ **Figure 8-30** ■ Location of the ulnar nerve as it passes through the cubital tunnel. A contraction of the flexor carpi ulnaris muscle can cause compression of the ulnar nerve between the two heads of the muscle, which are located on either side of the ulnar nerve at the elbow.

to be pulled inferiorly out of the annular ligament. This injury is common in young children younger than 5 years[115] and rare in adults.[116] Lifting a small child up into the air by one or both hands or yanking a child by the one hand is the usual causative mechanism, and therefore the injury is referred to as either **nursemaid's elbow** or "pulled elbow"[115] (Fig. 8–31).

■ **Varus/Valgus Injuries**

Distraction and compression forces are created if either one of the collateral ligaments is overstretched or torn. If one side of the joint is subjected to abnormal tensile stresses, the other side is subjected to abnormal compressive forces (Fig. 8–32).

For example, the MCL is subjected to tensile stress during the backswing or "cock-up" portion of throwing a ball (Fig. 8–33). If the stress on the MCL is repetitive, such as in baseball pitching, the ligament may become lax and unable to reinforce the medial aspect of the joint.[117–120] The resulting medial instability may cause an increase in the normal carrying angle and excessive compression on the lateral aspect of the joint so that the radial head impacts on the capitulum. If the abnor-

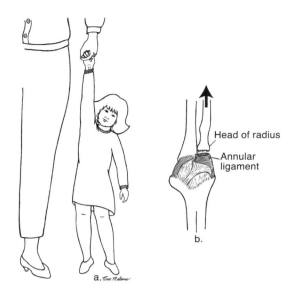

▲ **Figure 8-31** ■ Nursemaid's elbow. **A.** A pull on the hand creates tensile forces at the elbow. **B.** The radial head is shown being pulled out of the annular ligament.

mal compression forces on the articular cartilage are prolonged, these forces may interfere with the blood supply of the cartilage and result in avascular necrosis of the capitulum.

In a study of 40 uninjured professional baseball pitchers, Ellenbacher and colleagues found increased elbow laxity in players' pitching arms,[117] and in an MRI study, full-thickness tears of the MCL were found in over half of the elbows tested. In addition, 30 loose bodies were detected in the elbows of 14 subjects, and cartilaginous damage was present in 21 elbows.[119]

Other conditions that may occur in the throwing elbow include ulnar neuritis, flexor-pronator muscle strain or tendinitis, and medial epicondylitis.[120] Medial tendinitis or medial epicondylitis may be caused by forceful repetitive contractions of the pronator teres, the flexor carpi radialis, and, occasionally, the flexor carpi ulnaris. These muscles are involved in the tennis serve when the combined motion of elbow extension, pronation, and wrist flexion is used. High-speed video analysis shows that the elbow moves from 116° to 20° of flexion during serving. Ball impact occurs at an average of 35° of flexion. The forearm is in about 70° pronation at full impact.[121]

The classic tennis elbow (epicondylitis of the lateral epicondyle) appears to be caused by repeated forceful contractions of the wrist extensors, primarily the ECRB,[122] although Fairbank and Corelett suggested that the EDC muscles may also be involved.[123] The tensile stress created at the origin of the ECRB may cause microscopic tears that lead to inflammation of the lateral epicondyle.

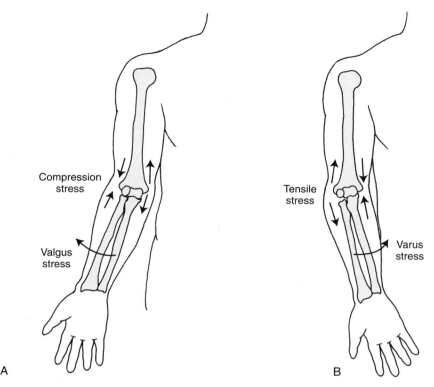

▲ **Figure 8-32** ■ **A.** The application of a valgus stress to the forearm produces a compression on the lateral aspect of the elbow joint and tensile strength on the medial joint aspect. **B.** The application of a varus stress to the forearm produces tensile stress on the lateral aspect of the elbow joint and compression on the medial joint aspect.

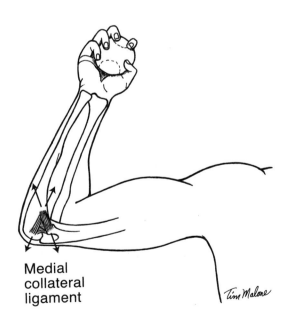

Medial
collateral
ligament

▲ **Figure 8-33** ■ Stretching of the medial collateral ligament during throwing.

Case Application 8-7: **Diagnosis and Treatment Options**

We have tentatively diagnosed James as having "tennis elbow"(lateral epicondylitis) even though we know that he is not a tennis player. A person does not have to be a tennis player to develop "tennis elbow." Any repetitive activity that causes tensile stresses on the lateral epicondyle may cause "tennis elbow."

Now we are faced with the challenge of determining which is the best treatment for James. Some treatment options include splinting, forearm support bands and taping,[123-129] ultrasound,[130,131] manipulation, exercise, and mobilization techniques.[132,133] Options that the physician may use to assist in reducing inflammation include oral nonsteroidal anti-inflammatory medications and corticosteroid injections.[134] Botulinum toxin injection and extracorporeal shock-wave treatments also have been employed.[135-137] Some evidence shows that ultrasound is more effective than a placebo, and some evidence shows that forearm support bands may offer some pain relief. Steroid injections are effective in relieving pain, but patients tend to return to normal activity too soon, before healing has occurred. Oral anti-inflammatory medications also may be helpful. Although many different options are available, more studies need to be performed to provide us sufficient evidence of the success of one method over another.

Summary

The interrelationship between the elbow complex and the wrist and hand complex makes normal functioning of the elbow vitally important. If elbow function is impaired, function of the hand also may be impaired. For example, if the elbow cannot be flexed, it is impossible for the hand to bring food to the mouth. Because many important vascular and neural structures that supply the hand are closely associated with the elbow, it is important to prevent excessive stress and to protect the elbow from injury. If the radial nerve is injured at the level of the epicondyle, the wrist extensors, supinator, thumb, and finger extensors will be affected. If the median nerve is injured at the level of the elbow, the pronators, flexor carpi radialis, finger flexors, thenar muscles, and lumbricales will be affected. In the following chapter, the reader will learn the specific functions of the hand muscles and will be better able to appreciate the significance of injury to some of the muscles.

Some of the interrelationships between the structure and function of elbow, shoulder, wrist, and hand have been introduced in this chapter. Muscles that have their primary actions at the wrist and hand also cross the elbow and contribute to its stability and function, whereas the stability and ROM at the shoulder and elbow help to enhance the function of the wrist and hand. Compensations at the elbow complex often are necessary when the ROM is limited at the shoulder or wrist. New relationships for the joints and muscles of the upper extremity will be introduced in the detailed study of the wrist and hand that follows in the next chapter.

Study Questions

1. Name and locate all of the articulating surfaces of the joints of the elbow complex. Describe the method of articulation at each joint, including axes of motion and degrees of freedom.
2. Explain the stabilizing function of the brachioradialis by diagramming the translatory and rotatory components at different joint angles.
3. Explain why active elbow flexion is more limited than passive flexion. Which structures limit extension?
4. Describe the "carrying angle" and explain why it is present.
5. Which structures limit supination and pronation?
6. If slow pronation of the forearm is attempted without resistance, which muscle will be used?
7. What does the term "concave incongruity" mean? Where is this condition found?
8. How does the structure and function of the annular ligament differ from that of the medial collateral ligament?
9. Describe the activity of the biceps brachii during a chin-up.
10. What is the mechanism of injury in tennis elbow?
11. Which position of the elbow is most stable? Why?
12. Compare the biceps brachii with the brachialis on the basis of structure and function.
13. Describe the mechanism of injury involved in cubital tunnel syndrome.

References

1. An KN, Hui FC, Morrey BF, et al.: Muscles across the elbow joint: A biomechanical analysis. J Biomech 14:659, 1981.
2. Morrey BF, Chao YS: Passive motion of the elbow joint. J Bone Joint Surg Am 58:501, 1976.
3. Williams PL (ed): Gray's Anatomy, 38th ed. New York, Churchill Livingstone, 1995.
4. Eckstein F, Lohe F, Muller-Gerbl M, et al.: Stress distribution in the trochlear notch. A model of bicentric load transmission through joints. J Bone Joint Surg Br 76:647, 1994.
5. Eckstein F, Lohe F, Hillebrand S, et al.: Morphomechanics of the humero-ulnar joint: I. Joint space width and contact area as a function of load and angle. Anat Rec 243:318, 1995.
6. Eckstein F, Merz B, Muller-Gerbl M, et al.: Morphomechanics of the humero-ulnar joint: II. Concave incongruity determines the distribution of load and subchondral mineralization. Anat Rec 243:327, 1995.
7. Milz S, Eckstein F, Putz R: Thickness distribution of the subchondral mineralization zone of the trochlear notch and its correlation with the cartilage thickness: An expression of functional adaptation to mechanical stress acting on the humeroulnar joint? Anat Rec 248:189, 1997.
8. Putz R, Milz S, Maier M, et al.: Functional morphology of the elbow joint. [Abstr] Orthopade 32:684, 2003.
9. Kapandji IA: The Physiology of the Joints, vol I. Edinburgh and London, E&S Livingstone, 1970.
10. Duparc F, Putz R, Michot C, et al.: The synovial fold of the humeroradial joint: Anatomical and histological features and clinical relevance in lateral

epicondylalgia of the elbow. Surg Radiol Anat 24:302, 2002.

11. Fuss F: The ulnar collateral ligament of the human elbow joint. Anatomy, function and biomechanics. J Anat 175:203, 1991.

12. Regan WD, Korinek SL, Morrey BF, et al.: Biomechanical study of ligaments around the elbow joint. Clin Orthop 271:170, 1991.

13. Bowling RW, Rockar PA: The elbow complex. In Malone TR, McPoil TG, Nitz AJ (eds): Orthopedic and Sports Physical Therapy, 3rd ed, p 382. St. Louis, Mosby-Year Book, 1996.

14. Sobel J, Nirschl RP: Elbow Injuries. In Zachazewski JE, Magee DJ, Quillen WS (eds): Athletic Injuries and Rehabilitation, p 544. Philadelphia, WB Saunders, 1996.

15. Richardson JK, Iglarsh ZA: Clinical Orthopaedic Physical Therapy, p 222. Philadelphia, WB Saunders, 1994.

16. Reid DC, Kushner S. The elbow. In Donatelli R, Wooden MJ (eds): Orthopaedic Physical Therapy, 2nd ed. New York, Churchill Livingstone, 1994.

17. Callaway GH, Field LD, Deng XH, et al.: Biomechanical evaluation of the medial collateral ligament of the elbow. J Bone Joint Surg Am 79:1223, 1997.

18. Petrie S, Collins JG, Solomonow M, et al.: Mechanoreceptors in the human elbow ligaments. J Hand Surg [Am] 23:512, 1998.

19. Sojbjerg JO, Ovesen J, Nielsen S: Experimental elbow instability after transection of the medial collateral ligament. Clin Orthop 218:1860, 1987.

20. Hotchkiss RN, Weiland AJ: Valgus stability of the elbow. J Orthop Res 5:372, 1987.

21. Olsen BS, Vaesel MT, Sojbjerg JO, et al.: Lateral collateral ligament of the elbow joint: Anatomy and kinematics. J Shoulder Elbow Surg 5:103, 1996.

22. Seki A, Olsen BS, Jensen SL, et al.: Functional anatomy of the lateral collateral ligament complex of the elbow: Configuration of the Y and its role. J Shoulder Elbow Surg 11:53, 2003.

23. Imatani J, Ogura T, Morito Y, et al.: Anatomic and histologic studies of collateral ligament complex of the elbow. J Shoulder Elbow Surg 8:625, 1999.

24. Morrey BF, An KN: Articular and ligamentous contributions to the stability of the elbow joint. Am J Sports Med 11:315, 1983.

25. O'Driscoll SW: Elbow instability. Acta Orthop Belg 65:404, 1999.

26. Olsen BS, Sojbjerg JO, Dalstra M, et al.: Kinematics of the lateral ligamentous constraints of the elbow joint. J Shoulder Elbow Surg 5:333, 1996.

27. Olsen BS, Sojbjerg JO, Nielsen KK, et al.: Posterolateral elbow joint instability: The basic kinematics. J Shoulder Elbow Surg 7:19, 1998.

28. Kim PT, Isogai S, Murakami G, et al.: The lateral collateral ligament complex and related muscles act as a dynamic stabilizer as well as a static supporting structure at the elbow joint: An anatomical and experimental study. Okajimas Folia Anat Jpn 79:55, 2002.

29. Dunning CE, Zarzour ZD, Patterson SD, et al.: Ligamentous stabilizers against poterolateral rotatory instability of the elbow. J Bone Joint Surg Am 83:1823, 2001.

30. Hannouche D, Begue T: Functional anatomy of the lateral collateral ligament complex of the elbow. Surg Radiol Anat 21:187, 1999.

31. Ball CM, Galatz LM, Yamaguchi K: Elbow instability: Treatment strategies and emerging concepts. Instr Course Lect 51:53, 2002.

32. McKee MD, Schemitsch EH, Sala MJ, et al.: The pathoanatomy of lateral ligamentous disruption in complex elbow instability. J Shoulder Elbow Surg 12:391, 2003.

33. Benjamin M, Kumai T, Milz S, et al.: The skeletal attachment of tendons—Tendon "entheses." Comp Biochem Physiol A Mol Integr Physiol 133:931, 2002.

34. Chard MD, Cawston TE, Riley GP, et al.: Rotator cuff degeneration and lateral epicondylitis: A comparative histological study. Ann Rheum Dis 53:30, 1994.

35. Galliani I, Burattini S, Mariani AR, et al.: Morphofunctional changes in human tendon tissue. Eur J Histochem 46:3, 2002.

36. Steinborn M, Heuck A, Jessel C, et al.: Magnetic resonance imaging of lateral epicondylitis of the elbow with a 0.2-T dedicated system. Eur Radiol 9:1376, 1999.

37. Ljung BO, Lieber RL, Friden J: Wrist extensor muscle pathology in lateral epicondylitis. J Hand Surg Br 24:177, 1999.

38. Mackay D, Rangan A, Hide G, et al.: The objective diagnosis of early tennis elbow by magnetic resonance imaging. Occup Med (Lond) 53:309, 2003.

39. Savnik A, Jensen B, Norregaard J, et al.: Magnetic resonance imaging in the evaluation of treatment response of lateral epicondylitis of the elbow. Eur Radiol 14:964, 2004.

40. Youm Y, Dryer RF, Thambyrajah K, et al.: Biomechanical analysis of forearm pronation-supination and elbow flexion-extension. J Biomech 12:245, 1979.

41. Deland JT, Garg A, Walker PS: Biomechanical basis for elbow hinge-distractor design. Clin Orthop 215:303, 1987.

42. Ericson A, Arndt A, Stark A, et al.: Variation in the position and orientation of the elbow flexion axis. J Bone Joint Surg Br 85:538, 2003.

43. Duck TR, Dunning CE, King GJ, et al.: Variability and repeatability of the flexion axis at the ulno-humeral joint. J Orthop Res 21:399, 2003.

44. Bottlang M, Madey SM, Steyers CM, et al.: Assessment of elbow joint kinematics in passive motion by electromagnetic tracking. J Orthop Res 18:195, 2000.

45. Amis AA, Dowson D, Wright V: Elbow joint force predictions for some strenuous isometric actions. J Biomech 13:765, 1980.

46. McGuigan FX, Bookout CB: Intra-articular fluid volume and restricted motion in the elbow. J Shoulder Elbow Surg 12:462, 2003.

47. O'Driscoll SW, Morrey BF, An KN: Interarticular pressure and capacity of the elbow. Arthroscopy 6:100, 1990.
48. Murray WM, Delp SL, Bucahnan TS: Variation of muscle moment arms with elbow and forearm position. J Biomech 28:513, 1995.
49. Murray WM, Buchanan TS, Delp SL: The isometric functional capacity of muscles that cross the elbow. J Biomech 33:943, 2000.
50. Zhang LQ, Nuber GW: Moment distribution among human elbow extensor muscles during isometric and submaximal extension. J Biomech 33:145, 2000.
51. Kasprisin JE, Grabiner MD: Joint angle-dependence of elbow flexor activation levels during isometric and isokinetic maximum voluntary contractions. Clin Biomech (Bristol, Avon) 15:743, 2000.
52. O'Sullivan LW, Gallwey TJ: Upper-limb surface electro-myography at maximum supination and pronation torques: The effect of elbow and forearm angle. J Electromyogr Kinesiol 12:275, 2002.
53. Naito A, Sun YJ, Yajima M, et al.: Electromyographic study of the flexors and extensors in a motion of forearm pronation/supination while maintaining elbow flexion in humans. Tohoku J Exp Med 186:267, 1998.
54. Nakazawa K, Kawakami Y, Fukunaga T, et al.: Differences in activation patterns in elbow flexor muscles during isometric, concentric and eccentric contractions. Eur J Applied Physiol Occup Physiol 66:214, 1993.
55. Provins KA, Salter N: Maximum torque exerted about the elbow joint. J Appl Physiol 7:393, 1955.
56. Currier DP: Maximal isometric tension of elbow extensors at varied positions. Phys Ther 52:1043, 1972.
57. Bohannon RW: Shoulder position influences elbow extension force in healthy individuals. J Orthop Sports Phys Ther 12:111, 1990.
58. Buchanan TS, Almdale DP, Lewis JL, et al.: Characteristics of synergistic relations during isometric contractions of human elbow muscles. J Neurophysiol 56:1225, 1986.
59. Dounskaia NV, Swinnen SP, Walter CB, et al.: Hierarchical control of different elbow/wrist coordination patterns. Exp Brain Res 121:239, 1998.
60. Prodoehl J, Gottlieb GL, Corocs DM: The neural control of single degree of freedom elbow movements. Effect of starting position. Exp Brain Res 153:7, 2003.
61. Mohiuddin A, Zanjua MZ: Form and function of radioulnar joint articular disc. Hand 14:61, 1982.
62. Linscheid RL: Biomechanics of the distal radioulnar joint. Clin Orthop 275:46, 1992.
63. Mikic Z: Detailed anatomy of the articular disc of the distal radioulnar joint. Clin Orthop 245:123, 1989.
64. Chiou HJ, Chang CY, Chou YH, et al.: Triangular fibrocartilage of wrist: Presentation on high resolu-

tion ultrasonography. J Ultrasound Med 17:41, 1998.
65. Chidgey LK, Dell PC, Bittar ES, et al.: Histologic anatomy of the triangular fibrocartilage. J Hand Surg [Am] 16:1084, 1991.
66. Ohmori M, Azuma H: Morphology and distribution of nerve endings in the human triangular fibrocartilage complex. J Hand Surg [Br] 23:522, 1998.
67. Palmer AK: The distal radioulnar joint. Orthop Clin North Am 15:321, 1984.
68. Palmer AK, Werner FW: Biomechanics of the distal radioulnar joint. Orthop Clin North Am 15:27, 1984.
69. Ekenstam F: Anatomy of the distal radioulnar joint. Clin Orthop 275:14, 1992.
70. Schind F, An KN, Berglund L, et al.: The distal radioulnar ligaments: A biomechanical study. J Hand Surg [Am] 16:1106, 1991.
71. Van Der Heijden ED, Hillen B: A two-dimensional kinematic analysis of the distal radioulnar joint. J Hand Surg [Br] 21:824, 1996.
72. Skahen JR 3rd, Palmer AK, Werner FW, et al.: The interosseous membrane of the forearm: Anatomy and function. J Hand Surg [Am] 22:981, 1997.
73. Pfaeffle HJ, Tomaino MM, Grewal R, et al.: Tensile properties of the interosseous membrane of the human forearm. J Orthop Res 14:842, 1996.
74. Nakamura T, Yabe Y, Horiuchi Y: Functional anatomy of the interosseous membrane of the forearm—Dynamic changes during rotation. Hand Surg 4:67, 1999.
75. McGinley JC, Heller JE, Fertala A, et al.: Biochemical composition and histologic structure of the foream interosseous membrane. J Hand Surg [Am] 28:503, 2003.
76. McGinley JC, Kozin SH: Interosseous membrane anatomy and functional mechanics. Clin Orthop 383:108, 2001.
77. Nakamura T, Yabe Y, Horiuchi Y, et al.: Normal kinematics of the interosseous membrane during forearm pronation-supination—A three-dimensional MRI study. Hand Surg 5:1, 2000.
78. Birkbeck DP, Failla JM, Hoshaw SJ, et al.: The interosseous membrane affects load distribution in the forearm. J Hand Surg [Am] 22:975, 1997.
79. Pfaeffle HJ, Fischer KJ, Manson TT, et al.: Role of the forearm interosseous ligament: Is it more than just longitudinal load transfer? J Hand Surg [Am] 25:683, 2000.
80. DeFrate LE, Li G, Zayontz SJ, et al.: A minimally invasive method for the determination of force in the interosseous ligament. Clin Biomech (Bristol, Avon) 16:895, 2001.
81. Gabl M, Zimmermann R, Angermann P, et al.: The interosseous membrane and its influence on the distal radioulnar joint. An investigation of the distal tract. J Hand Surg [Br] 23:179, 1998.
82. Kleinman WB, Graham JJ: The distal radioulnar joint capsule: Clinical anatomy and role in post

traumatic limitation of forearm rotation. J Hand Surg [Am] 23:588, 1998.

83. Johnson RK, Shrewsbury MM: The pronator quadratus in motions and in stabilization of the radius and ulna at the distal radioulnar joint. J Hand Surg [Am] 1:205, 1976.

84. Drobner WS, Hausman MR: The distal radioulnar joint. Hand Clin 8:631, 1992.

85. Haaugstvedt JR, Berger RA, Berglund LJ: A mechanical study of the moment-forces of the supinators and pronators of the forearm. Acta Orthop Scand 72:629, 2001.

86. Gordon KD, Pardo RD, Johnson JA, et al.: Electromagnetic activity and strength during maximum isometric pronation and supination efforts in healthy adults. J Orthop Res 22:208, 2004.

87. Askew LJ, An KN, Morrey BF, et al.: Isometric elbow strength in normal individuals. Clin Orthop 222:261, 1987.

88. Kihara H, Short WH, Werner FW, et al.. The stabilizing mechanisms of the distal radioulnar joint during pronation and supination. J Hand Surg [Am] 20:930, 1995.

89. Stuart PR: Pronator quadratus revisited. J Hand Surg [Am] 21:741, 1996.

90. Kauer JM: The distal radioulnar joint. Clin Orthop 275:37 1991.

91. Haahr P, Andersen, JH: Prognostic factors in lateral epicondylitis: A randomized trial with one-year follow-up in 266 new cases treated with minimal occupational intervention or the usual approach in general practice. Rheumatology (Oxford) 42:1216, 2003.

92. Adams BD, Holley KA: Strains in the articular disk of the triangular fibrocartilage complex: A biomechanical study. J Hand Surg [Am] 18:919, 1993.

93. Skahen JR 3rd, Palmer AK, Werner FW, et al.: Reconstruction of the interosseous membrane of the forearm in cadavers. J Hand Surg [Am] 22:986, 1997.

94. Markolf KL, Lamey D, Yang S, et al.: Radioulnar load-sharing in the forearm: A study in cadavera. J Bone Joint Surg Am 80:879, 1998.

95. Bade H, Koebke J, Schluter M: Morphology of the articular surfaces of the distal radio-ulnar joint. Anat Rec 246:410, 1996.

96. Morrey BF, Askew LJ, Chao EY: A biomechanical study of normal functional elbow motion. J Bone Joint Surg Am 63:872, 1981.

97. Safee-Rad R, Shwedyk E, Quanbury AO, et al.: Normal functional range of motion of upper limb joints during performance of three feeding activities. Arch Phys Med Rehabil 71:505, 1990.

98. Packer TL, Peat M, Wyss U, et al.: Examining the elbow during functional activities. Occup Ther J Res 10:323, 1990.

99. Davidson PA, Pink M, Perry J, et al.: Functional anatomy of the flexor pronator muscle group in relation to the medial collateral ligament of the elbow. Am J Sports Med 23:245, 1995.

100. Andersson GBJ, Schultz AB: Transmission of moments across the elbow joint and the lumbar spine. J Biomech 12:747, 1979.

101. Frontera WR, Hughes VA, Fielding RA, et al.: Aging of skeletal muscle: A 12-yr longitudinal study. J Appl Physiol 88:1321, 2000.

102. Hughes VA, Frontera WR, Wood M, et al.: Longitudinal muscle strength changes in older adults: Influence of muscle mass, physical activity, and health. J Gerontol A Biol Sci Med Sci 56:B209, 2001.

103. Lynch NA, Metter EJ, Lindle RS, et al.: Muscle quality. I. Age-associated differences between arm and leg muscle groups. J Appl Physiol 86:188, 1999.

104. Gallagher MA, Cuomo F, Polonsky L, et al.: Effects of age, testing speed, and arm dominance on isokinetic strength of the elbow. J Shoulder Elbow Surg 6:340, 1997.

105. Jakobi JM, Rice CL: Voluntary muscle activation varies with age and muscle group. J Appl Physiol 93:457, 2002.

106. Seghers J, Spaepen A, Delecluse C, et al.: Habitual level of physical activity and muscle fatigue of the elbow flexors muscles in older men. Eur J Appl Physiol 89:427, 2003.

107. Valour D, Pousson M: Compliance changes of the series elastic component of elbow flexor muscles with age in humans. Pflurgis Arch 445:712, 2003.

108. Klein CS, Marsh GD, Petrella RJ, et al.: Muscle fiber number in the biceps brachii of young and old men. Muscle Nerve 28:62, 2003.

109. Adrim TA, Cheng TL: Overview of injuries in the young athelete. Sports Med 33:75, 2003.

110. Werner SL, Fleisig GS, Dillman CJ, et al.: Biomechanics of the elbow during baseball pitching. J Orthop Sports Phys Ther 17:274, 1993.

111. Green JR, Rayan GM: The cubital tunnel: Anatomic, histologic and mechanical study. J Shoulder Elbow Surg 8:466, 1999.

112. Degeorges R, Masquelet AC: The cubital tunnel: Anatomical study of the distal part. Surg Radiol Anat 24:169, 2002.

113. Chen FS, Rokito AS, Jobe FW: Medial elbow problems in the overhead throwing athlete. J Am Acad Orthop Surg 9:99, 2001.

114. Gelberman RH, Yamaguchi K, Hollstien SB, et al.: Changes in the interstitial pressure and cross-sectional area of the cubital tunnel and of the ulnar nerve with flexion of the elbow. An experimental study in human cadavera. J Bone Joint Surg Am 80:492, 1998.

115. Choung W, Heinrich SD: Acute annular ligament interposition into the radiocapitellar joint in children (nursemaid's elbow). J Pediatr Orthop 15:454, 1995.

116. Obert L, Huot D, Lepage D, et al.: [Isolated traumatic luxation of the radial head in adults: Report of a case and review of the literature.] Chir Main 22:216, 2003.

117. Ellenbacher TS, Mattalino AJ, Elam EA, et al.: Medial elbow joint laxity in professional baseball pitchers. A bilateral comparison using stress radiography. Am J Sports Med 26:420, 1998.

118. Ireland ML, Andrews JR: Shoulder and elbow injuries in the young athlete. Clin Sports Med 7:473, 1988.

119. Sugimoto H, Mattalino AJ, Elam EA, et al.: Throwing injury of the elbow: Assessment with gradient three-dimensional Fourier transform gradient-echo and short tau inversion recovery images. J Magn Reson Imaging 8:487, 1998.

120. Cain EL Jr, Dugas JR, Wolf RS, et al.: Elbow injuries in the throwing athlete: A current concepts review. Am J Sports Med 31:621, 2003.

121. Kibler WB: Clinical biomechanics of the elbow in tennis: Implications for evaluation and diagnosis. Med Sci Sports Exerc 26:1203, 1994.

122. Priest JD, et al.: The elbow and tennis. Part 1: An analysis of players with and without pain. Phys Sports Med 8:4, 1980.

123. Fairbank SR, Corelett RJ: The role of the extensor digitorum communis muscle in lateral epicondylitis. J Hand Surg [Br] 27:405, 2002.

124. Meyer NJ, Pennington W, Haines B, et al.: The effect of the forearm support band on forces at the origin of the extensor carpi radialis brevis: A cadaveric study and review of literature. J Hand Ther 15:179, 2002.

125. Meyer NJ, Walter F, Haines B, et al.: Modeled evidence of force reduction at the extensor carpi radialis brevis origin with the forearm support band. J Hand Surg [Am] 28:279, 2003.

126. Chan HL, Ng GY: Effect of counterforce forearm bracing on wrist extensor muscle performance. Am J Phys Med Rehabil 82:290, 2003.

127. Vicenzino B, Brooksbank J, Minto J, et al.: Initial effects of elbow taping on pain-free grip strength and pressure pain. J Orthop Sports Phys Ther 33:400, 2003.

128. Knebel PT, Avery DW, Gebhardt TL, et al.: Effects of the forearm support band on wrist extensor muscle fatigue. J Orthop Sports Phys Ther 29:677, 1999.

129. Walther M, Kirschner S, Koenig A, et al.: Biomechanical evaluation of braces used for the treatment of epicondylitis. J Shoulder Elbow Surg 11:265, 2002.

130. Smidt N, Assendelft WJ, Arola H, et al.: Effectiveness of physiotherapy for lateral epicondylitis: A systematic review. Ann Med 35:51, 2003.

131. Ekstrom RA, Holden K: Examination of and intervention for a patient with lateral elbow pain with signs of nerve entrapment. Phys Ther 82:11, 2002.

132. Vincenzino B: Lateral epicondylalgia: A musculoskeletal physiotherapy perspective. Man Ther 8:66, 2003.

133. Abbott JH, Patla CE, Jensen RH: The initial effects of elbow mobilization with movement technique on grip strength in subjects with lateral epicondylalgia. Man Ther 6:163, 2001.

134. Mellor S: Treatment of tennis elbow: The evidence. BMJ 327:330, 2003.

135. Melikyan EY, Shahin E, Miles J, et al.: Extracorporeal shock-wave treatment for tennis elbow: A randomised double-blind study. J Bone Joint Surg Br 85:852, 2003.

136. Wang CJ: An overview of shock wave therapy in musculoskeletal disorders. Chang keng Med J 26:220, 2003.

137. Keizer SB, Rutten HP, Pilot P, et al.: Botulinum toxin injection versus surgical treatment for tennis elbow: A randomized pilot study. Clin Orthop 401:125, 2002.

Chapter **9**

The Wrist and Hand Complex

Noelle M. Austin, PT, MS, CHT

 Introduction

The human hand may well surpass all body parts except the brain as a topic of universal interest. The human hand has been characterized as a symbol of power,[1] as an extension of intellect,[2] and as the seat of the will.[3] The symbiotic relation of the mind and hand is exemplified by sociologists' claim that the brain is responsible for the design of civilization but the hand is responsible for its formation. The hand cannot function without the brain to control it; likewise, the encapsulated brain needs the hand as a primary tool of expression. The entire upper limb is subservient to the hand. Any loss of function in the upper limb, regardless of the segment, ultimately translates into diminished function of its most distal joints. It is the significance of this potential loss that has led to detailed study of the finely balanced intricacies of the normal upper limb and hand.

The Wrist Complex

The wrist (**carpus**) consists of two compound joints: the **radiocarpal** and the **midcarpal joints,** referred to collectively as the **wrist complex** (Fig. 9-1A and B). Each joint proximal to the wrist complex serves to broaden the placement of the hand in space and to increase the degrees of freedom available to the hand. The shoulder serves as a dynamic base of support; the elbow allows the hand to approach or extend away from the body; and the forearm adjusts the approach of the hand to an object. The carpus, unlike the more proximal joints, serves placement of the hand in space to only a minor degree. The major contribution of the wrist complex seems to be to control length-tension relationships in the multiarticular hand muscles and to allow fine adjustment of grip.[4] The wrist muscles appear to be designed for balance and control rather than for maximizing torque production.[5] The adjustments in the length-tension relationship of the extrinsic hand muscles that occur at the wrist cannot be replaced by compensatory movements of the shoulder, elbow, or forearm (radioulnar joint). The wrist has been called the most complex joint of the body, from both an anatomic and physiologic perspective.[6] The intricacy and variability of the interarticular and intra-articular relations within the wrist complex are such that the wrist has received a large amount of attention with agreement on relatively few points. Two points on which there appears to be consensus are that the structure and biomechanics of the wrist, as well as of the hand, vary tremendously from person to person and that even subtle variations can produce differences in how a given function occurs. The intent of this chapter, therefore, is less to provide details on what is "normal" and more to describe the wrist complex (and hand) in such a way that general structure is clear and a conceptual framework is developed within which normal function and pathology can be understood.

The wrist complex as a whole is considered to be biaxial, with motions of **extension/flexion** around a coronal axis and **ulnar deviation/radial deviation** around an anteroposterior axis. Some authors argue that some degree of **pronation/supination** may also be found, especially at the radiocarpal joint.[7] The ranges of motion (ROMs) of the entire complex are variable and reflect the differences in carpal kinematics that arise from such factors as ligamentous laxity, shape of articular surfaces, and constraining effects of muscles.[8] Normal ranges are cited as 65° to 85° of flexion, 60° to 85° of extension, 15° to 21° of radial deviation, and 20° to 45° of ulnar deviation.[9-12] The ranges are contributed in various proportions by the compound radiocarpal and midcarpal joints. Gilford and colleagues[13] proposed that the two-joint, rather than single-joint, system of the wrist complex (1) permitted large ROMs with less exposed articular surface and tighter joint capsules, (2) had less tendency for structural pinch at extremes of ranges, and (3) allowed for flatter multijoint surfaces that are more capable of withstanding imposed pressures.

 CONCEPT CORNERSTONE 9-1: *Nomenclature*

As is true at many other joints of the body, there are variations in nomenclature for the wrist and hand. Flexion/extension of the wrist may also be termed volar (palmar) flexion/dorsiflexion, respectively. Radial/ulnar deviation of the wrist may be also be called abduction/adduction, respectively. At both the wrist and with joints and structures in the hand, the terms volar and palmar are used virtually interchangeably, whereas reference to the posterior aspect of the hand is more consistently referred to as the dorsum. The terms medial/lateral may be used in lieu of ulnar/radial. We will use flexion/extension and radial/ulnar deviation for the wrist motions, although coronal plane motions of the fingers are referred to most commonly (and we will follow this convention) as abduction/adduction. The terms volar and palmar will be used interchangeably in order to accurately represent terms found in the cited literature.]

Radiocarpal Joint Structure

The radiocarpal joint is formed by the **radius** and **radioulnar disk** as part of the **triangular fibrocartilage com-**

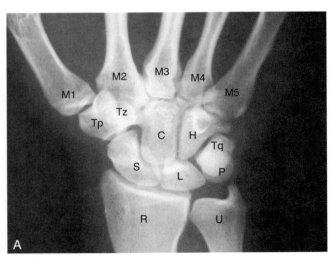
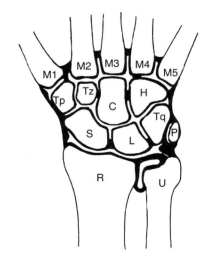

▲ **Figure 9-1** ■ Wrist complex as shown on radiograph (**A**) and in a schematic representation (**B**). The radiocarpal joint is composed of the radius and the radioulnar disk, with the scaphoid (S), lunate (L), and the triquetrum (Tq). The midcarpal joint is composed of the scaphoid, lunate, and triquetrum with the trapezium (Tp), the trapezoid (Tz), the capitate (C), and the hamate (H).

plex (**TFCC**) proximally and by the **scaphoid, lunate,** and **triquetrum** distally (see Fig. 9-1A and B).

■ Proximal and Distal Segments
of the Radiocarpal Joint

The distal radius has a single continuous, biconcave curvature that is long and shallow side to side (frontal plane) and shorter and sharper anteroposteriorly (sagittal plane). The proximal joint surface is composed of (1) the lateral radial facet, which articulates with the scaphoid; (2) the medial radial facet, which articulates with the lunate; and (3) the TFCC, which articulates predominantly with the triquetrum, although it also has some contact with the lunate in the neutral wrist. The radioulnar disk, a component of the TFCC, also serves as part of the distal radioulnar joint, as discussed in the previous chapter. As a whole, the compound proximal radiocarpal joint surface is oblique, angled slightly volarly and ulnarly. The average inclination of the distal radius is 23°. This inclination occurs because the radial length (height) is 12 mm greater on the radial side than on the ulnar side[14] (Fig. 9-2A). The distal radius is also tilted 11° volarly[14] (see Fig. 9-2B), with the posterior radius slightly longer than the volar radius.

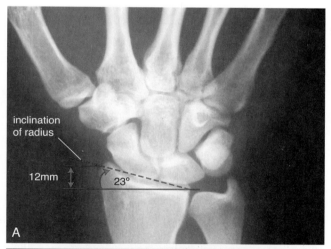

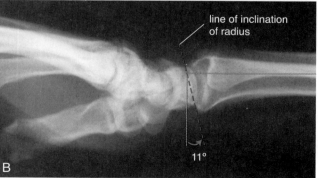

▲ **Figure 9-2** ■ **A.** A normal angle of 23° of inclination of the radius in the frontal plane, with the distal radius about 12 mm long on the radial side than on the ulnar side. **B.** A normal angulation of inclination of about 11° of the radius volarly in the sagittal plane.

The TFCC consists of the radioulnar disk and the various fibrous attachments that provide the primary support for the distal radioulnar joint (Fig. 9-3).[15] Although the attachments attributed to the TFCC vary somewhat, Mohiuddin and Janjua,[16] Benjamin and colleagues,[17] and Palmer[18] provided descriptions that represent a reasonable consensus. The articular disk is a fibrocartilaginous continuation of the articular cartilage of the distal radius. The disk is connected medially via two dense fibrous connective tissue laminae. The upper laminae include the **dorsal and volar radioulnar ligaments,** which attach to the ulnar head and ulnar styloid. The lower lamina has connections to the sheath of the **extensor carpi ulnaris** (ECU) tendon and to the **triquetrum, hamate,** and the base of the **fifth metacarpal** through fibers from the **ulnar collateral ligament.** The so-called **meniscus homolog** is a region of irregular connective tissue that lies within and is part of the lower lamina, which traverses volarly and ulnarly from the dorsal radius to insert on the triquetrum. Along its path, the meniscus homolog has fibers that insert into the ulnar styloid and contribute to the formation of the **prestyloid recess.**[19] The medial (ulnar) connective tissue structures may exist in lieu of more extensive fibrocartilage because connective tissue is more compressible than fibrocartilage and thus may contribute to ROM.[16] Overall, the TFCC should be considered to function at the wrist as an extension of the distal radius, just as it does at the distal radioulnar joint.

The scaphoid, lunate, and triquetrum compose the proximal carpal row (see Fig. 9-1A and B). The proximal carpal row articulates with the distal radius. These bones are interconnected by two ligaments that, like the carpals themselves, are covered with cartilage proximally.[20] They are the **scapholunate interosseous** and the **lunotriquetral interosseous ligaments,** respectively. The proximal carpal row and ligaments together appear to be a single biconvex cartilage-covered joint surface that, unlike a rigid segment, can change shape somewhat to accommodate to the demands of space between the forearm and hand.[21] The **pisiform,** anatomically part of the proximal row, does not participate in the radiocarpal articulation. The pisiform functions entirely as a sesamoid bone, presumably to increase the moment arm (MA) of the **flexor carpi ulnaris** (FCU) tendon that envelops it. The curvature of the distal radiocarpal joint surface is sharper than the proximal joint surface in both the sagittal and coronal planes, which makes the joint somewhat incongruent. The concept of articular incongruence is supported by the finding that the overall contact between the proximal and distal radiocarpal surfaces is typically only about 20% of available surface, with never more than 40% of available surface in contact at any one time.[22] Joint incongruence and the angulation of the proximal joint surface result in a greater range of flexion than extension[23] and in greater ulnar deviation than radial deviation for the radiocarpal joint.[20] The total range of flexion/extension is greater than the total range of radial/ulnar deviation. Incongruence and ligamentous laxity may account for as much as 45° of combined pas-

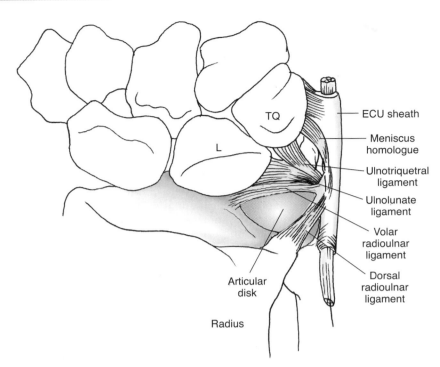

◀ **Figure 9-3** ■ The triangular fibrocartilage complex (TFCC), including the articular disk with its various fibrous attachments, which provide support to the distal radioulnar joint.

sive pronation/supination at the radiocarpal and midcarpal joints together,[7] although this motion is rarely considered to be an additional degree of freedom available to the wrist complex.

Not only do the curvature and inclination of the radiocarpal surfaces affect function, but the length of the ulna in relation to the radius is also a factor.[24,25] **Ulnar negative variance** is described as a short ulna in comparison with the radius at their distal ends, whereas in **ulnar positive variance,** the distal ulna is long in relation to the distal radius (Fig. 9-4).[26] When an axial (longitudinal compressive) load is applied to the wrist, the scaphoid and lunate receive approximately 80% of the load, whereas the TFCC receives approximately 20%.[15,22,27,28] At the distal radius, 60% of the contact is made with the scaphoid and 40% with the lunate.[22]

| 9-1 | **Patient Case: Distal Radius Fracture** |

Gail Angeles sustained a right distal radius fracture after a fall on an outstretched hand (known by the acronym FOOSH). The posteroanterior (P-A) view in the radiograph illustrates how there is a loss in length of the radius and the normal radial inclination is diminished (Fig. 9-5A). The normal volar inclination of the distal radius is now dorsally angulated in the postreduction lateral radiograph (see Fig. 9-5B). These changes would be likely to result in a loss of ROM and the likelihood of future joint degeneration. Restoring the articular surfaces to near-anatomic position (and correcting the relative lengths of the radius and ulna) would most like require open reduction and internal fixation (ORIF) with plate and screws.

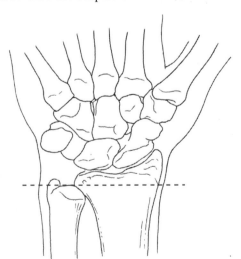

A

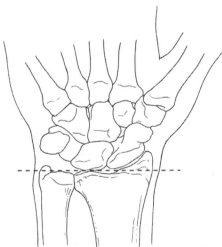

B

▲ **Figure 9-4** ■ Ulnar variance: negative (**A**) and positive (**B**).

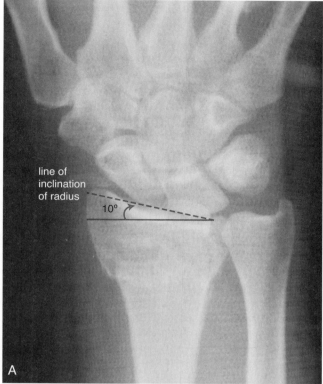

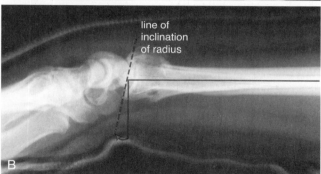

▲ **Figure 9-5** ■ A radial fracture from a fall on an outstretched hand resulting in diminished angulation (and length) of the distal radius (**A**). Relative shortening of the radius results in an increased ulnar variance, as well as a reversal of the normal volar inclination of the radius (**B**).

With an ulnar-positive variance, there is a potential for impingement of the TFCC structures between the distal ulna and the triquetrum.[24] Palmer et al. found an inverse relationship between the thickness of the TFCC and ulnar variance, with positive ulnar variance associated with a thinner TFCC and negative ulnar variance with a relatively thicker TFCC.[29] A relatively "long" ulna may be present after a distal radius fracture (see Fig. 9-5A) that healed in a shortened position. Pain is commonly present with end-range pronation and ulnar deviation because these motions increase the likelihood of impingement of the ulnar structures. Surgical intervention may include a joint-leveling procedure

such as ulnar shortening to unload the ulnar side of the wrist.[30]

In contrast to ulnar-positive variance, ulnar-negative variance (a relatively short ulna) may result in abnormal force distribution across the radiocarpal joint with potential degeneration at the radiocarpal joint.[25] **Avascular necrosis** of the lunate, **Kienbock's disease** (Fig. 9-6), has been associated with negative ulnar variance.[30,31] Treatment options include unloading of the radiocarpal joint by lengthening the ulna, shortening the radius, or fusing select carpal bones.[32]

■ Radiocarpal Capsule and Ligaments

The radiocarpal joint is enclosed by a strong but somewhat loose capsule and is reinforced by capsular and intracapsular ligaments. Most ligaments that cross the radiocarpal joint also contribute to stability at the midcarpal joint, and so all the ligaments will be presented together after introduction of the midcarpal joint. Similarly, the muscles of the radiocarpal joint also function at the midcarpal joint. In fact, the radiocarpal joint is not crossed by any muscles that act on the radiocarpal joint alone. The FCU is the only muscle that crosses the radiocarpal joint and attaches to any of the bones of the proximal carpal row. Although fibers of the FCU tendon end on the pisiform, the pisiform is only loosely connected to the triquetrum below.[33] Consequently, forces applied to the pisiform by the FCU muscle are translated not to the triquetrum on which it sits but to the hamate and fifth metacarpal via pisiform ligaments. Motions occurring at the radiocarpal joint are a result of forces applied by the abundant passive ligamentous structures and by muscles that are attached to the distal carpal row and metacarpals. Consequently, movements of the radiocarpal and midcarpal joints must be examined together.

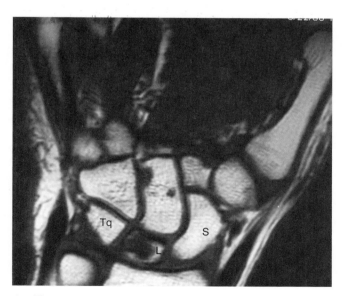

▲ **Figure 9-6** ■ Avascular necrosis of the lunate seen in this magnetic resonance image (MRI) is known as Kienbock's disease and has been associated with negative ulnar variance.

Midcarpal Joint Structure

The midcarpal joint is the articulation between the scaphoid, lunate, and triquetrum proximally and the distal carpal row composed of the **trapezium, trapezoid, capitate,** and hamate (see Fig. 9-1B). The midcarpal joint is a functional rather than anatomic unit because it does not form a single uninterrupted articular surface. However, it is anatomically separate from the radiocarpal joint and has a capsule and synovial lining that is continuous with each intercarpal articulation and may be continuous with some of the carpometacarpal (CMC) articulations.[20] The midcarpal joint surfaces are complex, with an overall reciprocally concave-convex configuration. The complexity of surfaces and ligamentous connections, however, simplify its movements. Functionally, the carpals of the distal row (with their attached metacarpals) move as an almost fixed unit. The capitate and hamate are most strongly bound together with, at most, a small amount of play between them.[34–36] The union of the distal carpals also results in nearly equal distribution of loads across the scaphoid-trapezium-trapezoid, the scaphoid-capitate, the lunate-capitate, and the triquetrum-hamate articulations.[22,37] Together the bones of the distal carpal row contribute two degrees of freedom to the wrist complex, with varying amounts of radial/ulnar deviation and flexion/extension credited to the joint. The excursions permitted by the articular surfaces of the midcarpal joint generally favor the range of extension over flexion and radial deviation over ulnar deviation—the opposite of what was found for the radiocarpal joint.[20,23,38] The functional union of the distal carpals with each other and with their contiguous metacarpals not only serve the wrist complex but also are the foundation for the transverse and longitudinal arches of the hand, which will be addressed in detail later.[35]

■ Ligaments of the Wrist Complex

The tremendous individual differences that exist in the structure of the carpus can, perhaps, best be appreciated after a review of the ligaments of the wrist. There are substantive differences in names, anatomic descriptions, and ascribed functions from investigator to investigator.[39–42] We will present the work of Taleisnik to organize and describe the wrist ligamentous anatomy.[43,44] Although there may not be universal agreement as to the structure and function of individual ligaments, there is consensus that the ligamentous structure of the carpus is responsible not only for articular stability but also for guiding and checking motion between and among the carpals.[45] When we examine the function of the wrist complex, we shall see that the variability of ligaments will, among other factors, translate into substantial and widely acknowledged differences among individuals in movement of the joints of the wrist complex. In general, the dorsal wrist ligaments are described as thin, whereas the more numerous volar ligaments are thicker and stronger.[43,44]

The ligaments of the wrist complex are designated either extrinsic or intrinsic.[39,43,44] The **extrinsic ligaments** are those that connect the carpals to the radius or ulna proximally or to the metacarpals distally; the **intrinsic ligaments** are those that interconnect the carpals themselves and are also known as intercarpal or interosseous ligaments. Nowalk and Logan[39] found the intrinsic ligaments to be stronger and less stiff than the extrinsic ligaments. They concluded that the intrinsic ligaments lie within the synovial lining and, therefore, must rely on synovial fluid for nutrition rather than contiguous vascularized tissues, as do the extrinsic ligaments. The extrinsic ligaments, therefore, are more likely to fail but also have better potential for healing and help protect the slower to heal intrinsic ligaments by accepting forces first.[39]

Volar Carpal Ligaments

On the volar surface of the wrist complex, the numerous intrinsic and extrinsic ligaments are variously described by either composite or separate names, depending on the investigator. Taleisnik organized the volar extrinsic ligaments into two groupings: the radiocarpal and the ulnocarpal ligaments. The composite ligament known as the **volar radiocarpal ligament** is described most commonly as having three distinct bands: the **radioscaphocapitate** (**radiocapitate**), short and long **radiolunate** (**radiolunotriquetral**), and **radioscapholunate ligaments** (Fig. 9-7A).[43–45] The radioscapholunate ligament was once described as the most important stabilizer of the proximal pole of the scaphoid, and disruption of it may lead to issues of scaphoid instability[44]; however, current research reveals that this structure offers little support to the joint but acts as a conduit for neurovascularity to the scapholunate joint.[45] The **radial collateral ligament** may be considered an extension of the volar radiocarpal ligament and capsule.[46] Nowalk and Logan[39] identified the radiocapitate as an extrinsic ligament, whereas Blevens and colleagues[41] identified it as part of the "palmar intracapsular radiocarpal ligaments." The **ulnocarpal ligament complex** is composed of the TFCC (including the articular disk and meniscus homolog), the **ulnolunate ligament,** and the **ulnar collateral ligament**.[19,46]

Two volar intrinsic ligaments have received particular attention and acknowledgment of their importance to wrist function. The first of these, the scapholunate interosseous ligament, is generally, although not universally,[47] credited with being a key factor in maintaining scaphoid stability and, therefore, stability of much of the wrist.[41,48–50] Studies have shown that the dorsal portion of this ligament is the most important in terms of contributing to stability.[45] Injury to this ligament appears to contribute largely to scaphoid instability and, therefore, to one of the most common wrist problems. As an intrinsic ligament, however, the scapholunate interosseous ligament is largely avascular and, therefore, may be susceptible to degenerative change.[51] The second key intrinsic ligament is the lunotriquetral interosseous ligament. This ligament is credited with maintaining stability between the lunate and triquetrum. Injury to this ligament appears to contribute to lunate instability, another problematic wrist pathology.[52,53] However, this instability pattern will most likely not occur without concomitant injury to the extrinsic ligaments. In general, the volar wrist ligaments are placed on stretch with wrist extension.[54]

Dorsal Carpal Ligaments

Dorsally, the major wrist ligament is the **dorsal radiocarpal ligament** (Fig. 9-7B). This ligament, as is true of the volar radiocarpal, varies somewhat in description but is obliquely oriented.[43,44] Essentially, the ligament as a whole converges on the triquetrum from the distal radius, with possible attachments along the way to the lunate and lunotriquetral interosseous ligament.[42,55,56] Garcia-Elias suggested that the obliquity of the volar and dorsal radiocarpal ligaments helps offset the sliding of the proximal "carpal condyle" on the inclined radius.[57] A second dorsal ligament is the **dorsal intercarpal ligament,** which courses horizontally from the triquetrum to the lunate, scaphoid, and trapezium.[46,55] The two dorsal ligaments together form a horizontal V that contributes to radiocarpal stability, notably stabilizing the scaphoid during wrist ROM.[43,55,56] The dorsal wrist ligaments are taut with wrist flexion.[54]

 CONCEPT CORNERSTONE 9-2: *Summary of Ligaments*

Extrinsic Ligaments
  Radiocarpal
    Radial Collateral
    Volar Collateral
      Superficial
      Deep
        Radioscaphocapitate
        Radiolunate (radioluntotriquetral)
        Radioscaphoid-lunate
  Ulnocarpal
    Triangular fibrocartilage complex
    Meniscus homolog
    Ulnolunate
    Ulnar collateral
  Dorsal radiocarpal (radiotriquetral)
Intrinsic Ligaments
  Short
    Volar
    Dorsal
    Interosseous
  Intermediate
    Lunotriquetral
    Scapholuante
    Scaphotrapezium
  Long
    Volar intercarpal (v-ligament, deltoid)
    Dorsal intercarpal

Function of the Wrist Complex

■ Movements of the Radiocarpal and Midcarpal Joints

Motions at the radiocarpal and midcarpal joints are caused by a rather unique combination of active muscular and passive ligamentous and joint reaction forces. Although there are abundant passive forces on the proximal carpal row, no muscular forces are applied directly to the articular bones of the proximal row, given that the FCU muscle applies its force via the pisiform to the more distal bones. The proximal carpals, therefore, are effectively a mechanical link between the radius and the distal carpals and metacarpals to which

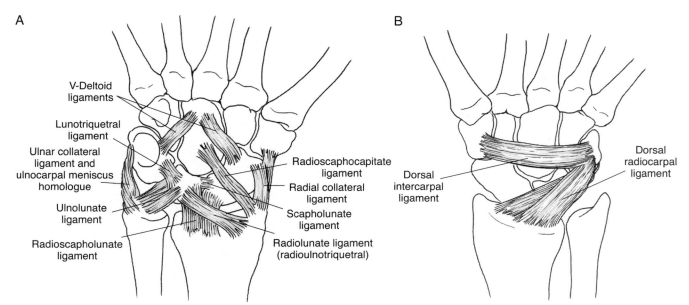

▲ **Figure 9-7** ■ A. Volar ligaments of the wrist complex, including the three bands of the volar radiocarpal ligament: radioscaphocapitate, radiolunate, and radioscapholunate. The two intrinsic ligaments (scapholunate and lunotriquetral) are credited with maintaining scaphoid stability. **B.** Dorsal wrist ligaments form a horizontal V, adding to radiocarpal stability.

the muscular forces are actually applied. Gilford and colleagues[13] suggested that the proximal carpal row is an **intercalated segment,** a relatively unattached middle segment of a three-segment linkage. Ruby and associates concurred, hypothesizing that the proximal carpal row functions as an intercalated segment between the distal radius/TFCC and the relatively immobile distal row.[58] When compressive forces are applied across an intercalated segment, the middle segment tends to collapse and move in the opposite direction from the segments above and below. For example, application of compressive muscular extensor forces across the biarticular wrist complex would cause an unstable proximal scaphoid to collapse into flexion while the distal carpal row extended. An intercalated segment requires some type of stabilizing mechanism to normalize combined midcarpal/radiocarpal motion and prevent collapse of the middle segment (the proximal carpal row). The stabilization mechanism appears to involve the scaphoid and its functional and anatomic (ligamentous) connections both to the adjacent lunate and to the distal carpal row.

Garcia-Elias[57] supported the hypothesis that the stability of the proximal carpal row depends on the interaction of two opposite tendencies when the carpals are axially loaded (compression across a neutral wrist); the scaphoid tends to flex, whereas the lunate and triquetrum tend to extend. These counterrotations within the proximal row are prevented by the ligamentous structure (including the key scapholunate interosseous and lunotriquetral interosseous ligaments). Linking the scaphoid to the lunate and triquetrum through ligaments, according to Garcia-Elias,[57] will cause the proximal carpals to "collapse synchronously" into flexion and pronation, whereas the distal carpals move into extension and supination. Garcia-Ellis proposed that the counterrotation between proximal and distal carpal rows and the resulting ligamentous tension increase coaptation of midcarpal articular surfaces and add to stability.

Although the carpal stability mechanism proposed by Garcia-Elias appears to hold as a conceptual framework, findings of other investigators differ in detail if not in substance. Advances in technology, including computer modeling, suggest that intercarpal motion is far more complex and individualistic than was once thought.[59,60] There is general agreement that the three bones of the proximal carpal row do not move as a unit but that motions of the three carpals vary both in magnitude and in direction with axial loading, with radiocarpal flexion/extension, and with radial/ulnar deviation.[6,44,57,61,62] In fact, Short and colleagues[63] found that carpal motions differed not only with individual osteoligamentous configuration and position but also with direction of motion; that is, relations in the carpus differed when the wrist reached neutral position, depending on whether the position was reached from full flexion, full extension, or deviation.

Controversy remains in terms of the existence of an actual "center of rotation" of the wrist complex. Much of the literature proposes that the head of the capitate, frequently referred to as the "keystone" of the wrist,

may serve as the location of the coronal axis for wrist extension/flexion and the A-P axis for radial/ulnar deviation,[38] as well as providing the rigid center of the fixed carpal arch.[54] Neu and associates studied the kinematics of the capitate with wrist motion in both planes and concluded that the axes of motion are not constant, which further supports the premise that carpal kinematics are complex and vary depending on the individual.[64]

Flexion/Extension of the Wrist

During flexion/extension of the wrist, the scaphoid seems to show the greatest motion of the three proximal carpal bones, whereas the lunate moves least.[6,36] Some investigators found that flexion and extension of the radiocarpal joint occurs almost exclusively as flexion and extension, respectively, of the proximal carpal row,[49,63] whereas others found simultaneous but lesser amounts of radial/ulnar deviation and pronation/supination of two or all three proximal carpal bones during radiocarpal flexion/extension.[6,20,54] Motion of the more tightly bound distal carpals and their attached metacarpals during midcarpal flexion/extension appears to be a fairly simple corresponding flexion and extension, with movement of the distal segments proportional to movement of the hand.[61]

In view of the apparent variability of findings, a conceptual framework for flexion/extension of the wrist is in order. The following sequence of events (Fig. 9-8A) was proposed by Conwell[65] and provides an expla-

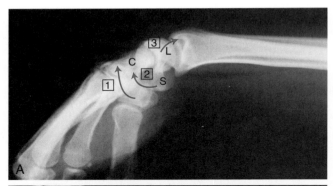

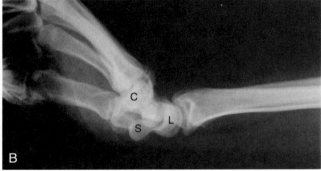

▲ **Figure 9-8** ■ **A.** As wrist extension is initiated from full flexion, (1) the distal carpal row moves on the proximal carpal row; (2) the scaphoid and distal row move on the lunate/triquetrum; and (3) the carpals move as a unit on the radius and TFCC to achieve **B.** Full wrist extension. C, capitate; L, lunate; S, scaphoid.

nation of the relative motions of the various segments and of their interdependence. It can easily be appreciated, however, that the conceptual framework is oversimplified and ignores some of the simultaneous interactions that occur among the key carpal bones.

1. The motion begins with the wrist in full flexion. Active extension is initiated at the distal carpal row and at the firmly attached metacarpals by the wrist extensor muscles attached to those bones. The distal carpals (capitate, hamate, trapezium, and trapezoid) glide on the relatively fixed proximal bones (scaphoid, lunate, and triquetrum). Although the surface configurations of the midcarpal joint are complex, the distal carpal row effectively glides in the same direction as motion of the hand. When the wrist complex reaches neutral (long axis of the third metacarpal in line with the long axis of the forearm), the ligaments spanning the capitate and scaphoid draw the capitate and scaphoid together into a close-packed position.

2. Continued extensor force now moves the combined unit of the distal carpal row and the scaphoid on the relatively fixed lunate and triquetrum. At approximately 45° of extension of the wrist complex, the scapholunate interosseous ligament brings the scaphoid and lunate into close-packed position. This unites all the carpals and causes them to function as a single unit.

3. Completion of wrist complex extension (see Fig. 9-8B) occurs as the proximal articular surface of the carpals move as a relatively solid unit on the radius and TFCC. All ligaments become taut as full extension is reached and the entire wrist complex is close-packed.[66]

Wrist motion from full extension to full flexion occurs in the reverse sequence. In the context of this conceptual framework, the scaphoid (through mediation of the wrist ligaments) participates at different times in scaphoid-capitate, scaphoid-lunate, or radio-scaphoid motion. Crumpling of the proximal carpal row (intercalated segment) is prevented, and full ROM is achieved. Interestingly, computer modeling and cadaver study of radiocarpal intra-articular contact patterns showed that radiocarpal extension is accompanied by increased contact dorsally. One would expect extension of the hand to be accompanied by sliding of the convex proximal carpal surface volarly in a direction opposite to hand motion. If this contact pattern exists *in vivo*, it likely reflects the complexity of radiocarpal motion and may contradict assumptions about movement between convex and concave surfaces.[22]

Radial/Ulnar Deviation of the Wrist

Radial and ulnar deviation of the wrist seems to be an even more complex, but perhaps less varied, motion than flexion/extension. The proximal carpal row displays a unique "reciprocal" motion with radial and ulnar deviation.[11] In radial deviation, the carpals slide ulnarly on the radius (Fig. 9-9A). The carpal motion not only produces deviation of the proximal and distal carpals radially, but simultaneous flexion of the proximal carpals and extension of the distal carpals (with observations of accompanying pronation/supination components varying among investigators).[6,21,27,63,67] The opposite motions of the proximal and distal carpals occur with ulnar deviation (see Fig. 9-9B). During radial/ulnar deviation, the distal carpals, once again, move as a relatively fixed unit, although the

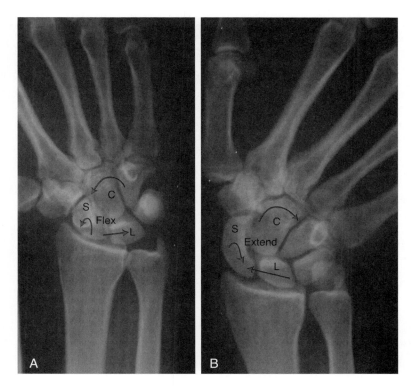

◀ **Figure 9-9** ■ With radial deviation of the wrist (**A**), the flexion of the scaphoid makes the scaphoid appear shorter than when the scapoid extends during ulnar deviation (**B**). C, capitate; L, lunate; S, scaphoid.

magnitude of motion between the bones of the proximal carpal row may differ.[6,36] Garcia-Elias and colleagues[8] found that the magnitude of scaphoid flexion during radial deviation (and extension during ulnar deviation) was related to ligamentous laxity. Volunteer subjects with ligamentous laxity showed more scaphoid flexion/extension and less radial/ulnar deviation than did others. Ligamentous laxity was more common among women than among men. The investigators proposed that ligamentous laxity led to less binding of the scaphoid to the distal carpal row and, therefore, more out-of-plane motion for the scaphoid.

In full radial deviation, both the radiocarpal and midcarpal joints are in close-packed position.[38,68–70] The ranges of wrist complex radial and ulnar deviation are greatest when the wrist is in neutral flexion/extension. When the wrist is extended and is in close-packed position, the carpals are all locked, and very little radial or ulnar deviation is possible. In wrist flexion, the joints are loose-packed and the bones are splayed. Further movement of the proximal row cannot occur, and, as in extreme extension, little radial or ulnar deviation is possible in the fully flexed position.[71]

Continuing Exploration: Functional Range of Motion

What appears to be a redundancy in function at the midcarpal and radiocarpal joints ensures maintenance of the minimum ROM required for activities of daily living. Brumfield and Champoux[72] found that a series of hand activities necessary for independence required a functional wrist motion of 10° of flexion and 35° of extension. Ryu and colleagues[12] included a wide range of hand functions in their test battery and determined that all could be completed with minimum wrist motions of 60° extension, 54° flexion, 40° ulnar deviation, and 17° radial deviation. There is consensus that wrist extension and ulnar deviation are most important for wrist activities. Wrist extension and ulnar deviation were also found to constitute the position of maximum scapholunate contact.[22] Given the key role of the scaphoid in wrist stability—acting as a link between the proximal and distal carpal rows—this extended and ulnarly deviated wrist position will provide a stable base that allows for maximum hand function distally. When deciding on the position of fusion for the wrist, the surgeon commonly chooses an optimal functional position of approximately 20° of extension and 10° of ulnar deviation.[54] This extended position also positions the long digital flexors for maximal force generation in prehension activities.

■ Wrist Instability

Injury to one or more of the ligaments attached to the scaphoid and lunate may diminish or remove the synergistic stabilization of the lunate and scaphoid. When this occurs, the scaphoid behaves as an unconstrained segment, following its natural tendency to collapse into flexion on the volarly inclined surface of the distal radius (potentially including some out-of-plane motion as well). The base of the flexed scaphoid slides dorsally on the radius and subluxes. Released from scaphoid stabilization, the lunate and triquetrum together act as an unconstrained segment, following their natural tendency to extend. The muscular forces that bypass the proximal carpals and apply force to the distal carpals cause the distal carpals to flex on the extended lunate and triquetrum. The flexed distal carpals glide dorsally on the lunate and triquetrum, accentuating the extension of the lunate and triquetrum. This zigzag pattern of the three segments (the scaphoid, the lunate/triquetrum, and the distal carpal row) is known as intercalated segmental instability.[21,27] When the lunate assumes an extended posture, the presentation is referred to as **dorsal intercalated segmental instability** (**DISI**) (Fig. 9-10A). The scaphoid subluxation may be dynamic, occurring only with compressive loading of the wrist with muscle forces, or the subluxation may become fixed or static.[73] With subluxation of the scaphoid, the contact pressures between the radius and scaphoid increase because the contact occurs over a smaller area.[22,41] A DISI problem, therefore, may result over time in degenerative changes at the radioscaphoid joint and then, ultimately, at the other intercarpal joints.[40] With sufficient ligamentous laxity, the capitate may sublux dorsally off the extended lunate or, more commonly, migrate into the gap between the flexed scaphoid and extended lunate. The progressive degenerative problem from an untreated DISI is known as **scapholunate advanced collapse** (**SLAC wrist**).[41,74] The progressive stages have been identified radiographically

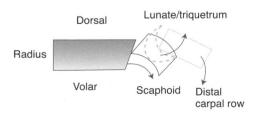

A   B

▲ **Figure 9-10** ■ **A.** Dorsal intercalated segmental instability (DISI). The lunate, released from the flexed scaphoid, extends on the radius. The capitate moves in the opposite direction (flexion) on top of the lunate. **B.** Volar intercalated segmental instability (VISI). The lunate and scaphoid flex on the radius, whereas the triquetrum extends. The distal carpal row (capitate shown) follows the triquetrum into extension.

on the basis of the time lapse from injury.[74,75] Although it is arguable whether the load between the scaphoid and the lunate increases or decreases with DISI,[22,33,49] there is agreement that the radiolunate articulation is less likely to show degenerative changes than is the radioscaphoid joint. The lesser tendency toward degenerative changes in the radiolunate joint has been attributed to a more spherical configuration of the radiolunate facets that better center applied loads across the articular surfaces.[41]

The other common form of carpal instability occurs when the ligamentous union of the lunate and triquetrum is disrupted through injury.[21,73] The lunate and triquetrum together normally tend to move toward extension and offset the tendency of the scaphoid to flex. When the lunate is no longer linked with the triquetrum, the lunate and scaphoid together fall into flexion, and the triquetrum and distal carpal row extend (see Fig. 9-10B). This ulnar perilunate instability is known as **volar intercalated segmental instability** (**VISI**).[44] This condition is not as common as DISI. The problems of VISI and DISI illustrate the importance of proximal carpal row stabilization to wrist function and of maintenance of the scaphoid as the bridge between the distal carpal row and the two other bones of the proximal carpal row.

9-2	**Patient Case: Scapholunate ligament injury**

Jeff O'Brien, playing in a men's softball league, sustained a fall on an outstretched hand (FOOSH) that resulted in pain and swelling on the dorsum of the wrist. A radiograph taken in a walk-in clinic a week later showed a separation between his scaphoid and lunate (Fig. 9-11A) that was indicative of ligamentous damage, including tear of the scapolunate interosseous ligament. It was recommended that Mr. O'Brien see a hand specialist. A follow-up radiograph with the hand surgeon showed dorsal intercalated segmental instability (DISI) (see Fig. 9-11B). Jeff made the decision not to pursue any kind of treatment beyond a period of immobilization. The problem appeared to resolve with time. Five years later, however, pain in Jeff's wrist increased to the point at which he sought medical attention from the hand surgeon once again. The hand surgeon diagnosed scapholunate advanced collapse (SLAC). Repetitive loading of the wrist (grasping, lifting) caused degenerative bony changes in the wrist complex, wrist instability marked by proximal migration of the capitate into the space between the scaphoid and lunate, and degenerative changes in the radioscaphoid and capitate-lunate joints (see Fig. 9-11C). A partial wrist fusion (scaphocapitate arthrodesis) was recommended to improve stability (and remove one source of pain) while allowing limited wrist mobility, to minimize loss of function.

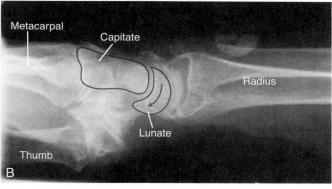

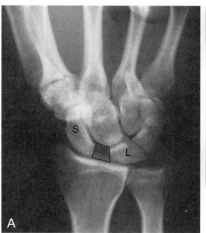

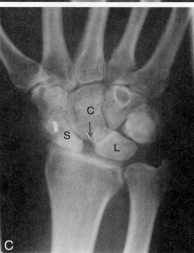

◀ **Figure 9-11** ■ **A.** With disruption of the scapholunate ligaments through trauma, the scaphoid and lunate migrate apart, leaving a gap (diastasis). **B.** Dorsal intercalated segmental instability (DISI) results in dorsal tilt of the lunate (shown), as well as less evident volar tilt of the scaphoid and capitate. **C.** Scapholunate advance collapse (SLAC) with migration of the capitate proximally and erosion of the radioscaphoid and capitate-lunate joints.

■ Muscles of the Wrist Complex

The primary role of the muscles of the wrist complex is to provide a stable base for the hand while permitting positional adjustments that allow for an optimal length-tension relationship in the long finger muscles.[4,54] Information on a muscle's cross-sectional area and length of moment arm will help facilitate understanding of a muscle's specific action, force, and torque potential. Many researchers investigated the peak force that could be exerted at the interphalangeal (IP) joints of the fingers by the long finger flexors during different wrist positions. Some studies found that the greatest IP flexor force occurs with ulnar deviation of the wrist (neutral flexion/extension), whereas the least force occurred with wrist flexion (neutral deviation).[2,76] Other studies concluded that 20° to 25° of wrist extension with 5° to 7° of ulnar deviation was the optimal range to maximize grip strength output.[77,78] The muscles of the wrist, however, are not structured merely to optimize the force of finger flexion. If optimizing finger flexor force outweighed other concerns, one might expect the wrist extensors to be stronger than the wrist flexors. Rather, the work capacity (ability of a muscle to generate force per unit of cross-section) of the wrist flexors is more than twice that of the extensors. Again contrary to expectation if optimizing finger flexor force was the goal, the work capacity of the radial deviators slightly exceeds that of the ulnar deviators.[79] The function of the wrist muscles cannot be understood by looking at any one factor or function; it should be assessed by electromyography (EMG) in various patterns of use against the resistance of gravity and external loads. Although we will describe the wrist muscles here, their function is best understood in the context of later discussion of the synergies between hand and wrist musculature.

Volar Wrist Musculature

Six muscles have tendons crossing the volar aspect of the wrist and, therefore, are capable of creating a wrist flexion movement (Fig. 9-12A). These are the **palmaris longus (PL)**, the **flexor carpi radialis (FCR)**, the FCU, the **flexor digitorum superficialis (FDS)**, **flexor digitorum profundus (FDP)**, and the **flexor pollicis longus (FPL)** muscles. The first three of these muscles are primary wrist muscles. The last three are flexors of the digits with secondary actions at the wrist. At the wrist level, all of the volar wrist muscles pass beneath the **flexor retinaculum** along with the median nerve except the PL and the FCU muscles (Fig. 9-12B). The flexor retinaculum prevents bowstringing of the long flexor tendons, thereby contributing to maintaining an appropriate length-tension relationship. The flexor retinaculum is often considered to have a proximal portion and a distal portion, with the distal portion more commonly known as the **transverse carpal ligament (TCL)**.

The positions of the FCR and FCU tendons in relation to the axis of the wrist indicate that these muscles can, respectively, radially deviate and ulnarly deviate the wrist, as well as flex. However, the FCR muscle does not appear to be effective as a radial deviator of the

wrist in an isolated contraction. Its distal attachment on the bases of the second and third metacarpals places it in line with the long axis of the hand. Along with the PL muscle, the FCR muscle functions as a wrist flexor with little concomitant deviation.[10] The FCR muscle is active during radial deviation, however. The FCR muscle either augments the strong radial deviating force of the **extensor carpi radialis longus (ECRL)** or offsets the extension also produced by the ECRL muscle. The PL muscle is a wrist flexor without producing either radial or ulnar deviation. The PL muscle and tendon are absent unilaterally or bilaterally in approximately 14% of people without any apparent strength or functional deficit.[80] Given its apparent redundancy with other muscles, the PL tendon (when present) may be "sacrificed" for surgical reconstruction of other structures.[30]

The FCU muscle envelops the pisiform, a sesamoid bone that increases the MA of the FCU muscle for flexion. The FCU muscle can act on the hamate and fifth metacarpal indirectly through the pisiform's ligaments,[33] effectively producing flexion and ulnar deviation of the wrist complex. The FCU tendon crosses the wrist at a greater distance from the axis for wrist radial/ulnar deviation than does the FCR muscle, so the FCU muscle is more effective in its ulnar deviation function than is the FCR muscle is in its radial deviation function.[4] The FCU muscle is able to exert the greatest tension of all the wrist muscles, giving it particular functional relevance, especially with activities requiring high ulnar deviation forces such as chopping wood.[4]

The FDS and FDP muscles are predominantly flexors of the fingers, and the FPL muscle is predominantly the flexor of the thumb. As multijoint muscles, their capacity to produce an effective wrist flexion force depends on synergistic stabilization by the extensor muscles of the more distal joints that these muscles cross to prevent excessive shortening of the muscles over multiple joints. If these muscles attempt to shorten over both the wrist and the more distal joints, the muscles will become actively insufficient. The FDS and FDP muscles show varied activity in wrist radial/ulnar deviation, as might be anticipated from the central location of the tendons. The FDS muscle seems to function more consistently as a wrist flexor than does the FDP muscle.[81] This is logical, because the FDP muscle is a longer, deeper muscle, crosses more joints, and is therefore more likely to become actively insufficient. The effect of the FPL muscle on the wrist has received relatively little attention. The position of the tendon suggests the ability to contribute to both flexion and radial deviation of the wrist if its more distal joints are stabilized.

Dorsal Wrist Musculature

The dorsum of the wrist complex is crossed by the tendons of nine muscles (Fig. 9-13). Three of the nine muscles are primary wrist muscles: the ECRL and **extensor carpi radialis brevis (ECRB)** and the ECU. The other six are finger and thumb muscles that may act secondarily on the wrist; these are the **extensor digitorum communis (EDC)**, the **extensor indicis proprius (EIP)**, the **extensor digiti minimi (EDM)**, the **extensor**

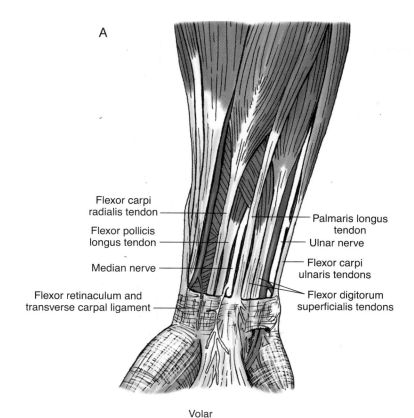

A

Flexor carpi radialis tendon

Flexor pollicis longus tendon

Median nerve

Flexor retinaculum and transverse carpal ligament

Palmaris longus tendon

Ulnar nerve

Flexor carpi ulnaris tendons

Flexor digitorum superficialis tendons

B

Volar

Palmaris longus

Median nerve

Transverse carpal ligament

Flexor pollicus longus

Ulnar artery and nerve

Flexor carpi radialis

Tp

Tz

C

H

Four stacked tendons of the flexor digitorum superficialis

Flexor carpi ulnaris

Four side-by-side tendons of the flexor digitorum profundus

Dorsal

◄ **Figure 9-12** ■ **A.** The tendons and nerves of the primary and secondary wrist flexors lie on the volar aspect of the wrist. All but the palmaris longus tendon, the ulnar nerve, and the flexor carpi ulnaris muscle pass beneath the flexor retinaculum. **B.** On cross-section, the relationship of the tendons and nerves to the transverse carpal ligament is more evident. The flexor pollicis longus is encased in its own tendon sheath (or radial bursa), whereas the four deep tendons of the flexor digitorum profundus and the four more superficial stacked tendons of the flexor digitorum superficialis are wrapped by folds in the ulnar bursa.

pollicis longus (**EPL**), the **extensor pollicis brevis** (**EPB**), and the **abductor pollicis longus** (**APL**). The EDC and the EIP muscles are also known, more simply, as the extensor digitorum and the extensor indicis, respectively. The tendons of all nine muscles pass under the **extensor retinaculum,** which is divided into six distinct tunnels by septa. As the tendons pass deep to the retinaculum, each tendon is encased within its own tendon sheath to prevent friction between tendons and friction on the retinaculum. The septa of the retinacu-

lum through which the tendons pass are attached to the dorsal carpal ligaments and help maintain stability of the extensor tendons on the dorsum, as well as allowing those muscles to contribute to wrist extension and preventing bowstringing of the tendons with active contraction.[46,82]

The ECRL and ECRB muscles together make up the predominant part of the wrist extensor mass.[83] The ECRB muscle is somewhat smaller than the ECRL muscle but has a more central location, inserting into the

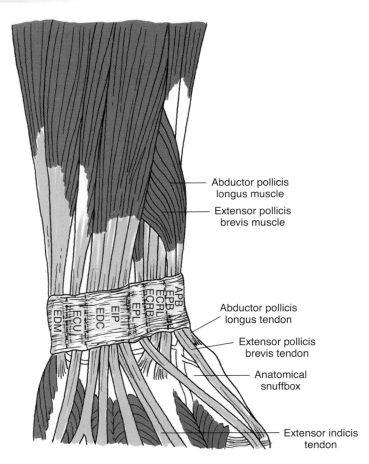

— Abductor pollicis
longus muscle

— Extensor pollicis
brevis muscle

— Abductor pollicis
longus tendon

— Extensor pollicis
brevis tendon

— Anatomical
snuffbox

— Extensor indicis
tendon

◀ **Figure 9-13** ■ The dorsally located extensor tendons pass beneath the extensor retinaculum, where the tendons are compartmentalized. From the radial to the ulnar side, the abductor pollicis longus (APL) and extensor pollicis brevis (EPB) muscles share a compartment; the extensor carpi radialis brevis (ECRB) and the extensor carpi radialis longus (ECRL) muscles share a compartment; the extensor pollicis longus (EPL) muscle has a compartment of its own; the four tendons of the extensor digitorum communis (EDC) muscle share a compartment with the extensor indicis proprius (EIP) muscle; the extensor digiti minimi (EDM) muscle has its own compartment; and the extensor carpi ulnaris (ECU) muscle has its own compartment.

third metacarpal, and generally shows more activity during wrist extension activities.[10,84] One study found the ECRB muscle to be active during all grasp-and-release hand activities, except those performed in supination.[85] The ECRL muscle inserts into the more radial second metacarpal and, therefore, has a smaller MA for wrist extension than does the ECRB muscle.[6] The ECRL muscle shows increased activity when either radial deviation or support against ulnar deviation is required or when forceful finger flexion motions are performed.[66,84] The ongoing activity of the ECRB muscle makes it vulnerable to overuse and is more likely than the quieter ECRL muscle to be inflamed in lateral epicondylitis.[86] The literature has questioned the role of the EDC muscle in development of this pathology.[87,88]

The ECU muscle extends and ulnarly deviates the wrist. It is active not only in wrist extension but frequently in wrist flexion as well.[84] Backdahl and Carlsoo[81] hypothesized that the ECU muscle activity in wrist flexion adds an additional component of stability to the structurally less stable position of wrist flexion. This is not needed on the radial side of the wrist, which has more developed ligamentous and bony structural checks. The connection of the ECU tendon sheath to the TFCC also appears to help tether the ECU muscle and prevent loss of excursion efficiency with bowstringing.[19] Tang and colleagues[89] found a 30% increase in excursion of the ECU muscle after release of the TFCC from the distal ulna. The effectiveness of the ECU mus-

cle as a wrist extensor is also affected by forearm position. When the forearm is pronated, the crossing of the radius over the ulna causes a reduction in the MA of the ECU muscle, making it less effective as a wrist extensor.[4,83,85]

The EDM and the EIP muscles insert into the tendons of the EDC muscle and, therefore, have a common function with the EDC muscle.[90] The EIP and EDM muscles are capable of extending the wrist, but wrist extension is credited more to the EDC muscle. The EDC muscle is a finger extensor muscle but functions also as a wrist extensor (without radial or ulnar deviation). There appears to be some reciprocal synergy of the EDC muscle with the ECRB muscle in providing wrist extension, because less ECRB muscle activity is seen when the EDC muscle is active.[84]

Three extrinsic thumb muscles cross the wrist. Both the APL and the EPB muscles are capable of radially deviating the wrist and may serve a minor role in that function.[80] However, radial deviation of the wrist may detract from their prime action on the thumb. A synergistic contraction of the ECU muscle may be required to offset the unwanted wrist motion when the APL and EPB muscles act on the thumb. When muscles producing ulnar deviation are absent, the thumb extrinsic muscles may produce a significant radial deviation deformity at the wrist. Little evidence has been found to indicate that the more centrally located EPL muscle has any notable effect on the wrist.

Now that we have examined the wrist complex, let us look at the hand complex that the wrist serves.

The Hand Complex

The hand consists of five digits: four fingers and a thumb (Fig. 9-14). Each digit has a CMC joint and a **metacarpophalangeal** (**MP**) joint. The fingers each have two **IP** joints, the proximal (**PIP**) and distal (**DIP**), and the thumb has only one. There are 19 bones and 19 joints distal to the carpals that make up the hand complex. Although the joints of the fingers and the joints of the thumb have structural similarities, function differs significantly enough that the joints of the fingers shall be examined separately from those of the thumb. In examining the joints of the fingers, however, one should be cautious about generalizations that we will make. Ranney[91] pointed out that each digit of the hand is unique and that models proposed for and conclusions drawn about one finger may not be accurate for all.

Carpometacarpal Joints of the Fingers

The CMC joints of the fingers are composed of the articulations between the distal carpal row and the bases of the second through fifth metacarpal joints (see Fig. 9-1). The distal carpal row also, of course, is part of the midcarpal joint. The proximal portion of the four metacarpals of the fingers articulate with the distal carpals to form the second through fifth CMC joints (see Fig. 9-14). The second metacarpal articulates primarily with the trapezoid and secondarily with the trapezium and capitate. The third metacarpal articulates primarily with the capitate, and the fourth metacarpal articulates with the capitate and hamate. Last, the fifth metacarpal articulates with the hamate. Each of the metacarpals also articulates at its base with the contiguous metacarpal or metacarpals, with the exception of the second metacarpal, which articulates at its base with the third but not the first metacarpal. All finger CMC joints are supported by strong transverse and weaker longitudinal ligaments volarly and dorsally.[92,93]

The **deep transverse metacarpal ligament** spans the heads of the second through fourth metacarpals volarly. The deep transverse metacarpal ligament tethers together the metacarpal heads and effectively prevents the attached metacarpals from any more than minimal abduction at the CMC joints. Although the transverse metacarpal ligament contributes directly to CMC stability, it also is structurally part of the MP joints of the fingers and will be discussed again in that context. The ligamentous structure is primarily responsible for controlling the total ROM available at each CMC joint, although some differences in articulations also exist.

One attribute of the distal carpals that affects CMC and hand function but not wrist function is the volar concavity, or **proximal transverse (carpal) arch,** formed by the trapezoid, trapezium, capitate, and hamate (Fig. 9-15). The carpal arch persists even when the hand is fully opened and is created not only by the curved shape of the carpals but also by the ligaments that maintain the concavity. The ligaments that maintain the arch are the TCL and the transversely oriented **intercarpal ligaments.** The TCL is the portion of the flexor retinaculum that attaches to the pisiform and hook of the hamate

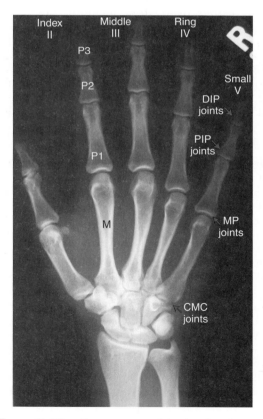

▲ **Figure 9-14** ■ Bony anatomy of the thumb and fingers. DIP, distal interphalangeal; PIP, proximal interphalangeal; MP, metacarpophalangeal; CMC, carpometacarpal; M, metacarpal; P1, proximal phalanx; P2, middle phalanx; P3, distal phalanx.

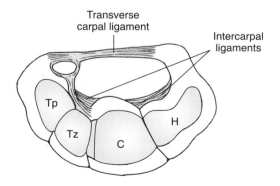

▲ **Figure 9-15** ■ The proximal transverse arch, or carpal arch, forms the tunnel through which the median nerve and long finger flexors travel. The transverse carpal ligament and intercarpal ligaments assist in maintaining this concavity. C, capitate; H, hamate; Tp, trapezium; Tz, trapezoid.

medially and to the scaphoid and trapezium laterally; the more proximal portion of the flexor retinaculum is continuous with the fascia overlying the forearm muscles. The TCL and intercarpal ligaments that link the four distal carpals maintain the relatively fixed concavity that will contribute to the arches of the palm. These structures also form the **carpal tunnel.** The carpal tunnel contains the median nerve and nine flexor tendons: the extrinsic finger and thumb flexors (see Fig. 9-12B). A number of intrinsic hand muscles attach to the TCL and bones of the distal carpal row. These may also contribute to maintaining the carpal arch.

9-3	**Patient Case: Carpal Tunnel Syndrome**

Carl George has been a computer programmer for over 20 years. He spends the majority of his day typing. He reports that he began waking with numbness in his right hand 5 years ago, specifically the thumb, index finger, and middle and radial half of the ring finger. He was evaluated by a hand surgeon, who found that tapping on the median nerve over the carpal tunnel reproduced Carl's paresthesias (tingling) in the median nerve distribution (positive Tinel's sign), as did placing Carl's wrist in sustained flexion for 1 minute (positive Phalen's test). The physician prescribed night splinting and patient education regarding proper ergonomics at work.[94] The splint held the wrist in a neutral position at night, which decreased the pressure on the median nerve.[95,96] In the subsequent 6 months, Carl noted progressive difficulty with completing fine motor tasks such as buttoning shirts and handling coins. Carl was referred to a neurologist who performed nerve conduction studies that revealed significant slowing in the median nerve conduction velocity, which was consistent with nerve compression at the wrist level. Also evident was atrophy of median nerve innervated thenar (thumb) muscles, a presentation commonly known as "ape hand" (Fig. 9-16).

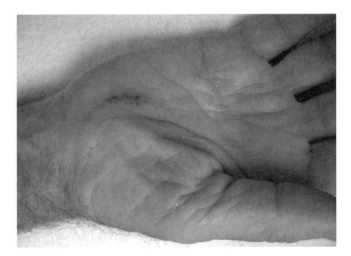

▲ **Figure 9-16 ■** Long-term median nerve compression can lead to atrophy of the median nerve innervated muscles in the thenar eminence, a presentation known as "ape hand" because of the flattening of the palm and the adducted position of the thumb. (The incision is from a surgical release of the transverse carpal ligament to relieve median nerve compression.)

Continuing Exploration: **Carpal Tunnel Syndrome**

When the median nerve becomes compressed within the carpal tunnel, a neuropathy known as **carpal tunnel syndrome** (**CTS**) may develop. Cobb and colleagues[97] proposed that the proximal edge of the TCL is the most common site for wrist flexion-induced median nerve compression. The tunnel is narrowest, however, at the level of the hook of the hamate, where median nerve compression is unlikely to be affected by changes in wrist position.[97] When the TCL is cut to release median nerve compression, the carpal arch may widen somewhat, but investigators found that the arch would maintain its dorsovolar stiffness as long as the stronger transverse intercarpal ligaments were intact.[98]

■ **Carpometacarpal Joint Range of Motion**

The range of CMC motion of the second through fifth metacarpals is observable most readily at the metacarpal heads, and shows increasing mobility from the radial to the ulnar side of the hand.[54,99] The second through fourth CMC joints are plane synovial joints with one degree of freedom: flexion/extension. Although structured to permit flexion/extension, the second and third CMC joints are essentially immobile and may be considered to have "zero degrees of freedom."[38,91] The fourth CMC joint has perceptible flexion/extension. The fifth CMC joint is a saddle joint with two degrees of freedom, including flexion/extension, some abduction/adduction, and a limited amount of opposition.[10,91,100] The immobile second and third metacarpals provide a fixed and stable axis about which the fourth and fifth metacarpals and the very mobile first metacarpal (thumb) can move.[34,91,101] The motion of the fourth and fifth metacarpals facilitates the ability of the ring and little fingers to oppose the thumb.

■ **Palmar Arches**

The function of the finger CMC joints and their segments overall is to contribute (with the thumb) to the **palmar arch system.** The concavity formed by the carpal bones results in the proximal transverse arch of the palm of the hand. The other palmar arches can easily be visualized as occurring transversely across the palm (often considered to be inclusive of the thumb and fourth finger) and longitudinally down the palm (inclusive of the fingers) (Fig. 9-17). The adjustable positions of the first, fourth, and fifth metacarpal heads around the relatively fixed second and third metacarpals form a mobile **distal transverse arch** at the level of the metacarpal heads that augments the fixed proximal transverse arch of the distal carpal row. The **longitudinal arch** traverses the length of the digits from proximal to distal. The deep transverse metacarpal ligament contributes to stability of the mobile arches during grip functions.[102] The palmar arches allow the palm and the digits to conform optimally to the shape of the object being held. This maximizes the amount of surface contact, enhancing stability as well as increasing sensory feedback.

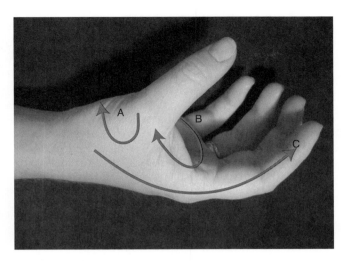

▲ **Figure 9-17** ■ The palmar arch system assists with functional grasp. The proximal transverse arch (A) is fixed, while the distal transverse arch (B) and longitudinal arch (C) are mobile.

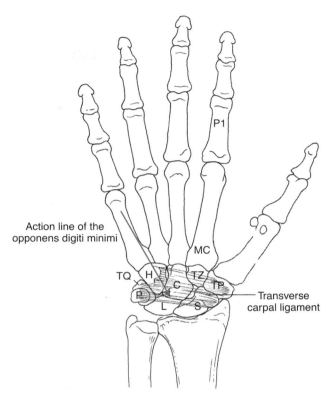

▲ **Figure 9-18** ■ The opponens digiti minimi (ODM) is the only muscle that acts exclusively on a CMC joint. As indicated by its action line, it is effective at flexion of the fifth metacarpal joint and rotation of the metacarpal joint around its long axis. The ODM muscle's attachment to the transverse carpal ligament may also contribute to supporting the proximal palmar arch.

Muscles that cross the CMC joints will contribute to palmar cupping (conformation of the palm to an object) by acting on the mobile segments of the palmar arches. Hollowing of the palm accompanies finger flexion, and relative flattening of the palm accompanies finger extension. The fifth CMC joint is crossed and acted on by the **opponens digiti minimi (ODM)** muscle. This oblique muscle is attached proximally to the hamate and TCL and distally to the ulnar side of the fifth metacarpal. It is optimally positioned, therefore, to flex and rotate the fifth metacarpal about its long axis (Fig. 9-18). No other muscles cross or act on the finger CMC joints alone. However, increased arching occurs with activity of the FCU muscle attached to the pisiform and with activity of the intrinsic hand muscles that insert on the TCL.[9,103] The radial wrist muscles (FCR, ECRL, and ECRB) cross the second and third CMC joints to insert on the bases of those metacarpals but produce little or no motion at these relatively fixed articulations. The stability of the second and third CMC joints can be viewed as a functional adaptation that enhances the efficiency of the FCR, ECRL, and ECRB muscles. If the second and third CMC joints were mobile, the radial flexor and extensors would act first on the CMC joints and, consequently, would be less effective at the midcarpal and radiocarpal joints, given the loss in length-tension.

Metacarpophalangeal Joints of the Fingers

Each of the four MP joints of the fingers is composed of the convex metacarpal head proximally and the concave base of the first phalanx distally (see Fig. 9-14). The MP joint is condyloid with two degrees of freedom: flexion/extension and abduction/adduction. The large metacarpal head has 180° of articular surface in the sagittal plane, with the predominant portion lying volarly. This is apposed to approximately 20° of articular surface on the base of the phalanx. In the frontal plane, there is less articular surface than in the sagittal plane, and the articular surfaces are more congruent.

The MP joint is surrounded by a capsule that is generally considered to be lax in extension. Given the incongruent articular surfaces, capsular laxity in extension allows some passive axial rotation of the proximal phalanx.[91] Two collateral ligaments at the volarly located transverse metacarpal ligament enhance joint stability. As we noted previously, incongruent joints often have an accessory joint structure to enhance stability. At the MP joint, this function is served by the volar plate.

■ Volar Plates

The **volar plate** (or palmar plate) at each of the MP joints is a unique structure that increases joint congruence. It also provides stability to the MP joint by limiting hyperextension and, therefore, providing indirect support to the longitudinal arch.[54] The volar plate is composed of fibrocartilage and is firmly attached to the base of the proximal phalanx distally but not to the metacarpal proximally.[52] The plate becomes membranous proximally to blend with the volar capsule that then attaches to the metacarpal head just proximal to the articular surface (Fig. 9-19A). The volar plate can also be visualized as a fibrocartilage impregnation of the volar portion of the capsule just superficial to the metacarpal head. The inner surface of the volar plate is effectively a continuation of the articular surface of the base of the proximal phalanx. In extension, the plate adds to the amount of surface in contact with the large metacarpal head. The fibrocartilage composition of the plate is consistent with its ability to resist both tensile stresses in restricting MP hyperextension and compressive forces needed to protect the volar articular surface of the metacarpal head from objects held in the palm.[104] The flexible attachment of the plate to the phalanx permits the plate to glide proximally down the volar surface of the metacarpal head in flexion without restricting motion, while also preventing pinching of the long flexor tendons in the MP joint (see Fig. 9-19B).

In addition to their connection to their respective proximal phalanges, the four volar plates and their respective capsules of the MP joints of the fingers also blend with and are interconnected superficially by the deep transverse metacarpal ligament that, as we noted earlier, tethers together the heads of the metacarpals of the four fingers (Fig. 9-20). Dorsal to the deep transverse metacarpal ligament are **sagittal bands** on each side of the metacarpal head that connect each volar plate (via the capsule and deep transverse metacarpal ligament) to the EDC tendon and **extensor expansion** (Fig. 9-21). The sagittal bands help stabilize the volar plates over the four metacarpal heads.[20,91,102]

The Collateral Ligaments

The radial and ulnar collateral ligaments of the MP joint are composed of two parts: the collateral ligament proper, which is cordlike, and the accessory collateral ligament (see Fig. 9-19). Minami and associates quantified the length changes in the different parts of the collateral ligament at the MP joint with varying degrees of motion.[105] They found that the more dorsally located collateral ligament proper was lengthened 3 to 4 mm with MP joint flexion from 0° to 80°, whereas the more volarly located accessory collateral ligament was shortened 1 to 2 mm. Conversely, with MP joint hyperextension, the accessory portion was lengthened and the proper portion was placed on slack. Tension in the collateral ligaments at full MP joint flexion (the close-packed position for the MP joint) is considered to account for the minimal amount of abduction/adduction that can be obtained at the MP joint in full flexion. Shultz and associates[106] concluded that the collateral ligaments provided stability throughout the MP joint ROM with parts of the fibers taut at various points in the range. They proposed that the bicondylar shape of the volar surface of the metacarpal head provided a bony block to abduction/adduction at about 70° of MP joint flexion, rather than collateral ligamentous tension.

Fisher and associates[107] completed a series of dissections of fingers, seeking an explanation for the relatively small incidence of osteoarthritis (OA) in MP joints in comparison with the fairly common changes seen in the DIP joints and, to a lesser extent, in the PIP joints. They found fibrocartilage that projected into the MP, PIP, and DIP joints from the inner surface of the dorsally located **extensor hood,** from the volar plates, and from the collateral ligaments. The fibrocartilage projections were most impressive in the MP joints and

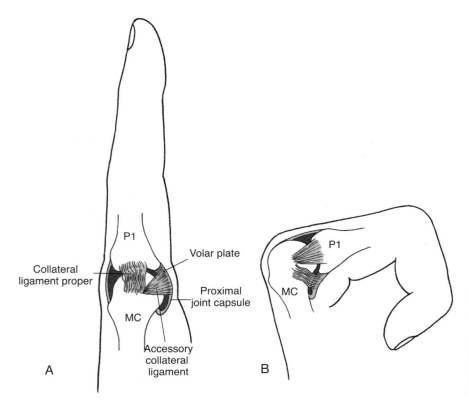

◀ **Figure 9-19** ■ **A.** The volar plate at the MP joint attaches to the base of the proximal phalanx. The plate blends with and lies deep to the MP joint capsule and the deep transverse metacarpal ligament volarly. **B.** In MP joint flexion, the flexible attachments of the plate allow the plate to slide proximally on the metacarpal head without impeding motion. The collateral ligament proper is loose in MP joint extension, whereas the accessory collateral ligament is taut. The reverse occurs in MP joint flexion.

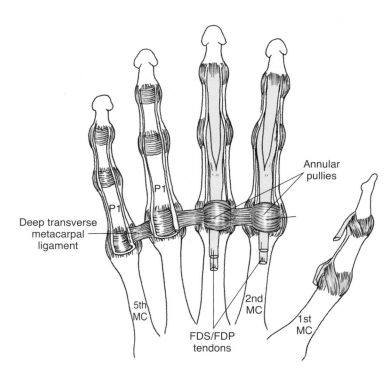

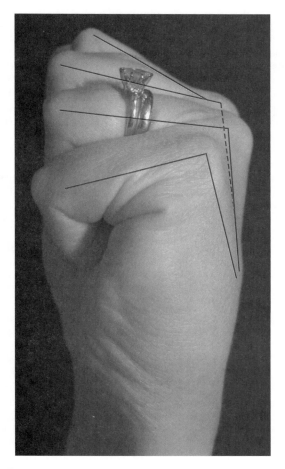

◀ **Figure 9-20** ■ The deep transverse metacarpal ligament (TML) runs transversely across the heads of the four MP joints of the fingers. The fibers of the TML blend with each MP joint capsule and with the deeper volar plates. The superficial aspect of the TML at each metatarsal head is grooved (shown on fourth and fifth MP joints) for the long finger flexors that pass over the TML and through the annular ligaments (shown on second and third MP joints).

may, like the volar plate itself, increase the surface area on the small base of the phalange for contact with the large metacarpal (and phalangeal) heads.

■ **Range of Motion**

The total ROM available at the MP joint varies with each finger. Flexion/extension increases radially to ulnarly, with the index finger having approximately 90° of MP joint flexion and the little finger approximately 110°[54] (Fig. 9-22). Hyperextension is fairly consistent between fingers but varies widely among individuals.

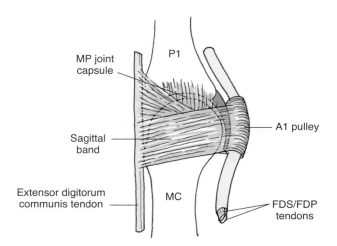

▲ **Figure 9-21** ■ The connections of the sagittal bands to each side of the volar plate, the collateral ligaments of the MP joint (via the capsule), and the extensor digitorum communis (EDC) muscle via the extensor expansion help stabilize the volar plates on the four metacarpal heads volarly and the EDC tendons over the MP joints dorsally.

▲ **Figure 9-22** ■ The available range of motion at the MP joints of the fingers increases from the radial to the ulnar side, with the greatest MP finger range at the fifth MP joint.

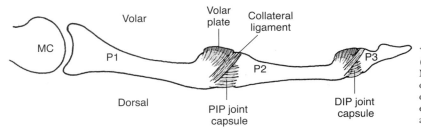

◀ **Figure 9-23** ■ The proximal interphalangeal (PIP) and distal interphalangeal (DIP) joints, like the MP joints, have volar plates that blend with the volar capsule portion of the capsule. The orientation of the collateral ligaments at the PIP and DIP joints, however, differs from the orientation of the collateral ligaments at the MPT joints.

The range of passive hyperextension has been used as a measure of generalized body flexibility.[9] The range of abduction/adduction is maximal in MP joint extension; the index and little fingers have more frontal plane mobility than do the middle and ring fingers. As previously noted, abduction/adduction is most restricted in MP joint flexion.[106] Passive rotation of the MP joints has been measured, which supports the contention that this mobility allows for adaptation of grasp for different size objects.[108]

Interphalangeal Joints of the Fingers

Each of the PIP and DIP joints of the fingers is composed of the head of a phalanx and the base of the phalanx distal to it. Each IP joint is a true synovial hinge joint with one degree of freedom (flexion/extension), a joint capsule, a volar plate, and two collateral ligaments (Fig. 9-23). The base of each middle and distal phalanx has two shallow concave facets with a central ridge. The distal phalanx sits on the pulley-shaped head of the phalanx proximal to it. The joint structure is similar to that of the MP joint in that the proximal articular surface is larger than the distal articular surface. Unlike the MP joints, there is little posterior articular surface at the PIP or DIP joint and, therefore, little hyperextension. The DIP joint may have some passive hyperextension, but the PIP joint has essentially none in most individuals.

Volar plates reinforce each of the joint capsules and enhance stability, limiting hyperextension.[109] The plates at the IP joints are structurally and functionally identical to those at the MP joint, except that the plates are not connected by a deep transverse ligament. Fisher and associates[107] found fibrocartilage projections from the extensor mechanism, the volar plate, and the collateral ligaments attached to the bases of the phalanges at both the PIP and the DIP joints, with the structures more obvious at the PIP joints. The collateral ligaments of the IP joints are not fully understood but are described to have cord and accessory parts similar to those of the MP joint.[54] Stability is provided by this collateral ligament complex because some portions remain taut and provide support throughout PIP and DIP joint motion.[54,110,111] Injuries to the collateral ligaments of the PIP joint are common, particularly in sports and workplace injuries, with the radial or lateral collateral twice as likely to be injured as the ulnar or medial collateral.[112,113] Dzwierzynski and colleagues[112] found the lateral collateral of the index finger to be the

strongest of the PIP collateral ligaments, whereas the fifth PIP joint had the weakest collateral ligaments. Because the thumb is most likely to oppose the lateral side of the index (creating a varus stress at the PIP joint) and least likely to do so at the fifth, the relative strengths of the lateral collateral ligaments meet functional expectations.

The total range of flexion/extension available to the index finger is greater at the PIP joint (100° to 110°) than it is at the DIP joint (80°). The ranges for PIP and DIP flexion at each finger increase ulnarly, with the fifth PIP and DIP joints achieving 135° and 90°, respectively. The pattern of increasing flexion/extension ROM from the radial to the ulnar side of the hand is consistent at the CMC, MP, and PIP joints and, to a lesser degree, at the DIP joints.[114] The additional range allocated to the more ulnarly located fingers results in angulation of the fingers toward the scaphoid and facilitates opposition of the fingers with the thumb (Fig. 9-24). The greater available range ulnarly also produces a grip that is tighter, or has greater closure, on the ulnar

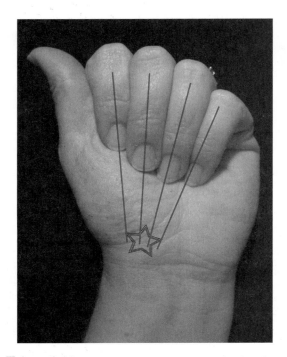

▲ **Figure 9-24** ■ With flexion of digits to the palm, there is a convergence toward the scaphoid tubercle (star burst) and toward the thumb. This obliquity is due to the increased flexion mobility of the MP and PIP joints from the radial to the ulnar side of the hand.

side of the hand. Many objects are constructed so that the shape is narrower at the ring and small fingers and widens toward the middle and index fingers to fit the ROM pattern.

Continuing Exploration: **Anti-Deformity Positioning**

After trauma to the hand, a custom-fabricated splint is commonly provided to immobilize the injured structures. The purpose of this device is to provide support and protection to the injured region during the healing process, while attempting to minimize the problems at the joints created by immobilization. Because the collateral ligaments of the MP joints are slack with extension, immobilization in MP extension in a splint would place the collateral ligaments at risk for adaptive shortening. Adaptive shortening of the collateral ligaments would limit MP joint flexion, with concomitant disruption of the longitudinal arch leading to impairments in grasp and functional use. Optimally, an immobilization splint should place the MP joints in flexion so that the collateral ligaments are on stretch; the IP joints should be held in extension to reduce the risk of flexion contractures from shortening of the volar plates. The thumb should be placed in some degree of CMC abduction to prevent a first web space contracture (Fig. 9-25). This position of MP joint flexion with IP extension is known as the "anti-deformity position."[115]

Extrinsic Finger Flexors

The muscles (also referred to as "motors") of the fingers and thumb that have proximal attachments above (proximal to) the wrist (radiocarpal joint) are known as extrinsic muscles, whereas those with all attachments distal to the radiocarpal joint are known as intrinsic muscles. Functionally, the extrinsic muscles are also divided into flexors and extensors. The intrinsic muscles are typically not referred to as flexor or extensor groups because several will flex one joint while extending another. We will first consider the extrinsic muscles of the fingers, then the intrinsic muscles of the fingers, and conclude with the extrinsic and intrinsic muscles of the thumb before discussing coordinated function of all the elements together.

There are two muscles originating outside the

hand (extrinsic) that contribute to finger flexion. These are the FDS and the FDP muscles. The FDS muscle primarily flexes the PIP joint, but it also contributes to MP joint flexion. The FDP muscle can flex the MP, PIP, and the DIP joints and is considered to be the more active of the two muscles.[4] With gentle pinch or grasp, the FDP muscle alone will be active. As greater flexor force is needed or when finger flexion with wrist flexion is desired, the FDS muscle joins the FDP muscle by increasing its activity.[81,90,116,117]

The FDS muscle can produce more torque at the MP joint than can the FDP muscle. Not only does the FDS muscle cross fewer joints (making it less likely to lose tension as it shortens over multiple joints), but also the FDS tendon is superficial to the FDP tendon at the MP joint. Because the FDS muscle is farther from the MP joint flexion/extension axis, it has a greater MA for MP joint flexion.[3] Although it is often thought that the FDS muscle is stronger at PIP flexion because the FDS muscle crosses few joints, this is not the case. In contrast to what is found at the MP joint, the FDS tendon lies deep to the FDP tendon at the PIP joint and, therefore, has a lesser MA.[91] The switch in position between the FDS and FDP tendons occurs just proximal to the PIP joint, where the FDP tendon emerges through the split in the FDS tendon (**Camper's chiasma**) so the that FDS tendon can attach to the base of the middle phalanx deep to the FDP tendon. Although the MA of the FDS tendon may not be optimal at the PIP joint, the FDS tendon is important for balance at the PIP joint. When the FDS tendon is absent, forceful pinch (thumb to fingertip) activity of the FDP muscle may create PIP *extension* along with DIP flexion (Fig. 9-26), rather than flexion at both joints.[118] This phenomenon can be observed in many normal hands because

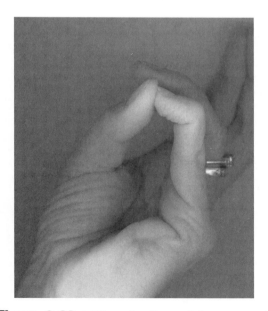

▲ **Figure 9-26** ■ When the flexor digitorum superficialis (FDS) muscle is not present (as is occasionally the case in the little finger), forcefully pressing the thumb and finger tip together produces DIP flexion with PIP *extension*, rather than flexion. Without the stabilization of the PIP joint by the FDS muscle, the FDP muscle is not able to flex both joints.

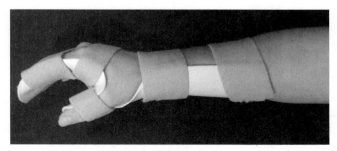

▲ **Figure 9-25** ■ Splinting the hand in the "anti-deformity" position minimizes the risk of dysfunctional changes to the immobilized joints.

the FDS tendon of the little finger is commonly absent or may have anomalous distal attachments.[118,119]

Both the FDS and FDP muscles are dependent on wrist position for an optimal length-tension relationship.[4] If there is no counterbalancing extensor torque at the wrist, the volarly located torques of the FDS and FDP muscles will cause wrist flexion to occur. If the finger flexor muscles are permitted to shorten over the wrist, there will be a concomitant loss of tension at the more distal joints. In fact, it is almost impossible to fully flex the fingers actively if the wrist is also flexed. Although the poor length-tension relationship in the FDS and FDP muscles accounts for some of this, the inability to complete the flexion ROM is also attributable to the concomitant passive tension in the finger extensors. During active finger flexion (as in grasp activities), the counterbalancing wrist extensor force is usually supplied by an active wrist extensor such as the ECRB muscle or, in some instances, the EDC muscle.

Continuing Exploration: **Finger Flexor Grasp**

The greater available range of MP and IP joint flexion in the ring and little fingers in comparison with the index or long fingers means that the long flexors of the ring and little fingers must shorten over a greater range, resulting in a loss of tension in the muscles of those fingers. If the object to be held by the fingers is heavy or requires strong grip, the object may be shaped so that it is wider ulnarly than radially, a so-called pistol grip (Fig. 9-27A). The pistol grip limits MP/IP joint flexion in the ring and little fingers, and the wrist extensors stabilize the wrist against a strong contraction of the finger flexors. The loss of tension in the long finger flexors is not a problem if strong grip is not required (e.g.,

holding a glass); then the object may be tapered at the ring and little fingers to accommodate the greater ROM (see Fig. 9-27B). Notice that the wrist in both forceful and gentle grips tends to assume a position of ulnar deviation that maximizes efficiency of the long finger flexors.[2,76]

■ Mechanisms of Finger Flexion

Optimal function of the FDS and FDP muscles depends not only on stabilization by the wrist musculature but also on intact flexor gliding mechanisms.[120] The gliding mechanisms consist of the flexor retinaculae, **bursae**, and **digital tendon sheaths**. The fibrous retinacular structures (proximal flexor retinaculum, TCL, and extensor retinaculum) tether the long flexor tendons to the hand; the bursae and tendon sheaths facilitate friction-free excursion of the tendons on the fibrous retinaculae. The retinaculae prevent bowstringing of the tendons that would result in loss of excursion and work efficiency in the contracting muscles that pass under them. The tendons must be anchored without interfering with their excursion and without creating frictional forces that would cause degeneration of the tendons over time.

As the tendons of the FDS and FDP muscles cross the wrist to enter the hand, they first pass beneath the proximal flexor retinaculum and through the carpal tunnel under the TCL (see Fig. 9-12A and B). Friction between the tendons themselves and friction of the tendons on the overlying TCL are prevented by the radial and ulnar bursae that envelop the flexor tendons at this level. All eight tendons of the FDP and FDS muscles are invested in a common bursa known as the **ulnar bursa** (Fig. 9-28A). The bursa is compartmentalized to prevent friction of tendon on tendon. The FPL muscle that

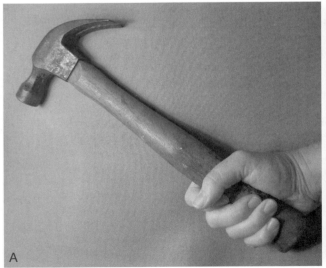
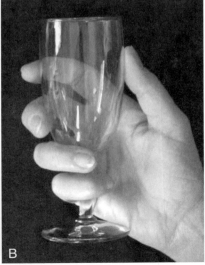

▲ **Figure 9-27** ■ **A.** The so-called "pistol grip" of the hammer allows the FDS and FDP muscles to work more forcefully at the ring and little fingers because the range of motion in the more mobile MP and IP joints in these fingers is restricted by the shape of the object. The shape also encourages wrist ulnar deviation that further enhances force production in the long finger flexors. **B.** When force is not needed, the shape of an object is often tapered to accommodate to the greater range of the ring and little fingers, allowing the long finger flexors to close the fingers fully around the object.

accompanies the FDS and FDP muscles through the carpal tunnel is encased in its own **radial bursa** (see Figs. 9-12 and 9-28A). The radial and ulnar bursae contain a synovial-like fluid that minimizes frictional forces. The pattern of bursae and tendon sheaths may vary among individuals. The most common representation shows the ulnar bursa to be continuous with the digital tendon sheath for the little finger (see Fig. 9-28A). However, Phillips and colleagues[121] found continuity between the ulnar bursa and tendon sheath of the little finger in only 30% of 60 specimens. The ulnar bursa is typically not continuous with the digital tendon sheaths for the index, middle, and ring fingers. Rather, for these fingers, the ulnar bursa ends just distal to the proximal palmar crease, and the digital tendon sheaths begin at the middle or distal palmar creases.[10] The radial bursa encases the FPL muscle and is continuous with its digital tendon sheath. The extent and communication of the digital tendon sheaths is functionally relevant because infection within a sheath will travel its full length, producing painful tenosynovitis. If a sheath is continuous with the ulnar or radial bursa, the infection may spread from the sheath into the palm (or vice versa).[30,80] The tendon sheaths for each finger end proximal to the insertion of the FDP muscle, effectively ending at the distal aspect of the middle phalanx. Consequently, puncture wounds or injuries to the pad (distal phalanx) of the fingers that are a fairly common site of trauma are unlikely to introduce infection into the digital tendon sheaths.

The FDS and FDP tendons of each finger pass through a fibro-osseous tunnel that comprises five transversely oriented **annular pulleys** (or **vaginal ligaments**), as well as three obliquely oriented **cruciate pulleys**.[20,122] The first two annular pulleys lie closely together, with one (designated the A1 pulley) at the head of the metacarpal and a second larger one (A2) along the volar midshaft of the proximal phalanx. The floor of the first pulley is formed by the flexor groove in the deep transverse metacarpal ligament, whereas all the other annular pulleys attach directly to bone. The third annular pulley (A3) lies at the distal-most part of the proximal phalanx, and the fourth (A4) lies centrally on the middle phalanx (see Fig. 9-28B). A fifth pulley (A5) may lie at the base of the distal phalanx. The base of each of the pulleys on the bone is longer than the roof superficially, and the roof has a slight concavity volarly. This shape prevents the pulleys from pinching each other at extremes of flexion, forming nearly one continuous tunnel.[20] The shorter roof of the fibro-osseous tunnel also minimizes the pressure on the tendon under tension, distributing pressure throughout the tunnel rather than just at the edges during finger flexion[122] (see Fig. 9-28B). The three cruciate (crisscrossing) pulleys also tether the long flexor tendons. One is located between the A2 and A3 pulleys and is designated as C1; the next cruciate pulley (C2) lies between the A3 and A4 pulleys; and the last cruciate pulley (C3) lies between the A4 and A5 pulleys. The A4, A5, and C3 structures contain only the FDP tendon because the FDS muscle inserts on the middle phalanx proximal to these structures. The annular pulleys and cruciate liga-

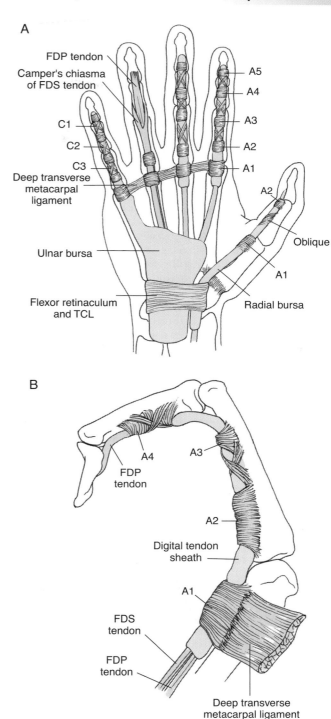

▲ **Figure 9-28** ■ **A.** The flexor mechanisms of the fingers and thumb include the fibro-osseous tunnels formed by the flexor retinaculum and transverse carpal ligament (TCL) at the wrist, the annular pulleys (A1 to A5), and the cruciate pulleys (C1 to C3). The tendons are protected within the tunnels by the radial and ulnar bursae and the digital tendon sheaths. The pulleys and the tendon sheath have been removed from the ring finger to show how the deep FDP tendon emerges through Camper's chiasma in the FDS tendon to pass on to the distal phalanx, and the split FDS tendon rejoins and inserts on the base of the middle phalanx. **B.** The shape of the pulleys allows finger flexion without pinching of the pulleys while more evenly distributing pressure on the tendon and sheath across the roof of the fibro-osseous tunnels.

ments vary among individuals in both number and extent.[122] More recently, an additional annular pulley found proximal to the A1 has also been described and has been named the palmar aponeurosis (PA) pulley.[123] The thumb has a distinct pulley system, including two annular and one oblique pulley (see Fig. 9-28A).[124]

Friction of the FDS and FDP tendons on the annular pulleys and cruciate ligaments is minimized by the digital tendon sheaths that envelop the tendons from the point at which the tendons pass into the most proximal annular pulley (PA or A1) to the point at which the tendon of the FDP muscle passes through the most distal cruciate pulley (C3 or A5) (see Fig. 9-28B). The synovial-like fluid contained in each of the digital tendon sheaths permits gliding of the tendons beneath their ligamentous constraints and between each other. This is particularly important over the proximal phalanx, where the FDS tendon splits to either side of the FDP tendon and rejoins *beneath* the FDP tendon to insert on the middle phalanx. The FDP tendon, consequently, must pass through Camper's chiasma (see ring finger of Fig. 9-28A). Once the FDP tendon is distal to the last annular pulley, the tendon sheath ends because lubrication of the tendon is no longer needed. Vascular supply to the gliding mechanism is critical to maintaining synovial fluid and tendon nutrition. Direct vascularization of each tendon occurs through vessels that reach the tendon via the **vincula tendinum.** These are folds of the synovial membrane (usually four in number) that carry blood vessels to the body of the tendon and to the tendinous insertions of the FDS and FDP muscles of each finger.[20,125] The tendons also receive some of their nutrition directly from the synovial fluid within the sheath and, through that mechanism, can withstand at least partial loss of direct vascularization.[125,126]

The function of the annular pulleys is to keep the flexor tendons close to the bone, allowing only a minimum amount of bowstringing and migration volarly from the joint axes.[127,128] This sacrifices the increase in MA that might occur with substantial bowstringing of the tendons but enhances both tendon excursion efficiency and work efficiency of the long flexors.[118,129] Any interruption in either the annular pulleys or the digital tendon sheaths can result in substantial impairment of FDS and FDP muscle functioning or in structural deformity. **Trigger finger** is one example of the disability that can be created when repetitive trauma to a flexor tendon results in the formation of nodules on the tendon and thickening of an annular pulley. Finger flexion may be prevented completely, or the finger may be unable to reextend.[9] Of the potential six annular pulleys (PA, A1 through A5), integrity of pulleys A2 and A4 is credited with being most critical to maintaining FDS/FDP muscle efficiency.[124,129,130]

 CONCEPT CORNERSTONE 9-3: *Flexor Gliding Mechanism at the MP Joint*

The flexor gliding mechanism at the MP joint is particularly complex because of its multilayered structure. From deep to superficial at each of the MP joints of the fingers, there are (1) the fibrocartilaginous volar plate, which is in contact with the metacarpal head; (2) the fibrous longitudinal fibers of the MP joint capsule, which blends with the volar aspect of the plate; (3) the fibers of the deep transverse metacarpal ligament (oriented perpendicularly to those of the longitudinal fibers of the capsule), which has grooves on its volar surface for the long flexor tendons of the fingers and form the floor of a fibro-osseous tunnel; (4) the FDP tendon, which lies in the groove of the transverse metacarpal ligament; (5) the FDS tendon, which lies just superficial to the FDP tendon; (6) the digital tendon sheath that envelops both the FDP and FDS tendons; and (7) the A1 annular pulley that forms the roof of the fibro-osseous tunnel and lies most superficially in this set of interconnected layers.

Extrinsic Finger Extensors

The extrinsic finger extensors are the EDC, the EIP, and the EDM muscles. Each of these muscles passes from the forearm to the hand beneath the extensor retinaculum, which maintains proximity of the tendons to the joints and improves excursion efficiency. Each of these six tendons is contained within a compartment of the extensor retinaculum and is enveloped by an isolated bursa or tendon sheath that generally ends as soon as the tendons emerge distal to the extensor retinaculum (Fig. 9-29). At approximately the MP joint, the EDC tendon of each finger merges with a broad aponeurosis known interchangeably as the **extensor expansion,** the **dorsal hood,** or the **extensor hood.** The EIP and EDM

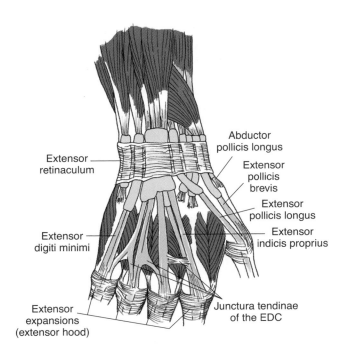

▲ **Figure 9-29** ■ Dorsal view of the hand, illustrating the six dorsal compartments of the extensor retinaculum at the wrist, the synovial sheaths, and the finger extensors (EDC, EIP, and EDM muscles) that merge with the extensor expansion at the MP joint. The juncturae tendinum of the EDC muscle lies just proximal to the MP joints.

tendons insert into the EDC tendons of the index and little fingers, respectively, at or just proximal to the extensor hood. Given the attachments of the EIP and EDM tendons to the EDC structure, the EIP and EDM muscles add independence of action to the index and ring fingers, rather than additional actions.

The tendons of the EDC, EIP, and EDM muscles show a good deal of variability on the dorsum of the hand. Most of the time, the index finger has one EDC tendon leading to the extensor hood and one EIP tendon inserting into the hood on the ulnar side of the EDC tendon.[131-133] At the little finger, the EDM tendon alone may merge with the extensor hood, with no EDC tendon to the little finger in as many as 30% of specimens.[134] The middle and ring fingers do not have their own auxiliary extensor muscles but frequently have two or even three EDC tendons leading to the hood.[133] The EDC tendons of one finger may also be connected to the tendon or tendons of an adjacent finger by **junctura tendinae** (see Fig. 9-29). These fibrous interconnections (frequently visible along with the extensor tendons on the dorsum of the hand) cause active extension of one finger to be accompanied by passive extension of the adjacent finger—with the patterns of interdependence varying with the connections.[82] In general, the EDC, EIP, EDM, and junctura tendinae connections result in the index finger's having the most independent extension, with extension of the little, middle, and ring fingers in declining order of independence.[91]

The EDC, EIP, and EDM are the only muscles capable of extending the MP joints of the fingers. These muscles extend the MP joint via their connection to the extensor hood and sagittal bands that (as we saw in discussion of the volar plates of the MP joint) interconnect the volar plates and the EDC tendon or extensor hood.[82] Active tension on the extensor hood from one or more of these muscles will extend the MP joint even though there are no direct attachments to the proximal phalanx.[135] The extrinsic extensors are also wrist extensors by continued action. Because the EIP and EDM muscles share innervation, insertion, and function with the EDC muscle to which each attaches, discussion of the EDC muscle from this point on should be assumed to include contributions from the EIP or the EDM muscles. For the sake of clarity and brevity, all three muscles will not be named each time.

Distal to the extensor hood (and therefore after the EIP and EDM tendons have joined the EDC tendon), the EDC tendon at each finger splits into three bands: the **central tendon,** which inserts on the base of the middle phalanx, and two **lateral bands,** which rejoin as the **terminal tendon** to insert into the base of the distal phalanx (Fig. 9-30).[82] Although tension on the hood can produce MP joint extension, the central tendon and terminal tendon distal to the extensor expansion cannot be tightened sufficiently by the extrinsic extensor muscles alone to produce extension at either the PIP or DIP joints. In order to also produce active IP extension, the EDC muscle requires the assistance of two intrinsic muscle groups that also have attachments to the extensor hood and the lateral bands. The EDC tendon and all its complicated active

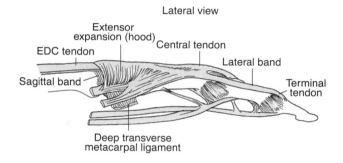

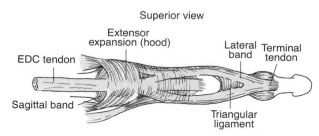

▲ **Figure 9-30** ■ The building blocks of the extensor mechanism are the EDC tendon, which merges with the extensor hood and sagittal bands and then continues distally to split into a central tendon inserting into the middle phalanx, and two lateral bands that merge into a terminal tendon that inserts into the distal phalanx. The two lateral bands are stabilized dorsally by the triangular ligament.

and passive interconnections at and distal to the MP joint are known together as the **extensor mechanism.**

Extensor Mechanism

The foundation of the extensor mechanism is formed by the tendons of the EDC muscle (with EIP and EDM muscles), the extensor hood, the central tendon, and the lateral bands that merge into the terminal tendon. The first two components that we will add to the extensor mechanism are the passive components of the **triangular ligament** and the sagittal bands (see Fig. 9-30). The lateral bands are interconnected dorsally by a triangular band of superficial fibers known as the triangular, or **dorsal retinacular,** ligament.[82] The triangular ligament helps stabilize the bands on the dorsum of the finger. The sagittal bands connect the volar surface of the hood to the volar plates and transverse metacarpal ligament. The sagittal bands aid in stabilization not only of the volar plates but also of the hood at the MP joint. The sagittal bands help to prevent bowstringing of the extensor mechanism during active MP joint extension, as well as transmitting force that will extend the proximal phalanx.[82] The sagittal bands are also responsible for centralizing the EDC tendon over the MP joint, preventing tendon subluxation.[136]

The **dorsal interossei (DI), volar interossei (VI),** and **lumbrical** muscles are the active components of the extensor mechanism (Fig. 9-31). The DI and VI muscles arise proximally from the sides of the metacarpal joints. Distally, some muscle fibers go deep to insert directly into the proximal phalanx, whereas others join with and become part of the hood that wraps around the proximal phalanx. The interossei muscles may also contribute fibers to the central tendon and both lateral bands. The lumbrical muscles attach proximally to the FDP tendons and distally to the lateral band. With the addition of the **oblique retinacular ligaments** (ORLs), the structure of the extensor mechanism for each finger is complete.

A final passive element that contributes to the extensor mechanism are the ORLs. The ORLs arise from both sides of the proximal phalanx and from the sides of the annular and cruciate pulleys volarly. The ORLs continue distally as slender bands to insert on the lateral bands distal to the PIP joint and conclude the building of the extensor mechanism (see Fig. 9-31).[137,138] The ORLs lie volar to the axis of the PIP joint and dorsal to the axis of the DIP joint through its attachment to the lateral bands. Function of the extensor mechanism can now be presented by looking in more detail at the active and passive elements that compose it and by referencing the relation of relevant segments to each joint individually.

■ Extensor Mechanism Influence on Metacarpophalangeal Joint Function

The EDC tendon passes dorsal to the MP joint axis. An active contraction of the muscle creates tension on the sagittal bands of the extensor mechanism, pulls the bands proximally over the MP joint, and extends the proximal phalanx. In order to simultaneously extend the PIP and DIP joints, the EDC muscle requires active assistance. The other active forces that are part of the extensor mechanism are the DI, VI, and lumbrical muscles. Each of these muscles passes volar to the MP joint axis and, therefore, creates a flexor force at the joint. However, when the EDC, interossei, and lumbrical muscles all contract simultaneously, the MP joint will extend (as will the IP joints) because the torque produced by the EDC muscle at the MP joint exceeds the MP joint flexor torque of the intrinsic muscles. An isolated contraction of the EDC muscle will result in MP joint hyperextension with IP flexion.[139–141] The flexion is produced by passive tension in the FDS and FDP muscles when the MP joint is extended. This position of the fingers (MP joint hyperextension with passive IP flexion) is known as **clawing.** Similar to what we saw at the proximal carpal row of the wrist complex, clawing is the classic zigzag pattern that occurs when a compressive force is exerted across several linked segments, one of which is an unstable "intercalated" segment. In the instance of clawing of the finger, the proximal phalanx hyperextends on the metacarpal below while the middle and distal phalanx flex over it. Normally the "collapse" (excessive extension) of the proximal phalanx is prevented by active tension in the lumbrical or interossei muscles that

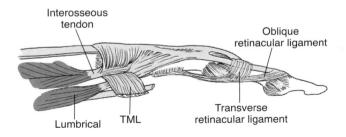

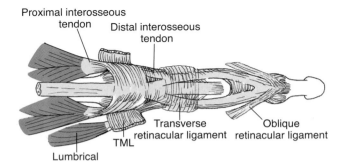

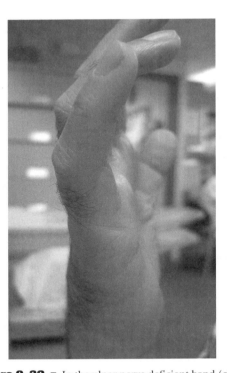

▲ **Figure 9-31** ■ The interossei muscles pass dorsal to the transverse metacarpal ligament (TML) and may attach directly to the extensor hood or may have fibers that attach more distally to the central tendon and lateral bands. The lumbrical muscles attach to the FDP tendon volarly and to the lateral bands. The oblique retinacular ligament (ORL) is attached to the annular pulley proximally and to the lateral bands distally, lying just deep to the transverse retinacular ligament.

▲ **Figure 9-32** ■ In the ulnar nerve-deficient hand (claw hand) at rest, the MP joints of the ring and little fingers are hyperextended because of relatively unopposed passive tension in the intact EDC muscle resulting from the loss of the interossei and lumbrical muscles; the IP joints are flexed because of increased passive tension in the long flexors caused by the MP joint position. The index and middle fingers are less affected because these fingers still have intact lumbrical and FDP muscles.

pass volar to the MP joint axis.[142] When the intrinsic muscles are weak or paralyzed (as in a low ulnar nerve injury), the EDC muscle is unopposed, and the fingers claw not only with active MP joint extension but also at rest (Fig. 9-32). The clawing at rest demonstrates that the passive tension in the intact EDC muscle exceeds the passive tension in the remaining MP joint flexors. The clawed position is also known as an **intrinsic minus position** because it is attributed to the absence of the finger intrinsic muscles (the interossei and lumbrical muscles).

■ **Extensor Mechanism Influence on Interphalangeal Joint Function**

The PIP and DIP joints are joined by active and passive forces in such a way that the DIP extension and PIP extension are interdependent. When the PIP joint is actively extended, the DIP joint will also extend. Similarly, active DIP extension will create PIP extension. The interdependence can be understood by examining structural relationships in the extensor mechanism.

Each PIP joint is crossed dorsally by the central tendon and lateral bands of the extensor mechanism (see Fig. 9-30). The EDC, interossei, and lumbrical muscles all have attachments to the hood, central tendon, or lateral bands at or proximal to the PIP joint (see Fig. 9-31). Consequently, the EDC, interossei, and lumbrical muscles are each capable of producing at least some tension in each of the following: the central tendon, the lateral bands, and (via the lateral bands) the terminal tendon, resulting in each contributing to some extensor force at both the PIP and DIP joints. An EDC muscle contraction alone will not produce effective IP extension. An active contraction of a DI, VI, or lumbrical muscle alone *is* capable of extending the PIP and DIP joints completely because of their more direct attachments to the central tendon and lateral bands. However, if one or more of the intrinsic muscles (DI, VI, or lumbrical) contracts without a simultaneous contraction of the EDC muscle of that finger, the MP joint will flex because each intrinsic muscles passes *volar* to the MP joint axis. Although it may appear that the intrinsic muscles are independently extending the IP joints, passive tension in the extensor mechanism may be assisting the active intrinsic muscles.

Stack[143] proposed that the interossei and lumbrical muscles would not be able to generate sufficient tension to cause independent IP extension if the EDC tendon was completely slack or severed. *Two* sources of tension in the extensor expansion appear to be necessary to fully extend the IP joints. Source 1 is normally an active contraction of one or more of the intrinsic finger muscles. Source 2 may be either an *active contraction* of the EDC muscle (with active MP joint extension) or *passive stretch* of the EDC muscle (created by MP joint flexion resulting from an active contraction of the intrinsic muscles).

Continuing Exploration: **Extension in the Absence of Intrinsic Muscles**

When the intrinsic musculature is paralyzed, as in an ulnar nerve injury, the interossei and lumbrical muscles of the ring and little fingers cannot provide the active assistance that the EDC muscle needs to fully extend the IP joints. The EDC muscle may be able to extend the IP joints "independently" but *only* if the MP joint is maintained in flexion by some external force. If some passive tension in the EDC muscle can be attained with MP joint flexion (source 1), additional tension can then be provided by an active contraction of the EDC muscle (source 2). These two sources (simultaneous active and passive tension in the EDC muscle) may be sufficient to produce full or nearly full PIP and DIP extension in the absence of intact intrinsic muscles.[140] An external splint or surgical fixation of the MP joints in a semiflexed position (Fig. 9-33A) is necessary to maintain some MP joint flexion to stretch the EDC muscle; it also provides adequate resistance to the active MP joint extensor force of the EDC muscle.[144] This can also be thought of as providing the means for the EDC muscle to strongly contract without the concomitant loss of tension that would happen if permitted to complete the MP joint extension ROM. The arrangement of the splint shown here restricts MP joint extension when the hand is actively opened, without restricting the ability of the intact FDS muscle (and the intact FDP muscle, depending on the level of ulnar nerve injury) to actively flex the PIP joints of the ring and little fingers (see Fig. 9-33B).

Some of the linkage between PIP and DIP joint extension may be attributed to passive tension in the ORLs. The ORLs pass just volar to the PIP joint axis and attach distally to the lateral bands (see Fig. 9-31). Tension will increase in the ORLs as the PIP joint is extended (actively or passively) *if* the lateral bands and their terminal tendon are already tensed by DIP flexion. Consequently, PIP extension may make a contribution to DIP extension through passive tension in the ORLs. The lengths of the ORLs are such, however, that the contribution of PIP extension to DIP extension via the ORLs may be significant only during the first half of the DIP joint's return from flexion (90° to 45° flexion), when the ORLs are most stretched.[137,143] Overall, the complex structure of the extensor expansion and its contributing active and passive elements result in a relative linking between PIP and DIP extension.[9,10,139,141]

Flexion of the DIP joint produces flexion of the PIP joint by a similar complex combination of active and passive forces that link PIP and DIP joint extension. When the DIP joint is flexed by the FDP muscle, a simultaneous flexor force is applied over both joints crossed by the FDP muscle, and so simultaneous DIP and PIP joint flexion are not surprising. However, the active force of the FDP muscle on the distal phalanx might *not* be sufficient to produce simultaneous PIP

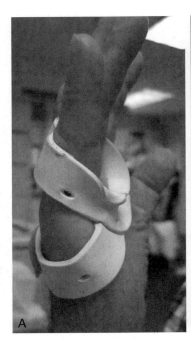

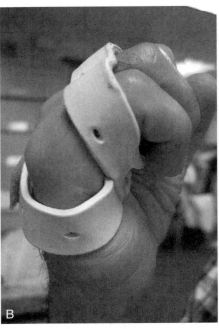

◀ **Figure 9-33** ■ **A.** In the ulnar nerve-deficient hand, the EDC muscle alone can extend the IP joints of the ring and little fingers in the absence of the interossei and lumbrical muscles if full MP joint extension is prevented by a splint during an active EDC muscle contraction. **B.** The splint is shaped so that the intact long finger flexor or flexors can flex the fingers with minimal interference by the splint.

flexion if extensor restraining forces at the PIP joint were not released at the same time.

When DIP flexion is initiated by the FDP muscle, the terminal tendon and its lateral bands are stretched over the dorsal aspect of the DIP joint. The stretch in the lateral bands pulls the extensor hood (from which the lateral bands arise) distally. The distal migration in the extensor hood causes the central tendon of the extensor expansion to relax, releasing its extensor influence at the PIP joint and facilitating PIP flexion. The simultaneous flexor torque and release of extensor torque still might not be adequate for the FDP muscle to flex the PIP joint if the lateral bands remained taut on the dorsal aspect of the PIP joint. The bands, however, are permitted to separate somewhat by the elasticity of the interconnecting triangular ligament and are assisted by passive tension in the **transverse retinacular ligament** (see Fig. 9-31). Although the example used here was initiated by an active contraction of the FDP muscle, the same set of mechanisms will tie passive DIP flexion (produced by an external flexor force) to passive PIP flexion.

Continuing Exploration: **Finger Tricks: DIP Flexion with PIP Extension**

The normal coupling of DIP flexion with PIP flexion can be overridden by some individuals; that is, some people can actively flex a DIP joint (using the FDP muscle) while maintaining the PIP joint in extension (Fig. 9-34). This "trick" is due to the influence of the ORLs and requires some PIP hyperextension of the finger. When the PIP joint can be sufficiently hyperextended, the ORLs that ordinarily lie *just* volar to the PIP joint axis will migrate *dorsal* to the PIP joint axis. At that point, tension in the ORLs produced by active DIP flexion (stretch of the terminal tendon and lateral bands to which the ORLs attach) will

accentuate PIP *extension* because the ORLs function as passive PIP joint extensors. The trick of active DIP flexion and PIP extension serves no functional purpose and can be accomplished only in fingers in which PIP hyperextension is available. The "trick" does, however, highlight the necessity of releasing extensor tension at the PIP joint before the FDP muscle can effectively flex that joint.

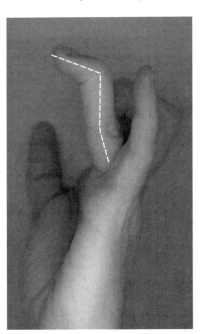

▲ **Figure 9-34** ■ Some individuals can actively flex the DIP joint in the presence of PIP extension. This generally requires that the individual have PIP joint hyperextension, so that in the extended finger, the ORLs migrate dorsal to the PIP joint axis. With initiation of DIP flexion, tension in the terminal tendon and lateral bands caused by the DIP flexion tenses the ORLs that serve as PIP extensors rather than flexors.

The functional coupling of PIP/DIP joint action can be demonstrated by one other PIP/DIP joint relation.[54] When the PIP joint is fully flexed actively (by the FDS muscle) or passively (by an external force), the DIP joint cannot be actively extended. When the PIP joint is flexing, the dorsally located central tendon is becoming stretched. The increasing tension in the central tendon pulls the extensor hood (from which the central tendon arises) distally. This distal migration of the hood releases some of the tension in the lateral bands. The tension in the lateral bands is further released as the bands separate slightly at the flexing PIP joint. Releasing tension in the lateral bands releases tension in the terminal tendon on the distal phalanx. As 90° of PIP flexion is reached, loss of tension in the terminal tendon completely eliminates any extensor force at the DIP joint, including any potential contribution from the ORLs that have also been released by PIP flexion.[145] Although the DIP joint can be actively flexed by the FDP muscle when the PIP is already flexed, the distal phalanx cannot be actively reextended as long as the PIP joint remains flexed.

 CONCEPT CORNERSTONE 9-4: *Summary of Coupled Actions of the PIP and DIP Joints*

■ Active extension of the PIP joint will normally be accompanied by extension of the DIP joint.
■ Active or passive flexion of the DIP joint will normally initiate flexion of the PIP joint.
■ Full flexion of the PIP joint (actively or passively) will prevent the DIP joint from being actively extended.

Intrinsic Finger Musculature

■ Dorsal and Volar Interossei Muscles

The DI and VI muscles, as already noted, arise from between the metacarpals and are an important part of the extensor mechanism. There are four DI muscles (one to each finger) and three to four VI muscles. Many (but not all) anatomy texts describe the thumb as having the first VI muscle. Mardel and Underwood[146] suggested that the discrepancy may be in whether the controversial muscle is considered a separate VI muscle or as part of the **flexor pollicis brevis** (**FPB**). Although we will consider the thumb as having the first VI muscle, at this time we will consider only the action of the VI and DI muscles of the fingers. Because the DI and VI muscles are alike in location and in some of their actions, these two muscle groups are often characterized by their ability to produce MP joint abduction and adduction, respectively. More recently, additional detail on the variable attachments of these muscles, as well as studies revealing multiple muscle heads, has increased our understanding of their contribution to hand function.[147] We will now look at how the attachments of the interossei muscles affect their role as MP joint flexors or stabilizers and as IP extensors.

The interossei muscle fibers join the extensor expansions in two locations. Some fibers attach *proximally* to the proximal phalanx and to the extensor hood; some fibers attach more *distally* to the lateral bands and central tendon (see Fig. 9-31). Although individual variations in muscle attachments exist, studies have found some consistency in the point of attachment of the different interossei muscles.[138,143,148] The first DI muscle has the most consistent attachment of its group, inserting entirely into the bony base of the proximal phalanx and the extensor hood. The DI muscles of the middle and ring fingers (with the middle finger having a DI muscle on each side) each have both proximal and distal attachments (to the proximal phalanx/hood and to the lateral bands/central tendon). The little finger does not have a DI muscle. The abductor digiti minimi (ADM) muscle is, in effect, a DI muscle and typically has only a proximal attachment (proximal phalanx/hood)[91] The three VI muscles consistently appear to have distal attachments only (attachments to the lateral bands/central tendon). Conceptually, then, we can establish a frame of reference in which we can summarize the DI and VI attachments as follows: the first DI muscle has only a proximal attachment; the second, third, and fourth DI muscles have both proximal and distal attachments, the "fifth DI" muscle (the ADM) has only a proximal attachment; and the three VI muscles of the fingers have only distal attachments.

Given the particular proximal or distal attachment patterns of the DI, VI, and ADM muscles, these muscles can be characterized not only as abductors or adductors of the MP joint but also as proximal or distal interossei according to the pattern of attachment. Proximal interossei will have their predominant effect at the MP joint alone, whereas the distal interossei will produce their predominant action at the IP joints, with some effect by continued action at the MP joint.

All of the DI and VI muscles (regardless of their designation as proximal or distal) pass *dorsal* to the transverse metacarpal ligament but just volar to the axis for MP joint flexion/extension. All the interossei muscles, therefore, are potentially flexors of the MP joint. The ability of the interossei muscles to flex the MP joint, however, will vary somewhat with MP joint position.

Role of the Interossei Muscles at the Metacarpophalangeal Joint in Metacarpophalangeal Joint Extension

When the MP joint is in extension, the MA (and rotatory component) of all the interossei muscles for MP joint flexion is so small that little flexion torque is produced. Given that the action lines of the interossei muscles pass almost directly through the coronal axis in MP joint extension, the interossei muscles are not very effective flexors when the MP joint is extended, although they can be effective stabilizers (joint compressors). In spite of their poor flexor torque, the interossei muscles appear to be important in helping to prevent clawing (MP joint hyperextension) of the finger.[91,139]

There is typically no EMG activity recorded in the interossei muscles when the hand is at rest, when there is isolated EDC muscle activity, or when there is combined EDC/FDP muscle activity. However, when these activities are performed in a hand with long-standing ulnar nerve paralysis (therefore, no interossei muscles), an exaggerated MP joint extension or hyperextension (clawing) results. In a low ulnar nerve injury, the index and middle fingers retain a lumbrical muscle as well as both the FDS and FDP muscles. The loss of the interossei muscles is reflected by a resting MP joint posture of neutral flexion/extension, rather than slight flexion, as is usually observed. The ring and little fingers, missing both interossei and lumbrical muscles in a hand with ulnar nerve deficit, will assume an MP joint hyperextended and IP flexed posture at rest (clawing) even in the presence of intact FDS and FDP muscles.[9,10,79,139] Clawing is not evident at rest in the ulnar nerve-deficient hand until the viscoelastic tension in the interossei muscles has been lost through atrophy and the volar plates have stretched out. Once such atrophy occurs, the predominance of EDC muscle tension even in relaxation is evidenced by the MP joint posture assumed by each finger of the hand at rest (see Fig. 9-32). The role of the interossei muscles in balancing passive tension in the extrinsic extensors at the MP joints at rest appears, therefore, to be provided by *passive* viscoelastic tension in the muscle.

Continuing Exploration: **Wartenberg's Sign**

In addition to the clawing evident in the ring and little fingers in the ulnar nerve-deficient hand, the little finger may also assume an MP joint abducted position with loss of the intrinsic muscles. Abduction of the little finger (**Wartenberg's sign**) may be the result of the unbalanced pull of the EDM muscle among those individuals having a direct connection of the EDM muscle to the abductor tubercle of the proximal phalanx—the only one of the extensor tendons that has an insertion directly on to the proximal phalanx in any substantial number of people.[131]

When the MP joint is extended, the interossei (and ADM) muscles lie at a relatively large distance from the A-P axis for MP joint abduction/adduction. Consequently, in the MP joint extended position, the interossei (and ADM) muscles are effective abductors or adductors of the MP joint without the loss of tension that would occur if the muscles were simultaneously producing MP joint flexion. The interossei muscles that insert proximally (on the proximal phalanx/hood) are better as MP joint abductors/adductors, whereas the interossei muscles with more distal insertions (lateral bands/central tendon) are less effective at the MP joint because they must act on the MP joint by continued action. In our conceptual framework, all the DI muscles (MP joint abductors) have proximal insertions, and the VI muscles (MP joint adductors) have only distal insertions. Therefore, MP joint abduction is stronger than MP joint adduction. The DI muscles also have twice the muscle mass of the VI muscles. In a progressive ulnar nerve paralysis, the relatively ineffective MP joint adduction component of the VI muscles is the first to show weakness.

Role of the Interossei Muscles at the Metacarpo-phalangeal Joint in Metacarpophalangeal Joint Flexion. As the MP joint flexes from extension, the tendons and action lines of the interossei muscles migrate volarly away from the MP joint's coronal axis, increasing the MA for MP flexion. In fact, in full MP joint flexion, the action lines of the interossei muscles are nearly perpendicular to the moving segment (proximal phalanx) (Fig. 9-35). Consequently, the ability of the interossei muscles to create an MP joint flexion torque increases as the MP joint moves toward full flexion. As the MP joint approaches full flexion, the volar migration of the interossei muscles is restricted by the location of the interossei tendons dorsal to the deep transverse metacarpal ligament. Although the transverse metacarpal ligament limits the MA of the interossei muscles, the ligament also both prevents the loss of active tension that would occur with bowstringing and serves as an anatomic pulley. With increased MP joint flexion, the collateral ligaments of the MP joint also become increasingly taut. The increasing tension in the collateral ligaments helps prevent the loss of MP joint flexor force that would occur if the interossei muscles concomitantly produced MP joint abduction/adduction. In full MP joint flexion, MP joint abduction and adduction are completely restricted by tight collateral ligaments, by the shape of the condyles of the metacarpal head, and by active insufficiency of the fully shortened interossei muscles. The net effect of these combined mechanisms is that the ability of the interossei muscles to produce an MP joint flexion torque (in the MP flexed position) makes them powerful MP joint flexor muscles[149] that contribute to grip when a strong pinch or grip is required.[117,150]

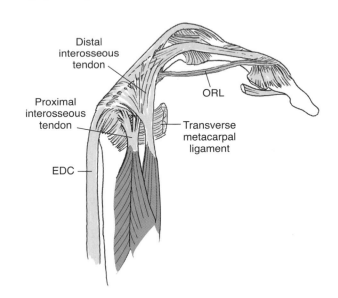

▲ **Figure 9-35** ■ When the MP joint is flexed, the interossei muscles (those with both proximal and distal attachments) migrate volarly away from the MP joint axis for flexion/extension, which results in a relatively large moment arm and a line of pull that is nearly perpendicular to the proximal phalanx. The volar migration of the interossei muscles is limited by the deep transverse metacarpal ligament, which prevents loss of tension and serves as an anatomic pulley.

Role of the Interossei Muscles at the Interphalangeal Joint in Interphalangeal Joint Extension. The ability of the interossei muscles to produce IP joint extension is influenced by their attachments. To create sufficient tension in the extensor mechanism to contribute effectively to IP extension, the muscles must attach to the central tendon or lateral bands. All the interossei muscles have distal attachments except the two "outside" abductors on the first and fourth fingers (first DI and ADM muscles).

When the MP joint is extended, the action lines of the distal interossei are ineffective in producing MP joint flexion (because of the poor MA) but capable of extending the IP joints because the distal interossei attach directly to the central tendon and lateral bands. The IP extension produced by the distal interossei is stronger than the MP joint abduction/adduction action because that is produced by continued action. We have already noted that when the MP joint flexes, the tendons of the interossei muscles migrate volarly at the MP joint but are restricted in their volar excursion by the deep transverse metacarpal ligament. The transverse metacarpal ligament prevents the interosseous tendons from becoming slack through volar migration and has a pulley effect on the distal tendons. The anatomic pulley effect of the deep transverse metacarpal ligament may enhance the function of the distal interossei muscles, because IP extension appears to be more effective in MP joint flexion than in MP joint extension.

The index and little fingers each have only one interosseous muscle with a distal insertion (second VI and fourth VI muscles, respectively). The middle and ring fingers each have two distal tendons (second and third DI muscles for the middle finger, and fourth VI and fourth DI muscles for the ring finger). The index and little fingers, therefore, are weaker in IP extension than are the middle and ring fingers because they have fewer distal interossei muscles.[148]

Overall, in approaching or holding the position of MP flexion and IP extension, both proximal and distal insertions of the interossei muscles contribute to the MP joint flexion torque. The proximal components are effective MP joint flexors, and the distal components are effective as both MP joint flexors and IP extensors. The most consistent activity of the interossei muscles appears to occur when the MP joints are being flexed and the IP joints are simultaneously extended,[139,151] a position that takes advantage of optimal biomechanics for both the proximal and the distal interossei muscles.

■ Lumbrical Muscles

The lumbrical muscles are the only muscles in the body that attach at both ends to tendons of other muscles. Each muscle arises from a tendon of the FDP muscle in the palm, passes volar to the transverse metacarpal ligament, and attaches to the lateral band of the extensor mechanism on the radial side (see Fig. 9-31).[152] Like the interossei muscles, the lumbrical muscles cross the MP joint volarly and the IP joints dorsally. Differences in function in the two muscle groups can be attributed to the more distal insertion of the lumbrical muscles on the lateral band, to their FDP tendon origin, and to their great contractile range.

The insertion of the lumbrical muscles on the lateral bands of the extensor mechanism distal to the attachment of the distal interossei muscles makes them consistently effective IP extensors, regardless of MP joint position. Studies have found the lumbrical muscles to be more frequently active as IP extensors in the MP joint extended position than are the interossei muscles.[139,153] The deep transverse metacarpal ligament prevents the volarly located lumbrical muscle from migrating dorsally and losing tension as the MP and IP joints extend. When a lumbrical muscle contracts, it pulls not only on its distal attachment (the lateral band) but also on its proximal attachment (the FDP tendon). Because the proximal attachment of the lumbrical muscle is on a somewhat movable tendon, shortening of the lumbrical muscle not only increases tension in the lateral bands to extend the IP joints but also pulls the FDP tendon distally in the palm. The distal migration of the FDP tendon releases much of the passive flexor force of the inactive FDP muscle at the MP and IP joints (Fig. 9-36). Ranney and Wells[142] confirmed this, finding that the lumbrical muscles did not begin to extend the IP joints until the tension within the lumbrical muscle equaled the tension in the FDP tendon (produced by the lumbrical muscle's distal pull on the FDP tendon). Given these circumstances, the lumbrical muscles might be considered to be both agonists and synergists for IP extension. Tension in the lumbrical muscles on the lateral bands produces IP extension, while the lumbrical muscle simultaneously releases antagonistic tension in the FDP tendon.[154] The distal insertion of the interossei muscles can also extend the IP joints. However, they are less effective as IP extensors in the absence of the lumbrical muscles, because the interossei muscles do not have the same ability to release the passive resistance of the FDP tendon to IP extension.

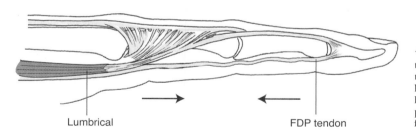

Lumbrical   FDP tendon

◀ **Figure 9-36** ■ The lumbrical muscle attaches to the FDP tendon proximally and to the lateral band of the extensor expansion distally. A contraction of the lumbrical muscle will create tension in the lateral band, leading to PIP/DIP joint extension, while concomitantly pulling the FDP tendon distally and releasing the passive flexor tension that could impede IP extension.

The complexity of the interconnections of the intrinsic muscles with the extensor mechanism can be highlighted not only by the interrelationships of the interossei muscles but also by the lumbrical muscle interdependent on the FDP and extensor muscle expansion to produce IP extension. Although active IP extension is facilitated by the active lumbrical muscle's effective release of passive FDP tendon tension, the lumbrical muscle is also dependent upon FDP tendon tension; that is, *some* tension in the FDP tendon is critical to lumbrical function. If passive tension were not present in the tendon of the inactive FDP muscle (if the FDP tendon were cut), an active lumbrical contraction would pull the FDP tendon so far distally that the muscle would become actively insufficient and ineffective as an IP extensor. Similarly, active or passive tension in the EDC tendon and extensor expansion are necessary before the second source of tension, the active lumbrical muscle, can be effective in fully extending both IP joints.[143] The lumbrical muscles may also assist the FDP muscle indirectly with hand closure. When the FDP muscle contracts, the FDP tendon moves proximally, carrying its associated (presumably passive) lumbrical muscle along with it. This creates a passive pull of the lumbrical muscle on the lateral band during hand closure that may assist the FDP muscle in flexing the MP joint *before* the IP joints, which avoids the problem of catching the fingertips in the palm during grasp as occurs in the intrinsic minus hand.[149]

The lumbrical muscles' role as an MP joint flexor is relatively minimal. The lumbrical muscles actually have a greater MA for MP joint flexion than do the interossei muscles because the lumbrical muscles lie volar to the interossei muscles. Functionally, however, this component of lumbrical action is weaker in the lumbrical muscles than in the interossei muscles.[139,148,149,153,155] This relative weakness may be attributed to the small cross-section of the lumbrical muscles in comparison with the interossei muscles. However, it may also have to do with the moving attachment of the lumbrical muscle on the FDP tendon. A contraction of a lumbrical muscle causes the associated FDP tendon to migrate distally and carries the lumbrical muscle along with it. The distal migration of the FDP tendon and lumbrical muscle has the effect both of releasing passive tension in the inactive FDP tendon that might contribute to MP joint flexion and of minimizing the active force of the lumbrical muscle at the MP joint. Although the lumbrical muscles do not contribute much force to MP joint flexion, MP flexion does not appear to weaken their effectiveness as IP extensors. The unusually large contractile range of the lumbrical muscles seems to prevent the lumbrical muscles from becoming actively insufficient when shortening both over the MP joints and at the IP joints.

 CONCEPT CORNERSTONE 9-5: *Intrinsic Muscles Summary*

The complex functions of the interossei muscles are summarized in Table 9-1. The function of the lumbrical muscles is simpler than that of the interossei muscles. The lumbrical muscles are strong extensors of the IP joints, regardless of MP joint position. The lumbrical muscles are also relatively weak MP joint flexors, regardless of MP joint position. The ability of the lumbrical muscles to extend the IPs appears to depend only on intact tension in the extensor mechanism and in the FDP tendons. When the lumbrical and interossei muscles contract together without any extrinsic finger muscle activity, these muscles produce flexion and IP extension, the so-called **intrinsic plus** position of the hand (Fig. 9-37A). When the extrinsic finger flexors and extensors are active without any concomitant activity of the intrinsic muscles, the hand assumes an intrinsic minus position (see Fig. 9-37B).

Table 9-1	Summary of Interossei Muscle Action			
		Action		
Muscle	Attachments	MP Extended		MP Flexed
		First Finger		
DI	Proximal only	MP abduction		MP flexion
VI	Distal only	IP extension and MP adduction*		IP extension and MP flexion*
		Second Finger		
DI	Proximal and distal	MP abduction and IP extension		MP flexion and IP extension
DI	Proximal and distal	MP abduction and IP extension		MP flexion and IP extension
		Third Finger		
DI	Proximal and distal	MP abduction and IP extension		MP flexion and IP extension
VI	Distal only	IP extension and MP adduction*		IP extension and MP flexion*
		Fourth Finger		
DI	Proximal only	MP abduction		MP flexion
VI	Distal only	IP extension and MP adduction*		IP extension and MP flexion*

*Occurs indirectly by continued action.
DI, dorsal interossei; IP, interphalangeal; MP, metacarpophalangeal; VI, volar interossei.

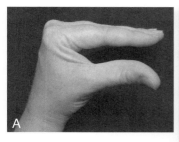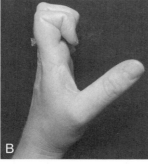

▲ **Figure 9-37** ■ **A.** Activity of the lumbrical and interossei muscles without any extrinsic finger flexors or extensors produces the "intrinsic plus" position of the hand. **B.** Activity of the extrinsic finger flexors and extensors without any activity of intrinsic finger muscles produces the "intrinsic minus" position of the hand.

Structure of the Thumb

■ Carpometacarpal Joint of the Thumb

The CMC (or trapeziometacarpal [TM]) joint of the thumb is the articulation between the trapezium and the base of the first metacarpal. Unlike the CMC joints of the fingers, the first CMC joint is a saddle joint with two degrees of freedom: flexion/extension and abduction/adduction (Fig. 9-38). The joint also permits some axial rotation, which occurs concurrently with the other motions. The net effect at this joint is a circumduction motion commonly termed **opposition.** Opposition permits the tip of the thumb to oppose the tips of the fingers.

First Carpometacarpal Joint Structure

Zancolli and associates[156] proposed that the first CMC joint surfaces consist not only of the traditionally described saddle-shaped surfaces but also of a spherical portion located near the anterior radial tubercle of the trapezium. The saddle-shaped portion of the trapezium is concave in the sagittal plane (abduction/adduction) and convex in the frontal plane (flexion/extension). The spherical portion is convex in all directions. The base of the first metacarpal has a reciprocal shape to that of the trapezium (see Fig. 9-38). Flexion/extension and abduction/adduction are proposed to occur on the saddle-shaped surfaces, whereas the axial rotation of the metacarpal that accompanies opposition is proposed to occur on the spherical surfaces.[156] Flexion/extension of the joint occurs around a somewhat oblique A-P axis, whereas abduction/adduction occurs around an oblique coronal axis. This is a reversal of what is found at most other joints, with flexion/extension usually occurring around a coronal axis and abduction/adduction around an A-P axis. The change in the CMC joint motions occurs because of the orientation of the trapezium, which effectively rotates the volar surface of the thumb medially. As a consequence, flexion/extension occurs nearly parallel to the palm, with abduction/adduction occurring nearly per-

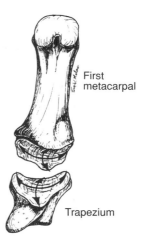

▲ **Figure 9-38** ■ The saddle-shaped portion of the trapezium is concave in the sagittal plane (abduction/adduction) and convex in the frontal plane (flexion/extension). The spherical portion found near the anterior radial tubercle is convex in all directions. The base of the first metacarpal joint has a shape reciprocal to that of the trapezium.

pendicular to the palm. Cooney and associates[157] measured the first CMC joint ROM as an average of 53° of flexion/extension, 42° of abduction/adduction, and 17° of rotation.

The capsule of the CMC joint is relatively lax but is reinforced by radial, ulnar, volar, and dorsal ligaments. There is also an **intermetacarpal ligament** that helps tether the bases of the first and second metacarpals, preventing extremes of radial and dorsal displacement of the base of the first metacarpal joint.[156,158] The **dorsoradial** and **anterior oblique ligaments** are reported to be key stabilizers of the CMC joint.[159,160] Although some investigators hold that the axial rotation seen in the metacarpal during opposition is a function of incongruence and joint laxity,[10,161] Zancolli and associates[156] theorized that it is a result of the congruence of the spherical surfaces and resultant tensions encountered in the supporting ligaments. It seems, however, that some incongruence must exist at the joint. Osteoarthritic changes with aging are common at the first CMC joint and may be attributable to the cartilage thinning in high-load areas imposed on this joint by pinch and grasp across incongruent surfaces.[162] Ateshian and colleagues[163] found gender differences in the fit of the trapezium with the metacarpal, with the trapezium of women showing more incongruence than that of men in a group of older individuals. This matches an increased incidence of OA of the first CMC joint among older women, but it does not address whether the incongruence of the trapezium is a cause or effect of degenerative changes. The first CMC joint is close-packed both in extremes of abduction and adduction, with maximal motion available in neutral position.[100]

First Carpometacarpal Joint Function

It is the unique range and direction of motion at the first CMC joint that produces opposition of the thumb.

Opposition is, sequentially, abduction, flexion, and adduction of the first metacarpal, with simultaneous rotation. These movements change the orientation of the metacarpal, bringing the thumb out of the palm and positioning the thumb for contact with the fingers. The functional significance of the CMC joint of the thumb and of the movement of opposition can be appreciated when one realizes that use of the thumb against a finger occurs in almost all forms of **prehension** (grasp and dexterity activities). When the first CMC joint is fused in extension and adduction, opposition cannot occur. The importance of opposition is such that fusion of the first CMC joint may be followed over time by an adaptation of the trapezioscaphoid joint that develops a more saddle-shaped configuration to restore some of the lost opposition.[103] This amazing shift in joint function is an excellent example of the body's ability to replace essential functions whenever possible.

9-4	Patient Case: CMC Osteoarthritis

Marilyn Ferrier is a 78-year-old woman referred to a hand surgeon by her primary care physician after she reported progressive onset of thumb pain. Her symptoms of aching and tenderness were exacerbated by activities such as turning keys, opening jars, and writing. Manual longitudinal compressing of the first metacarpal joint into the trapezium produced pain and crepitation (positive **Grind test**), indicative of CMC OA. Osteoarthritic changes and subluxation of the metacarpal were evident on radiograph (Fig. 9-39). A custom thumb splint was fabricated, and the patient was instructed in activity modifications along with general joint protection principles, including avoiding forceful, repetitive, and sustained pinching, along with utilizing pens and kitchen utensils with larger handles.

■ Metacarpophalangeal and Interphalangeal Joints of the Thumb

The MP joint of the thumb is the articulation between the head of the first metacarpal and the base of its proximal phalanx. It is considered to be a condyloid joint with two degrees of freedom: flexion/extension and abduction/adduction.[91] There is an insignificant amount of passive rotation.[103] The metacarpal head is not covered with cartilage dorsally or laterally, and it more closely resembles the head of the proximal phalanx, without its central groove. The joint capsule, the reinforcing volar plate, and the collateral ligaments are similar to those of the other MP joints. The main functional contribution of the first MP joint is to provide additional flexion range to the thumb in opposition and to allow the thumb to grasp and contour to objects. Despite the structural similarities between the MP joints, the first MP joint is far more restricted in motion than those of the fingers. Although the available range varies significantly among individuals, the first MP joint rarely has more than half the flexion available at the fingers and little if any hyperextension. Abduction/adduction and rotation are extremely limited. This lim-

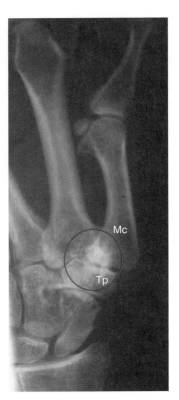

▲ **Figure 9-39** ■ Degenerative changes between the trapezium and first metacarpal joint (first CMC joint) cause painful opposition.

itation to motion is probably attributable to the major structural difference between the MP joints of the thumb and fingers. The first MP joint is reinforced extracapsularly on its volar surface by two sesamoid bones (Fig. 9-40). These are maintained in position by fibers from the collateral ligaments and by an intersesamoid ligament. Goldberg and Nathan[164] proposed that the sesamoid bones are the result of friction and pressure on the tendons in which the sesamoid bones are embedded. They support this by noting that the sesamoid bones of the first MP joint do not appear until around 12 years of age and that sesamoid bones in

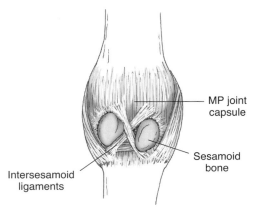

▲ **Figure 9-40** ■ The MP joint of the thumb has two sesamoid bones secured to the volar aspect of the joint capsule by intersesamoid ligaments.

some investigations have also been found in as many as 70% of fifth MP joints and 50% of second MP joints.

The IP joint of the thumb is the articulation between the head of the proximal phalanx and the base of the distal phalanx. It is structurally and functionally identical to the IP joints of the fingers.

Thumb Musculature

The muscles of the thumb have been compared to guy wires supporting a flagpole, in which there must be a continuous effective pull in every direction to maintain stability. The metacarpal joint and the proximal and distal phalanges form an articulated shaft that sits on the trapezium. As in the flagpole, tension from the muscular guy wires must be provided in every direction for stability to be maintained. Because the stability comes from the muscles more than from articular constraints (at least at the CMC joint), the majority of muscles that attach to the thumb tend to be active during most thumb motions. There is also substantial individual variability in motor strategies among normal subjects.[165] Consequently, exploration of muscle function in the thumb (and, to a somewhat lesser extent, function through the hand) is largely an issue not of when a muscle functions but when the preponderance of muscle activity might be expected with shifting tasks. The role of the extrinsic and intrinsic thumb muscles will be presented as generalizations (conceptual frameworks), as will the final section of this chapter, on hand prehension.

■ Extrinsic Thumb Muscles

There are four extrinsic thumb muscles: the FPL, EPB, EPL, and APL muscles. The FPL muscle is located volarly (see Fig. 9-12A). The FPL muscle inserts on the distal phalanx and is the correlate of the FDP muscles of the fingers. The FPL tendon at the wrist is invested by the radial bursa, which is continuous with its digital tendon sheath (see Fig. 9-28A). The FPL muscle is unique in that it functions independently of other muscles and is the only muscle responsible for flexion of the thumb IP joint.[5] Its tendon sits between the sesamoid bones and appears to derive some protection from those bones.

Three of the thumb extrinsic muscles are located dorsoradially. The EPB and APL muscles run a common course from the dorsal forearm, traversing through the first dorsal compartment and crossing the wrist on its radial aspect (see Fig. 9-29) to their insertion. The APL muscle inserts on the base of the metacarpal joint, whereas the EPB muscle inserts on the base of the proximal phalanx. Both muscles abduct the CMC joint. The EPB muscle also extends the MP joint. The APL and EPB muscles also radially deviate the wrist slightly.

The EPL muscle originates in the forearm by the APL and EPB muscle but crosses the wrist closer to the dorsal midline before using the dorsal radial (**Lister's**) tubercle as an anatomic pulley to turn toward the

thumb; the EPL muscle inserts on the base of the distal phalanx. At the level of the proximal phalanx, the EPL tendon is joined by expansions from the **abductor pollicis brevis** (APB) muscle, the first VI muscle, and the **adductor pollicis** (AdP) muscle.[20] There is no further elaboration of the extensor expansion at the MP joint of the thumb, but we see the same balance of MP joint abductors and adductors contributing to resting tension in the MP joint and to stabilization of the long extensor tendon. The more volarly located APB and AdP muscles that attach to the EPL tendon can extend the thumb IP joint to neutral but cannot complete the range into hyperextension in individuals who have that range available. The EPL is the only muscle that can complete the full range of hyperextension at the IP joint, as well as applying an extensor force at the MP joint along with the EPB muscle.[82] The EPL muscle can also extend and adduct the CMC joint of the thumb. In contrast to the fingers, there is a separate extensor tendon for each joint of the thumb. The APL muscle attaches to the base of the metacarpal joint, the EPB muscle to the base of the proximal phalanx, and the EPL muscle to the base of the distal phalanx.

As is true for other extrinsic hand muscles, wrist positioning is an essential factor in providing an optimal length-tension relationship for the extrinsic muscles of the thumb.[4] The FPL muscle is less effective as an IP flexor in wrist flexion. The EPL muscle cannot complete IP extension when the wrist, CMC, and MP joints are simultaneously extended. The APL and EPB muscles require the synergy of an ulnar deviator of the wrist to prevent the muscles from creating wrist radial deviation, which thus affects their ability to generate tension over the joints of the thumb.

■ Intrinsic Thumb Muscles

There are five **thenar,** or intrinsic thumb, muscles that originate primarily from the carpal bones and the flexor retinaculum (or TCL). The **opponens pollicis** (OP) is the only intrinsic thumb muscle to have its distal attachment on the first metacarpal. Its action line is nearly perpendicular to the long axis of the metacarpal joint and is applied to the lateral side of the bone. The OP muscle, therefore, is very effective in positioning the metacarpal in an abducted, flexed, and rotated posture. The APB, FPB, AdP, and first VI muscles all insert on the proximal phalanx. The FPB muscle has two heads of insertion. Its larger lateral head attaches distally with the APB muscle and also applies some abductor force. The FPB muscle crosses the sesamoid bones at the MP joint, increasing the MA of the FPB muscle for MP joint flexion. The medial head of the FPB muscle attaches distally with the AdP muscle and assists in thumb adduction. The first VI muscle arises from the first metacarpal and attaches to the ulnar sesamoid bone and then attaches distally to the proximal phalanx.

Although not generally considered a thenar muscle, the first DI muscle may make a contribution to thumb function, along with its contribution to MP flexion and IP extension of the index finger. The first DI muscle is a bipennate muscle arising from both the first and second metacarpals and from the intercarpal ligament that joins the metacarpal bases. Brand and Hollister[149] proposed that the first DI muscle is a CMC joint distractor, rather than, as is typically found, a joint compressor, because it pulls the first metacarpal distally toward the first DI muscle's insertion on the base of the index proximal phalanx (Fig. 9-41). These investigators also argued that thumb attachment of the first DI muscle has little or no ability to move the thumb but it is important in offsetting the compressive and dorsoradially directed forces that the flexor/adductor muscles create across the CMC joint in lateral pinch and power grip. When these forces were created in laboratory specimens without tension in the first DI muscle, the CMC joint subluxed.[149] Belanger and Noel[166] suggested that the first DI muscle can assist with thumb adduction.

The thenar muscles are active in most grasping activities, regardless of the precise position of the thumb as it participates. The OP muscle works together most frequently with the APB and the FPB muscles, although the intensity of the relation varies. When the thumb is gently brought into contact with any of the other fingers, activity of the OP muscle predominates in the thumb, and APB activity exceeds that of the FPB muscle. When opposition to the index finger or middle finger is performed firmly, activity of the FPB muscle exceeds that of the OP muscle. With firm opposition to the ring and little fingers, however, the relation changes; OP activity increases with firm opposition to the ring finger, equaling activity of the FPB muscle with firm opposition to the little finger.[66] The change in bal-

ance of muscle activity with firm opposition and with increasingly ulnar opposition can be accounted for by the increased need for abduction and metacarpal rotation. Increased pressure in opposition additionally appears to bring in activity of the AdP muscle. The AdP muscle stabilizes the thumb against the opposed finger. In firm opposition to the index and middle fingers, AdP activity exceeds the very minimal activity of the APB muscle. With a more ulnarly located position, the increased need for abduction results in simultaneous activity of the abductor and adductor.[66] Activity of the extrinsic thumb musculature in grasp appears to be partially a function of helping to position the MP and IP joints. The main function of the extrinsic muscles, however, is in returning the thumb to extension from its position in the palm. Although release of an object is essentially an extrinsic function, some OP and abductor brevis activity have been identified.[66] This muscular activity would assist in maintaining the thumb in abduction and in maintaining the metacarpal rotation that facilitates the next move of the thumb back into opposition.

The joint structure and musculature of the wrist complex, the fingers, and the thumb have each been examined. Some instances of specific muscle activity have been presented to clarify the potential function of the muscle. A summary of wrist and hand function, however, can best be presented through the assessment of purposeful hand activity. Because the entire upper limb is geared toward execution of movement of the hand, it is appropriate to complete the description of the upper limb by looking at an overview of the wrist and hand in prehension activities.

◆ Prehension

Prehension activities of the hand involve the grasping or taking hold of an object between any two surfaces in the hand; the thumb participates in most but not all prehension tasks. There are numerous ways that objects of varying sizes and shapes may be grasped, with strategies also varying among individuals. Consequently, the nomenclature related to these functional patterns also varies,[167] although there has evolved a broad classification system for grasp that will permit general observations about the coordinated muscular function necessary to produce or maintain common forms of grasp.

Prehension can be categorized as either **power grip** (full hand prehension) (Fig. 9-42A) or **precision handling** (finger-thumb prehension) (see Fig. 9-42B).[168] Each of these two categories has subgroups that further define the grasp. Power grip is generally a forceful act resulting in flexion at all finger joints. When the thumb is used, it acts as a stabilizer to the object held between the fingers and, most commonly, the palm. Precision handling, in contrast, is the skillful placement of an object between fingers or between finger and thumb.[169] The palm is not involved. Landsmeer[170] suggested that power grip and precision handling can be differenti-

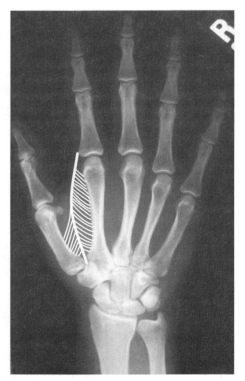

▲ **Figure 9-41** ■ Brand and Hollister[149] proposed that the first DI muscle is a distractor of the first CMC joint, which helps offset the strong compressive forces that occur across the first CMC joint.

ated on the basis of the dynamic and static phases. Power grip is the result of a sequence of (1) opening the hand, (2) positioning the fingers, (3) bringing the fingers to the object, and (4) maintaining a static phase that actually constitutes the grip. This is in contrast to precision handling, which shares the first three steps of the sequence but does not contain a static phase at all. In power grip, the object is grasped so that the object can be moved through space by the more proximal joints; in precision handling, the fingers and thumb grasp the object for the purpose of manipulating it within the hand.

In assessment of the muscular function during each type of grasp, synergy of the hand muscles results in almost constant activity of all intrinsic and extrinsic muscles.[150,171,172] The task becomes more one of identifying when muscles are *not* working or when the balance of activity between muscles might change. It should also be emphasized that the muscular activity documented by EMG studies is specific to the activity as performed in a given study. Even in studies using similar forms of prehension, variables such as size of object, firmness of grip, timing, and instructions to the subject can cause substantial changes in reported muscle activity. However, as indications of general muscular activity patterns, the studies are useful in the development of a conceptual framework within which hand function can be understood.

Power Grip

The fingers in power grip usually function in concert to clamp on and hold an object into the palm. The fingers assume a position of sustained flexion that varies in degree with the size, shape, and weight of the object. The palm is likely to contour to the object as the palmar arches form around it. The thumb may serve as an additional surface to the finger-palm vise by adducting against the object, or it may be removed from the object. When the thumb is involved, it generally is adducted to clamp the object to the palm. This is in contrast to precision handling, in which the thumb is more likely to assume a position of abduction.[173] Four varieties of power grip studied by Long and associates[116] exemplify the similarities and differences seen in power grip. These are cylindrical grip, spherical grip, hook grip, and lateral prehension.

■ Cylindrical Grip

Cylindrical grip (Fig. 9-43A) almost exclusively involves use of the flexors to carry the fingers around and maintain grasp on an object. The function in the fingers is performed largely by the FDP muscle, especially in the dynamic closing action of the fingers. In the static phase, the FDS muscle assists when the intensity of the grip requires greater force. Although power grip traditionally has been thought of as an extrinsic muscle activity, studies have indicated considerable interosseous (intrinsic) muscle activity. The interossei muscles are considered to be functioning primarily as MP joint flexors and abductors/adductors. In strong grip, however, the magnitude of torque production of the interossei muscles for metacarpal flexion was found to nearly equal that of the extrinsic flexors.[150,155,169] Because both the MP and the IP joints are being flexed during cylindrical grip, the MP joint flexion task most likely falls to the proximal (dorsal) interossei muscles because their attachments to the proximal phalanx and

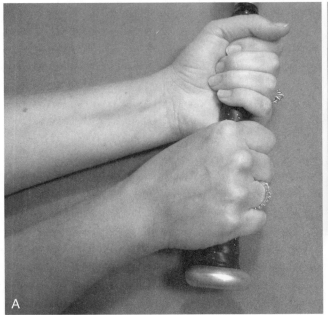

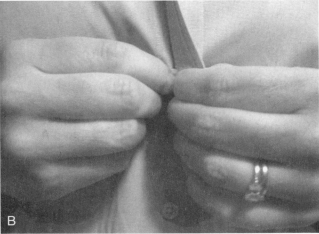

▲ **Figure 9-42** ■ Prehension generally consists of either (**A**) power grip, in which the object makes full contact with the palm and is moved through space, or (**B**) precision handling, in which the thumb and fingers dynamically manipulate the object.

hood do not have a significant (and antagonistic) IP extension influence. The interossei muscles may also ulnarly deviate the MP joint to direct the distal phalanges of the fingers toward the thumb. The combination of MP joint flexion and ulnar deviation (adduction for the index finger and abduction for the middle, ring, and little fingers) (see Fig. 9-43B) points the fingers toward the thumb but also tends to produce ulnar subluxation forces on the MP joints and on the tendons of the long flexors at the MP joint. The subluxing forces are ordinarily counteracted by the radial collateral ligaments, by the annular pulleys that anchor the flexor long tendons in place, and by the sagittal bands that connect the volar structures to the extensor mechanism. Active or passive tension in the EDC muscle can further stabilize the restraining mechanisms, as well as increase joint compression and enhance overall joint stability during power grip.[169] Although the location of the lumbrical muscles indicates a possible contribution to MP joint flexion in power grip, their lack of EMG activity, regardless of strength grip, is consistent with their role as IP extensors.[116]

Thumb position in cylindrical grip is the most variable of the digits. The thumb usually comes around the object, then flexes and adducts to close the vise. The FPL and thenar muscles are all active. The activity of the thenar muscles will vary with the width of the web space, with the CMC rotation required, and with increased pressure or resistance. A distinguishing characteristic of power grip over precision handling is, in general, the greater magnitude of activity in the AdP muscle during power grip. The EPL muscle may be variably active as an MP joint stabilizer or as an adductor.

Muscles of the hypothenar eminence usually are active in cylindrical grip. The ADM functions as a proximal interosseous muscle to flex and abduct (ulnarly deviate) the fifth MP joint. The ODM and the flexor digiti minimi (FDM) muscles are more variable but frequently are active in direct proportion to the amount of abduction and rotation of the first metacarpal. In fact, increased activity of the OP muscle automatically results in increased activity of the ODM and FDM muscles.

Cylindrical grip is typically performed with the wrist in neutral flexion/extension and slight ulnar deviation. Ulnar deviation also puts the thumb in line with the long axis of the forearm (see Fig. 9-43A); this alignment better positions the object in the hand to be turned by pronation/supination of the forearm[173] as, for example, in turning a door knob. Ulnar deviation of the wrist is the position that optimizes force of the long finger flexors. The least flexion force is generated at these joints in wrist flexion.[2] The heavier an object is, the more likely it is that the wrist will ulnarly deviate. In addition, a strong contraction of the FCU muscle at the wrist will increase tension on the TCL. This provides a more stable base for the active hypothenar muscles that originate from that ligament. It is interesting to note that regardless of wrist position, the percentage of total IP flexor force allocated to each finger is relatively constant. The ring and little fingers can generate only 70% of the flexor force of the index and middle fingers.[2] The ring and little fingers seem to serve as weaker but more mobile assists to the more stable and stronger index and middle fingers. The contribution of the ring and little finger to grip can be improved if full flexion

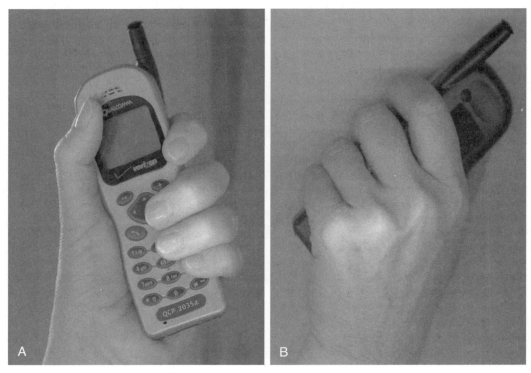

▲ **Figure 9-43** ■ **A.** Cylindrical grip may orient the finger tips toward the thumb. This is accomplished by ulnarly deviating the MP joints using the interossei muscles (**B**).

of the joints in those fingers (and concomitant loss of tension) is prevented by an object that is wider ulnarly than radially (the pistol-grip shape).

■ **Spherical Grip**

Spherical grip (Fig. 9-44A) is similar in most respects to cylindrical grip. The extrinsic finger and thumb flexors and the thenar muscles follow similar patterns of activity and variability. The main distinction can be made by the greater spread of the fingers to encompass the object. This evokes more interosseous activity than is seen in other forms of power grip.[116] The MP joints do not deviate in the same direction (e.g., ulnarly) but tend to abduct. The phalanges are no longer parallel to each other, as they commonly are in cylindrical grip. The MP joint abductors must be joined by the adductors to stabilize the joints that are in the loose-packed position of semiflexion. Although flexor activity predominates in the digits as it does in all forms of power grip, the extensors do have a role. The extensors not only provide a balancing force for the flexors but also are essential for smooth and controlled opening of the

hand and release of the object. Opening the hand during object approach and object release is primarily an extensor function, calling in the lumbrical, EDC, and thumb extrinsic muscles.

■ **Hook Grip**

Hook grip (see Fig. 9-44B) is actually a specialized form of prehension. It is included in power grip because it has more characteristics of power grip than of precision handling. It is a function primarily of the fingers. It may include the palm but never includes the thumb. It can be sustained for prolonged periods of time, as anyone who has carried a briefcase or books at his side or hung onto a commuter strap on a bus or train can attest. The major muscular activity is provided by the FDP and FDS muscles. The load may be sustained completely by one muscle or the other or by both muscles in concert. This depends on the position of the load in relation to the phalanges. If the load is carried more distally so that DIP flexion is mandatory, the FDP muscle must participate. If the load is carried more in the middle of the fingers, the FDS muscle may be sufficient. Some

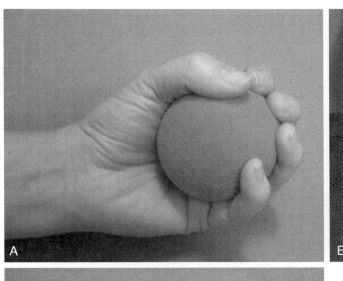

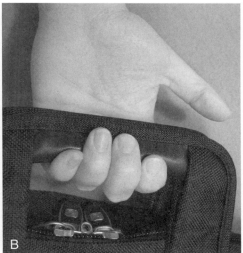

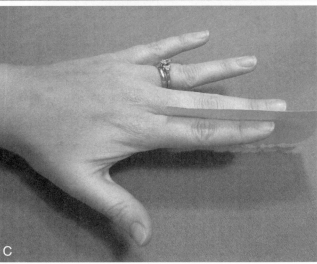

◀ **Figure 9-44** ■ A. Spherical grip. B. Hook grip. C. Lateral prehension.

interosseous muscle activity has been demonstrated on EMG, but its purpose is not fully understood. It may help prevent clawing in the MP joints, although the activity is not evident in every finger.[116] In hook grip, the thumb is held in moderate to full extension by thumb extrinsic muscles.

■ Lateral Prehension

Lateral prehension (see Fig. 9-44C) is a rather unique form of grasp. Contact occurs between two adjacent fingers. The MP and IP joints are usually maintained in extension as the contiguous MP joints simultaneously abduct and adduct. This is the only form of prehension in which the extensor musculature predominate in the maintenance of the posture; the EDC and the lumbrical muscles are active to extend the MP and IP joints, and MP joint abduction and adduction are performed by the interossei muscles. Lateral prehension is included here as a form of power grip because lateral grip involves the static holding of an object that is then moved by the more proximal joints of the upper extremity. Although not a "powerful" grip, neither is lateral prehension used to manipulate objects in the hand. It is generally typified by the holding of a cigarette.

Precision Handling

The positions and muscular requirements of precision handling are somewhat more variable than those of power grip, require much finer motor control, and are more dependent on intact sensation. The thumb serves as one "jaw" of what has been termed a "two-jaw chuck"; the thumb is generally abducted and rotated from the palm. The second and opposing "jaw" is formed by the distal tip, the pad, or the side of a finger. When two fingers oppose the thumb, it is called a three-jaw chuck. The three varieties of precision handling that exemplify this mode of prehension are **pad-to-pad prehension,** **tip-to-tip prehension,** and **pad-to-side prehension.** Each tends to be a dynamic function with relatively little static holding.

■ Pad-to-Pad Prehension

Pad-to-pad prehension involves opposition of the pad, or pulp, of the thumb to the pad, or pulp, of the finger (Fig. 9-45A). The pad of the distal phalanx of each digit has the greatest concentration of tactile corpuscles found in the body. Of all forms of precision handling, 80% are considered to fall into the category of pad-to-pad.[1] The finger used in two-jaw chuck is usually the index; in three-jaw chuck, the middle finger is added. The MP and PIP joints of the fingers are partially flexed, with the degree of flexion being dependent on the size of the object being held. The DIP joint may be fully extended or in slight flexion. When the DIP joint is extended, the FDS muscle can perform the function alone, without the assistance of the FDP muscle. Extension of the DIP joint in this instance is caused by flexion of the middle phalanx (FDS muscle) against the

upward force of the object or thumb on the distal phalanx in what is effectively a closed chain. When partial DIP flexion is required by the pad-to-pad task, the FDP muscle must be active. Interosseous activity is often present both to supplement MP joint flexor force and to provide the MP joint abduction or adduction required in object manipulation. In dynamic manipulation, the VI and DI muscles tend to work reciprocally, rather than in the synergistic co-contraction pattern observed during power grip. In a static but firm pad-to-pad pinch, the interossei muscles may again co-contract.[116]

The thumb in pad-to-pad prehension is held in CMC flexion, abduction, and rotation (opposition). The first MP and IP joints may be partially flexed or fully extended. The thenar muscle control is provided by the OP, FPB, and APB muscles, each of which is innervated by the median nerve. The AdP activity (ulnar nerve) increases with increased pressure of pinch. In ulnar nerve paralysis, loss of AdP function (as well as loss of function of the first DI and first VI muscles) makes the thumb less stable and affects the precision of the grasp activity.

Fine adjustments in the flexion angle of the DIP joint of the finger and the IP joint of the thumb control the points of contact on the pads of the digits. In full-finger DIP and thumb IP extension, contact occurs on the more proximal portion of the distal phalanx (see Fig. 9-45A). As flexion of the finger DIP and thumb IP joints increases, the contact moves distally toward the nails. Flexion of the distal phalanx, when required, is provided by the FDP muscle for the finger and by the FPL muscle for the thumb. DIP flexion in the finger is accompanied by a proportional flexion in the PIP joint.

As is found in power grip, the extensor musculature is used for opening the hand to grasp, for release, and for stabilization when necessary. In the thumb, the EPL muscle may be used to maintain the IP joint in extension when contact is light and on the proximal pad. Synergistic wrist activity must also occur to balance the forces created by the FDS and FDP muscles. The wrist is more typically held in neutral radial/ulnar deviation and slight extension.[171]

■ Tip-to-Tip Prehension

Although the muscular activity found in tip-to-tip prehension (see Fig. 9-45B) is nearly identical to that of pad-to-pad prehension,[116] there are some key differences. In tip-to-tip prehension, the IP joints of the finger and thumb must have the range and available muscle force to create nearly full joint flexion. The MP joint of the opposing finger must also be ulnarly deviated (with fingertip pointed radially) to present the tip of the finger to the thumb. In the first finger, the ulnar deviation occurs as MP joint adduction. In the remaining fingers, MP abduction produces ulnar deviation. If the flexion range for the distal phalanx in either the opposing finger or the thumb is not available, or if the active force for IP flexion and MP joint ulnar deviation cannot be provided, tip-to-tip prehension cannot be performed effectively. As the most precise form of grasp, it is also the most easily disturbed. Tip-to-tip pre-

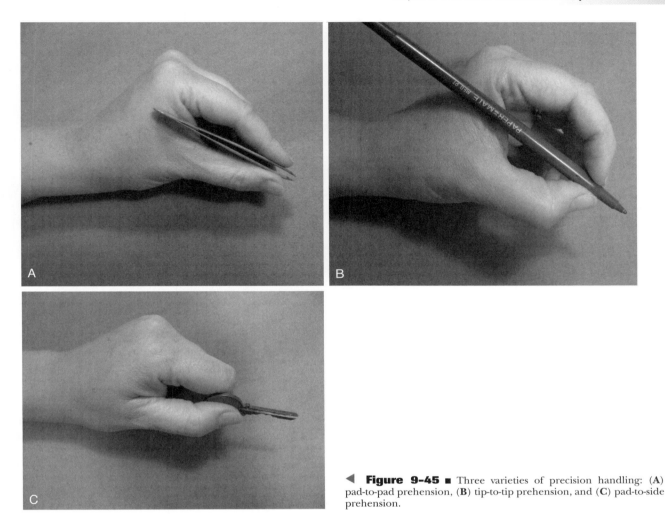

◀ **Figure 9-45** ■ Three varieties of precision handling: (**A**) pad-to-pad prehension, (**B**) tip-to-tip prehension, and (**C**) pad-to-side prehension.

hension has all the same muscular requirements as pad-to-pad prehension in both fingers and thumb. In addition, however, activity of the FDP, FPL, and interossei muscles is a necessity in tip-to-tip prehension, whereas they are not in pad-to-pad prehension.

■ **Pad-to-Side Prehension**

Pad-to-side prehension is also known as **key grip** (or lateral pinch) because a key is held between the pad of the thumb and side of the index finger (see Fig. 9-45C). Pad-to-side prehension differs from the other forms of precision handling only in that the thumb is more adducted and less rotated. The activity level of the FPB muscle increases and that of the OP muscle decreases, in comparison with tip-to-tip prehension. Activity of the AdP muscle also increases over that seen in either tip-to-tip or pad-to-pad prehension.[13] Slight flexion of the distal phalanx of the thumb is required. If the pad-to-side prehension is being used for something like turning a key, the wrist will again assume neutral flexion/extension and drop into slight ulnar deviation to put the key in line with the forearm so that pronation or supination can be used to turn the key.

Pad-to-side prehension is the least precise of the forms of precision handling; it can actually be performed by a person with paralysis of all hand muscles. If the hand muscles are paralyzed as they would be in a person with a spinal cord injury above the C7 level, active wrist extensors (assuming they are present) can create pad-to-side prehension. Wrist extension provided by the intact and active ECU, ECRL, and ECRB muscles create the force needed to flex the MP and IP joints of the fingers and thumb by generating passive tension in the extrinsic finger flexor tendons (FDS and FDP) as the tendons are stretched over the extending wrist. The grip may be released by relaxing the wrist extensor muscles and allowing gravity to flex the wrist. As the wrist flexes, the tendons of the FDS and FDP muscles become slack, and the tendons of the EDC (with the related EIP and EDM tendons) and EPL tendons become stretched. The passive tension in the long finger extensors in a dropped (flexed) wrist is adequate for partially extending both MP and IP joints. The phenomenon of using active wrist extension to close the fingers and passive wrist flexion to open the fingers is known as **tenodesis**. The same tenodesis action can achieve a cylindrical grip if the proper balance of tension exists in the extrinsic flexors. The flexors must be loose enough to permit the partially flexed fingers of the "open" hand to surround the object in wrist flexion while still being tight enough to hold onto the object when the wrist is extended. Active control of at least one wrist extensor muscle is the minimal requirement for functional use of tenodesis in a person without any active control of finger or thumb musculature. Tenodesis was described in Chapter 3 when we first discussed passive insufficiency. As was noted then, tenodesis can and does also occur in the fully intact hand, although the presence of balancing muscles permits us to override it.

◆ Functional Position of The Wrist And Hand

Although it is difficult to isolate any one joint or function as being singularly important among all those examined, grasp would have to take precedence. There can be little doubt that the hand cannot function either as a manipulator or as a sensory organ unless an object can enter the palmar surface and unless moderate finger flexion and thumb opposition are available to allow sustained contact. Application of either an active muscular or passive tendinous flexor force to the digits requires the wrist to be stabilized in moderate extension and ulnar deviation. Delineation of the so-called functional position of the wrist and hand takes into account these needs and is the position from which optimal function is most likely to occur. It is *not necessarily* the position in which a hand should be immobilized. Position for immobilization depends on the disability.

The functional position is (1) wrist complex in slight extension (20°) and slight ulnar deviation (10°) and (2) fingers moderately flexed at the MP joints (45°) and PIP joints (30°) and slightly flexed at the DIP joints (Fig. 9-46).[1] The wrist position optimizes the power of the finger flexors so that hand closure can be accomplished with the least possible effort. It is also the position in which all wrist muscles are under equal tension. With similar considerations for the position of the joints of the digits, the functional position provides the best opportunity for the disabled hand to interact with the brain that controls it.

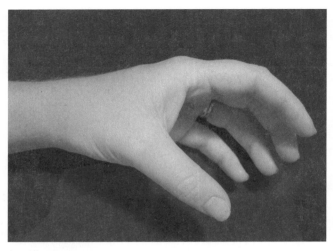

▲ **Figure 9-46** ■ Functional position of the hand: wrist extension and ulnar deviation with moderate flexion of the MP and IP joints of the finger and thumb.

Summary

Despite the many articulations that make up the hand and wrist complex, the bony and ligamentous components of these joints have less potential for problems than the musculotendinous structures that cross and act on other joints. The motor control of and sensory feedback from the wrist and hand alone occupy more space topographically on the primary motor and sensory cortices of the brain than does the entire lower extremity. As we proceed to examine the joints of the lower extremity, an analogy to the corresponding joints of the upper extremity can and should be made. However, the primary weight-bearing function of the lower extremities does not require the complexity and delicate balance of muscular control that can so profoundly affect functional performance in the hand.

Acknowledgment

Many thanks to Richard Bernstein, MD, whose invaluable feedback aided in the reworking of this chapter.

 Study Questions

1. Name the bones of the wrist complex; describe the articulations that occur between these bones and the functional joints that are formed.
2. Describe the components and role of the triangular fibrocartilage complex in wrist function.
3. What is the total ROM normally available at the wrist complex? How are the motions distributed between the radiocarpal and midcarpal joints of the complex?
4. Describe the sequence of carpal motion occurring from full wrist flexion to full extension and radial to ulnar deviation, emphasizing the role of the scaphoid.
5. What effect does release of the scapholunate stabilizers or of the lunotriquetral stabilizers have on bony positions?

(Continued on following page)

6. Identify the muscles that can extend the wrist; include the joints crossed, actions produced, and activity levels of each.
7. Describe the transverse carpal ligament, its attachments, and its role in wrist and hand function.
8. What is the function of the CMC joints of the fingers? How do the variations in ROM among the four CMC joints of the fingers contribute to function?
9. What role does the transverse metacarpal ligament play at the CMC joint? What role at the MP joint?
10. Describe the locations and functions of the volar (palmar) fibrocartilage plates.
11. What MP joint position is most prone to injury and why?
12. Compare the joint structure of the MP joints with that of the IP joints of the fingers. Identify both similarities and differences.
13. Describe the mechanisms, joint motions, and muscles that are necessary for the fingers to gently close into the palm without friction or loss of the length-tension relationship.
14. How does the "pistol-grip" design of most tools (larger ulnarly) relate to the MP joint ROM and muscular function of the four fingers?
15. When is the FDS muscle active as the primary finger flexor? When does it back up the FDP muscle?
16. What muscles are active in gentle closure of the normal hand? What role, if any, do the intrinsic muscles play in this activity?
17. What wrist position is assumed when a person needs to optimize finger flexion strength? Which wrist position is least effective for grasp?
18. What are annular pulleys and cruciate ligaments in the digits? Where are they found, and what functions do they serve?
19. Identify the bursae of the hand. What are their functions and how are they most typically related to the digital tendon sheaths?
20. Describe the active and passive elements that make up the extensor mechanism.
21. What role do the EDC, EIP, and EDM muscles play in active extension of the PIP and DIP joints of the hand?
22. How do the proximal and distal attachments of the interossei muscles affect function at the MP and IP joints?
23. Describe the attachments of the lumbrical muscles to the extensor mechanism. How do these muscles contribute to IP extension? What is their role at the MP joint?
24. Why is active DIP flexion normally accompanied by PIP flexion at the same time?
25. Explain why the DIP cannot be actively extended if the PIP joint is fully flexed.
26. Why will an isolated contraction of the EDC muscle produce flexion of the PIP and DIP joints? What is this finger position called?
27. How are the extrinsic flexors and extensors stabilized at the MP joints?
28. Why is finger extension weaker in the index and little fingers?
29. Why does MP joint adduction weaken more quickly than abduction in a progressive ulnar nerve problem?
30. Which are stronger flexors of the MP joint, the lumbrical or the interossei muscles?
31. Compare and contrast the MP joint structure of the thumb with the MP joint structure of the fingers.
32. What does the motion of thumb opposition require in terms of joint function and musculature?
33. What are the primary muscles of release in the wrist and hand?
34. In general, what is the difference between power grip and precision handling at the wrist, in the fingers, and in the thumb? What do these two forms of prehension have in common?
35. Cylindrical grip is generally referred to as an extrinsic hand function. Why is this true?
36. What requirement does spherical grip have that differentiates it from cylindrical grip?
37. Which form of prehension requires only intrinsic musculature?
38. Which forms of prehension do not require the thumb?
39. What roles do interossei muscles play in precision handling?
40. What requirements does tip-to-tip prehension have that are not necessary for pad-to-pad prehension?
41. What is the finest (most precise) form of prehension that can be accomplished by someone without intact hand musculature, assuming availability of an active wrist extensor?
42. What is the functional position of the wrist and hand? Why is this the optimal resting position when there is no specific hand problem?
43. Why is an ulnar nerve injury called "claw hand"? What deficiency causes the clawing, and in which fingers does it occur?

◆ References

1. Harty M: The hand of man. Phys Ther 51:777, 1974.
2. Hazelton F, Smidt GL, Flatt AE, et al.: The influence of wrist position on the force produced by the finger flexors. J Biomech 8:301, 1975.
3. Simpson D: The functioning hand, the human advantage. J R Coll Surg Edinb 21:329, 1976.
4. Brand P, Hollister A: Clinical Mechanics of the Hand, 3rd ed. St. Louis, Mosby-Year Book, 1999.
5. Lieber R, Friden J: Musculoskeletal balance of the human wrist elucidated using intraoperative laser diffraction. J Electromyogr Kinesiol 8:93–100, 1998.
6. Kobayashi M, Berger R, Linscheid R, et al.: Intercarpal kinematics during wrist motion. Hand Clin 13:143–149, 1997.
7. Ritt M, Stuart P, Berglund L, et al.: Rotational stability of the carpus relative to the forearm. J Hand Surg [Am] 20:305–311, 1995.
8. Garcia-Elias M, Ribe M, Rodriguez J, et al.: Influence of joint laxity on scaphoid kinematics. J Hand Surg [Br] 20:379–382, 1995.
9. Cailliet R: Hand Pain and Impairment, 4th ed. Philadelphia, FA Davis, 1994.
10. Kapandji I: The Physiology of the Joints, 5th ed. Edinburgh, Churchill Livingstone, 1982.
11. Berger R: Anatomy and kinesiology of the wrist. In Mackin E, Callahan AD, Skirven T, et al. (eds): Rehabilitation of the Hand and Upper Extremity, 5th ed. St. Louis, Mosby-Year Book, 2002.
12. Ryu J, Cooney W, Askey L, et al.: Functional ranges of motion of the wrist joint. J Hand Surg [Am] 16:409–419, 1991.
13. Gilford V, Bolton RH, Lambrinudi C: The mechanism of the wrist joint. Guy's Hosp Rep 92:52, 1943.
14. Szabo RM, Weber SC: Comminuted intraarticular fractures of the distal radius. Clin Orthop 230: 39–48, 1988.
15. Palmer AK, Werner FW: Biomechanics of the distal radioulnar joint. Clin Orthop 187:26–35, 1984.
16. Mohiuddin A, Janjua M: Form and function of the radioulnar disc. Hand 14:61, 1982.
17. Benjamin M, Evans E, Pemberton D: Histological studies on the triangular fibrocartilage complex of the wrist. J Anat 172:59–67, 1990.
18. Palmer AK: The distal radioulnar joint. Anatomy, biomechanics, and triangular fibrocartilage complex abnormalities. Hand Clin 3:31–40, 1987.
19. Jaffe R, Chidgey LK, LaStayo PC: The distal radioulnar joint: Anatomy and management of disorders. J Hand Ther 9:129–138, 1996.
20. Williams P: Gray's Anatomy, 38th ed. New York, Churchill Livingstone, 1995.
21. Taleisnik J: Current concepts review: Carpal instability. J Bone Joint Surg Am 70:1262–1268, 1988.
22. Patterson R, Viegas S: Biomechanics of the wrist. J Hand Ther 8:97–105, 1995.
23. Viegas S, Patterson R: Load mechanics of the wrist. Hand Clin 13:109–128, 1997.
24. Taleisnik J: Pain on the ulnar side of the wrist. Hand Clin 3:51–68, 1987.
25. Drobner WS, Hausman MR: The distal radioulnar joint. Hand Clin 8:631–644, 1992.
26. Palmer AK, Glisson RR, Werner FW: Ulnar variance determination. J Hand Surg [Am] 7:376–79, 1982.
27. Linscheid RL: Kinematic considerations of the wrist. Clin Orthop 202:27–39, 1986.
28. Schuind F, Cooney W, Linscheid R, et al.: Force and pressure transmission through the normal wrist. A theoretical two-dimensional study in the posteroanterior plane. J Biomech 28:587–601, 1995.
29. Palmer A, Glisson RR, Werner FW: Relationship between ulnar variance and triangular fibrocartilage complex thickness. J Hand Surg [Am] 9: 681–682, 1984.
30. Green D, Hotchkiss RN, Pederson WC: Operative Hand Surgery, 4th ed. New York, Churchill Livingstone, 1999.
31. Bonzar M, Firrell JC, Hainer M, et al.: Kienbock disease and negative ulnar variance. J Bone Joint Surg Am 80:1154–1157, 1998.
32. Allan CH, Joshi A, Lichtman DM: Kienbock's disease: Diagnosis and treatment. J Am Acad Orthop Surg 9:128–136, 2001.
33. Pevny T, Rayan G, Egle D: Ligamentous and tendinous support of the pisiform, anatomy and biomechanical study. J Hand Surg [Am] 20:299–304, 1995.
34. Ritt M, Berger R, Kauer J: The gross and histologic anatomy of the ligaments of the capitohamate joint. J Hand Surg [Am] 21:1022–1028, 1996.
35. Ritt M, Berger R, Bishop A, et al.: The capitohamate ligaments. J Hand Surg [Br] 21:451–454, 1996.
36. Li G, Ryu J, Rowen B, et al.: Carpal kinematics of lunotriquetral dissociations. Biomed Sci Instrum 27:273–281, 1991.
37. Viegas S, Patterson R, Todd P, et al.: Load mechanics of the midcarpal joint. J Hand Surg [Am] 18:14, 1993.
38. Youm Y, McMurthy RY, Flatt AE, et al.: Kinematics of the wrist. I. An experimental study of radial-ulnar deviation and flexion-extension. J Bone Joint Surg Am 60:423, 1978.
39. Nowalk M, Logan S: Distinguishing biomechanical properties of intrinsic and extrinsic human wrist ligaments. J Biomech Eng 113:85–93, 1991.
40. Mayfield J: Wrist ligamentous anatomy and pathogenesis of carpal instability. Orthop Clin North Am 15:209–216, 1984.
41. Blevens A, Light T, Jablonsky W, et al.: Radiocarpal articular contact characteristics with scaphoid instability. J Hand Surg [Am] 14:781–790, 1989.
42. Mayfield J, Johnson RP, Kilcoyne RF: The ligaments

of the human wrist and their functional significance. Anat Rec 186:417, 1976.

43. Taleisnik J: The ligaments of the wrist. J Hand Surg [Am] 1:110–118, 1976.

44. Taleisnik J: The Wrist. New York, Churchill Livingstone, 1985.

45. Berger RA, Kauer JM, Landsmeer JM: Radio-scapholunate ligament: A gross anatomic and histologic study of fetal and adult wrists. J Hand Surg [Am] 16:350–355, 1991.

46. Mizuseki T, Ikuta Y: The dorsal carpal ligaments: Their anatomy and function. J Hand Surg [Br] 14:91–98, 1989.

47. Boabighi A, Kuhlmann J, Kenesi C: The distal ligamentous complex of the scaphoid and the scapholunate ligament. An anatomic, histological and biomechanical study. J Hand Surg [Br] 18: 65–69, 1993.

48. Kauer J: The interdependence of the carpal articulation chains. Acta Anat (Basel) 88:481–501, 1976.

49. Short W, Werner F, Fortino M, et al.: A dynamic biomechanical study of scapholunate ligament sectioning. J Hand Surg [Am] 20:986–999, 1995.

50. Short WH, Werner FW, Green JK, et al.: Biomechanical evaluation of ligamentous stabilizers of the scaphoid and lunate. J Hand Surg [Am] 27:991–1002, 2002.

51. Berger R: The gross and histologic anatomy of the scapholunate interosseous ligament. J Hand Surg [Am] 21:170–178, 1996.

52. Shin AY, Battaglia MJ, Bishop AT: Lunotriquetral instability: Diagnosis and treatment. J Am Acad Orthop Surg 8:170–179, 2000.

53. Viegas SF, Patterson RM, Peterson PD, et al.: Ulnar-sided perilunate instability: An anatomic and biomechanic study. J Hand Surg [Am] 15: 268–278, 1990.

54. Tubiana R, Thomine J, Mackin E: Examination of the Hand and Wrist, 2nd ed. St. Louis, CV Mosby, 1996.

55. Viegas S, Yamaguchi S, Boyd N, et al.: The dorsal ligaments of the wrist: Anatomy, mechanical properties, and function. J Hand Surg [Am] 24: 456–468, 1999.

56. Viegas SF: The dorsal ligaments of the wrist. Hand Clin 17:65–75, 2001.

57. Garcia-Elias M: Kinetic analysis of carpal stability during grip. Hand Clin 13:151–158, 1997.

58. Ruby LK, Cooney WP 3rd, An KN, et al.: Relative motion of selected carpal bones: A kinematic analysis of the normal wrist. J Hand Surg [Am] 13:1–10, 1988.

59. Moojen TM, Snel JG, Ritt MJ, et al.: Three-dimensional carpal kinematics *in vivo*. Clin Biomech (Bristol, Avon) 17:506–514, 2002.

60. Crisco JJ, Wolfe SW, Neu CP, et al.: Advances in the *in vivo* measurement of normal and abnormal carpal kinematics. Orthop Clin North Am 32: 219–231, 2001.

61. Savelberg H, Otten J, Kooloos J, et al.: Carpal bone kinematics and ligament lengthening studied for the full range of joint movement. J Biomech 26: 1389–1402, 1993.

62. Kobayahsi M, Garcia-Elias M, Nagy L, et al.: Axial loading induces rotation of the proximal carpal row bones around unique screw-displacement axes. J Biomech 30:1165–1167, 1997.

63. Short W, Werner F, Fortino M, et al.: Analysis of the kinematics of the scaphoid and lunate in the intact wrist joint. Hand Clin 13:93–108, 1997.

64. Neu CP, Crisco JJ, Wolfe SW: *In vivo* kinematic behavior of the radio-capitate joint during wrist flexion-extension and radio-ulnar deviation. J Biomech 34:1429–1438, 2001.

65. Conwell H: Injuries to the Wrist. Summit, NJ, CIBA Pharmaceutical, 1970.

66. MacConaill M, Basmajian J: Muscles and Movement: A Basis for Human Kinesiology. Baltimore, Williams & Wilkins, 1969.

67. Kauer J: The mechanism of the carpal joint. Clin Orthop 202:16–26, 1986.

68. Wright R: A detailed study of movement of the wrist joint. J Anat 70:137, 1935.

69. Sarrafian S, Melamed J, Goshgarian F: Study of wrist motion in flexion and extension. Clin Orthop 126:153, 1977.

70. Fisk G: Carpal instability and the fractured scaphoid. Ann R Coll Surg Engl 46:63–76, 1970.

71. MacConaill M: The mechanical anatomy of the carpus and its bearing on some surgical problems. J Anat 75:166, 1941.

72. Brumfield RH, Champoux JA: A biomechanical study of normal functional wrist motion. Clin Orthop 187:23, 1984.

73. Cooney W, Linscheid R, Dobyns J: The Wrist: Diagnosis and operative treatment. St. Louis, Mosby-Year Book, 1998.

74. Watson HK, Ballet FL: The SLAC wrist: Scapholunate advanced collapse pattern of degenerative arthritis. J Hand Surg [Am] 9:358–365, 1984.

75. Stabler A, Heuck A, Reiser M: Imaging of the hand: Degeneration, impingement and overuse. Eur J Radiol 25:118–128, 1997.

76. Lamoreaux L, Hoffer M: The effect of wrist deviation on grip and pinch strength. Clin Orthop 314:152–155, 1995.

77. Li ZM: The influence of wrist position on individual finger forces during forceful grip. J Hand Surg [Am] 27:886–896, 2002.

78. O'Driscoll S, Horii E, Ness R, et al.: The relationship between wrist position, grasp size, and grip strength. J Hand Surg [Am] 17:169–177, 1992.

79. Steindler A: Kinesiology of the Human Body. Springfield, IL, Charles C Thomas, 1955.

80. Moore K, Dalley AI: Clinically Oriented Anatomy, 4th ed. Philadelphia, Lippincott Williams & Wilkins, 1999.

81. Backdahl M, Carlsoo S: Distribution of activity in muscles acting on the wrist (an electromyographic study). Acta Morphol Neerl Scand 4:136, 1961.

82. Rosenthal E: Extensor tendons: Anatomy and management. In Mackin E, Callahan AD, Skirven T, et al. (eds): Rehabilitation of the Hand and Upper Extremity, 5th ed. St. Louis, Mosby-Year Book, 2002.

83. Ketchum L, Brand PW, Thompson D, et al.: The determination of moments for extension of the wrist generated by muscles of the forearm. J Hand Surg [Am] 3:205–210, 1978.

84. Radonjic F, Long C: Kinesiology of the wrist. Am J Phys Med 50:57, 1971.

85. Perry J: Normal upper extremity kinesiology. Phys Ther 58:265, 1978.

86. Ljung BO, Lieber RL, Friden J: Wrist extensor muscle pathology in lateral epicondylitis. J Hand Surg [Br] 24:177–183, 1999.

87. Fairbank SR, Corelett RJ: The role of the extensor digitorum communis muscle in lateral epicondylitis. J Hand Surg [Br] 27:405–409, 2002.

88. Greenbaum B, Itamura J, Vangsness CT, et al.: Extensor carpi radialis brevis. An anatomical analysis of its origin. J Bone Joint Surg Br 81:926–929, 1999.

89. Tang J, Ryu J, Kish V: The triangular fibrocartilage complex: An important component of the pulley for the ulnar wrist flexor. J Hand Surg [Am] 23:986–991, 1998.

90. Boivin J, Wadsworth GE, Landsmeer JM, et al.: Electromyographic kinesiology of the hand: Muscles driving the index finger. Arch Phys Med Rehabil 50:17–26, 1969.

91. Ranney D: The hand as a concept: Digital differences and their importance. Clin Anat 8:281–287, 1995.

92. Nakamura K, Patterson RM, Viegas SF: The ligament and skeletal anatomy of the second through fifth carpometacarpal joints and adjacent structures. J Hand Surg [Am] 26:1016–1029, 2001.

93. Dzwierzynski WW, Matloub HS, Yan JG, et al.: Anatomy of the intermetacarpal ligaments of the carpometacarpal joints of the fingers. J Hand Surg [Am] 22:931–934, 1997.

94. Hayes E, Carney K, Wolf J, et al.: Carpal tunnel syndrome. In Mackin E, Callahan AD, Skirven T, et al. (eds): Rehabilitation of the Hand and Upper Extremity, 5th ed. St. Louis, Mosby-Year Book, 2002.

95. Kruger V, Kraft GH, Deitz JC, et al.: Carpal tunnel syndrome: Objective measures and splint use. Arch Phys Med Rehabil 72:517–520, 1991.

96. Walker WC, Metzler M, Cifu DX, et al.: Neutral wrist splinting in carpal tunnel syndrome: A comparison of night-only versus full-time wear instructions. Arch Phys Med Rehabil 81:424–429, 2000.

97. Cobb T, Dalley B, Posteraro R, et al.: Anatomy of the flexor retinaculum. J Hand Surg [Am] 18:91–99, 1993.

98. Garcia-Elias M, An K, Cooney W, et al.: Stability of the transverse carpal arch: An experimental study. J Hand Surg [Am] 14:277–282, 1989.

99. El-Shennawy M, Nakamura K, Patterson RM, et al.: Three-dimensional kinematic analysis of the second through fifth carpometacarpal joints. J Hand Surg [Am] 26:1030–1035, 2001.

100. Batmanabane M, Malathi S: Movements at the carpometacarpal and metacarpophalangeal joints of the hand and their effect on the dimensions of the articular ends of the metacarpal bones. Anat Rec 213:102–110, 1985.

101. Joseph R, Linscheid RL, Dobyns JH, et al.: Chronic sprains of the carpometacarpal joints. J Hand Surg [Am] 6:172–180, 1981.

102. Al-Qattan M, Robertson G: An anatomical study of the deep transverse metacarpal ligament. J Anat 12:443–446, 1993.

103. Kaplan E: The participation of the metacarpophalangeal joint of the thumb in the act of opposition. Bull Hosp Joint Dis 27:39, 1966.

104. Benjamin M, Ralphs J, Shibu M, et al.: Capsular tissues of the proximal interphalangeal joint: Normal composition and effects of Dupuytren's disease and rheumatoid arthritis. J Hand Surg [Br] 18:370–376, 1993.

105. Minami A, An KN, Cooney WP 3rd, et al.: Ligamentous structures of the metacarpophalangeal joint: A quantitative anatomic study. J Orthop Res 1:361–368, 1984.

106. Shultz R, Storace A, Krishnamurthy S: Metacarpophalangeal joint motion and the role of the collateral ligaments. Int Orthop 11:149–155, 1987.

107. Fisher D, Elliott S, Cooke TD, et al.: Descriptive anatomy of fibrocartilaginous menisci in the finger joints of the hand. J Orthop Res 3:484–491, 1985.

108. Krishnan J, Chipchase L: Passive axial rotation of the metacarpophalangeal joint. J Hand Surg [Br] 22:270–273, 1997.

109. Bowers WH, Wolf JW Jr, Nehil JL, et al.: The proximal interphalangeal joint volar plate. I. An anatomical and biomechanical study. J Hand Surg [Am] 5:79–88, 1980.

110. Minamikwa Y, Horii E, Amadio P, et al.: Stability and constraint of the proximal interphalangeal joint. J Hand Surg [Am] 18:198–204, 1993.

111. Rhee R, Reading G, Wray R: A biomechanical study of the collateral ligaments of the proximal interphalangeal joint. J Hand Surg [Am] 17:157–163, 1992.

112. Dzwierzynski W, Pintar F, Matloub H, et al.: Biomechanics of the intact and surgically repaired proximal interphalangeal joint collateral ligaments. J Hand Surg [Am] 21:679–683, 1996.

113. Campbell P, Wilson R: Management of joint injuries and intraarticular fractures. In Mackin E, Callahan AD, Skirven T, et al. (eds): Rehabilitation of the Hand and Upper Extremity, 5th ed. St. Louis, Mosby-Year Book, 2002.

114. Mallon WJ, Brown HR, Nunley JA: Digital ranges of motion: Normal values in young adults. J Hand Surg [Am] 16:882–887, 1991.

115. Jacobs M, Austin N: Splinting the Hand and Upper Extremity: Principles and Process. Baltimore, Lippincott Williams & Wilkins, 2002.

116. Long C 2nd, Conrad PW, Hall EA, et al.: Intrinsic-extrinsic muscle control of the hand in power grip and precision handling. An electromyographic study. J Bone Joint Surg Am 52:853–867, 1970.
117. Brook N, Mizrahi J, Shoham M, et al.: A biomechanical model of index finger dynamics. Med Eng Phys 17:54–63, 1993.
118. Hamman J, Sli A, Phillips C, et al.: A biomechanical study of the flexor digitorum superficialis: Effects of digital pulley excision and loss of the flexor digitorum profundus. J Hand Surg [Am] 22:328–335, 1997.
119. Baker D, Gaul JS Jr, Williams VK, et al.: The little finger superficialis—Clinical investigation of its anatomic and functional shortcomings. J Hand Surg [Am] 6:374–378, 1981.
120. Idler RS: Anatomy and biomechanics of the digital flexor tendons. Hand Clin 1:3–11, 1985.
121. Phillips C, Falender R, Mass D: The flexor synovial sheath anatomy of the little finger: A macroscopic study. J Hand Surg [Am] 20:636–641, 1995.
122. Lin G, Amadio P, An K, et al.: Functional anatomy of the human digital flexor pulley system. J Hand Surg [Am] 14:949–956, 1989.
123. Phillips C, Mass D: Mechanical analysis of the palmar aponeurosis pulley in human cadavers. J Hand Surg [Am] 21:240–244, 1996.
124. Doyle JR, Blythe WF: Anatomy of the flexor tendon sheath and pulleys of the thumb. J Hand Surg [Am] 2:149–151, 1977.
125. Manske P, Lesker P: Diffusion as a nutrient pathway to the flexor tendon. In Hunter J, Schneider LH, Mackin E (eds): Tendon Surgery in the Hand. St. Louis, CV Mosby, 1987.
126. Hunter J, Mackin E, Callahan A: Rehabilitation of the Hand: Surgery and Therapy, 4th ed. St. Louis, CV Mosby, 1995.
127. Mester S, Schmidt B, Derczy K, et al.: Biomechanics of the human flexor tendon sheath investigated by tenography. J Hand Surg [Br] 20:500–504, 1995.
128. Doyle JR: Palmar and digital flexor tendon pulleys. Clin Orthop 383:84–96, 2001.
129. Rispler D, Greenwald D, Shumway S, et al.: Efficiency of the flexor tendon pulley system in human cadaver hands. J Hand Surg [Am] 21:444–450, 1996.
130. Manske P, Lesker P: Palmar aponeurosis pulley. J Hand Surg [Am] 8:259–263, 1983.
131. Gonzalez M, Weinzweig N, Kay T, et al.: Anatomy of the extensor tendons to the index finger. J Hand Surg [Am] 21:988–991, 1996.
132. von Schroeder H, Botte M: Anatomy of the extensor tendons of the fingers: Variations and multiplicity. J Hand Surg [Am] 20:27–34, 1995.
133. El-Badawi M, Butt M, Al-Zuhair A, et al.: Extensor tendons of the fingers: Arrangement and variations—II. Clin Anat 8:391–398, 1995.
134. Gonzalez M, Gray T, Ortinau E, et al.: The extensor tendons to the little finger: An anatomic study. J Hand Surg [Am] 20:844–847, 1995.
135. Van Sint Jan S, Rooze M, Van Audekerke J, et al.: The insertion of the extensor digitorum tendon on the proximal phalanx. J Hand Surg [Am] 21:69–76, 1996.
136. Young CM, Rayan GM: The sagittal band: Anatomic and biomechanical study. J Hand Surg [Am] 25:1107–1113, 2000.
137. El-Gammal T, Steyers C, Blair W, et al.: Anatomy of the oblique retinacular ligament of the index finger. J Hand Surg [Am] 18:717–721, 1993.
138. Salisbury C: The interosseous muscles of the hand. J Anat 71:395, 1936.
139. Long C: Intrinsic-extrinsic muscle control of the fingers. J Bone Joint Surg Am 50:973, 1968.
140. von Schroeder H, Botte M: The functional significance of the long extensors and juncturae tendinum in finger extension. J Hand Surg [Am] 18:641–647, 1993.
141. Brand P: Paralytic claw hand. J Bone Joint Surg Br 40:618, 1958.
142. Ranney D, Wells R: Lumbrical muscle function as revealed by a new and physiological approach. Anat Rec 222:110–114, 1988.
143. Stack H: Muscle function in the fingers. J Bone Joint Surg Br 44:899, 1962.
144. Bell-Krotoski J: Preoperative and postoperative management of tendon transfers after median- and ulnar-nerve injury. In Mackin E, Callahan AD, Skirven T, et al. (eds): Rehabilitation of the Hand and Upper Extremity, 5th ed. St. Louis, Mosby-Year Book, 2002.
145. Landsmeer J: The anatomy of the dorsal aponeurosis of the human fingers and its functional significance. Anat Rec 104:31, 1949.
146. Mardel S, Underwood M: Adductor pollicis. The missing interosseous. Surg Radiol Anat 13:49–52, 1991.
147. Eladoumikdachi F, Valkov PL, Thomas J, et al.: Anatomy of the intrinsic hand muscles revisited: Part I. Interossei. Plast Reconstr Surg 110:1211–1224, 2002.
148. Eyler D, Markee J: The anatomy and function of the intrinsic musculature of the fingers. J Bone Joint Surg Am 36:1, 1954.
149. Brand P, Hollister A: Clinical Mechanics of the Hand, 2nd ed. St. Louis, CV Mosby Year Book, 1993.
150. Kozin S, Porter S, Clark P, et al.: The contribution of the intrinsic muscles to grip and pinch strength. J Hand Surg [Am] 24:64–72, 1999.
151. Close J, Kidd C: The functions of the muscles of the thumb, the index and the long fingers. J Bone Joint Surg Am 51:1601, 1969.
152. Eladoumikdachi F, Valkov PL, Thomas J, et al.: Anatomy of the intrinsic hand muscles revisited: Part II. Lumbricals. Plast Reconstr Surg 110:1225–1231, 2002.
153. Backhouse K, Catton W: An experimental study of the functions of the lumbrical muscles in the human hand. J Anat 88:133, 1954.
154. Leijnse H, Kalker J: A two-dimensional kinematic model of the lumbrical in the human finger. J Biomech 28:237–249, 1995.

155. Ketchum L, Thompson D, Pocock G, et al.: A clinical study of the forces generated by the intrinsic muscles of the index finger and extrinsic flexor and extensor muscles of the hand. J Hand Surg [Am] 3:571–578, 1978.

156. Zancolli E, Ziadenberg C, Zancolli E: Biomechanics of the trapeziometacarpal joint. Clin Orthop 220:14–26, 1987.

157. Cooney WP 3rd, Lucca MJ, Chao EY, et al.: The kinesiology of the thumb trapeziometacarpal joint. J Bone Joint Surg Am 63:1371–1381, 1981.

158. Pagalidis T, Kuczynski K, Lamb DW: Ligamentous stability of the base of the thumb. Hand 13:29–35, 1981.

159. Bettinger PC, Linscheid RL, Berger RA, et al.: An anatomic study of the stabilizing ligaments of the trapezium and trapeziometacarpal joint. J Hand Surg [Am] 24:786–798, 1999.

160. Bettinger PC, Berger RA: Functional ligamentous anatomy of the trapezium and trapeziometacarpal joint (gross and arthroscopic). Hand Clin 17:151–168, 2001.

161. Kauer J: Functional anatomy of the carpometacarpal joint of the thumb. Clin Orthop 220:7–13, 1987.

162. Koff MF, Ugwonali OF, Strauch RJ, et al.: Sequential wear patterns of the articular cartilage of the thumb carpometacarpal joint in osteoarthritis. J Hand Surg [Am] 28:597–604, 2003.

163. Ateshian G, Rosenwasser M, Mow V: Curvature characteristics and congruence of the thumb carpometacarpal joint: Differences between female and male joints. J Biomech 25:591–607, 1992.

164. Goldberg I, Nathan H: Anatomy and pathology of the sesamoid bones. Int Orthop 11:141–147, 1987.

165. Johanson M, Skinner S, Lamoreux L: Phasic relationships of the intrinsic and extrinsic thumb musculature. Clin Orthop 322:120–130, 1996.

166. Belanger A, Noel G: Force-generating capacity of thumb adductor muscles in the parallel and perpendicular plane of adduction. J Orthop Sports Phys Ther 21:139–146, 1995.

167. Casanova J, Grunert B: Adult prehension: Patterns and nomenclature for pinches. J Hand Ther 2: 231–243, 1989.

168. Melvin J: Rheumatic Disease in the Adult and Child, 3rd ed. Philadelphia, FA Davis, 1989.

169. Chao E, Opgrande JD, Axmeare FE: Three-dimensional force analysis of the finger joints in selected isometric hand functions. J Biomech 9:387, 1976.

170. Landsmeer J: Power grip and precision handling. Ann Rheum Dis 22:164, 1962.

171. Kamper D, George Hornby T, Rymer WZ: Extrinsic flexor muscles generate concurrent flexion of all three finger joints. J Biomech 35:1581–1589, 2002.

172. Milner TE, Dhaliwal SS: Activation of intrinsic and extrinsic finger muscles in relation to the fingertip force vector. Exp Brain Res 146:197–204, 2002.

173. Bejjani F, Landsmeer J: Biomechanics of the hand. In Nordin M, Frankel V (eds): Basic Biomechanics of the Musculoskeletal System, 2nd ed. Philadelphia, Lea & Febiger, 1989.

Section 4

Hip Joint

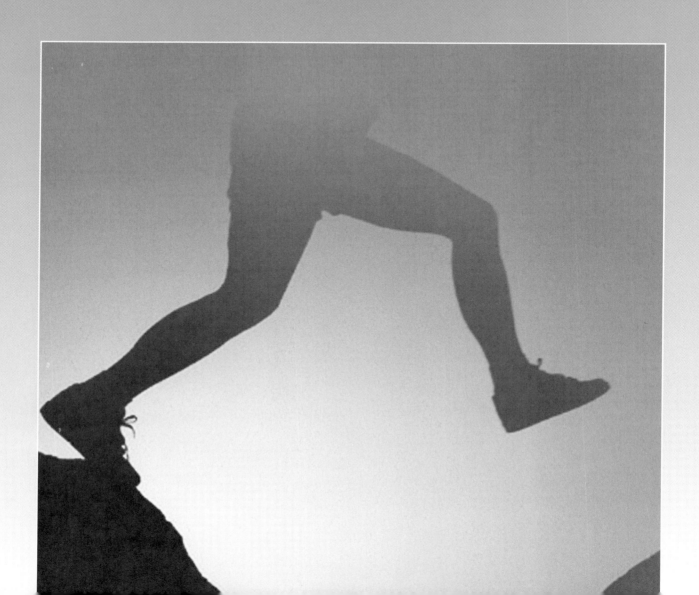

Introduction

The hip joint, or **coxofemoral joint,** is the articulation of the acetabulum of the pelvis and the head of the femur (Fig. 10-1). These two segments form a diarthrodial ball-and-socket joint with three degrees of freedom: flexion/extension in the sagittal plane, abduction/adduction in the frontal plane, and medial/lateral rotation in the transverse plane. Although the hip joint and the shoulder complex have a number of common features, the functional and structural adaptations of each to its respective roles have been so extensive that such comparisons are more of general interest than of functional relevance. The role of the shoulder

complex is to provide a stable base on which a wide range of mobility for the hand can be superimposed. Shoulder complex structure gives precedence to open-chain function. The primary function of the hip joint is to support the weight of the head, arms, and trunk (HAT) both in static erect posture and in dynamic postures such as ambulation, running, and stair climbing. The hip joint, like the other joints of the lower extremity that we will examine, is structured primarily to serve its weight-bearing functions. Although we examine hip joint structure and function as if the joint were designed to move the foot through space in an open chain, hip joint structure is more influenced by the demands placed on the joint when the limb is bearing weight. As we shall see later in this chapter, weight-bearing

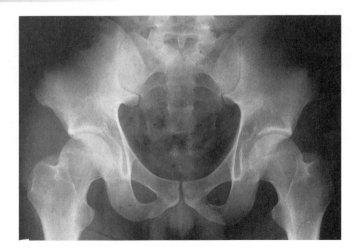

▲ **Figure 10-1** ■ The hip joint is formed by the head of the femur and the acetabulum of the innominate bone (one half) of the pelvis.

function of the hip joint and its related weight-bearing responses are basic to understanding the hip joint and the interactions that occur between the hip joint and the other joints of the spine and lower extremities.

| 10-1 | **Patient Case** |

Gloria Martinez is a 78-year-old woman who retired from teaching second grade after 40 years of service. Over the past few years, she has had increasing problems with hip pain, predominantly on the left, that interferes with climbing the stairs to her second-floor apartment and with caring for her 3-year-old great-granddaughter, for whom she provides daycare 3 days a week. Gloria reports that she has had problems with her left hip since her childhood in Guatemala. Her family moved to the United States when she was 8 years old. She remembers being told by a physician when she was in her teens that she would probably have problems with the hip when she got older. New radiographs and magnetic resonance imaging (MRI) showed a valgus anteverted femur and a shallow acetabulum on the left. On the basis of imaging, a diagnosis of left developmental hip dysplasia with osteoarthritic changes was made. Gloria localizes her primary pain to her left groin, although the lateral hip area is tender to palpation. On clinical examination, Gloria is observed to walk with asymmetrical toe-out, with the right greater than the left. She has a slight left lateral lean during left stance. There is a 1-inch leg length discrepancy, with the left leg shorter. Gloria finds passive hip flexion with medial rotation painful on the left. In the supine position, medial rotation of the left hip is much greater than lateral rotation. This asymmetry is not evident on the right.

◆ **Structure of the Hip Joint**

Proximal Articular Surface

The cuplike concave socket of the hip joint is called the **acetabulum** and is located on the lateral aspect of the pelvic bone (**innominate** or **os coxa**). Three bones form the pelvis: the ilium, the ischium, and the pubis. Each of the three bones contributes to the structure of the acetabulum (Fig. 10-2A). The pubis forms one fifth of the acetabulum, the ischium forms two fifths, and the ilium forms the remainder. Until full ossification of the pelvis occurs between 20 and 25 years of age, the separate segments of the acetabulum may remain visible on radiograph[1] (see Fig. 10-2B).

The acetabulum appears to be a hemisphere, but only its upper margin has a true circular contour,[2] and the roundness of the acetabulum as a whole decreases

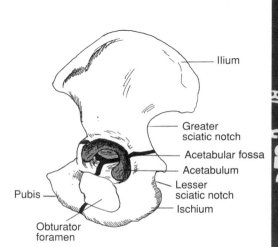

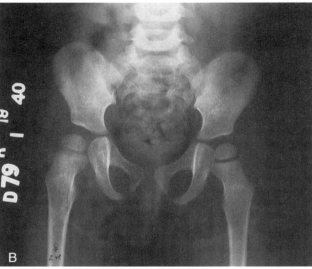

▲ **Figure 10-2** ■ **A.** The acetabulum is formed by the union of the three bones of the pelvis, with only the upper horseshoe-shaped area being articular. **B.** In this radiograph of a 2-year-old without impairments, the cartilaginous rather than bony union of the acetabulum is clearly evident.

with age.[3] In actuality, only a horseshoe-shaped portion of the periphery of the acetabulum (the **lunate surface**) is covered with hyaline cartilage and articulates with the head of the femur (see Fig. 10-2A). The inferior aspect of the lunate surface (the base of the horseshoe) is interrupted by a deep notch called the **acetabular notch.** The acetabular notch is spanned by a fibrous band, the **transverse acetabular ligament,** that connects the two ends of the horseshoe. The transverse acetabular ligament also spans the acetabular notch to create a fibro-osseous tunnel, called the **acetabular fossa,** beneath the ligament, through which blood vessels may pass into the central or deepest portion of the acetabulum. The acetabulum is deepened by the fibrocartilaginous **acetabular labrum,** which surrounds the periphery. The acetabular fossa is nonarticular; the femoral head does not contact this surface (Fig. 10-3). The acetabular fossa contains fibroelastic fat covered with synovial membrane.

■ Center Edge Angle of the Acetabulum

Each acetabulum, in addition to its obvious lateral orientation, is oriented on each innominate bone somewhat inferiorly and anteriorly. The magnitude of inferior orientation is assessed on radiograph by using a line connecting the lateral rim of the acetabulum and the center of the femoral head. This line forms an angle with the vertical known as the **center edge (CE) angle** or the **angle of Wiberg** (see Fig. 10-3) and is the amount of inferior tilt of the acetabulum. The inferior tilt is essentially a measure of the amount of coverage or "roof" there is over the femoral head. Using computed tomography (CT), Adna and associates[4] found CE angles in adults to average 38° in men and 35° in women (with ranges in both sexes to be about 22° to

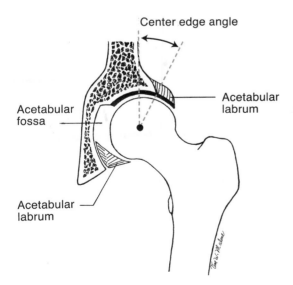

▲ **Figure 10-3** ■ The center edge (CE) angle of the acetabulum is formed between a vertical line through the center of the femoral head and a line connecting the center of the femoral head and the bony edge of the acetabulum. The acetabular labrum deepens the acetabulum.

42°). Other investigators, using radiographs, have found the CE angles to be similar between men and women,[5,6] and across ages groups in women (25 to 65 years old).[6] The similarity of the CE angle between men and women is somewhat surprising, given the increased diameter and more vertical orientation of the sides of the female pelvis.[7] There is also evidence that the CE angle increases from childhood to skeletal maturity.[8] The implication is that young children have relatively less coverage over the head of the femur and, therefore, relatively decreased joint stability than do adults. Genda and colleagues used radiographs and modeling to conclude that there was a significant positive correlation ($r = 0.678$) between CE angle and joint contact area.[6]

■ Acetabular Anteversion

The acetabulum faces not only somewhat inferiorly but also anteriorly. The magnitude of anterior orientation of the acetabulum may be referred to as the **angle of acetabular anteversion.** Adna and associates[4] found the average value to be 18.5° for men and 21.5° for women, although Kapandji[9] cited larger values of 30° to 40°. Pathologic increases in the angle of acetabular anteversion are associated with decreased joint stability and increased tendency for anterior dislocation of the head of the femur.

■ Acetabular Labrum

Given the need for stability at the hip joint, it is not surprising to find an accessory joint structure. The entire periphery of the acetabulum is rimmed by a ring of wedge-shaped fibrocartilage called the acetabular labrum (see labrum cross-section in Fig. 10-3). The labrum is attached to the periphery of the acetabulum by a zone of calcified cartilage with a well-defined tidemark.[10] The acetabular labrum not only deepens the socket but also increases the concavity of the acetabulum through its triangular shape and grasps the head of the femur to maintain contact with the acetabulum. Although the labrum appears to broaden the articular surface of the acetabulum, experimental evidence suggests that load distribution in the acetabulum is not affected by removal of the labrum.[11] Histological examination demonstrated free nerve endings and sensory receptors in the superficial layer of the labrum,[11] as well as vascularization from the adjacent joint capsule only in the superficial third of the labrum.[12] The evidence suggests that the labrum is not load-bearing but serves a role in proprioception and pain sensitivity that may help protect the rim of the acetabulum. Ferguson and colleagues found that hydrostatic fluid pressure within the intra-articular space was greater within the labrum than without, which suggests that the labrum may also enhance joint lubrication if the labrum adequately fits the femoral head.[13]

The transverse acetabular ligament is considered to be part of the acetabular labrum, although, unlike the labrum, it contains no cartilage cells.[7] Although it is positioned to protect the blood vessels traveling beneath it to reach the head of the femur, experimental data do not support the notion of the transverse acetabular ligament as a load-bearing structure.[11] Konrath and colleagues[11] supported the hypothesis of others that the ligament served as a tension band between the anteroinferior and posteroinferior aspects of the acetabulum (the "feet" of the horseshoe-shaped articular surface) but were not able to corroborate this from their data.

Continuing Exploration: **Acetabular Labrum in the Aging Hip**

Acetabular labral tears are increasingly recognized as a source of hip pain and as a starting point for degenerative changes at the acetabular rim.[10,14–18] Damage to the labrum was evident in 96% of postmortem and cadaveric hip joints in persons 61 to 98 years of age, with 74% showing damage in the anterosuperior quadrant.[10] Findings were quite similar among those examined surgically after femoral neck fractures and among those with asymptomatic, painful, or dysplastic hips examined on MRI.[14,17,19] The causative factor is hypothesized to be impingement of the femur on the acetabular rim, which creates microtrauma over time, or tears caused by a sudden twisting injury. Although apparently not always symptomatic, labral tears are associated with the possibility of persistent hip pain or disabling mechanical symptoms progressing to acetabular chondral defects and osteoarthritis.[14–16]

Case Application 10-1: **Labral Damage**

Gloria's left groin pain was provoked by passive hip flexion and medial rotation. This clinical finding and her age are consistent with damage of the anterosuperior labrum, most likely also a site of osteoarthritic changes.[17,20] Although impingement of the femur on the labrum remains a hypothetical cause, that mechanism is consistent with Gloria's 40 years as a second-grade teacher, in which she spent a great deal of her time on the floor with the children or in small chairs that required excessive hip flexion. It also may be consistent with her history of hip dysplasia.[15,19]

Distal Articular Surface

The head of the femur is a fairly rounded hyaline cartilage-covered surface that may be slightly larger than a true hemisphere or as much as two thirds of a sphere, depending on body type.[9] The head of the femur is considered to be circular, unlike the more irregularly shaped acetabulum.[3] The radius of curvature of the femoral head is smaller in women than in men in comparison with the dimensions of the pelvis.[5,6] Just inferior to the most medial point on the femoral head is a small roughened pit called the **fovea** or **fovea**

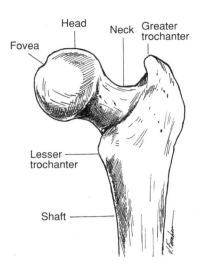

▲ **Figure 10-4** ■ Posterior view of the proximal portion of the right femur shows the relationship between the head, neck, trochanters, and femoral shaft.

capitis (Fig. 10-4). The fovea is not covered with articular cartilage and is the point at which the ligament of the head of the femur is attached.

The femoral head is attached to the femoral neck; the femoral neck is attached to the shaft of the femur between the greater trochanter and the lesser trochanter. The femoral neck is, in general, only about 5 cm long.[7] The femoral neck is angulated so that the femoral head most commonly faces medially, superiorly, and anteriorly. Although the angulation of the femoral head and neck on the shaft is more consistent across the population than is angulation of the humeral head and neck on its shaft, there are still substantial individual differences and differences from side to side in the same individual.

■ Angulation of the Femur

There are two angulations made by the head and neck of the femur in relation to the shaft. One angulation (**angle of inclination**) occurs in the frontal plane between an axis through the femoral head and neck and the longitudinal axis of the femoral shaft. The other angulation (**angle of torsion**) occurs in the transverse plane between an axis through the femoral head and neck and an axis through the distal femoral condyles. The origin and variability of these angulations can be understood in the context of the embryonic development of the lower limb. In the early stages of fetal development, both upper extremity and lower extremity limb buds project laterally from the body as if in full abduction. During the seventh and eighth weeks of gestational age and before full definition of the joints, adduction of the buds begins. At the end of the eighth week, the "fetal position" has been achieved, but the upper and lower limbs are no longer positioned similarly. Although the upper limb buds have undergone torsion somewhat laterally (so that the ventral surface of the limb bud faces anteriorly), the lower limb buds have undergone torsion medially, so that the ventral surface faces posteriorly.[7] The result for the lower limb is critical to understanding function. The knee flexes in the opposite direction from the elbow, and the extensor (dorsal) surface of the lower limb is anteriorly rather than posteriorly located. Although the head and neck of the femur retain the original position of the limb bud, the femoral shaft is inclined medially and undergoes medial torsion with regard to the head and neck. The magnitude of medial inclination and torsion of the distal femur (with regard to the head and neck) is dependent on embryonic growth and, presumably, fetal positioning during the remaining months of uterine life. The development of the angulations of the femur appear to continue after birth and through the early years of development.

Angle of Inclination of the Femur

The angle of inclination of the femur averages 126° (referencing the medial angle formed by the axes of the head/neck and the shaft), ranging from 115° to 140° in the unimpaired adult[1,21] (Fig. 10-5). As with the angle of inclination of the humerus, there are variations not only among individuals but also from side to side. In women, the angle of inclination is somewhat smaller than it is in men, owing to the greater width of the female pelvis.[7] With a normal angle of inclination, the greater trochanter lies at the level of the center of the femoral head.[22] The angle of inclination of the femur changes across the life span, being substantially greater in infancy and childhood (see Fig. 10-2B) and gradually declining to about 120° in the normal elderly person.[23,24] A pathologic increase in the medial angulation between the neck and shaft is called **coxa**

valga (Fig. 10-6A), and a pathologic decrease is called **coxa vara** (see Fig. 10-6B).

Angle of Torsion of the Femur

The angle of torsion of the femur can best be viewed by looking down the length of the femur from top to bottom. An axis through the femoral head and neck in the transverse plane will lie at an angle to an axis through the femoral condyles, with the head and neck torsioned anteriorly (laterally) with regard to an angle through the femoral condyles (Fig. 10-7). This angulation reflects the medial rotatory migration of the lower limb bud that occurred during fetal development. The apparent contradiction between medial torsion of the embryonic limb bud and lateral torsion of the femoral head and neck simply reflects a shift in reference. In medial torsion of the limb bud, the proximal end is fixed and the distal end migrates medially. When torsion of the femur is assessed in a child or adult, the reference is an axis through the femoral condyles (the knee joint axis) that is generally presumed to lie in the frontal plane. If the axis through the femoral condyles lies in the frontal plane (as it functionally should), then the head and neck of the femur are torsioned anteriorly, relatively speaking, on the femoral condyles. The angle of torsion decreases with age. In the newborn, the angle of torsion has been estimated to be 40°, decreasing substantially in the first 2 years.[25] Svenningsen and associates[8] found a decrease of approximately 1.5° per year until cessation of growth among children with both normal and exaggerated angles of anteversion. In the adult, the normal angle of torsion is considered to be 10° to 20°.[7,9,26] Noble and colleagues[21] used three-dimensional analysis of CT scans on 54 women without

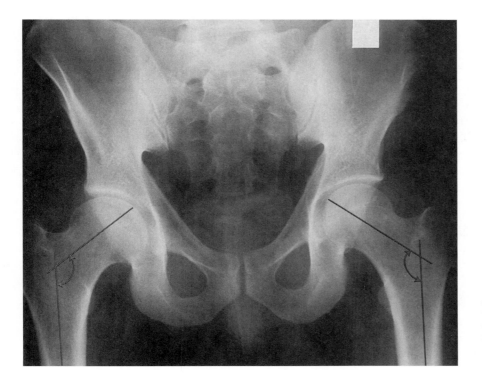

◀ **Figure 10-5** ■ The axis of the femoral head and neck forms an angle with the axis of the femoral shaft called the **angle of inclination**. In this adult subject without impairments, the angles are slightly less than 130°, with a couple of degrees of variation from side to side.

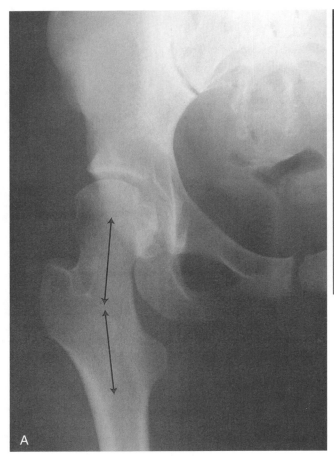

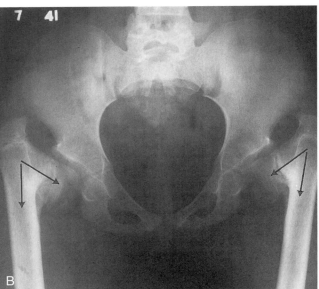

◀ **Figure 10-6** ■ Abnormal angles of inclination found in two young adults with developmental hip dysplasia. **A.** A pathologic increase in the angle of inclination is called coxa valga. **B.** A pathologic decrease in the angle is called coxa vara.

impairments whose ages ranged from 18 to 82 years. These investigators found an average anterior torsion of 35.6° (±13.7°), which indicated a greater variation than is ordinarily appreciated.

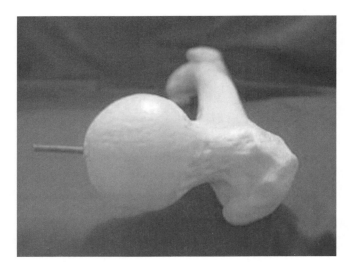

▲ **Figure 10-7** ■ A line parallel to the posterior femoral condyles and a line through the head and neck of the femur normally make an angle with each other that averages 15° to 20° in the adult without impairments. The femoral head and neck are in torsion anteriorly (medially) with respect to the femoral condyles.

A pathologic increase in the angle of torsion is called **anteversion** (Fig. 10-8A and 10-8B), and a pathologic decrease in the angle or reversal of torsion is known as **retroversion** (see Fig. 10-8 C). There may not be one angulation at which pathologic femoral torsion may be diagnosed, given the substantial normal variability. Heller and colleagues used an angle of 30° to model effects of anteversion, acknowledging that children with cerebral palsy have demonstrated angles of 60° or more.[27] Noble and colleagues found an average angle of 42.3° (±16°) among 154 women diagnosed with developmental hip dysplasia who had not had surgical intervention.[21]

It should be recognized that both normal and abnormal angles of inclination and torsion of the femur are *properties of the femur alone* (i.e., both can be measured or assessed independently of the continuous bones, as in Fig. 10-8). However, abnormalities in the angulations of the femur can cause compensatory hip changes and can substantially alter hip joint stability, the weight-bearing biomechanics of the hip joint, and muscle biomechanics.

Although some structural deviations such as femoral anteversion and coxa valga are commonly found together, each may occur independently of the other. Each structural deviation warrants careful consideration as to the impact on hip joint function *and* function of the joints both proximal and distal to the hip joint.

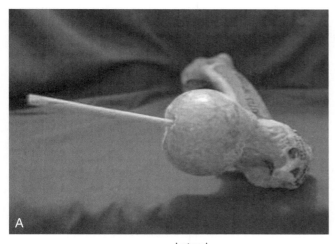

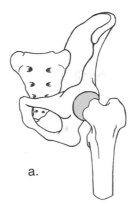 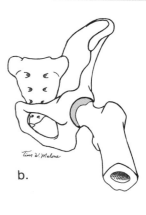

a. b.

▲ **Figure 10-9** ■ **A.** In the neutral hip joint, articular cartilage from the head of the femur is exposed anteriorly and, to a lesser extent, superiorly. **B.** Maximum articular contact of the head of the femur with the acetabulum is obtained when the femur is flexed, abducted, and laterally rotated slightly.

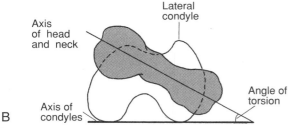

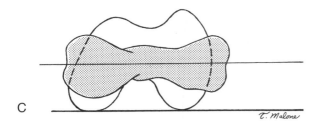

▲ **Figure 10-8** ■ Abnormal angles of torsion in a right femur. **A.** and **B.** A pathologic increase in the angle of torsion is called **anteversion. C.** A pathologic decrease in the normal angle of torsion is called **retroversion.**

As shall be evident when the knee and foot are discussed in subsequent chapters, femoral anteversion is often implicated in dysfunction at both the knee and at the foot. The other pathologic angulations of the femur (retroversion, coxa vara, and coxa valga) similarly affect the hip joint and other joints proximally and distally. The impact of abnormal angulations of the femur on hip joint function will continue to be discussed in this chapter.

Articular Congruence

The hip joint is considered to be a congruent joint. However, there is substantially more articular surface on the head of the femur than on the acetabulum. In the neutral or standing position, the articular surface of the femoral head remains exposed anteriorly and somewhat superiorly (Fig. 10-9A). The acetabulum

does not fully cover the head superiorly, and the anterior torsion of the femoral head (angle of torsion) exposes a substantial amount of the femoral head's articular surface anteriorly. Articular contact between the femur and the acetabulum can be increased in the normal non–weight-bearing hip joint by a combination of flexion, abduction, and slight lateral rotation[9] (see Fig. 10-9B). This position (also known as the frog-leg position) corresponds to that assumed by the hip joint in a quadruped position and, according to Kapandji,[9] is the true physiologic position of the hip joint.

Konrath and colleagues[11] concluded both from their work and from evidence in the literature that the hip joint actually functions as an incongruent joint in non–weight-bearing, given the larger femoral head. In weight-bearing, the elastic deformation of the acetabulum increases contact with the femoral head, with primary contact at the anterior, superior, and posterior articular surfaces of the acetabulum.[11] An additional contribution to articular congruence and coaptation of joint surfaces may be made by the nonarticular and non–weight-bearing acetabular fossa. The acetabular fossa may be important in setting up a partial vacuum in the joint so that atmospheric pressure contributes to stability by helping maintain contact between the femoral head and the acetabulum. Wingstrand and colleagues[28] concluded that atmospheric pressure in hip flexion activities played a stronger role in stabilization than capsuloligamentous structures. It is also true that the head and acetabulum will remain together in an anesthetized patient even after the joint capsule has been opened. The pressure within the joint must be broken before the hip can be dislocated.[9]

Case Application 10-2: **Articular Contact in the Dysplastic Hip**

Gloria's structural deviations of femoral anteversion, coxa valga, and a shallow acetabulum (decreased CE angle) can result in increased articular exposure of the femoral head, less congruence, and reduced stability of the hip joint in the neutral weight-bearing position. If Gloria's hip dysplasia had been diagnosed in infancy, frog-leg positioning might have been maintained using something like a Frejka pillow or Pavlik harness[29] (Fig. 10-10) to decrease the deformities by increasing the contact between the femoral head and acetabulum. The position of combined flexion, abduction, and rotation is commonly used for immobilization of the hip joint when the goal is to improve articular contact and joint congruence in conditions such as congenital dislocation of the hip and in Legg-Calvé-Perthes disease.[30] Whether this was done or not, Gloria's deformities of the femur and acetabulum persisted. Considering the reduction in CE angle alone, investigators have demonstrated that the stress distribution within the joint is concentrated in a smaller weight-bearing area throughout the gait cycle.[31] That increase in stress alone is likely to lead to degenerative changes over time. One estimate is that 25% of all cases of adult osteoarthritis are related to the residual effects of developmental hip dysplasias.[1]

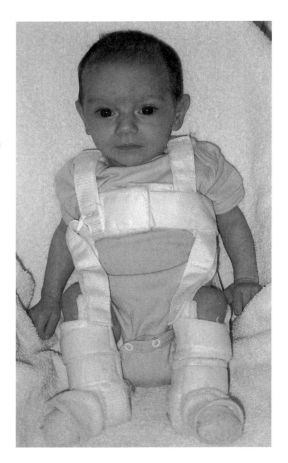

▲ **Figure 10-10** ■ An infant can easily be maintained the hip joint position of flexion, abduction, and external rotation (frog-leg position) by using a positioning device.

Hip Joint Capsule and Ligaments

■ Hip Joint Capsule

Unlike the relatively weak articular capsule of the shoulder, the hip joint capsule is a substantial contributor to joint stability. The articular capsule of the hip joint is an irregular, dense fibrous structure with longitudinal and oblique fibers and with three thickened regions that constitute the capsular ligaments.[7,32] The capsule is attached proximally to the entire periphery of the acetabulum beyond the acetabular labrum.[7] Fibers near the proximal attachment are aligned in a somewhat circumferential manner.[7,32] The capsule itself is thickened anterosuperiorly, where the predominant stresses occur; it is relatively thin and loosely attached posteroinferiorly,[7] with some areas of the capsule thin enough to be nearly translucent.[32] The capsule covers the femoral head and neck like a cylindrical sleeve and attaches to the base of the femoral neck. The femoral neck is intracapsular, whereas both the greater and lesser trochanters are extracapsular. The synovial membrane lines the inside of the capsule. Anteriorly, there are longitudinal retinacular fibers deep in the capsule that travel along the neck toward the femoral head.[7] The retinacular fibers carry blood vessels that are the major source of nutrition to the femoral head and neck.[1] The retinacular blood vessels arise from a vascular ring located at the base of the neck and formed by the medial and lateral circumflex arteries (branches of the deep femoral artery).

As with the other joints already described, there are numerous bursae associated with the hip joint. Although as many as 20 bursae have been described, there are commonly recognized to be three primary or important bursae.[15,33,34] Because the bursae are more strongly associated with the hip joint muscles rather than its capsule, the bursae will be described with their corresponding musculature.

■ Hip Joint Ligaments

The **ligamentum teres** is an intra-articular but extrasynovial accessory joint structure. The ligament is a triangular band attached at one end to both sides of the peripheral edge of the acetabular notch. The ligament then passes under the transverse acetabular ligament (with which it blends) to attach at its other end to the fovea of the femur; thus, it is also called the **ligament of the head of the femur** (Fig. 10-11). The ligamentum teres is encased in a flattened sleeve of synovial membrane so that it does not communicate with the synovial cavity of the joint. The material properties of the ligament of the head are similar to those of other ligaments,[35] and it is tensed in semiflexion and adduction.[7] However, it does not appear to play a significant role in joint stabilization regardless of joint position.[36] Rather, the ligamentum teres appears to function primarily as a conduit for the secondary blood supply from the obturator artery and for the nerves that travel along the ligament to reach the head of the femur through the fovea.

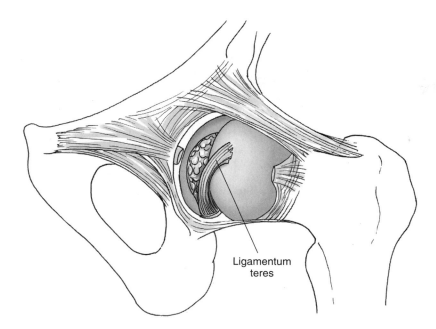

◄ **Figure 10-11** ■ Anterior view of a right hip shows the centrally located ligamentum teres arising from the fovea on the femoral head. The joint capsule and other structures have been removed.

Continuing Exploration: **Blood Supply to the Femoral Head**

The importance of the secondary blood supply carried by the ligamentum teres will vary across the life span, with a greater contribution to be made in childhood. While a child is still growing, the primary retinacular vessels (the medial and lateral circumflex arteries) cannot travel through the avascular cartilaginous epiphysis but must travel across the surface, where the vessels are more vulnerable to disruption. Crock[37] proposed that the femoral head was supplied predominantly by the blood vessels of the ligamentum teres until bony maturation and epiphyseal closure. However, Tan and Wong[38] found the ligament absent in 10% of their examined specimens. The vessels of the ligament of the head are commonly sclerosed in elderly persons.[1] In elderly persons, therefore, the secondary blood supply cannot be counted on to back up the primary retinacular supply when that supply is disrupted by such problems as femoral neck fracture.[38] The absence of a secondary blood supply to the head increases the risk of avascular necrosis of the femoral head with femoral neck trauma.

The hip joint capsule is typically considered to have three reinforcing capsular ligaments (two anteriorly and one posteriorly), although some investigators have further divided or otherwise renamed the ligaments.[9,36] For purposes of understanding hip joint function, the following three traditional descriptions appear to suffice. The two anterior ligaments are the **iliofemoral ligament** and the **pubofemoral ligament**. The iliofemoral ligament is a fan-shaped ligament that resembles an inverted letter Y (Fig. 10-12). It often is referred to as the **Y ligament of Bigelow**. The apex of the ligament is attached to the anterior inferior iliac spine, and the two arms of the Y fan out to attach along the intertrochanteric line of the femur. The superior band of the iliofemoral ligament is the strongest and thickest of the hip joint ligaments.[9] The pubofemoral ligament (see Fig. 10-12) is also anteriorly located, arising from the

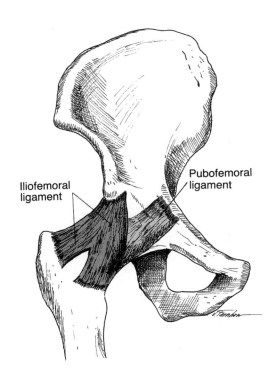

▲ **Figure 10-12** ■ Anterior view of the right hip joint shows the two bands of the iliofemoral (Y) ligament and the more inferiorly located pubofemoral ligament.

anterior aspect of the pubic ramus and passing to the anterior surface of the intertrochanteric fossa. The bands of the iliofemoral and the pubofemoral ligaments form a Z on the anterior capsule, similar to that of the glenohumeral ligaments. The **ischiofemoral ligament** is the posterior capsular ligament. The ischiofemoral ligament (Fig. 10-13) attaches to the posterior surface of the acetabular rim and the acetabulum labrum. Some of its fibers spiral around the femoral neck and blend with the fibers of the circumferential fibers of the capsule. Other fibers are arranged horizontally and attach to the inner surface of the greater trochanter.

There is at the hip joint, as at other joints, some disagreement as to the roles of the joint ligaments. Fuss and Bacher[36] provided an excellent summary of the similarities and discrepancies to be found among of a number of investigators. It may be sufficient to conclude, however, that each of the hip joint motions will be checked by at least one portion of one of the hip joint ligaments[36] and that the forces transmitted by the ligaments (and capsule) are dependent on orientation of the femur in relation to the acetabulum.[32] There is consensus that the hip joint capsule and the majority of its ligaments are quite strong and that each tightens with full hip extension (hyperextension). However, there is also evidence that the anterior ligaments are stronger (stiffer and withstanding greater force at failure) than the ischiofemoral ligament.[39] The capsule and ligaments permit little or no joint distraction even under strong traction forces. When a dysplastic hip is completely dislocated, the capsule and ligaments are

strong enough to support the femoral head in weight-bearing. In these unusual conditions, the stresses on the capsule imposed by the femoral head may lead to impregnation of the capsule with cartilage cells that contribute to a sliding surface for the head.[40]

Under normal circumstances, the hip joint, its capsule, and ligaments routinely support two thirds of the body weight (the weight of head, arms, and trunk, or HAT). In bilateral stance, the hip joint is typically in neutral position or slight extension. In this position, the capsule and ligaments are under some tension.[9] The normal line of gravity (LoG) in bilateral stance falls behind the hip joint axis, creating a gravitational extension moment. Further hip joint extension creates additional passive tension in the capsuloligamentous complex that is sufficient to offset the gravitation extension moment. As long as the LoG falls behind the hip joint axis, the capsuloligamentous structures are adequate to support the superimposed body weight in symmetrical bilateral stance without active or passive assistance from the muscles crossing the hip.

■ Capsuloligamentous Tension

Hip joint extension, with slight abduction and medial rotation, is the close-packed position for the hip joint.[7] With increased extension, the ligaments twist around the femoral head and neck, drawing the head into the acetabulum. In contrast to most other joints in the body, the close-packed and stable position for the hip joint is *not* the position of optimal articular contact (congruence). As already noted, optimal articular contact occurs with combined flexion, abduction, and lateral rotation. Under circumstances in which the joint surfaces are *neither* maximally congruent *nor* close-packed, the hip joint is at greatest risk for traumatic dislocation. A position of particular vulnerability occurs when the hip joint is flexed and adducted (as it is when sitting with the thighs crossed). In this position, a strong force up the femoral shaft toward the hip joint (as when the knee hits the dashboard in a car accident) may push the femoral head out of the acetabulum.[9,30]

The capsuloligamentous tension at the hip joint is least when the hip is in moderate flexion, slight abduction, and midrotation. In this position, the normal intra-articular pressure is minimized, and the capacity of the synovial capsule to accommodate abnormal amounts of fluid is greatest.[28] This is the position assumed by the hip when there is pain arising from capsuloligamentous problems or from excessive intra-articular pressure caused by extra fluid (blood or synovial fluid) in the joint. Extra fluid in the joint may be a result of such conditions as synovitis of the hip joint or bleeding in the joint from tearing of blood vessels with femoral neck fracture. Wingstrand and colleagues[28] proposed that minimizing intra-articular pressure not only decreases pain in the joint but also prevents the excessive pressure from compressing the intra-articular blood vessels and interfering with the blood supply to the femoral head.

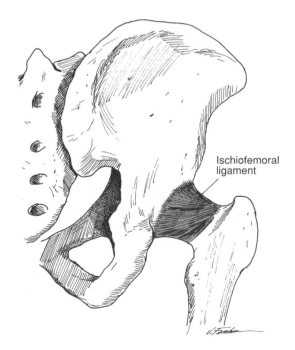

Ischiofemoral ligament

▲ **Figure 10-13** ■ Posterior view of a right hip joint shows that the spiral fibers of the ischiofemoral ligament are tightened during hyperextension and therefore limit hyperextension.

Structural Adaptations to Weight-Bearing

The internal architecture of the pelvis and femur reveal the remarkable interaction between mechanical stresses and structural adaptation created by the transmission of forces between the femur and the pelvis. The trabeculae (calcified plates of tissue within the cancellous bone) line up along lines of stress and form systems that normally adapt to stress requirements. The trabeculae are quite evident on bony cross-section, as seen in Figure 10-14, along with some of the other structural elements of the hip joint.

In Chapter 4, we followed the line of weight-bearing through the vertebrae of the spinal column to the sacral promontory and on through the sacroiliac joints. Most of the weight-bearing stresses in the pelvis pass from the sacroiliac joints to the acetabulum.[7] In standing or upright weight-bearing activities, at least half the weight of the HAT (the gravitational force) passes down through the pelvis to the femoral head, whereas the ground reaction force (GRF) travels up the shaft. These two forces, nearly parallel and in opposite directions, create a force couple with a moment arm (MA) equal to the distance between the superimposed body weight on the femoral head and the GRF up the shaft. These forces create a bending moment (or set of shear forces) across the femoral neck[41] (Fig. 10-15). The bending stress creates a tensile force on the superior aspect of

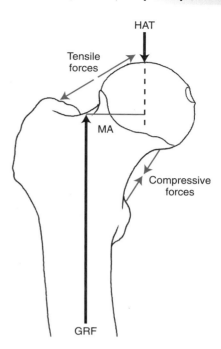

▲ **Figure 10-15** ■ The weight-bearing line of the head, arms, and trunk (HAT) loads the head of the femur, whereas the ground reaction force (GRF) comes up the shaft of the femur, resulting in a force couple that creates a bending moment, with a moment arm (MA) that is dependent on the length and angle of the neck of the femur. The bending moment creates tensile stress on the superior aspect of the femoral neck and compressive stress on the inferior aspect.

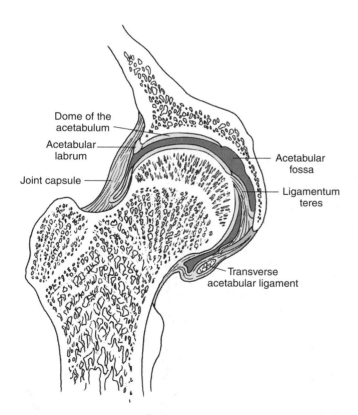

▲ **Figure 10-14** ■ The trabeculae of the femur line up along lines of stress in the cancellous bone and can be seen on cross-section.

the femoral neck and a compressive stress on the inferior aspect. A complex set of forces prevents the rotation and resists the shear forces that the force couple causes; among these forces are the structural resistance of two major and three minor **trabecular systems** (Fig. 10-16).

The medial (or principal compressive) trabecular system arises from the medial cortex of the upper femoral shaft and radiates through the cancellous bone to the cortical bone of the superior aspect of the femoral head. The medial system of trabeculae is oriented along the vertical compressive forces passing through the hip joint.[9] The lateral (or principal tensile) trabecular system of the femur arises from the lateral cortex of the upper femoral shaft and, after crossing the medial system, terminates in the cortical bone on the inferior aspect of the head of the femur. The lateral trabecular system is oblique and may develop in response to parallel (shear) forces of the weight of HAT and the GRF.[9] There are two accessory (or secondary) trabecular systems, of which one is considered compressive and the other is considered tensile.[42] Another secondary trabecular system is confined to the trochanteric area femur.[9,42] Heller and colleagues used data from instrumented *in vivo* hip prostheses and mathematical modeling to conclude that the loading environment in the femur during activity was largely compressive, with relatively small shear forces.[27]

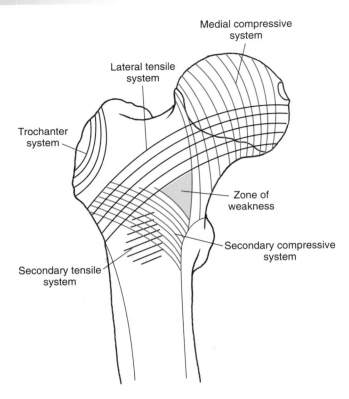

▲ **Figure 10-16** ■ Two major (the medial compressive and lateral tensile) trabecular systems show the primary transmission of forces. Additional lines of stress are evident at the secondary compressive and tensile systems and at the trochanteric system.

The areas in which the trabecular systems cross each other at right angles are areas that offer the greatest resistance to stress and strain. There is an area in the femoral neck in which the trabeculae are relatively thin and do not cross each other. This **zone of weakness** has less reinforcement and thus more potential for failure. The zone of weakness of the femoral neck is particularly susceptible to the bending forces across the area and can fracture either when forces are excessive or when compromised bony composition reduces the tissue's ability to resist typical forces.

Continuing Exploration: **Femoral Neck Stresses**

Although the zone of weakness in the cancellous bone has received a great deal of attention as a factor in hip fracture, Crabtree and colleagues[43] used data from patients and cadavers with a hip fracture to conclude that the cortical bone in the femoral neck supports at least 50% of the load placed on the proximal femur. They suggested that compromise of cortical bone may be more of a factor in fracture than diminished cancellous bone. A more detailed description of the problems of hip fracture will be presented later in the chapter.

The primary weight-bearing surface of the acetabulum, or **dome** of the acetabulum, is located on the superior portion of the lunate surface[44,45] (see Fig. 10-14). In the normal hip, the dome lies directly over the cen-

ter of rotation of the femoral head.[45] Genda and colleagues,[6] using radiographs and modeling, found peak contact pressures during unilateral stance to be located near the dome but with some variation that was positively correlated with CE angle. They also found that the contact area was significantly smaller in women than in men and that the peak contact forces were higher in women. The dome shows the greatest prevalence of degenerative changes in the acetabulum.[44] The primary weight-bearing area of the femoral head is, correspondingly, its superior portion.[44] Although the primary weight-bearing area of the acetabulum is subject to the most degenerative changes, degenerative changes in the femoral head are most common around or immediately below the fovea or around the peripheral edges of the head's articular surface.

Athanasiou and colleagues[44] proposed that the variations in material properties, creep characteristics, and thickness may explain the differences in response of articular cartilage in the acetabular and femoral primary weight-bearing areas. If loading of the hip joint is necessary to achieve congruence and optimize load distribution between the larger femoral head and the acetabulum,[11] persisting incongruence in the dome of the acetabulum in the moderately loaded hip (especially in young adults) could result in incomplete compression of the dome cartilage and, therefore, inadequate fluid exchange to maintain cartilage nutrition.[44] The superior femoral head receives compression not only from the dome in standing but also from the posterior acetabulum in sitting and the anterior acetabulum in extension. The more frequent and complete compression of the cartilage of the superior femoral head, according to this premise, accounts for better nutrition within the cartilage. It must be remembered, however, that avascular articular cartilage is dependent on both *compression* and *release* to move nutrients through the tissue; both too little compression and excessive compression can lead to compromise of the cartilage structure.

The forces of HAT and GRF that act on the articular surfaces of the hip joint and on the femoral head and neck also act on the femoral shaft. The shaft of the femur is not vertical but lies at an angle that varies considerably among individuals. However, the vertical loading on the oblique femur results in bending stresses in the shaft.[9,46] The medial cortical bone in the shaft (diaphysis) must resist compressive stresses, whereas the lateral cortical bone must resist tensile stresses (Fig. 10-17).

◆ Function of the Hip Joint

Motion of the Femur on the Acetabulum

The motions of the hip joint are easiest to visualize as movement of the convex femoral head within the concavity of the acetabulum as the femur moves through its three degrees of freedom: flexion/extension, abduction/adduction, and medial/lateral rotation. The femoral head will glide within the acetabulum in a

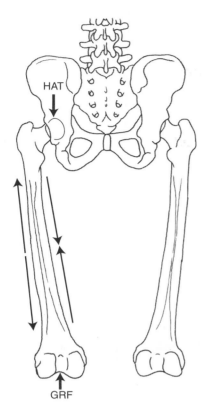

▲ **Figure 10-17** ■ The weight-bearing line (HAT) from the center of rotation of the femoral head and the ground reaction force (GRF) causes a bending force on the shaft of the femur that results in compressive forces medially and tensile forces laterally.

direction opposite to motion of the distal end of the femur. Flexion and extension of the femur occur from a neutral position as an almost pure spin of the femoral head around a coronal axis through the head and neck of the femur. The head spins posteriorly in flexion and anteriorly in extension. However, flexion and extension from other positions (e.g., in abduction or medial rotation) must include both spinning and gliding of the articular surfaces, depending on the combination of motions. The motions of abduction/adduction and medial/lateral rotation must include both spinning and gliding of the femoral head within the acetabulum, but the intra-articular motion again occurs in a direction opposite to motion of the distal end of the femur.

As is true at most joints, the joint's range of motion (ROM) is influenced by structural elements, as well as by whether the motion is performed actively or passively and whether passive tension in two-joint muscles is encountered or avoided. The following ranges of passive joint motion are typical of the hip joint.[47] Flexion of the hip is generally about 90° with the knee extended and 120° when the knee is flexed and when passive tension in the two-joint **hamstrings** muscle group is released. Hip extension is considered to have a range of 10° to 30°. Hip extension ROM appears to diminish somewhat with age, whereas flexion remains relatively unchanged.[48] When hip extension is combined with knee flexion, passive tension in the two-joint **rectus femoris** muscle may limit the movement. The femur

can be abducted 45° to 50° and adducted 20° to 30°. Abduction can be limited by the two-joint **gracilis** muscle and adduction limited by the **tensor fascia lata (TFL)** muscle and its associated **iliotibial (IT) band**. Medial and lateral rotation of the hip are usually measured with the hip joint in 90° of flexion; the typical range is 42° to 50°. Femoral anteversion is correlated with decreased range of lateral rotation and less strongly with increased range of medial rotation.[8] When the femoral head is torsioned anteriorly more than normal (Fig. 10-18), lateral rotation of the femur turns the head out even more, both risking subluxation and encountering capsuloligamentous and muscular restrictions on the anterior aspect of the joint as the head presses forward. Hip joint rotation can correspondingly be affected by retroversion of the femur, as well as by acetabular anteversion and laxity of the joint capsule.[26]

Normal gait on level ground requires at least the following hip joint ranges: 30° flexion, 10° hyperextension, 5° of both abduction and adduction, and 5° of both medial and lateral rotation.[27,28] Walking on uneven terrain or stairs will increase the need for joint range beyond that required for level ground, as will activities such as sitting in a chair or sitting cross-legged.

Case Application 10-3: **Range of Motion in the Dysplastic Hip**

What we know of Gloria's findings on passive ROM testing and her gait correspond to her femoral anteversion on the left. In the supine position on the examination table (hip extended), she has more hip joint medial than lateral rotation (although medial rotation with hip flexion is limited by pain). In her case, her shallow acetabulum increases the tendency for joint subluxation with lateral rotation of the hip. In walking, Gloria's left foot is toed

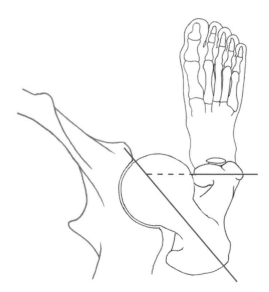

▲ **Figure 10-18** ■ In the supine position with the femoral condyles parallel to the supporting surface, the anteverted femoral head is exposed anteriorly. Lateral rotation will be limited, but medial rotation is relatively excessive.

out less than her right. With an anteverted femur, the hip joint in weight-bearing commonly rotates medially (Fig. 10-19). This may be the body's way of maximizing congruence on the weight-bearing joint, or it may be to minimize stretch on the proprioceptor-rich anterior capsule. The "penalty" for increased hip joint congruence is that the femoral condyles (and the patella that sits on the condyles) are medially rotated as well. When the torsional deformity of the femur is recognized by the deviant positioning of the patella and femoral condyles, the pathology is often referred to as medial femoral torsion.[49] Gloria's foot would be more toed-in than she demonstrates, but it appears that Gloria, like many persons with femoral anteversion (medial femoral torsion), has also developed an excessive lateral tibial torsion.

Motion of the Pelvis on the Femur

Whenever the hip joint is weight-bearing, the femur is relatively fixed, and, in fact, motion of the hip joint is produced by movement of the pelvis on the femur. At all joints, the motion between articular surfaces is the same whether the distal lever moves or the proximal lever moves. However, the proximal lever and distal lever move in opposite directions to produce the same articular motion. For example, elbow flexion can be a rotation of the distal forearm upward or, conversely, a rotation of the proximal humerus downward. In examinations of the upper extremity joint complexes thus far, motion of the distal lever functionally tended to predominate, and so this apparent reversal of motions was not a point of discussion. At the hip joint, this reversal of motion of the lever is further complicated by the

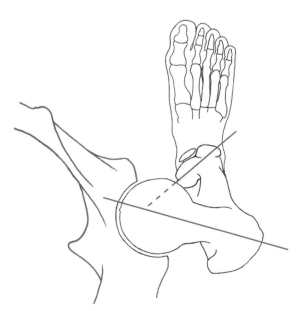

▲ **Figure 10-19 ■** In standing, the anteverted femur tends to medially rotate within the acetabulum, resulting in medial rotation of the femoral condyles in relation to the plane of progression. The torsional deformity of the femur, when assessed in standing, is referred to as medial femoral torsion. If there is an accompanying lateral tibial torsion, the expected toe-in may be minimized or reversed.

horizontal orientation and shape of the pelvis (the "levers" of the hip are not in line but lie essentially perpendicular to each other). In contrast to other joints, there is also a new set of terms to identify joint motion when the pelvis (rather than femur) is the moving segment. The terms for pelvic motions are used with weight-bearing hip motion because the motions of the pelvis are more apparent to the eye of the examiner and are, in fact, key to what occurs at the joints above and below the pelvis. It must be emphasized, however, that the motion of the pelvis presented in the next sections are *not new motions of the hip joint* but are simply how the same three degrees of freedom for the joint are accomplished by the pelvis rather than the femur.

■ Anterior and Posterior Pelvic Tilt

Anterior and posterior pelvic tilt are motions of the entire pelvic ring in the sagittal plane around a coronal axis. In the normally aligned pelvis, the anterosuperior iliac spines (ASISs) of the pelvis lie on a horizontal line with the posterior superior iliac spines and on a vertical line with the symphysis pubis[50] (Fig. 10-20A). Anterior and posterior tilting of the pelvis on the fixed femur produce hip flexion and extension, respectively. Hip joint extension through posterior tilting of the pelvis brings the symphysis pubis up and the sacrum of the pelvis closer to the femur, rather than moving the femur posteriorly on the pelvis (see Fig. 10-20B). Hip flexion through anterior tilting of the pelvis moves the ASISs anteriorly and inferiorly; the inferior sacrum moves farther from the femur, rather than moving the femur away from the sacrum (see Fig. 10-20C). Anterior and posterior tilting will result in flexion and extension of both hip joints simultaneously in bilateral stance or can occur at the stance hip joint alone if the opposite limb is non–weight-bearing.

CONCEPT CORNERSTONE 10-1: *Anterior/Posterior Pelvic Tilt versus Torsion*

Clinicians who evaluate and treat sacroiliac joint dysfunction may attempt to diagnose someone as having asymmetry in the sagittal plane between the two halves of the pelvis (ilia or innominate bones). There are a number of terms used to label this imbalance that are beyond this discussion. However, when the imbalance is referred to as anterior or posterior torsion—or, more confusingly, anterior or posterior tilt—the potential for confusion for the novice is great. When the terms anterior/posterior torsion or anterior/posterior tilt are used in reference to the sacroiliac joint and sacroiliac joint dysfunction, these terms generally need to be distinguished as different from anterior/posterior tilt of the entire pelvis, in which the pelvis is considered to, in effect, move as a single fixed unit. In this chapter and through this text, **anterior/posterior tilt** of the pelvis will be used exclusively to refer to the pelvis as a fixed unit.

■ Lateral Pelvic Tilt

Lateral pelvic tilt is a frontal plane motion of the entire pelvis around an anteroposterior axis. In the normally aligned pelvis, a line through the ASISs is horizontal. In

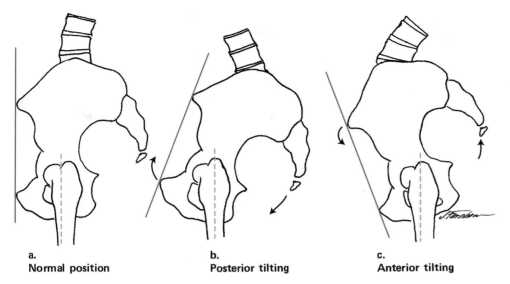

◀ **Figure 10-20** ■ Flexion and extension of the hip occurring as tilting of the pelvis in the sagittal plane. **A.** The pelvis is shown in its normal position in erect stance. **B.** Posterior tilting of the pelvis moves the symphysis pubis superiorly on the fixed femur. The hip joint extends. **C.** In anterior tilting, the anterior superior iliac spines move inferiorly on the fixed femur. The hip joint flexes.

a. **Normal position** b. **Posterior tilting** c. **Anterior tilting**

lateral tilt of the pelvis in unilateral stance, one hip joint is the pivot point or axis for motion of the *opposite* side of the pelvis as it elevates (pelvic hiking) or drops (pelvic drop). If a person stands on the left limb and hikes the pelvis, the left hip joint is being abducted because the medial angle between the femur and a line through the ASISs increases (Fig. 10-21A). If a person stands on the left leg and drops the pelvis, the left hip joint will adduct because the medial angle formed by the femur and a line through the ASISs will decrease (see Fig. 10-21B).

In descriptions of the hip joint motions that occur in unilateral stance, the hip joint of the non–weight-bearing limb is in an open chain and has no motions on it. However, the non–weight-bearing leg typically hangs straight down as the pelvis moves.

 Concept Cornerstone 10-2: *Pelvic Hike and Pelvic Drop*

Identifying the motions of pelvic hike or pelvic drop in lateral pelvic tilt often confuses the examiner because the eye tends to follow the iliac crest on the *same* side as the supporting hip joint rather than the opposite side. Because the hip joint is not at the end of

the pelvic lever but is offset quite a bit (more medially located), the eye can be fooled because the end of the pelvis opposite the supporting hip joint moves in the opposite direction to the end of the pelvis nearest the supporting hip joint. In Figure 10-21A and B, the gray arrows indicate the side of the pelvis that the eye might be tempted to follow, but the arrows are also "crossed" out to indicate that the wrong side of the pelvis is being referenced. Although it may not have been necessary to specify this previously, it should also be kept in mind that, in naming motions of levers, the motion of the end of the lever *farthest from the joint axis* is *always* referenced. Lateral pelvic tilt is named (and should be observed) by what is happening to the side of the pelvis opposite the supporting hip in unilateral stance. The weightbearing hip in unilateral stance will always be the axis of rotation, and the opposite side of the pelvis will always identify the movement. If a woman is standing on her right leg and hikes her pelvis, it should not be necessary to specify that the left side of the pelvis is the one that is rising. Because the right hip joint is the axis, the motion is defined by movement of the left side of the pelvis.

Lateral Shift of the Pelvis

Lateral pelvic tilt can also occur in bilateral stance. If both feet are on the ground and the hip and knee of

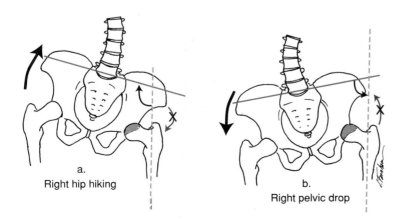

a. **Right hip hiking** b. **Right pelvic drop**

◀ **Figure 10-21** ■ Lateral tilting of the pelvis around the left can occur either as hip hiking (elevation of the opposite side of the pelvis) or as pelvic drop (drop of the opposite side of the pelvis). **A.** Hiking of the pelvis around the left hip joint results in left hip abduction. **B.** Dropping of the pelvis around the left hip joint results in left hip joint adduction. Although it is visually tempting to name the direction of lateral tilt by the motion of the side of the pelvis *nearest* the hip (gray arrows that are "crossed out"), this is incorrect.

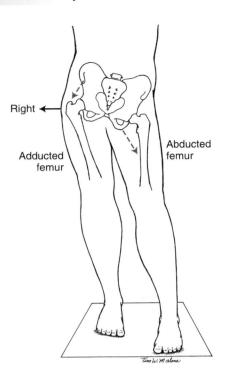

▲ **Figure 10-22** ■ When the pelvis is shifted to the right in bilateral stance, the right hip joint will be adducted and the left hip joint will be abducted. To return to neutral position while continuing to bear weight on both feet, the right abductor and left adductor muscles work synergistically to shorten and shift the weight back to center.

one limb are flexed, the opposite limb is largely the weight-bearing limb and the terminology is the same as for unilateral stance. However, if both limbs are weight-bearing, lateral tilt of the pelvis will cause the pelvis to shift to one side or the other. With pelvic shift, the pelvis cannot hike but can only drop. Because there is a closed chain between the two weight-bearing feet and the pelvis, both hip joints will move in the frontal plane in a predictable way as the pelvic tilt (or pelvic shift) occurs. If the pelvis is shifted to the right in bilateral stance, the left side of the pelvis will drop, the right hip joint will be adducted, and the left hip joint will be abducted (Fig. 10-22).

■ Anterior and Posterior Pelvic Rotation

Pelvic rotation is motion of the entire pelvic ring in the transverse plane around a vertical axis. Although rotation can occur around a vertical axis through the middle of the pelvis in bilateral stance, it most commonly and more importantly occurs in single-limb support around the axis of the supporting hip joint. Forward rotation of the pelvis occurs in unilateral stance when the side of the pelvis *opposite to the supporting hip* joint moves anteriorly (Fig. 10-23A). Forward rotation of the pelvis produces medial rotation of the supporting hip joint. Backward rotation of the pelvis occurs when the side of the pelvis opposite the supporting hip moves posteriorly (see Fig. 10-23C). Posterior rotation of the pelvis produces lateral rotation of the supporting hip joint.

Pelvic rotation can occur in bilateral stance as well as unilateral stance, as is true for lateral pelvic tilt. If both feet are bearing weight and the axis of motion occurs around a vertical axis through the center of the pelvis, the terms forward rotation and backward rotation must be used by referencing a side (e.g., forward rotation on the right and backward rotation on the left).

 CONCEPT CORNERSTONE 10-3: *Pelvic Rotation and Hip Joint Rotation*

In referencing forward and backward rotation, we must again make sure that the *opposite* side of the pelvis from the axis of rotation is the reference. In Figure 10-23, the gray arrows again indicate the side the eye often erroneously follows (and so are "crossed out"). If it is known which leg a person is standing on in unilateral stance, identifying forward or backward rotation of the pelvis around that hip should not also require naming the side of the pelvis that is referenced.

The relative rotation of the hip that occurs with forward or backward rotation of the pelvis in unilateral stance is often difficult for the novice to identify. The rotation of the hip joint that occurs during rotation of the pelvis can best be appreciated by performing the motion yourself. Standing on one leg and rotating the pelvis and trunk forward as much as possible will give a clear "feeling" of the relative medial rotation of the supporting limb. Similarly, rotating the pelvis backward as far as possible will give the feeling of the relative lateral rotation of the stance hip joint.

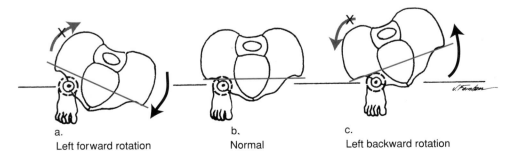

a.
Left forward rotation

b.
Normal

c.
Left backward rotation

◀ **Figure 10-23** ■ A superior view of rotation of the pelvis in the transverse plane. **A.** Forward rotation of the pelvis around the right hip joint results in medial rotation of the right hip joint. **B.** Neutral position of the pelvis and the right hip joint. **C.** Backward rotation of the pelvis around the right hip joint results in lateral rotation of the right hip joint. The reference for forward and backward rotation is the side *opposite* the supporting hip, although the eye often erroneously catches the opposite motion of the pelvis on the same side (gray crossed-out arrows).

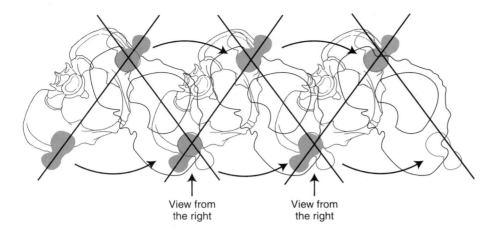

View from
the right   View from
the right

◀ **Figure 10-24** ■ This schematic representation of a superior view of the pelvis is shown forwardly rotating sequentially around the left and right hips during gait (the rotation is exaggerated to make the point more clearly). Observation of the right side of the pelvis alone will give the illusion of the pelvis forwardly and backwardly rotating sequentially.

Continuing Exploration: **Pelvic Rotation in Gait**

One exception to the convention of naming pelvic rotation as the side opposite the supporting hip may occur in observational gait analysis. In normal gait, the pelvis forwardly rotates around the weight-bearing hip while the other limb prepares for or is in swing.[51] Because this happens first on one leg and then on the other, it appears to the eye as if the pelvis is forwardly rotating and then backwardly rotation (Fig. 10-24). Because gait is often observed for one side of the body (the referent side) at a time, the pelvis may be identified as forwardly rotating during swing of the referent side and backwardly rotating during stance of the referent limb.[52] This terminology, although useful during observation, is misleading and misrepresents both the pelvic and hip joint motions during normal gait.

Coordinated Motions of the Femur, Pelvis, and Lumbar Spine

When the pelvis moves on a relatively fixed femur, there are two possible outcomes to consider. Either the head and trunk will follow the motion of the pelvis (moving the head through space) or the head will continue to remain relatively upright and vertical despite the pelvic motions. These are open- and closed-chain responses, respectively. Each of these two situations produces very different reactions from the joints and segments proximal and distal to the hip joints and pelvis and must be examined separately.

■ Pelvifemoral Motion

When the femur, pelvis, and spine move in a coordinated manner to produce a larger ROM than is available to one segment alone, the hip joint is participating in what will predominantly (but not exclusively) be an open-chain motion termed **pelvifemoral motion**. Pelvifemoral motion can be considered analogous to scapulohumeral motion because the combination of motions at several joints serves to increase the range available to the distal segment. In the case of scapulo-

humeral motion, the joints are serving the hand. In the case of pelvifemoral motion, the joints may serve either end of the chain: the foot or head.

Example 10-1

Moving the Head and Arms through Space

If the goal is to bend forward to bring the hands (and head) toward the floor, isolated flexion at the hip joints (anteriorly tilting the pelvis on the femurs) is generally insufficient to reach the ground. *If* the knees remain extended, the hips will typically flex no more than 90° (and often less, depending on extensibility of the hamstrings). The addition of flexion of the lumbar spine (and, perhaps, flexion of the thoracic spine) will add to the total ROM (Fig. 10-25). The combination of hip

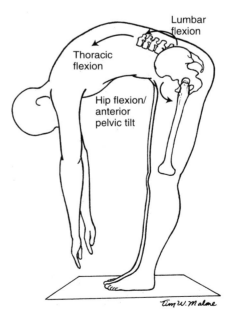

Lumbar flexion

Thoracic flexion

Hip flexion/ anterior pelvic tilt

Tim W. Malone

▲ **Figure 10-25** ■ Pelvifemoral motion can increase the range of forward flexion of the head and arms by combining hip flexion, anterior pelvic tilt, and flexion of the lumbar spine. This combination permits the hands to maximize the reach toward the ground.

and trunk flexion is generally sufficient for the hands to reach the ground—as long as the hamstrings and lumbar extensors allow sufficient lengthening. The combination of hip motion and lumbar motion to achieve a greater ROM for the hands and head is an example of a largely open-chain response in the hips and trunk. [*Side-bar:* Please note that this is *not* an example of how to reach the floor to pick up an object!] The open-chain response (the ability of each joint in the chain to move independently) is somewhat constrained (largely at the ankles) by the need to keep the LoG within the base of support.

Example 10-2

Moving the Foot through Space

When a person is lying on the right side, the left foot may be moved through an arc of motion approaching 90° (Fig. 10-26). This is clearly not all from the left hip joint, which can typically abduct only to 45°; motion of the foot through space also includes lateral tilting of the pelvis (hiking around the right hip joint) and lateral flexion of the lumbar spine to the left. The abducting limb is in an open chain; the lumbar spine (and thoracic spine) are constrained by the body weight and contact with the ground.

Pelvifemoral motion has also been referred to as **pelvifemoral "rhythm,"** which implies a continuous relationship between the two segments, which is arguable because the relative contributions can vary among individuals and in different activities. Bohannon and colleagues determined that pelvic rotation contributed between 30% and 46% of the total range of a passive straight leg raise.[53] During active maximal hip flexion (knee flexed) in standing, Murray and colleagues found that the pelvis contributed between 8% and 32% of the total motion, with an even greater variability among individuals (9% to 53%) when a 4.53-kg ankle weight was added.[54] The link between hip, pelvis, and lumbar motion is the basis of using pain with active straight-leg raising as a test for severity of dysfunction in persons with low back pain.[55,56]

■ Closed-Chain Hip Joint Function

The joints of the right and left lower limbs are part of a true closed chain when both lower limbs are weight-bearing and the chain is defined as all the segments between the right foot, up through the pelvis, and down through the left foot. A true closed chain is formed because both ends of the chain (both feet in this example) are "fixed" and movement at any one joint in the chain invariably involves movement at one or more other links in the chain. It is also common usage to consider that the joints of one or both lower limbs are part of a closed chain whenever a person is standing (weight-bearing) on one or both lower limbs, which leads to inappropriately considering the terms "weight-bearing" and "closed chain" to be interchangeable.[57] The lower limbs were weight-bearing in Example 10-1 but were effectively part of an open chain. Consequently, weight-bearing and closed chain cannot be synonymous. How, then, do the joints of the lower extremity function in a closed chain in standing?

For the hips (and other lower limb joints) to be in a closed chain in standing, both ends of the chain (the head and the feet) must be fixed. The feet are, in fact, fixed by weight-bearing. The head, however, is often (but not necessarily) functionally "fixed." Although the head is certainly free to move in space, the head most often remains upright and vertically oriented during upright activities. The drive to keep the head upright is due, in part, to the influence of the tonic labyrinthine and optical righting reflexes that are normally evident almost immediately at birth[58] and continue to operate throughout life. The drive to keep the head upright and over the sacrum will effectively *fix the head in relative space* even though this is not structurally the case; that is, the head is functionally rather than structurally fixed. When the head (one end of the chain) is held

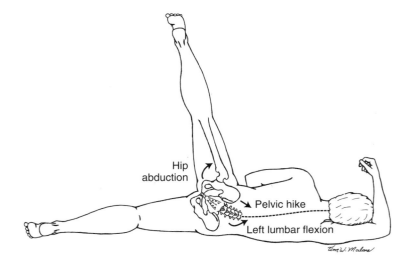

Hip abduction

Pelvic hike

Left lumbar flexion

◀ **Figure 10-26** ■ Pelvifemoral motion increases the range through which the foot can be moved in space by combining left hip abduction, lateral pelvic tilt (left hike), and flexion of the lumbar spine to the left.

upright and over the feet (the other end of the chain), all the segments in the axial skeleton and lower limbs function as part of a closed chain; movement at one joint will create movement in at least one other linkage in the chain. Consequently, in our functional closed-chain premise, hip flexion does not occur independently (which would move the head forward in space) but is accompanied by motion in one or more interposed segments to ensure that the head remains upright over the base of support and that the body does not become unstable.

Example 10-3

Closed-Chain Hip Joint Function

A common example of closed-chain versus open-chain function is seen when the hip flexor musculature is tight and the hip joint is maintained in flexion. A person standing with fixed hip flexion is shown in Figure 10-27A (an open-chain response) and B (a closed-chain response). A true open-chain response to isolated hip flexion would displace the head and trunk forward, with the LoG falling in front of the supporting feet. More commonly, hip flexion in stance is not isolated to the hips but is accompanied by compensatory movements of the vertebral column (including extension or lordosis of the lumbar spine) that maintain the head in the upright position and keep the LoG well within the

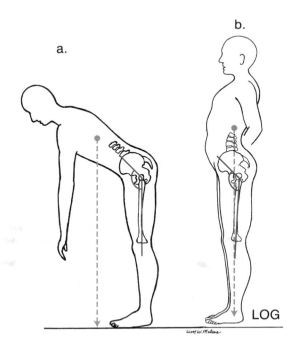

▲ **Figure 10-27** ■ **A.** In an open-chain response to tight hip flexors that is isolated to the hip joints, the trunk will be inclined forward. The line of gravity (LoG) will fall outside the base of support if no other adjustments are made. **B.** In a functional closed-chain response to tight hip flexors, the head seeks to maintain a vertical position; the lumbar spine will extend (become lordotic) to return the head to a position over the sacrum and maintain the LoG within the base of support.

base of support). In a functional closed chain, motion at the hip (one link in the chain) is accompanied by an essentially mandatory lumbar *extension* to maintain the head over the sacrum (see Fig. 10-27B). In contrast, hip flexion in open-chain pelvifemoral motion is accompanied by *lumbar flexion* because the goal is to achieve more range for the head in space (see Fig. 10-25).

Case Application 10-4: **The Hip and Leg Length Discrepancy**

Skeletal shortening of the limb with a developmental hip dysplasia is not unusual. As Gloria stands with her weight evenly distributed between her feet, her pelvis will be laterally tilted (down on the left) as a result of the 1-inch shortening of her left leg. To keep the LoG within the center of her base of support in bilateral stance, Gloria's lumbar spine will be slightly laterally flexed to the right (away from the side of shortening). This is the opposite lumbar motion to what we saw in Example 10-2 because Gloria's goal is to keep her head upright, not to gain range. The lateral flexion of the spine with asymmetrical leg lengths puts a person at risk for low back pain, although this is not one of Gloria's presenting complaints. Interesting, the relative abduction of the left leg that occurs in stance with shortening of Gloria's dysplastic limb may reduce stress on the hip. The abducted position of the hip has the potential to increases congruence slightly, diminishing the peak pressure at the hip joint by distributing the forces over a larger contact area.

In any instance in which there is normal or abnormal pelvic motion during weight-bearing and the head must remain upright, compensatory motions of the lumbar spine will occur if available. This does not rule out the need for compensation at additional joints as well, but the lumbar spine tends to be the "first line of defense." As we examine the other joints of the lower extremity and move on to posture and gait, other compensatory motions will be encountered and discussed. Table 10-1 presents the compensatory motions of the lumbar spine that accompany given motions of the pelvis and hip joint in a functional closed chain.

Hip Joint Musculature

There have been numerous studies of the muscles of the hip joint. Most confirm underlying principles of muscle physiology seen at the other joints we have examined so far. That is, hip joint muscles work best in the middle of their contractile range or on a slight stretch (at so-called optimal length-tension); two-joint muscles generate greatest force when not required to shorten over both joints simultaneously; and tension generation is optimal with eccentric contractions, followed by isometric and then concentric contractions.

The muscles of the hip joint make their most important contributions to function during weight-

Table 10-1	Relationship of Pelvis, Hip Joint, and Lumbar Spine during Right Lower Extremity Weight-Bearing and Upright Posture	
Pelvic Motion	**Accompanying Hip Joint Motion**	**Compensatory Lumbar Spine Motion**
Anterior pelvic tilt	Hip flexion	Lumbar extension
Posterior pelvic tilt	Hip extension	Lumbar flexion
Lateral pelvic tilt (pelvic drop)	Right hip adduction	Right lateral flexion
Lateral pelvic tilt (pelvic hike)	Right hip abduction	Left lateral flexion
Forward rotation	Right hip medial rotation	Rotation to the left
Backward rotation	Right hip lateral rotation	Rotation to the right

bearing. In weight-bearing, the muscles are called on to move or support the HAT (approximately two thirds of body weight) rather than the weight of one lower limb (approximately one sixth of body weight). Consequently, the hip joint muscles adapt their structure to the required function, as can be seen in their large areas of attachment, their length, and their large cross-section. The alignment of the hip joint muscles and the large ROM available at the hip joint result in muscle functions that are strongly influenced by hip joint position. For example, the adductor muscles may be hip flexors in the neutral hip joint but will be hip extensors when the hip joint is already flexed.[59] Delp and colleagues[60] used computer modeling to determine that the torque-generating capability of the medial rotators increased with increased hip flexion, whereas the torque-generating capacity of the lateral rotators decreased with increasing hip flexion. They similarly determined that the **piriformis muscle** was a lateral rotator at 0° of hip flexion but a medial rotator at 90° of hip flexion. Such inversions of function are found in a few muscles at the shoulder (the clavicular portion of the pectoralis major, for example), but are fairly common in the hip joint. As a consequence, results of various studies may appear to be contradictory, but, in fact, testing conditions explain differing results. Some gender-related differences also have been found that explain differential findings.[61]

It is best to examine muscle action at the hip joint in the context of specific functions such as single-limb support, posture, and gait. The next section will briefly review muscle function, but we will leave more detailed analyses for later in this and other chapters. Although the traditional action of each muscle on the distal femoral segment is described for the most part, it must be emphasized that any of the muscles is as likely (or more likely) to produce joint action by moving the proximal pelvic segment instead.

■ Flexors

The flexors of the hip joint function primarily as mobility muscles in open-chain function; that is, they function primarily to bring the swinging limb forward during ambulation or in various sports. The flexors may function secondarily to resist strong hip extension forces that occur as the body passes over the weight-bearing foot. Nine muscles have action lines crossing

the anterior aspect of the hip joint. Of these, the primary muscles of hip flexion are the **iliopsoas,** rectus femoris, TFL, and **sartorius.** The iliopsoas muscle is considered to be the most important of the primary hip flexors. It consists of two separate muscles, the **iliacus** muscle and the **psoas major** muscle, both of which attach to the femur by a common tendon. The two components of the iliopsoas muscle have many points of origin, including the iliac fossa and the disks, bodies, and transverse processes of the lumbar vertebrae. Given the attachments of the psoas major muscle to the anterior vertebrae and the iliacus muscle to the iliac fossa, activity of or passive tension in these muscles would anteriorly tilt the pelvis (iliacus muscle) and, apparently, pull the lumbar vertebrae anteriorly into flexion (psoas major muscle). In closed-chain function (head vertical), however, these muscles seem to create a paradoxical lumbar lordosis (lumbar extension) that results from the body's attempt to keep the head over the sacrum with anterior pelvic tilt and lower lumbar flexion. The role of the iliopsoas muscle in hip flexion may be particularly critical when hip flexion from a sitting position is required. Smith and colleagues[62] proposed that the hip cannot be flexed beyond 90° when the iliopsoas muscle is paralyzed, because the other hip flexor muscles are effectively actively insufficient in that position. Basmajian and DeLuca[59] summarized the often contradictory evidence of many investigations by concluding that both segments of the iliopsoas muscle are active in various stages of hip flexion. The moment arm (MA) of the iliopsoas muscle for medial or lateral rotation is very small and probably not functionally relevant.[59,60]

The rectus femoris muscle is the only portion of the quadriceps muscle that crosses both the hip joint and knee joint. It originates on the anterior inferior iliac spine and inserts by way of a common tendon into the tibial tuberosity. The rectus femoris muscle flexes the hip joint and extends the knee joint. Because it is a two-joint hip flexor, the position of the knee during hip flexion will affect its ability to generate force at the hip. Simultaneous hip flexion and knee extension considerably shorten this muscle and increase the likelihood of active insufficiency. Consequently, the rectus femoris muscle makes its best contribution to hip flexion when the knee is maintained in flexion.

The sartorius muscle is a straplike muscle originating on the ASIS. It crosses the anterior aspect of the femur to insert into the upper portion of the medial aspect of the tibia. The sartorius muscle is considered to be a flexor, abductor, and lateral rotator of the hip, as well as a flexor and medial rotator of the knee. Wheatley and Jahnke[63] proposed that the sartorius muscle, although a two-joint muscle, should be relatively unaffected by the position of the knee, given the relatively small proportional change in length with increased knee flexion. Its function is probably most important when the knee and hip need to be flexed simultaneously (as in climbing stairs), but its small cross-section argues against a unique or critical role at the hip joint.[7]

The TFL muscle originates more laterally than the sartorius muscle. Its origin is on the anterolateral lip of the iliac crest. The muscle fibers extend only about one fourth of the way down the lateral aspect of the thigh before inserting into the IT band. The IT band or IT tract is the thickened lateral portion of the fascia lata of the hip and thigh. The IT band attaches proximally to the iliac crest lateral to the TFL muscle. After the tensor attaches to the IT band, the IT band continues distally on the lateral thigh to insert into the lateral condyle of the tibia. The TFL muscle is considered to flex, abduct, and medially rotate the femur at the hip,[59] although the TFL's contribution to hip abduction may be dependent on simultaneous hip flexion.[64] The most important contribution of the TFL muscle may be in maintaining tension in the IT band. The IT band assists in relieving the femur of some of the tensile stresses imposed on the shaft by weight-bearing forces.[25,64] Because bone more effectively resists compressive than tensile stresses, reduction of tensile stresses is important in maintaining integrity of the bone.[46]

Functionally, it appears that the TFL muscle and IT band are expendable. The IT band may be removed and used for autogenous fascial transplants without any evident change in active or passive hip or knee function.[64] Excessive tension in the IT band may also contribute to reduced hip adduction ROM when the hip is extended. Gajdosik and colleagues[65] performed the Ober test, presumed to test tension in the IT band, on men and women without impairments. They found an average passive hip adduction of 9° for men and 4° for women when both the hip and knee were extended. When the knee was flexed during the maneuver, the hip remained in 4° of abduction for men and 6° of abduction for women, which implied that there was greater tension in the lateral hip joint structures (potentially with the IT band as a key factor) when the knee was flexed.[65] The Ober test presumably moves the IT band from its position anterior to the greater trochanter to a position posterior to the greater trochanter by extending the hip. Movement of the IT band anteriorly and posteriorly over the greater trochanter during functional activities has been implicated in **"snapping hip" syndrome** and in inflammation of the **trochanteric bursa.**[15]

The secondary hip flexors are the **pectineus, adductor longus, adductor magnus,** and the **gracilis** muscles. These muscles are described in the next section because they are predominantly adductors of the hip. Each, however, is capable of contributing to hip joint flexion, but that contribution is dependent on hip joint position. Kapandji[9] noted that these muscles contribute to flexion only up to 40° to 50° of hip flexion. Once the femur is superior to the point of origin of a muscle, the muscle will become an extensor of the hip joint. The gracilis, a two-joint muscle, is active as a hip flexor when the knee is extended but not when the knee is flexed.[63]

■ Adductors

The hip adductor muscle group is generally considered to include the pectineus, **adductor brevis,** adductor longus, adductor magnus, and the gracilis muscles. The adductors are located anteromedially. The adductors longus, brevis, and magnus muscles arise in a group from the body and inferior ramus of the pubis to insert along the linea aspera. The gracilis muscle is the only two-joint adductor. It originates on the symphysis pubis and pubic arch and inserts on the medial surface of the shaft of the tibia.

The contribution of the adductor muscles to hip joint function has been debated for many years. One of the reasons for debate is a question as to the degree to which the flexed, adducted, and medially rotated posture assumed by many individuals with cerebral palsy is attributable to adductor spasticity. Arnold and Delp[26] (using kinematic data from children with cerebral palsy and excessive medial rotation of the hip, and a "deformable femur" model) concluded that, in the normal hip in standing, the adductor brevis, adductor longus, pectineus, and posterior adductor magnus muscles had only small MAs for medial rotation, whereas the gracilis and anterior adductor magnus muscles had small MAs for lateral rotation. With excessive femoral anteversion, the MAs of the adductor brevis, pectineus and the middle gluteus magnus muscles switched from medial rotatory to lateral rotatory lines of pull. After examining the changes in MAs with femoral anteversion or combined hip medial rotation and knee flexion, the investigators concluded that the adductors were unlikely to have a strong influence on the medially rotated hip position during the gait cycle.[26]

Basmajian and DeLuca[59] believed that the variability in study findings for the adductors supported the theory of Janda and Stará[65a] that the adductors function not as prime movers but by reflex response to gait activities. As shall be seen in our discussion of muscle function in bilateral stance, the adductors may be synergists to the abductor muscles when both feet are on the ground, enhancing side-to-side stabilization of the pelvis. Although the role of the adductor muscles may be less clear than that of other hip muscle groups, the relative importance of the adductors should not be underestimated. The adductors as a group contribute 22.5% to the total muscle mass of the lower extremity, in comparison with only 18.4% for the flexors and 14.9% for the abductors.[66] The adductors are also capable of generating a maximum isometric torque greater than that of the abductors.[67]

■ Extensors

The one-joint **gluteus maximus** muscle and the two-joint hamstrings muscle group are the primary hip joint extensors. These muscles may receive assistance from the posterior fibers of the gluteus medius, from the posterior adductor magnus muscle, and from the piriformis muscle. The gluteus maximus is a large, quadrangular muscle that originates from the posterior sacrum, dorsal sacroiliac ligaments, sacrotuberous ligament, and a small portion of the ilium. The gluteus maximus crosses the sacroiliac joint before its most superior fibers insert into the IT band (as do the fibers of the TFL muscle) and its inferior fibers insert into the gluteal tuberosity. The gluteus maximus is the largest of the lower extremity muscles; this muscle alone constituting 12.8% of the total muscle mass of the lower extremity.[66] The maximus is a strong hip extensor that appears to be active primarily against a resistance greater than the weight of the limb. Its MA for hip extension is considerably longer than that of either the hamstrings or the adductor magnus muscles and is maximal in the neutral hip joint position.[61] A favorable length-tension relationship, however, allows it to exert its peak extensor moment at 70° of hip flexion.[68] The segments of the maximus have a substantial capacity to laterally rotate the femur, although the MAs for lateral rotation diminish with increased hip flexion.[60]

The three two-joint extensors are the long head of the **biceps femoris,** the **semitendinosus,** and the **semimembranosus** muscles, known collectively as the hamstrings. Each of these three muscles originates on the ischial tuberosity. The biceps femoris crosses the posterior femur to insert into the head of the fibula and lateral aspect of the lateral tibial condyle. The other two hamstrings insert on the medial aspect of the tibia. All three muscles extend the hip with or without resistance, as well as serving as important knee flexors. The hamstrings increase their MA for hip extension as the hip flexes to 35° and decrease it thereafter. This is somewhat in contrast to the MA of the gluteus maximus that is maximal at neutral position and decreases with any hip flexion thereafter.[61] Regardless of these changes in MA with joint position, the MA of the combined hamstrings for hip extension is smaller than that of the gluteus maximus at all points in the hip flexion/extension ROM. As two-joint muscles, the role of the hamstrings in hip extension is also strongly influenced by knee position. Chleboun and colleagues (using ultrasonography) determined that the MA for the long head of the biceps femoris was greater for hip extension than for knee flexion, with hip position affecting its excursion capability more than did knee position.[69] Although these investigators reported only on the long head of the biceps femoris, the anatomy of the medial hamstrings (semimembranosus and semitendinosus) makes it likely that these muscles have similar attributes. If the hip is extended and the knee is flexed to 90° or more, the hamstrings may not be able to contribute much to hip extension force because of active insufficiency or approaching active insufficiency. Extension forces in the hip increase by 30% if the knee is extended during hip extension.[68] The optimal length-tension relationship for the long head of the biceps is estimated to be at 90° of hip flexion and 90° of knee flexion,[69] and it is likely that the medial hamstrings show similar behavior. The medial hamstrings have a small MA for medial rotation in the neutral hip but appear to switch to lateral rotators with hip flexion or knee flexion.[26] The biceps femoris appears to contribute to lateral rotation of the hip.[59]

■ Abductors

Active abduction of the hip is brought about predominantly by the **gluteus medius** and the **gluteus minimus** muscles. The superior fibers of the gluteus maximus and the sartorius muscles may assist when the hip is abducted against strong resistance. The TFL muscle is given variable credit for its contribution and may be effective as an abductor only during simultaneous hip flexion. The gluteus medius originates on the lateral surface of the wing of the ilium and inserts into the greater trochanter, beneath the gluteus maximus. The gluteus medius has anterior, middle, and posterior parts that function asynchronously during movement at the hip.[70] Analogous to the deltoid muscle of the glenohumeral joint, the anterior fibers of the gluteus medius are active in hip flexion, whereas the posterior fibers function during extension. In the neutral hip, the posterior portion of the medius will produce a lateral rotatory moment, whereas the middle and anterior have small medial rotatory moments. In hip flexion, all portions medially rotate the hip.[60] All portions of the muscle abduct, regardless of hip joint position.

The gluteus minimus muscle lies deep to the gluteus medius, arising from the outer surface of the ilium with its fibers converging on an aponeurosis that ends in a tendon on the greater trochanter. The minimus is consistently an abductor and flexor of the hip, with its rotator function dependent on hip position. However, the minimus is a medial rotator in hip flexion.[71] There appears to be consensus that the gluteus minimus commonly has a tendinous insertion into the joint capsule as it passes to the greater trochanter. It is hypothesized that this attachment retracts the capsule during hip abduction to prevent entrapment[72] or tightens the capsule to add to the gluteus minimus's primary function of stabilizing the femoral head in the acetabulum.[71]

The gluteus minimus and medius muscles function together to either abduct the femur (distal level free) or, more important, to stabilize the pelvis (and superimposed HAT) in unilateral stance against the effects of gravity. As will be presented later, the gluteus medius and minimus muscles will offset the gravitation adduction torque on the pelvis (pelvis drop) around the stance hip. The abductors are physiologically designed to work most effectively in a neutral or slightly adducted hip (slightly lengthened abductors).[73,74] Isometric abduction torque in the neutral hip position is 82% greater than abduction torque when the hip is in 25° of abduction (shortened abductors).[67]

Continuing Exploration: **Trochanteric Bursae**

The greater trochanter has become the focus of increased interest as lateral hip pain syndromes among both the elderly and athletes are diagnosed more often.[15,30,33,34] Although a number of possible pathologies of both intra-articular and extra-articular origin are probably involved, there is consensus that the bursae around the greater trochanter are commonly involved. There does not appear to be consensus on how many discrete bursae there are or how to name them. Pfirrmann and colleagues[33] used MRI, bursography, and conventional radiography to study the greater trochanter and its bursae in cadavers and asymptomatic volunteers. They concluded that the greater trochanter consisted of four facets. The gluteus minimus attached to the anterior facet, with the subgluteus minimus bursa beneath the tendon; the gluteus medius attached to the superoposterior and lateral facets, with the subgluteus medius bursa beneath the tendon at the lateral facet; and the large trochanteric bursa covered the posterior facet, which was free of tendinous attachments (Fig. 10-28). Presumably, the trochanteric bursa serves to reduce friction between the posterior facet and the overlying gluteus maximus, as well as between the IT band and the trochanter.

Case Application 10-5: **Lateral Hip Pain**

In addition to her other problems, Gloria was complaining of lateral hip pain that was tender to palpation. Although other explanations for her pain exist, greater trochanter pain syndrome is common among middle-aged and elderly women (with a 4:1 ratio of women to men).[15,34] Trochanteric bursitis and lesions of the abductor (gluteus medius and gluteus minimus) tendons commonly coexist and have been analogized to rotator cuff tears and bursitis in the shoulder.[15,33,34] As we continue to explore the role of the hip abductors in standing and the possible effects of hip dysplasia on the hip abductors, it will become clear that Gloria's hip abductors and associated bursae are likely at risk for overuse injury and degenerative changes.

■ **Lateral Rotators**

Six short muscles have lateral rotation as a primary function. These muscles are the **obturator internus** and **externus,** the **gemellus superior** and **inferior,** the **quadratus femoris,** and the **piriformis** muscles. Other muscles that have fibers posterior to the axis of motion at the hip (the posterior fibers of the gluteus medius and minimus and the gluteus maximus) may produce lateral rotation combined with the primary action of the muscle (although it has already been noted that the lateral rotatory function of these muscles decreases or becomes medial with increased hip flexion)[60]. Of the primary lateral rotators, each inserts either on or in the vicinity of the greater trochanter (Fig. 10-29). The obturator internus muscle originates from the inside (posterior aspect) of the obturator foramen and emerges through the lesser sciatic foramen to insert on the medial aspect (inside) of the greater trochanter. The gemellus superior and gemellus inferior muscles arise from the ischium of the pelvis, just above and just below the point at which the obturator internus passes through the lesser sciatic notch. Both gemelli follow and blend with the obturator internus tendon to insert with the internus tendon into the greater trochanter.

The obturator externus muscle is sometimes considered to be an anteromedial muscle of the thigh because it originates on the external (anterior) surface of the obturator foramen. However, it crosses the posterior aspect of the hip joint and inserts on the medial aspect of the greater trochanter in the trochanteric fossa. The quadratus femoris muscle is a small quadrangular

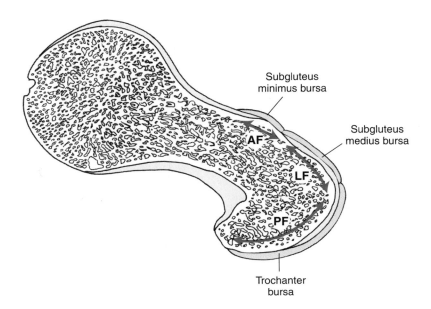

◀ **Figure 10-28** ■ The greater trochanter has four facets, three of which can be seen in this horizontal cross-section: the anterior facet (AF), the lateral facet (LF), and the posterior facet (PF). The superoposterior facet is not seen. Also seen on cross-section are three bursae. (From Pfirrmann C, Chung C, Theumann B, et al.: Greater trochanter of the hip: Attachment of the abductor mechanism and a complex of three bursae—MR imaging and MR bursography in cadavers and MR imaging in asymptomatic volunteers. Radiology 221:469–477, 2001.)

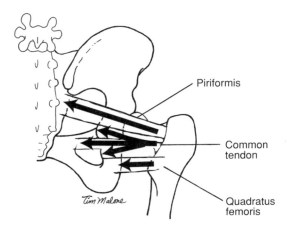

▲ **Figure 10-29** ■ The lateral rotators of the hip joint have action lines that lie nearly perpendicular to the femoral shaft (making them excellent rotators) and parallel to the head and neck of the femur (making them excellent compressors). The common tendon is the shared insertion of the gemellus superior, gemellus inferior, and the obturator internus muscles. The obturator externus muscle is not shown.

muscle that originates on the ischial tuberosity and inserts on the posterior femur between the greater and lesser trochanters. The piriformis muscle originates largely on the anterior surface of the sacrum, passes through the greater sciatic notch, and follows the inferior border of the posterior gluteus medius to insert above the other lateral rotators into the medial aspect of the greater trochanter. The piriformis and gluteus maximus are the only two muscles that cross the sacroiliac joint. The sciatic nerve, the largest nerve in the body, enters the gluteal region just inferior to the piriformis muscle.

The lateral rotator muscles are positioned to perform their rotatory function effectively, given the nearly perpendicular orientation to the shaft of the femur (see Fig. 10-29). However, exploration of function of these muscles has been restricted because of the relatively limited access to electromyography (EMG) surface or wire electrodes. Like their rotator cuff counterpart at the glenohumeral joint, these muscles would certainly appear to be effective joint compressors because their combined action line parallels the head and neck of the femur. Using modeling, Delp and colleagues[60] determined that the obturator internus, like the gluteal muscles, decreased its MA for lateral rotation with increased hip flexion. The piriformis was estimated to have a large MA for lateral rotation with the hip joint at 0° but switched to a medial rotator with half the MA when the hip reached 90° of flexion. The obturator externus and quadratus femoris were the only lateral rotators that did not diminish their MA for lateral rotation with increased hip joint flexion.[60] Hypothetically, the lines of pull of the deep one-joint lateral rotators should make them ideal tonic stabilizers of the joint during most weight-bearing and non–weight-bearing hip joint activities. Although their ability to perform lateral rotation may decrease with hip flexion in some instances, the action lines of these muscles should remain largely compressive (parallel to the femoral neck) throughout the hip joint ROM.

■ **Medial Rotators**

There are no muscles with the primary function of producing medial rotation of the hip joint. The more consistent medial rotators are the anterior portion of the gluteus medius, gluteus minimus, and the TFL muscles. Although controversial, the weight of evidence appears to support the adductor muscles as medial rotators of the joint,[59,62] with the possible exception of the gracilis muscle.[26] The ability of hip joint muscles to shift function with changing position of the hip joint is evident when medial rotation of the hip is examined. There is a trend toward increased medial rotation torques (or decreased lateral rotation torques) with increased hip flexion among many of the hip joint muscles,[26,60] with three times more medial rotation torque in the flexed hip than in the extended hip.[62] Delp and colleagues,[60] although clear as to the limitations of their modeling, suggested that the medial rotation that accompanies a "crouched" gait seen in many individuals with cerebral palsy may be attributable more to hip flexion than to adductor spasticity.

◆ **Hip Joint Forces and Muscle Function in Stance**

Bilateral Stance

In erect bilateral stance, both hips are in neutral or slight hyperextension, and weight is evenly distributed between both legs. The LoG falls just posterior to axis for flexion/extension of the hip joint. The posterior location of the LoG creates an extension moment of force around the hip that tends to posteriorly tilt the pelvis on the femoral heads. The gravitational extension moment is largely checked by passive tension in the hip joint capsuloligamentous structures, although slight or intermittent activity in the iliopsoas muscles in relaxed standing may assist the passive structures.[59]

In the frontal plane during bilateral stance, the superincumbent body weight is transmitted through the sacroiliac joints and pelvis to the right and left femoral heads. Hypothetically, the weight of the HAT (two thirds of body weight) should be distributed so that each femoral head receives approximately half of the superincumbent weight.[75] As shown in Figure 10-30, the joint axis of each hip lies at an equal distance from the LoG of HAT; that is, the gravitational MAs for the right hip (DR) and the left hip (DL) are equal. Because the body weight (W) on each femoral head is the same (WR = WL), the magnitude of the gravitational torques around each hip must be identical (WR × DR = WL × DL). The gravitational torques on the right and left hips, however, occur in opposite directions. The weight of the body acting around the right hip tends to drop

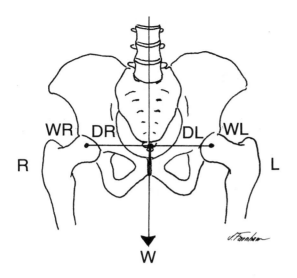

▲ **Figure 10-30** ■ An anterior view of the pelvis in normal erect bilateral stance. The weight acting on the right hip joint (WR) multiplied by the distance from the right hip joint axis to the body's center of gravity (DR) is equal to the weight acting at the left hip joint (WL) multiplied by the distance from the left hip to the body's center of gravity (DL). Therefore, WR × DR = WL × DL.

the pelvis down on the left (right adduction moment), whereas the weight acting around the left hip tends to drop the pelvis down on the right (left adduction moment). These two opposing gravitational moments of equal magnitude balance each other, and the pelvis is maintained in equilibrium in the frontal plane without the assistance of active muscles. Assuming that muscular forces are not required to maintain either sagittal or frontal plane stability at the hip joint in bilateral stance, the compression across each hip joint in bilateral stance should simply be half the superimposed body weight (or one third of HAT to each hip).

Example 10-4

Calculating Hip Joint Compression in Bilateral Stance

Using a hypothetical case of someone weighing 825 N (~185 lb), the weight of HAT (2/3 body weight) will be 550 N (~124 lb). Of that 550 N, half will presumably be distributed through each hip. Because we are assuming no additional compressive force produced by hip muscle activity, the total hip joint compression at each hip in bilateral stance is estimated to be 225 N (~50 lb); that is, total hip joint compression through each hip in bilateral stance is one third of body weight.

The rationale presented in Example 10-4 for assuming that each hip received one third of body weight in bilateral stance is reasonable. However, Bergmann and colleagues[76] showed in several subjects

with an instrumented pressure-sensitive hip prosthesis that the joint compression across each hip in bilateral stance was 80% to 100% of body weight, rather than one third (33%) of body weight, as commonly proposed. When they added a symmetrically distributed load to the subject's trunk, the forces at both hip joints increased by the full weight of the load, rather than by half of the superimposed load as might be expected. Although the mechanics of someone standing who has a prosthetic hip may not fully represent normal hip joint forces, the findings of Bergmann and colleagues call into question the simplistic view of hip joint forces in bilateral stance. The slight activity in the iliopsoas muscle may account for more joint compression than previously thought. Alternatively, capsuloligamentous tension may contribute to joint compression.

When bilateral stance is not symmetrical, frontal plane muscle activity will be necessary to either control the side-to-side motion or to return the hips to symmetrical stance. In Figure 10-22, the pelvis is shifted to the right, resulting in relative adduction of the right hip and abduction of the left hip. To return to neutral position, an active contraction of the right hip abductors would be expected. However, a contraction of the left hip adductors would accomplish the same goal. [In bilateral stance, the contralateral abductors and adductors may function as synergists to control the frontal plane motion of the pelvis.] *Under the condition that both extremities bear at least some of the superimposed body weight,* the adductors may assist the abductors in control of the pelvis against the force of gravity or the GRF. In unilateral stance, activity of the adductors either in the weight-bearing or non–weight-bearing hip *cannot* contribute to stability of the stance limb. Hip joint stability in unilateral stance is the sole domain of the hip joint abductors. In the absence of adequate hip abductor function, the adductors can contribute to stability—but only in bilateral stance.

Unilateral Stance

In Figure 10-31, the left leg has been lifted from the ground and the full superimposed body weight is being supported by the right hip joint. Rather than sharing the compressive force of the superimposed body weight with the left limb, the right hip joint must now carry the full burden. In addition, the weight of the non–weight-bearing left limb that is hanging on the left side of the pelvis must be supported along with the weight of HAT. Of the one-third portion of the body weight found in the lower extremities, the nonsupporting limb must account for half of that, or one sixth of the full body weight.[77] The magnitude of body weight (W) compressing the right hip joint in right unilateral stance, therefore, is:

$$\text{Right hip joint compression}_{\text{body weight}} = [2/3 \times W] + [1/6 \times W]$$

$$\text{Right hip joint compression}_{\text{body weight}} = 5/6 \times W$$

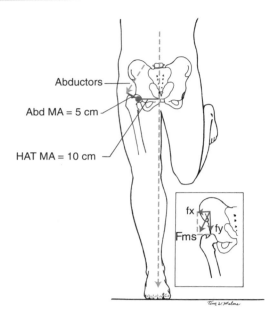

▲ **Figure 10-31** ■ In right unilateral stance, the weight of HAT acts 10 cm from the right hip joint. The 10 cm moment arm slightly underestimates the location of the LoG because it does not account for the weight of the hanging left limb. The hip abductors have a moment arm of approximately 5 cm. **Inset.** The pull of the abductors (F_{ms}) on the horizontally oriented pelvis will resolve into a parallel component (Fx) that will pull the acetabulum into the center of the femoral head and a perpendicular component (Fy) that will pull the pelvis down on the superior aspect of the femoral head, as well as pull the ilium closer to the femur, producing a hip abduction torque.

In our hypothetical subject from Example 10-4 who weighs 825 N, HAT in this individual weighs 550 N. One lower extremity weighs one sixth of body weight, or 137.5 N. Therefore, when this individual lifts one leg off the ground, the supporting hip joint will undergo 687.5 N (or five sixths of body weight)[6] of compression *from body weight alone.*

Although we have accounted for the increase in hip joint compression from body weight as a person moves from double-limb support (bilateral stance) to single-limb support, the problem is more complex. Not only is the hip joint in unilateral stance being compressed by body weight (gravity), but also that body weight is concomitantly creating a torque around the hip joint.

The force of gravity acting on HAT and the non–weight-bearing left lower limb (HATLL) will create an adduction torque around the supporting hip joint; that is, gravity will attempt to drop the pelvis around the right weight-bearing hip joint axis. The abduction countertorque will have to be supplied by the hip abductor musculature. The result will be joint compression or a joint reaction force that is a combination of both body weight and abductor muscular compression. The total joint compression can be calculated for our hypothetical 825-N subject. The LoG of HATLL can be estimated to lie 10 cm (0.1 m, or ~4 inches) from the right hip joint axis (that is, MA = 0.1 m), although the actual distance will vary among indi-

viduals.[78] The 10-cm estimate of the gravitational MA is for symmetrical stance. The actual MA is likely to be slightly greater because the weight of the hanging left leg will pull the center of gravity of the superimposed weight slightly to the left, although the LoG will simultaneously be shifted slightly right to get the LoG within the single foot base of support.

Calculating Hip Joint Compression in Unilateral Stance

For simplicity, the possible increase in the MA of HATLL from the non–weight-bearing limb will be ignored, but our torque calculation here is likely to *underestimate* the actual gravitational torque. In our simplified hypothetical example, the magnitude of the gravitational adduction torque at the right hip will be as follows:

HATLL torque$_{adduction}$: 687.5 N × 0.1 m = 68.75 Nm

To maintain the single-limb support position, there must be a countertorque (abduction moment) of equivalent magnitude. The countertorque must be produced by the force of the hip abductors (gluteus medius, minimus, and tensor fascia lata muscles) acting on the pelvis. Assuming that the abductor muscles act through a typical MA of 5 cm (0.05 m, or 2 inches)[78] and knowing that the muscles must generate an abduction torque equivalent to the adduction torque of gravity (68.75 Nm), we can solve for the magnitude of muscle contraction (F_{ms}) needed to maintain equilibrium in our hypothetical example.

Torque$_{abduction}$: 68.75 Nm = F_{ms} × 0.05 m

F_{ms} = 68.75 Nm ÷ 0.05 m = 1375 N

Assuming that all the abductor muscular force is transmitted through the acetabulum to the femoral head, the 1375-N abductor muscular compressive force is now added to the 687.5 N of compression caused by body weight passing through the supporting hip. Thus, the total hip joint compression, or joint reaction force, at the stance hip joint in unilateral support can be estimated for our hypothetical subject at:

1375 N abductor joint compression
+ 687.5 N body weight (HATLL) compression
2062.5 N total joint compression

The location of the 2062.5 N total hip joint reaction force computed in Example 10-5 can be further defined by knowing the angle of pull of the hip abductors. The action line of the abductors has been estimated to average 10° to 30° (±2 standard deviations) from vertical.[6] Assuming an angle of pull of approximately 30° from vertical (see Fig. 10-31 inset), we can estimate that nearly two thirds of the total hip abductor force (>917 N) acting on the pelvis will bring the pelvis vertically downward on the femoral head, and one third of the force (>454 N) will pull the pelvis laterally into the femoral head. The vertically directed downward force of 917 N will fall into the same line as the vertical force of the body weight (687.5 N), which results in a net force of approximately 1605 N (>361 lb) through the primary weight-bearing areas of the acetabulum and femoral head.[6] The remaining 454 N of the total 2062.5 N of hip joint compression should be distributed more uniformly around the periphery of the acetabulum[11] as the femur and acetabulum are snugged together, and the acetabulum widens with load.[11] It should be recalled that the acetabular fossa and fovea of the femur are nonarticular and, therefore, non–weight-bearing.

The hypothetical figures used above oversimplify the forces involved in hip joint stresses as already noted. Total hip joint compression or joint reaction forces are generally considered to be 2.5 to 3 times body weight in static unilateral stance.[68,75,78] Investigators have calculated or measured forces of four and seven times body weight in, respectively, the beginning and end of the stance phase of gait[79] and seven times the body weight in activities such as stair climbing.[80] Although weight loss can reduce the hip joint reaction force, the larger component of the joint reaction force is generated by the contraction of muscles, primarily presumed to be the hip abductors. The magnitude of hip abductor force required can be affected by individual differences in the angle of pull of the abductor muscles in particular, although peak pressures may not vary within the normal variations in abductor angle of pull.[6] Presuming that muscle force requirements are unchanged, substantial changes in the angle of inclination of the femoral head or in the angle of femoral torsion can affect the contact areas within the hip joint, thereby resulting in the potential for increased pressures in certain segments of the femoral head or acetabulum.[27,31,81] Krebs and colleagues[82] (evaluating a subject with an instrumented hip prosthesis over time) found that gluteus medius EMG activity, hip adduction torque, and acetabular contact pressures peak most often during single-limb support phase of gait. Acetabular contact pressures peaked before torque and GRFs, which implies that preparatory muscle activity rather than gravity and GRFs are a chief factor in hip joint contact forces. They also found that walking relatively slowly (60 beats per minute) reduced vertical GRFs, torques, and ROM but increased hip joint contact pressures. They hypothesized that the slower gait required increased muscle activity at the slower speeds, more than offsetting the reduction in external forces on the hip joint.[82] In addition, physiologic and biomechanical factors that lead to increases in force production by the hip abductor or other hip muscles may, over time, accelerate joint deterioration as a result of the abnormally large joint compressive forces that prevent normal compression and release of cartilage or that are concentrated in too small an area for the cartilage to sustain itself.

Reduction of Muscle Forces in Unilateral Stance

If the hip joint undergoes osteoarthritic changes that lead to pain on weight-bearing, the joint reaction force must be reduced to avoid pain. If total joint compression in unilateral stance is approximately three times body weight, a loss of 1 N (~4.5 lb) of body weight will reduce the joint reaction force by 3 N (13.5 lb). For most painful hip joints, however, the reductions in compression generally required are greater than can be realistically achieved through weight loss. The solution must be in a reduction of abductor muscle force requirements. If less muscular countertorque is needed to offset the effects of gravity, there will be a decrease in the amount of muscular compression across the joint, although the body weight compression will remain unchanged. The need to diminish abductor force requirements also occurs when the abductor muscles are weakened through paralysis, through structural changes in the femur that reduce biomechanical efficiency of the muscles, or through degenerative changes producing tears at the greater trochanter. Hip abductor muscle weakness will inevitably affect gait, whereas paralysis of other hip joint muscles in the presence of intact abductors will permit someone to walk or even run with relatively little disability.

Several options are available when there is a need to decrease abductor muscle force requirements. Some compression reduction strategies occur automatically, but at a cost of extra energy expenditure and structural stress. Other strategies require intervention such as assistive devices but minimize the energy cost.

■ Compensatory Lateral Lean of the Trunk

Gravitational torque at the pelvis is the product of body weight and the distance that the LoG lies from the hip joint axis (MA). If there is a need to reduce the torque of gravity in unilateral stance and if body weight cannot be reduced, the MA of the gravitational force can be reduced by laterally leaning the trunk over the pelvis *toward the side of pain or weakness* when in unilateral stance on the painful limb. Although leaning toward the side of pain might appear counterintuitive, the compensatory lateral lean of the trunk toward the painful stance limb will swing the LoG closer to the hip joint, thereby reducing the gravitational MA. Because the weight of HATLL must pass through the weight-bearing hip joint regardless of trunk position, leaning toward the painful or weak supporting hip does not increase the joint compression caused by body weight. However, it does reduce the gravitational torque. If there is a smaller gravitational adduction torque, there will be a proportional reduction in the need for an abductor countertorque. Although it is theoretically possible to laterally lean the trunk enough to bring the LoG *through* the supporting hip (reducing the torque to zero) or to the *opposite side* of the supporting hip (reversing the direction of the gravitational torque), these are relatively extreme motions that require high energy expenditure and would result in excessive wear and tear on the lumbar spine. More energy efficient and less structurally stressful compensations can still yield dramatic reductions in the hip abductor force.

Example 10-6

Calculating Hip Joint Compression with Lateral Lean

Returning to our hypothetical subject weighing 825 N, let us assume that he can laterally lean to the right enough to bring the LoG within 2.5 cm (0.025 m) of the right hip joint axis (Fig. 10-32). The gravitational adduction torque would now be:

$$\text{HATLL torque}_{\text{adduction}} = [5/6\ (825\ \text{N})] \times 0.25\ \text{m}$$

$$\text{HATLL torque}_{\text{adduction}} = 17.2\ \text{Nm}$$

If only 17.2 Nm of adduction torque were produced by the superimposed weight, the abductor force needed would be as follows:

$$\text{Torque}_{\text{abduction}}: 17.2\ \text{Nm} = F_{ms} \times 0.05\ \text{m}$$

$$F_{ms}: 17.2\ \text{Nm} \div 0.05\ \text{m} = 343.75\ \text{N}$$

If only ~344 N (~77 lb) of abductor force were required, the total hip joint compression in unilateral

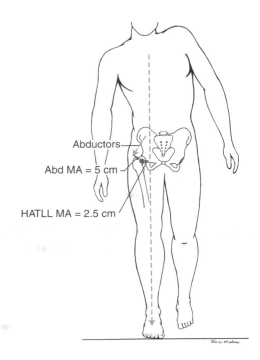

Abductors
Abd MA = 5 cm
HATLL MA = 2.5 cm

▲ **Figure 10-32** ■ When the trunk is laterally flexed toward the stance limb, the moment arm of HATLL is substantially reduced (e.g., 2.5 cm, in comparison with 10 cm with the neutral trunk), whereas that of the abductors remains unchanged (e.g., 5 cm). The result is a substantially diminished torque from HATLL and, consequently, a substantially decreased need for hip abductor force to generate a countertorque.

stance using the compensatory lateral lean would now be:

> 343.75 N abductor joint compression
> + 687.5 N body weight (HATLL) compression
> 1031.25 N total joint compression

The 1031.25-N joint reaction force estimated in Example 10-6 is half the 2062.5 N of hip joint compression previously calculated for our hypothetical subject in single-limb support. This 50% reduction in joint compression is enough to relieve some of the pain symptoms experienced by a person with arthritic changes in the hip joint or to provide some relief to a weak or painful set of abductors. The compensatory lean is instinctive and commonly seen in people with hip joint disability.

Continuing Exploration: **Pathologic Gaits**

When a lateral trunk lean is seen during gait and is due to hip abductor muscle weakness, it is known as **a gluteus medius gait.** If the same compensation is due to hip joint pain, it is known as an **antalgic gait.** In some instances, the 344-N abductor force we calculated as necessary to stabilize the pelvis in Example 10-6 is still beyond the work capacity of very weak or completely paralyzed hip abductors. In such cases of extreme abductor muscle weakness, the pelvis will drop to the unsupported side even in the presence of a lateral trunk lean to the supported side. If lateral lean and pelvic drop occur during walking, the gait deviation is commonly referred to as a **Trendelenburg gait.** The lateral lean that accompanies the drop of the pelvis must be sufficient to keep the LoG within the supporting foot.

Whether a lateral trunk lean is due to muscular weakness or pain, a lateral lean of the trunk during walking still uses more energy than ordinarily required for single-limb support and may result in stress changes within the lumbar spine if used over an extended time period. Use of a cane or some other assistive device offers a realistic alternative to the person with hip pain or weakness.

■ Use of a Cane Ipsilaterally

Pushing downward on a cane held in the hand on the *side of pain or weakness* should reduce the superimposed body weight by the amount of downward thrust; that is, some of the weight of HATLL would follow the arm to the cane, rather than arriving on the sacrum and the weight-bearing hip joint. Inman et al.[68] suggested that it is realistic to expect that someone can push down on a cane with approximately 15% of his body weight. The proportion of body weight that passes through the cane will not pass through the hip joint and will not create an adduction torque around the supporting hip joint.

Example 10-7

Calculating Hip Joint Compression with a Cane Ipsilaterally

If our 825-N subject can push down on the cane with 15% of his body weight, 123.75 N of body weight (825 N × 0.15) will pass through the cane. The magnitude of HATLL is thereby reduced to 563.75 N (687.5 N – 123.75 N). If the gravitational force of HATLL works through our estimated MA of 10 cm or 0.10 m (remember, the cane is intended to prevent the trunk lean), the torque of gravity is reduced to 56.38 Nm (563.75 N × 0.10 m). With a gravitational adduction torque of 56.38 Nm, the required force of the abductors acting through the usual 5 cm (0.05 m) MA is reduced to 1127.6 N (56.38 Nm ÷ 0.05 m). The new hip joint reaction force using a cane *ipsilaterally* would then be:

1127.6 N abductor joint compression
+ 563.75 N body weight (HATLL-cane) compression
1691.35 N total joint compression

Total hip joint compression of 1691.35 N calculated in Example 10-7 when a cane is used ipsilaterally provides some relief over the total hip joint compression of 2062.5 N ordinarily experienced in unilateral stance. The total hip joint compression when the cane is used ipsilaterally is still greater, however, than the total joint compression of 1031.25 N found with a compensatory lateral trunk lean. Although a cane used ipsilaterally provides some benefits in energy expenditure and structural stress reduction, it is not as effective in reducing hip joint compression as the undesirable lateral lean of the trunk. *Moving the cane to the opposite hand produces substantially different and better results.*

▪ Use of a Cane Contralaterally

When the cane is moved to the side *opposite the painful or weak hip joint,* the reduction in HATLL is the same as it is when the cane is used on the same side as the painful hip joint; that is, the superimposed body weight passing through the weight-bearing hip joint is reduced by approximately 15% of body weight. However, the cane is now substantially farther from the painful supporting hip joint (Fig. 10-33) than it would be if the cane is used on the same side; that is, in addition to relieving some of the superimposed body weight, the cane is now in a position to assist the abductor muscles in providing a countertorque to the torque of gravity.[83] A classic description of the benefit of using a cane in the hand opposite to the hip impairment presumes that the downward force on the cane acts through the full distance between the hand and the stance (impaired) hip joint.[83] We will first look at an example using the classic analysis and then determine how this analysis might be misleading.

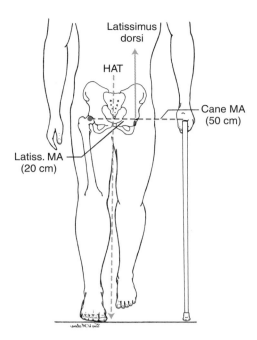

▲ **Figure 10-33** ▪ When a cane is placed in the hand opposite the painful supporting hip, the weight passing through the left hip is reduced, and activation of the right latissimus dorsi provides a countertorque to that of HATLL and diminishes the need for a contraction of the left hip abductors. The moment arm of the cane is estimated to be 25 cm, whereas the moment arm of the latissimus dorsi is estimated to be 20 cm.

Example 10-8

Classic Calculation of Hip Joint Compression with a Cane Contralaterally

Our sample 825-N patient has a superimposed body weight (HATLL) of 687.5 N, of which 123.75 N (W × 0.15) passes through the cane. Consequently, 563.75 N of body weight will pass through the right stance hip joint and the gravitation adduction torque will be:

HATLL torque$_{adduction}$: 563.75 N × 0.10 m = 56.38 Nm.

The downward force on the cane of 123.75 N acts through an estimated MA of 50 cm (0.5 m) between the cane in the right hand and the right weight-bearing hip joint (see Fig. 10-31). The cane, therefore, would generate an opposing abduction torque as follows:

Cane torque$_{abduction}$: 123.75 N × 0.5 m = 61.88 Nm

The torque around the right stance hip produced by a cane in the left hand (61.88 Nm) exceeds the torque produced by the remaining weight of HATLL (56.38 Nm). Because the gravitational torque (HATLL) may be underestimated, let us assume that the gravitational adduction torque and the countertorque provided by the cane offset each other. If the cane completely offset the effect of gravity, there would be no need for hip abductor muscle force. The total hip joint compression in unilateral stance when a cane is used in the opposite hand would be:

$$
\begin{array}{r}
0 \text{ N abductor joint compression} \\
+ \text{ } 563.75 \text{ N body weight (HATLL-cane) compression} \\
\hline
563.75 \text{ N total joint compression}
\end{array}
$$

According to the classic analysis of the value of a cane in the opposite hand in Example 10-8, the hip joint reaction force would be due exclusively to body weight (563.75 N). This is, of course, an improvement over our calculated total hip compression with a lateral lean (1031.25 N) and a greater improvement yet over joint compression in normal unilateral stance (2062.5 N) for a person weighing 825 N. Unfortunately, the classic treatment of biomechanics of cane use appears to substantially overestimate the effects of the cane. Krebs and colleagues[82] (monitoring the patient with an instrumented hip prosthesis) found reductions in peak pressure magnitudes of 28% to 40% during cane-assisted gait. Although they reported pressures rather than forces, these values do not match the nearly 75% reduction in force that the classic calculation would indicate. Furthermore, Krebs and colleagues found a 45% reduction in gluteus medius EMG, not an elimination of activity.[82] The discrepancy in the classic analysis and laboratory and modeling data can be resolved by examining *how* the force applied to the cane by a person provides a countertorque to gravity.

Hip Joint Compression with Contralateral Cane Use: A Hypothesis

The classic description of how using a cane in the hand opposite to a painful or weak hip affects forces across that joint can be found in numerous texts and journal articles. However, few publications address the question of *how* the downward thrust of the arm on the cane actually acts on the pelvis. As we saw in Chapter 1, the equilibrium of an object (such as the pelvis) can be affected only by forces actually applied to that object. The explanation for the effect of the cane is not logical unless we can explain how the force on the cane translates to a force applied to the pelvis. Although this is conjectural, we propose that the force of the downward thrust on the cane arrives on the pelvis through a contraction of the latissimus dorsi muscle.

It is well established that the latissimus dorsi is a depressor of the humerus[59] through both its humeral attachment and its more variable scapular attachment[7] and has been classically defined as the "crutch-walking muscle."[62,84] Because the downward thrust on the cane is accomplished through shoulder depression just as crutch walking is, it is logical to assume that the latissimus dorsi is active when a cane is used. The latissimus dorsi attaches to the iliac crest of the pelvis. A contraction of the latissimus dorsi would result in an upward pull on the iliac crest on the side of the cane (opposite the weak or painful weight-bearing hip), as shown in Figure 10-31. An upward pull on the side of the pelvis opposite the supporting hip joint axis (hip hiking

force) creates an abduction torque around the supporting hip joint. This abduction torque can offset the gravitational adduction torque around the same hip joint.

It is reasonable to estimate that the magnitude of a latissimus dorsi muscle contraction should be approximately the same as the downward thrust on the cane on the same side (123.75 N in our examples) under the supposition that this muscle initiates the thrust. Measures of the MA of the pull of the latissimus dorsi muscle on the pelvis are not readily available. However, the latissimus dorsi muscle has an attachment to the pelvis on the posterior iliac crest, lateral to the erector spinae.[7] Given this attachment site, the line of pull of the muscle can be approximated to have a point of application on the pelvis above the ipsilateral acetabulum. In our sample MA for HAT of 10 cm between the LoG and the hip joint axis, the line of pull of, for example, the left latissimus dorsi muscle (presuming the subject is using a cane in the left hand) should lie twice that distance (about 20 cm, or 0.20 m) from the right weight-bearing and impaired hip joint (see Fig. 10-31). Now let us use the estimated upward pull of the latissimus dorsi muscle and its estimated MA to calculate the total hip joint compression for our hypothetical hip patient using a cane in the contralateral hand.

Example 10-9

Hypothesized Calculation of Hip Joint Compression with a Cane Contralaterally

We have already established in Example 10-8 that the adduction torque of the body weight when a cane is used (HATLL – cane) is 56.38 N (563.75 N × 0.10 m). The countertorque (abduction around the stance right hip) produced by a contraction of the left latissimus dorsi is given as follows:

Left latissimus dorsi torque$_{abduction}$: 123.75 N × 0.20 m
$$= 24.75 \text{ Nm}$$

If the gravitational adduction torque at the right hip is 56.38 Nm and the abduction torque produced by the left latissimus dorsi at the right hip is 24.75 Nm, there is still an unopposed adduction torque around the stance right hip of 31.63 Nm. Consequently, a contraction of the right hip abductors is still needed. The magnitude of required abductor force (continuing to use the estimated abductor MA of 5 cm (0.05 m) will be as follows:

Torque$_{abduction}$: 31.63 Nm = F_{ms} × 0.05 m

F_{ms}: 31.63 ÷ 0.05 = 632.6 N

Given both a contraction of the right latissimus dorsi and the left hip abductors, total hip joint compression at the left stance hip would be:

$$
\begin{array}{r}
632.6 \text{ N abductor joint compression} \\
+ \text{ } 563.75 \text{ N body weight (HATLL-cane) compression} \\
\hline
1193.35 \text{ N total joint compression}
\end{array}
$$

In Example 10-9, body weight compression and abductor muscle compression were used to compute total joint compression on the right stance hip without taking into consideration any compression from the contraction of the contralateral latissimus dorsi. The latissimus dorsi, unlike the hip abductor muscles, does not cross the hip and cannot create compression across the hip joint.

The estimated total hip joint compression in right stance when a cane is used in the left hand and with an assumed contraction of the left latissimus dorsi (Example 10-9) was 1196.35 N. The estimate is a 42% reduction from the estimated joint compression of 2062.5 N for unaided unilateral stance (Example 10-5). This reduction is well in line with the findings of Krebs and colleagues[82] that use of a cane opposite a painful hip can relieve the affected hip of as much as 40% of its load and reduce gluteus medius activity by 45%.

■ **Adjustment of a Carried Load**

When someone with hip joint pain or weakness carries a load in the hand or on the trunk (as with a backpack or purse), there is a potential for increasing the demands on the hip abductors and increasing the hip joint compression. The added external load will increase the superimposed weight acting through the affected supporting hip in unilateral stance. Concomitantly, the gravitational torque *may* increase, resulting in an increased demand on the supporting hip abductors to prevent drop of the pelvis. Although the increase in superimposed weight when a load is carried cannot be avoided, it is possible to minimize the demand on the abductor muscles on the side of a painful or weak hip. If the external load is carried in the arm or on the side of the trunk *ipsilateral* to the painful or weak hip, the asymmetrical external load will cause a shift in the combined force of HAT/external load center of mass (CoM) *toward* the painful hip. Any shift of the combined CoM (or resulting LoG) toward the painful hip will reduce the MA of the HAT/external load. *If the external load is not too great*, the reduction in MA of the HAT/external load can result in a reduction in adduction torque not only of the combined load but also of HAT alone around the stance hip joint. With a reduction in adduction torque, the demand on the hip abductors is reduced. Of course, the reverse effect will occur if the load is carried on the side *opposite* to the weak or painful hip. In that scenario, the external load both increases superimposed body weight *and* increases the gravitational MA around the weak or painful hip when in unilateral stance on that hip.

Neumann and Cook[85] measured EMG activity in the gluteus medius during varying load-carrying conditions. They found that a load of 10% of body weight carried on the right reduced the need for hip abductor activity in right unilateral stance; that is, the increase in superimposed body weight was more than offset by the decrease in the MA of HAT/external load, which resulted in a diminished adduction torque and a reduced need for abductor muscle contraction. When the load on the right was increased to 20% of body weight, the right abductor activity was statistically similar to the activity before the load was added. That is, the reduction in the MA of HAT/external load resulted in the same adduction torque as was found in the no-load condition; the abductor activity did not change from the no-load condition because the adduction torque did not change. When the load was carried in the left hand, there was a substantial increase in right abductor activity during right stance. This load condition increased the magnitude of HAT/external load *and* displaced the combined CoM (and LoG) *away* from the stance hip joint, increasing the gravitational torque and increasing the need for hip abductor activity.

Neumann and Cook[85] looked at gluteus medius activity as a measure of the impact of a carried load on the stance hip joint. Bergmann and colleagues[76] estimated hip joint reaction forces in several subjects and measured actual forces in one subject with an instrumented femoral head prosthesis. They found that most of their subjects could carry loads of up to 25% of body weight in the right hand and still show a slight reduction in hip joint compression over the no-load condition when in right unilateral stance. They pointed out, however, that a typical compensatory shift of the trunk away from the load should be avoided if the goal is to reduce hip joint compression.

Case Application 10-6: **Strategies to Reduce Hip Pain**

Gloria has osteoarthritic changes in her left hip that, if sufficient, can be a source of her pain. Furthermore, her lateral hip pain and lateral lean during left stance may be at least partially attributable to degenerative changes in the gluteus medius/minimus tendons and trochanteric bursal inflammation. There is little doubt that Gloria can benefit from reducing the demands on her left hip abductor muscles. Reduction in demand may both minimize aggravation of any tears or inflammation and reduce hip joint compressive force that, with her hip dysplasia, are likely to be carried over a reduced area of articular contact. Using a cane in her right hand whenever possible is appropriate. Although a lateral lean actually reduces the demands on the hip abductors a bit more, the energy expenditure and structural stress on the spine must be considered. When Gloria carries her great-granddaughter or groceries, she should always carry on the left. In fact, carrying a moderate load (less than 25% of body weight) on the side of hip pain or hip abductor weakness may be a reasonable alternative for reducing hip joint pain or a gluteus medius gait if a person is resistant to using a cane. Carrying a load on the side opposite a weak or painful hip should be avoided.

◆ **Hip Joint Pathology**

The very large active and passive forces crossing the hip joint make the joint's structures susceptible to wear and tear of normal components and to failure of weakened components. Small changes in the biomechanics of the femur or the acetabulum can result in increases in passive forces above normal levels or in weakness of the dynamic joint stabilizers. Some of the more common problems and the underlying mechanisms are discussed in this section.

Arthrosis

The most common painful condition of the hip is due to deterioration of the articular cartilage and to subsequent related changes in articular tissues.[78] It is known as **osteoarthritis, degenerative arthritis,** or perhaps most appropriately as **hip joint arthrosis,** and its prevalence rates are about 10% to 15% in those older than 55 years, with approximately equal distribution among men and women.[86] Although trauma or malalignment such as femoral anteversion may be associated with occurrence,[27,87] 50% of the cases are considered to be idiopathic[5]; that is, half of the cases of hip joint arthrosis have no evident underlying pathology. Changes may be due to subtle deviations present from birth, to tissue changes inherent in aging, to the repetitive mechanical stress of loading the body weight on the hip joint over a prolonged period, to impingement between the femur and labrum or adjacent acetabulum,[15–17] or to interactions of each of these factors. The factors most closely associated with idiopathic hip joint arthrosis are increased age and increased weight/height ratio.[88] Lane and colleagues found no association between osteoarthritic changes and running status among older subjects.[89]

The mechanism for cartilaginous degeneration in the hip joint is not clear-cut. When a biomechanical problem is not evident, degenerative changes may be due not to excessive forces at the hip joint but to inadequate forces. This would explain why there is little or no association between increased activity level with sports or recreational activities and hip arthrosis.[89,90]

It may be that forces in excess of half the body weight are needed to fully compress the femoral head into congruent contact with the dome of the acetabulum.[3] Using a number of other studies as a base, Bullough and associates[3] hypothesized that we typically spend no more than 5% to 25% of our time in unilateral lower extremity weight-bearing activities in which the load may be sufficient to compress the articular cartilage of the dome of the acetabulum. Lower loads and infrequent high joint forces may be inadequate to maintain flow of nutrients and wastes through the avascular cartilage. The theory of inadequate compression as a contributing factor to hip joint degeneration is supported by the fact that the more common degenerative changes in the femur are at the periphery of the head and the perifoveal area, rather than at the superior primary weight-bearing area.[3,44] The periphery of the head receives only about one third the compressive force of the superior portion of the head,[75] whereas the superior portion of the head is compressed not only in standing but is also in contact with the posterior acetabulum during sitting activities.[44] The area of the femoral head around the fovea is most commonly in the non–weight-bearing acetabular notch and would undergo compression relatively infrequently. Wingstrand and colleagues[28] proposed that excessive intra-articular fluid from relatively benign synovitis or trauma may reduce articular congruence and the stabilizing effect of atmospheric pressure, resulting in microinstability and unfavorable cartilage loads.

Fracture

Although the weight-bearing forces coming through the hip joint may cause deterioration of the articular cartilage, the bony components must also be of sufficient strength to withstand the forces that are acting around and through the hip joint. As noted in the section on the weight-bearing structure of the hip joint, the vertical weight-bearing forces that pass down through the superior margin of the acetabulum in both unilateral and bilateral stance act at some distance from GRF up the shaft of the femur. The result is a bending force across the femoral neck (see Fig. 10-15). Normally the trabecular systems are capable of resisting the bending forces, but abnormal increases in the magnitude of the force or weakening of the bone can lead to bony failure. The site of failure is likely to be in areas of thinner trabecular distribution such as the zone of weakness (see Fig. 10-16). Crabtree and colleagues used both patients and cadavers with a fracture to conclude that a loss in cortical bone, not cancellous bone (trabeculae), may be the source of the problem. Although cancellous bone mass was similar for cases and controls in similar age groups, there was a 25% reduction in cortical bone mass in the fracture cases.[43]

Bony failure in the femoral neck is uncommon in the child or young adult, even with large applied loads. However, femoral neck fractures occur at the rate of about 98/100,000 people in the United States, with the average age at occurrence being in the seventies. There is a predominance of fractures in women, although this is certainly influenced by their greater longevity. Of middle-aged people, women actually suffer fewer hip fractures than do men, although the fractures in this age group are usually attributable to substantial trauma.[91]

In 87% of cases of hip fracture among the elderly population, the precipitating factor appears to be moderate trauma such as that caused by a fall from standing, from a chair, or from a bed. There is consensus that hip fracture is associated with, but not exclusively due to, diminished bone density.[86] Bone density decreases about 2% per year after age 50 and trabeculae clearly thin and disappear with aging.[92] Cummings and Nevitt[92] believed the exponential increase in hip fractures with age could not be accounted for by decreased bone density alone and proposed that the slowed gait characteristic of the elderly may play an important part. They contended that the slowing of gait makes it less likely that momentum will carry the body forward in a fall (generally onto an outstretched hand) and more likely that the fall will occur backward on to the hip area weakened by bone loss and no longer padded by the fat and muscle bulk of youth.

Hip fracture will continue to receive considerable attention because of the high health care costs of both conservative and operative treatment. Of all fall-related fractures, hip fractures cause the greatest number of deaths and lead to the most severe health problems and reduced quality of life. In 1999 in the United States, hip fractures resulted in approximately 338,000 hospital admissions.[93] Not only is the condition painful, but malunion of the fracture can lead to joint instability or cartilaginous deterioration (or both) as a result of poorly aligned bony segments. Although the femoral head may receive some blood supply via the ligament of the femoral head, an absent or diminished supply through the ligament of the head (as occurs with aging) means reliance on anastomoses from the circumflex arteries. This circumflex arterial supply may be disrupted by femoral neck fracture, which leaves the femoral head susceptible to avascular necrosis and necessitates replacement of the head of the femur with an artificial implant. Femoral neck fracture also has an associated mortality rate that may be as high as 20%.[91]

Bony Abnormalities of the Femur

When the bony structure of the femur is altered through abnormal angles of torsion or inclination, subsequent changes in the direction and magnitude of the forces acting around the hip can lead to other pathologic conditions such as increased likelihood of joint arthrosis, increased likelihood of femoral neck fracture, or muscular weakness. The normal angles of inclination and torsion appear to represent optimal balance of stresses and muscle alignment. Alterations may actually appear to result in advantages in relation to some functions but are always accompanied by concomitant disadvantages in relation to others.

■ Coxa Valga/Coxa Vara

In coxa valga (see Fig. 10-6A), the angle of inclination in the femur is greater than the normal adult angle of 125°. The increased angle brings the vertical weight-bearing line closer to the shaft of the femur, diminishing the shear, or bending, force across the femoral neck. The reduction in force is actually reflected in a reduction in density of the lateral trabecular system.[45] However, the decreased distance between the femoral head and the greater trochanter also decreases the length of the MA of the hip abductor muscles. The decreased muscular MA results in an increased demand for muscular force generation to maintain sufficient abduction torque to counterbalance the gravitational adduction moment acting around the supporting hip joint during single-limb support. Either the additional muscular force requirement will increase the total joint reaction force within the hip joint or the abductor muscles will be unable to meet the increased demand and will be functionally weakened. Although the abductors may be otherwise normal, the reduction in biomechanical effectiveness may produce the compensations typical of primary abductor muscle weakness. Coxa valga

also decreases the amount of femoral articular surface in contact with the dome of the acetabulum. As the femoral head points more superiorly, there is a decreasing amount of coverage from the acetabulum superiorly. Consequently, coxa valga decreases the stability of the hip and predisposes the hip to dislocation.[9,23,46]

Coxa vara is considered to give the advantage of improved hip joint stability (if angle reduction is not too extreme). The apparent improvement in congruence occurs because the decreased angle between the neck and shaft of the femur will turn the femoral head deeper into the acetabulum, decreasing the amount of articular surface exposed superiorly and increasing coverage from the acetabulum. A varus femur, if not caused by trauma, may also increase the length of the MA of the hip abductor muscles by increasing the distance between the femoral head and the greater trochanter.[22] The increased MA decreases the amount of force that must be generated by the abductor muscles in single-limb support and reduces the joint reaction force. However, coxa vara has the disadvantage of increasing the bending moment along the femoral head and neck. This increase in bending force can actually be seen by the increased density of trabeculae laterally in the femur, caused by the increase in tensile stresses.[45] The increased shear force along the femoral neck will increase the predisposition toward femoral neck fracture.[23,46]

Coxa vara may increase the likelihood in the adolescent child that the femoral head will slide on the cartilaginous epiphysis of the head of the femur. In childhood, the epiphysis is fairly horizontal.[7] Consequently, the superimposed weight merely compresses the head into the epiphyseal plate. In adolescence, growth of the bone results in a more oblique orientation of the epiphyseal plate. The epiphyseal obliquity makes the plate more vulnerable to shear forces at a time when the plate is already weakened by the rapid growth that occurs during this period of life.[91] Weight-bearing forces may slide the femoral head inferiorly, resulting in a slipped capital femoral epiphysis. As is true for a hip fracture, the altered biomechanics and at-risk blood supply necessitate restoration of normal alignment before secondary degenerative changes can occur.

■ Anteversion/Retroversion

Variations in the angle of torsion also affect hip biomechanics and function. Anteversion of the femoral head reduces hip joint stability because the femoral articular surface is more exposed anteriorly. The line of the hip abductors may fall more posterior to the joint, reducing the MA for abduction.[87] As is true for coxa valga, the resulting need for additional abductor muscle force may predispose the joint to arthrosis or may functionally weaken the joint, producing energy-consuming and wearing gait deviations. The effect of femoral anteversion may also be seen at the knee joint. When the femoral head is anteverted, pressure from the anterior capsuloligamentous structures and the anterior musculature may push the femoral head back into the acetabulum, causing the entire femur to rotate medially. Although the medial rotation of the femur improves the congruence in the acetabulum, the knee joint axis through the femoral condyles is now turned medially, altering the plane of knee flexion/extension and resulting, at least initially, in a toe-in gait. The toe-in position of the foot may appear to diminish over time, because it is not uncommon to see a compensatory lateral tibial torsion develop. Although the foot placement looks better, the underlying hip problem generally remains (with some developmental reduction). As noted earlier, the abnormal position of the knee joint axis is commonly labeled medial femoral torsion. Medial femoral torsion and femoral anteversion are the *same* abnormal condition of the femur. The label designates whether the exaggerated twist in the femur is altering the mechanics at the hip joint (femoral anteversion) or at the knee joint (medial femoral torsion). As shall be seen in the next two chapters, an anteverted femur will also affect the biomechanics of the patellofemoral joint at the knee and of the subtalar joint in the foot.

Femoral retroversion is the opposite of anteversion and creates opposite problems from femoral anteversion.

Case Application 10-7: **Hip Dysplasia**

Although we have probably covered the potential sources of Gloria's problems fairly well at this point, it is worth taking note of the most likely underlying cause. Gloria's persisting coxa valga and femoral anteversion are the likely source of many, if not all, her problems, although aging alone is a factor. With a valgus and anteverted femur, the articular contact within Gloria's hip joint is substantially reduced, increasing the contact pressures and locating them atypically within the acetabulum and on the head of the femur. The mechanical disadvantage to her hip abductors is likely to have contributed to overuse and degenerative lesions of the abductor mechanism, further affecting abductor function and resulting in what might be referred to either as a gluteus medius or antalgic gait. Both her hip dysplasia and the many years of working on a floor level with young children have exacerbated the likelihood of anterior impingement of the labrum, resulting in probable tear and chondral lesions. As is the case for many people in her situation, Gloria may find that a total hip joint replacement is offered to her as a way to restore function and reduce pain.

Summary

The normal hip joint is well designed to withstand the forces that act through and around it, assisted by the trabecular systems, cartilaginous coverings, muscles, and ligaments. Alterations in the direction or magnitude of forces acting around the hip create abnormal concentrations of stress that predispose the joint structures to injury and degenerative changes. The degenerative changes, in turn, can create additional alterations in function that not only affect the hip joint's ability to support the body weight in standing, in locomotor activities, and in other activities of daily living but may also result in adaptive changes at more proximal and distal joints. Consequently, the reader must understand both the dysfunction that might occur at the hip *and* the associated dysfunctions that may result in or from dysfunction elsewhere in the lower extremity and spine. The remaining chapters of this text will focus not only on primary dysfunction at a joint complex but also on associated dysfunction related to proximal and distal joint problems.

Study Questions

1. Which side of the femoral neck and which side of the femoral shaft are subjected to compressive stresses during weight-bearing? How does the bone respond to these stresses?
2. What is the primary weight-bearing area of the femoral head? Of the acetabulum? Where are degenerative changes most commonly found in the femoral head and acetabulum?
3. Describe why using a cane on the side opposite hip joint pain or weakness is more effective than using the cane on the same side.
4. Demonstrate how variations in the angle of inclination affect the MA of the hip abductors by drawing the following: a normal angle of inclination at the hip, the angle in coxa vara, and the angle in coxa valga. Please include the action line and the MA of the hip abductors in the diagram.
5. Describe what would happen to the pelvis in left unilateral stance when the left hip abductors are paralyzed. How is equilibrium maintained in this situation?
6. Describe motion at the right and left hip joints and at the lumbar spine during hiking of the pelvis in right limb stance, assuming that the person is to remain upright.
7. Contrast the close-packed versus maximally congruent position for the hip joint.

(Continued on following page)

8. Calculate the minimum joint reaction force (total hip joint compression) at the right hip joint that would occur for a 200-lb person standing symmetrically on both legs versus one leg (assuming a gravitational MA of 4 inches and the abductor muscle MA of 2 inches).

9. Under what circumstances does the hip joint participate as part of an open chain? As part of a closed chain?

10. What bony abnormality or abnormalities of the femur or pelvis predispose the hip joint to the possibility of dislocation? Why?

11. Which structures at the hip joint, given their location, appear likely to limit the extremes of motion in flexion? In extension? In lateral rotation? In medial rotation? In abduction and adduction?

12. Which muscles of the hip joint are affected by knee joint position? Which position of the knee makes these muscles less effective at the hip joint?

13. If someone were in a unilateral stance on the left limb, what hip joint motion would result from forward rotation of the pelvis?

14. If a person has a painful right hip, in which direction should she lean her trunk to reduce the forces on the right hip during right unilateral support? Explain the reasons for your answer.

15. What position does the hip joint tend to assume when there is joint pain? Why is this?

16. Identify several factors that might predispose someone to a femoral neck fracture.

17. How does the femoral head receive its blood supply? What problems might jeopardize that supply?

18. Relate femoral anteversion to medial femoral torsion.

19. Under what circumstances might the hip adductors work synergistically with the hip abductors?

20. Why is the acetabular notch nonarticular? In what ways does this serve hip joint function?

21. How would you advise a woman with hip joint pain to carry her purse? Why?

◆ References

1. Moore K, Dalley AI: Clinically Oriented Anatomy, 4th ed. Philadelphia, Lippincott Williams & Wilkins, 1999.

2. Brinckmann P, Frobin W, Hierholzer E: Stress on the articular surface of the hip joint in healthy adults and persons with idiopathic osteoarthrosis of the hip joint. Biomechanics 14:149–156, 1981.

3. Bullough P, Goodfellow J, O'Connor J: The relationship between degenerative changes and load-bearing in the human hip. J Bone Joint Surg Br 55:746–758, 1973.

4. Anda S, Svenningsen S, Dale LG, et al.: The acetabular sector angle of the adult hip determined by computed tomography. Acta Radiol Diagn (Stockh) 27:443–447, 1986.

5. Brinckmann P, Hoefert H, Jongen HT: Sex differences in the skeletal geometry of the human pelvis and hip joint. Biomechanics 1:427–430, 1981.

6. Genda E, Iwasaki N, Li G, et al.: Normal hip joint contact pressure distribution in single-leg standing—Effect of gender and anatomic parameters. J Biomech 34:895–905, 2001.

7. Williams P: Gray's Anatomy, 38th ed. New York, Churchill Livingstone, 1999.

8. Svenningsen S, Apalset K, Terjesen T, et al.: Regression of femoral anteversion. A prospective study of intoeing children. Acta Orthop Scand 60:170–173, 1989.

9. Kapandji I: The Physiology of the Joints, 5th ed. Baltimore, Williams & Wilkins, 1987.

10. Seldes RM, Tan V, Hunt J, et al.: Anatomy, histo-logic features, and vascularity of the adult acetabular labrum. Clin Orthop 382:232–240, 2001.

11. Konrath G, Hamel A, Olson S, et al.: The role of the acetabular labrum and the transverse acetabular ligament in load transmission of the hip. J Bone Joint Surg Am 80:1781–1788, 1998.

12. Petersen W, Petersen F, Tillmann B: Structure and vascularization of the acetabular labrum with regard to the pathogenesis and healing of labral lesions. Arch Orthop Trauma Surg 123:283–288, 2003.

13. Ferguson SJ, Bryant JT, Ganz R, et al.: An in vitro investigation of the acetabular labral seal in hip joint mechanics. J Biomech 36:171–178, 2003.

14. Leunig M, Beck M, Woo A, et al.: Acetabular rim degeneration: A constant finding in the aged hip. Clin Orthop 413:201–207, 2003.

15. Bencardino J, Palmer W: Imaging of hip disorders in athletes. Radiol Clin North Am 40:267–287, 2002.

16. McCarthy JC: The diagnosis and treatment of labral and chondral injuries. Instr Course Lect 53: 573–577, 2004.

17. Notzli H, Wyss T, Stoecklin C, et al.: The contour of the femoral head-neck junction as a predictor for the risk of anterior impingement. J Bone Joint Surg Br 84:556–560, 2002.

18. Ito K, Minka Mn, Leunig M, et al.: Femoro-acetabular impingement and the cam-effect. A MRI-based quantitative anatomical study of the femoral head-neck offset. J Bone Joint Surg Br 83: 171–176, 2001.

19. Leunig M, Podeszwa D, Beck M, et al.: Magnetic resonance arthrography of labral disorders in hips with dysplasia and impingement. Clin Orthop 418: 74–80, 2004.

20. Narvani AA, Tsiridis E, Kendall S, et al.: A preliminary report on prevalence of acetabular labrum tears in sports patients with groin pain. Knee Surg Sports Traumatol Arthrosc 11:403–408, 2003.

21. Noble PC, Kamaric E, Sugano N, et al.: Three-dimensional shape of the dysplastic femur: Implications for THR. Clin Orthop 417:27–40, 2003.

22. Iglic A, Antolic V, Srakar F, et al.: Biomechanical study of various greater trochanter positions. Arch Orthop Trauma Surg 114:76–78, 1995.

23. Singleton M, LeVeau B: Stability and stress. A review. Phys Ther 55:9, 1975.

24. Rosse C: The Musculoskeletal System in Health and Disease. Hagerstown, MD, Harper & Row, 1980.

25. Radin E: Biomechanics of the human hip. Clin Orthop 152:28–34, 1980.

26. Arnold A, Delp S: Rotational moment arms of the medial hamstrings and adductors vary with femoral geometry and limb position: Implications for the treatment of internally rotated gait. J Biomech 34:437–447, 2001.

27. Heller M, Bergmann G, Deuretzbacher G, et al.: Influence of femoral anteversion on proximal femoral loading: Measurement and simulation in four patients. Clin Biomech (Bristol, Avon) 16:644–649, 2001.

28. Wingstrand H, Wingstrand A, Krantz P: Intracapsular and atmospheric pressure in the dynamics and stability of the hip. Acta Orthop Scand 61:231–235, 1990.

29. O'Sullivan S, Schmitz T: Physical Rehabilitation: Assessment and Treatment, 4th ed. Philadelphia, FA Davis, 2000.

30. D'Ambrosia R: Musculoskeletal Disorders: Regional Examination and Differential Diagnosis, 2nd ed. Philadelphia, JB Lippincott, 1986.

31. Mavcic B, Pompe B, Antolic V, et al.: Mathematical estimation of stress distribution in normal and dysplatic human hips. J Orthop Res 20:1025–1030, 2002.

32. Stewart K, Edmonds-Wilson R, Brand R, et al.: Spatial distribution of hip capsule structural and material properties. J Biomech 35:1491–1498, 2002.

33. Pfirrmann C, Chung C, Theumann B, et al.: Greater trochanter of the hip: Attachment of the abductor mechanism and a complex of three bursae—MR imaging and MR bursography in cadavers and MR imaging in asymptomatic volunteers. Radiology 221:469–477, 2001.

34. Bird P, Oakley S, Shnier R, et al.: Prospective evaluation of magnetic resonance imaging and physical examination findings in patients with greater trochanteric pain syndrome. Arthritis Rheum 44: 2138–2145, 2001.

35. Chen H-H, Li A-Y, Li K-C, et al.: Adaptations of ligamentum teres in ischemic necrosis of the human femoral head. Clin Orthop 328:268–275, 1996.

36. Fuss F, Bacher A: New aspects of the morphology and function of the human hip joint ligaments. Am J Anat 192:1–13, 1991.

37. Crock H: An atlas of the arterial supply of the head and neck of the femur in man. Clin Orthop 152:17–27, 1980.

38. Tan C, Wong W: Absence of the ligament of the head of femur in the human hip joint. Singapore Med J 31:360–363, 1990.

39. Hewitt JD, Glisson RR, Guilak F, et al.: The mechanical properties of the human hip capsule ligaments. J Arthroplasty 17:82–89, 2002.

40. Yutani Y, Yano Y, Ohashi H, et al.: Cartilaginous differentiation in the joint capsule. J Bone Miner Metab 17:7–10, 1999.

41. Kummer B: Is the Pauwels' theory of hip biomechanics still valid? A critical analysis, based on modern methods. Ann Anat 175:203–210, 1993.

42. Greenspan A: Orthopedic Radiology: A Practical Approach. 2nd ed. New York, Raven Press, 1992.

43. Crabtree N, Loveridge N, Parker M, et al.: Intracapsular hip fracture and the region-specific loss of cortical bone: Analysis by peripheral quantitative computed tomography. J Bone Miner Res 16:1318–1328, 2001.

44. Athanasiou K, Agarwal A, Dzida F: Comparative study of the intrinsic mechanical properties of the human acetabular and femoral head cartilage. J Orthop Res 12:340–349, 1994.

45. Bombelli R, Santore RF, Poss R: Mechanics of the normal and osteoarthritic hip: A new perspective. Clin Orthop 182:69–78, 1984.

46. Radin E (ed): Practical Biomechanics for the Orthopedic Surgeon. New York, John Wiley & Sons, 1979.

47. Norkin C, White D: Measurement of Joint Motion: A Guide to Goniometry, 3rd ed. Philadelphia, FA Davis, 2003.

48. Nonaka H, Mita K, Watakabe M, et al.: Age-related changes in the interactive mobility of the hip and knee joints: A geometrical analysis. Gait Posture 15:236–243, 2002.

49. Valmassy R: Clinical Biomechanics of the Lower Extremities. St. Louis, CV Mosby, 1996.

50. Kendall F, McCreary E, Provance P: Muscles: Testing and Function, 4th ed. Baltimore, Williams & Wilkins, 1993.

51. Perry J: Gait Analysis: Normal and Pathological Function. Thorofare, NJ, Slack, 1992.

52. Observational Gait Analysis Handbook. Downey, CA, Rancho Los Amigos Hospital, 2002.

53. Bohannon R, Gajdosik R, LeVeau B: Contribution of pelvic and lower limb motion to increases in the angle of passive straight leg raising test. Phys Ther 65:474–476, 1985.

54. Murray R, Bohannon R, Tiberio D, et al.: Pelvifemoral rhythm during unilateral hip flexion in standing. Clin Biomech (Bristol, Avon) 17:147–151, 2002.

55. Mens J, Vleeming A, Snijders C, et al.: Validity of the active straight leg raise test for measuring dis-

ease severity in patients with posterior pelvic pain after pregnancy. Spine 27:196–200, 2002.

56. Hahne A, Keating J, Wilson S: Do within-session changes in pain intensity and range of motion predict between-session changes in patients with low back pain? Aust J Physiother 50:17–23, 2004.

57. Schmidt G: Current open and closed kinetic chain concepts—Clarifying or confusing? J Orthop Sports Phys Ther 20:235, 1994.

58. Gowitzke B, Milner M: Scientific Bases of Human Movement, 3rd ed. Baltimore, Williams & Wilkins, 1988.

59. Basmajian J, DeLuca C: Muscles Alive, 5th ed. Baltimore, Williams & Wilkins, 1985.

60. Delp S, Hess W, Hungerford D, et al.: Variation of rotation moment arms with hip flexion. J Biomech 32:493–501, 1999.

61. Nemeth G, Ohlsen H: *In vivo* moment arm lengths for hip extensor muscles at different angles of hip flexion. J Biomech 18:129–140, 1985.

62. Smith L, Weiss E, Lehmkuhl L: Brunnstrom's Clinical Kinesiology, 5th ed. Philadelphia, FA Davis, 1996.

63. Wheatley M, Jahnke W: Electromyographic study of the superficial thigh and hip muscles in normal individuals. Arch Phys Med 32:508, 1951.

64. Kaplan E: The iliotibial tract. J Bone Joint Surg Am 40:825–832, 1958.

65. Gajdosik R, Sandler M, Marr H: Influence of knee positions and gender on the Ober test for length of the iliotibial band. Clin Biomech (Bristol, Avon) 18:77–79, 2003.

65a. Janda V, Stará V: The role of the thigh adductors in movement patterns of the hip and knee joint. Courrier (Centre Internat de l'Enfance), 15:1–3.

66. Ito J: Morphological analysis of the human lower extremity based on the relative muscle weight. Okajimas Folia Anat Jpn 73:247–252, 1996.

67. Murray M, Sepic S: Maximum isometric torque of hip abductor and adductor muscles. Phys Ther 48:2, 1968.

68. Inman V, Ralston HJ, Todd F: Human Walking. Baltimore, Williams & Wilkins, 1981.

69. Chleboun G, France A, Crill M, et al.: *In vivo* measurement of fascicle length and pennation angle of the human biceps femoris muscle. Cells Tissues Organs 169:401–409, 2001.

70. Soderburg G, Dostal W: Electromyographic study of three parts of the gluteus medius muscle during functional activities. Phys Ther 58:6, 1978.

71. Beck M, Sledge J, Gautier E, et al.: The anatomy and function of the gluteus minimus muscle. J Bone Joint Surg Br 82:358–363, 2000.

72. Walters J, Solomons M, Davies J: Gluteus minimus; observations on its insertion. J Anat 198(Pt 2):239–242, 2001.

73. Jensen R, Smidt GL, Johnston RC: A technique for obtaining measurements of force generated by hip muscles. Arch Phys Med 52:207, 1971.

74. Olson V, Smidt GL, Johnston RC: The maximum torque generated by the eccentric, isometric and concentric contractions of the hip abductor muscles. Phys Ther 52:2, 1972.

75. Nordin M, Frankel V: Basic Biomechanics of the Skeletal System, 2nd ed. Philadelphia, Lea & Febiger, 1989.

76. Bergmann G, Graichen F, Rohlmann A, et al.: Hip joint forces during load carrying. Clin Orthop 335:190–201, 1997.

77. LeVeau B: Williams and Lissner's Biomechanics of Human Motion, 3rd ed. Philadelphia, WB Saunders, 1992.

78. Cailliet R: Soft Tissue Pain and Disability, 3rd ed. Philadelphia, FA Davis, 1996.

79. Paul J, McGrouther D: Forces transmitted at the hip and knee joint of normal and disabled persons during a range of activities. Acta Orthop Belg (Suppl) 41:78–88, 1975.

80. Crowninshield RD, Johnston RC, Andrews JG, et al.: A biomechanical investigation of the human hip. J Biomech 11:75, 1976.

81. Kummer F, Shah S, Iyer S, et al.: The effect of acetabular cup orientations on limiting hip rotation. J Arthoplasty 14:509–513, 1999.

82. Krebs D, Robbins C, Lavine L, et al.: Hip biomechanics during gait. J Orthop Sports Phys Ther 28:51–59, 1998.

83. Blount W: Don't throw away the cane. J Bone Joint Surg Am 18:3, 1956.

84. Schenkman M, DeCartaya V: Kinesiology of the shoulder complex. J Orthop Sports Phys Ther 8:438–450, 1987.

85. Neumann D, Cook T: Effect of load and carrying position on the electromyographic activity of the gluteus medius muscle during walking. Phys Ther 65:305–311, 1985.

86. Kelsey J: The epidemiology of diseases of the hip: A review of the literature. Int J Epidemiol 6:269–280, 1977.

87. Clark J, Haynor D: Anatomy of the abductor muscles of the hip as studied by computed tomography. J Bone Joint Surg Am 69:1021–1031, 1987.

88. Pogrund H, Bloom R, Mogle P: Normal width of the adult hip joint: The relationship to age, sex and obesity. Skel Radiol 10:10–12, 1983.

89. Lane N, Hochberg M, Pressman A, et al.: Recreational physical activity and the risk of osteoarthritis of the hip in elderly women. J Rheumatol 26:849–854, 1999.

90. Panush R, Brown D: Exercise and arthritis. Sports Med 4:54–64, 1987.

91. Lewinnek G, Kelsey J, White AA 3rd, et al.: The significance and a comparative analysis of the epidemiology of hip fractures. Clin Orthop 152:35–43, 1980.

92. Cummings S, Nevitt M: A hypothesis: The causes of hip fracture. J Gerontol Med Sci 44:M107-M111, 1989.

93. Falls and hip fractures among older adults. National Center for Injury Prevention and Control. Atlanta, Centers for Disease Control and Prevention, 2004. Accessed 11/7/04 at http://www.cdc.gov/ncipc/factsheets/falls.htm

Introduction

The knee complex is one of the most often injured joints in the human body. The myriad of ligamentous attachments, along with numerous muscles crossing the joint, provide insight into the joint's complexity. This anatomic complexity is necessary to allow for the elaborate interplay between the joint's mobility and stability roles. The knee joint works in conjunction with the hip joint and ankle to support the body's weight during static erect posture. Dynamically, the knee complex is responsible for moving and supporting the body during a variety of both routine and difficult activities. The fact that the knee must fulfill major stability as well as major mobility roles is reflected in its structure and function.

The knee complex is composed of two distinct articulations located within a single joint capsule: the tibiofemoral joint and the patellofemoral joint. The tibiofemoral joint is the articulation between the distal femur and the proximal tibia. The patellofemoral joint is the articulation between the posterior patella and the femur. Although the patella enhances the tibiofemoral mechanism, the characteristics, responses, and problems of the patellofemoral joint are distinct enough from the tibiofemoral joint to warrant separate attention. The superior tibiofibular joint is not considered to be a part of the knee complex because it is not contained within the knee joint capsule and is functionally related to the ankle joint; it will therefore be discussed in Chapter 12.

Tina Mongelli is a 43-year-old female patient who presents to your clinic with complaints of knee pain with increased activity. Tina's chief complaint is significant pain in and around her knee during tennis and during stair ascents and descents. She has pain in the medial aspect of her tibiofemoral joint and anteriorly around her patella, which she describes as being laterally, behind her patella. She is currently unable to jog, play tennis, and walk for more than 1 mile without discomfort. When Tina was 24 years old, she tore her anterior cruciate ligament (ACL), medial collateral ligament (MCL), and medial meniscus. After 4 months of exercise in an attempt to delay surgery, she subsequently underwent surgical stabilization of the ACL with a patellar tendon autograft and a partial medial meniscectomy. The MCL was left to heal on its own. Weight-bearing radiographs of Tina's lower extremity reveal genu varum with moderate joint space narrowing in the patellofemoral and medial tibiofemoral compartments. Clinical testing revealed increased laxity with a valgus stress test, full tibiofemoral range of motion (ROM), a hypomobile medial patellar glide, and diminished quadriceps strength. What structural abnormalities do you think are contributing to the atypical function at her knee, and could be contributing to her pain?

◆ Structure of the Tibiofemoral Joint

The **tibiofemoral,** or knee, joint is a double condyloid joint with three degrees of freedom of angular (rotatory) motion. Flexion and extension occur in the sagittal plane around a coronal axis through the epicondyles of the distal femur,[1] medial/lateral (internal/external) rotation occur in the transverse plane about a longitudinal axis through the lateral side of the medial tibial condyle,[2] and abduction and adduction can occur in the frontal plane around an anteroposterior axis. The double condyloid knee joint is defined by its medial and lateral articular surfaces, also referred to as the **medial** and **lateral compartments** of the knee. Careful examination of the articular surfaces and the relationship of the surfaces to each other are necessary for a full understanding of the knee joint's movements and of both the functions and dysfunctions common to the joint.

Femur

The proximal articular surface of the knee joint is composed of the large medial and lateral condyles of the distal femur. Because of the obliquity of the shaft of the femur, the femoral condyles do not lie immediately below the femoral head but are slightly medial to it (Fig. 11-1A). As a result, the lateral condyle lies more directly in line with the shaft than does the medial condyle. The medial condyle therefore must extend further distally, so that, despite the angulation of the femur's shaft, the distal end of the femur remains essentially horizontal.

In the sagittal plane, the condyles have a convex shape, with a smaller radius of curvature posteriorly (see Fig. 11-1B).[2,3] Although the distal femur as a whole has very little curvature in the frontal plane, both the medial and lateral condyles individually exhibit a slight convexity in the frontal plane. The lateral femoral condyle is shifted anteriorly in relation to the medial femoral condyle.[4] In addition, the articular surface of the lateral condyle is shorter than the articular surface of the medial condyle.[3] When the femur is examined through an inferior view (Fig. 11-2), the lateral condyle appears at first glance to be longer. However, when the patellofemoral surface is excluded, it can be seen that the lateral tibial surface ends before the medial condyle. The two condyles are separated inferiorly by the **intercondylar notch** through most of their length but are joined anteriorly by an asymmetrical, shallow

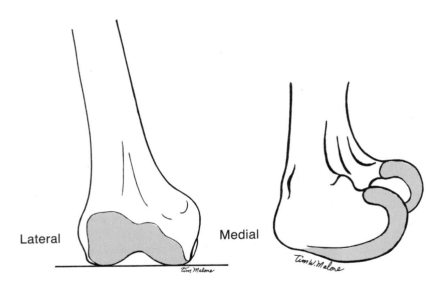

A   B

◀ **Figure 11-1** ■ **A.** Because of the obliquity of the shaft of the femur, the lateral femoral condyle lies more directly in line with the shaft than does the medial condyle. The medial condyle is more prominent, however, which results in a horizontal distal femoral surface despite the oblique shaft. **B.** The anteroposterior convexity of the condyles is not consistently spherical, having a smaller radius of curvature posteriorly.

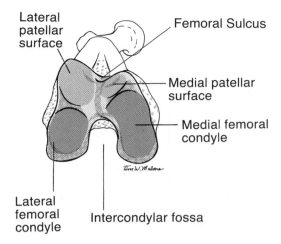

Lateral patellar surface

Femoral Sulcus

Medial patellar surface

Medial femoral condyle

Lateral femoral condyle

Intercondylar fossa

▲ **Figure 11-2** ■ The patellar surface (shaded light pink) is separated from the femur's tibial articular surface (shaded darker pink) by two slight grooves that run obliquely across the condyles. The medial femoral condyle is longer than the lateral femoral condyle; the lateral lip of the patellar surface is larger than the medial lip of the patellar surface.

groove called the **patellar groove** or **surface** that engages the patella during early flexion.

Tibia

The asymmetrical medial and lateral tibial condyles or plateaus constitute the distal articular surface of the knee joint (Fig. 11-3A). The medial tibial plateau is longer in the anteroposterior direction than is the lateral plateau[3,5]; however, the lateral tibial articular cartilage is thicker than the articular cartilage on the medial side.[5] The proximal tibia is larger than the shaft and, consequently, overhangs the shaft posteriorly (see Fig. 11-3B). Accompanying this posterior overhang, the tibial plateau slopes posteriorly approximately 7° to 10°.[3,4] The medial and lateral tibial condyles are separated by a roughened area and two bony spines called the **intercondylar tubercles** (Fig. 11-4). These tubercles become lodged in the intercondylar notch of the femur during knee extension. The tibial plateaus are predominantly flat, with a slight convexity at the anterior and posterior margins,[2] which suggests that the bony architecture of the tibial plateaus does not match up well with the convexity of the femoral condyle. Because of this lack of bony stability, accessory joint structures (**menisci**) are necessary to improve joint congruency.

Tibiofemoral Alignment and Weight-Bearing Forces

The **anatomic (longitudinal) axis** of the femur, as already noted, is oblique, directed inferiorly and medially from its proximal to distal end. The anatomic axis of the tibia is directed almost vertically. Consequently, the femoral and tibial longitudinal axes normally form an angle medially at the knee joint of 180° to 185°; that

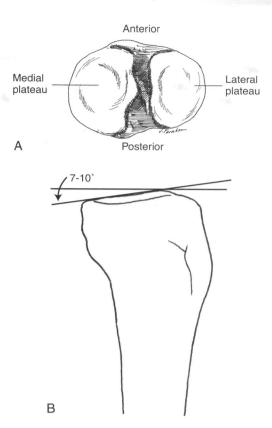

Anterior

Medial plateau

Lateral plateau

A

Posterior

7-10°

B

▲ **Figure 11-3** ■ **A.** A superior view of the articulating surfaces on the tibia illustrates differences in size and configuration between the medial and lateral tibial plateaus. **B.** The tibial plateau overhangs the shaft of the tibia posteriorly and is inclined posteriorly 7° to 10°.

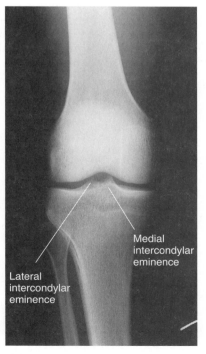

Medial intercondylar eminence

Lateral intercondylar eminence

▲ **Figure 11-4** ■ A radiograph of the right knee shows how the medial and lateral intercondylar eminences of the tibia lodge in the intercondylar notch of the femur in the extended knee.

is, the femur is angled up to 5° off vertical, creating a slight physiologic (normal) valgus angle at the knee (Fig. 11-5). If the medial tibiofemoral angle is greater than 185°, an abnormal condition called **genu valgum** ("knock knees") exists. If the medial tibiofemoral angle is 175° or less, the resulting abnormality is called **genu varum** ("bow legs"). Each condition alters the compressive and tensile stresses on the medial and lateral compartments of the knee joint.

An alternative method of measuring tibiofemoral alignment is performed by drawing a line from the center of the femoral head to the center of the head of the talus (see Fig. 11-5). This line represents the **mechanical axis**, or **weight-bearing line,** of the lower extremity, and in a normally aligned knee, it will pass through the center of the joint between the intercondylar tubercles.[6] The weight-bearing line can be used as a simplification of the ground reaction force as it travels up the lower extremity. In bilateral stance, the weight-bearing stresses on the knee joint are, therefore, equally distributed between the medial and lateral condyles (or medial and lateral compartments).[6] However, once unilateral stance is adopted or dynamic forces are applied to the joint, compartmental loading is altered. In the case of unilateral stance (e.g., during the stance phase of gait), the weight-bearing line must shift medially across the knee to account for the now smaller base of support below the center of mass (Fig. 11-6A). This shift increases the compressive forces on the medial compartment[7] (see Fig. 11-6B). Abnormal compartmental loading may be also be caused by frontal plane malalignment (genu varum or genu valgum). Genu valgum, for instance, shifts the weight-bearing line onto the lateral compartment, increasing the lateral compressive force while increasing the tensile forces on the medial structures (Fig. 11-7A). In the case of genu varum, the weight-bearing line is shifted medially, increasing the compressive force on the medial condyle,

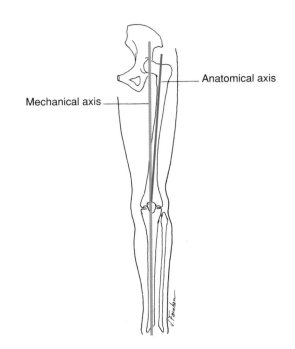

▲ **Figure 11-5** ■ The anatomic axes of the femur and tibia result in a normal physiologic valgus angulation of approximately 185°. The mechanical axis (weight-bearing line) of the lower extremity passes from the center of the hip to the center of the ankle joint and, in a neutrally aligned limb, results in weight-bearing forces that are distributed about equally between the medial and lateral condyles of the knee joint.

whereas the tensile stresses are increased laterally (see Fig. 11-7B). The presence of genu valgum or genu varum creates a constant overload of the lateral or medial articular cartilage, respectively, which may result in damage to the cartilage and the development of frontal plane laxity. Genu varum, for instance, may contribute to the progression of medial compartment knee

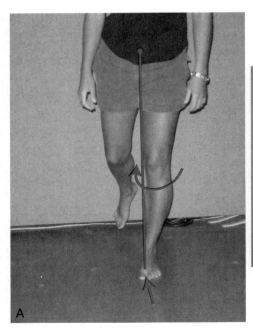

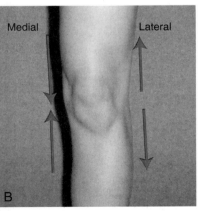

◄ **Figure 11-6** ■ **A.** During dynamic activities, such as gait, the line of force shifts medially to the knee joint center. **B.** This medial shift increases the compressive stresses medially and increases the tensile stresses laterally.

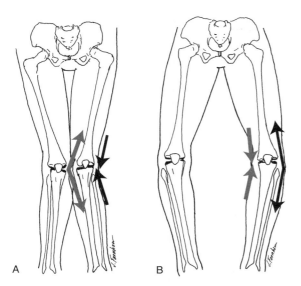

▲ **Figure 11-7** ■ **A.** An increase in the normal tibiofemoral angle results in genu valgum, or "knock knees." Arrows on the lateral aspect of the left tibiofemoral joint indicate the presence of compression forces, whereas the arrows on the medial aspect indicate the presence of distraction (tensile) forces. **B.** A decrease in the normal tibiofemoral angle results in genu varum, or "bow legs." Arrows on the lateral aspect of the left tibiofemoral joint indicate the presence of distraction (tensile) forces, whereas arrows on the medial aspect of the joint indicate the presence of compression forces.

osteoarthritis and lead to excessive medial joint laxity as the medial capsular ligament's attachment sites are gradually approximated through the erosion of the medial compartment's articular cartilage.

> *Continuing Exploration:* **Effects and Corrections of Malalignment**
>
> In the presence of severe frontal plane malalignment and osteoarthritis, some orthopedic surgeons will perform a realignment procedure at the knee, called a high tibial osteotomy. This procedure functions to realign the limb to lessen the compressive force on the damaged painful tibiofemoral compartment. In the case of either significant genu varum or genu valgum, the surgery creates a surgical fracture in the tibia (or sometimes in the femur) in order to realign the limb to a more neutral position. Other, less invasive methods of attempting to diminish compartmental loads in the presence of malalignment include lateral/medial heel wedges or a knee brace that shifts weight-bearing to the uninvolved compartment (so-called "unloading" braces).

Menisci

Tibiofemoral congruence is improved by the medial and lateral menisci, forming concavities into which the femoral condyles sit (Fig. 11-8). In addition to enhancing joint congruence, these accessory joint structures play an important role in distributing weight-bearing forces, in reducing friction between the tibia and the

femur, and in serving as shock absorbers.[8,9] The menisci are fibrocartilaginous disks with a semicircular shape. The medial meniscus is C-shaped, whereas the lateral meniscus forms four fifths of a circle.[8] Lying within the tibiofemoral joint, the menisci are located on top of the tibial condyles, covering one half to two thirds of the articular surface of the tibial plateau (Fig. 11-9).[9] Both menisci are open toward the intercondylar tubercles, thick peripherally and thin centrally. The lateral meniscus covers a greater percentage of the smaller lateral tibial surface than the medial meniscus.[10] As a result of its larger exposed surface, the medial condyle has a greater susceptibility to the enormous compressive loads that pass through the medial condyle during routine daily activities. Although compressive forces in the knee may reach one to two times body weight during gait and stair climbing[11,12] and three to four times body weight during running,[13] the menisci assume 50% to 70% of this imposed load.[8] These loads, however, can be influenced by the presence of frontal plane malalignment. The greater the degree of genu varum, for instance, the greater is the compression on the medial meniscus.

■ **Meniscal Attachments**

The open anterior and posterior ends of the menisci are called the **anterior** and **posterior horns**, each of which is firmly attached to the tibia below.[8] Meniscal motion on the tibia is consequently limited by multiple attachments to surrounding structures, some common to both menisci and some unique to each. The medial meniscus has greater ligamentous and capsular restraints, limiting translation to a greater extent than

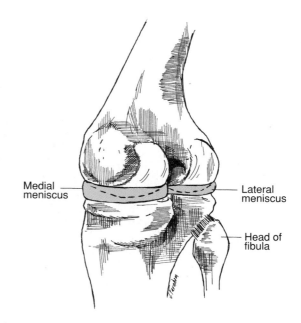

▲ **Figure 11-8** ■ A posteromedial view of an extended right tibiofemoral joint, showing the menisci tightly interposed between the femur and the tibia. The dotted lines indicate the wedge shape of the menisci and show how the menisci deepen and contour the tibial articulating surface to accommodate the femoral condyles.

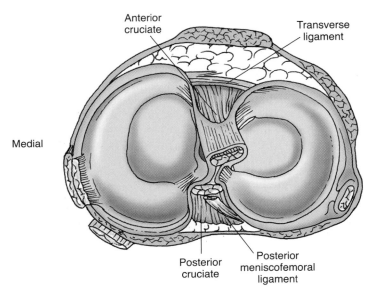

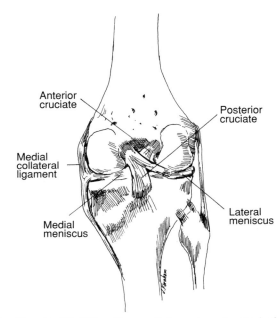

◀ **Figure 11-9** ■ Structure of the menisci. A superior view of the menisci illustrates differences in size and configuration between the medial and lateral menisci. The medial meniscus is C-shaped, whereas the lateral meniscus is shaped like a nearly complete ring or circle. The location of the attachments of the ACL and PCL on the tibial plateau are also shown.

the lateral meniscus. The relative lack of mobility of the medial meniscus may contribute to its greater incidence of injury.[10,14]

Anteriorly, the menisci are connected to each other by the **transverse ligament.**[9,10] Both menisci are also attached directly or indirectly to the patella via the **patellomeniscal ligaments,** which are anterior capsular thickenings.[15] At the periphery, the menisci are connected to the tibial condyle by the **coronary ligaments,** which are composed of fibers from the knee joint capsule. Some of these connections can be seen in Figure 11-9. The medial meniscus has less relative motion than does the lateral meniscus, and it is more firmly attached to the joint capsule through medial thickening of the joint capsule that extends distally from the femur to the tibia. This capsular thickening, referred to as the deep portion of the **medial collateral ligament** (**MCL**), further restricts the motion of the medial meniscus.[10] The anterior and posterior horns of the medial meniscus are attached to the **anterior cruciate ligament** (**ACL**) and **posterior cruciate ligament** (**PCL**), respectively. Through capsular connections, the **semimembranosus muscle** connects to the medial meniscus.[16] Posteriorly, the lateral meniscus attaches to the PCL and the medial femoral condyle through the **meniscofemoral ligaments.**[9,17,18] Some of the ligamentous attachments are shown in Figure 11-10. In much the same way that the semimembranosus tendon is attached to the medial meniscus, the tendon of the **popliteus muscle** attaches to the lateral meniscus.[9,19] The attachment to the popliteus tendon helps restrain or control the motion of the lateral meniscus.[20]

■ **Role of the Menisci**

The strong attachments to the menisci prevent them from being squeezed out during compression of the tibiofemoral joint, allowing for greater contact area between the menisci and the femur. If the femoral condyles sat directly on the relatively flat tibial plateau,

▲ **Figure 11-10** ■ The medial meniscus is attached to the medial collateral, anterior cruciate, and posterior cruciate ligaments. The lateral meniscus is also attached to the posterior cruciate ligament (the joint capsule has been removed for visualization).

there would be little contact between the bony surfaces. With the addition of the menisci, the contact at the tibiofemoral joint is increased and joint stress (force per unit area) is, therefore, reduced on the joint's articular cartilage (Fig. 11-11).[8] After the removal of a meniscus, the contact area in the tibiofemoral joint is decreased, which thus increases joint stress. Specifically, removal of the menisci nearly doubles the articular cartilage stress on the femur and multiplies the forces by six or seven times on the tibial plateau.[21] The increase in joint stress may contribute to degenerative changes within the tibiofemoral joint. For this reason, total meniscectomies are rarely performed after a meniscal

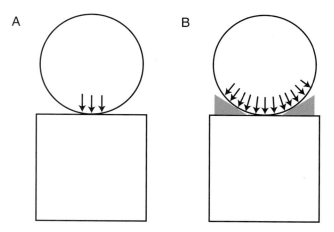

▲ **Figure 11-11** ■ **A.** If the round block (the femoral condyles) sits on the flat block (the tibial plateau), the stress (force per unit area) is high because of the limited contact. **B.** With the addition of the soft chocks or wedges (menisci), the contact area is increased, and the stress between the blocks (bony surfaces) is reduced.

tear; instead, care is taken to preserve as much of the meniscus as possible, either through débridement (removal of damaged tissue) or repair.[22]

Case Application 11-1: **Alignment**

Our patient, Tina, was shown to have genu varum, according to measurements taken from her radiographs. The presence of this frontal plane malalignment could be increasing the magnitude of the compressive force through the medial tibiofemoral joint, promoting the breakdown of the medial compartment's articular cartilage. With the genu varum's generating greater force through the medial compartment, the partial removal of the medial meniscus in her initial surgery becomes more detrimental. The partial removal of Tina's medial meniscus diminishes the contact area within the medial tibiofemoral compartment. The force is, therefore, focused through a smaller area, creating significantly higher joint stress and raising the potential for degenerative articular cartilage changes within the joint. This can be picked up as joint space narrowing on her radiographs and could explain at least some of her medial pain.

■ **Meniscal Nutrition and Innervation**

The location of a meniscal lesion and the age of the patient influence the options available after injury because of the capacity of the meniscus to heal. During the first year of life, the meniscus contains blood vessels throughout the meniscal body. Once weight-bearing is initiated, vascularity begins to diminish until only the outer 25% to 33% is vascularized by capillaries from the joint capsule and the synovial membrane.[23] After 50 years of age, only the periphery of the meniscal body is vascularized.[23] Therefore, the peripheral portion obtains its nutrition through blood vessels, but the central portion must rely on the diffusion of synovial fluid.[14]

The process of fluid diffusion to support nutrition requires intermittent loading of the meniscus by either weight-bearing or muscular contractions.[23] Subsequently, during prolonged periods of immobilization or conditions of non–weight-bearing, the meniscus may not receive appropriate nutrition. The avascular nature of the central portion of the meniscus reduces the potential for healing after an injury.[24] In adults, only the peripheral vascularized region of the meniscus is capable of inflammation, repair, and remodeling after a tearing injury.

The horns of the menisci and the peripheral vascularized portion of the meniscal bodies are well innervated with free nerve endings (nociceptors) and three different mechanoreceptors (Ruffini corpuscles, pacinian corpuscles, and Golgi tendon organs).[23,25,26] The presence of nociceptors in the meniscus could explain some of the pain felt by patients after a meniscal tear, at least for tears located in the periphery.[26] Proprioceptive deficits may potentially occur after meniscal injury as a result of injury to the mechanoreceptors within the meniscus.

Joint Capsule

Given the incongruence of the knee joint, even with the improvements provided by the menisci, joint stability is heavily dependent on the surrounding joint structures. The delicate balance between stability and mobility varies as the knee is flexed from full extension toward increased flexion. Bony congruence and overall ligament tautness are maximal in full extension, representing the close-packed position of the knee joint. In knee flexion, the periarticular passive structures tend to be lax, and the relative bony incongruence of the joint permits greater anterior and posterior translations, as well as rotation of the tibia beneath the femur.[27]

The joint capsule that encloses the tibiofemoral and patellofemoral joints is large and lax. It is grossly composed of an exterior or superficial fibrous layer and a thinner internal synovial membrane that is even more complex than the already complex fibrous portion. In general, the outer or fibrous portion of the capsule is firmly attached to the inferior aspect of the femur and the superior portion of the tibia.[28] Posteriorly, the capsule is attached proximally to the posterior margins of the femoral condyles and intercondylar notch and distally to the posterior tibial condyle.[29] The patella, the tendon of the quadriceps muscles superiorly, and the **patellar tendon** inferiorly complete the anterior portion of the joint capsule. The anteromedial and anterolateral portions of the capsule, as we shall see, are often separately identified as the **medial** and **lateral patellar retinaculae** or together as the **extensor retinaculum**.[30] The joint capsule is reinforced medially, laterally, and posteriorly by capsular ligaments.

The knee joint capsule and its associated ligaments are critical in restricting excessive joint motions to maintain joint integrity and normal function. Although muscles clearly play a dominant role in stabilization (as we shall examine more closely later in the chapter), it is difficult to stabilize the knee with active muscular forces alone in the presence of substantial disruption of passive restraining mechanisms of the capsule and ligaments. The joint capsule plays a role beyond that of a simple passive structure, however. The joint capsule is strongly innervated by both nociceptors as well as pacinian and Ruffini corpuscles. These mechanoreceptors may contribute to muscular stabilization of the knee joint by initiating reflex-mediated muscular responses. In addition, the joint capsule is responsible for providing a tight seal for keeping the lubricating synovial fluid within the joint space.[28]

■ Synovial Layer of the Joint Capsule

The synovial membrane forms the inner lining in much of the knee joint capsule.[31,32] The roles of the synovial tissue are to secrete and absorb synovial fluid into the joint for lubrication and to provide nutrition to avascular structures, such as the menisci. The synovial lining of the joint capsule is quite complex and is among the most extensive and involved in the body (Fig. 11-12). Posteriorly, the synovium breaks away from the inner wall of the fibrous joint capsule and invaginates anteriorly between the femoral condyles. The invaginated synovium adheres to the anterior aspect and sides of the ACL and the PCL.[32–34] Therefore, both the ACL and the PCL are contained within the fibrous capsule (intracapsular) but lie outside of the synovial sheath (extrasynovial).[32–34] Posterolaterally, the synovial lining delves between the popliteus muscle and lateral femoral condyle, whereas posteromedially it may invaginate between the semimembranosus tendon, the medial head of the **gastrocnemius** muscle, and the medial femoral condyle. The intricate folds of the synovium exclude several fat pads that lie within the fibrous capsule,

making them intracapular but extrasynovial, like the cruciate ligaments.[35] The anterior and posterior suprapatellar fat pads lie posterior to the **quadriceps tendon** and anterior to the distal femoral epiphysis, respectively. The infrapatellar (Hoffa's) fat pad lies deep to the patellar tendon[35] (see Fig. 11-9).

Patellar Plicae

Formation of the knee joint's synovial membrane occurs in early embryonic development.[36] Initially, the synovial membrane may separate the medial and lateral articular surfaces into separate joint cavities. By 12 weeks of gestation, the synovial septae are resorbed to some degree, which results in a single joint cavity but with retention of the posterior invagination of the synovium that forms some separation of the condyles.[32] The failure of the synovial membrane to become fully resorbed results in persistent folds in specific regions of the membrane. These folds are called **patellar plicae**.[36,37] There are four potential locations where patellar plicae may be found. Because size, shape, and frequency of these plicae vary among individuals, descriptions also vary among authors. The most frequent locations for the plicae, in descending order of incidence, are inferior (infrapatellar plica), superior (suprapatellar plica), and medial (mediopatellar plica)[37] (Fig. 11-13). There is also the potential for a lateral plica, although finding this lateral plica is relatively rare.[36] Synovial plicae, when they exist, are generally composed of loose, pliant, and elastic fibrous connective tissue that easily passes back and forth over the femoral condyles as the knee flexes and extends.[36] On occasion, a plica may become irritated and inflamed, which leads to pain, effusion, and changes in joint structure and function, called **plica syndrome**.[36]

Continuing Exploration: **Patellar Plicae**

The locations of the most commonly found patellar plicae are shown in Figure 11-13. The inferior plica, also called the **ligamentum mucosum**, is located anterior to the ACL in the intercondylar area, passes through the infrapatellar fat pad (of Hoffa), and attaches to the inferior pole of the patella.[35,36,38] A superior plica is generally located superior to the patella, between the suprapatellar bursa and the superior portion of the patella. It connects the posterior aspect of the quadriceps tendon above to the synovial pouch at the anterior aspect of the distal femoral shaft. Despite its location above the patella, the superior plica rarely gets impinged upon between the patella and the femur.[36] The medial plica is found less frequently (in only 25% to 30% of knees) than either the superior or inferior plica (found in 50% to 65% of knees), but it may be more clinically important. The medial plica arises from the medial wall of the pouch of the extensor retinaculum and runs parallel to the medial edge of the patella to attach to the infrapatellar fat pad and synovium of the inferior plicae.[36] The plica syndrome generally arises not from the most common infrapatellar plica but from either the medial or superior plica.[36,39] The great deal of pain that occurs from the

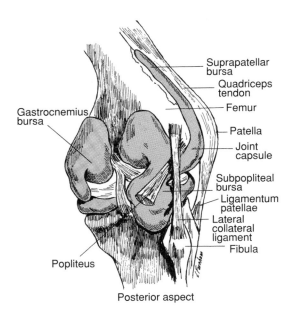

▲ **Figure 11-12** ■ This view of the posterolateral aspect of the knee complex (with the fibrous outer layer of the capsule removed) shows the complex course of the synovial layer of the knee joint capsule, including the related bursae.

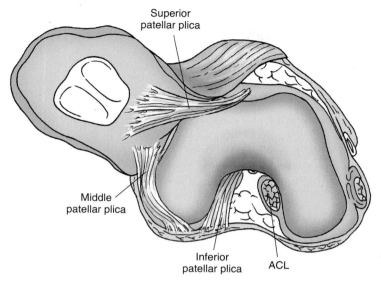

Superior
patellar plica

Middle
patellar plica

Inferior
patellar plica   ACL

◀ **Figure 11-13** ■ The knee joint may contain an inferior, superior, or medial patellar plica or a combination of these. These plicae are folds within the synovial layer of the joint capsule and can become irritated through repetitive trauma.

irritated synovial membrane can be attributed to its rich supply of pacinian corpuscles and free nerve endings.[31]

■ Fibrous Layer of the Joint Capsule

Superficial to the synovial lining of the knee joint lies the fibrous joint capsule, which provides passive support for the joint. The fibrous joint capsule itself is composed of two or three layers, depending on location. Additional structural support to the incongruent knee joint is provided by several capsular thickenings (or

capsular ligaments), as well as both intracapsular and extracapsular ligaments.

The anterior portion of the knee joint capsule is called the extensor retinaculum. A fascial layer covers the distal quadriceps muscles and extends inferiorly. Deep to this layer, the **medial** and **lateral retinacula** are composed of a series of transverse and longitudinal fibrous bands connecting the patella to the surrounding structures (Fig. 11-14). Medially, the thickest and clinically most important band within the medial retinaculum is the **medial patellofemoral ligament** (MPFL).[40,41] Its fibers, oriented in a transverse manner, course ante-

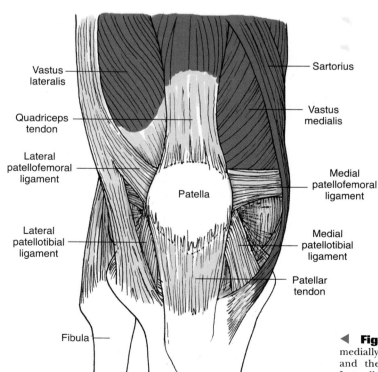

Vastus
lateralis

Quadriceps
tendon

Lateral
patellofemoral
ligament

Lateral
patellotibial
ligament

Fibula

Sartorius

Vastus
medialis

Patella

Medial
patellofemoral
ligament

Medial
patellotibial
ligament

Patellar
tendon

◀ **Figure 11-14** ■ The extensor retinaculum is reinforced medially by the transversely oriented medial patellofemoral ligament and the longitudinally oriented medial patellotibial ligament. Laterally, the lateral patellofemoral ligament and lateral patellotibial ligament help resist an excessive medial glide of the patella.

riorly from the adductor tubercle of the femur to blend with the distal fibers of the **vastus medialis** and eventually insert onto the superomedial border of the patella.[40,42] The transversely oriented fibers within the lateral retinaculum, called the **lateral patellofemoral ligament,** travel from the **iliotibial (IT) band** to the lateral border of the patella.[19,30] The remainder of the retinacular bands include the obliquely oriented **medial patellomeniscal ligament** and the longitudinally positioned **medial** and **lateral patellotibial ligaments**[19,30,41] (see Fig. 11-14).

The medial portion of the joint capsule is composed of the deep and superficial portions of the MCL. The most superficial layer of the joint capsule on the medial side of the knee joint is a fascial layer that covers the vastus medialis muscle anteriorly and the **sartorius** muscle posteriorly.[43] Laterally, the joint capsule is composed superficially of the IT band and its thick **fascia lata.**[19] The capsule is reinforced posterolaterally by the **arcuate ligament**[44,45] and posteromedially by the **posterior oblique ligament (POL).**[43]

Ligaments

The roles of the various ligaments of the knee have received extensive attention, which reflects their importance for knee joint stability and the frequency with which function is disrupted through injury. Given the lack of bony restraint to virtually any of the knee motions, the knee joint ligaments are variously credited with resisting or controlling:

1. excessive knee extension
2. varus and valgus stresses at the knee (attempted adduction or abduction of the tibia, respectively)
3. anterior or posterior displacement of the tibia beneath the femur
4. medial or lateral rotation of the tibia beneath the femur
5. combinations of anteroposterior displacements and rotations of the tibia, together known as **rotatory stabilization** of the tibia

CONCEPT CORNERSTONE 11-1: *Weight-Bearing/Non–Weight-Bearing versus Open/Closed Chain*

Although the ligamentous checks just described were defined by the tibia's motions, it is also possible that stresses may occur on the femur while the tibia is fixed (as in weight-bearing). Such weight-bearing activities (often called "closed-chain" activities) involve motion of the femur moving on a relatively fixed tibia. In contrast, non–weight-bearing activities (often termed "open-chain" activities) involve a moving tibia on a relatively fixed femur. As noted in earlier chapters, weight-bearing activities result in true closed-chain effects only when the position of the head (or trunk) is relatively fixed in space, generally to maintain the line of gravity (LoG) within the base of support (BoS). Consequently, we will refer to activities as weight-bearing or non–weight-bearing, rather than as "closed-chain" or "open-chain." The difference between weight-bearing and non–weight-bearing motions is important because the displacements and rotations of the tibia and the femur will reverse.

For example, anterior displacement of the tibia on the femur (during non–weight-bearing) is equivalent to posterior displacement of the femur on the tibia (during weight-bearing) and so forth.

The large body of literature available on ligamentous function of the knee joint can be confusing and appears contradictory. This may be due to some confusion in terms as to whether the tibia or the femur is being referenced, but it is more likely due to complex and variable functioning and to dissimilar testing conditions. It is clear that ligamentous function can change, depending on the position of the knee joint, on how the stresses are applied, and on what active or passive structures are concomitantly intact.

■ Medial Collateral Ligament

The MCL can be divided into a superficial portion and a deep portion that are separated by a bursa. The superficial portion of the MCL arises proximally from the medial femoral epicondyle and travels distally to insert into the medial aspect of the proximal tibia distal to the pes anserinus (Fig. 11-15). The deep portion of the MCL is continuous with the joint capsule, originates from the inferior aspect of the medial femoral condyle, and inserts on the proximal aspect of the medial tibial plateau. Throughout its course of travel, the deep portion of the MCL is rigidly affixed to the medial border of the medial meniscus[43,46] (see Fig. 11-10).

The MCL, specifically the superficial portion, is the primary restraint to excessive abduction (valgus) and lateral rotation stresses at the knee.[46,47] The knee joint is best able to resist a valgus stress at full extension because the MCL is taut in this position. As joint flexion is increased, the MCL becomes more lax and greater joint space opening is allowed (medially gapping).[47] With the knee flexed, the MCL plays a more critical role in resisting valgus stress despite the permitted joint gapping. Grood et al. determined that at close to full extension, the MCL accounted for 57% of the restraining force against valgus opening, but at 25° of knee flexion,

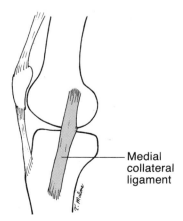

▲ **Figure 11-15** ■ The superficial portion of the medial collateral ligament (MCL) runs inferiorly from the medial femoral condyle to the anteromedial tibial condyle.

the MCL accounted for 78% of the load.[48] This difference is likely due to the greater bony congruence and inclusion of other soft tissue structures (e.g., posteromedial capsule, ACL) that at full extension can more effectively assist with checking a valgus stress. The MCL also plays a supportive role in resisting anterior translation of the tibia on the femur in the absence of the primary restraints against anterior tibial translation.[49] The MCL has the capacity to heal when ruptured or damaged, because of its rich blood supply. An isolated injury, therefore, does not often necessitate surgical stabilization but is often left to heal on its own, although this remodeling process can take up to a year.[50]

■ Lateral Collateral Ligament

The **lateral collateral ligament** (**LCL**) is located on the lateral side of the tibiofemoral joint, beginning proximally from the lateral femoral condyle. The LCL then travels distally to the fibular head (Fig. 11-16), where it joins with the tendon of the **biceps femoris** muscle to form the conjoined tendon.[19,51] Unlike the MCL, the LCL is not a thickening of the capsule but is separate throughout much of its length and is thereby considered to be an extracapsular ligament. The LCL is primarily responsible for checking varus stresses, and like the MCL, limits varus motion most successfully at full extension.[47,48] Grood et al.[48] reported that at 5° of knee flexion, the LCL accounted for 55% of the restraining force against varus stress. This capacity increased to 69% with the knee flexed to 25°. Although the LCL's primary role is to resist varus stresses, its orientation enables the LCL to limit excessive lateral rotation of the tibia as well.

■ Anterior Cruciate Ligament

The relatively high rate of injury of the ACL by athletes and other active individuals has resulted in the ACL's being one of the most highly researched ligaments in the human body. The ACL is attached to the anterior tibial spine (see Fig. 11-9), where it extends superiorly and posteriorly to attach to the posteromedial aspect of the lateral femoral condyle (Fig. 11-17).[33] The ACL courses posteriorly, laterally, and superiorly from tibia to femur. In addition, the ACL twists inwardly (medially) as it travels proximally.[33] The ACL may also be considered to consist of two separate bands that wrap around each other. Each of these bands is thought to have a different role in controlling tibiofemoral motion. The **anteromedial band** (**AMB**) and the **posterolateral band** (**PLB**) are each named for their origins on the tibia.[33] The major blood supply to the ACL arises primarily from the middle genicular artery.[33]

The ACL functions as the primary restraint against anterior translation (anterior shear) of the tibia on the femur.[34] This role, however, belongs to either the AMB or the PLB, depending on the knee flexion angle. With the knee in full extension, the PLB is taut; as knee flexion increases, the PLB loosens and the AMB becomes tight, as demonstrated by the data plotted in Figure 11-18.[33,52] This shift in tension between the bands allows some portion of the ACL to remain tight at all times. In the intact joint, forces producing an anterior translation of the tibia will result in maximal excursion of the tibia at about 30° of flexion[53] when neither of the ACL bands are particularly tensed. The ACL is also responsible for resisting hyperextension of the knee.[54] There

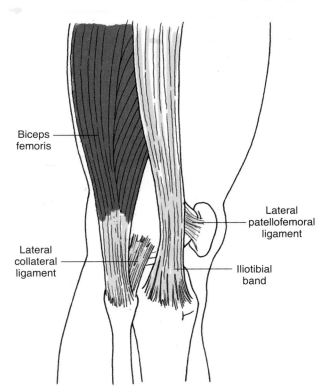

▲ **Figure 11-16** ■ Lateral collateral ligament joins the biceps femoris muscle in a common attachment to the fibular head, whereas the iliotibial band is also attached distally to the anterolateral tibia.

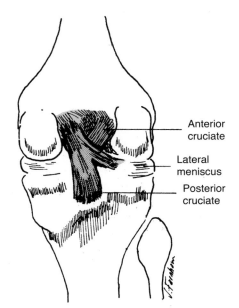

▲ **Figure 11-17** ■ A posterior view of the knee joint shows the femoral condyles to which the ACL and PCL each attach.

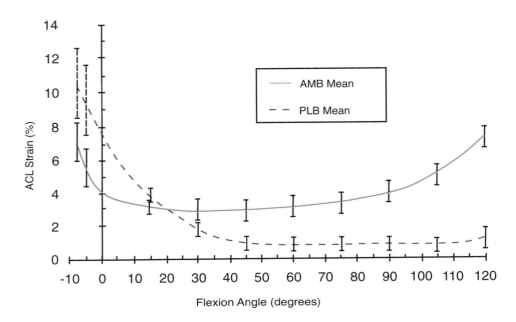

◀ **Figure 11-18** ■ Although the anteromedial band of the ACL is slack in extension and the postero-lateral band is slack in flexion, there is a continuum between the two, so that some portion of the ACL remains fairly taut throughout the range of motion.

appears to be essentially no anterior translation of the tibia possible in full extension when many of the supporting passive structures of the knee are taut (including the PLB of the ACL).

In addition to its primary restraint against anterior shear, the ACL can act as a secondary restraint against either varus or valgus motions (adduction and abduction rotations respectively) at the knee.[54-57] With valgus loading, the lengths of both bands of the ACL increase as knee flexion increases. After injury to the MCL, a valgus moment will increase the strain on the ACL throughout the flexion range. Although the ACL may not make an important contribution to limiting medial rotation of the tibia, medial rotation of the tibia on the femur increases the strain on the AMB of the ACL, with the peak strain occurring between 10° and 15°.[57-59] This is most likely due to the orientation of the ACL, inasmuch as it winds its way medially around the PCL, becoming tighter with medial rotation.

Continuing Exploration: Loading the ACL through Combined Motions

Markolf et al.[58] found that the conditions that individually stress the ACL can in combination generate even greater stress on the ligament. They determined that a combination of either varus or valgus forces with anterior translation increases the strain on the ACL, as did the combination of a valgus force and medial rotation. A combination of medial rotation and anterior translation increased the force on the ACL during a knee flexion range of −5° to 10° beyond that of isolated anterior translation. The inclusion of tibial lateral rotation with anterior tibial translation reduced the force on the ACL at all knee flexion angles greater than 10°.

Regardless of the rotational effect on the ACL's loading pattern, injury to the ACL appears to occur most commonly when the knee is slightly flexed and the tibia is rotated in either direction in weight-bearing. In flexion and medial rotation, the ACL is tensed as it winds around the PCL. In flexion and lateral rotation, the ACL is tensed as it is stretched over the lateral femoral condyle.[60]

The muscles surrounding the knee joint are capable of either inducing or minimizing strain in the ACL. With the tibiofemoral joint in nearly full extension, a quadriceps muscle contraction is capable of generating an anterior shear force on the tibia,[57,61,62] thereby increasing stress on the ACL. Fleming et al. reported that the gastrocnemius muscle similarly has the potential to translate the tibia anteriorly and strain the ACL because the proximal tendon of the gastrocnemius wraps around the posterior tibia,[63] effectively pushing the tibia forward when the muscle becomes tense through active contraction or passive stretch. The hamstring muscles are capable of inducing a posterior shear force on the tibia throughout the range of knee flexion,[64,65] becoming more effective in this role at greater knee flexion angles.[66] The hamstrings, therefore, have the potential to relieve the ACL of some of the stress of checking anterior shear of the tibia on the femur. With the foot on the ground, the soleus muscle may also have the ability to posteriorly translate the tibia and assist the ACL in restraining anterior tibial translation (Fig. 11-19).[67]

Given the potential of individual muscles to either increase or decrease loads on the ACL, it is not surprising that co-contraction of multiple muscles across the knee can influence the strain on the ACL. For example, co-contraction of the hamstrings and quadriceps muscles will allow the hamstrings to counter the anterior translatory effect of the quadriceps and reduce the strain on the ACL. In contrast, activation of both the gastrocnemius and the quadriceps muscles results in greater strain on the ACL than either muscle alone would produce,[63] unless the hamstrings also co-contract

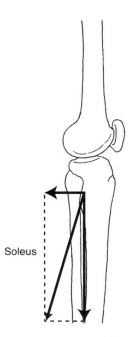

▲ **Figure 11-19** ■ A contraction of the soleus muscle acting on the tibia in weight-bearing has a component that will produce posterior tibial translation at the knee.

Soleus

to mitigate the anterior translation imposed by the gastrocnemius.[63] Although muscular co-contraction will limit the strain imposed on the ligaments of the knee, it comes at a price. Co-contraction will reduce the anterior shear force on the tibia, but it increases joint compressive loads.[64]

Case Application 11-2: ACL Injury and Tibial Shear

The ACL tear that our patient, Tina, experienced resulted in excessive anterior translation of the tibia on the femur. Patients will often experience episodes of giving way, including buckling, shifting, or slipping of the knee with weight-bearing, inasmuch as there appears to be an anterior shift of the tibia as the knee is loaded.[68,69] Because of the greater shearing forces across the tibiofemoral joint, there is the potential for creating more damage to the joint with each episode of instability. To avoid these episodes of giving way, early surgical stabilization is typically recommended. However, Tina chose to delay surgery and was called upon to resist excessive anterior tibial translation through active muscular co-contractions. She was given an exercise program that includes hamstring-dominant exercises throughout the range of knee motion, as well as quadriceps exercises with the knee flexed beyond 60°. This program minimizes ACL strain, according to data from Beynnon and Fleming, who identified the amount of ACL strain that occurred with various exercises (Fig. 11-20).[70]

■ **Posterior Cruciate Ligament**

The PCL attaches distally to the posterior tibial spine (see Fig. 11-9) and travels superiorly and somewhat

anteriorly to attach to the lateral aspect of the medial femoral condyle (see Fig. 11-17). Like the ACL, the PCL is intracapsular but extrasynovial.[34] The PCL is a shorter and less oblique structure than the ACL, with a cross-sectional area 120% to 150% greater than that of the ACL.[71] The PCL blends with the posterior capsule and periosteum as it crosses to its tibial attachment.[72] The PCL, again like the ACL, is typically divided into an AMB and a PLB that are each named for their tibial origins.[71] When the knee is close to full extension, the larger and stronger AMB is lax, whereas the PLB becomes taut. At 80° to 90° of flexion, the AMB is maximally taut and the PLB is relaxed.[73]

The PCL serves as the primary restraint to posterior displacement, or posterior shear, of the tibia beneath the femur.[74] In the fully extended knee, the PCL will absorb 93% of a posteriorly directed load applied to the tibia. This ability of the PCL to assume such a large load in full extension restricts posterior displacement to very minimal amounts.[75] Unlike the ACL, which resists force better at full extension, the PCL is more adept at restraining motion with the knee flexed.[54] Maximal posterior displacement of the tibia occurs at 75° to 90° of flexion, however, because with greater knee flexion, the secondary restraints against posterior translation become ineffective. Sectioning of the PCL, therefore, increases posterior translation at all angles of knee flexion.[76] Like the ACL, the PCL has a role in restraining varus and valgus stresses at the knee[75] and appears to play a role in both restraining and producing rotation of the tibia. The orientation of the PCL may result in a concomitant lateral rotation of the tibia when posterior translational forces are applied to the tibia. The PCL resists tibial medial rotation at 90° but less so in full extension.[54] The PCL does not resist lateral rotation very well.[54]

In the absence of the PCL, muscles must be recruited to actively stabilize against excessive posterior tibial translation. The popliteus muscle shares the role of the PCL in resisting posteriorly directed forces on the tibia and can contribute to knee stability when the PCL is absent.[77] In contrast, an isolated hamstring contraction might destabilize the knee joint in the absence of the PCL because of its posterior shear on the tibia in the flexed knee. Contraction of the gastrocnemius muscle also significantly strains the PCL at flexion angles greater than 40°, whereas quadriceps contraction reduces the strain in the PCL at knee flexion angles between 20° and 60°.[62]

■ **Ligaments of the Posterior Capsule**

Several structures reinforce the "corners" of the posterior knee joint capsule (Fig. 11-21). The posteromedial corner of the capsule is reinforced by the semimembranosus muscle, by its tendinous expansion called the oblique popliteal ligament, and by the stronger and more superficial POL.[78] The posterolateral corner of the capsule is reinforced by the arcuate ligament, the LCL, and the popliteus muscle and tendon. The arcuate ligament is a Y-shaped capsular thickening found in nearly 70% of knees.[45] (Attachments of these ligaments

ACL Strain During Rehabilitation Activities

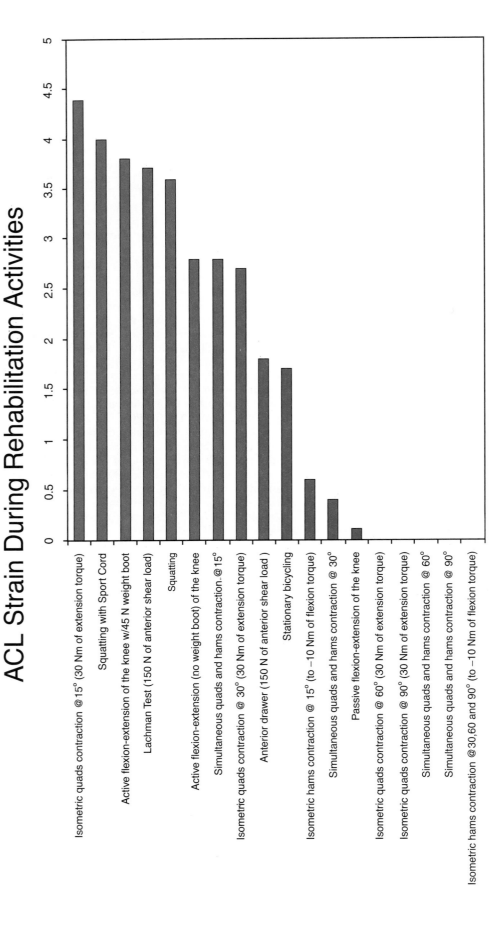

▲ **Figure 11-20** ■ Various activities are routinely prescribed to improve muscle strength and joint function after ACL tear or reconstruction. This graph provides information on the magnitude of strain on the ACL during various activities. It should be noted, however that it is currently unclear as to how much strain can be detrimental to an already damaged ACL or a healing graft.

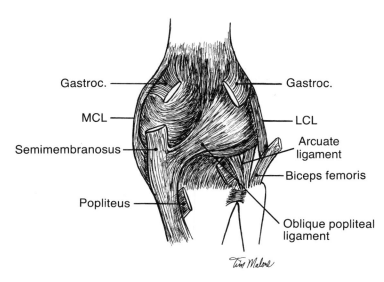

◀ **Figure 11-21** ■ A view of the posterior capsule of the knee joint shows the reinforcing oblique popliteal ligament. Also seen are the collateral ligaments (MCL and LCL), the arcuate ligament, and some of the reinforcing posterior musculature (semimembranosus, biceps femoris, medial and lateral heads of the gastrocnemius, and the upper and lower sections of the popliteus muscles). The medially located posterior oblique (POL) muscle is not shown because it lies superficial to the other medial capsular structures.

are given in Table 11-1.) Both the POL and the arcuate ligaments are taut in full extension and assist in checking hyperextension of the knee; the POL and arcuate ligaments also check valgus and varus forces, respectively.[79] The orientation of the lateral branch of the arcuate ligament allows it to become tight in tibial lateral rotation.[80,81]

Continuing Exploration: **Meniscofemoral Ligaments**

There are two potential portions of the meniscofemoral ligaments that have a variable presence in the human knee. These meniscofemoral ligaments are not true ligaments because they attach bone to meniscus, rather than bone to bone. When present, however, both originate from the posterior horn of the lateral meniscus and insert on the lateral aspect of the medial femoral condyle either anterior to the PCL on the tibia (ligament of Humphry) or posterior to the PCL on the tibia (ligament of Wrisberg).[8,17,18] In a review of the literature, Gupte et

al. reported that at least one of the meniscofemoral ligaments are present in 91% of knees, with approximately 30% of knees having both of the meniscofemoral ligaments. The incidence of the posterior meniscofemoral ligament is greater than the occurrence of the anterior ligament.[18] Although the cross-sectional area of the meniscofemoral ligaments is only about 14% of that of the PCL, they may assist the PCL in restraining posterior translation of the tibia on the femur.[17] The meniscofemoral ligaments can also assist the popliteus muscle by checking tibial lateral rotation.

Iliotibial Band

The IT band (or ITB) or IT tract is formed proximally from the fascia investing the tensor fascia lata, the gluteus maximus, and the gluteus medius muscles. The IT band continues distally to attach to the lateral intermuscular septum and inserts into the anterolateral tibia

Table 11-1	**Ligaments of the Posterior Knee Joint Capsule**		
Ligament	Proximal Attachment	Distal Attachment	Function
Oblique popliteal ligament [43]	The central part of the posterior aspect of the joint capsule	Posterior medial tibial condyle	Reinforces the posteromedial knee joint capsule obliquely on a lateral-to-medial diagonal from proximal to distal
Posterior oblique ligament [79]	Near the proximal origin of the MCL and adductor tubercle	Posteromedial tibia, posterior capsule and posteromedial aspect of the medial meniscus	Reinforces the posteromedial knee joint capsule obliquely on a medial-to-lateral diagonal from proximal to distal
Arcuate ligament: lateral branch [29, 44, 45, 80, 81].	The tendon of the popliteus muscle and the posterior capsule	The posterior aspect of the head of the fibula	Reinforces the posterolateral knee joint capsule obliquely on a medial to lateral diagonal from proximal to distal
Arcuate ligament: medial branch [29, 44]		The medical branch inserts into the oblique popliteal ligament on the medial side of the joint	

(Gerdy's tubercle), reinforcing the anterolateral aspect of the knee joint (see Fig. 11-16).[51,80] Despite the muscular attachments to the IT band, it remains an essentially passive structure at the knee joint; a contraction of the tensor fascia lata (TFL) or the gluteus maximus muscles that attach to the IT band proximally produce only minimal longitudinal excursion of the band distally. The IT band moves anterior to the knee joint axis as the knee is extended, and posteriorly over the lateral femoral condyle as the knee is flexed[80,81] (Fig. 11-22). The IT band, therefore, remains consistently taut, regardless of the hip or knee's position. The fibrous connections of the IT band to the biceps femoris and **vastus lateralis** muscles form a sling behind the lateral femoral condyle, assisting the ACL in checking posterior femoral (or anterior tibial) translation when the knee joint is nearly full extension.[51,82] With the knee in flexion, the combination of the IT band, the LCL, and the popliteal tendon crossing over each other increases the stability of the lateral side of the joint[80] and even more effectively assists the ACL in resisting anterior displacement of the tibia on the femur (see Fig. 11-22). Despite its lateral location, the IT band alone provides only minimal resistance to lateral joint space opening.[48] The IT band also attaches to the patella via the lateral patellofemoral ligament of the lateral retinaculum. As we shall see, this attachment of the IT band to the lateral border of the patella may affect patellofemoral function.

Bursae

The extensive array of ligaments and muscles crossing the tibiofemoral joint, in combination with the large excursions of bony segments, sets up the potential for substantial frictional forces among muscular, ligamentous, and bony structures. Numerous bursae, however, prevent or limit such degenerative forces. Three of the knee joint's bursae, the suprapatellar bursa, the subpopliteal bursa, and the gastrocnemius bursa, are not separate entities but either are invaginations of the capsule's synovium or communicate with the synovial lining of the joint capsule through small openings (see Fig. 11-12). The anteriorly located suprapatellar bursa lies between the quadriceps tendon and the anterior femur, superior to the patella. The posteriorly located

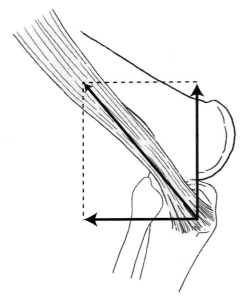

▲ **Figure 11-22** ■ The IT band provides lateral support to the knee joint. In the flexed knee, the IT band tends to migrate posteriorly, increasingly its ability to restrict excessive anterior translation of the tibia under the femur.

subpopliteal bursa lies between the tendon of the popliteus muscle and the lateral femoral condyle, and the gastrocnemius bursa lies between the tendon of the medial head of the gastrocnemius muscle and the medial femoral condyle. The gastrocnemius bursa continues beneath the tendon of the semimembranosus muscle to protect it from the medial femoral condyle.

The three bursae that are connected to the synovial lining of the joint capsule allow the lubricating synovial fluid to move from recess to recess during flexion and extension of the knee. In extension, the posterior capsule and ligaments are taut, and the gastrocnemius and subpopliteal bursae are compressed. This shifts the synovial fluid anteriorly[83] (Fig. 11-23A). In flexion, the suprapatellar bursa is compressed anteriorly and the fluid is forced posteriorly (see Fig. 11-23B). When the knee joint is in the semiflexed position, the synovial fluid is under the least amount of pressure (see Fig. 11-23C). Clinically, when there is excess fluid within the joint cavity as a result of injury or disease (termed **joint**

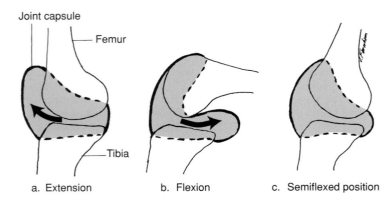

Joint capsule

Femur

Tibia

a. Extension   b. Flexion   c. Semiflexed position

◄ **Figure 11-23** ■ **A.** The synovial fluid is forced anteriorly during extension. **B.** In flexion, the synovial fluid is forced posteriorly. **C.** In the semiflexed position, the capsule is under the least amount of tension, and therefore this is the most comfortable position when joint effusion is present.

Chapter 11: **The Knee** ■ 409

effusion), the semiflexed knee position helps to relieve tension in the capsule and, therefore, minimizes discomfort.

Besides the bursae that communicate with the synovial capsule, there are several other bursae associated with the knee joint (Fig. 11-24). The prepatellar bursa, located between the skin and the anterior surface of the patella, allows free movement of the skin over the patella during flexion and extension. The infrapatellar bursa lies inferior to the patella, between the patellar tendon and the overlying skin. Both the infrapatellar bursa and the prepatellar bursa may become inflamed as a result of direct trauma to the front of the knee or through activities such as prolonged kneeling. The deep infrapatellar bursa, located between the patellar tendon and the tibial tuberosity, helps to reduce friction between the patellar tendon and the tibial tuberosity.[84] This bursa is separated from the synovial cavity of the joint by the **infrapatellar** (Hoffa's) **fat pad**.[84] There are also several small bursae that are associated with the ligaments of the knee joint. There is commonly a bursa between the LCL and the biceps femoris tendon.[85] On the medial side of the joint, small bursae can be found both superficial and deep to the superficial portion of the MCL to protect it from the deep portion of the MCL and the tendons of the **semitendinosus** and **gracilis** muscles, respectively.[43]

◆ Tibiofemoral Joint Function

Joint Kinematics

The primary angular (or rotatory) motion of the tibiofemoral joint is flexion/extension, although both medial/lateral (internal/external) rotation and varus/valgus (adduction/adduction) motions can also occur to a lesser extent. These motions occur about changing but definable axes. In addition to the angular motions,

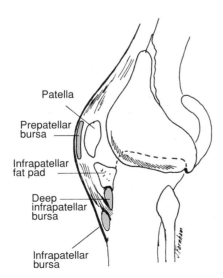

▲ **Figure 11-24** ■ The prepatellar bursa, deep infrapatellar bursa, and infrapatellar bursa are separate from the knee joint cavity.

translation in an anteroposterior direction is common on both the medial and lateral tibial plateaus; to a lesser extent, medial and lateral translations can occur in response to varus and valgus forces. The small amounts of anteroposterior and medial/lateral displacements that occur in the normal knee are the result of joint incongruence and variations in ligamentous elasticity. Although these translations may be seen as undesirable, they are necessary for normal joint motions to occur. Excessive translational motions, however, should be considered abnormal and generally indicate some degree of ligamentous incompetence. We will focus on here on the normal knee joint motions, including both osteokinematics and arthrokinematics.

■ Flexion/Extension

The axis for tibiofemoral flexion and extension can be simplified as a horizontal line passing through the femoral epicondyles.[1] Although this transepicondylar axis represents an accurate estimate of the axis for flexion and extension, it should be appreciated that this axis is not truly fixed but rather shifts throughout the ROM. Much of the shift in the axis can be attributed to the incongruence of the joint surfaces.

The large articular surface of the femur and the relatively small tibial condyle create a potential problem as the femur begins to flex on the fixed tibia. If the femoral condyles were permitted to roll posteriorly on the tibial plateau, the femur would run out of tibia and limit the flexion excursion (Fig. 11-25). For the femoral condyles to continue to roll as flexion increases without leaving the tibial plateau, the femoral condyles must simultaneously glide anteriorly (Fig. 11-26A). The initiation of knee flexion (0° to 25°), therefore, occurs primarily as rolling of the femoral condyles on the tibia that brings the contact of the femoral condyles posteriorly on the tibial condyle. As flexion continues, the rolling of the femoral condyles is accompanied by a simultaneous anterior glide that is just sufficient to create a nearly pure spin of the femur on the posterior tibia with little linear displacement of the femoral condyles after 25° of flexion. Extension of the knee from flexion is essentially a reversal of this motion. Tibiofemoral extension occurs initially as an anterior rolling of the femoral condyles on the tibial plateau, displacing the femoral condyles back to a neutral position on the tibial plateau. After the initial forward rolling, the femoral condyles glide posteriorly just enough to continue extension of the femur as an almost pure spin of the femoral condyles on the tibial plateau (see Fig. 11-26B). This description of the interdependent osteokinematics and arthrokinematics indicates that the femur was moving on a fixed tibia (e.g., during a squat). The tibia, of course, is also capable of moving on a fixed femur (e.g., during a seated knee extension or the swing phase of gait). In this case, the movements would be somewhat different. When the tibia is flexing on a fixed femur, the tibia both rolls and glides posteriorly on the relatively fixed femoral condyles. Extension of the tibia on a fixed femur incorporates an anterior roll and glide of the tibial plateau on the fixed femur.

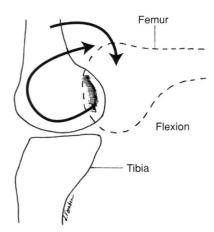

▲ **Figure 11-25** ■ Schematic illustration of pure rolling of the femoral condyles on a fixed tibia shows the femur rolling off the tibia.

Role of the Cruciate Ligaments and Menisci in Flexion/Extension

The arthrokinematics associated with tibiofemoral flexion and extension are somewhat dictated by the presence of the cruciate ligaments. If the cruciate ligaments are assumed to be rigid segments with a constant length,[86] posterior rolling of the femur during knee flexion would cause the "rigid" ACL to tighten (or serve as a check rein). Continued rolling of the femur would result in the taut ACL's simultaneously creating an anterior translational force on the femoral condyles (Fig. 11-27A). During knee extension, the femoral condyles roll anteriorly on the tibial plateau until the "rigid" PCL checks further anterior progression of the femur, creating a posterior translational force on the femoral condyles (see Fig. 11-27B).

The anterior glide of the femur during flexion may be further facilitated by the shape of the menisci. The wedge shape of the menisci posteriorly forces the femoral condyle to roll "uphill" as the knee flexes. The oblique contact force of the menisci on the femur helps guide the femur anteriorly during flexion while the

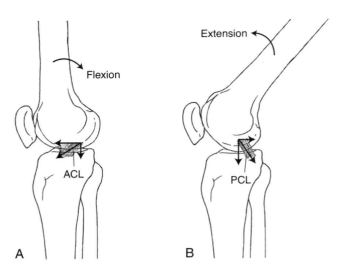

▲ **Figure 11-27** ■ **A.** In flexion of the femur, posterior rolling of the femoral condyles creates tension in the "rigid" ACL that results in an anterior translational force imposed by the ACL on the femur. **B.** In extension of the femur, anterior rolling of the femoral condyles creates tension in the "rigid" PCL that results in a posterior translational force imposed by the PCL on the femur.

reaction force of the femur on the menisci deforms the menisci posteriorly on the tibial plateau[87] (Fig. 11-28). Posterior deformation occurs because the rigid attachments at the meniscal horns limit the ability of the menisci to move in its entirety.[87] Posterior deformation also allows the menisci to remain beneath the rounded femoral condyles as the condyles move on the relatively flat tibial plateau. As the knee joint begins to return to extension from full flexion, the posterior margins of the menisci return to their neutral position. As extension continues, the anterior margins of the menisci deform anteriorly with the femoral condyles.

The motion (or distortion) of the menisci is an important component of tibiofemoral flexion and extension. Given the need of the menisci to reduce friction and absorb the forces of the femoral condyles that are imposed on the relatively small tibial plateau, the menisci must remain beneath the femoral condyles to

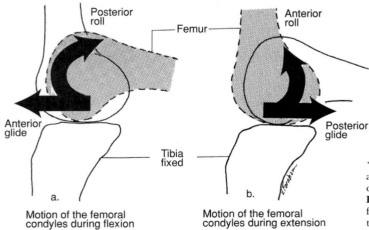

Motion of the femoral condyles during flexion

Motion of the femoral condyles during extension

◄ **Figure 11-26** ■ **A.** A schematic representation of rolling and gliding of the femoral condyles on a fixed tibia. The femoral condyles roll posteriorly while simultaneously gliding anteriorly. **B.** Motion of the femoral condyles during extension. The femoral condyles roll anteriorly while simultaneously gliding posteriorly.

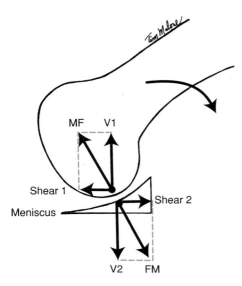

▲ **Figure 11-28** ■ Schematically represented, the oblique contact of the femur with the wedge-shaped meniscus results in the forces of **meniscus-on-femur** (MF) and **femur-on-meniscus** (FM). These can be resolved into vertical and shear components. Shear 1 assists the femur in its forward glide during flexion, and shear 2 assists in the posterior migration of the menisci that occurs with knee flexion.

continue their function. The posterior deformation of the menisci is assisted by muscular mechanisms to ensure that appropriate meniscal motion occurs. During knee flexion, for example, the semimembranosus exerts a posterior pull on the medial meniscus[16] (Fig. 11-29), whereas the popliteus assists with deformation of the lateral meniscus.[20]

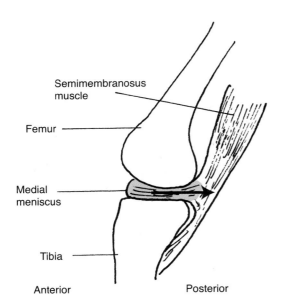

▲ **Figure 11-29** ■ A schematic representation of the semimembranosus muscle and its attachment to the medial meniscus is shown. The arrow represents the direction of pull of the muscle on the medial meniscus during flexion.

Case Application 11-3: **Meniscal Entrapment**

Failure of the menisci to distort in the proper direction can result in limitations of joint motion and/or damage to the menisci. If the femur literally rolls up the wedge-shaped menisci in flexion (without either the anterior glide of the femur or the posterior distortion of the menisci), the increasing thickness of the menisci and the threat of rolling off the posterior margin will cause flexion to be limited. Alternatively, the stress on the meniscus (especially the less mobile medial meniscus) may cause the meniscus to tear. Similarly, failures of the menisci to distort anteriorly during extension causes the thick anterior margins to become wedged between the femur and tibia as the segments are drawn together in the final stages of extension, thus limiting extension. The failure of the meniscus or femoral condyles to move appropriately on each other may be part of the explanation for Tina's original injury to her medial meniscus, although it is likely that additional stresses to the meniscus contributed.

Flexion/Extension Range of Motion

Passive range of knee flexion is generally considered to be 130° to 140°.[88] During an activity such as squatting, knee flexion may reach as much as 160° as the hip and knee are both flexed and the body weight is superimposed on the joint. Normal gait on level ground requires approximately 60° to 70° of knee flexion, whereas ascending stairs requires about 80°, and sitting down into and arising from a chair requires 90° of flexion or more.[88] Knee joint extension (or hyperextension) up to 5° is considered within normal limits. Excessive knee hyperextension (i.e., beyond 5° of hyperextension) is termed **genu recurvatum**.[89]

Many of the muscles acting at the knee are two-joint muscles crossing not only the knee but also the hip or ankle. Therefore, the hip joint's position can influence the knee joint's ROM. Passive insufficiency of the **rectus femoris** could limit knee flexion to 120° or less if the hip joint is simultaneously hyperextended. When the lower extremity is in weight-bearing, ROM limitations at other joints such as the ankle may cause restrictions in knee flexion or extension.

Example 11-1

Ski boots generally hold the ankle in dorsiflexion, preventing full knee extension when the foot is on the ground (see Fig. 11-30A). The choice is either to walk with flexed knees or to walk on the heels. The same problem may be created by a fixed dorsiflexion deformity in the ankle/foot complex. The opposite situation happens with a limitation in dorsiflexion. A limitation to ankle dorsiflexion (e.g., caused by tight plantarflexors) may limit the amount of knee flexion that can be performed without lifting the heel off the ground. If there is a fixed plantarflexion deformity at the ankle, the inability to bring the tibia forward in weight-bearing may result in a hyperextension deformity (genu recurvatum) at the knee (Fig. 11-30B). The relationship between ankle and knee motions when the foot is on the ground can be exploited by intentionally altering ankle joint motion (e.g., through a heel lift or an ankle-foot orthosis) to prevent or control undesired knee motions.

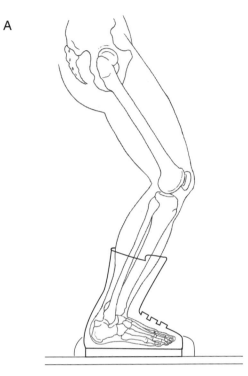

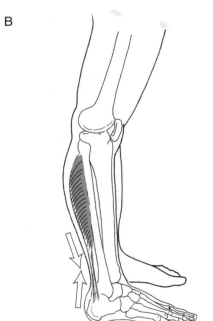

▲ **Figure 11-30** ■ **A.** With the ankle fixed in dorsiflexion by the ski boot, the knee cannot be fully extended without the forefoot's being lifted from the ground. **B.** With a fixed plantarflexion deformity of the ankle/foot, the knee is forced into hyperextension when the foot is flat on the ground.

■ Medial/Lateral Rotation

Medial and lateral rotation of the knee joint are angular motions that are named for the motion (or relative motion) of the tibia on the femur. These **axial rotations** of the knee joint occur about a longitudinal axis that runs through or close to the medial tibial intercondylar tubercle.[2,90] Consequently, the medial condyle acts as the pivot point while the lateral condyles move through a greater arc of motion, regardless of the direction of rotation (Fig. 11-31). As the tibia laterally rotates on the femur, the medial tibial condyle moves only slightly anteriorly on the relatively fixed medial femoral condyle, whereas the lateral tibial condyle moves a larger distance posteriorly on the relatively fixed lateral femoral condyle. During tibial medial rotation, the medial tibial condyle moves only slightly posteriorly, whereas the lateral condyle moves anteriorly through a larger arc of motion. During both medial and lateral rotation, the knee joint's menisci will distort in the direction of movement of the corresponding femoral condyle and, therefore, maintain their relationship to the femoral condyles just as they did in flexion and extension. For example, as the tibia medially rotates (femur laterally rotates on the tibia), the medial meniscus will distort anteriorly on the tibial condyle to remain beneath the anteriorly moving medial femoral condyle, and the lateral meniscus will distort posteriorly to remain beneath the posteriorly moving lateral femoral condyle. In this way, the menisci continue to reduce friction and distribute forces without restricting motion of the femur, as more solid or rigidly attached structures would do.

Axial rotation is permitted by articular incongruence and ligamentous laxity. Therefore, the range of knee joint rotation depends on the flexion/extension position of the knee. When the knee is in full exten-

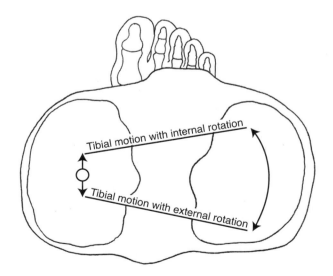

Tibial motion with internal rotation

Tibial motion with external rotation

▲ **Figure 11-31** ■ With internal/external rotation of the tibia, there is more motion of the lateral tibial condyle than of the medial tibial condyle in both directions; that is, the longitudinal axis for medial/lateral rotation appears to be located on the medial tibial plateau.

sion, the ligaments are taut, the tibial tubercles are lodged in the intercondylar notch, and the menisci are tightly interposed between the articulating surfaces; consequently, very little axial rotation is possible. As the knee flexes toward 90°, capsular and ligamentous laxity increase, the tibial tubercles are no longer in the intercondylar notch, and the condyles of the tibia and femur are free to move on each other. The maximum range of axial rotation is available at 90° of knee flexion. The magnitude of axial rotation diminishes as the knee approaches both full extension and full flexion. At 90°, the total medial/lateral rotation available is approximately 35°, with the range for lateral rotation being slightly greater (0° to 20°) than the range for medial rotation (0° to 15°).[91]

■ Valgus (Abduction)/Varus (Adduction)

Frontal plane motion at the knee, although minimal, does exist and can contribute to normal functioning of the tibiofemoral joint. Frontal plane ROM is typically only 8° at full extension, and 13° with 20° of knee flexion.[27,92] Excessive frontal plane motion could indicate ligamentous insufficiency. There is evidence that the muscles that cross the knee joint have the ability both to generate and control substantial valgus and varus torques.[93,94] When there is ligamentous laxity, the excessive varus/valgus motion or increased dynamic activity of muscles attempting to control this excessive motion could precipitate greater peak stresses across the joint.[7]

■ Coupled Motions

Typical tibiofemoral motions are, unfortunately, not as straightforward as we have described. In fact, biplanar intra-articular motions can occur because of the oblique orientation of the axes of motion with respect to the bony levers. The true flexion/extension axis is not perpendicular to the shafts of the femur and tibia.[95] Therefore, flexion and extension do not occur as pure sagittal plane motions but include frontal plane components termed "coupled motions" (similar to coupling that occurs with lateral flexion and rotation in the vertebral column). As already noted, the medial femoral condyle lies slightly distal to the lateral femoral condyle, which results in a physiologic valgus angle in the extended knee that is similar to the physiologic valgus angle that exists at the elbow. With knee flexion around the obliquely oriented axis, the tibia moves from a position oriented slightly lateral to the femur to a position slightly medial to the femur in full flexion; that is, the foot approaches the midline of the body with knee flexion just as the hand approaches the midline of the body with elbow flexion. Flexion is, therefore, considered to be coupled to a varus motion, while extension is coupled with valgus motion.

Automatic or Locking Mechanism of the Knee

There is an obligatory lateral rotation of the tibia that accompanies the final stages of knee extension that is not voluntary or produced by muscular forces. This coupled motion (lateral rotation with extension) is referred to as **automatic** or **terminal rotation.** We have already noted that the medial articular surface of the knee is longer (has more articular surface) than does the lateral articular surface (see Fig. 11-3). Consequently, during the last 30° of knee extension (30° to 0°), the shorter lateral tibial plateau/femoral condyle pair completes its rolling-gliding motion before the longer medial articular surfaces do. As extension continues (referencing non–weight-bearing motion of the tibia), the longer medial plateau continues to roll and to glide anteriorly after the lateral side of the plateau has halted. This continued anterior motion of the medial tibial condyle results in lateral rotation of the tibia on the femur, with the motion most evident in the final 5° of extension. Increasing tension in the knee joint ligaments as the knee approaches full extension may also contribute to the obligatory rotational motion, bringing the knee joint into its close-packed or locked position. The tibial tubercles become lodged in the intercondylar notch, the menisci are tightly interposed between the tibial and femoral condyles, and the ligaments are taut. Consequently, automatic rotation is also known as the **locking** or **screw home mechanism** of the knee. To initiate knee flexion from full extension, the knee must first be unlocked; that is, the laterally rotated tibia cannot simply flex but must medially rotate concomitantly as flexion is initiated. A flexion force will automatically result in medial rotation of the tibia because the longer medial side will move before the shorter lateral compartment. If there is a lateral restraint to unlocking or derotation of the femur, the joint surfaces, ligaments, and menisci can become damaged as the tibia or femur is forced into flexion. This automatic rotation or locking of the knee occurs in both weight-bearing and non–weight-bearing knee joint function. In weight-bearing, the freely moving femur medially rotates on the relatively fixed tibia during the last 30° of extension. Unlocking, consequently, is brought about by lateral rotation of the femur on the tibia before flexion can proceed.

The motions of the knee joint, exclusive of automatic rotation, are produced to a great extent by the muscles that cross the joint. We will complete our examination of the tibiofemoral joint by first examining the individual contribution of the muscles, emphasizing their role in producing and controlling knee joint motion. We will then reexamine both the passive knee joint structures and the muscles in their combined role as stabilizers of this very complicated joint.

Muscles

The muscles that cross the knee are typically thought of as either flexors or extensors, because flexion and extension are the primary motions occurring at the tibiofemoral joint. Each of the muscles that flex and extend the knee has a moment arm (MA) that is capable of generating both frontal and transverse plane motions, although the MAs for these latter motions are generally small. Therefore, each of the muscles, although grouped as flexors and extensors, will also be discussed with regard to its role in controlling frontal and transverse plane motions.

■ Knee Flexor Group

There are seven muscles that flex the knee. These are the semimembranosus, semitendinosus, biceps femoris (long and short heads), sartorius, gracilis, popliteus, and gastrocnemius muscles. The **plantaris** muscle may be considered an eighth knee flexor, but it is commonly absent. With the exception of the short head of the biceps femoris and the popliteus, all of the knee flexors are two-joint muscles. As two-joint muscles, the ability to produce effective force at the knee is influenced by the relative position of the other joint over which that muscle crosses. Five of the flexors (the popliteus, gracilis, sartorius, semimembranosus, and semitendinosus muscles) have the potential to medially rotate the tibia on a fixed femur, whereas the biceps femoris has a MA capable of laterally rotating the tibia.[96] The lateral muscles (biceps femoris, lateral head of the gastrocnemius, and the popliteus) are capable of producing valgus moments at the knee, whereas those on the medial side of the joint (semimembranosus, semitendinosus, medial head of the gastrocnemius, sartorius, and gracilis) can generate varus moments.[93]

The semitendinosus, semimembranosus, and the long and short heads of the biceps femoris muscles are collectively known as the hamstrings. These muscles each attach proximally to the ischial tuberosity of the pelvis, except the short head of the biceps, which has a proximal attachment on the posterior femur. The semitendinosus muscle attaches distally to the anteromedial aspect of the tibia by way of a common tendon with the sartorius and the gracilis muscles. The common tendon is called the pes anserinus because of its shape (pes anserinus means "goose's foot") (Fig. 11-32). The semimembranosus muscle inserts posteromedially on the tibia (and, as noted earlier, has fibers that attach to the medial meniscus that can facilitate posterior distortion of the medial meniscus during knee flexion[16]). Both heads of the biceps femoris muscle attach distally to the head of the fibula, with a slip to the lateral tibia. The short head of the biceps femoris muscle does not cross the hip joint and, therefore, acts uniquely at the knee joint. The rest of the hamstring muscles cross both the hip (as extensors) and the knee (as flexors); therefore, their efficacy in producing force at the knee is dictated by the angle of the hip joint. Greater hamstring force is produced with the hip in flexion when the hamstrings are lengthened over that joint, regardless of knee position.[97] When the two-joint hamstrings are required to contract with the hip extended and the knee flexed to 90° or more, the hamstrings must shorten over both the hip and over the knee. The hamstrings will weaken as knee flexion proceeds because not only are they approaching maximal shortening capability,[97] but also the muscle group must overcome the increasing tension in the rectus femoris muscle that is approaching passive insufficiency. In non–weight-bearing activities, the hamstrings generate a posterior shearing force of

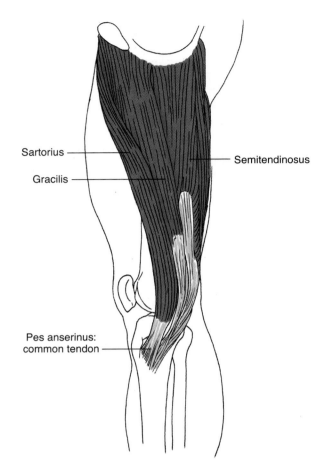

▲ **Figure 11-32** ■ The semitendinosus, sartorius, and gracilis muscles form a common tendon (the pes anserinus) that inserts into the anteromedial tibia.

the tibia on the femur that increases as knee flexion increases,[98] peaking between 75° and 90° of knee flexion. This posterior shear or posterior translational force can reduce strain on the ACL, although conceivably increasing strain on the PCL.

The gastrocnemius muscle originates by two heads from the posterior aspects of the medial and lateral condyles of the femur and attaches distally to the calcaneal (or Achilles) tendon. Except for the small and often absent plantaris muscle, the gastrocnemius muscle is the only muscle that crosses both the knee joint and the ankle joint. Much like the hamstrings' interaction with the hip joint, the gastrocnemius muscle quickly weakens as a knee flexor as it loses tension with the ankle in simultaneous plantarflexion. The gastrocnemius muscle (capable of generating a large plantarflexor torque at the ankle) makes a relatively small contribution to knee flexion, producing the most knee flexion torque when the knee is in full extension.[99] As the knee is flexed, the ability of the gastrocnemius muscle to produce a knee flexion torque is significantly diminished.[99] The gastrocnemius muscle does, however, work synergistically with the quadriceps[63] and, during gait, may be capable of increasing the stiffness of the knee joint.[67] At the knee, therefore, the gastrocnemius muscle appears to be less of a mobility muscle than a dynamic stabilizer.

The sartorius muscle arises anteriorly from the anterosuperior iliac spine (ASIS) and crosses the femur to insert into the anteromedial surface of the tibial shaft (most often as part of the common pes anserinus tendon). Variations in the distal attachment of the sartorius muscle are not uncommon and may be functionally relevant. When attached just anterior to its typical location, the sartorius muscle may fall anterior to the knee joint axis, serving as a mild knee joint extensor rather than as a knee flexor. Typically, however, the sartorius muscle functions as a flexor and medial rotator of the tibia. Despite its potential actions at the knee, activity in the sartorius muscle is more common with hip motion rather than with knee motion. During gait, the sartorius muscle is typically active only during the swing phase.[100]

The gracilis muscle arises from the symphysis pubis and attaches distally to the common pes anserinus tendon. The gracilis muscle functions primarily as a hip joint flexor and adductor, as well as having the capability to flex the knee joint and produce slight medial rotation of the tibia. The three muscles of the pes anserinus appear to function effectively as a group to resist valgus forces and provide dynamic stability to the anteromedial aspect of the knee joint.

The popliteus muscle is a relatively small single-joint muscle that attaches to the posterolateral lateral femoral condyle[45] and courses inferiorly and medially to attach to the posteromedial surface of the proximal tibia.[101] The primary function of the popliteus muscle is as a medial rotator of the tibia on the femur.[96] Because medial rotation of the tibia is required to unlock the knee, the role of unlocking the knee has been attributed to the popliteus muscle. However, it should be noted that unlocking is part of automatic rotation and is due in part to the obliquity of the joint axis and the anatomy of the articular surfaces. The obligatory medial rotation of the knee joint during early flexion is a coupled motion that would likely occur even with paralysis of the popliteus muscle. The popliteus muscle does, however, play a role in deforming the lateral meniscus posteriorly[9] during active knee flexion, given its attachment to the lateral meniscus. Activity of both the semimembranosus and the popliteus muscles will generate a flexion torque at the knee, as well as contribute to the posterior movement and deformation of their respective menisci on the tibial plateau. The menisci will move posteriorly on the tibial condyle even during passive flexion. However, active assistance of the semimembranosus and popliteus muscles ensures that tibiofemoral congruence is maximized throughout the range of knee flexion as the menisci remain beneath the femoral condyles, while also minimizing the chance that the menisci will become entrapped, thus limiting knee flexion and risking meniscal injury. The soleus and gluteus maximus muscles do not cross the knee joint. However, we would be remiss if we did not mention their function at the knee during weight-bearing activities. The soleus muscle attaches proximally to the proximal posterior aspect of the tibia and fibula and

attaches distally to the calcaneal tendon. With the foot fixed on the ground by weight-bearing, a soleus muscle contraction can assist with knee extension by pulling the tibia posteriorly (Fig. 11-33). As noted earlier, the posterior pull of the soleus on the weight-bearing leg can also assist the hamstrings in restraining excessive anterior displacement of the tibia.[67] The gluteus maximus muscle, like the soleus muscle, is capable of assisting with knee extension in a weight-bearing position. It is well known that the large muscle mass of the gluteus maximus functions well as a hip extensor. With the foot flat on the ground and the knee bent, a contraction of the gluteus maximus must influence each of the joints below it. In this case, the contraction generates knee extension and ankle plantarflexion (see Fig. 11-33). The gluteus maximus, however, would produce, if anything, a posterior shear of the femur on the tibia (or a relative anterior shear of the tibia on the femur) that would increase tension in the ACL without offsetting co-contraction of other muscles.

■ **Knee Extensor Group**

The four extensors of the knee are known collectively as the quadriceps femoris muscle. The only portion of the quadriceps that crosses two joints is the rectus femoris muscle, which crosses the hip and knee from its

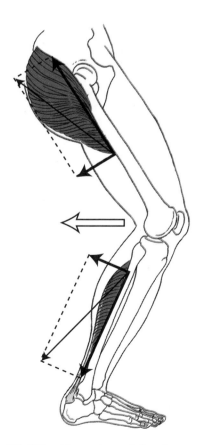

▲ **Figure 11-33** ■ The actions of the gluteus maximus and soleus muscles can influence knee motion in weight-bearing. Although they do not cross the knee joint, these muscles are capable of assisting with knee extension.

attachment on the anterior inferior iliac spine. The **vastus intermedius**, vastus lateralis, and vastus medialis muscles originate on the femur and merge with the rectus femoris muscle into a common tendon, called the quadriceps tendon. The quadriceps tendon inserts into the proximal aspect of the patella and then continues distally past the patella, where it is known as the patellar tendon (or **patellar ligament**). The patellar tendon runs from the apex of the patella into the proximal portion of the tibial tuberosity. The vastus medialis and vastus lateralis also insert directly into the medial and lateral aspects of the patella by way of the retinacular fibers of the joint capsule (see Fig. 11-14).

Together, the four components of the quadriceps femoris muscle function to extend the knee. In 1968, Lieb and Perry[102] examined the direction of pull of each of the components of the quadriceps. The pull of the vastus lateralis muscle alone was found to be 12° to 15° lateral to the long axis of the femur, with the distal fibers the most angled. The pull of the vastus intermedius muscle was parallel to the shaft of the femur, making it the purest knee extensor of the group. The angulation of the pull of the vastus medialis muscle depended on which segment of the muscle was assessed. The upper fibers were angled 15° to 18° medially to the femoral shaft, whereas the distal fibers were angled as much as 50° to 55° medially.[102,103] Powers et al., using more current technology, reported that the resultant pull of vastus lateralis muscle was 35° laterally, whereas the resultant pull of the vastus medialis muscle was 40° medially (Fig. 11-34A).[104] Because of the drastically different orientation of the upper and lower fibers of the vastus medialis muscle, the upper fibers are commonly referred to as the vastus medialis longus (VML), and the lower fibers are referred to as the vastus medialis oblique (VMO). The obliquity of the distal portion of the vastus medialis muscle has become the focus of attention in patients with patellofemoral pain as clinicians and researchers have attempted to try to preferentially recruit the VMO to maximize its medial pull on the patella. It should be noted, however, that despite the different orientation of the fibers of the VMO and VML, these fibers are simply portions of the same muscle.[103,105] Lieb and Perry[102] found the resultant pull of the four portions of the quadriceps muscle to be 7° to 10° in the lateral direction and 3° to 5° anteriorly in relation to the long axis of the femur. Powers et al., however, used a multiplane analysis and noted that the relatively large vastus lateralis and vastus medialis muscles have a posterior attachment site, which results in a net posterior or compressive force that averages 55° in the extended knee (see Fig 11-34B). The compressive force from these muscles is present throughout the ROM but is minimized at full extension and increases as knee flexion continues.

Patellar Influence on Quadriceps Muscle Function

Function of the quadriceps muscle is strongly influenced by the patella (which, in turn, is strongly influenced by the quadriceps, as we shall see shortly). From the perspective of mechanical efficiency, the patella lengthens the MA of the quadriceps by increasing the

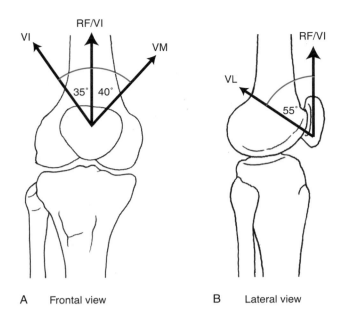

A　Frontal view　　　　　B　Lateral view

▲　**Figure 11-34** ■ With the data from Powers et al.,[104] the orientation of the four components of the quadriceps muscle are shown (**A**), and the posteriorly directed vector of the VL and VM were found to result in net compression of the patella against the tibia even in full extension (**B**).

distance of the quadriceps tendon and patellar tendon from the axis of the knee joint. The patella, as an anatomic pulley, deflects the action line of the quadriceps femoris muscle away from the joint center, increasing the angle of pull and the ability of the muscle to generate an extension torque. The patella does not, however, function as a simple pulley because in a simple pulley the tension is equal on either side of the pulley. In contrast, the tension in the patellar tendon on the inferior aspect of the patella is less than the tension in the quadriceps tendon at the superior aspect of the patella.[106]

The knee joint's geometry and the patella together dictate the quadriceps angle of pull on the tibia as the knee flexes and extends. During early flexion, the patella is primarily responsible for increasing the quadriceps angle of pull. In full knee flexion, however, the patella is fixed firmly inside the intercondylar notch of the femur, which effectively eliminates the patella as a pulley. Despite this, the quadriceps maintains a fairly large MA because the rounded contour of the femoral condyles deflects the muscle's action line and because the axis of rotation has shifted posteriorly into the femoral condyle. Consequently, the quadriceps maintains a reasonable ability to produce torque in full knee flexion, although the patella is not contributing to its MA. During knee extension from full flexion, the MA of the quadriceps muscle lengthens as the patella leaves the intercondylar notch and begins to travel up and over the rounded femoral condyles. At about 50° of knee flexion, the femoral condyles have pushed the patella as far as it will go from the axis of rotation. The influence of the changing MA on quadriceps torque production is readily apparent when knee extension strength is measured throughout the ROM. Peak torques are often observed at approximately 45° to 60° of knee flexion, a region in which both the MA and the length-tension relationship of the muscle are maximized.[107] Finally, with continued extension, the MA will once again diminish.[108]

Although the patella's effect on the quadriceps' MA is diminished in the final stages of knee extension, the small improvement in joint torque provided by the patella may be most important here. Near end range extension, the quadriceps is in a shortened position, which reduces its ability to generate active tension. The decreased ability of the quadriceps to produce active force makes the relative size of the MA critical to torque production in the last 15° of knee extension. In this range, the quadriceps must increase motor unit activity to offset the loss in active tension-generating ability and the decrease in MA.

Continuing Exploration: **Quadriceps Lag**

If there is substantial quadriceps weakness or if the patella has been removed because of trauma (a procedure known as a **patellectomy**), the quadriceps may not be able to produce adequate torque to complete the last 15° of non–weight-bearing knee extension. This can be seen clinically in a patient who demonstrates a "quad lag" or "extension lag." For example, the patient may have difficulty maintaining full knee extension while performing a straight leg raise (Fig. 11-35). With the tibiofemoral joint in greater flexion, removal of the patella or quadriceps weakness will have less effect on the ability of the quadriceps to generate extension torque because the femoral condyles also serve as a pulley, and the total muscle tension of the quadriceps will be greater than in the muscle's shortened state. The patient will not have a "quad lag" in weight-bearing because the soleus and gluteus maximus muscles can assist the quadriceps with knee extension once the foot is fixed.

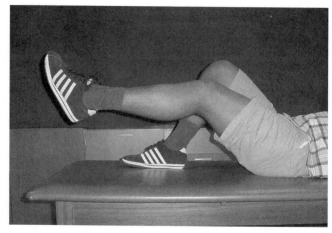

▲ **Figure 11-35** ■ Severe quadriceps weakness can result in a quadriceps lag ("quad lag") during a straight-leg–raise exercise. Near full extension, the patella increases the MA only slightly, and the decreased length-tension relationship of the already weakened quadriceps renders it incapable of generating sufficient torque to complete the range of motion.

The patella's role in increasing the angle of pull of the quadriceps enhances the quadriceps' torque production but at a cost. Increasing the quadriceps' MA also, by definition, increases the rotatory (Fy) component of the pull of the quadriceps on the tibia. The Fy component not only produces extension torque but also creates an anterior shear of the tibia on the femur (Fig. 11-36A). This anterior translational force must be resisted by active or passive forces capable of either producing a posterior tibial translation or passively resisting the anterior tibial translation imposed by the quadriceps. The ACL represents the most prominent passive restraint to the imposed anterior tibial translation of the quadriceps. Increases and decreases in the angle of pull of the quadriceps are accompanied by concomitant increases and decreases in stress in the

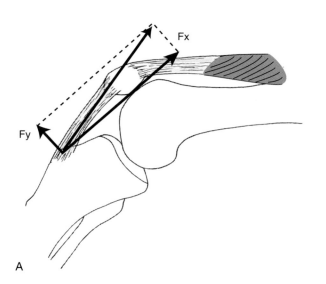

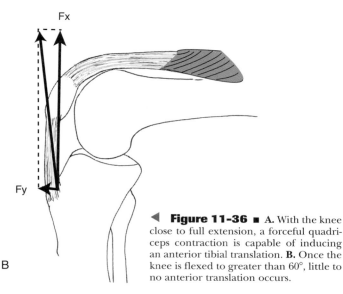

A   B

◀ **Figure 11-36** ■ **A.** With the knee close to full extension, a forceful quadriceps contraction is capable of inducing an anterior tibial translation. **B.** Once the knee is flexed to greater than 60°, little to no anterior translation occurs.

ACL. The strain on both bands of the ACL ordinarily increases as the knee joint approaches full extension. In the absence of passive stabilizers such as the ACL, a quadriceps contraction near full extension has the potential (even with a relatively small Fy component) to generate a large anterior tibial translation,[61] which the patient may describe as "giving way." The strain on the ACL evoked by a quadriceps contraction is substantially diminished as the knee is flexed beyond 60° and as the Fy component of the quadriceps diminishes from its maximum value (see Fig. 11-36B).

Case Application 11-4: **Muscular Consequences of ACL Deficiency**

Although Tina's ACL has been reconstructed, she had to go for some time without an ACL. During that time, she had to restrain excessive anterior tibial translation caused by a forceful quadriceps contraction or ground reaction forces with muscles, such as the hamstrings, gastrocnemius, and soleus muscles. All these muscles can help restrain the tibia or, along with the gluteus maximus, stiffen the knee to minimize movement. Although this can be helpful for maintaining knee joint stability, there are detrimental consequences. Large amounts of co-contraction in muscles crossing the knee joint will increase tibiofemoral compression, given that force of most muscles produce substantially larger joint compression (Fx) than rotation or shear (Fy) components. In addition, tendinitis can develop in muscles that are overworked from trying to actively maintain joint stability. The moderate joint space narrowing in the medial tibiofemoral compartment evident in Tina's weight-bearing radiographs may be associated (along with other factors) with excessive shear and compressive forces during her 4-month period without an ACL.

During weight-bearing activities, the quadriceps' activity in knee extension is influenced by a number of other factors. Muscles such as the soleus and gluteus maximus muscles are capable of assisting with knee joint extension. When an erect posture is attained, activity of the quadriceps is minimal because the line of gravity passes just anterior to the knee axis for flex-ion/extension, which results in a gravitational extension torque that maintains the joint in extension. The posterior joint capsule, ligaments, and largely passive posterior muscles maintain equilibrium by offsetting the gravitational torque and preventing hyperextension. In weight-bearing with the knee somewhat flexed, as during a squat or when someone cannot fully extend the knee (as in the case of a flexion contraction), the line of gravity will pass posterior to the knee joint axis. The gravitational torque will now tend to promote knee flexion, and activity of the quadriceps is necessary to counterbalance the gravitational torque and maintain the knee joint in equilibrium. Because the quadriceps femoris muscle has the responsibility of supporting the body weight and resisting the force of gravity, it is about twice as strong as the hamstring muscles. Although the hamstrings perform a similar function in supporting the body weight when there is a gravitational flexion moment at the hip, the hamstrings are assisted in this function by the large gluteus maximus while the quadriceps are the primary knee joint extensor.

Clearly, the quadriceps functions differently, depending on the activity or the exercise condition. In non–weight-bearing knee extension, the MA of the resistance (i.e., weight of the leg plus external resistance) is minimal when the knee is flexed to 90° but increases as knee extension progresses (Fig. 11-37). Therefore, greater quadriceps force is required as the knee approaches full extension. The opposite happens during weight-bearing activities. In a standing squat, the MA of the resistance (i.e., the superimposed body weight) is minimal when the knee is extended and yet increases with increasing knee flexion (Fig. 11-38). Therefore, during weight-bearing activities such as a squat, the quadriceps muscle must produce more force with greater knee flexion.[109]

Continuing Exploration: **Quadriceps Strengthening: Weight-Bearing versus Non–Weight-Bearing**

Wilk and coworkers[110] investigated anteroposterior shear force, compression force, and extensor torque at the knee in weight-bearing versus non–weight-bearing exercises that are used for quadriceps muscle strengthening. These authors found that the

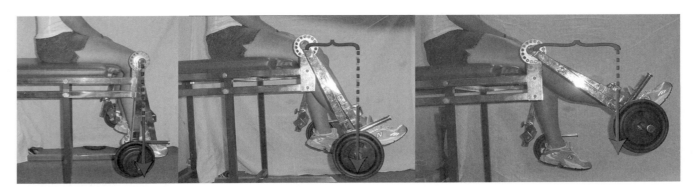

▲ **Figure 11-37** ■ During non–weight-bearing exercises, the quadriceps muscle must generate more torque (and more force) as the knee approaches full extension to overcome the increasing MA (and torque) of the resistance.

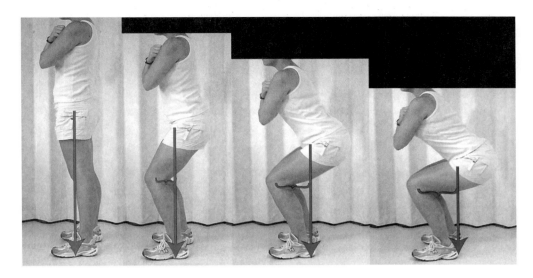

◀ **Figure 11-38** ■ In a weight-bearing exercise, the quadriceps must generate more torque (and more force) as knee flexion increases to control the increasing MA (and torque) of the superimposed body weight at the knee joint.

weight-bearing quadriceps exercises of a squat and leg press resulted in a posterior shear force at the knee throughout the entire ROM, peaking between 83° and 105° of knee flexion.[110,111] The posterior shear would presumably stress the PCL. There was no anterior shear anywhere in the ROM. In contrast, there was an anterior shear force in a non–weight-bearing knee extension exercise when the quadriceps actively extended the knee from 40° to 10°, with the maximal anterior shear occurring between 20° and 10°. One might assume that the ACL was a key element in resisting the anterior shear that was found. A posterior shear force was also found during non–weight-bearing exercise, but this force was present only between 60° and 101° of flexion. Weight-bearing exercises are often prescribed after ACL or PCL injury on the premise that they are less stressful, more like functional movements, and safer than non–weight-bearing exercises. This study demonstrated that the stress on the PCL that is present during some types of weight-bearing exercises may actually be detrimental to the healing process if this ligament is damaged.

Stabilizers of the Knee

Since the beginning of this chapter, we have identified the role of both passive (capsuloligamentous) and active (muscular) forces in contributing to stability of the tibiofemoral joint. However, attempting to credit structures with contributing primarily to one type of stabilization is extremely difficult and generally requires oversimplification. The contribution of both muscles and capsuloligamentous structures to maintaining appropriate joint stability are dependent on the position not only of the knee joint but also of the surrounding joints, the magnitude and direction of the applied force, and the availability of secondary restraints. There can also be considerable variation among individuals (as well as between knees in the same individual) that contributes to the diversity of findings observed by both clinicians and researchers. Although admittedly an oversimplification, Table 11-2 summarizes the potential contribution of the different structures that limit: anteroposterior translation or knee joint hyperextension, varus/valgus rotation, and medial/lateral rotation of the knee joint.

Table 11-2	Summary of Knee Joint Stabilizers*	
	Structures	Function
A-P/hyperextension stabilizers	Anterior cruciate ligament Iliotibial band Hamstring muscles Soleus muscle (in weight-bearing) Gluteus maximus muscle (in weight-bearing)	Limit anterior tibial (or posterior femoral) translation
	Posterior cruciate ligament Meniscofemoral ligaments [17] Quadriceps muscle Popliteus muscle Medial and lateral heads of gastrocnemius [64]	Limit posterior tibial (or anterior femoral) translation

(Continued on following page)

Table 11-2	Summary of Knee Joint Stabilizers* *(Continued)*		
	Structures		Function
Varus/valgus stabilizers	Medial collateral ligament Anterior cruciate ligament Posterior cruciate ligament Arcuate ligament Posterior oblique ligament Sartorius muscle Gracilis muscle Semitendinosus muscle Semimembranosus muscle Medial head of gastrocnemius muscle	} Pes anserinus	Limits valgus of tibia
	Lateral collateral ligament Iliotibial band Anterior cruciate ligament Posterior cruciate ligament Arcuate ligament Posterior oblique ligament Biceps femoris muscle Lateral head of gastrocnemius muscle		Limit varus of tibia
Internal/external rotational stabilizers	Anterior cruciate ligament Posterior cruciate ligament Posteromedial capsule [80] Meniscofemoral ligament Biceps femoris		Limit medial rotation of tibia
	Posterolateral capsule [80] Medial collateral ligament Lateral collateral ligament Popliteus muscle Sartorius muscle Gracilis muscle Semitendinosus muscle Semimembranosus muscle	} Pes anserinus	Limit lateral rotation of tibia

*The contribution of both muscles and capsuloligamentous structures depends on the position of both the knee and contiguous joints, the magnitude and direction of the applied force, and the availability of secondary restraints. Findings vary among investigators, given the testing conditions. (A-P, anteroposterior.)

Table 11-2 describes stability in terms of straight plane movements. In reality, there are more complicated motions that are possible. Therefore, stability is often described as coupled stability, or as rotatory stability (a combination of uniplanar motions) (Table 11-3). For example, injury to the posterolateral corner (i.e., posterolateral joint capsule, popliteus muscle, arcuate ligament) can yield posterior instability and excessive lateral tibial rotation. This is termed **posterolateral instability.** In contrast, damage to the POL, medial hamstrings, MCL, and posteromedial joint capsule contribute to **posteromedial instability.** The extensor retinaculum, which is composed of fibers from the quadriceps femoris muscle, fuses with fibers of the joint capsule to provide dynamic support for the anteromedial and anterolateral aspects of the knee.

✦ Patellofemoral Joint

Embedded within the quadriceps muscle, the flat, triangularly shaped patella is the largest sesamoid bone in the body. The patella is an inverted triangle with its apex directed inferiorly. The posterior surface is divided by a vertical ridge and covered by articular cartilage (Fig. 11-39). This ridge is situated approximately in the center of the patella, dividing the articular surface into approximately equally sized medial and lateral facets. Both the medial and lateral facets are flat to slightly convex side to side and top to bottom. Most patellae also have a second vertical ridge toward the medial border that separates the medial facet from an extreme medial edge, known as the odd facet of the patella[112] (see Fig. 11-39). The posterior surface of the patella in the extended knee sits on the femoral sulcus (or patellar surface) of the anterior aspect of the distal femur (Fig. 11-40). The femoral sulcus has a groove that corresponds to the ridge on the posterior patella and divides the sulcus into medial and lateral facets. The lateral facet of the femoral sulcus is slightly more convex than the medial facet and has a more highly developed lip than does the medial surface (see Fig. 11-2). The patella is attached to the tibial tuberosity by the patellar tendon. Given the shape of the articular surfaces and the fact that the patella has a much smaller

Table 11-3	Components to Rotary Stability	
	Medial	Lateral
	Anteromedial stability*	Anterolateral stability†
Anterior	Medial collateral ligament (MCL) Posterior oblique ligament (POL) Posteromedial capsule Anterior cruciate ligament (ACL)	Anterior cruciate ligament (ACL) Lateral collateral ligament (LCL) Posterolateral capsule Arcuate complex/popliteus Iliotibial band
	Posteromedial stability	Posterolateral stability
Posterior	Posterior cruciate ligament (PCL) Posterior oblique ligament (POL) Medial collateral ligament (MCL) Semimembranosis Posteromedial capsule Anterior cruciate ligament (ACL)	Posterior cruciate ligament (PCL) Arcuate complex/popliteus Lateral collateral ligament (LCL) Biceps femoris Posterolateral capsule

*Indicates that the following active and passive stabilizers are capable of resisting one or more of the following: anterior translation, valgus, or external rotation of the tibia.
†Indicates that the following active and passive stabilizers are capable of resisting one or more of the following: anterior translation, varus, or internal rotation of the tibia.

articular surface area than its femoral counterpart, the patellofemoral joint is one of the most incongruent joints in the body.

The patella functions primarily as an anatomic pulley for the quadriceps muscle. Interposing the patella between the quadriceps tendon and the femoral condyles also reduces friction as the femoral condyles contact the hyaline cartilage–covered posterior surface of the patella rather than the quadriceps tendon. The ability of the patella to perform its functions without restricting knee motion depends on its mobility. Because of the incongruence of the patellofemoral joint, however, the patella is dependent on static and dynamic structures for its stability. We must closely

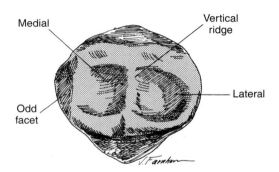

▲ **Figure 11-39** ■ Articulating surfaces on the posterior aspect of the patella.

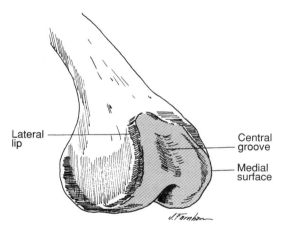

▲ **Figure 11-40** ■ Articulating surfaces on the femoral sulcus. Note the well-developed lateral lip on the lateral aspect of the articulating surface.

examine the oddly shaped patella and the uneven surface on which it sits in order to understand the normal motions of the patella that accompany knee joint motion and the tremendous forces to which the patella and patellofemoral surfaces are susceptible. The goal of such examination is to understand the many potential problems encountered by the patella in performing what appears to be a relatively simple function. A comprehension of the structures and forces that influence patellofemoral function leads readily to an understanding of the common clinical problems found at the patellofemoral joint as it attempts to meet its contradictory demands for both mobility and stability.

Patellofemoral Articular Surfaces and Joint Congruence

In the fully extended knee, the patella lies on the femoral sulcus. Because the patella has not yet entered the intercondylar groove, joint congruency in this position is minimal, which suggests that there is a great potential for patellar instability. Stability of the patella is affected by the vertical position of the patella in the femoral sulcus, because the superior aspect of the femoral sulcus is less developed than the inferior aspect. The vertical position of the patella, in turn, is related to the length of the patellar tendon. Ordinarily, the ratio of the length of the patellar tendon to the length of the patella is approximately 1:1 and is referred to as the Insall-Salvati index.[113] A markedly long tendon produces an abnormally high position of the patella on the femoral sulcus known as **patella alta**, which increases the risk for patellar instability. The interaction of the height of the lateral lip of the femoral sulcus with patella alta may also be a factor in patellar instability. In this condition, the lateral lip is not necessarily underdeveloped (although it may be), but the high position of the patella places the patella proximal to the high lateral wall, rendering the patella less stable and easier to sublux. In patients with patella alta, the tibiofemoral joint must be flexed more before the patella translates inferiorly enough to engage the intercondylar groove. This leaves a larger knee ROM within which the patella is relatively unstable.

Given the incongruence of the patella, the contact between the patella and the femur changes throughout the knee ROM (Fig. 11-41). When the patella sits in the femoral sulcus in the extended knee, only the inferior pole of the patella is making contact with the femur.[114] As the knee begins to flex, the patella slides down the femur, increasing the surface contact area. In this manner, the first consistent contact between the patella and the femur occurs along the inferior margin of both the medial and lateral facets of the patella at 10° to 20° of knee flexion. As tibiofemoral flexion progresses, the contact area increases and shifts from the initial inferior location on the patella to a more superior position.[114] As the contact area shifts superiorly along the posterior aspect of the patella, it also spreads outward to cover the medial and lateral facet. By 90° of knee flexion, all portions of the patella have experienced some (although inconsistent) contact, with the exception of the odd facet. As flexion continues beyond 90°, the area of contact begins to migrate inferiorly once again as the smaller odd facet makes contact with the medial femoral condyle for the first time. At full flexion, the patella is lodged in the intercondylar groove, and contact is on the lateral and odd facets, with the medial facet completely out of contact.[115,116]

Motions of the Patella

As the contact between the patella and the femur changes with knee joint motion, the patella simultaneously translates and rotates on the femoral condyles. These movements are influenced by and reflect the patella's relationship to both the femur and the tibia. Consequently, the description of motions can appear quite complicated. When the femur is fixed and the tibia is flexing, the patella (fixed to the tibial tuberosity via the patellar tendon) is pulled down and under the femoral condyles, ending with the apex of the patella pointing posteriorly in full knee flexion. This sagittal plane rotation of the patella as the patella travels (or "tracks") down the intercondylar groove of the femur is termed **patellar flexion.** Knee extension brings the patella back to its original position in the femoral sulcus, with the apex of the patella pointing inferiorly at the end of the normal ROM. This patellar motion is referred to as **patellar extension.**

In addition to patellar flexion and extension, the patella rotates around a longitudinal (or nearly vertical) axis and tilts around an anteroposterior axis. Rotation about the longitudinal axis is termed **medial** or **lateral patellar tilt** and is named for the direction in which the anterior surface of the patella is moving (Fig. 11-42). When the tibia medially rotates beneath the femur during axial rotation, the patella must remain in the intercondylar groove during the relative lateral rotation of the femur. This relative motion of the femur forces the patella to face more laterally; this is termed lateral rotation. Patellar tilt is also dictated somewhat by the asym-

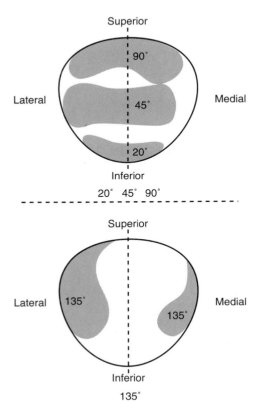

▲ **Figure 11-41** ■ Near full extension, only the inferior pole of the patella makes contact with the femur. As flexion continues, the contact area moves superiorly and then laterally along the patella. By full flexion, only the lateral and odd facets are making contact with the femur.

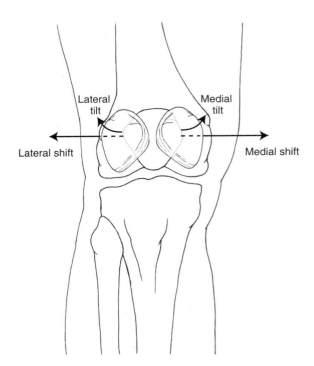

▲ **Figure 11-42** ■ Patellar motions with respect to the femur. Medial/lateral shift is named on the basis of the direction in which the patella is moving; medial/lateral tilt is named for the direction toward which the anterior surface of the patella is moving.

metrical nature of the femoral condyles. For instance, the more anteriorly protruding lateral femoral condyle forces the anterior surface of the patella to tilt medially during much of knee flexion.[117-119]

Rotation of the patella about an anteroposterior axis (termed **medial** or **lateral rotation** of the patella) is, like patellar tilt, necessary in order for the patella to remain seated between the femoral condyles as the femur undergoes axial rotation on the tibia. Because the inferior aspect of the patella is "tied" to the tibia via the patellar tendon, the inferior patella continually points toward the tibial tuberosity while moving with the femur[120] (Fig. 11-43). Therefore, when the knee is in some flexion and there is medial rotation of the tibia on the fixed femur, the inferior pole of the patella will point medially; this is termed medial rotation of the patella. In lateral rotation of the patella, the inferior patellar pole follows the laterally rotated tibia. The patella laterally rotates approximately 5° as the knee flexes from 20° to 90°,[118] given the asymmetrical configuration of the femoral condyles.

The patella, although firmly attached to soft tissue stabilizers (for example, the extensor retinaculum), undergoes translational motions that are dependant on the point in the tibiofemoral ROM. The patella translates superiorly and inferiorly with knee extension and flexion, respectively. During active extension, the patella glides superiorly. If this glide is restricted, quadriceps function is compromised, and passive knee extension may be lost. During active tibiofemoral flexion, the patella glides inferiorly. A restricted inferior glide could therefore limit knee flexion. There is a sim-

ultaneous medial-lateral translation of the patella that accompanies the superior-inferior glide that is referred to as patellar shift[118] (see Fig. 11-42). The patella is typically situated slightly laterally in the femoral sulcus with the knee in full extension. As knee flexion is initiated, the patella shifts medially as it is pushed by the larger lateral femoral condyle and as the tibial medially rotates with unlocking of the knee. As knee flexion proceeds past 30°, the patella may shift slightly laterally or remain fairly stable, inasmuch as the patella is now firmly engaged within the femoral condyles (Fig. 11-44). Consequently, the patella shifts as the knee moves from full extension into flexion. Failure of the patella to slide, tilt, rotate, or shift appropriately can lead to restrictions in knee joint ROM, to instability of the patellofemoral joint, or to pain caused by erosion of the patellofemoral articular surfaces. Therefore, passive mobility of the patella is often assessed clinically to determine the presence of hypermobility or hypomobility of the patella with respect to the femur.

Patellofemoral Joint Stress

The patellofemoral joint can undergo very high stresses during typical activities of daily living.[106,121] Joint stress (force per unit area) can be influenced by any combination of large joint forces or small contact areas, both of which are present during routine flexion and extension of the tibiofemoral joint. The patellofemoral joint reaction (contact) force is influenced by both the quadriceps force and the knee angle. As the knee flexes

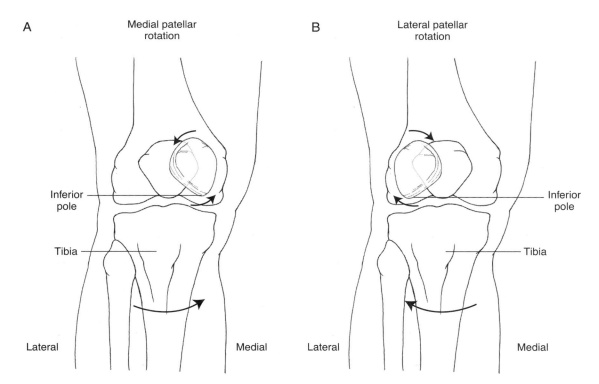

▲ **Figure 11-43** ■ **A.** Medial rotation of the patella. The inferior pole of the patella follows the tibial tuberosity during medial rotation of the tibia. **B.** Lateral rotation of the patella. The inferior pole of the patella follows the tibial tuberosity during lateral rotation of the tibia.

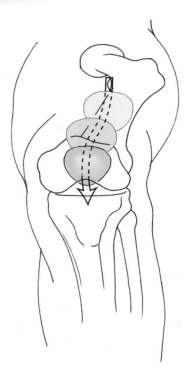

▲ **Figure 11-44** ■ The patella shifts medially during early flexion and then either remains there or shifts slightly laterally with deeper flexion.

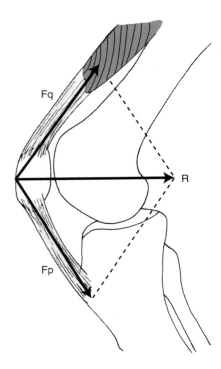

▲ **Figure 11-45** ■ Patellofemoral joint reaction forces are partially explained by the knee flexion angle. As the knee is flexed further, the patellofemoral compressive load is increased.

and extends, the patella is pulled by the quadriceps tendon superiorly and simultaneously by the patella tendon inferiorly. The combination of these pulls produces a posterior compressive force of the patella on the femur that varies with knee flexion. At full extension, the quadriceps posterior compressive force on the patella is minimized and due exclusively to the origin of the vastus medialis and vastus lateralis muscles on the posterior femur.[104] Despite the small contact area that the patella has with the femur in full extension, the minimal posterior compressive vector of the vastus lateralis and vastus medialis muscles maintains low joint stress at full extension. This is the rationale for the use of straight-leg–raising exercises as a way of improving quadriceps muscle strength without creating or exacerbating patellofemoral pain.

As knee flexion progresses from full extension, the angle of pull between the quadriceps tendon and the patellar tendon decreases, creating greater joint compression (Fig. 11-45). This increased compression occurs whether the muscle is active or passive. If the quadriceps muscle is inactive, then elastic tension alone increases with increased knee joint flexion. If the quadriceps muscle is active, then both the active tension and passive elastic tension will contribute to increasing the joint compression. This compression, of course, creates a joint reaction force across the patellofemoral joint. The total joint reaction force is therefore influenced by the magnitude of active and passive pull of the quadriceps, as well as by the angle of knee flexion. Although the compressive force arising from the quadriceps increases as the knee flexes from 0° to 90°,

the patellar contact area also increases.[104] The increase in contact area with increased compressive force functions to minimize patellofemoral joint stress until approximately 90° of flexion. As knee flexion continues beyond 90°, the contact area once again diminishes and patellofemoral stress increases as only the lateral and odd facets make contact with the femoral condyles.

Patellofemoral joint reaction forces can become very high during routine daily activities. During the stance phase of walking, when peak knee flexion is only approximately 20°, the patellofemoral compressive force is approximately 25% to 50% of body weight.[121] With greater knee flexion and greater quadriceps activity, as during running, patellofemoral compressive forces have been estimated to reach between five and six times body weight.[122] Deep knee flexion exercises that require large magnitudes of quadriceps activity can increase this compressive force further. Although reaction forces at other lower extremity joints may reach these same magnitudes, they do so over much more congruent joints; that is, the compressive forces are distributed over larger areas. At the normal patellofemoral joint, the medial facet bears the brunt of the compressive force. Several mechanisms help minimize or dissipate the patellofemoral joint compression on the patella in general and on the medial facet specifically. In full extension, there is minimal compressive force on the patella; therefore, no compensatory mechanisms are necessary. As knee joint flexion proceeds, the area of patella contact gradually increases, spreading out the increased compressive force. From 30° to 70° of flexion, the magnitude of contact force is higher at the thick cartilage of the medial facet near the central ridge. This articular cartilage is among the thickest hyaline cartilage in the human body. The presence of this thick cartilage is better able to withstand the substantial compressive forces transmitted across the medial facet of the patella. Within this same ROM, the patella has its greatest effect as a pulley, maximizing the MA of the quadriceps. With a larger MA, less quadriceps muscle force is needed to produce the same torque, minimizing patellofemoral joint compression. As flexion proceeds, the MA diminishes, which necessitates an increase in force production by the quadriceps. Beyond 90°, however, the patella is no longer the only structure contacting the femoral condyles. At this point in the flexion range, the quadriceps tendon contacts the femoral condyles, helping to dissipate more of the compressive force on the patella.[123]

The vertical position of the patella can also significantly influence patellofemoral stress. Singerman and colleagues[123] demonstrated that in the presence of patella alta, the onset of contact between the quadriceps tendon and femoral condyles is delayed. As flexion increases, patellofemoral compressive forces will therefore continue to rise. In contrast to patella alta, the patella can also sit lower than normal. If the patella is positioned more inferiorly, it is termed **patella baja** and may be due to a shortened patellar tendon. With patella baja, the contact between the quadriceps tendon and the femoral condyles occurs earlier in the range, resulting in a concomitant reduction in the magnitude of the patellofemoral contact force.[123–125]

Frontal Plane Patellofemoral Joint Stability

The patellofemoral joint is unique in its potential for frontal plane instability near full knee extension, as well as for degenerative changes resulting from increased patellofemoral joint stresses (in flexion). This multifaceted problem makes understanding the control of the patella's frontal plane motion particularly important. In the extended knee, instability can be a problem because the patella sits on the shallow aspect of the superior femoral sulcus. There is less bony stability and less patellofemoral compression from the quadriceps. Because of the physiologic valgus that normally exists between the tibia and femur, the action lines of the quadriceps and the patellar tendon do not coincide. This results in the patella's being pulled slightly laterally by the two forces (Fig. 11-46). The presence of a resultant lateral pull on the patella suggests that soft tissue stabilizers must assume more responsibility for medial-lateral stability in the absence of suitable bony stability. Once knee flexion is initiated and the patella begins to slide down the femur and into the femoral sulcus (at about 20° of flexion), medial-lateral stability is increased by the addition of the bony stability of the femoral sulcus. However, the concomitant increased compression of the patella against the femoral condyles can present another problem. Whether the patella is at risk for instability or for increased medial-lateral compression,

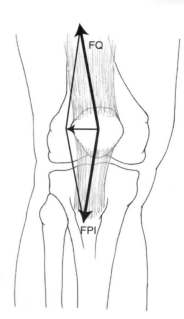

▲ **Figure 11-46** ■ Because of the obliquity (physiologic valgus angle) between the long axis of the femur and the tibia, the pull of the quadriceps (F_Q) and the pull of the patellar ligament (Fp_L) lie at a slight angle to each other, producing a slight lateral force on the patella.

the position, mobility, and control of the patella in the frontal plane are of utmost concern. These factors are determined by the relative tension in both the transverse and longitudinal stabilizers of the patella.

The longitudinal stabilizers of the patella consist of the patellar tendon inferiorly and the quadriceps tendon superiorly. The patellotibial ligaments that are part of the extensor retinaculum and reinforce the capsule also are longitudinal stabilizers[19,30,41] (see Fig. 11-14). The longitudinal stabilizers are capable of providing medial-lateral stability of the patella in knee flexion through increased patellofemoral compression (see Fig. 11-45). In the extended knee, this compression is minimal, however, leaving the patella relatively unstable in this position. When extension is exaggerated, as in genu recurvatum, the pull of the quadriceps muscle and patellar tendon may actually distract the patella somewhat from the femoral sulcus, further aggravating the relative patella instability.

The transverse stabilizers are composed of the superficial portion of the extensor retinaculum. This retinaculum connects the vastus medialis and vastus lateralis muscles directly to the patella for improved muscular stabilization. In addition, passive stabilizers such as the medial and lateral patellofemoral ligaments firmly attach the patella to the adductor tubercle medially[40,41], and the IT band laterally.[19,30] The role of the medial patellofemoral ligament in assisting normal patellar tracking should not be understated. As the thickest portion of the medial retinaculum, the medial patellofemoral ligament alone provides approximately 60% of the passive restraining force against lateral translation (lateral shift) of the patella.[41] An additional passive stabilizer that is sometimes overlooked is the large lateral lip of the femoral sulcus (see Fig. 11-2). The steep lateral facet acts as a buttress to excessive lateral patellar shift. Therefore, even large lateral forces can be prevented from subluxing or dislocating the patella, provided that the lateral lip of the femoral sulcus is of sufficient height. In the case of trochlear dysplasia, however, even relatively small lateral forces imposed on the patella can cause the patella to sublux or fully dislocate. Both the transverse and the longitudinal structures will influence the medial-lateral positioning of the patella within the femoral sulcus, as well as influence patellar tracking as the patella slides down the femoral condyles and into the intercondylar groove.

The passive mobility of the patella and its medial-lateral positioning are largely governed by the passive and dynamic pulls of the structures surrounding it. This is important because the presence of hypermobility could result in patellar subluxations or dislocations, whereas hypomobility could yield greater patellofemoral stresses. Passive mobility of the patella is maximal when the knee is fully extended and the musculature is relaxed. An imbalance in the passive tension or a change in the line of pull of the dynamic structures will substantially influence the orientation of the patella. This is predominantly true when the knee joint is in extension and the patella sits on the relatively shallow superior femoral sulcus. Abnormal forces, however, may influence the excursion of the patella even in its more secure location within the intercondylar groove with the knee in flexion.

As already noted, tension in the active and/or stretched quadriceps muscle helps create compression between the patella and the femur to increase patellofemoral stability. The force on the patella is determined by the resultant pull of the four muscles that constitute the quadriceps and by the pull of the patellar tendon. Each of the segments of the quadriceps can make some contribution to frontal plane mobility and stability. As noted earlier, the pull of the vastus lateralis muscle is normally 35° lateral to the long axis of the femur,[104] whereas the pull of the proximal portion of the vastus medialis muscle (VML) is approximately 15° to 18° medial to the femoral shaft with the distal fibers (VMO) oriented 50° to 55° medially[102] (see Fig. 11-34).

Because the vastus medialis and vastus lateralis muscles not only pull on the quadriceps tendon but also exert a pull on the patella through their retinacular connections, complementary function is critical. Relative weakness of the vastus medialis muscle may substantially increase the resultant lateral forces on the patella. The individual pulls of each respective portion of the quadriceps is impossible to measure *in vivo*, however. Although measurements of muscular force cannot be made, the literature supports the contention that muscle activity of the two portions of the vastus medialis (VMO and VML) and the vastus lateralis muscles are not selectively altered in patients with patellofemoral pain.[126–128] Anatomic variations may contribute to asymmetrical pulls on the patella. In general, the VMO inserts into the superomedial aspect of the patella

about one third to one half of the way down on the medial border. In instances of patellar malalignment, the VMO insertion site may be located less than a fourth of the way down on the patella's medial aspect, and as a result, the vastus medialis muscle cannot effectively counteract the lateral motion of the patella.[106]

Although individual components of the quadriceps may not necessarily be influenced by pain, the quadriceps muscle as a whole does appear to be susceptible to the inhibitory effects of the acute joint effusions caused by injury.[129] This inhibition can result in hypotonia and atrophy, minimizing the compressive role of the quadriceps and thus altering the resultant pull on the patella.

Case Application 11-5: **Quadriceps Inhibition**

Tina underwent an ACL reconstruction in which a graft from the central third of her patellar tendon was used. This disruption of her extensor mechanism could influence how she uses her quadriceps and may be contributing to her knee extensor weakness. With each quadriceps contraction, she is pulling on the patellar tendon, which, if sore, could cause her to minimize her quadriceps activity to avoid pain. The result is a weak, atrophied quadriceps muscle. The quadriceps weakness that Tina exhibits could clearly be contributing to the pain and dysfunction around her patella. Because her quadriceps has become weaker, Tina is now unable to provide adequate dynamic control of the patella. The distal portion of the vastus medialis (VMO) is thought to be partially responsible for frontal plane control of patellar motions. With quadriceps weakness, including weakness of the VMO, this role is diminished, and patellofemoral forces can increase laterally. Poor control of the patella can also lead to the presence of a hypomobile patella with limited medial-lateral glide.

Continuing Exploration: **Selective Strengthening of the VMO**

For years, therapists have assumed that a weak VMO contributed to diminished medial glide of the patella. Therefore, numerous authors have attempted to devise exercise regimens to strengthen the VMO. It is sometimes incorrectly assumed that the VMO can be selectively recruited in order to preferentially strengthen that particular component of the vastus medialis muscle. Both portions of the vastus medialis muscle, like the other components of the quadriceps, are innervated by the femoral nerve, making preferential recruitment quite difficult.[103] In the absence of evidence supporting differential recruitment of the VMO, strengthening of the VMO portion of the vastus medialis muscle should be accomplished through whole quadriceps strengthening, with techniques such as biofeedback or neuromuscular electrical stimulation if activation deficits exist. In this way, it can be ensured that the quadriceps, and specifically the VMO, is being sufficiently overloaded to promote muscle hypertrophy.

■ **Asymmetry of Patellofemoral Stabilization**

The orientation of the quadriceps resultant pull with respect to the pull of the patellar tendon provides information about the net force on the patella in the frontal plane. The net effect of the pull of the quadriceps and the patellar ligament can be assessed clinically using a measurement called the Q-angle (quadriceps angle). The Q-angle is the angle formed between a line connecting the ASIS to the midpoint of the patella and a line connecting the tibial tuberosity and the midpoint of the patella (Fig. 11-47). A Q-angle of 10° to 15° measured with the knee either in full extension or slightly flexed is considered normal.[130] Any alteration in alignment that increases the Q-angle is thought to increase the lateral force on the patella. This can be harmful because an increase in this lateral force may increase the compression of the lateral patella on the lateral lip of the femoral sulcus. In the presence of a large enough lateral force, the patella may actually sublux or dislocate over the femoral sulcus when the quadriceps muscle is activated on an extended knee. The Q-angle is usually measured with the knee at or near full extension because lateral forces on the patella may be more of a problem in these circumstances. With the knee flexed, the patella is set within the intercondylar notch, and even a very large lateral force on the patella is unlikely to result in dislocation. Furthermore, the Q-angle will reduce with knee flexion as the tibia rotates medially in relation to the femur.[131]

It has been postulated that women have a slightly greater Q-angle than do men because of the presence of a wider pelvis, increased femoral anteversion, and a relative knee valgus angle. However, other authors have disputed this, and the presence of a gender difference in the Q-angle is still a matter of debate.[130,132] Although an excessively large Q-angle of 20° or more is usually an indicator of some structural malalignment, an apparently normal Q-angle will not necessarily ensure the absence of problems. Large Q-angles are thought to create excessive lateral forces on the patella that may predispose the patella to pathologic changes. One problem with using the Q-angle as a measure of the lateral pull on the patella is that the line between the ASIS and the midpatella is only an estimate of the line of pull of the quadriceps and does not necessarily reflect the actual line of pull in the patient being examined. If a substantial imbalance exists between the vastus medialis and vastus lateralis muscles in a patient, the Q-angle may lead to an incorrect estimate of the lateral force on the patella because the actual pull of the quadriceps muscle is no longer along the estimated line. Furthermore, a patella that sits in an abnormal lateral position in the femoral sulcus because of imbalanced forces will yield a smaller Q-angle because the patella lies more in line with the ASIS and tibial tuberosity.

There are several abnormalities that can yield increased lateral forces. There is a potential for imbalance between the vastus lateralis and vastus medialis muscles, although, as identified earlier, this imbalance cannot be measured *in vivo*. The presence of a tight IT band could also limit the mobility of the patella and restrict its ability to shift medially during flexion, contributing to increased stress under the lateral facet of the patella.[81] When the IT band moves posteriorly with knee flexion, it exerts an even greater lateral pull on the patella, which results in a progressive lateral tilting as knee flexion increases.[81] The increased lateral tilt could further load the lateral facet, increasing joint stress. The frontal plane deviation of genu valgum increases the obliquity of the femur (see Fig. 11-7A) and, concomitantly, the obliquity of the pull of the quadriceps. In contrast, individuals with genu varum exhibit less obliquity of the femur (see Fig. 11-7B), and therefore should have a diminished lateral quadriceps pull. The transverse plane deviation of medial femoral torsion (or femoral aneversion) generally results in the femoral condyles being turned in (medially rotated), carrying the patella medially with the femoral condyles and increasing the Q-angle by increasing the obliquity of the pull of the quadriceps on the patella. Medial femoral torsion is often associated with lateral tibial torsion in the older child or adult, or it may exist independently. In lateral tibial torsion, the tibial tuberosity lies more lateral to the patella, increasing the Q-angle by increasing the obliquity of the patellar tendon. When medial femoral torsion and lateral tibial torsion coexist, the Q-angle will increase substantially, resulting in a substantial lateral force on the patella (Fig. 11-48). As we will see in Chapter 12, the presence of excessive or prolonged pronation in the foot can contribute to excessive or prolonged medial rotation of the lower extremity that moves the patella medially, increasing the Q-angle and promoting a greater lateral force on the patella in a way similar to that of medial femoral torsion. Each of these conditions can predispose the

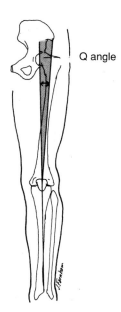

Figure 11-47 ■ The Q-angle is the angle between a line connecting the anterior superior iliac spine to the midpoint of the patella and the extension of a line connecting the tibial tubercle and the midpoint of the patella.

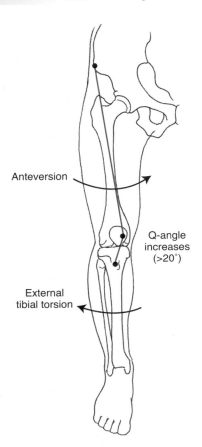

▲ **Figure 11-48** ■ Increased medial femoral torsion (femoral anteversion) and tibial lateral torsion will result in a larger Q-angle and an increased lateral force on the patella.

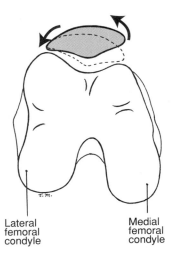

▲ **Figure 11-49** ■ Laxity in the medial extensor retinaculum or adaptive shortening of the lateral retinaculum may result in maintaining the patella in a laterally tilted position on the femoral sulcus (shown in a view up the femur from its distal end).

patella to excessive pressure laterally or to lateral subluxation or dislocation.

Forces other than the alignment and balance of the quadriceps muscle components may influence patellar positioning. Either laxity of the medial retinaculum or excessive tension in or adaptive shortening of the lateral retinaculum may contribute to a laterally tilted patella in the femoral sulcus (Fig. 11-49). In addition, a tight IT band may exert an excessive lateral pull on the patella through the lateral patellofemoral ligament.[81] Such deficits in the passive stabilizers, as well as weakness in the medial active stabilizers, result in increased lateral compressive forces. It is currently unknown whether such changes in the passive structures are primary or are secondary to abnormalities in the dynamic stabilizers.

Weight-Bearing versus Non–Weight-Bearing Exercises with Patellofemoral Pain

Both weight-bearing and non–weight-bearing exercises are often prescribed for patients with patellofemoral pain. Each mode of exercise influences the patellofem-

oral joint differently on the basis of the knee's position within the ROM. Effective quadriceps strengthening in a patient with pain must be performed in a pain-free range. This necessitates a complete understanding of how both weight-bearing and non–weight-bearing exercises influence the contact area and force across the patellofemoral joint. We already noted that in non–weight-bearing extension, such as the seated knee extension, the quadriceps must work harder as extension progresses (quadriceps force increases with decreasing knee flexion angle) (see Fig. 11-37). The increased work of the quadriceps near extension is necessary to compensate for the increased MA of the resistance. However, the greater compressive force generated by the increased quadriceps contraction can be detrimental for an individual with patellofemoral pain, especially if the degeneration is located on the inferior aspect of the patella that is in contact with the femur near extension. In contrast, a weight-bearing exercise requires greater quadriceps activity with greater knee flexion (e.g., at the bottom of a squat) as the MA of the resistance increases (see Fig. 11-38). During weight-bearing exercise, greater knee flexion will therefore increase the compressive force across the patellofemoral joint both because of increased force demands on the quadriceps muscle and because of the increased patellofemoral compression that occurs even with passive knee flexion. The substantial patellofemoral compression will aggravate patellofemoral pain. Exercise recommendations for the person with patellofemoral pain can be based on changing patellofemoral joint stress with weight-bearing and non–weight-bearing exercises and knee flexion angle (Fig. 11-50). It has been recommended that those with patellofemoral pain avoid deep flexion while doing weight-bearing extension exercises and avoid the final 30° of extension during non–weight-bearing knee extension exercises.[133]

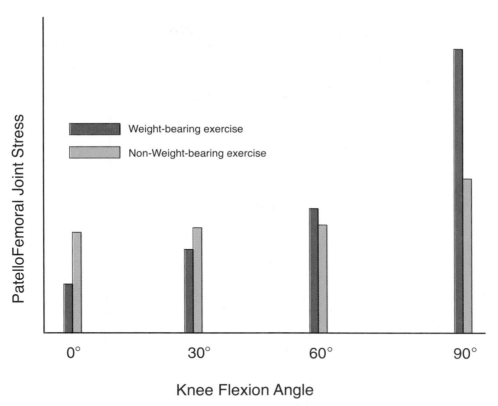

▲ **Figure 11–50** ■ Simulations showed patellofemoral joint stress to be greater during loaded non–weight-bearing exercises than weight-bearing exercises when the knee was closer to knee extension. Patellofemoral joint stress was higher, however, during weight-bearing exercises when knee flexion exceeds approximately 50°. [Data from Cohen ZA, Roglic H, Grelsamer RP, et al: Patellofemoral stresses during open and closed kinetic chain exercises. An analysis using computer simulation. Am J Sports Med 29:483–484, 2001.]

Continuing Exploration: **Weight-Bearing versus Non–Weight-Bearing Exercises**

The use of weight-bearing exercises has occasionally been promoted as safer and "more functional" than non–weight-bearing exercises.[133] There are, however, numerous activities performed throughout the day in a non–weight-bearing position. Although it is true that other muscles are forced to work together in a weight-bearing situation in order to control other joints, this is not always the best strategy for strengthening. The use of non–weight-bearing exercise isolates the targeted muscle, typically making strengthening more effective.[134,135] With regard to safety (e.g., patellofemoral joint stress, ACL strain), an understanding of how joint stress and tissue strain change throughout the knee ROM will assist with patient safety. For example, during quadriceps strengthening exercises, non–weight-bearing exercises produce large anterior shear forces near full extension, which diminishes with increased flexion, and produce larger patellofemoral joint stress closer to full extension. In contrast, during weight-bearing extension exercises, patellofemoral joint stress is minimal near full extension but increases with increasing flexion, whereas anterior shearing forces are similar to those produced during non–weight-bearing exercises throughout the ROM.

Effects of Injury and Disease

The joints of the knee complex, like other joints in the body, are subject to developmental defects, injury, and disease processes. A number of factors, however, make the knee joint unique in its development of various pathologies. The knee, unlike the shoulder, elbow, and wrist, must support the body weight and at the same time provide considerable mobility. Although the hip and ankle joints similarly support the body's weight, the knee is a more complex structure than either the hip or ankle. The anatomic complexity is necessary to dissipate the enormous forces applied through the joint as two of the longest levers in the body meet at the knee complex.

Tibiofemoral Joint Injury

The tremendous forces applied through the knee have the potential to contribute to numerous injuries and degenerative damage. In addition, participation in physical fitness and sports activities that involve jumping, pivoting, cutting, or repetitive cyclic loading among all age groups and both sexes can subject the knee complex to risk of injury. Injuries to the knee complex may involve the menisci, the ligaments, the bones, or the musculotendinous structures.

Meniscal injuries are common and usually occur as a result of sudden rotation of the femur on the fixed tibia when the knee is in flexion. The pivot point during axial rotation in the flexed knee occurs through the medial meniscus. Therefore, the more rigidly attached medial meniscus may tear under the sudden load. Ligamentous injuries may occur as a result of a force that causes the joint to exceed its normal ROM, usually the translational ROM. Although excessive forces may cause ligamentous tears, lower-level forces may similarly cause disruption in ligaments weakened by aging, disease, immobilization, steroids, or vascular insufficiency. Cyclic loading (whether short term and intense or over a prolonged period) may also affect viscoelasticity and stiffness. A weakened ligament may take 10 months or more to return to normal stiffness once the underlying problem has been resolved. After a ligament injury or reconstruction, the new or damaged tissue must be protected to minimize excessive stress through the healing tissue. Absence of tissue stress, however, is also detrimental, because the new tissue will not adapt and become stronger under unloaded conditions. Rehabilitation of the repaired or reconstructed ligament, therefore, is a balance between too much applied stress and too little.

The bony and cartilaginous structures of the tibiofemoral joint may be injured either by the application of a large direct force, such as during a twist or fall, or by forces exerted by abnormal ligamentous and muscular forces. Knee osteoarthritis is often seen in older adults and is particularly common in women. This progressive erosion of articular cartilage may be initiated by a previous traumatic joint injury, obesity, malalignment, instability, or quadriceps muscle weakness, to name just a few of the many suspected contributors to the development of osteoarthritis. Tibial plateau fractures can occur when large magnitudes of force are applied through the joint. Knee joint instability, as frequently seen in the knee after ACL injury, can lead to progressive changes in the articular cartilage, in the menisci, and in the other ligaments attempting to restrain the increased joint mobility. The presence of ligamentous instability induces abnormal forces through the joint, inasmuch as excessive shearing can often occur. In addition, this excessive laxity must be controlled in order to avoid episodes of giving way. Because the knee has poor bony congruency, the muscles must provide greater control of all fine movements of the tibiofemoral joint in the absence of ligaments. Increased muscular co-contraction, however, may generate greater compressive forces through the joint, contributing to articular cartilage degeneration. An improved method of providing dynamic stability to a lax joint, therefore, is to generate isolated muscle contractions as needed, rather than a massive co-contraction to stiffen the joint.

The numerous bursae and tendons at the knee are also subject to injury. The cause of injuries to these structures may be either a direct blow or prolonged compressive or tensile stresses. Bursitis is common after either blunt trauma or repetitive low-level compressions, which can irritate the tissue. The prepatellar bursa, the superficial infrapatellar bursa (known as housemaid's knee when it is inflamed), and the bursa beneath the pes anserinus are common locations for injury. Tendinitis results from repetitive low-level stresses to the tissues of the tendon. Frequently this is caused by an overworking of the muscle and can occur in response to a previous ligamentous injury. Another potential source of pain and dysfunction in the knee joint is the irritation of a patellar plica. Classic symptoms include pain with prolonged sitting, with stair climbing, and during resisted extension exercises. In flexion, the medial patellar plica is drawn over the medial femoral condyle and can become pressed beneath the patella. The resulting tension in the band may cause plica to become inflamed. If the inflamed plica becomes fibrotic, it may create a secondary synovitis around the femoral condyle, and deterioration of the condylar cartilage may occur. A thickened or inflamed superior plica may erode the superior aspect of the medial facet of the patella.

Patellofemoral Joint Injury

We have presented the mechanics of a number of problems that may predispose the knee to patellofemoral dysfunction. Any one problem in isolation or various combinations of problems may lead to excessive pressure on the lateral facets of the patella, to lateral subluxation, or to lateral dislocation. Both patellar instability and increased patellofemoral compression are commonly associated with knee pain, poor tolerance of sustained passive knee flexion (as in sitting for long periods), "giving way" of the knee, and exacerbation of symptoms by repeated use of the quadriceps on a flexed knee. Often this results in diminished use of the quadriceps, leading to atrophy and subsequently a further deterioration of patellar control. As muscle function declines, patellofemoral dysfunction may progress, necessitating a reversal of muscle function under a series of controlled situations to generate hypertrophy of the quadriceps, while minimizing discomfort.

Among the causes of increased patellar compression include a tight IT band, large Q-angle (e.g., as in genu valgum or femoral anteversion with lateral tibial torsion), relative vastus medialis muscle weakness, or patellar hypomobility. With patellar hypermobility, lax medial structures, and a short lateral femoral condyle, the risk of lateral patellar subluxation or dislocation is increased. After a lateral patellar subluxation or dislocation, the medial retinaculum is stretched as the patella deviates toward or slips over the lateral lip of the femoral sulcus or condyle. The return of the patella into the intercondylar notch may affect the medial patella (occasionally causing an osteochondral fracture). There are a host of other pathologies that can occur around the patellofemoral joint, including pain from the lateral patellofemoral ligament, inflammation of the medial patellar plica (discussed previously), and pain from the quadriceps tendon above or the patellar ligament below. Patellofemoral pain is most often observed in adolescents and may resolve spontaneously. In addition, patellar subluxation is more often seen in younger patients, who may have a less developed patella and lateral condyle to resist an excessive lateral force on the patella.

Cartilaginous changes seen on the lateral patellar facet were once considered to be diagnostic of patellofemoral dysfunction, and the term chondromalacia patella (softening of the cartilage) was assigned. With the knowledge that similar cartilaginous changes can be found in asymptomatic knees and that the medial patellar facet can show greater change without symptoms or progressive cartilage deterioration, more general diagnoses have been used, including patellofemoral arthralgia or patellofemoral pain syndrome. The use of this more general terminology suggests that the damage extends beyond the articular cartilage. Cartilage is aneural and therefore cannot be the cause of pain.[136] Instead, patients with patellofemoral pain can experience discomfort from damage to subchondral bone, the synovial membrane, and ligamentous or musculotendinous structures.

Case Application 11-6: **Case Summary**

Tina's initial injury (in which she tore her ACL, MCL, and medial meniscus) has likely led to the development of the problems that we are now observing. Tina went for 4 months without several of her passive tibiofemoral stabilizers (ACL and MCL). During that time, greater muscular control was necessary to dynamically stabilize the knee, but the excessive muscle activity contributed to greater compressive forces across the joint. As a result of the tear of the medial meniscus, these greater compressive forces became focused on a smaller surface area within the medial compartment. The increased force per unit area increased joint stress and likely led to the gradual erosion of Tina's medial compartment articular cartilage, leading in turn to the development of genu varum. The joint space narrowing observed on the weight-bearing radiographs is indicative of medial compartment osteoarthritis; however, her medial joint pain may be attributed to other causes. For instance, Tina may have overworked the medial muscles trying to control exces-

sive laxity, which resulted in tendinitis. It is also possible that Tina has further damaged the already injured medial meniscus, which contributed to medial joint pain.

After her ACL reconstruction, the discomfort that she felt around the patellar tendon donor site led to disuse atrophy of her quadriceps muscle. As the muscle atrophied, she became less adept at controlling the tracking of her patella, which led to increased lateral patellar compression. The repetitive compression of the lateral patellar facet against the lateral femoral condyle has gradually resulted in patellofemoral degenerative changes on the lateral facet. This lateral patellofemoral joint space narrowing was observed on her radiographs and likely was influenced by her long-standing quadriceps weakness, as well as by potential structural abnormalities. The presence of a tight IT band, excessive Q-angle, excessive or prolonged foot pronation or hip medial rotation, or patella baja are but a few of the contributing factors that could have contributed to Tina's excessive lateral patellofemoral compression and must be screened for to determine the cause of her patellar pain. A complete understanding of the structures and relevant functioning of the tibiofemoral and the patellofemoral joints allows for appropriate diagnosis and treatment of these joints.

Summary

Given the range of possible problems that can occur in the knee joint, an exhaustive discussion is beyond the scope of this text. A thorough knowledge of normal structure and function, however, can be used to predict or understand the immediate impact of a specific injury and the secondary effects on intact structures. The variety of forces transmitted through the knee complex arises from gravity (weight-bearing forces), muscles, ligaments, and other passive soft-tissue structures. Any alteration of the knees anatomy can substantially influence these forces and can have a dramatic impact on the function of the knee joint. Damage to the tibiofemoral joint or the patellofemoral joint can result from either a large rapid load or the accumulation of smaller repetitive loads. An understanding of both the primary and secondary effects of injury is important in order to gain a full appreciation for the pathogenesis of knee disorders.

Study Questions

1. Describe the congruency of the tibiofemoral joint. What factors add to or detract from stability?
2. Describe the menisci of the knee, including their function, shape, and attachments.
3. Describe the intra-articular movement of the femur on the tibia, as the femur moves from full extension into flexion.
4. Describe the automatic axial mechanism of the knee, including the structure or structures responsible.
5. What happens to the menisci during motions of the knee? How do their attachments contribute to the movement?

(Continued on following page)

Study Questions *(Continued)*

6. Identify the bursae of the knee joint. Which of these are generally separate from and which are parts of the capsule?
7. Which knee joint ligaments contribute to anterior-posterior stability of the knee joint?
8. Which ligaments contribute to medial-lateral stability of the knee joint?
9. What are the dynamic stabilizers of the knee, and in what plane or planes do they contribute to stability?
10. At which point in the knee's ROM is axial rotation greatest? Which muscles produce active medial rotation? Lateral rotation?
11. What is the patella plica, and what implications does it have for knee joint dysfunction?
12. Describe the patellofemoral articulation, including the number and shape of the surfaces.
13. What function or functions does the patella serve at the knee joint?
14. How does the patella move in relation to the femur in normal motions? How would function be affected if the patella could not slide on the femur?
15. Describe the contact of the patella with the femur at rest in full extension. Describe the contact as knee flexion proceeds.
16. Is the patella equally effective as an anatomic pulley at all points in the knee ROM? At which point or points is it most effective? Least effective?
17. Which facet of the patella is most likely to undergo excessive degenerative changes when there is malalignment? Describe the malalignment and the condition or conditions that may predispose these changes.
18. What is the Q-angle of the knee joint? How is it measured, and what implications does it have for patellofemoral problems?
19. What changes will the condition of genu recurvatum produce at the patellofemoral joint?
20. Why is ascending stairs commonly cited as producing knee pain? Relate this to patellofemoral joint compression.

References

1. Churchill DL, Incavo SJ, Johnson CC, et al.: The transepicondylar axis approximates the optimal flexion axis of the knee. Clin Orthop 356: 111–118, 1998.
2. Iwaki H, Pinskerova V, Freeman MA: Tibiofemoral movement 1: The shapes and relative movements of the femur and tibia in the unloaded cadaver knee. J Bone Joint Surg Br 82:1189–1195, 2000.
3. Martelli S, Pinskerova V: The shapes of the tibial and femoral articular surfaces in relation to tibiofemoral movement. J Bone Joint Surg Br 84:607–613, 2002.
4. Siu D, Rudan J, Wevers HW, et al.: Femoral articular shape and geometry. A three-dimensional computerized analysis of the knee. J Arthroplasty 11: 166–173, 1996.
5. Cicuttini FM, Wluka AE, Wang Y, et al.: Compartment differences in knee cartilage volume in healthy adults. J Rheumatol 29:554–556, 2002.
6. Johnson F, Leitl S, Waugh W: The distribution of load across the knee. A comparison of static and dynamic measurements. J Bone Joint Surg Br 62: 346–349, 1980.
7. Andriacchi TP: Dynamics of knee malalignment. Orthop Clin North Am 25:395–403, 1994.
8. Messner K, Gao J: The menisci of the knee joint. Anatomical and functional characteristics, and a rationale for clinical treatment. J Anat 193(Pt 2): 161–178, 1998.
9. Rath E, Richmond JC: The menisci: Basic science and advances in treatment. Br J Sports Med 34:252–257, 2000.
10. Greis PE, Bardana DD, Holmstrom MC, et al.: Meniscal injury: I. Basic science and evaluation. J Am Acad Orthop Surg 10:168–176, 2002.
11. Robon MJ, Perell KL, Fang M, et al.: The relationship between ankle plantar flexor muscle moments and knee compressive forces in subjects with and without pain. Clin Biomech (Bristol, Avon) 15: 522–227, 2000.
12. Riener R, Rabuffetti M, Frigo C: Stair ascent and descent at different inclinations. Gait Posture 15:32–44, 2002.
13. Kuitunen S, Komi PV, Kyrolainen H: Knee and ankle joint stiffness in sprint running. Med Sci Sports Exerc 34:166–173, 2002.
14. McCarty EC, Marx RG, DeHaven KE: Meniscus repair: Considerations in treatment and update of clinical results. Clin Orthop 402:122–134, 2002.
15. Tuxoe JI, Teir M, Winge S, et al.: The medial patellofemoral ligament: A dissection study. Knee Surg Sports Traumatol Arthrosc 10:138–140, 2002.
16. Beltran J, Matityahu A, Hwang K, et al.: The distal semimembranosus complex: Normal MR anatomy, variants, biomechanics and pathology. Skeletal Radiol 32:435–445, 2003.
17. Kusayama T, Harner CD, Carlin GJ, et al.: Anatom-

ical and biomechanical characteristics of human meniscofemoral ligaments. Knee Surg Sports Traumatol Arthrosc 2:234–237, 1994.

18. Gupte CM, Bull AM, Thomas RD, et al.: A review of the function and biomechanics of the meniscofemoral ligaments. Arthroscopy 19:161–171, 2003.

19. Fulkerson JP, Gossling HR: Anatomy of the knee joint lateral retinaculum. Clin Orthop 153: 183–188, 1980.

20. Simonian PT, Sussmann PS, Wickiewicz TL, et al.: Popliteomeniscal fasciculi and the unstable lateral meniscus: Clinical correlation and magnetic resonance diagnosis. Arthroscopy 13:590–596, 1997.

21. Radin EL, de Lamotte F, Maquet P: Role of the menisci in the distribution of stress in the knee. Clin Orthop 185:290–294, 1984.

22. Ihn JC, Kim SJ, Park IH: *In vitro* study of contact area and pressure distribution in the human knee after partial and total meniscectomy. Int Orthop 17:214–218, 1993.

23. Gray JC: Neural and vascular anatomy of the menisci of the human knee. J Orthop Sports Phys Ther 29:23–30, 1999.

24. Hauger O, Frank LR, Boutin RD, et al.: Characterization of the "red zone" of knee meniscus: MR imaging and histologic correlation. Radiology 217: 193–200, 2000.

25. Zimny ML, Albright DJ, Dabezies E: Mechanoreceptors in the human medial meniscus. Acta Anat (Basel) 133:35–40, 1988.

26. Mine T, Kimura M, Sakka A, et al.: Innervation of nociceptors in the menisci of the knee joint: An immunohistochemical study. Arch Orthop Trauma Surg 120:201–204, 2000.

27. Markolf KL, Graff-Radford A, Amstutz HC: *In vivo* knee stability. A quantitative assessment using an instrumented clinical testing apparatus. J Bone Joint Surg Am 60:664–674, 1978.

28. Ralphs JR, Benjamin M: The joint capsule: Structure, composition, ageing and disease. J Anat 184(Pt 3):503–509, 1994.

29. Terry GC, LaPrade RF: The posterolateral aspect of the knee. Anatomy and surgical approach. Am J Sports Med 24:732–739, 1996.

30. Starok M, Lenchik L, Trudell D, et al.: Normal patellar retinaculum: MR and sonographic imaging with cadaveric correlation. AJR Am J Roentgenol 168:1493–1499, 1997.

31. Berumen-Nafarrate E, Leal-Berumen I, Luevano E, et al.: Synovial tissue and synovial fluid. J Knee Surg 15:46–48, 2002.

32. Lee SH, Petersilge CA, Trudell DJ, et al.: Extrasynovial spaces of the cruciate ligaments: Anatomy, MR imaging, and diagnostic implications. AJR Am J Roentgenol 166:1433–1437, 1996.

33. Dodds JA, Arnoczky SP: Anatomy of the anterior cruciate ligament: A blueprint for repair and reconstruction. Arthroscopy 10:132–139, 1994.

34. Petersen W, Tillmann B: Structure and vascularization of the cruciate ligaments of the human knee joint. Anat Embryol (Berl) 200:325–334, 1999.

35. Jacobson JA, Lenchik L, Ruhoy MK, et al.: MR imaging of the infrapatellar fat pad of Hoffa. Radiographics 17:675–691, 1997.

36. Dupont JY: Synovial plicae of the knee. Controversies and review. Clin Sports Med 16:87–122, 1997.

37. Garcia-Valtuille R, Abascal F, Cerezal L, et al.: Anatomy and MR imaging appearances of synovial plicae of the knee. Radiographics 22:775–784, 2002.

38. Kosarek FJ, Helms CA: The MR appearance of the infrapatellar plica. AJR Am J Roentgenol 172: 481–484, 1999.

39. Biedert RM, Sanchis-Alfonso V: Sources of anterior knee pain. Clin Sports Med 21:335–347, vii, 2002.

40. Feller JA, Feagin JA Jr, Garrett WE Jr: The medial patellofemoral ligament revisited: An anatomical study. Knee Surg Sports Traumatol Arthrosc 1: 184–186, 1993.

41. Desio SM, Burks RT, Bachus KN: Soft tissue restraints to lateral patellar translation in the human knee. Am J Sports Med 26:59–65, 1998.

42. Nomura E, Horiuchi Y, Inoue M: Correlation of MR imaging findings and open exploration of medial patellofemoral ligament injuries in acute patellar dislocations. Knee 9:139–143, 2002.

43. De Maeseneer M, Van Roy F, Lenchik L, et al.: Three layers of the medial capsular and supporting structures of the knee: MR imaging–anatomic correlation. Radiographics 20(Spec No):S83-S89, 2000.

44. Sekiya JK, Jacobson JA, Wojtys EM: Sonographic imaging of the posterolateral structures of the knee: Findings in human cadavers. Arthroscopy 18: 872–881, 2002.

45. Kim YC, Chung IH, Yoo WK, et al.: Anatomy and magnetic resonance imaging of the posterolateral structures of the knee. Clin Anat 10:397–404, 1997.

46. Warren LA, Marshall JL, Girgis F: The prime static stabilizer of the medial side of the knee. J Bone Joint Surg Am 56:665–674, 1974.

47. Harfe DT, Chuinard CR, Espinoza LM, et al.: Elongation patterns of the collateral ligaments of the human knee. Clin Biomech (Bristol, Avon) 13:163–175, 1998.

48. Grood ES, Noyes FR, Butler DL, et al.: Ligamentous and capsular restraints preventing straight medial and lateral laxity in intact human cadaver knees. J Bone Joint Surg Am 63:1257–1269, 1981.

49. Kanamori A, Sakane M, Zeminski J, et al.: *In-situ* force in the medial and lateral structures of intact and ACL-deficient knees. J Orthop Sci 5:567–571, 2000.

50. Frank CB, Hart DA, Shrive NG: Molecular biology and biomechanics of normal and healing ligaments—A review. Osteoarthritis Cartilage 7: 130–140, 1999.

51. Recondo JA, Salvador E, Villanua JA, et al.: Lateral stabilizing structures of the knee: Functional anatomy and injuries assessed with MR imaging. Radiographics 20(Spec No):S91-S102, 2000.

52. Bach JM, Hull ML, Patterson HA: Direct measurement of strain in the posterolateral bundle of the anterior cruciate ligament. J Biomech 30:281–283, 1997.

53. Torzilli PA, Greenberg RL, Insall J: An *in vivo* biomechanical evaluation of anterior-posterior motion of the knee. Roentgenographic measurement technique, stress machine, and stable population. J Bone Joint Surg Am 63:960–968, 1981.

54. Wascher DC, Markolf KL, Shapiro MS, et al.: Direct *in vitro* measurement of forces in the cruciate ligaments. Part I: The effect of multiplane loading in the intact knee. J Bone Joint Surg Am 75:377–386, 1993.

55. Inoue M, McGurk-Burleson E, Hollis JM, et al.: Treatment of the medial collateral ligament injury. I: The importance of anterior cruciate ligament on the varus-valgus knee laxity. Am J Sports Med 15:15–21, 1987.

56. Shapiro MS, Markolf KL, Finerman GA, et al.: The effect of section of the medial collateral ligament on force generated in the anterior cruciate ligament. J Bone Joint Surg Am 73:248–256, 1991.

57. Arms SW, Pope MH, Johnson RJ, et al.: The biomechanics of anterior cruciate ligament rehabilitation and reconstruction. Am J Sports Med 12:8–18, 1984.

58. Markolf KL, Burchfield DM, Shapiro MM, et al.: Combined knee loading states that generate high anterior cruciate ligament forces. J Orthop Res 13:930–935, 1995.

59. Markolf KL, Gorek JF, Kabo JM, et al.: Direct measurement of resultant forces in the anterior cruciate ligament. An *in vitro* study performed with a new experimental technique. J Bone Joint Surg Am 72:557–567, 1990.

60. Feagin JA Jr, Lambert KL: Mechanism of injury and pathology of anterior cruciate ligament injuries. Orthop Clin North Am 16:41–45, 1985.

61. Hirokawa S, Solomonow M, Lu Y, et al.: Anterior-posterior and rotational displacement of the tibia elicited by quadriceps contraction. Am J Sports Med 20:299–306, 1992.

62. Durselen L, Claes L, Kiefer H: The influence of muscle forces and external loads on cruciate ligament strain. Am J Sports Med 23:129–136, 1995.

63. Fleming BC, Renstrom PA, Ohlen G, et al.: The gastrocnemius muscle is an antagonist of the anterior cruciate ligament. J Orthop Res 19:1178–1184, 2001.

64. MacWilliams BA, Wilson DR, DesJardins JD, et al.: Hamstrings cocontraction reduces internal rotation, anterior translation, and anterior cruciate ligament load in weight-bearing flexion. J Orthop Res 17:817–822, 1999.

65. O'Connor JJ: Can muscle co-contraction protect knee ligaments after injury or repair? J Bone Joint Surg Br 75:41–48, 1993.

66. Pandy MG, Shelburne KB: Dependence of cruciate-ligament loading on muscle forces and external load. J Biomech 30:1015–1024, 1997.

67. Elias JJ, Faust AF, Chu YH, et al.: The soleus muscle acts as an agonist for the anterior cruciate ligament: An *in vitro* experimental study. Am J Sports Med 31:241–246, 2003.

68. Fleming BC, Renstrom PA, Beynnon BD, et al.: The effect of weightbearing and external loading on anterior cruciate ligament strain. J Biomech 34:163–170, 2001.

69. Torzilli PA, Deng X, Warren RF: The effect of joint-compressive load and quadriceps muscle force on knee motion in the intact and anterior cruciate ligament–sectioned knee. Am J Sports Med 22:105–112, 1994.

70. Beynnon BD, Fleming BC: Anterior cruciate ligament strain *in-vivo*: A review of previous work. J Biomech 31:519–525, 1998.

71. Harner CD, Xerogeanes JW, Livesay GA, et al.: The human posterior cruciate ligament complex: An interdisciplinary study. Ligament morphology and biomechanical evaluation. Am J Sports Med 23:736–745, 1995.

72. Saddler SC, Noyes FR, Grood ES, et al.: Posterior cruciate ligament anatomy and length-tension behavior of PCL surface fibers. Am J Knee Surg 9:194–199, 1996.

73. Kurosawa H, Yamakoshi K, Yasuda K, et al.: Simultaneous measurement of changes in length of the cruciate ligaments during knee motion. Clin Orthop 265:233–240, 1991.

74. Ritchie JR, Bergfeld JA, Kambic H, et al.: Isolated sectioning of the medial and posteromedial capsular ligaments in the posterior cruciate ligament–deficient knee. Influence on posterior tibial translation. Am J Sports Med 26:389–394, 1998.

75. Piziali RL, Seering WP, Nagel DA, et al.: The function of the primary ligaments of the knee in anterior-posterior and medial-lateral motions. J Biomech 13:777–784, 1980.

76. Li G, Gill TJ, DeFrate LE, et al.: Biomechanical consequences of PCL deficiency in the knee under simulated muscle loads—An *in vitro* experimental study. J Orthop Res 20:887–892, 2002.

77. Harner CD, Hoher J, Vogrin TM, et al.: The effects of a popliteus muscle load on *in situ* forces in the posterior cruciate ligament and on knee kinematics. A human cadaveric study. Am J Sports Med 26:669–673, 1998.

78. Loredo R, Hodler J, Pedowitz R, et al.: Posteromedial corner of the knee: MR imaging with gross anatomic correlation. Skeletal Radiol 28:305–311, 1999.

79. Aronowitz ER, Parker RD, Gatt CJ: Arthroscopic identification of the popliteofibular ligament. Arthroscopy 17:932–939, 2001.

80. Muhle C, Ahn JM, Yeh L, et al.: Iliotibial band friction syndrome: MR imaging findings in 16 patients and MR arthrographic study of six cadaveric knees. Radiology 212:103–110, 1999.

81. Puniello MS: Iliotibial band tightness and medial patellar glide in patients with patellofemoral dysfunction. J Orthop Sports Phys Ther 17:144–148, 1993.

82. Terry GC, Hughston JC, Norwood LA: The anatomy of the iliopatellar band and iliotibial tract. Am J Sports Med 14:39–45, 1986.

83. Rauschning W: Anatomy and function of the communication between knee joint and popliteal bursae. Ann Rheum Dis 39:354–358, 1980.

84. LaPrade RF: The anatomy of the deep infrapatellar bursa of the knee. Am J Sports Med 26:129–132, 1998.

85. LaPrade RF, Hamilton CD: The fibular collateral ligament–biceps femoris bursa. An anatomic study. Am J Sports Med 25:439–443, 1997.

86. Fuss FK: Anatomy of the cruciate ligaments and their function in extension and flexion of the human knee joint. Am J Anat 184:165–176, 1989.

87. Thompson WO, Thaete FL, Fu FH, et al.: Tibial meniscal dynamics using three-dimensional reconstruction of magnetic resonance images. Am J Sports Med 19:210–215, 1991; discussion, 19:215–216, 1991

88. Rowe PJ, Myles CM, Walker C, et al.: Knee joint kinematics in gait and other functional activities measured using flexible electrogoniometry: How much knee motion is sufficient for normal daily life? Gait Posture 12:143–155, 2000.

89. Loudon JK, Goist HL, Loudon KL: Genu recurvatum syndrome. J Orthop Sports Phys Ther 27:361–367, 1998.

90. Bull AM, Amis AA: Knee joint motion: Description and measurement. Proc Inst Mech Eng [H] 212: 357–372, 1998.

91. Almquist PO, Arnbjornsson A, Zatterstrom R, et al.: Evaluation of an external device measuring knee joint rotation: An *in vivo* study with simultaneous Roentgen stereometric analysis. J Orthop Res 20:427–432, 2002.

92. Markolf KL, Bargar WL, Shoemaker SC, et al.: The role of joint load in knee stability. J Bone Joint Surg Am 63:570–585, 1981.

93. Zhang LQ, Xu D, Wang G, et al.: Muscle strength in knee varus and valgus. Med Sci Sports Exerc 33:1194–1199, 2001.

94. Buchanan TS, Lloyd DG: Muscle activation at the human knee during isometric flexion-extension and varus-valgus loads. J Orthop Res 15:11–17, 1997.

95. Piazza SJ, Cavanagh PR: Measurement of the screw-home motion of the knee is sensitive to errors in axis alignment. J Biomech 33:1029–1034, 2000.

96. Buford WL Jr, Ivey FM Jr, Nakamura T, et al.: Internal/external rotation MAs of muscles at the knee: MAs for the normal knee and the ACL-deficient knee. Knee 8:293–303, 2001.

97. Mohamed O, Perry J, Hislop H: Relationship between wire EMG activity, muscle length, and torque of the hamstrings. Clin Biomech (Bristol, Avon) 17:569–579, 2002.

98. Shelburne KB, Pandy MG: A musculoskeletal model of the knee for evaluating ligament forces during isometric contractions. J Biomech 30: 163–176, 1997.

99. Li L, Landin D, Grodesky J, et al.: The function of gastrocnemius as a knee flexor at selected knee and ankle angles. J Electromyogr Kinesiol 12: 385–390, 2002.

100. Johnson CE, Basmajian JV, Dasher W: Electromyography of sartorius muscle. Anat Rec 173: 127–130, 1972.

101. Ullrich K, Krudwig WK, Witzel U: Posterolateral aspect and stability of the knee joint. I. Anatomy and function of the popliteus muscle-tendon unit: An anatomical and biomechanical study. Knee Surg Sports Traumatol Arthrosc 10:86–90, 2002.

102. Lieb FJ, Perry J: Quadriceps function. An anatomical and mechanical study using amputated limbs. J Bone Joint Surg Am 50:1535–1548, 1968.

103. Hubbard JK, Sampson HW, Elledge JR: Prevalence and morphology of the vastus medialis oblique muscle in human cadavers. Anat Rec 249: 135–142, 1997.

104. Powers CM, Lilley JC, Lee TQ: The effects of axial and multi-plane loading of the extensor mechanism on the patellofemoral joint. Clin Biomech (Bristol, Avon) 13:616–624, 1998.

105. Glenn LL, Samojla BG: A critical reexamination of the morphology, neurovasculature, and fiber architecture of knee extensor muscles in animal models and humans. Biol Res Nurs 4:128–141, 2002.

106. Grelsamer RP, Weinstein CH: Applied biomechanics of the patella. Clin Orthop 389:9–14, 2001.

107. Murray MP, Gardner GM, Mollinger LA, et al.: Strength of isometric and isokinetic contractions: Knee muscles of men aged 20 to 86. Phys Ther 60:412–419, 1980.

108. Kellis E, Baltzopoulos V: *In vivo* determination of the patella tendon and hamstrings MAs in adult males using videofluoroscopy during submaximal knee extension and flexion. Clin Biomech (Bristol, Avon) 14:118–124, 1999.

109. Escamilla RF, Fleisig GS, Zheng N, et al.: Biomechanics of the knee during closed kinetic chain and open kinetic chain exercises. Med Sci Sports Exerc 30:556–569, 1998.

110. Wilk KE, Escamilla RF, Fleisig GS, et al.: A comparison of tibiofemoral joint forces and electromyographic activity during open and closed kinetic chain exercises. Am J Sports Med 24:518–527, 1996.

111. Stuart MJ, Meglan DA, Lutz GE, et al.: Comparison of intersegmental tibiofemoral joint forces and muscle activity during various closed kinetic chain exercises. Am J Sports Med 24:792–799, 1996.

112. Kwak SD, Colman WW, Ateshian GA, et al.: Anatomy of the human patellofemoral joint articular cartilage: Surface curvature analysis. J Orthop Res 15:468–472, 1997.

113. Schlenzka D, Schwesinger G: The height of the patella: An anatomical study. Eur J Radiol 11:19–21, 1990.

114. Komistek RD, Dennis DA, Mabe JA, et al.: An *in vivo* determination of patellofemoral contact positions. Clin Biomech (Bristol, Avon) 15:29–36, 2000.
115. Goodfellow J, Hungerford DS, Zindel M: Patellofemoral joint mechanics and pathology. 1. Functional anatomy of the patello-femoral joint. J Bone Joint Surg Br 58:287–290, 1976.
116. Nakagawa S, Kadoya Y, Kobayashi A, et al.: Kinematics of the patella in deep flexion. Analysis with magnetic resonance imaging. J Bone Joint Surg Am 85:1238–1242, 2003.
117. Lin F, Makhsous M, Chang AH, et al.: *In vivo* and noninvasive six degrees of freedom patellar tracking during voluntary knee movement. Clin Biomech (Bristol, Avon) 18:401–409, 2003.
118. Mizuno Y, Kumagai M, Mattessich SM, et al.: Q-angle influences tibiofemoral and patellofemoral kinematics. J Orthop Res 19:834–840, 2001.
119. Moro-oka T, Matsuda S, Miura H, et al.: Patellar tracking and patellofemoral geometry in deep knee flexion. Clin Orthop 394:161–8, 2002.
120. Hefzy MS, Jackson WT, Saddemi SR, et al.: Effects of tibial rotations on patellar tracking and patellofemoral contact areas. J Biomed Eng 14:329–343, 1992.
121. Heino Brechter J, Powers CM: Patellofemoral stress during walking in persons with and without patellofemoral pain. Med Sci Sports Exerc 34:1582–1593, 2002.
122. Flynn TW, Soutas-Little RW: Patellofemoral joint compressive forces in forward and backward running. J Orthop Sports Phys Ther 21:277–282, 1995.
123. Singerman R, Davy DT, Goldberg VM: Effects of patella alta and patella infera on patellofemoral contact forces. J Biomech 27:1059–1065, 1994.
124. Meyer SA, Brown TD, Pedersen DR, et al.: Retropatellar contact stress in simulated patella infera. Am J Knee Surg 10:129–138, 1997.
125. Hirokawa S: Three-dimensional mathematical model analysis of the patellofemoral joint. J Biomech 24:659–671, 1991.
126. Powers CM: Patellar kinematics, part I: The influence of vastus muscle activity in subjects with and without patellofemoral pain. Phys Ther 80:956–964, 2000.
127. Karst GM, Willett GM: Onset timing of electromyographic activity in the vastus medialis oblique and vastus lateralis muscles in subjects with and without patellofemoral pain syndrome. Phys Ther 75:813–823, 1995.
128. Sheehy P, Burdett RG, Irrgang JJ, et al.: An electromyographic study of vastus medialis oblique and vastus lateralis activity while ascending and descending steps. J Orthop Sports Phys Ther 27:423–429, 1998.
129. Spencer JD, Hayes KC, Alexander IJ: Knee joint effusion and quadriceps reflex inhibition in man. Arch Phys Med Rehabil 65:171–177, 1984.
130. Livingston LA, Mandigo JL: Bilateral within-subject Q angle asymmetry in young adult females and males. Biomed Sci Instrum 33:112–117, 1997.
131. Hvid I: The stability of the human patello-femoral joint. Eng Med 12:55–59, 1983.
132. Horton MG, Hall TL: Quadriceps femoris muscle angle: Normal values and relationships with gender and selected skeletal measures. Phys Ther 69:897–901, 1989.
133. Fitzgerald GK: Open versus closed kinetic chain exercise: Issues in rehabilitation after anterior cruciate ligament reconstruction surgery. Phys Ther 77:1747–1754, 1997.
134. Snyder-Mackler L, Delitto A, Bailey SL, et al.: Strength of the quadriceps femoris muscle and functional recovery after reconstruction of the anterior cruciate ligament. A prospective, randomized clinical trial of electrical stimulation. J Bone Joint Surg Am 77:1166–1173, 1995.
135. Mikkelsen C, Werner S, Eriksson E: Closed kinetic chain alone compared to combined open and closed kinetic chain exercises for quadriceps strengthening after anterior cruciate ligament reconstruction with respect to return to sports: A prospective matched follow-up study. Knee Surg Sports Traumatol Arthrosc 8:337–342, 2000.
136. Dye SF, Vaupel GL, Dye CC: Conscious neurosensory mapping of the internal structures of the human knee without intraarticular anesthesia. Am J Sports Med 26:773–777, 1998.

Chapter 12

The Ankle and Foot Complex

Michael J. Mueller, PT, PhD, FAPTA

Introduction

The ankle/foot complex is structurally analogous to the wrist-hand complex of the upper extremity but has a number of distinct differences to optimize its primary role to bear weight. The complementing structures of the foot allow the foot to sustain large weight-bearing stresses under a variety of surfaces and activities that maximize stability and mobility. The ankle/foot complex must meet the stability demands of (1) providing a stable base of support for the body in a variety of weight-bearing postures without excessive muscular activity and energy expenditure and (2) acting as a rigid lever for effective push-off during gait. The stability requirements can be contrasted to the mobility demands of (1) dampening rotations imposed by the more proximal joints of the lower limbs, (2) being flexible enough to absorb the shock of the superimposed body weight as the foot hits the ground, and (3) permitting the foot to conform to a wide range of changing and varied terrain.[1] The ankle/foot complex meets these diverse requirements through the integrated movements of its 28 bones that form 25 component joints. These joints include the proximal and distal tibiofibular joints; the talocrural, or ankle, joint; the talocalcaneal, or subtalar, joint; the talonavicular and the calcaneocuboid joints (transverse tarsal joints); the five tarsometatarsal joints; five metatarsophalangeal joints; and nine interphalangeal joints.

To facilitate description and understanding of the ankle/foot complex, the bones of the foot are traditionally divided into three functional segments. These are the **hindfoot** (posterior segment), composed of the talus and calcaneus; the **midfoot** (middle segment), composed of the navicular, cuboid, and three cuneiform bones; and the **forefoot** (anterior segment), composed of the metatarsals and the phalanges (Fig. 12-1). These terms are commonly used in descriptions of ankle or foot dysfunction or deformity and are similarly useful in understanding normal ankle and foot function.

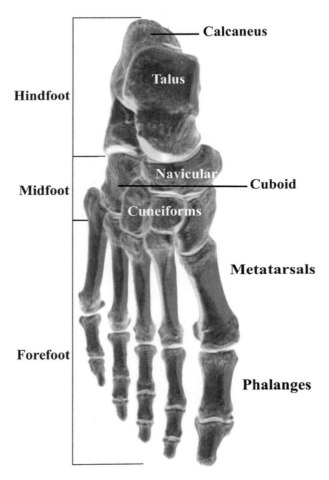

▲ **Figure 12-1** ■ Functional segments and bones of the foot.

The frequency of many ankle or foot problems can be traced readily to the complex structure of the foot and their participation in all weight-bearing activities. Structural abnormalities can lead to altered movements between joints and contribute to excessive stresses on tissues of the foot and ankle that result in injury.[2]

| 12-1 | **Patient Case** |

Arnold Benson is a 63-year-old man seeking intervention for pain in his right knee and foot. Three weeks ago, at the suggestion of his physician, Mr. Benson (who is quite overweight) started a walking program. Mr. Benson reports that after about a week, he had pain at his right heel that was greatest when he first got out of bed in the morning. He reports that this pain eases after a few steps but increases again when he walks more than 2 blocks, at which point he also reports pain around the area of his "knee cap." Despite having a sedentary job, Mr. Benson identifies that his feet often ache at the end of the day and that his knee hurts after prolonged sitting. He also reports that occasionally his "bunion" on his right foot will flare up and he has pain in the region of his big toe. He says that he has had very "flat feet" since he was young.

Mr. Benson stands with his hips positioned in medial rotation so that both knees are pointing medially. He has a low arch and a valgus positioning of his calcaneus when viewed from behind (more noticeable on the right than the left). He reports that he starts to feel a pain in a line behind his right medial malleolus that increases when he points his foot down and in (plantarflexion and inversion). Finally, Mr. Benson feels a strong pulling behind his knee and into the calf when he sits and is asked to extend his knee and pull his toes up (dorsiflexion), with the discomfort on the right side being more evident than on the left.

◆ Definitions of Motions

A unique set of terms is used to refer to motion of the foot and ankle. The same terms are used at most of the joints of the ankle and foot, and, consequently, it is useful to describe them at the outset. As we have seen at other joint complexes, few if any of the joint axes lies in the cardinal planes; more commonly, the joint axes are oblique and cut across all three planes of motion. The obliquity of the axes and implications for motion and function will be described in detail as we present individual joints.

The three motions of the ankle/foot complex that *approximate* cardinal planes and axes are **dorsiflexion/plantarflexion, inversion/eversion,** and **abduction/adduction** (Fig. 12-2). Dorsiflexion and plantarflexion are motions that occur approximately in the sagittal plane around a coronal axis. Dorsiflexion decreases the angle between the leg and the dorsum of the foot, whereas plantarflexion increases this angle. At the toes, motion around a similar axis is termed extension (bringing the toes up), whereas the opposite motion is flexion (bringing the toes down or curling them). Inversion and eversion occur approximately in the frontal plane around a longitudinal (anteroposterior [A-P]) axis that runs through the length of the foot.

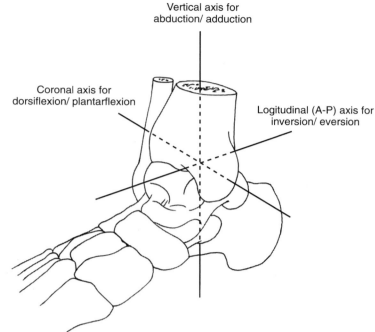

Vertical axis for
abduction/ adduction

Coronal axis for
dorsiflexion/ plantarflexion

Logitudinal (A-P) axis for
inversion/ eversion

◀ **Figure 12-2** ■ "Cardinal" axes for the motions of the ankle/foot complex.

Inversion occurs when the plantar surface of the segment is brought toward the midline; eversion is the opposite. Abduction and adduction occur approximately in the transverse plane around a vertical axis. Abduction is when the distal aspect of a segment moves away from the midline of the body (or away from the midline of the foot in the case of the toes); adduction is the opposite.

Pronation/supination in the foot are motions that occur around an axis that lies at an angle to each of the axes for "cardinal" motions of dorsiflexion/plantarflexion, inversion/eversion, and abduction/adduction. Consequently, pronation and supination are terms used to describe "composite" motions that have components of, or are coupled to, each of the cardinal motions. Pronation is motion about an axis that results in coupled motions of dorsiflexion, eversion, and abduction. Supination is a motion about an axis that results in coupled motions of plantarflexion, inversion, and adduction. The proportional contribution that each of the coupled motions makes to pronation/supination is dependent on and varies with the angle of the pronation/supination joint axis.

Valgus and **varus** are terms that may be used for the ankle/foot complex in several ways, depending on the context. The definitions that we used throughout discussion of other joints in other chapters will not change. That is, valgus refers to a reduction in the medial angle between two bones (or movement of the distal segment away from the midline); varus refers to the opposite. However, valgus and varus are sometimes used to refer to *fixed deformities* in the ankle/foot complex, whereas at other times the terms are used to describe or as synonyms for other normal motions. An example of common usage is to describe the fixed or weight-bearing position of the posterior calcaneus in relation to the

posterior midline of the leg, with an increase in the medial angle between the two reference lines being valgus of the calcaneus (or calcaneovalgus) and a decrease being varus of the calcaneus (or calcaneovarus) (Fig. 12-3). We will define use and context as we encounter these terms in descriptions of ankle/foot structure and function.

CONCEPT CORNERSTONE 12-1: *Ankle/Foot Terminology*

As we have seen at other joints, terminology used to describe motions around a joint or of a segment are often not consistent among investigators. This is very much the case for the ankle/foot complex. Because the anterior surface of the leg and the top of the foot are embryologically dorsal surfaces,[3] dorsiflexion may also be referred to as extension, and plantarflexion may be referred to as flexion. Although the flexion/extension terminology is commonly used for the toes, it may also be applied to the ankle. Some resources reverse the terminology applied to the "composite"

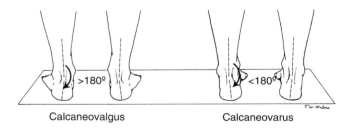

Calcaneovalgus >180°   Calcaneovarus <180°

▲ **Figure 12-3** ■ The term valgus (or calcaneovalgus) refers to an increase in the medial angle between the calcaneus and posterior leg. The term varus (or calcaneovarus) refers to an decrease in the medial angle between the calcaneus and posterior leg.

movement of pronation/supination and the coupled (component) movement of inversion/eversion; that is, inversion/eversion is used to refer to the composite motion, and pronation/supination is used to refer to the component (coupled) motion. As we proceed to describe the joints and their motions, we will see that some of these terminology differences are not really as problematic as they might initially seem.

◆ Ankle Joint

The term **ankle** refers specifically to the **talocrural joint:** that is, the articulation between the distal tibia and fibula proximally and the body of the talus distally (Fig. 12-4). The ankle is a synovial hinge joint with a joint capsule and associated ligaments. It is generally considered to have a single oblique axis with one degree of freedom around which the motions of dorsiflexion/plantarflexion occur.

Ankle Joint Structure

■ Proximal Articular Surfaces

The proximal segment of the ankle is composed of the concave surface of the distal tibia and of the tibial and fibular malleoli. These three facets form an almost continuous concave joint surface that extends more distally on the fibular (lateral) side than on the tibial (medial) side (see Fig. 12-4) and more distally on the posterior margin of the tibia than on the anterior margin. The structure of the distal tibia and the malleoli resembles and is referred to as a **mortise.** A common example of

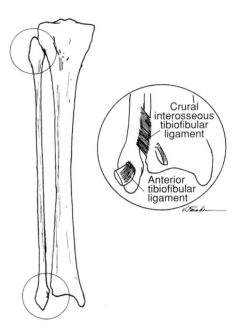

▲ **Figure 12-5** ■ Proximal and distal tibiofibular joints.

a mortise is the gripping part of a wrench. Either the wrench can be fixed (fitting a bolt of only one size) or it can be adjustable (permitting use of the wrench on a variety of bolt sizes). The adjustable mortise is more complex than a fixed mortise because it combines mobility and stability functions. The mortise of the ankle is adjustable, relying on the **proximal** and **distal tibiofibular joints** to both permit and control the changes in the mortise.

The proximal and distal tibiofibular joints (Fig. 12-5) are anatomically distinct from the ankle joint, but these two linked joints function exclusively to serve the ankle. Unlike their upper extremity counterparts, the proximal and distal radioulnar joints, the tibiofibular joints do not add any degrees of freedom to the more distal ankle and foot. However, fusion of the radioulnar joints would have little effect on wrist range of motion (ROM), whereas fusion of the tibiofibular joints may impair normal ankle function by limiting the ability of the talus to move within the ankle mortise.

Proximal Tibiofibular Joint

The proximal tibiofibular joint is a plane synovial joint formed by the articulation of the head of the fibula with the posterolateral aspect of the tibia. Although the facets of the proximal tibiofibular joint are fairly flat and vary in configuration among individuals, a slight convexity of the tibial facet and a slight concavity of the fibular facet seem to predominate.[4] The inclination of the facets may vary from nearly vertical to nearly horizontal in orientation.[4,5] Each proximal tibiofibular joint is surrounded by a joint capsule that is reinforced by **anterior** and **posterior tibiofibular ligaments.** Most typically, the proximal tibiofibular joint is anatomically separate from the knee joint.[4] Motion at the proximal

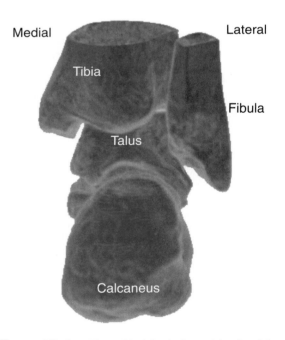

▲ **Figure 12-4** ■ The ankle joint is formed by the tibia and fibular (mortise) proximally and by the talus distally.

tibiofibular joint is variable but consistently small; it has been described as superior and inferior sliding of the fibula and as fibular rotation.[5,6] The relevance of motion at the proximal and distal tibiofibular joints will be seen when the ankle joint motion is discussed.

Distal Tibiofibular Joint

The distal tibiofibular joint is a syndesmosis, or fibrous union, between the concave facet of the tibia and the convex facet of the fibula. The distal tibia and fibula do not actually come into contact with each other but are separated by fibroadipose tissue. Although there is no joint capsule, there are several associated ligaments at the distal tibiofibular joint. Because the proximal and distal joints are linked (the tibia, fibular, and tibiofibular joints are part of a closed chain), all the ligaments that lie between the tibia and fibular contribute to stability at both joints.

The ligaments of the distal tibiofibular joint are primarily responsible for maintaining a stable mortise. The ligamentous structures that support the distal tibiofibular joint are the **anterior** and **posterior tibiofibular ligaments** and the **interosseous membrane.**[7] The interosseous membrane directly supports both proximal and distal tibiofibular articulations. The distal tibiofibular joint is an extremely strong articulation. Stresses that tend to move the talus excessively in the mortise (e.g., falling onto the side of the foot) often tear an ankle collateral ligament before the tibiofibular ligaments. Continued force may fracture the fibula proximal to the distal tibiofibular ligaments before the tibiofibular ligaments will tear.[8]

The function of the ankle (talocrural) joint is dependent on stability of the tibiofibular mortise. The tibia and fibula would be unable to grasp and hold on to the talus if the tibia and fibular were permitted to separate or if one side of the mortise were missing. The analogous mortise of a wrench could not perform its function of grasping a bolt if the two pincer segments moved apart every time a force was applied to the wrench. Conversely, the ankle mortise must have some mobility function to serve; otherwise, a single fused arch would better serve ankle joint function. The mobility role of the mortise belongs primarily to the fibula. The fibula has, in fact, little weight-bearing function; no more than 10% of the weight that comes through the femur is transmitted through the fibula.[9,10] Given the relatively small weight-bearing function of the fibula, the hyaline cartilage of the synovial proximal tibiofibular joint appears to be dependent on joint motion (rather than weight-bearing) to maintain nutrition of the cartilage. That is, the proximal tibiofibular joint must be mobile; if the proximal tibiofibular joint is mobile, so too must the distal tibiofibular joint be, because the two joints are mechanically linked.

■ Distal Articular Surface

The **body** of the talus (Fig. 12-6) forms the distal articulation of the ankle joint. The body of the talus has three articular surfaces: a large lateral (fibular) facet, a

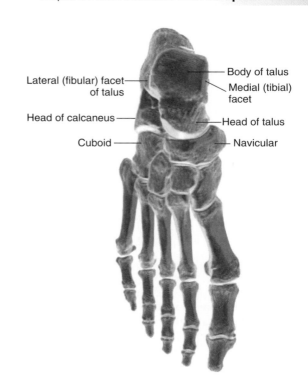

▲ **Figure 12-6** ■ The body of the talus with its trochlear (superior) surface, medial (tibial) facet, and lateral (fibular) facet form the distal aspect of the ankle joint.

smaller medial (tibial) facet, and a **trochlear** (superior) facet. The large, convex trochlear surface has a central groove that runs at a slight angle to the head and neck of the talus. The body of the talus also appears wider anteriorly than posteriorly, which gives it a wedge shape. The degree of wedging may vary among individuals, with no wedging at all in some and a 25% decrease in width anteriorly to posteriorly in others.[11] The articular cartilage covering the trochlea is continuous with the cartilage covering the more extensive lateral facet and the smaller medial facet.

The structural integrity of the ankle joint is maintained throughout the ROM of the joint by a number of important ligaments.

■ Capsule and Ligaments

The capsule of the ankle joint is fairly thin and especially weak anteriorly and posteriorly. Therefore, the stability of the ankle depends on an intact ligamentous structure. The ligaments that support the proximal and distal tibiofibular joints (the crural tibiofibular interosseous ligament, the anterior and posterior tibiofibular ligaments, and the tibiofibular interosseous membrane) are important for stability of the mortise and, therefore, for stability of the ankle. Two other major ligaments maintain contact and congruence of the mortise and talus and control medial-lateral joint stability. These are the **medial collateral ligament** (**MCL**) and the **lateral collateral ligament** (**LCL**). Both of these ligaments also provide key support for the **subtalar** (or

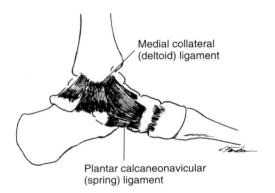

▲ **Figure 12-7** ■ Medial ligaments of the posterior ankle/foot complex.

talocalcaneal) **joint** that they also cross. The function of the collaterals at the ankle joint, therefore, are difficult to separate from the function at the subtalar joint. Portions of the **extensor** and **peroneal retinaculae** of the ankle are also credited with contributing to stability at the ankle joint.

The MCL is most commonly called the **deltoid ligament**. As its name implies, the deltoid ligament is a fan-shaped. It has superficial and deep fibers that arise from the borders of the tibial malleolus and insert in a continuous line on the navicular bone anteriorly and on the talus and calcaneus distally and posteriorly (Fig. 12-7). The deltoid ligament as a whole is extremely strong. Valgus forces that would open the medial side of the ankle may actually fracture and displace (avulse) the tibial malleolus before the deltoid ligament tears. This ligament helps control medial distraction stresses on the ankle joint and also helps check motion at the extremes of joint range, particularly with calcaneal eversion.

The LCL is composed of three separate bands that are commonly referred to as separate ligaments. These are the **anterior** and **posterior talofibular** ligaments and the **calcaneofibular** ligament (Fig. 12-8). The anterior and posterior ligaments run in a fairly horizontal position, whereas the longer calcaneofibular ligament is nearly vertical.[7] The LCL helps control varus stresses that result in lateral distraction of the joint and helps

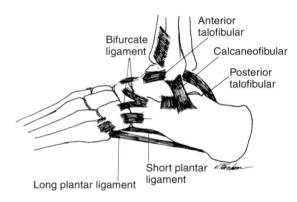

▲ **Figure 12-8** ■ Lateral ligaments of the posterior ankle/foot complex.

check extremes of joint ROM, particularly calcaneal inversion. In general, the components of the LCL are weaker and more susceptible to injury than are those of the MCL. As a result, the relative contributions of the LCL to ankle stability have been studied extensively, with (as we often find) some differing conclusions.

CONCEPT CORNERSTONE 12-2: *Summary of Studies Investigating Stresses Applied to the LCL*

1. The contribution of the various segments of the LCL to checking motion of the talus in the mortise depends on the position of the ankle joint.[12–16]
2. The anterior talofibular ligament is the weakest and most commonly torn of the LCLs. This ligament is most easily stressed when the ankle is in a plantarflexed and inverted position, such as when a basketball player lands on another player's foot. Rupture of the anterior talofibular ligament often results in anterolateral rotatory instability of the ankle.[7,15,17,18]
3. The posterior talofibular ligament is the strongest of the collateral ligaments and is rarely torn in isolation.[17,18]
4. There appears to be poor correlation between clinical ligament stress tests and the degree of ligamentous disruption.[19]

The **inferior extensor retinaculum** (Fig. 12-9) may also contribute to stability of the ankle joint.[20] Two additional structures that lie close and parallel to the calcaneofibular ligament appear to reinforce that ligament and serve a similar function. These are the inferior band of the **superior peroneal retinaculum** (see Fig. 12-9) and the much more variable **lateral talocalcaneal ligament.**[12,20,21] The ankle collateral ligaments and the retinaculae also contribute to stability of the subtalar joint and will be discussed again in that context.

The ankle joint classically is considered to have one degree of freedom, with dorsiflexion/plantarflexion occurring between the talus and the mortise. At the ankle, dorsiflexion refers to a motion of the head of the talus (see Fig. 12-6) dorsally (or upward) while the body of the talus moves posteriorly in the mortise. Plantarflexion is the opposite motion of the head and body of the talus. However, many investigators have concluded from both *in vivo* and *in vitro* investigations that the talus may rotate slightly within the mortise in both the transverse plane around a vertical axis (**talar rotation** or **talar abduction/adduction**) and in the frontal plane around an A-P axis (**talar tilt** or **talar inversion/eversion**).[17,22,23] Such motions result in a moving or instantaneous axis of rotation for the ankle joint. In comparison with motions of dorsiflexion and plantarflexion, these motions are quite small, with a maximum of 7° of medial rotation and 10° of lateral rotation in the transverse plane. Talar tilt (A-P axis) averages 5° or less.[17,23–25]

Although there is some disagreement regarding the excursion of the joint axis during ankle joint motion, there is consensus among investigators that the primary ankle motion of dorsiflexion/plantarflexion occurs around an oblique axis that causes the foot to move across all three planes.

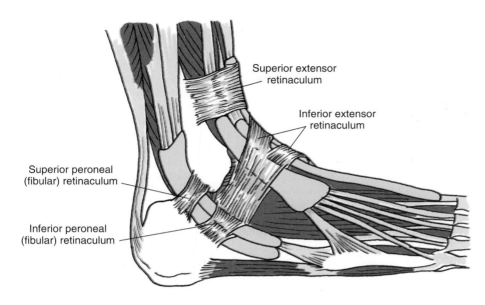

Superior extensor
retinaculum

Inferior extensor
retinaculum

Superior peroneal
(fibular) retinaculum

Inferior peroneal
(fibular) retinaculum

◀ **Figure 12-9** ■ The superior and inferior extensor retinacula; the superior and inferior peroneal retinacula.

■ Axis

In neutral position of the ankle joint, the joint axis passes approximately through the fibular malleolus and the body of the talus and through or just below the tibial malleolus.[26] The fibular malleolus and its associated fibular facet on the talus are located more distally (Fig. 12-10A) and posteriorly (see Fig. 12-10B) than the tibial malleolus and its associated tibial facet. The more posterior position of the fibular malleolus is due to the normal torsion or twist that exists in the distal tibia in relation to the tibia's proximal plateau. This twisting may be referred to as **tibial torsion**[27] (or **tibiofibular torsion** because both the tibia and fibula are involved with the rotation in the transverse plane[28]) and accounts for the toe-out position of the foot in normal standing. The torsion in the tibia is similar to the torsion found in the shaft of the femur, although normally reversed in direction. Reports of the position of the ankle joint axis in relation to the frontal plane (torsion) are highly variable, ranging from a low of $6° \pm 7°$[29] to a high of $32° \pm 7°$.[30] An average value for this axis angle taken from several studies would be $23° \pm 9°$.[29,31,32]

Because of the lower position of the fibular malleolus, the axis of the ankle is inclined down on the lateral side between $10° \pm 4°$[29] and $18° \pm 4°$, which yields an average of $14° \pm 4°$.[5,33] Individual variation is high, however, with the magnitudes varying as much as 30° from the average inclination values.[34] Stiehl used a simple hinged model with a level indicator to demonstrate how an axis inclined more distally and more posteriorly on the lateral side will create a motion across three planes (triplanar motion) while still around a single fixed axis.[34] He showed that dorsiflexion of the foot around a typically inclined ankle axis will not only bring the foot up but will also simultaneously bring it slightly lateral to the leg and appear to turn the foot longitudinally away from the midline. Conversely, plantarflexion around the same single oblique ankle axis will result in the foot's going down, moving medial to the leg and appearing to turn the foot longitudinally toward the

midline. When the foot is weight-bearing, the same relative pattern of motion exists when the tibia and fibular move on the foot. In weight-bearing ankle dorsiflexion, the leg (tibia and fibula) will move toward and medial to the foot, as well as appear to rotate medially in the transverse plane. The opposite occurs during weight-bearing ankle plantarflexion.

Continuing Exploration: **Tibial (Tibiofibular) Torsion**

Tibial torsion may be defined as the torsion, or twisting, between the upper and lower ends of the tibiofibular unit. Lateral tibial torsion increases between $1\frac{1}{2}$ and 8 years of age. Valmassy and Stanton[27] reported that lateral tibial torsion increased from $5.5° (\pm1.2°)$ at 18 months of age to $11.2° (\pm2.7°)$ at 6 years of age, with an average rate of increase of $1.4°$ per year. Methods of measuring and reported averages of tibial torsion in adults are highly variable.[35] Seber et al. used computed tomography to measure tibial torsion in men without impairments and reported a mean tibiofibular torsion of about 30° (range, 16° to 50°).[28] As tibial torsion increased, the axis of the ankle joint also was positioned more laterally in the transverse plane. The increased displacement laterally of the ankle joint axis would exaggerate the change in alignment of the foot and leg.

Ankle Joint Function

The primary motions allowed at the ankle joint are dorsiflexion and plantarflexion. Normal ankle joint ranges of motion are reported to be 10° to 20° for dorsiflexion and 20° to 50° for plantarflexion.[6,17,24,36,37] The large variation in magnitudes of ankle motion is due to differences in measurement techniques, subject populations, and even which joints are included in the measure of dorsiflexion or plantarflexion. If ankle joint range of motion measurement includes other joints of the foot

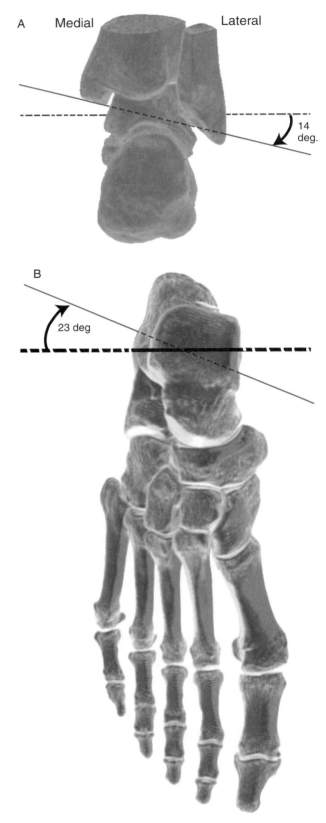

A   Medial   Lateral

14 deg.

B

23 deg

▲ **Figure 12-10** ■ The axis of the ankle joint. **A.** Posterior view showing the mortise around the body of the talus and the average 14° inclination of the of the ankle axis from the transverse plane. **B.** Superior view showing the ankle axis rotated, on average, 23° from the frontal plane.

(i.e., subtalar joint or transverse tarsal joints), greater ROM values will be obtained. Isolating motion to the tibia and talus will yield lower ROM values (10° dorsiflexion and 20° plantarflexion[37]). Ten degrees of ankle dorsiflexion often is considered the minimal amount needed to ambulate without deviations or injury.[38]

During ankle joint dorsiflexion/plantarflexion, the shape of the body of the talus facilitates joint stability. The trochlear (superior) surface of the talus is wider anteriorly than posteriorly (see Fig. 12-10B). When the foot is weight-bearing, dorsiflexion occurs by the tibia's rotating over the talus. As the tibia rotates over the talus, the concave tibiofibular segment slides forward on the trochlear surface of the talus. Therefore, the wider anterior portion of the talus "wedges" into the mortise formed by the spreading tibia and fibula, enhancing stability of the ankle joint. The enhanced stability at the ankle joint in dorsiflexion allows the ankle to withstand compression forces of as much as 450% of body weight, with little incidence of primary (nontraumatic) degenerative arthritis over time.[39,40] The sliding of the tibia on the talus during ankle motion contributes to a changing instantaneous center of rotation and also changes contact areas across the joint surfaces. This motion between the mortise and the talus, including some incongruence in the ankle joint, may be necessary for normal load distribution, cartilage nutrition, and lubrication of the ankle joint.[41] The loosepacked position of the ankle joint is in plantarflexion when only the relatively narrow posterior body of the talus is in contact with the mortise. The ankle is considered to be less stable when in plantarflexion; there is a higher incidence of ankle sprains when the ankle is plantarflexed than when dorsiflexed.

The asymmetry in size and orientation of the lateral and medial facets of the ankle joint contribute to changes in the ankle mortise that occur during ankle dorsiflexion. The lateral (fibular) facet is substantially larger than the medial (tibial) facet, and its surface is oriented slightly obliquely to that of the medial facet (see Fig. 12-10). Inman and Mann[32] proposed that the body of the talus can be thought of as a segment of a cone lying on its side with its base directed laterally. The cone should be visualized as "truncated" or cut off on either end at slightly different angles[28] (Fig. 12-11). The asymmetry in size and orientation of the facets means that the distal fibula moving on the larger lateral facet of the talus must undergo a greater displacement (in a slightly different plane) than the tibial malleolus as the tibia and fibular move together during dorsiflexion. The greater arc of motion for the fibula malleolus than for the tibial malleolus results in superior/inferior motion and medial/lateral rotation of the fibula that requires mobility of the fibula at both the proximal and the distal tibiofibular joints. Johnson, in reviewing the research literature, found the motions to be consistently small in magnitude but variable in direction among individuals and with different loading conditions.[42] Individual differences in fibular motion may be related to orientation of the proximal tibiofibular facet, with more mobility available in the facets that are more

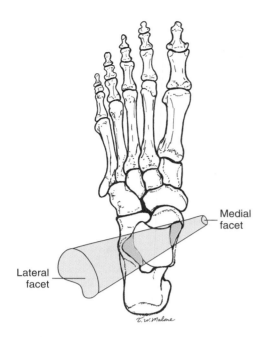

▲ **Figure 12-11** ■ The three articular surfaces of the talus (the trochlea, smaller medial facet, and larger lateral facet) can be pictured as part of a cone-shaped surface, with ends of the cone cut off (the larger end of the cone facing laterally).

Medial facet

Lateral facet

vertical, or to factors such as tibiofibular ligamentous elasticity. Such individual differences may account for the variations in effect on ankle dorsiflexion/plantarflexion ROM that are seen when surgical tibiofibular fixation is necessary.[42] Effectively, however, mobility of the fibula at the tibiofibular joints should be considered a component of normal ankle motion. One might also expect that the magnitude of proximal tibiofibular joint motion should exceed that of the distal tibiofibular joint, given that small motion at the distal fibula would be magnified at the opposite (proximal) end. This presumably accounts for the proximal joint's being synovial, whereas the distal joint is a comparatively less mobile syndesmosis joint.

Continuing Exploration: **Tibiofibular and Ankle Joint Linkage**

Some mobility of the fibula appears to be required at the proximal and distal tibiofibular joints to allow the talus to posteriorly rotate fully into the ankle mortise during ankle dorsiflexion. After ankle injury and prolonged immobilization, restoration of some movement at the tibiofibular joints may facilitate recovery of full ankle dorsiflexion. The functional implications of restriction of the fibula (or of the mortise) are unclear, because some studies have shown that fixation of the mortise does not affect ankle dorsiflexion range.[43]

Ankle dorsiflexion and plantarflexion movements are limited primarily by soft tissue restrictions. Active or passive tension in the triceps surae (**gastrocnemius** and **soleus muscles**) is the primary limitation to dorsiflex-

ion. Dorsiflexion is more limited typically with the knee in extension than with the knee in flexion (as demonstrated in the patient case) because the gastrocnemius muscle is lengthened over two joints when the knee is extended.[44] Tension in the **tibialis anterior, extensor hallucis longus,** and **extensor digitorum longus** muscles is the primary limit to plantarflexion. Although the ligaments of the ankle assist in checking dorsiflexion and plantarflexion,[44] a more important function appears to be in minimizing side-to-side movement or rotation of the mortise on the talus. The ligaments are assisted in that function by the muscles that pass on either side of the ankle. The **tibialis posterior, flexor hallucis longus,** and **flexor digitorum longus** muscles help protect the medial aspect of the ankle; the **peroneus longus** and **peroneus brevis** muscles protect the lateral aspect. Bony checks of any of the potential ankle motions are rarely encountered unless there is extreme hypermobility (as may be found among gymnasts or dancers) or a failure of one or more of the other restraint systems. A more complete analysis of the function of the muscles crossing the ankle will be presented later, because all muscles of the ankle cross at least two and generally three or more joints of the ankle and foot.

◆ The Subtalar Joint

The **talocalcaneal,** or **subtalar, joint** is a composite joint formed by three separate plane articulations between the talus superiorly and the calcaneus inferiorly. Together, the three surfaces provide a triplanar movement around a single joint axis. Function at the weight-bearing subtalar joint is critical for dampening the rotational forces imposed by the body weight while maintaining contact of the foot with the supporting surface.

Subtalar Joint Structure

The subtalar joint articulating surfaces are highly variable, but the posterior articulation is consistently the largest of the three articulations found between the talus and calcaneus. The posterior articulation is formed by a concave facet on the undersurface of the body of the talus and a convex facet on the body of the calcaneus; the smaller anterior and medial talocalcaneal articulations are formed by two convex facets on the inferior body and neck of the talus and two concave facets on the calcaneus (Fig. 12-12). The anterior and medial articulations, therefore, have an intra-articular configuration that is the reverse of that found at the posterior facet. Between the posterior articulation and the anterior and medial articulations, there is a bony tunnel formed by a **sulcus** (concave groove) in the inferior talus and superior calcaneus. This funnel-shaped tunnel, known as the **tarsal canal,** runs obliquely across the foot. Its large end (the **sinus tarsi**) lies just anterior to the fibular malleolus (Fig. 12-13); its small end lies posteriorly below the tibial malleolus and above a bony

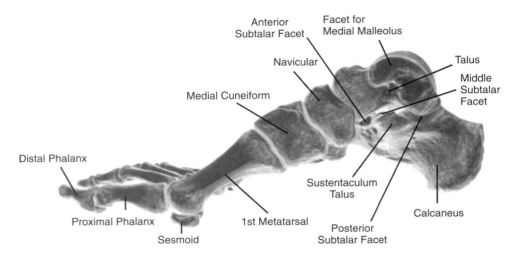

◀ **Figure 12-12** ■ Medial view of the foot, showing the talus sitting on the calcaneus (the subtalar joint).

outcropping on the calcaneus called the **sustentaculum tali** (see Fig. 12-12). The tarsal canal and ligaments running the length of the tarsal canal divide the posterior articulation and the anterior and medial articulations into two separate noncommunicating joint cavities.[45] The posterior articulation has its own capsule; the anterior and medial articulations share a capsule with the **talonavicular joint.**

Wang and colleagues[40] found that the subtalar articular surfaces, although smaller than those of the ankle joint surfaces, showed a similar proportion of contact across surfaces under similar conditions. These investigators found that the posterior facet received 75% of the force transmitted through the subtalar joint. They also determined that the pressure in the posterior facet was similar to that at the medial and anterior facets, given the larger contact area of the posterior facet. Like the ankle joint, the subtalar joint rarely undergoes degenerative change unless damaged by high stresses (e.g., fracture).

■ Ligaments

The subtalar joint is a stable joint that rarely dislocates. It receives ligamentous support from the ligamentous structures that support the ankle,[13] as well as from ligamentous structures that cross the subtalar joint alone. Harper[46] described a number of structures contributing to the lateral support of the subtalar joint. These included, from superficial to deep, the calcaneofibular ligament and the lateral talocalcaneal ligament (variously present[21]), the **cervical ligament,** and the **interosseous talocalcaneal ligament.** The cervical ligament (Fig. 12-14) is the strongest of the talocalcaneal structures.[20,46] It lies in the anterior sinus tarsi and joins the *neck* of the talus to the *neck* of the calcaneus (hence its name). The interosseous talocalcaneal ligament lies more medially within the tarsal canal, is more oblique (see Fig. 12-14), and has been described as having anterior and posterior bands.[6] Harper[46] also described the fairly complex connections of the inferior extensor

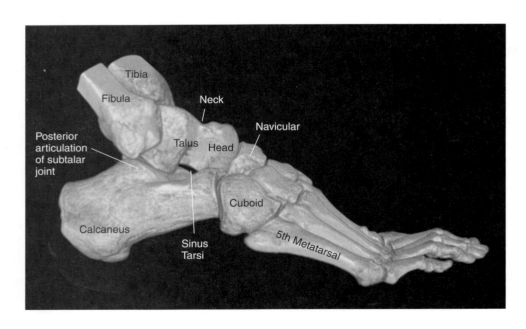

◀ **Figure 12-13** ■ Lateral view of the foot, showing the talus sitting on the calcaneus (the subtalar joint). The sinus tarsi is the lateral opening of the tarsal canal.

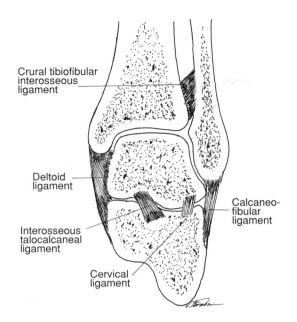

▲ **Figure 12-14** ■ The ligaments of the subtalar joint (in a posterior cross-sectional view).

Crural tibiofibular interosseous ligament

Deltoid ligament

Interosseous talocalcaneal ligament

Cervical ligament

Calcaneofibular ligament

retinaculum, which provides subtalar support superficially and within the tarsal canal. Although the roles of the cervical and interosseous ligaments in maintaining talocalcaneal stability are obvious, the contributions of the collateral ligaments should not be underestimated.[12,21,47]

Subtalar Joint Function

Although the subtalar joint is composed of three articulations, the alternating convex-concave facets limit the potential mobility of the joint. When the talus moves on the posterior facet of the calcaneus, the articular surface of the talus should, theoretically, slide in the *same* direction as the bone moves—a concave surface moving on a stable convex surface. However, at the middle and anterior joints, the talar surfaces (again, theoretically) should glide in a direction opposite to movement of the bone—a convex surface moving on a stable concave surface. Motion of the talus on the calcaneus, therefore, is a complex twisting or screwlike motion that can proceed only as long as the facets can accommodate simultaneous and opposite motions across the surfaces. The result is a triplanar motion of the talus around a single oblique joint axis, producing the motion of supination/pronation.

■ The Subtalar Axis

The axis for subtalar supination/pronation has been the subject of many investigations that indicate substantial variability, even among healthy individuals without impairments. Manter[48] reported that the average subtalar axis was (1) inclined 42° upward and anteriorly from the transverse plane (with a broad interindividual range of 29° to 47°) (Fig. 12-15A), and (2) inclined

medially 16° from the sagittal plane (with a broad interindividual range of 8° to 24°) (see Fig. 12-15B). Clearly, motion about this oblique axis will cross all three planes. Supination/pronation, like the triplanar ankle joint motion, can be modeled by a single oblique hinge joint.[49,50] Although the triplanar motions of pronation/supination can be described by its three component (cardinal) motions, these subtalar component motions are coupled and cannot occur independently. The coupled motions must occur simultaneously as the calcaneus (or talus) twists across the subtalar joint's three articular surfaces.

To understand the components of subtalar pronation/supination, we can consider how the subtalar axis varies from the cardinal axes shown in Figure 12-2. If the subtalar joint axis were vertical, the motion around that axis would be as abduction/adduction; if the subtalar axis were longitudinal, the motion would be inversion/eversion; and if the subtalar axis were coronal, the motion would be plantarflexion/dorsiflexion. In reality, the subtalar axis lies about halfway between being longitudinal and being vertical. Consequently, pronation/supination includes about equal magnitudes of eversion/inversion and abduction/adduction. The subtalar axis is inclined only very slightly toward being a coronal axis (~16°) and therefore has only a small component of dorsiflexion/plantarflexion. The contribution of each of the coupled movements to supination or pronation will depend greatly on individual differences in inclination of the subtalar axis. As one example, if the subtalar axis is inclined upwardly only 30° (rather than the average of 42°), the relative amount of inversion/eversion will be much greater than the relative amount of adduction/abduction because the axis is closer to being longitudinal. We will now examine how the subtalar joint's component motions are coupled to constitute the complex motions of pronation/supination in both non–weight-bearing and weight-bearing positions.

■ Non–Weight-Bearing Subtalar Joint Motion

In non–weight-bearing supination and pronation, subtalar motion is described by motion of its distal segment (the calcaneus) on the stationary talus and lower leg, where the reference point on the calcaneus is its anteriorly located head (see Fig. 12-6). Non–weightbearing supination is composed of the coupled calcaneal motions of adduction, inversion, and plantarflexion; pronation of the non–weight-bearing calcaneus on the fixed talus and lower leg is composed of the coupled motions of abduction, eversion, and dorsiflexion (Table 12-1). The most readily observable of the coupled motions of the calcaneus during pronation and supination are eversion and inversion, respectively. These motions of the calcaneus are often observed at the posterior calcaneus with the subject prone and the foot and lower leg over the end of the plinth. Eversion (Fig. 12-16A) may also be referred to as valgus movement of the calcaneus. Inversion (see Fig. 12-16B) may also be referred to as varus movement of the calcaneus. The eversion and inversion components of prona-

A

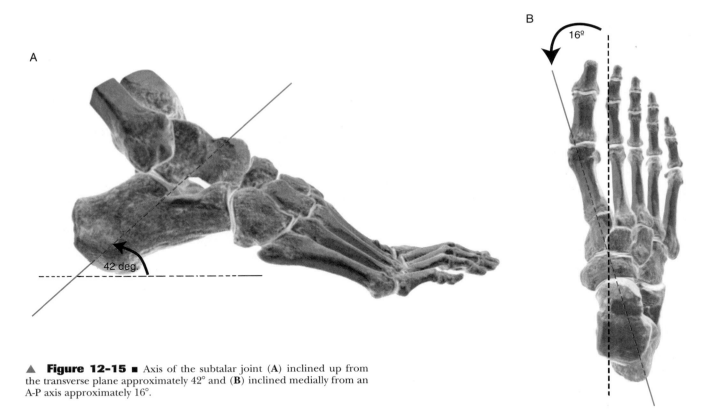

B

16°

42 deg.

▲ **Figure 12-15** ■ Axis of the subtalar joint (**A**) inclined up from the transverse plane approximately 42° and (**B**) inclined medially from an A-P axis approximately 16°.

tion/supination appear as if they are occurring in isolation. However, the coupled components of calcaneal abduction and dorsiflexion must simultaneously accompany eversion, and the coupled components of calcaneal adduction and plantarflexion must simultaneously accompany inversion.

 CONCEPT CORNERSTONE 12-3: *Terminology Revisited*

Although the apparent interchangeable use of the terms pronation/supination and eversion/inversion to describe the composite

uniaxial motions of the subtalar joint appears contradictory, the "disagreement" in terminology is not as discrepant as it first appears. When the composite term "pronation" is used to describe subtalar motion, the coupled calcaneal component of "eversion" will always be part of the motion. When the composite term "eversion" is used to describe subtalar motion, the coupled calcaneal component of "pronation" will always be part of the motion. Consequently, "pronation" and "eversion" are invariably linked, regardless of the terminology frame of reference. The same is true of supination and inversion; whether used as a composite

Table 12-1	Summary of Coupled Subtalar Motions: Coupled Movements of Subtalar Pronation/Supination	
	Non–Weight-Bearing	Weight-Bearing
Supination	Calcaneal inversion (or varus)	Calcaneal inversion (or varus)
	Calcaneal adduction	Talar abduction (or lateral rotation)
	Calcaneal plantarflexion	Talar dorsiflexion
		Tibiofibular lateral rotation
Pronation	Calcaneal eversion (or valgus)	Calcaneal eversion (or valgus)
	Calcaneal abduction	Talar adduction (or medial rotation)
	Calcaneal dorsiflexion	Talar plantarflexion
		Tibiofibular medial rotation

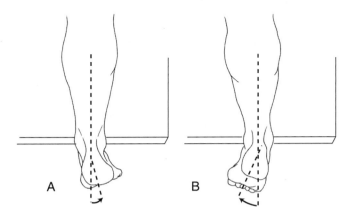

A   B

▲ **Figure 12-16** ■ Non–weight-bearing motion at the right subtalar joint. **A.** Pronation of the subtalar joint is observable as eversion (valgus movement) of the calcaneus, although the coupled motions of dorsiflexion and abduction of the calcaneus must also be occurring. **B.** Supination of the subtalar joint is observable as inversion (varus movement) of the calcaneus, although the coupled motions of plantarflexion and adduction of the calcaneus must also be occurring.

term or a component term, "supination" and "inversion" are invariably linked. It would certainly be less troublesome if a universal definitional framework were accepted. However, the wary reader who understands the association between supination/pronation and inversion/eversion may be able to infer definitions when they are not overtly offered by authors.

■ **Weight-Bearing Subtalar Joint Motion**

When an individual is weight-bearing, the calcaneus is on the ground and generally free to move around a longitudinal axis (inversion/eversion) but limited in its ability to move around a coronal axis (plantarflexion/dorsiflexion) and vertical axis (adduction/abduction) because of the superimposed body weight. Consequently, the coupled motions that contribute to pronation/supination cannot be accomplished exclusively by the calcaneus. Although the weight-bearing calcaneus will continue to contribute the inversion/ eversion component of subtalar motion, the other two coupled components of the subtalar motion (abduction/adduction and dorsiflexion/plantarflexion) will be accomplished by movement of the talus (whereby the head of the talus is used as the reference) on the more fixed calcaneus rather than by movement of the calcaneus on the relatively fixed talus. The motion accomplished at any joint around a given axis remains unchanged whether the distal segment of the joint moves or whether the proximal segment moves. When the proximal segment moves on the distal segment, however, the motion of the proximal segment will be the opposite of what was described as occurring to the distal segment. In weight-bearing subtalar motion, the direction of the component movement contributed by the talus is the opposite of what the calcaneus would contribute, although the same relative motion occurs between the segments.

In weight-bearing supination, the calcaneus continues to contribute the component of inversion. However, the calcaneus cannot adduct and plantarflex in weight-bearing, and so the remaining coupled components of subtalar supination are accomplished by abduction and dorsiflexion of the head of the *talus*. Weight-bearing subtalar supination (see Table 12-1), therefore, is observable as inversion (or varus movement) of the calcaneus, whereas the dorsiflexion and abduction of the head of the talus are reflected in elevation of the medial longitudinal arch and a convexity on the dorsal lateral midfoot. Although subtalar joint supination is a normal foot motion, a foot that appears fixed in this position often is called a "supinated" or **cavus foot.**

Weight-bearing subtalar pronation is accomplished by the coupled component movements of eversion of the calcaneus and plantarflexion and adduction of the head of the talus (see Table 12-1). In standing, the calcaneus can be observed to move into eversion (or valgus movement), whereas talar adduction and plantarflexion are reflected in a lowering of the medial longitudinal arch and a bulging or convexity in the plantar medial midfoot. Although subtalar joint pronation is a normal foot motion, a foot that appears fixed in this position often is called "pronated," **pes planus,** or **flat foot.**

The most critical functions of the foot occur in weight-bearing. When the foot is weight-bearing and the head remains relatively positioned over one or both feet, the joints of the lower extremity effectively form a closed chain. Consequently, the kinematics and kinetics of the subtalar joint will affect and be affected by more proximal and distal joints. An important consequence of closed-chain subtalar function can be seen in its interdependence with lower extremity or leg rotation.

Weight-Bearing Subtalar Joint Motion and Its Effect on the Leg

During weight-bearing subtalar supination/pronation, the coupled component motions of dorsiflexion/plantarflexion and abduction/adduction of the talar head require that the body of the talus move as well. The body of the talus is, of course, lodged within the superimposed mortise. Dorsiflexion the head of the talus requires the body of the talus to slide posteriorly within the mortise (Fig. 12-17A), whereas plantarflexion of the head of the talus requires the body of the talus to move anteriorly within the mortise. The tibia (leg) remains unaffected by the talar dorsiflexion/plantarflexion as long as the ankle joint is free to move. However, the ankle joint cannot absorb the coupled component motions of talar abduction/adduction without affecting the leg.

When the head of the talus abducts in weight-bearing subtalar supination, the body of the talus must rotate laterally in the transverse plane (see Fig. 12-17B). When the head of the talus adducts in weight-bearing subtalar pronation, the body of the talus must rotate medially in the transverse plane. Because the body of the talus can rotate only minimally at most *within* the mortise, rotation of the body of the talus can occur in weight-bearing only if the superimposed mortise moves *with* the talus. When the subtalar joint supinates in a weight-bearing position, the coupled component of talar abduction carries the mortise (the tibia and fibula) laterally, producing lateral rotation of the leg. Correspondingly, weight-bearing subtalar joint pronation causes talar adduction, with the body of the talus rotating medially and carrying the superimposed tibia and fibula into medial rotation.

Through the component movements of abduction and adduction of the talus, weight-bearing subtalar joint motion directly influences the segments and joints superior to it. A weight-bearing subtalar joint maintained in a pronated position (e.g., a flat foot) can create a medial rotation force on the leg that may influence the knee and hip joints. Just as subtalar pronation and supination may impose rotatory forces on the leg in weight-bearing, so too may rotation of the leg influence the subtalar joint. When a lateral rotatory force is imposed on the weight-bearing leg (as when you rotate to the right around a planted right foot), the lateral motion of the leg carries the mortise and its mated body of the talus laterally. Lateral rotation of the body of the talus (adduction of the head of the talus) cannot occur without its coupled components of talar dorsiflexion and calcaneal inversion, which produce supination of the subtalar joint. A medial rotatory force

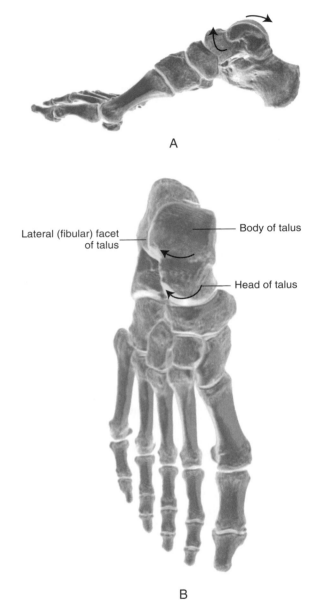

A

Lateral (fibular) facet of talus

Body of talus

Head of talus

B

▲ **Figure 12-17** ■ **A.** Dorsiflexion of the head of the talus during weight-bearing subtalar supination slides the body of the talus posteriorly within the tibiofibular mortise. **B.** Abduction of the head of the talus during weight-bearing subtalar supination rotates the body of the talus laterally, potentially taking the tibiofibular mortise along with it.

imposed on the weight-bearing leg will necessarily result in subtalar pronation as the talus is medially rotated (adducted) by the rotating tibiofibular mortise and carries with it the coupled components of talar plantarflexion and calcaneal eversion. The interdependence of the leg and talus were mechanically represented by Inman and Mann,[32] who used the concept of the subtalar joint as a mitered hinge. This mitered hinge concept (Fig. 12-18) presents a good visualization of the concept of the interdependence of the leg and foot through the oblique subtalar axis.

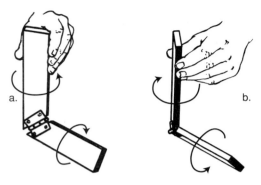

a.

b.

▲ **Figure 12-18** ■ The subtalar joint can be visualized as a mitered hinge between the leg and the foot. **A.** Medial rotation of the weight-bearing leg imposes pronation on the distally located subtalar joint. **B.** Lateral rotation of the leg proximally imposes supination on the distally located subtalar joint. (From Mann, RA: Biomechanics of running. In Mann RA [ed]: Surgery of the Foot, 5th ed, p 19. St. Louis, CV Mosby, 1986, with permission.)

Case Application 12-1: **Hip Rotation and Subtalar Joint Position**

When the foot is maintained in a more pronated position during weight-bearing, as is true for Mr. Benson, there can be a sustained medial rotation force on the lower extremity. That force may create a rotatory stress at the knee joint in weight-bearing, or it may cause medial rotation at the hip joint. Although it is difficult to determine whether the evident subtalar pronation is causing the medially rotated position of the right extremity or a result of the medial rotation, the hip joint position is likely to be related to the somewhat medially facing right patella, can increase the Q-angle, and potentially contributes to the patellofemoral pain that Mr. Benson appears to be reporting.[51]

■ Range of Subtalar Motion and Subtalar Neutral

The range of subtalar supination and pronation is difficult to determine objectively because of the triplanar nature of the movement and because the component contributions vary with the inclination of the subtalar axis. The calcaneal inversion/eversion (varus/valgus) component of subtalar motion is relatively easy to measure in both weight-bearing and non–weight-bearing positions by using the posterior calcaneus and posterior midline of the leg as reference points and assuming that neutral position (0°) is when the two posterior lines coincide (see Fig. 12-16). For individuals without impairments, 5° to 10° of calcaneal eversion (valgus) and 20° to 30° of calcaneal inversion (varus) have been reported for a total range of 25° to 40°.[21,52,53]Although it is acknowledged that the ranges of calcaneal inversion/eversion are not equivalent in magnitude to those of subtalar supination/pronation, the ranges should be directly proportional.

The variability in the inclination of the subtalar axis described by Manter[48] directly affects the range of the coupled components of subtalar motion. If the axis is inclined upward less than the average of 42° (see Fig. 12-15A), the subtalar axis will more closely approximate a longitudinal axis; the proportion of inversion/eversion of the calcaneus that is part of subtalar motion will increase, whereas the proportion of coupled abduction/adduction of the calcaneus (or talus) will decrease. Because the change in inclination of the subtalar axis will affect both the foot and leg position in weight-bearing, a considerable amount of attention has been given to determining how an individual's subtalar axis might differ from the average (or standard) axis. This has led to an attempt to define an individual's **subtalar neutral** position of the subtalar joint, under the presumption that an individual's neutral subtalar joint position may deviate from the point at which the midlines of the posterior calcaneus and the posterior leg coincide, with a medial increase in that angle referred to as valgus and an decrease referred to as varus (see Fig. 12-3).

The subtalar neutral position has been defined differently by various investigators, with some issues raised as to the appropriateness of the concept or the measurement techniques. Root and colleagues[52] defined subtalar neutral position as the point from which the calcaneus will invert twice as many degrees as it will evert. Bailey and colleagues[54] used radiographic evidence to demonstrate that the neutral position of the subtalar joint was not always found two thirds of the way from maximum supination, although the average neutral subtalar position for their subjects was close to this value. Elveru and colleagues[55] proposed palpating the medial head and neck of the talus while supinating and pronating the subtalar joint, with subtalar neutral as the point where the talus is equally positioned between the fingers. This technique is fairly subjective, and the interrater reliability generally is poor[56] but can be improved with standardized methods and practice between the testers.[57] Åstrom and Arvidson[53] used the technique of Elveru and colleagues[55] to find subtalar neutral in 121 subjects without impairments and found the average position of the calcaneus in the palpated subtalar neutral position to be 2° of calcaneal valgus angle (in relation to the midline of the calf). When Åstrom and Arvidson used the method of Root and colleagues, the "subtalar neutral" position was 1° of calcaneal varus. McPoil and Cornwall[58] used palpation of the talar head to determine subtalar neutral among normal subjects and found an average position of 1.5° of calcaneal varus angle.

The work of Cornwall and McPoil[59] can be used to indicate some of the controversy that exists around the definition and application of the term "subtalar neutral." Cornwall and McPoil described calcaneal motion during walking in 153 subjects between 18 and 41 years old with no history of foot impairments. They reported that the calcaneus is inverted 3.0° (±2.7°) at heel strike relative to the tibia and then everts to 2.2° (±2.4°) of inversion by 55% of stance phase. After a period of eversion, the motion is reversed and achieves a maximum value of 5.5° (±3.2°) of inversion just before the foot leaves the ground.[59] These findings are in agreement with their previous study, which refuted the notion that a subtalar joint neutral position is reached during mid-

stance.[58] They concluded that the "neutral" position of the rear foot during the walking cycle was better represented by the resting position of the calcaneus with respect to the lower leg than the palpated subtalar joint neutral position. The resting position of the calcaneus in relaxed bilateral stance averaged approximately 3.5° of calcaneal valgus angle (eversion) in their subjects. Their data appear to support the conclusion of Åstrom and Arvidson that the normal weight-bearing foot is more pronated than previously thought and that reliance on the palpated subtalar neutral position could lead to overdiagnosis of excessive subtalar pronation.[53]

The calcaneal inversion/eversion components of subtalar motion have received a large amount of attention because of the availability of measurement strategies. The talar dorsiflexion/plantarflexion component of weight-bearing subtalar motion cannot be measured accurately except in static radiographs. The talar abduction/adduction component is also difficult to quantify, even on radiographs. Estimates of the degree of talar abduction/adduction have been made by measuring the tibial rotation that accompanies abduction/adduction of the talus in weight-bearing. One study[60] measured approximately 10° of tibial rotation during the stance phase of gait. Another study measured about 4° (±4°) of medial rotation and 6° (±5°) degrees of lateral rotation of the tibia with respect to the calcaneus, for a total of about 10° degrees of transverse plane motion.[59] This 10° range serves as a reasonable estimate of the amount of abduction/adduction of the talus that occurs during the weight-bearing portion of gait (although not necessarily all the talar abduction/adduction that is available at the subtalar joint).

 CONCEPT CORNERSTONE 12-4: *Subtalar Joint Neutral Summary*

Morton Root, a podiatrist, is credited with describing the theoretical management approach to foot and ankle problems that focused on the subtalar joint neutral position.[52,61] A basic premise of the approach is that the subtalar joint should be in a neutral position during midstance. The approach to intervention for several foot deformities includes use of an orthotic device to "balance the foot" and achieve a defined subtalar joint neutral position during midstance. However, a number of problems have been identified with this approach, such as data indicating that the subtalar joint does not approach neutral at midstance,[58] poor reliability of measures, and poor validity of static measures to predict subtalar neutral measures during walking or other functional outcomes.[61,62] Although the subtalar joint position may contribute to our understanding of foot structure and function, the influence of subtalar position must be considered with other interdependent factors, including structural deviations (i.e., femoral or tibial rotation); extrinsic factors such as footwear, running surface, and activity level (magnitude and change); and physiological factors such as obesity or disease.[2,62]

When the subtalar joint is non–weight-bearing, the motions of the subtalar joint and the leg are independent and do not influence each other. When the foot is weight-bearing, a primary function of the subtalar joint is to absorb the imposed lower extremity transverse plane rotations that occur during walking and other weight-bearing activities. Such rotations would otherwise spin the foot on the ground or disrupt the ankle joint by rotating the talus within the mortise. In supination, ligamentous tension draws the subtalar joint surfaces together, which results in locking (close-packing) of the articular surfaces. Conversely, the adduction and plantarflexion of the talus that occur in weight-bearing pronation cause a splaying (spreading) of the adjacent tarsal bones that permits some intertarsal mobility. The role of the ligaments in contributing to mobility or stability at the subtalar joint, however, is somewhat controversial. The cervical ligament and interosseous talocalcaneal ligament are variously credited with checking pronation or supination.[11,21,37,41,45,63,64] Sarrafian[21] believed that the position of the ligaments are along the subtalar axis, which causes the ligaments to remain tight in both positions. According to this premise, individual shifts in location of the axis or of the ligaments could account for discrepant findings of other investigators.

The subtalar joint is strategically located between the ankle joint proximally and the transverse tarsal joint distally. We have already discussed how motions at the subtalar joint are associated with motions of the leg and ankle joint in weight-bearing. We will now focus our attention on motion between the talus and the navicular bone and between the calcaneus and cuboid bones. These articulations are grouped differently according to various authors, but the approach of this chapter will focus on the **transverse tarsal joint** as the primary functional unit accounting for motion in the midfoot. We will also see how motion at the subtalar joint influences motion at the transverse tarsal joint.

◆ Transverse Tarsal Joint

The transverse tarsal joint, also called the midtarsal or Chopart joint,[31] is a compound joint formed by the talonavicular and **calcaneocuboid joints** (Fig. 12-19). The two joints together present an S-shaped joint line that transects the foot horizontally, dividing the hindfoot from the midfoot and forefoot. The navicular and the cuboid bones are considered, in essence, immobile in the weight-bearing foot. Transverse tarsal joint motion, therefore, is considered to be motion of the talus and of the calcaneus on the relatively fixed naviculocuboid unit.[31,65] Motion at the compound transverse tarsal joint, however, is more complex than the relatively simple joint line might suggest and occurs predominantly in response to motion at the subtalar joint.

Transverse Tarsal Joint Structure

■ Talonavicular Joint

The proximal portion of the talonavicular articulation is formed by the anterior portion of the head of the

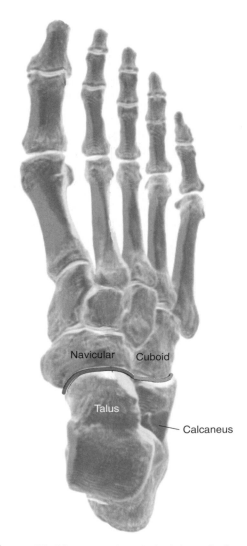

▲ **Figure 12-19** ■ The talonavicular joint and calcaneocuboid joint form a compound joint known as the transverse tarsal joint line that transects the foot.

talus, and the distal portion of the articulation, by the concave posterior aspect of the navicular bone. We also noted earlier that the talar head articulates inferiorly with the anterior and medial facets of the calcaneus as the anterior part of the subtalar joint. A single joint capsule encompasses the talonavicular joint facets and the anterior and medial facets of the subtalar joint. The inferior aspect of this joint capsule is formed by the **plantar calcaneonavicular ligament** (**spring ligament**) that spans the gap between the calcaneus and navicular bone below the talar head. The capsule is reinforced medially by the deltoid ligament and laterally by the **bifurcate ligaments.** Given these structural relationships, the large convexity of the head of the talus can be considered the "ball" that is received by a large "socket" formed anteriorly by the concavity of the navicular bone; inferiorly by the concavities of the anterior and medial calcaneal facets and by the plantar calcaneonavicular ligament; medially by the deltoid ligament; and laterally by the bifurcate ligament (Fig. 12-20).

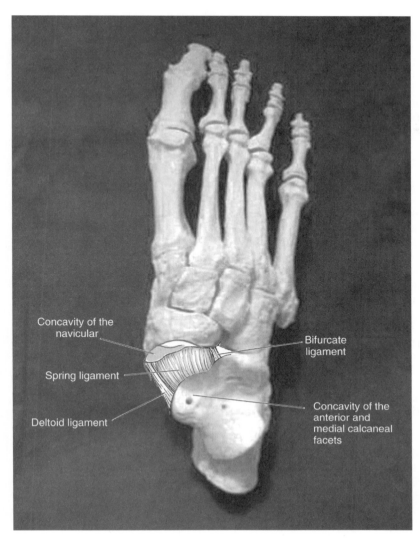

Concavity of the
navicular

Spring ligament

Deltoid ligament

Bifurcate
ligament

Concavity of the
anterior and
medial calcaneal
facets

◀ **Figure 12-20** ■ With the talus removed, this superior view shows the concavity ("socket") formed by the navicular bone anteriorly, the deltoid ligament medially, the medial band of the bifurcate ligament laterally, and the spring (plantar calcaneonavicular) ligament inferiorly.

The spring (plantar calcaneonavicular) ligament (see Fig. 12-7 and Fig. 12-20) is a triangular sheet of ligamentous connective tissue arising from the sustentaculum tali of the calcaneus and inserting on the inferior navicular bone. The spring ligament is continuous medially with a portion of the deltoid ligament of the ankle and joins laterally with the medial band of the bifurcate ligament. Davis and colleagues[66] found the spring ligament to have two distinct segments, each of which contributed to the talar "acetabulum." According to the authors, the more medially located segment of the spring ligament appeared to form a medial and plantar articular sling for the head of the talus rather than simply holding the calcaneus and navicular bone together, with a triangular- shaped avascular articular facet where the talar head rested on the ligament. The more laterally located segment of the spring ligament had a composition that suggested that its role was to resist tensile stresses only.[57] Besides the spring ligament's important role in supporting the head of the talus and the talonavicular joint, the ligament is critical in providing support for the medial longitudinal arch. Investigators agree, however, that the spring ligament has little or no elasticity.[66,67]

We already noted that the talonavicular facets and the anteriorly located talocalcaneal facets share a joint capsule. The large posterior facet of the subtalar joint is contained within its own capsule and is physically separated from the capsule containing the talonavicular joint by the tarsal canal and the ligaments within the canal. However, the talonavicular joint and the subtalar joint are linked in the weight-bearing foot. Weight-bearing dorsiflexion/plantarflexion and abduction/adduction of the talus on the calcaneus during subtalar supination/pronation necessarily involve simultaneous movement of the head of the talus on the relatively fixed navicular bone. In weight-bearing, therefore, the talonavicular joint and subtalar joint are both anatomically and functionally related.

 CONCEPT CORNERSTONE 12-5: *Talar Linkages*

Because of this anatomic and functional linkage of the talus to the structures below and anterior to it, the subtalar joint and talonavicular joint have been referred to by the compound term talocalcaneonavicular joint.[37] However, it might be argued that even this compound term is incomplete. The talus in weight-bearing also can be considered to act as a ball bearing between three joints: (1) the tibiofibular mortise (the ankle joint) superiorly, (2) the calcaneus (the subtalar joint) inferiorly, and (3) the navicular bone (the talonavicular joint) anteriorly. In weight-bearing supination/pronation, the talus dorsiflexes and plantarflexes within the mortise, as well as on the calcaneus and navicular bone. Abduction/adduction of the talus during supination/pronation not only occurs on the calcaneus and the navicular bone but also affects the position of the mortise as the body of the talus laterally and medially rotates.

The ligaments of the talonavicular joint include, of course, the ligaments that help compose it: the spring and bifurcate ligaments. The talonavicular articulation is also supported by the **dorsal talonavicular ligament** and receives support from the ligaments of the subtalar joint— including the MCL and LCL, the inferior extensor retinacular structures, and the cervical and interosseous talocalcaneal ligaments. Additional support is also received from the ligaments that reinforce the adjacent calcaneocuboid joint, which forms the remainder of the transverse tarsal joint and to which the talonavicular joint is linked functionally.

■ Calcaneocuboid Joint

The calcaneocuboid joint is formed proximally by the anterior calcaneus and distally by the posterior cuboid bone (see Fig. 12-19). The articular surfaces of both the calcaneus and the cuboid bone are complex, being reciprocally concave/convex both side to side and top to bottom. The reciprocal shape makes available motion at the calcaneocuboid joint more restricted than that of the ball-and-socket–shaped talonavicular joint. The calcaneocuboid joint, like the talonavicular joint, is linked in weight-bearing to the subtalar joint. In weight-bearing subtalar supination/pronation, the inversion/eversion of the calcaneus on the talus causes the calcaneus to move simultaneously on the relatively fixed cuboid bone. As the calcaneus moves at the subtalar joint during weight-bearing activities, it must meet the conflicting intra-articular demands of the opposing saddle-shaped surfaces, which results in a twisting motion.

The calcaneocuboid articulation has its own capsule that is reinforced by several important ligaments. The capsule is reinforced laterally by the lateral band of the bifurcate ligament (also known as the **calcaneocuboid ligament**), dorsally by the **dorsal calcaneocuboid ligament,** and inferiorly by the **plantar calcaneocuboid (short plantar)** and the **long plantar ligaments.** The long plantar ligament is the most important of these ligaments, because the inferiorly located long plantar ligament spans the calcaneus and the cuboid bone and then continues on distally to the bases of the second, third, and fourth metatarsals. The long plantar ligament makes a significant contribution both to transverse tarsal joint stability and to related support of the lateral longitudinal arch of the foot. The extrinsic muscles of the foot also provide important support for the transverse tarsal joint as they pass medial, lateral, and inferior to the joint.

■ Transversal Tarsal Joint Axes

Movements at the transverse tarsal joint are more difficult to study than movement at the ankle or subtalar joint, because multiple segments and axes are involved. Markers cannot easily be positioned about the joint to study movement. Because of the difficulties in studying movement at this joint, Elftman stated, "[The transverse tarsal joint] has yielded its secrets more reluctantly than the talocrural and subtalar joints."[31]

Although the talonavicular and calcaneocuboid joints have some independent movement, motion at one is generally accompanied by at least some motion of the other because of their functional, bony, and ligamentous connections. We continue to rely on the classic works of Elftman,[31] Manter,[48] and Hicks,[33] who proposed longitudinal and oblique axes around which the talus and calcaneus move on the relatively fixed naviculocuboid unit. The longitudinal axis is nearly horizontal, being inclined 15° upward from the transverse plane (Fig. 12-21A) and angled 9° medially from the sagittal plane[48] (see Fig. 12-21B). Motion around this axis is triplanar, producing supination/pronation with coupled components similar to those seen at the subtalar joint but now simultaneously including both the talus and calcaneus segments moving on the navicular and cuboid segments. Unlike the axis of the subtalar joint, the longitudinal axis of the transverse tarsal joint approaches a true A-P axis, and so the inversion/eversion components of the transverse tarsal movement predominate.

The oblique (transverse) axis of the transverse tarsal joint is positioned approximately 57° medial to the sagittal plane (Fig. 12-22A) and 52° superior to the transverse plane (see Fig. 12-22B).[48] This triplanar axis also provides supination/pronation with coupled component movements of the talus and calcaneus segments moving together on the navicular and cuboid bones, but dorsiflexion/plantarflexion and abduction/adduction components predominate over inversion/eversion motions. Motions about the longitudinal and oblique axes are difficult to separate and to quantify. The longitudinal and oblique axes together provide a total range of supination/pronation of the talus and calcaneus that is about one third to one half of the range available at the subtalar joint.[33]

Transverse Tarsal Joint Function

The proposed longitudinal and oblique axes for the transverse tarsal joint indicate a function similar to that of the subtalar joint. In fact, as already noted, the subtalar and the transverse tarsal joints are linked mechanically. Any weight-bearing subtalar motion includes talar abduction/adduction and dorsiflexion/plantarflexion that also causes motion at the talonavicular joint and calcaneal inversion/eversion that causes motion at the calcaneocuboid joint. Weight-bearing subtalar motion, therefore, must involve the entire transverse tarsal joint. As the subtalar joint supinates, its linkage to the transverse tarsal joint causes both the

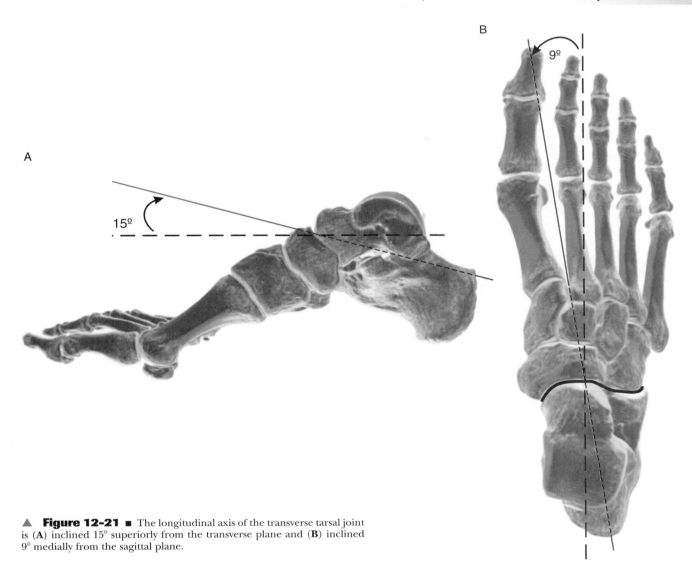

▲ **Figure 12-21** ▪ The longitudinal axis of the transverse tarsal joint is (**A**) inclined 15° superiorly from the transverse plane and (**B**) inclined 9° medially from the sagittal plane.

talonavicular joint and the calcaneocuboid joint to begin to supinate also. When the subtalar joint is fully supinated and locked (bony surfaces are drawn together), the transverse tarsal joint is also carried into full supination, and its bony surfaces are similarly drawn together into a locked position. When the subtalar joint is pronated and loose-packed, the transverse tarsal joint is also mobile and loose-packed.

The transverse tarsal joint is the transitional link between the hindfoot and the forefoot, serving to (1) add to the supination/pronation range of the subtalar joint and (2) compensate the forefoot for hindfoot position. Compensation in this context refers to the ability of the forefoot to remain flat on the ground (relatively immobile) while the hindfoot (talus and calcaneus) pronates or supinates in response to the terrain or the rotations imposed by the leg. The first of the transverse tarsal joint functions (adding range to supination/pronation) can occur either in the weight-bearing foot or in the non–weight-bearing foot. The second function requires closer analysis.

▪ Weight-Bearing Hindfoot Pronation and Transverse Tarsal Joint Motion

In the weight-bearing position, medial rotation of the tibia (as occurs, for example, if someone pivots on a fixed foot) imposes pronation on the subtalar joint. If the pronation force continued distally through the foot, the lateral border of the foot would tend to lift from the ground, diminishing the stability of the base of support, resulting in unequal weight-bearing, and imposing stress at multiple joints. This undesirable effect of weight-bearing subtalar joint pronation may be avoided if the forefoot remains flat on the ground. This can occur if the transverse tarsal joint is mobile and can effectively "absorb" the hindfoot pronation (allowing the hindfoot to move without passing the movement on to the forefoot). When the talus and calcaneus move on an essentially fixed naviculocuboid unit, there is a relative supination of the bony segments distal to the transverse tarsal joint, with the result that the forefoot remains relatively flat on the ground. The transverse

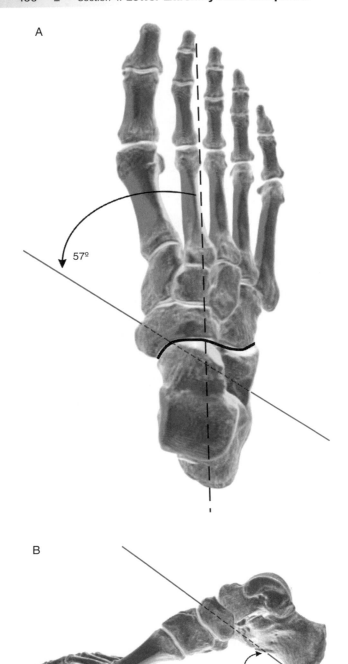

▲ **Figure 12-22** ■ The oblique axis of the transverse tarsal joint is (**A**) inclined 57° from the sagittal plane and (**B**) inclined 52° superiorly from the transverse plane.

tarsal joint maintains normal weight-bearing forces on the forefoot while allowing the hindfoot (subtalar joint) to absorb the rotation of the lower limb. Inman and Mann's[32] mechanical model (Fig. 12-23A) nicely represents how a medial rotatory force imposed on the leg acts through the oblique axis of the "subtalar joint" and through the "transverse tarsal joint" to maintain the forefoot in a relatively fixed position. Note that the

fixed "forefoot" has effectively moved in a direction opposite to that of the "hindfoot" segment.

Inman and Mann's model indicates that when the weight-bearing hindfoot (subtalar joint) is pronated, the transverse tarsal joint will supinate (move in a direction opposite to the hindfoot). However, in reality the transverse tarsal joint is relatively free to move either into pronation or supination (depending on the demands of the terrain) because both the subtalar and the transverse tarsal joints are loose-packed. In a bilateral standing position on level ground, both the subtalar joint and the transverse tarsal joints pronate slightly (see Fig. 12-23B), presumably to allow the foot to absorb the body's weight. As a result of the pronation, there will be a slight medial rotatory force on the leg. As a person moves into single-limb support and begins to walk, the subtalar joint will continue to pronate, whereas the transverse tarsal joint will move in the direction of supination approximately an equal amount to maintain proper weight-bearing in the forefoot. During walking on uneven terrain, as long as the hindfoot is in pronation, the forefoot can move either toward supination or pronation, depending on the demands of the terrain. If, for example, there is a rock under the medial forefoot during walking, the transverse tarsal joint may move into greater supination to maintain appropriate contact of the forefoot with the ground (see Fig. 12-23C). If the supination range is not available at the transverse tarsal joint, the rock may also force the hindfoot into a supinated position (putting the LCLs at risk). With other surface demands, such as standing sideways on a steep hill, the uphill foot must pronate substantially to maintain contact with the ground. Therefore, pronation may be required at both the subtalar and the transverse tarsal joints. As long as the subtalar joint is in some degree of pronation, both the subtalar joint and the transverse tarsal joint are relatively mobile and free to make compensatory changes (within the limits of the joints' ROM) to maintain contact of the foot with the ground.

■ **Weight-Bearing Hindfoot Supination and Transverse Tarsal Joint Motion**

As shown in the mechanical model of Inman and Mann,[32] a lateral rotatory force on the leg will create subtalar supination in the weight-bearing subtalar joint with a relative pronation of the transverse tarsal joint (opposite motion of the forefoot segment) to maintain appropriate weight-bearing on a level surface (Fig. 12-24A). Supination of the subtalar joint, however, can proceed to only a certain point before the transverse tarsal joint also begins to supinate. As bony and ligamentous structures of the subtalar joint draw the talus and calcaneus closer together (become increasingly close-packed), the navicular and cuboid bones are also drawn toward the talus and calcaneus; that is, transverse tarsal joint mobility is increasingly limited as the subtalar joint moves toward full supination. With increasing supination of the subtalar joint (caused either by the terrain or by an increased lateral rotatory force on the leg), the transverse tarsal joint cannot absorb the

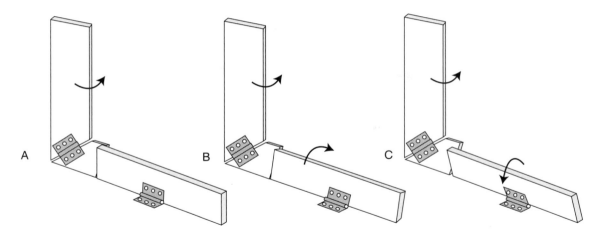

▲ **Figure 12-23** ■ With pronation occurring at the subtalar joint through medial rotation of the leg, the transverse tarsal joint is free to (**A**) supinate slightly to maintain the relatively fixed position of the forefoot segment; (**B**) pronate slightly as occurs in normal standing; or (**C**) supinate substantially to maintain appropriate weight-bearing of the forefoot segment on uneven terrain. (Adapted from Mann RA: Biomechanics of running. In Mann RA [ed]: Surgery of the Foot, 5th ed, p. 15. St. Louis, CV Mosby, 1986, with permission.)

additional rotation but begins to move toward supination as well (see Fig. 12-24B).

In full subtalar joint supination, such as when the tibia is maximally laterally rotated on the weight-bearing foot, supination locks not only the subtalar joint but also the transverse tarsal joint (see Fig. 12-14C). The fully supinated subtalar joint and transverse tarsal joint will tend to shift the weight-bearing in the forefoot fully to the lateral border of the foot. Barring other compensatory mechanisms or when the demands of the terrain exceed the foot's ability to compensate, the entire medial border of the foot may lift and, unless the muscles on the lateral side of the foot and ankle are active, a supination sprain of the lateral ligaments may occur. When the locked subtalar and transverse tarsal joints are unable to absorb the rotation superimposed by the weight-bearing limb or by uneven ground, the forces must be dissipated at the ankle, and excessive stresses

may result in injury to the ankle joint structures. The subtalar joint of a high-arched (pes cavus) foot tends to be set in a supinated position with limited pronation motion. This supinated position also limits the ability of the transverse tarsal joint to compensate. Therefore, a high-arched foot is thought to be relatively rigid and be more susceptible to impact-type injuries, especially on the lateral side of the foot.[68]

Case Application 12-2: **Flat Feet**

Mr. Benson, according to report and observation, has "flat feet." In flat foot (pes planus or pes valgus) deformity, a foot typically remains in a position of excessive pronation at the subtalar joint during weight-bearing. The slight pronation of both the subtalar and transverse tarsal joint seen in normal bilateral stance are

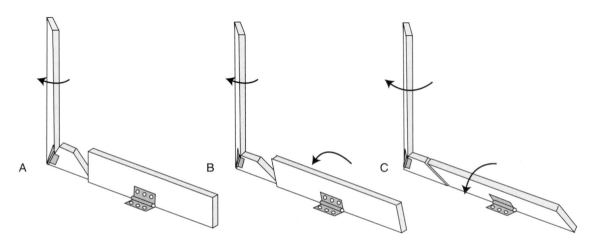

▲ **Figure 12-24** ■ With supination occurring at the subtalar joint through lateral rotation of the leg, the transverse tarsal joint has limited ability to pronate to maintain the relatively fixed position of the forefoot segment (**A**); will begin to supinate with a greater range of subtalar supination and lateral rotation of the leg (**B**); or will fully supinate along with a fully supinated subtalar joint and maximal lateral rotation of the superimposed leg (**C**).

exaggerated. Rather than seeing the transverse tarsal joint reverse to absorb the excessive pronation of the hindfoot, the navicular bone is pushed down by the pressure of the plantarflexed and adducted talar head, which produces a low medial arch with a medial bulge[52,69] Perhaps because the foot is too flexible, some evidence suggests that excessive pronation is associated with weakness in the plantarflexor muscles and decreased ability to push off.[70] People with severe or chronic pes planus often have inadequate push-off and a flat-footed gait pattern. We have already noted that the pronated position of the subtalar joint may be related to Mr. Benson's medially rotated knees. Although there is not a strong relationship between excessive pronation and tibial rotation during walking,[71] reducing excessive pronation at the foot and ankle by using orthotic devices has been shown to reduce tibial rotation during early stance phase[72] and helps to decrease pain in the patellofemoral region.[73]

The most common form of flat foot is termed a **flexible flat foot** and is marked by an arch that reappears when the foot is non–weight-bearing. It can be quickly ascertained that this is the form of flat foot that Mr. Benson has bilaterally. Treatment is focused on limiting excessive pronation by using footwear[74] or orthotic devices.[61,62,73] If excessive pronation can be reduced, the excessive stresses that may be related to his right knee pain may be reduced or eliminated.

◆ Tarsometatarsal Joints

Tarsometatarsal Joint Structure

The **tarsometatarsal TMT joints** are plane synovial joints formed by the distal row of tarsal bones (posteriorly) and the bases of the metatarsals (Fig. 12-25). The first (medial) TMT joint is composed of the articulation between the base of the first metatarsal and the medial cuneiform bone and has its own articular capsule. The second TMT joint is composed of the articulation of the base of the second metatarsal with a mortise formed by the middle cuneiform bone and the sides of the medial and lateral cuneiform bones. This joint is set more posteriorly than the other TMT joints; it is stronger and its motion is more restricted. The third TMT joint, formed by the third metatarsal and the lateral cuneiform, shares a capsule with the second TMT joint. The bases of the fourth and fifth metatarsals, with the distal surface of the cuboid bone, form the fourth and fifth TMT joints. These two joints also share a common joint capsule. Small plane articulations exist between the bases of the metatarsals to permit motion of one metatarsal on the next. Numerous dorsal, plantar, and interosseous ligaments reinforce each TMT joint. In addition, there is a **deep transverse metatarsal ligament** that spans the heads of the metatarsals on the plantar surface and is similar to that found in the hand. Just as the deep transverse metacarpal ligament contributed to stability of the more proximally located **carpometacarpal (CMC)** joints, the deep transverse

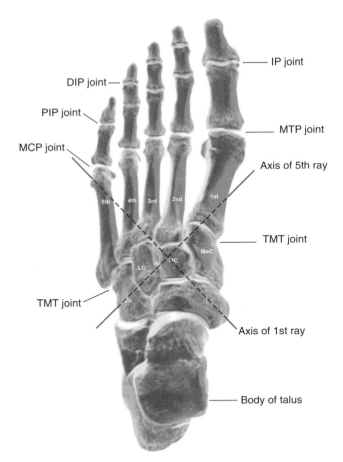

▲ **Figure 12-25** ■ Tarsometatarsal (TMT), metatarsophalangeal, and interphalangeal joints of the foot, showing the axes of the first and fifth TMT joints. CU, cuboid; LC, lateral cuneiform; MC, middle cuneiform; MeC, medial cuneiform.

metatarsal ligament contributes to stability of the proximally located TMT joints by preventing excessive motion and splaying of the metatarsal heads.[75].

■ Axes

Each TMT joint is considered to have a unique, although not fully independent, axis of motion. Hicks[33] examined the axes for the five rays. A **ray** is defined as a functional unit formed by a metatarsal and (for the first through third rays) its associated cuneiform bone. The cuneiform bones are included as parts of the movement units of the TMT rays because of the small and relatively insignificant amount of motion occurring at the cuneonavicular joints. The cuneonavicular motion, therefore, becomes functionally part of the available TMT motions. The fourth and fifth rays are formed by the metatarsal alone because these metatarsals share an articulation with the cuboid bone.

According to Hicks,[33] most motion at the TMT joints occurs at the first and fifth rays. The axes for the first and fifth rays are shown in Figure 12-25. Each axis is oblique and, therefore, triplanar. Of the TMT joints, the first has the largest ROM. The axis of the first ray is inclined in such as way that dorsiflexion of the first ray also includes inversion and adduction, whereas plantarflexion is accompanied by eversion and abduction. The abduction/adduction components normally are minimal. Movements of the fifth ray around its axis are more restricted and occur with the opposite arrangement of components: dorsiflexion is accompanied by eversion and abduction, and plantarflexion is accompanied by inversion and adduction.

The axis for the third ray nearly coincides with a coronal axis; the predominant motion, therefore, is dorsiflexion/plantarflexion. The axes for the second and fourth rays were not determined by Hicks[33] but were considered to be intermediate between the adjacent axes for the first and fifth rays, respectively. The second ray moves around an axis that is inclined toward, but is not as oblique as, the first axis. The fourth ray moves around an axis that is similar to, but not as steep as, the fifth axis. The second ray is considered to be the least mobile of the five.

Tarsometatarsal Joint Function

The motions of the TMT joints are interdependent, as are the motions of the CMC joints in the hand. Like the CMC joints of the hand, the TMT joints contribute to hollowing and flattening of the foot. In contrast to the hand, however, the greatest relevance of TMT joint motions is found during weight-bearing. In weight-bearing, the TMT joints function primarily to augment the function of the transverse tarsal joint; that is, the TMT joints attempt to regulate position of the metatarsals and phalanges (the forefoot) in relation to the weight-bearing surface. As long as transverse tarsal joint motion is adequate to compensate for the hindfoot position, considerable TMT joint motion is not required. However, when the hindfoot position is at an end point in its available ROM or the transverse tarsal joint is inadequate to provide full compensation, the TMT joints may rotate to provide further adjustment of forefoot position.[52]

■ Supination Twist

When the hindfoot pronates substantially in weight-bearing, the transverse tarsal joint generally will supinate to some degree to counterrotate the forefoot and keep the plantar aspect of the foot in contact with the ground. If the range of transverse tarsal supination is not sufficient to meet the demands of the pronating hindfoot (or if the transverse tarsal joint is prevented from effectively serving this function), the medial forefoot will press into the ground, and the lateral forefoot will tend to lift. The first and second ray will be pushed into dorsiflexion by the ground reaction force, and the muscles controlling the fourth and fifth rays will plantarflex the TMT joints in an attempt to maintain contact with the ground. Both *dorsiflexion* of the first and second rays and *plantarflexion* of the fourth and fifth rays include the component motion of *inversion* of the ray. Consequently, the entire forefoot (each ray and its associated toe) undergoes an inversion rotation around

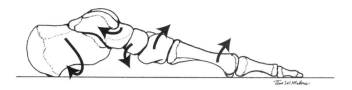

▲ **Figure 12-26** ■ Extreme pronation at the subtalar joint is accompanied by adduction and plantarflexion of the head of the talus, eversion of the calcaneus, and (in some instances) pronation at the transverse tarsal joint as a result of the navicular bone's being forced down by the talus. If the forefoot is to remain on the ground, the tarsometatarsal joints must undergo a counteracting supination twist.

a hypothetical axis at the second ray. This rotation is referred to as **supination twist** of the TMT joints.[33]

As an example of supination twist of the forefoot, Figure 12-26 shows the response of the segments of the foot to a strong pronation torque across the subtalar joint that may be caused either by a strong medial rotatory force from the leg or by inadequate support of the arch. The calcaneus everts, and the talus plantarflexes and adducts. With sufficient pronation, the navicular bone is pushed downward with the motion of the head of the talus, limiting the ability of the transverse tarsal joint to supinate adequately. The first and second rays will dorsiflex and invert, whereas the fourth and fifth rays will plantarflex and invert, which results in a supination (inversion) twist of the TMT joints to attempt to adequately adjust the forefoot. Because the five TMT joints have some independence, the configuration of the forefoot in a supination twist can vary according to the weight-bearing needs of the foot and the terrain.

■ Pronation Twist

When both the hindfoot and the transverse tarsal joints are locked in supination, the adjustment of forefoot position must be left entirely to the TMT joints. With hindfoot supination, the forefoot tends to lift off the ground on its medial side and press into the ground on its lateral side. The muscles controlling the first and second rays will cause the rays to plantarflex in order to maintain contact with the ground, whereas the fourth and fifth rays are forced into dorsiflexion by the ground reaction force. Because *eversion* accompanies both *plantarflexion* of the first and second rays and *dorsiflexion* of the fourth and fifth rays, the forefoot as a whole undergoes a **pronation twist**.[33]

Pronation twist, like supination twist, can vary in configuration. Although the pronation twist may provide adequate counterrotation for moderate hindfoot supination, it may be inadequate to maintain forefoot stability in extreme supination. In Figure 12-27, subtalar supination results in calcaneal inversion, with dorsiflexion and abduction of the talus. The transverse tarsal joint will have little if any ability to pronate, inasmuch as the navicular and cuboid bones are carried along with the hindfoot motion. The first and second rays will plantarflex and evert, whereas the fourth and fifth rays will dorsiflex and evert, which result in a

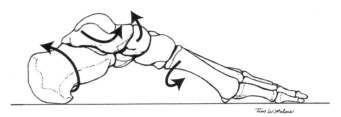

▲ **Figure 12-27** ■ Extreme supination at the subtalar joint is accompanied by abduction and dorsiflexion of the head of the talus, inversion of the calcaneus, and forced supination of the transverse tarsal joint. If the forefoot is to remain on the ground, the tarsometatarsal joints must undergo a counteracting pronation twist.

pronation (eversion) twist of the TMT joints in an attempt to adequately adjust the forefoot.

Pronation twist and supination twist of the TMT joints occur only when the transverse tarsal joint function is inadequate: that is, when the transverse tarsal joint is unable to counterrotate or when the transverse tarsal joint range is insufficient to fully compensate for hindfoot position.

Case Application 12-3: **Forefoot Varus**

Excessive pronation of the hindfoot has been associated with a **forefoot varus** deformity. With hindfoot pronation in weight-bearing, the forefoot must supinate at the TMT joints to maintain appropriate weight distribution across the metatarsal heads. If adaptive tissue changes result in a sustained TMT supination, the deformity is known as a **forefoot varus** (effectively the same as a fixed supination twist). Given that Mr. Benson has chronically pronated feet, it would be wise to look for adaptive changes in the forefoot. Forefoot varus can be identified by assessing the position of the forefoot in the frontal plane *in relation to* the subtalar neutral position of the hindfoot (typically in a non–weight-bearing position). A forefoot varus deformity is considered present if the forefoot is inverted in relation to the frontal plane when the subtalar joint (calcaneus) is manually held in its neutral position (Fig. 12-28). Identifying forefoot varus can be challenging, given the problems with ascertaining subtalar neutral in the pronated foot,[53,57,76] and may best be identified visually as simply present or not present.

◆ **Metatarsophalangeal Joints**

The five **metatarsophalangeal** (**MTP**) joints are condyloid synovial joints with two degrees of freedom: extension/flexion (or dorsiflexion/plantarflexion) and abduction/adduction. Although both degrees of freedom might be useful to the MTP joints in the rare instances when the foot participates in grasplike activities, flexion and extension are the predominant functional movements at these joints. During the late stance phase of walking, toe extension at the MTP joints

permits the foot to pass over the toes, whereas the metatarsal heads and toes help balance the superimposed body weight through activity of the intrinsic and extrinsic toe flexor muscles.

Metatarsophalangeal Joint Structure

The MTP joints are formed proximally by the convex heads of the metatarsals and distally by the concave bases of the proximal phalanges (see Fig. 12-25).

Continuing Exploration: **Metatarsal Length**

The lengths of the five metatarsals vary. In the majority of individuals, the second metatarsal is the longest of the metatarsals, followed by the first metatarsal and then followed in order by the third through fifth metatarsals. In approximately 25% of individuals, the first metatarsal is equivalent in length to the second metatarsal (see Fig. 12-25), and in 16% of individuals, the first metatarsal is longer than the second.[77] The pattern of metatarsal length may predispose an individual to a particular set of problems with the MTP joints and the toes by placing excessive stress on a particular structure.

The structure of the MTP joints is analogous to the structure of the metacarpophalangeal (MCP) joints of the hands, with a few exceptions. Unlike the MCP joints, the range of MTP extension exceeds the range

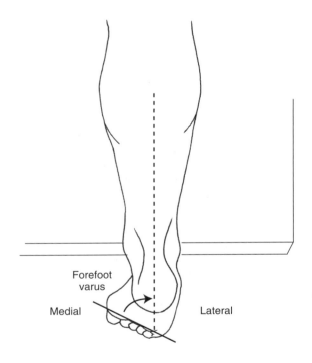

▲ **Figure 12-28** ■ A forefoot varus deformity is identified by manually placing the non–weight-bearing calcaneus in subtalar neutral position (manipulating hand not shown) and determining whether the forefoot is deviated in the frontal plane from a line bisecting the calcaneus.

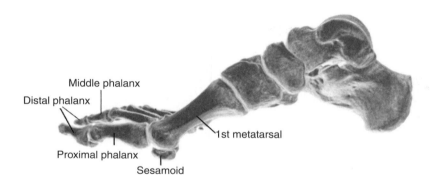

Middle phalanx

Distal phalanx

1st metatarsal

Proximal phalanx

Sesamoid

◄ **Figure 12-29** ■ In this radiograph, the two sesamoid bones can easily be seen sitting on the head of the first metatarsal.

of MTP flexion. All metatarsal heads bear weight in stance. Consequently, the articular cartilage must remain clear of the weight-bearing surface on the plantar aspect of the metatarsal head. This structural requirement restricts the available range of MTP flexion. Also in contrast to the hand, there is no opposition available at the first TMT joint; the first toe (**hallux**) moves exclusively in the same planes as the other four digits.

The first MTP joint has two sesamoid bones associated with it that are located on the plantar aspect of the first metatarsal head (Fig. 12-29). These are analogous to the sesamoid bones on the volar surface of the MCP joint. In the neutral position of the first MTP joint, the sesamoid bones lie in two grooves on the metatarsal head that are separated by the intersesamoid ridge. The ligaments associated with the sesamoid bones form a triangular mass that stabilizes the sesamoid bones within their grooves.[78] The sesamoid bones serve as anatomic pulleys for the **flexor hallucis brevis** muscle and protect the tendon of the **flexor hallucis longus** muscle from weight-bearing trauma as the flexor hallucis longus passes through a tunnel formed by the sesamoid bones and the intersesamoidal ligament that connects the sesamoid bones across their plantar surfaces.[78] Unlike the sesamoid bones of the thumb, the sesamoid bones of the first toe share in weight-bearing with the relatively large, quadrilaterally shaped head of the first metatarsal.[79,80] In toe extension greater than 10°, the sesamoid bones no longer lie in their grooves and may become unstable. Chronic lateral instability of the sesamoid bones may lead to MTP deformity.[79]

Continuing Exploration: Sesamoiditis

The sesamoid bones and their supporting structures can become traumatized with excessive loading, which results in pain and a condition known as **sesamoiditis.** Athletes with a prominent first metatarsal head who participate in prolonged running, jumping, or gymnastics are particularly susceptible to this condition of localized pain under the first metatarsal head.[81,82] Conservative treatment focuses on protecting the region from continued stresses by modifying activity, shoes, and orthotic devices. If a fracture is identified or the symptoms do not improve, surgical excision of part or all of the sesamoid bones may be necessary.[81,82]

Stability of the MTP joints is provided by a joint capsule, **plantar plates, collateral ligaments,** and the deep transverse metatarsal ligament. The plantar plates are structurally similar to the volar plates in the hand. These fibrocartilaginous structures in the four lesser toes are each connected to the base of the proximal phalange distally and blend with the joint capsule proximally. The plates of the four lesser toes are interconnected by the deep transverse metatarsal ligament and by the **plantar aponeurosis.** The collateral ligaments of the MTP joints, like those at the MCP joint, have two components: a phalangeal portion that parallels the metatarsal and phalange, and an accessory component that runs obliquely from the metatarsal head to the plantar plate.[83] The plantar plates protect the weight-bearing surface of the metatarsal heads and, with the collateral ligaments, contribute to stability of the MTP joints.[84] Deland and colleagues[83] noted that the plate and collaterals form a "substantial soft tissue box" connected to the sides of the metatarsal heads and supporting the MTP joints. They also noted that the long flexor tendons run in grooves in the plates that help maintain tendon position as the MTP joints are crossed. At the first MTP joint, the sesamoid bones and thick plantar capsule are in place of the plantar plates found at the other toes.[78]

Metatarsophalangeal Joint Function

The MTP joints have two degrees of freedom, but flexion/extension motion is much greater than abduction/adduction motion, and extension exceeds flexion. Although MTP motions can occur in weight-bearing or non–weight-bearing, the MTP joints serve primarily to allow the weight-bearing foot to rotate over the toes through MTP extension (known as the **metatarsal break**) when rising on the toes or during walking.

■ Metatarsophalangeal Extension and the Metatarsal Break

The metatarsal break derives its name from the hinge or "break" that occurs at the MTP joints as the heel rises and the metatarsal heads and toes remain weight-bearing. The metatarsal break occurs as MTP extension around a single oblique axis that lies through the second to fifth metatarsal heads (Fig. 12-30). The inclination of

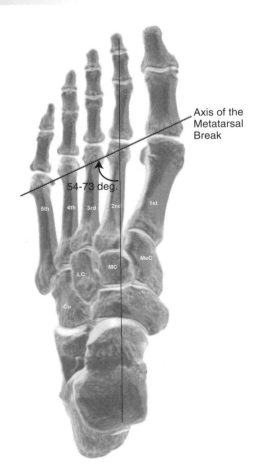

Axis of the
Metatarsal
Break

54-73 deg.

5th 4th 3rd 2nd 1st

MeC

LC MC

Cu

▲ **Figure 12–30** ■ The metatarsal break occurs around an oblique axis that passes through the heads of the four lesser toes, at an angle to the long axis of the foot that varies widely among individuals from 54° to 73°.

the axis is produced by the diminishing lengths of the metatarsals from the second through the fifth toes and varies among individuals. The angle of the axis around which the metatarsal break occurs may range from 54° to 73° with respect to the long axis of the foot.[1] The range of MTP extension will also vary somewhat, depending on the relative lengths of the metatarsals and whether the motions occur in weight-bearing or non–weight-bearing activities. One study reported that the first MTP joint had an average of 82° of extension and 17° of flexion,[85] with an average of 42° degrees of extension used during walking.[86] The ROM of the first MTP joint also may be influenced by the amount of dorsiflexion/plantarflexion motion at the TMT joints and is thought to be more restricted with increasing age.[85] Limited extension ROM at the first MTP joint will interfere with the metatarsal break and is known as **hallux rigidus.**

For the heel to rise while weight-bearing, there must be an active contraction of ankle plantarflexor musculature. Most of the plantarflexion muscles also contribute to supination of the subtalar and transverse tarsal joints. The plantarflexion musculature normally cannot lift the heel completely unless the joints of the hindfoot and midfoot are supinated and locked so that the foot can become a rigid lever from the calcaneus through the metatarsals. This rigid lever will then rotate ("break") around the MTP axis. As MTP joint extension occurs, the metatarsal heads glide in a posterior and plantar direction on the plantar plates and the phalanges that are stabilized by the supporting surface. The metatarsal heads and toes becomes the base of support, and the body's line of gravity (LoG) must move within this base to remain stable. The obliquity of the axis for the metatarsal break allows weight to be distributed across the metatarsal heads and toes more evenly than would occur if the axis were truly coronal. If the body weight passed forward through the foot and the metatarsal break occurred around a coronal MTP axis, an excessive amount of weight would be placed on the first and second metatarsal heads. These two toes would also require a disproportionately large extension range. The obliquity of the axis of the metatarsal break shifts the weight laterally, minimizing the large load on the first two digits.

Continuing Exploration: **Hammer Toe Deformity**

Excessive extension at the MTP joint in a resting position is called a hammer toe deformity. In one group of 20 healthy subjects averaging 56 (±11) years of age without foot problems, the resting MTP joint angle was 11° (±5°) of extension for the first MTP joint and 23° to 42° for the second through fifth MTP joints.[87] This MTP joint angle generally is higher in patients with diabetes and peripheral neuropathy (Fig. 12-31), possibly because of weakness in the intrinsic foot muscles that stabilize the MTP joint.[88] Presumably, because the toes cannot participate properly in weight-bearing, hammer toe deformity has been associated with increased pressures under the metatarsal heads that can result in pain or skin breakdown.[87]

■ Metatarsophalangeal Flexion, Abduction, and Adduction

Flexion ROM at the MTP joints can occur to a limited degree from neutral position but has relatively little purpose in the weight-bearing foot other than when the supporting terrain drops away distal to the metatarsal heads. Most MTP flexion occurs as a return to neutral position from extension. However, toe flexor musculature is quite important and should be distinguished from the functionally less relevant MTP flexion ROM. Abduction and adduction of the MTP joint appear to be helpful in absorbing some of the force that would be imposed on the toes by the metatarsals as they move in a pronation or supination twist. The first toe normally is adducted on the first metatarsal about 15° to 19°.[79,87] An increase in this normal valgus angulation of the first MTP joint is referred to as **hallux valgus** and may be associated with a varus angulation of the first

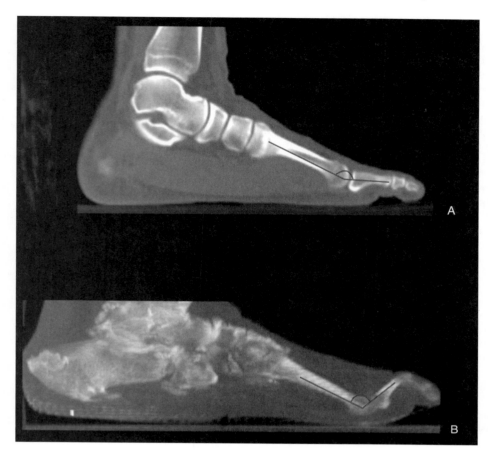

◀ **Figure 12-31** ■ Radiographic image of a foot from a healthy subject (**A**) and a foot from a subject with diabetes and peripheral neuropathy (**B**). The diabetic foot shows a hammer toe deformity (hyperextension at the MTP joint and flexion at the IP joint).

metatarsal at the TMT joint, known as **metatarsus varus** (Fig. 12-32).

Case Application 12-4: **Hallux Valgus**

Mr. Benson reported that he had a bunion that bothered him occasionally, along with periodic pain around his great toe. By inspection, he has an evident hallux valgus. Hallux valgus can result in or may be associated with a reduction in first MTP joint ROM, gradual lateral subluxation of the toe flexor tendons crossing the first MTP joint,[80] reduced weight-bearing on the great toe, and increased weight-bearing on the metatarsal head.[87] These structural changes can lead to pain and difficulty during walking. People with a pronated foot may push off during walking with a greater than normal adductor moment on the great toe that pushes the toe into a valgus (MTP joint adducted) position. Localized swelling and pain at the medial or dorsal aspect of the first MTP joint may be related to an inflamed medial bursa and is commonly called a bunion. The person with a flat foot and excessive pronation, like Mr. Benson, may have instability and excessive mobility of the first ray, which contributes to hallux valgus deformity.[89] A hallux valgus is not unique to a pronated foot but may be associated with various foot deformities.

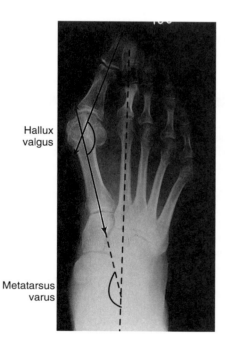

Hallux valgus

Metatarsus varus

▲ **Figure 12-32** ■ A radiograph showing both a hallux valgus at the first MTP joint, and a metatarsus varus at the first TMT joint. Excessive bony growth at the head of the first metatarsal is due to abnormal pressures from the malalignment.

Continuing Exploration: **Varus/Valgus Terminology**

Varus and valgus are consistently used to refer to a decrease or increase, respectively, in the medial angle. However, the reference line and the location of the angles keep changing. In the hindfoot, we already noted that varus/valgus either can be synonyms for inversion/eversion of the calcaneus (see Fig. 12-16) or may refer to fixed positioning of the subtalar joint in excessive supination or pronation (see Fig. 12-3). In both cases, the reference line was the posterior leg and a line bisecting the calcaneus. Now we refer to metatarsus varus as a deformity identified as a decrease in the medial angle between the long axis of the metatarsal and the long axis of the foot (or adduction of the metatarsal); hallux valgus is a deformity identified by an increase in the medial angle between the long axes of the metatarsal and proximal phalanx (adduction of the proximal phalanx) (see Fig. 12-32). We also defined forefoot varus as a fixed supination twist of the forefoot in relation to a neutral subtalar joint. In this instance, the medial angle is formed by a line through the metatarsal heads and a line bisecting the "neutral" subtalar joint (see Fig. 12-28). Unfortunately, here the terminology may conflict.

To someone who most often assesses deviations in an otherwise normal foot (as we have with Mr. Benson), a "forefoot varus" refers to a supinated forefoot. To someone who most often assesses paralytic or congenital deformities in the foot, the term "forefoot varus" may indicate a metatarsus varus of all the metatarsals and toes. The plane of the deviation differs in these two usages. Until the terminology is standardized, the context of the presentation will have to give the reader clues as to which usage is being applied.

◆ Interphalangeal Joints

The **interphalangeal (IP)** joints of the toes are synovial hinge joints with one degree of freedom: flexion/extension. The great toe has only one IP joint connecting two phalanges, whereas the four lesser toes have two IP joints (proximal and distal IP joints) connecting three phalanges (see Fig. 12-29). Each phalanx is virtually identical in structure to its counterpart in the hand, although substantially shorter in length. Consequently, the reader is referred to Chapter 9 for details on IP joint structure of the thumb and fingers to understand the structure of the IP joints of the toes.

The toes function to smooth the weight shift to the opposite foot in gait and help maintain stability by pressing against the ground in standing. The relative lengths of the toes may vary. The most common pattern is to find the first toe longer than the others (69% of individuals). The second toe may be longer than the first in 22% of the people, with 9% having first and second toes of equal lengths.[77] Each configuration may predispose the foot to different problems.[77]

◆ Plantar Arches

Although we have examined the function of the joints of the foot individually and discussed the effect of each joint on contiguous joints, combined function is best investigated by looking at the behavior of the archlike structures of the foot. The foot typically is characterized as having three arches: medial and lateral longitudinal arches and a transverse arch, of which the medial longitudinal arch is the largest. Although we may think of and refer to the two longitudinal and the transverse arches as if the arches were separate, the arches are fully integrated with one another (being more analogous to a segmented continuous vault) and enhance the dynamic function of the foot. The arches are not present at birth but evolve with the progression of weight-bearing. Gould and associates[90] described flattened longitudinal arches in all children examined between 11 and 14 months of age. By 5 years of age, as children approached gait parameters similar to those of adults, the majority of children had developed an adultlike arch.

Structure of the Arches

The longitudinal arches are anchored posteriorly at the calcaneus and anteriorly at the metatarsal heads. The longitudinal arch is continuous both medially and laterally through the foot, but because the arch is higher medially, the medial side usually is the side of reference. The lateral arch (Fig. 12-33A) is lower than the medial arch (see Fig. 12-33B). The talus rests at the top of the vault of the foot and is considered to be the "keystone" of the arch. All weight transferred from the body to the heel or the forefoot must pass through the talus.

The transverse arch, like the longitudinal arch, is a continuous structure. It is easiest to visualize in the midfoot at the level of the TMT joints. At the anterior tarsals (Fig. 12-34A), the middle cuneiform bone forms the keystone of the arch. The transverse arch still can be visualized at the distal metatarsals but with less curvature (see Fig. 12-34B). The second metatarsal, recessed into its mortise, is at the apex of this part of the arch. The transverse arch is completely reduced at the level of the metatarsal heads, with all metatarsal heads parallel to the weight-bearing surface.

The shape and arrangement of the bones are partially responsible for stability of the plantar arches. As illustrated in Figure 12-34A, the wedge-shaped midtarsal bones provide an inherent stability to the transverse arch. The inclination of the calcaneus and first metatarsal contribute to stability of the medial longitudinal arch, particularly in standing (see Fig. 12-33B). Although the structure of the tarsal bones provides a certain inherent stability to the arches, the arches would collapse without additional support from ligaments and muscles.

Because the three arches can be thought of as a segmented vault or one continuous set of interdependent linkages, support at one point in the system contributes

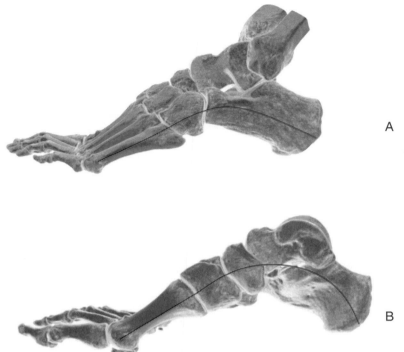

A

B

◀ **Figure 12-33** ■ The longitudinal arch viewed from (**A**) the lateral side of the foot is low in comparison with the view from (**B**) the medial side of the foot.

to support throughout the system. The plantar calcaneonavicular (spring) ligament, the interosseous talocalcaneal ligament, and the plantar aponeurosis have been credited with providing key passive support to the plate (Fig. 12-35).[91,92] The "articular" (superomedial portion) portion of the spring ligament provides particularly important support as it directly supports the head of the talus and the keystone of the longitudinal arch. Likewise, the cervical ligament is credited with contributing particularly important support of the posterior aspect of the longitudinal arch. According to one study conducted on cadavers, support from the more laterally located long and short plantar ligaments

(see Fig. 12-35) appeared to be important but less influential than support from the spring and cervical ligaments.[91]

Function of the Arches

Although the archlike structures of the foot are similar to the palmar arches of the hand, the purpose served by each of these systems is quite different. The arches of the hand are structured predominantly to facilitate grasping and manipulation but must also assist the hand in occasional weight-bearing functions. In contrast, the

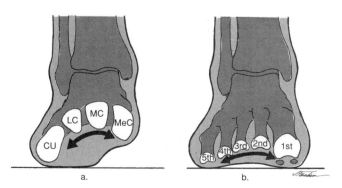

▲ **Figure 12-34** ■ The transverse arch. **A.** At the level of the anterior tarsals. **B.** At the level of the middle of the metatarsals. CU, cuboid; LC, lateral cuneiform; MC, middle cuneiform; MeC, medial cuneiform.

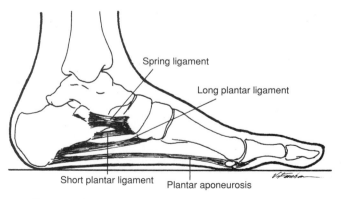

▲ **Figure 12-35** ■ The medial longitudinal arch with its associated ligamentous support, including the plantar aponeurosis. The more laterally located short plantar ligament would not ordinarily be seen in a medial view but is shown as if projected "through" the foot.

foot in most individuals is rarely called on to perform any grasping activities. The plantar arches are adapted uniquely to serve two contrasting mobility and stability weight-bearing functions. First, the foot must accept weight during early stance phase and adapt to various surface shapes. To accomplish this weight-bearing mobility function, the plantar arches must be flexible enough to allow the foot to (1) dampen the impact of weight-bearing forces, (2) dampen superimposed rotational motions, and (3) adapt to changes in the supporting surface. To accomplish weight-bearing stability functions, the arches must allow (1) distribution of weight through the foot for proper weight-bearing and (2) conversion of the flexible foot to a rigid lever. The mobility-stability functions of the arches of the weight-bearing foot may be examined by looking at the role of the plantar aponeurosis and by looking at the distribution of weight through the foot in different activities.

■ Plantar Aponeurosis

Although other passive structures contribute to arch support, the role of the plantar aponeurosis (the **plantar fascia**) is particularly important. The plantar aponeurosis is a dense fascia that runs nearly the entire length of the foot. It begins posteriorly on the medial tubercle of the calcaneus and continues anteriorly to attach by digitations to the plantar plates and then, via the plates, to the proximal phalanx of each toe[75,83] (see Fig. 12-35). From the beginning to the end of the stance phase of gait, tension on the plantar aponeurosis increases, with *in vivo* experiments using radiographic fluoroscopy to show that the plantar fascia deforms, or stretches, 9% to 12% during this time.[93] For this reason, the function of the aponeurosis in supporting the arches has been compared to the function of a tie-rod on a truss.[67] The truss and the tie-rod form a triangle (Fig. 12-36); the two struts of the truss form the sides of the triangle and the tie-rod is the bottom. The talus and calcaneus form the posterior strut, and the remaining tarsal and metatarsals form the anterior strut. The plantar aponeurosis, as the tie-rod, holds together the anterior and posterior struts when the body weight is loaded on the triangle. This structural design is efficient for the weight-bearing foot because

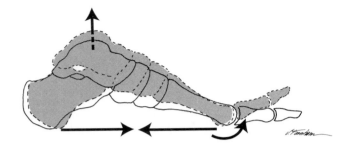

▲ **Figure 12-37** ■ Elevation of the arch with toe extension occurs as the plantar aponeurosis winds around the metatarsal heads and draws the two ends of the aponeurosis toward each other.

the struts (bones) are subjected to compression forces, whereas the tie-rod (aponeurosis) is subjected to tension forces. Bending moments to the bone that can cause injury are minimized. The fibrocartilaginous plantar plates of the MTP joints are organized not only to resist compressive forces from weight-bearing on the metatarsal heads but also to resist tensile stresses presumably applied through the tensed plantar aponeurosis.[83] Therefore, each biological structure is positioned to maximize its optimal loading pattern and minimize the opportunity for injury.

The plantar aponeurosis and its role in arch support are linked to the relationship between the plantar aponeurosis and the MTP joint. When the toes are extended at the MTP joints (regardless of whether the motion is active or passive, weight-bearing or non–weight-bearing), the plantar aponeurosis is pulled increasingly tight as the proximal phalanges glide dorsally in relation to the metatarsals or as the metatarsal heads glide in a relatively plantar direction on the fixed toes). The metatarsal heads act as pulleys around which the plantar aponeurosis is pulled and tightened (Fig. 12-37). As the plantar aponeurosis is tensed with MTP extension, the heel and MTP joint are drawn toward each other as the tie-rod is shortened, raising the arch and contributing to supination of the foot. This phenomenon allows the plantar aponeurosis to increase its role in supporting the arches as the heel rises and the foot rotates around the MTP joints in weight-bearing (during the metatarsal break).

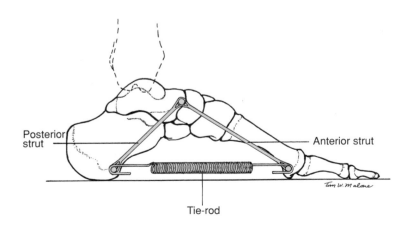

Posterior strut — Anterior strut

Tie-rod

◀ **Figure 12-36** ■ The foot can be considered to function as a truss and tie-rod, with the calcaneus and talus serving as the posterior strut, the remainder of the tarsals and the metatarsals serving as the anterior strut, and the plantar aponeurosis serving as a tensed tie-rod. Weighting the foot will compress the struts and create additional tension in the tie-rod.

The tension in the plantar aponeurosis (the tie-rod) in the loaded foot is evident if active or passive MTP extension is attempted while the triangle is flattened (that is, when the subtalar and transverse tarsal joint are pronated). The range of MTP extension will be limited. Alternatively, raising the height of the triangle by acting on the struts can unload the tie-rod. For example, when the tibia is subjected to a lateral rotatory force, the hindfoot will supinate, the posterior strut will become more oblique, the height of the medial longitudinal arch will increase, and the plantar aponeurosis (the tie-rod) will be relatively unloaded. The reduction in tension in the plantar aponeurosis will allow an increase in the range of MTP extension.

Through the pulley effect of the MTP joints on the plantar aponeurosis, the plantar aponeurosis acts interdependently with the joints of the hindfoot to contribute to increasing the longitudinal arch (supination of the foot) as the heel rises during the metatarsal break, thus contributing to converting the foot to a rigid lever for effective push-off. The tightened plantar aponeurosis also increases the passive flexor force at the MTP joints, preventing *excessive* toe extension that might stress the MTP joint or allow the LoG to move anterior to the toes. Finally, the passive flexor force of the tensed plantar aponeurosis also assists the active toe flexor musculature in pressing the toes into the ground to support the body weight on its limited base of support.

 CONCEPT CORNERSTONE 12-6: *Summary of Tie-Rod and Truss Relations*

- Tension in the plantar aponeurosis (the tie-rod) caused by MTP joint extension can draw the hindfoot and forefoot (the struts) together to raise the longitudinal arch (supinate the foot).

- Supination of the weight-bearing foot through lateral rotation of the leg or by applying a varus force to the calcaneus will decrease the angle between the struts (raise the apex of the triangle) and release tension in the tie-rod (plantar aponeurosis).

- Flattening of the triangle (pronation of the foot) in weight-bearing will increase tension in the plantar aponeurosis (the tie-rod) and limit MTP joint extension.

Case Application 12-5: **Plantar Fasciitis**

Mr. Benson reported heel pain that was greatest in the morning when he first got out of bed. The pain decreased after several steps but increased again with prolonged walking. These signs are classic for **plantar fasciitis** (inflammation of the plantar aponeurosis). The pain typically is localized at the medial calcaneal tubercle, where the plantar aponeurosis inserts, but the pain can spread distally down the fascia toward the toes. Toe extension may also increase pain because extending the toes places additional tension on the fascia. Mr. Benson's pronated foot may be contributing to excessive stress on the plantar fascia.[94] Providing an arch support to control excessive pronation has been shown to be effective at ameliorating this common problem.[94]

■ Weight Distribution

Because the foot is a flexible rather than fixed arch, the distribution of body weight through the foot depends on many factors, including the shape of the arch and the location of the LoG at any given moment. Distribution of superimposed body weight begins with the talus, because the body of the talus receives all the weight that passes down through the leg. In bilateral stance, each talus receives 50% of the body weight. In unilateral stance, the weight-bearing talus receives 100% of the superimposed body weight. In standing, at least 50% of the weight received by the talus passes through the large posterior subtalar articulation to the calcaneus, and 50% or less passes anteriorly through the talonavicular and calcaneocuboid joints to the forefoot. The pattern of weight distribution through the foot can be seen by looking at the trabeculae in the bones of the foot (Fig. 12-38). Because of the more medial location of the talar head, about twice as much weight passes through the talonavicular joint as through the calcaneocuboid joint. The somewhat lesser roles of the more laterally located long and short plantar ligaments in supporting the longitudinal arch may be attributable to the reduced weight-bearing compression through the calcaneocuboid joint in comparison with the more medially located talonavicular joint.[95]

In static standing, the distribution of weight-bearing on the plantar foot is highly variable and depends on a number of postural and structural factors.[96] In one heterogeneous sample of feet ($n = 107$), peak pressures under the heel (139 kPa) were, on average, 2.6 times greater than peak pressures under the forefoot (53 kPa). Furthermore, load distribution analysis during quiet standing showed that the heel carried 60%, the midfoot 8%, and the forefoot 28% of the weight-bearing load. The toes were minimally involved in bearing weight.

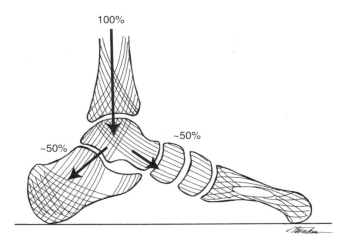

▲ **Figure 12-38** ■ Trabeculae of the bones on the medial aspect of the foot illustrating transfer of 100% of the force through the talus, with 50% passing posteriorly to the calcaneus and 50% anteriorly to the forefoot through the talonavicular and calcaneocuboid joints.

Plantar pressures are much greater during walking than during standing, with the highest pressures typically under the metatarsal heads and occurring during the push-off phase of walking (~80% of stance), when only the forefoot is in contact with the ground and is pushing to accelerate the body forward.[97] Excessive plantar pressures can contribute to pain and injury in otherwise healthy people or contribute to skin breakdown in patients with diabetes and peripheral neuropathy. Structural and functional factors such as hammer toe deformity, soft tissue thickness, hallux valgus, foot type, and walking speed have been shown to be important predictors of forefoot plantar pressures during walking in people without impairments and in people with diabetes.[87,98] In general, the increased extension of the MTP joint seen in hammer toe deformity reduces pressures on the toes and increases pressure under the metatarsal heads.[87] Pressure under the first metatarsal head also increases as arch height increases (as indicted by the inclination of the calcaneus or first metatarsal).[98] As one might expect, the soft tissue under the forefoot and the heel acts as a cushion, and as this soft tissue thickness decreases, pressures increase.[87,98]

The greatest stresses to the heel during walking occur at heelstrike and typically are 85% to 130% of body weight. Running with a heel contact pattern increases this force to 220% of body weight.[99] These large forces on the calcaneus are partially dissipated by the heel pad that lies on the plantar surface of the calcaneus. The heel pad is composed of fat cells that are located in chambers formed by fibrous septa attached to the calcaneus above and the skin below. The effectiveness of the cushioning action of the heel pad decreases with age and with concomitant loss of collagen, elastic tissue, and water. The change is evident in most people older than 40 years.[11,100]

Muscular Contribution to the Arches

Muscle activity appears to contribute little to arch support in the normal *static* foot.[101] The small intrinsic muscles of the foot (i.e., those that arise and insert within the foot) contract periodically during quiet stance, presumably to provide brief periods of unloading for the many ligaments supporting the foot. In gait, however, both the longitudinally and transversely oriented muscles become active and contribute support to the arches of the foot. Key muscular support is provided to the medial longitudinal arch during gait by the extrinsic muscles that pass posterior to the medial malleolus and inserting on the plantar foot: namely, the tibialis posterior, the flexor digitorum longus, and the flexor hallucis longus muscles.[102] The peroneus longus muscle provides important lateral stability as its tendon passes behind the lateral malleolus, glides along the lateral cuboid just behind the base of the fifth metatarsal, and then courses the entire length of the transverse arch to insert into the base of the first metatarsal.[92,102] These medial and lateral muscles provide a dynamic sling to support the arches of the foot during the entire stance phase of walking and enhance adaptation to uneven surfaces.

◆ Muscles of the Ankle and Foot

As discussed throughout this chapter, muscle activity is critical for the dynamic stability and integration of movement at multiple joints of the foot. There are no muscles in the ankle or foot that cross and act on one joint in isolation; all these muscles act on at least two joints or joint complexes. Muscle function is dependent upon the muscle's structure and, of course, where the muscle passes in relation to each joint axis the muscle crosses. The position of the ankle/foot muscles with respect to the talocrural joint axis and subtalar joint axis is represented in Figure 12-39. As illustrated in this figure, all muscles that pass anterior to the talocrural (ankle) joint will cause dorsiflexion torques or moments, while those that pass posterior to the axis will cause plantarflexion moments. Muscles that pass medial to the subtalar axis will create supination moments at the subtalar joint, whereas those that pass lateral to the subtalar axis will create pronation moments. A muscle, of course, can (and will) create both an ankle joint and a subtalar joint moment simultaneously. For example, the tibialis anterior muscle passes anterior to the talocrural axis *and* medial to the subtalar joint axis, and so it will create a simultaneous dorsiflexion moment at the ankle and a supination moment at the subtalar joint. An understanding of the position of the muscle with respect to the axis is critical for understanding its function.

A brief overview of muscle function is presented in this chapter with a more comprehensive description of the muscles described in Chapters 13 and 14. Extrinsic ankle/foot muscles are those that arise proximal to the ankle and insert onto the foot. Intrinsic foot muscles arise from within the foot (do not cross the ankle) and insert on the foot. Extrinsic muscles will be divided further into the three compartments of the lower leg: the posterior, lateral, and anterior compartments.

Extrinsic Musculature

■ Posterior Compartment Muscles

The posterior compartment muscles all pass posterior to the talocrural joint axis and, therefore, are all plantarflexors. The muscles in the posterior compartment are the gastrocnemius, soleus, tibialis posterior, flexor digitorum longus, and flexor hallucis longus muscles. The gastrocnemius muscle arises from two heads of origin on the condyles of the femur and inserts via the Achilles tendon into the most posterior aspect of the calcaneus. The soleus muscle is deep to the gastrocnemius, originating on the tibia and fibula and inserting with the gastrocnemius into the posterior calcaneus. The two heads of the gastrocnemius and the soleus muscles together are known as the **triceps surae** and are the strongest plantarflexors of the ankle. The large

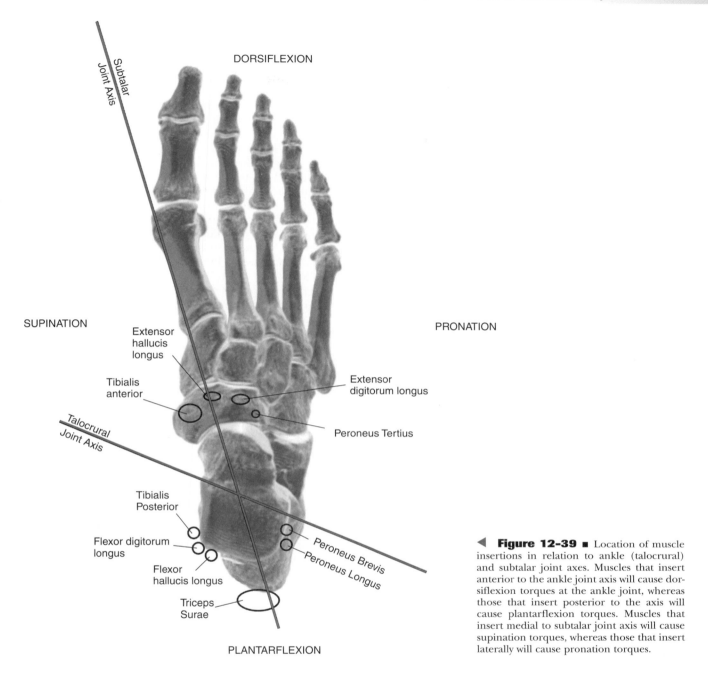

DORSIFLEXION

Subtalar Joint Axis

SUPINATION

PRONATION

Extensor hallucis longus

Tibialis anterior

Extensor digitorum longus

Peroneus Tertius

Talocrural Joint Axis

Tibialis Posterior

Flexor digitorum longus

Flexor hallucis longus

Peroneus Brevis
Peroneus Longus

Triceps Surae

PLANTARFLEXION

◀ **Figure 12-39** ■ Location of muscle insertions in relation to ankle (talocrural) and subtalar joint axes. Muscles that insert anterior to the ankle joint axis will cause dorsiflexion torques at the ankle joint, whereas those that insert posterior to the axis will cause plantarflexion torques. Muscles that insert medial to subtalar joint axis will cause supination torques, whereas those that insert laterally will cause pronation torques.

volume of the triceps surae is strongly associated with its ability to generate torque ($r^2 = .69$).[103] The Achilles tendon inserts perpendicularly on the calcaneus relatively far from the ankle joint axis (see Fig. 12-39). This efficient attachment provides a large moment arm to generate plantarflexion torque. The Achilles tendon also passes just medial to the subtalar joint. Although the moment arm for supination may be small, the large cross-section of the triceps surae makes it a strong supinator at the subtalar joint,[4,5,64,100,104] although individual variation in the location of the subtalar axis can affect the ability of the muscles to supinate.[105] Activity of the gastrocnemius and soleus on the weight-bearing foot helps lock the foot into a rigid lever both through

direct supination of the subtalar joint and through indirect supination of the transverse tarsal joint. Continued plantarflexion force will raise the heel and cause elevation of the arch (potentially assisted by the increased tension in the plantar aponeurosis as the MTP joints extend). Elevation of the arch by the triceps surae when the heel is lifted off the ground is observable in most people when they actively plantarflex the weight-bearing foot (Fig. 12-40).

The soleus and the gastrocnemius together eccentrically control dorsiflexion of the ankle while also supinating the subtalar joint after the foot is loaded in stance. These muscles provide supination torque that contributes to making the foot a rigid lever for push-off

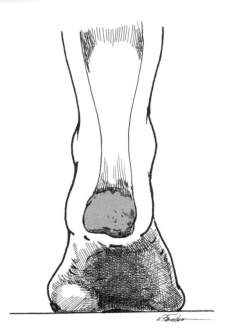

▲ **Figure 12-40** ■ Activity of the triceps surae muscles on the fixed foot will cause ankle plantarflexion, talocalcaneonavicular supination, and elevation of the longitudinal arch.

and continue to provide plantarflexion torque throughout heel rise and plantarflexion of the ankle as the ground reaction force moves to the metatarsal heads and toes.

Continuing Exploration: **Shortening of the Gastrocnemius and Soleus Muscles**

Because the gastrocnemius and soleus muscles pass behind the ankle joint, a limitation in the length of the muscles results in limited dorsiflexion ROM. Furthermore, the gastrocnemius also passes behind the knee joint, and so shortness in the gastrocnemius may further limit dorsiflexion ROM when the knee is extended. Mr. Benson had limited dorsiflexion ROM as a result of a short gastrocnemius muscle, as evidenced by the reported pulling sensation behind his knee when he sat and simultaneously extended his knee and dorsiflexed his ankle. Tight hamstring muscles also may contribute to this type of pulling sensation behind the knee and could be distinguished from a short gastrocnemius muscle by extending the hip (which relieves tension on the hamstrings but not the gastrocnemius muscle). Limited dorsiflexion ROM as a result of a short triceps surae muscle group is thought to contribute to excessive pronation at the subtalar joint and is associated with midfoot and forefoot pain.[38]

The other ankle plantarflexion muscles are the plantaris, the tibialis posterior, the flexor hallucis longus, the flexor digitorum longus, the peroneus longus, and the peroneus brevis muscles. Although each of these muscles passes posterior to the ankle axis,

the moment arm for plantarflexion for these muscles is so small that they provide only 5% of the total plantarflexor force at the ankle.[63] The plantaris muscle is so small that its function can essentially be disregarded.

The tendon of tibialis posterior muscle passes just behind the medial malleolus, medial to the subtalar joint (see Fig. 12-39), to insert into the navicular bone and plantar medial arch. The tibialis posterior muscle is the largest extrinsic foot muscle after the triceps surae and has a relatively large moment arm for both subtalar joint and transverse tarsal joint supination.[105] The tibialis posterior muscle is an important dynamic contributor to arch support and has a significant role in controlling and reversing pronation of the foot that occurs during gait.[64,92,105] When the foot is being loaded early in the stance phase of walking, the tibialis posterior muscle contracts eccentrically to control subtalar and transverse tarsal pronation. Tibialis posterior muscle activity continues to work concentrically as the foot moves toward supination and plantarflexion. Because of its insertion along the plantar medial longitudinal arch, tibialis posterior dysfunction is a key problem associated with acquired pes planus, or flat foot.[92]

The flexor hallucis longus and the flexor digitorum longus muscles pass posterior to the tibialis posterior muscles and the medial malleolus, spanning the medial longitudinal arch and helping support the arch during gait. Because the tendons pass medial to the subtalar joint, the extrinsic toe flexors also assist in subtalar joint supination. These muscles attach to the distal phalanges of each digit and, through their actions, cause the toes to flex. The flexor digitorum longus tendon courses around the medial malleolus before splitting and passing to the distal phalanx of the four lesser toes. The line of pull of the tendon is oblique and, without assistance, would cause the toes to simultaneously flex and deviate toward the medial aspect of the foot. The **quadratus plantae** muscle is an intrinsic muscle arising from either side of the inferior calcaneus that inserts into the lateral border and plantar surface of the flexor digitorum longus tendon.[3] This intrinsic muscle and the long toe flexors together form a concurrent force system with a resultant line of pull that flexes the toes with minimal deviation.

Although there is relatively little need for the toes to actually go into flexion, the toe flexors play an important role in balance when the LoG moves toward the metatarsal heads and toes. The toe flexors actively reinforce the passive role of the plantar aponeurosis during gait by eccentrically controlling the MTP extension (metatarsal break) at the end of stance phase, preventing the LoG from passing too far forward in the foot. In more static activities, the toes effectively lengthen the base of support for postural sway and during activities such as leaning forward to reach or pick up objects as long as the toe flexors are strong enough to resist MTP extension and press firmly into the ground.

Flexion of the IP joint of the hallux by the flexor hallucis longus muscles produces a press of the toe against the ground (Fig. 12-41A). Flexion of the distal

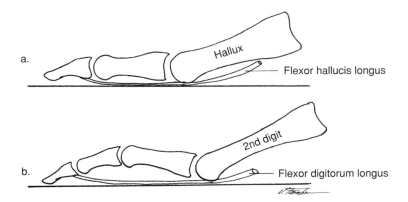

a.

Hallux

Flexor hallucis longus

b.

2nd digit

Flexor digitorum longus

◀ **Figure 12-41** ▪ **A.** Action of the flexor hallucis longus causes the distal phalanx of the hallux to press against the ground. **B.** Activity of the flexor digitorum longus causes the four lesser toes to grip the ground.

and proximal IP joints of the four lesser toes by the flexor digitorum longus causes clawing (MTP extension with IP flexion) similar to what occurs in the fingers when the proximal phalanx is not stabilized by intrinsic musculature (see Fig. 12-41B). As is true in the hand, activity of the interossei muscles can stabilize the MTP joint and prevent MTP hyperextension. Pathologies (such as peripheral neuropathy) that cause weakness of the interossei muscles can contribute to destabilization of the MTP joint, hammer toe deformity (hyperextension at the MTP joint), and excessive stresses under the metatarsal heads.[88] These excessive stresses can contribute to pain under the metatarsal heads (i.e., **metatarsalgia**) or skin breakdown in persons who lack protective sensation (i.e., those with peripheral neuropathy).

▪ Lateral Compartment Muscles

The peroneus longus and brevis muscles pass lateral to the subtalar joint and, because of their significant moment arms, are the primary pronators at the subtalar joint.[105] Their tendons pass posterior but close to the ankle axis and thus are weak plantar flexors. The tendon of the peroneus longus muscle passes around the lateral malleolus, under the cuboid bone, and across the transverse arch and inserts into the medial cuneiform bone and base of the first metatarsal (Fig. 12-42). Muscle contraction during late stance phase of gait facilitates transfer of weight from the lateral to the medial side of the foot and stabilizes the first ray as the ground reaction force attempts to dorsiflex it,[102] actively facilitating pronation twist of the TMT joints while the hindfoot moves into increased supination. Because of its path across the arches, the peroneus longus tendon is credited with support of the transverse and lateral longitudinal arches.[104]

The stability of each of the peroneal tendons at the lateral malleolus depends on integrity of the superior and inferior peroneal retinacula located just superior and inferior to the ankle joint respectively (see Fig. 12-9). Sprains of the lateral ankle structures may affect the peroneal retinacula that contribute to lateral ankle and subtalar support. Laxity of the superior retinaculum in particular may lead to subluxation of peroneal tendons

and to splitting of the peroneus brevis from its unchecked excursion over the fibular malleolus.[12]

▪ Anterior Compartment Muscles

The muscles of the anterior compartment of the leg are the tibialis anterior, the extensor hallucis longus, the extensor digitorum longus, and the peroneus tertius muscles. All muscles in the anterior compartment of the lower leg pass under the extensor retinaculum (see Fig. 12-9) and insert well anterior to the talocrural joint axis (see Fig. 12-39); these muscles are strong ankle dorsiflexors. Besides being a strong dorsiflexor muscle at the ankle joint, the tibialis anterior muscle passes medial to the subtalar axis and is a key supinator of the subtalar and transverse tarsal joints. The tendon of the extensor hallucis longus muscle inserts near the subtalar joint axis and is, at best, a weak supinator of the foot. The tibialis anterior and extensor hallucis longus muscles are active in gait when the heel first contacts the ground to control the strong plantarflexion moment at

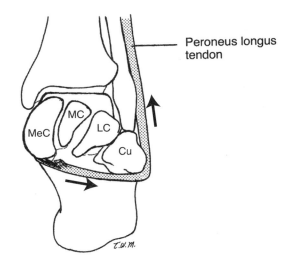

Peroneus longus tendon

MC

MeC

LC

Cu

▲ **Figure 12-42** ▪ The tendon of the peroneus longus passes transversely beneath the foot to insert into the base of the first metatarsal. An active contraction of the muscle can support the transverse arch and the first ray of the foot.

the ankle created by the ground reaction force. The tibialis anterior muscle also contributes to control of the strong pronation force on the hindfoot during the early part of stance.[102] Both the tibialis anterior and extensor hallucis longus muscles are active in dorsiflexing the ankle as the foot leaves the ground and in holding the foot up against the plantarflexion torque of gravity. The extensor hallucis longus muscle also prevents the toes from dragging by extending (or preventing flexion) of the MTP joints of the hallux.

The tendons of the extensor digitorum longus and the peroneus tertius muscles pass beneath the extensor retinaculum and insert anterior to the ankle joint axis and lateral to the subtalar joint axis; consequently, these muscles are dorsiflexors of the ankle and pronators of the hindfoot. The extensor digitorum longus muscle also extends the MTP joints of the lesser toes, working with the extensor hallucis longus muscle to hold the toes up when the foot is off the ground. The structure and function of the extensor digitorum longus muscle at the MTP and IP joints are identical to those of the extensor digitorum communis of the hand.

The extrinsic musculature producing supination of the foot is stronger than that producing pronation. This phenomenon is likely to be attributable to the fact that the LoG in weight-bearing most often falls medial to the subtalar joint, creating a strong pronation torque that must be controlled.[100] Similarly, the plantarflexors are stronger than the dorsiflexors because the LoG in weight-bearing is most often anterior to the ankle joint axis.

Intrinsic Musculature

The most important functions of the intrinsic muscles of the foot are their roles as (1) stabilizers of the toes and (2) dynamic supporters of the transverse and longitudinal arches during gait. The intrinsic muscles of the hallux attach either directly or indirectly to the sesamoid bones and contribute to the stabilization of these weight-bearing bones.[78] The extensor mechanism of the toes is similar to that of the fingers. The extensor digitorum longus and brevis muscles are MTP extensors. Activity in the **lumbrical** and the **dorsal** and **plantar interossei muscles** stabilizes the MTP joints and maintains or produces IP extension. Stabilization of the MTP joints is critical during walking to allow the toes to remain weight-bearing and reduce loading on the metatarsal heads. The small intrinsic flexor muscles contract eccentrically to assist in control of toe extension as the foot and body roll over the forefoot during late stance phase.[106] Furthermore, many of the intrinsic muscles arise on the posterior strut (calcaneus) and insert on the anterior strut (metatarsals) of the longitudinal arch, thereby serving to actively augment the tie-rod function of the plantar aponeurosis. Periodic contraction during standing and consistent contraction during the stance phase of walking dynamically help relieve stress on the passive connective tissue structures supporting the longitudinal arch.

Case Application 12-6: **Achy, Flat Feet**

Mr. Benson has flat feet, and he complained that his feet often ache at the end of the day. Although there can be several reasons for this type of generalized foot pain, a primary reason may be that the intrinsic muscles have to work harder and longer to stabilize the arches of the flat foot in comparison with a normal or high-arched foot. The high-arched foot in particular receives substantial passive support (i.e., bony alignment and ligaments), whereas the flat foot may rely more on the active contraction of the intrinsic muscles, which results in overuse, fatigue, and an "achy feeling" at the end of the day that could lead to an inflammatory response over time.

The specific function of the intrinsic muscles of the foot can be understood and appreciated by comparing each foot muscle with its corresponding hand muscle. Although most people are not able to use the muscles of the foot with the ability of those in the hand, the potential for similar function is limited only by the unopposable hallux and the length of the digits. Table 12-2 summarizes the specific functions of the intrinsic muscles of the foot.

◆ Deviations from Normal Structure and Function

The complex interdependency of the foot and ankle joints makes it almost impossible to have dysfunction or abnormality in only one joint or structure. Once present, deviations from neutral positions will affect both proximal and distal joints. The large number of congenital and acquired ankle/foot problems cannot each be described, although several have already been referenced in the chapter. The key is the "domino effect" that an ankle or foot problem has on the joints proximal and distal to the problem.

Example 12-1

Supinated Foot (Pes Cavus)

In a cavus foot, (1) the calcaneus is noticeably inverted, (2) the medial longitudinal arch height is noticeably high, and (3) a lateral dorsal bulge is present at the talonavicular joint that is associated with talar abduction and dorsiflexion.[52,69] The subtalar and transverse tarsal joints are excessively supinated and may be locked into full supination, which prohibits these joints from participating in shock absorption or in adapting to uneven terrain. Hindfoot supination often is associated with a lateral rotation stress on the leg. The inability to absorb additional lower limb rotations at the hindfoot may place a strain on the ankle joint structures, especially the LCLs. Some evidence indicates that

Table 12-2	Intrinsic Muscles of the Foot	
Muscle	Function	Analog in Hand
Extensor digitorum brevis	Extends the MTP joints	None
Abductor hallucis	Abducts and flexes MTP of hallux	Abductor pollicis brevis
Flexor digitorum brevis	Flexes PIP of four lesser toes	Flexor digitorum superficialis*
Abductor digiti minimi	Abducts and flexes small toe	Abductor digiti minimi
Quadratus plantae	Adjusts oblique pull of flexor digitorum longus into line with long axes of digits	None
Lumbricals	Flex MTPs, extend IPs of four lesser toes	Lumbricals
Flexor hallucis brevis	Flexes MTP of hallux	Flexor pollicis brevis
Adductor hallucis	Oblique head: adducts and flexes MTP of hallux Transverse head: adducts metatarsal heads transversely	Adductor pollicis
Flexor digiti minimi	Flexes MTP of small toe	Flexor digiti minimi
Plantar interossei	Adduct MTPs of 3rd–5th toes, flex MTPs, extend IPs of four lesser toes	Volar interossei
Dorsal interossei	Abduct MTPs of 2nd toe (either way), abduct MTPs, 3rd and 4th toes, flex MTPs, extend IPs of four lesser toes	Dorsal interossei

*The flexor digitorum superficialis is an extrinsic muscle, whereas the flexor digitorum brevis is an intrinsic foot muscle. IP, interphalangeal; MTP, metatarsophalangeal; PIP, proximal interphalangeal:

the inverted, or varus, position of the calcaneus places the ankle in a more susceptible position for ankle sprains.[68] Because the transverse tarsal joint is locked along with the subtalar joint, the TMT joints are solely responsible with attempting to maintain the forefoot on the ground by doing a pronation twist . If the sustained pronation twist results in adaptive tissue changes, the deformity known as a **forefoot valgus** will develop.[52,76] The excessive pronation and plantarflexion of the first ray that accompanies a pronation twist may create a valgus stress at the first MTP joint and contribute to the formation of a hallux valgus. Hallux valgus, in turn, changes the line of pull of the flexor muscles of the first toe and may affect the power of push-off in the final stages of stance.[77]

Case Application 12-7: **Case Summary**

We already established that the heel pain that Mr. Benson is experiencing is most likely from inflammation of his plantar fascia (or aponeurosis). His pronated foot may be placing excessive stress on his plantar fascia during walking, especially at the end of stance phase when the metatarsal break pulls the plantar fascia tight. His walking program has added an additional level of stress to an already susceptible structure, with the stress on this tissue crossing the threshold for injury.[2] The pain behind his medial malleolus that increases when he plantarflexes and inverts his toe may be an inflammation of the posterior tibialis tendon. The posterior tibialis may be "overworking" trying to control his excessive pronation during walking. The pulling behind his knee and calf when he dorsiflexes his foot likely is from a shortened

triceps surae that is being stretched with dorsiflexion. A shortened triceps surae is thought to be a contributing factor to excessive pronation and stress to the plantar fascia.[94] One study validated the clinical impression that isolated contracture of the gastrocnemius (dorsiflexion limited with knee extended but not with knee flexed) is an important contributing factor to forefoot and midfoot pain and pathology.[38]

Mr. Benson's pronated feet are probably also responsible for the medially located position of his patellae, inasmuch as the lower extremities have followed the talus into medial rotation. The pain that Mr. Benson complains of in his right knee is consistent with the patellofemoral stress associated with an increased Q-angle. The asymmetrical foot pronation noted in Mr. Benson's examination (right greater than left) makes his right knee slightly more vulnerable to lateral patellofemoral compression problems.

Treatment for Mr. Benson should be directed at reducing the stresses on the plantar fascia and posterior tibialis muscle by limiting excessive pronation during walking.[2,62] Stretching the triceps surae, wearing footwear with a good heel counter,[74] wearing a good arch support,[94] or using an orthotic device[61,62,73] may help Mr. Benson to reduce pronation and stress on his plantar fascia. If, in fact, the pronated foot is the primary problem, these interventions should also help with Mr. Benson's knee pain. Although there is not a strong relationship between excessive pronation and tibial rotation during walking,[71] reducing excessive pronation at the foot and ankle by using orthotic devices has been shown to reduce tibial rotation during early stance phase[72] and helps decrease pain in the patellofemoral region.[73]

Summary

The foot and ankle consist of a complex arrangement of structures and joints that allow the foot to be flexible and accommodating during early stance phase and relatively rigid during late stance phase. The complexity of the interrelationships makes it easy to disrupt normal function or exceed the limitations of the active and passive tissues that make up the ankle/foot complex. Studies that have investigated the relationship between various foot types or alignments and lower extremity injury often show little or no correlation.[2,68,69,107,108]

This should not be surprising, given the many factors that may contribute to health or injury of a given tissue.[2] An important point of this chapter, however, has been to consider how various structures and structural deviations can affect movement and stresses on adjacent structures and tissues. Although group studies may minimize the apparent influence of a given structural problem in dysfunction, the problem should not be ruled out as a factor in, or even primary cause of, pain or dysfunction in an individual case. The kinesiologic impact of a given set of alignments and apparent forces in producing maladaptive stresses should be placed in the full context of the individual person, his or her health status, and his or her activity level and activity goals.[2]

Study Questions

1. Identify the proximal and distal articular surfaces that constitute the ankle (talocrural) joint. What is the joint classification?
2. Describe the proximal and distal tibiofibular joints, including classification and their composite function.
3. Identify the ligaments that support the tibiofibular joints.
4. Describe the ligaments that support the ankle joint, including the names of components when relevant.
5. Why is ankle joint motion considered triplanar?
6. Why does the fibula move during dorsiflexion/plantarflexion of the ankle?
7. What are the primary checks of ankle joint motion?
8. Which muscles crossing the ankle are single-joint muscles?
9. Describe the three articular surfaces of the subtalar joint, including the capsular arrangement.
10. Which ligaments support the subtalar joint?
11. Describe the axis for subtalar motion. What movements take place around that axis, and how are these motions defined?
12. When the foot is weight-bearing, the calcaneus (the distal segment) of the subtalar joint is not free to move in all directions. Describe the movements that take place during weight-bearing subtalar supination/pronation.
13. What is the close-packed position for the subtalar joint? Which motion of the tibia will lock the weight-bearing subtalar joint?
14. Describe the relationship between the subtalar and the talonavicular joint with regard to articular surfaces, axes, and available motion.
15. Describe the articulations of the transverse tarsal joint.
16. What is the general function of the transverse tarsal joint in relation to the subtalar joint?
17. What are the TMT rays? Describe the axis for the first and fifth ray and the movements that occur around each axis.
18. What is the function of the TMT joints in relation to the subtalar and the transverse tarsal joints?
19. How does pronation twist of the TMT joints relate to supination of the subtalar joint?
20. What ligaments contribute to support of the medial longitudinal arch of the foot?
21. What is the weight distribution through the various joints from the ankle through the metatarsal heads in unilateral stance?
22. How does extension of the MTP joints contribute to stability of the foot?
23. In terms of structure, compare the MTP joints of the foot with the MCP joints of the fingers.
24. What is the metatarsal break? When does this occur, and how is it related to support of the longitudinal arch?
25. What is the role of the triceps surae muscle group at each joint it crosses?
26. What is the non–weight-bearing posture of the subtalar and transverse tarsal joints?
27. What other muscles besides the triceps surae exert a plantarflexion influence at the ankle? What is the primary function of each of these muscles?
28. Which muscles may contribute to support of the arches of the foot?
29. What is the function of the quadratus plantae? What is the analog of this muscle in the hand?

(Continued on following page)

30. Drawing an analogy between the foot and the hand, describe the function of each of the intrinsic and extrinsic foot muscles.
31. If a person has a pes planus, describe two possible causes for this condition.
32. Identify at least three possible effects of pes planus.
33. Identify three primary signs to identify an excessively supinated or pronated foot.

◆ References

1. Morris J: Biomechanics of the foot and ankle. Clin Orthop 122:10, 1977.
2. Mueller M, Maluf K: Tissue adaptation to physical stress: A proposed "physical stress theory" to guide physical therapist practice, education, and research. Phys Ther 2:383–403, 2002.
3. Williams P: Gray's Anatomy, 38th ed. New York, Churchill Livingstone, 1999.
4. Eichenblat M, Nathan H: The proximal tibio fibular joint. An anatomical study with clinical and pathological considerations. Int Orthop 7:31–39, 1983.
5. Barnett C, Napier J: The axis of rotation at the ankle joint in man: Its influence upon the form of the talus and mobility of the fibula. J Anat 86:1, 1952.
6. Kapandji I: The Physiology of the Joints, 5th ed. Baltimore, Williams & Wilkins, 1987.
7. Masciocchi C, Barile A: Magnetic resonance imaging of the hindfoot with surgical correlations. Skeletal Radiol 31:131–142, 2002.
8. Rasmussen O, Tovborg-Jensen I, Boe S: Distal tibiofibular ligaments. Acta Orthop Scand 53:681–686, 1982.
9. Takebe K, Nakagawa A, Minami H, et al.: Role of the fibula in weight-bearing. Clin Orthop 184:289–292, 1984.
10. Segal D, Pick RY, Klein HA, et al.: The role of the lateral malleolus as a stabilizing factor of the ankle joint: Preliminary report. Foot Ankle 2:25–29, 1981.
11. Nuber G: Biomechanics of the foot and ankle during gait. Clin Sports Med 7:1–12, 1988.
12. Geppert M, Sobel M, Bohne W: Lateral ankle instability as a cause of superior peroneal retinacular laxity: An anatomic and biomechanical study of cadaveric feet. Foot Ankle 14:330–334, 1993.
13. Kjaersgaard-Anderson P, Wethelund J, Nielsen S: Lateral talocalcaneal instability following section of the calcaneofibular ligament: A kinesiologic study. Foot Ankle 7:355–361, 1987.
14. Johnson E, Markolf K: The contribution of the anterior talofibular ligament to ankle laxity. J Bone Joint Surg Am 44:81–88, 1983.
15. Rasmussen O, Kromann-Andersen C: Experimental ankle injuries. Acta Orthop Scand 54:356–362, 1983.
16. Bahr R, Pena F, Shine J, et al.: Ligament force and joint motion in the intact ankle: A cadaveric study. Knee Surg Sports Traumatol Arthrosc 6:115–121, 1998.
17. Rasmussen O, Tovborg-Jensen I: Mobility of the ankle joint: Recording of rotatory movements in the talocrural joint in vitro with and without the lateral collateral ligaments of the ankle. Acta Orthop Scand 53:155–160, 1982.
18. Rasmussen O, Tovberg-Jensen I, Hedeboe J: An analysis of the function of the posterior talofibular ligament. Int Orthop 7:41–48, 1983.
19. Fujii T, Luo ZP, Kitaoka HB, et al.: The manual stress test may not be sufficient to differentiate ankle ligament injuries. Clin Biomech (Bristol, Avon) 15:619–623, 2000.
20. Stephens M, Sammarco G: The stabilizing role of the lateral ligament complex around the ankle and subtalar joints. Foot Ankle 13:130–136, 1992.
21. Sarrafian S: Biomechanics of the subtalar joint. Clin Orthop 290:17–26, 1993.
22. Siegler S, Chen, J, Schneck, CD: The three dimensional kinematics and flexibility characteristics of the human ankle and sutalar joints—Part I. Biomech Eng 110:364–373, 1988.
23. Lundberg A, Svensson O, Bylund C, et al.: Kinematics of the ankle/foot complex—Part 3: Influence of leg rotation. Foot Ankle 9:304–309, 1989.
24. Lundberg A: Kinematics of the ankle/foot complex: Plantarflexion and dorsiflexion. Foot Ankle 9: 194–200, 1989.
25. Lundberg A, Svensson OK, Bylund C, et al.: Kinematics of the ankle/foot complex—Part 2: Pronation and supination. Foot Ankle 9:248–253, 1989.
26. Lundberg A, Svensson OK, Nemeth G, et al.: The axis of rotation of the ankle joint. J Bone Joint Surg Br 71:194–199, 1989.
27. Valmassy R, Stanton B: Tibial torsion. Normal values in children. J Am Podiatr Med Assoc 79:432–435, 1989.
28. Seber S, Hazer B, Kose N, et al.: Rotational profile of the lower extremity and foot progression angle: Computerized tomographic examination of 50 male adults. Arch Orthop Trauma Surg 120: 255–258, 2000.
29. Isman R, Inman V: Anthropometric studies of the human foot and ankle. Bull Prosthet Res 10/11: 97–129, 1969.
30. Elftman H: The orientation of the joints of the lower extremity. Bull Hosp Joint Dis 6:139–143, 1945.
31. Elftman H: The transverse tarsal joint and its control. Clin Orthop 16:41–45, 1960.
32. Inman V, Mann R: Biomechanics of the foot and ankle. In Mann R (ed): DuVries Surgery of the Foot, 4th ed. St. Louis, CV Mosby, 1978.

33. Hicks J: Mechanics of the foot I: The joints. J Anat 87:345, 1953.

34. Stiehl J: Biomechanics of the ankle joint. In Stiehl J (ed): Inman's Joints of the Ankle, 2nd ed. Baltimore, Willliams & Wilkins, 1991.

35. Milner CE, Soames RW: A comparison of four *in vivo* methods of measuring tibial torsion. J Anat 193(Pt 1):139–144, 1998.

36. Sammarcho W, Burstein AH, Frankel VH: Biomechanics of the ankle: A kinematic study. Orthop Clin North Am 4:76, 1973.

37. Williams P: Gray's Anatomy, 38th ed. New York, Churchill Livingstone, 1995.

38. DiGiovanni CW, Kuo R, Tejwani N, et al.: Isolated gastrocnemius tightness. J Bone Joint Surg Am 84:962–970, 2002.

39. Stauffer R, Chao EYS, Brewster RC: Force and motion analysis of normal, diseased and prosthetic ankle joints. Clin Orthop 127:189, 1977.

40. Wang C, Cheng C, Chen S, et al.: Contact areas and pressure distributions in the subtatar joint. J Biomech 28:269–279, 1995.

41. Greenwald A, Matejczyk M: Pathomechanics of the human ankle joint. Bull Hosp Joint Dis 38:105, 1977.

42. Johnson J: Shape of the trochlea and mobility of the lateral malleolus. In Stiehl J (ed): Inman's Joints of the Ankle, 2nd ed. Baltimore, Williams & Wilkins, 1991.

43. Tornetta P 3rd, Spoo JE, Reynolds FA, et al.: Overtightening of the ankle syndesmosis: Is it really possible? J Bone Joint Surg Am 83:489–492, 2001.

44. Hornsby T, Nicholson GG, Gossman MR, et al.: Effect of inherent muscle length on isometric plantar flexion torque in healthy women. Phys Ther 67:1191–1197, 1987.

45. Viladot A, Lorenzo JC, Salazar J, et al.: The subtalar joint: Embryology and morphology. Foot Ankle 5:54–66, 1984.

46. Harper MC: The lateral ligamentous support of the subtalar joint. Foot Ankle 11:354–358, 1991.

47. Martin L, Wayne J, Monahan T, et al.: Elongation behavior of the calcaneofibular and cervical ligaments during inversion loads applied in an open kinetic chain. Foot Ankle Int 19:232–239, 1998.

48. Manter J: Movements of the subtalar and transverse tarsal joints. Anat Rec 80:397, 1941.

49. Sangeorzan B: Biomechanics of the subtalar joint. In Stiehl J (ed): Inman's Joints of the Ankle, 2nd ed. Baltimore, Williams & Wilkins, 1991.

50. Scott S, Winter D: Talocrural and talocalcaneal joint kinematics and kinetics during the stance phase of walking. J Biomech 24:743–752, 1991.

51. Fulkerson JP: Diagnosis and treatment of patients with patellofemoral pain. Am J Sports Med 30:447–456, 2002.

52. Root M, Orien WP, Weed JH: Normal and Abnormal Function of the Foot: Clinical Biomechanics, vol II. Los Angeles, Clinical Biomechanics Corp., 1977.

53. Åstrom M, Arvidson T: Alignment and joint motion in the normal foot. J Orthop Sports Phys Ther 22:216–222, 1995.

54. Bailey D, Perillo JT, Forman M: Subtalar joint neutral. A study using tomography. J Am Podiatr Assoc 74:59–64, 1984.

55. Elveru R, Rothstein J, Lamb R: Goniometric reliability in a clinical setting. Subtalar and ankle joint measurements. Phys Ther 6:672–677, 1988.

56. Smith-Oricchio K, Harris B: Interraterreliability of subtalar neutral, calcaneal inversion and evesion. J Orthop Sports Phys Ther 12:10–15, 1990.

57. Diamond JE, Mueller MJ, Delitto A, et al.: Reliability of a diabetic foot evaluation. Phys Ther 69:797–802, 1989.

58. McPoil T, Cornwall M: Relationship between neutral subtalar joint position and pattern of rearfoot motion during walking. Foot Ankle 15:141–145, 1994.

59. Cornwall MW, McPoil TG: Motion of the calcaneus, navicular, and first metatarsal during the stance phase of walking. J Am Podiatr Med Assoc 92:67–76, 2002.

60. Close J, Inman V, Poor P, et al.: The function of the subtalar joint. Clin Orthop 50:59, 1967.

61. Ball KA, Afheldt MJ: Evolution of foot orthotics—Part 2: Research reshapes long-standing theory. J Manipulative Physiol Ther 25:125–134, 2002.

62. McPoil TG, Hunt GC: Evaluation and management of foot and ankle disorders: Present problems and future directions. J Orthop Sports Phys Ther 21:381–388, 1995.

63. Leardini A, Stagni R, O'Connor JJ: Mobility of the subtalar joint in the intact ankle complex. J Biomech 34:805–809, 2001.

64. Cailliet R: Foot and Ankle Pain, 3rd ed. Philadelphia, FA Davis, 1997.

65. Lewis O: The joints of the evolving foot. Part II: The intrinsic joints. J Anat 130:833–857, 1980.

66. Davis W, Sobel M, DiCarlo E, et al.: Gross, histological, and microvascular anatomy and biomechanical testing of the spring ligament complex. Foot Ankle 17:95–102, 1996.

67. Lapidus P: Kinesiology and mechanical anatomy of the transverse tarsal joints. Clin Orthop 30:20, 1963.

68. Williams DS 3rd, McClay IS, Hamill J: Arch structure and injury patterns in runners. Clin Biomech (Bristol, Avon) 16:341–347, 2001.

69. Dahle L, Mueller MJ, Delitto A, et al.: Visual assessment of foot type and relationship of foot type to lower extremity. J Orthop Sports Phys Ther 14:70–74, 1991.

70. Snook AG: The relationship between excessive pronation as measured by navicular drop and isokinetic strength of the ankle musculature. Foot Ankle Int 22:234–240, 2001.

71. Reischl SF, Powers CM, Rao S, et al.: Relationship between foot pronation and rotation of the tibia and femur during walking. Foot Ankle Int 20:513–520, 1999.

72. Nawoczenski DA, Cook TM, Saltzman CL: The effect of foot orthotics on three-dimensional kinematics of the leg and rearfoot during running. J Orthop Sports Phys Ther 21:317–327, 1995.

73. Eng JJ, Pierrynowski MR: Evaluation of soft foot

orthotics in the treatment of patellofemoral pain syndrome. Phys Ther 73:62–68, 1993; discussion, 73:68–70, 1993.

74. Clarke TE, Frederick EC, Hamill CL: The effects of shoe design parameters on rearfoot control in running. Med Sci Sports Exerc 15:376–381, 1983.

75. Stainsby G: Pathological anatomy and dynamic effect of the displaced plantar plate and the importance of the integrity of the plantar plate-deep transverse metatarsal ligament tie-bar. Ann R Coll Surg Engl 79:58–68, 1997.

76. Garbalosa J, McClure M, Catlin P, et al.: The frontal plane relationship of the forefoot to the rearfoot in an asymptomatic population. J Orthop Sports Phys Ther 20:200–206, 1994.

77. Viladot A: Metatarsalgia due to biomechanical alterations of the forefoot. Orthop Clin North Am 4:165–178, 1973.

78. McCarthy D, Grode SE: The anatomical relationships of the first metatarsophalangeal joint: A cryomicrotomy study. J Am Podiatr Assoc 70:493–504, 1980.

79. Yoshioka Y, Siu DW, Cooke TD, et al.: Geometry of the first metatarsophalangeal joint. J Orthop Res 6:878–885, 1988.

80. Shereff M: Pathophysiology, anatomy and biomechanics of hallux valgus. Orthopedics 13:939–945, 1990.

81. Saxena A, Krisdakumtorn T: Return to activity after sesamoidectomy in athletically active individuals. Foot Ankle Int 24:415–419, 2003.

82. Biedert R, Hintermann B: Stress fractures of the medial great toe sesamoids in athletes. Foot Ankle Int 24:137–141, 2003.

83. Deland J, Lee K, Sobel M, et al.: Anatomy of the plantar plate and its attachments in the lesser metatarsal phalangeal joint. Foot Ankle 16: 480–486, 1995.

84. Bhatia E, Myerson M, Curtis M, et al.: Anatomical restraints to dislocation of the second metatarsophalangeal joint and assessment of a repair technique. J Bone Joint Surg Am 76:1371–1375, 1994.

85. Buell T, Green DR, Risser J: Measurement of the first metatarsophalangeal joint range of motion. J Am Podiatr Med Assoc 78:439–448, 1988.

86. Nawoczenski DA, Baumhauer JF, Umberger BR: Relationship between clinical measurements and motion of the first metatarsophalangeal joint during gait. J Bone Joint Surg Am 81:370–376, 1999.

87. Mueller M, Hastings M, Commean PK, et al.: Forefoot structural predictors of plantar pressure during walking in people with diabetes and peripheral neuropathy. J Biomech 36:1009–1017, 2003.

88. Robertson DD, Mueller MJ, Smith KE, et al.: Structural changes in the forefoot of individuals with diabetes and a prior plantar ulcer. J Bone Joint Surg Am 84:1395–1404, 2002.

89. Glasoe WM, Allen MK, Saltzman CL: First ray dorsal mobility in relation to hallux valgus deformity and first intermetatarsal angle. Foot Ankle Int 22:98–101, 2001.

90. Gould N, Moreland M, Alvarez R, et al.: Develop-

ment of the child's arch. Foot Ankle 9:241–245, 1989.

91. Thordarson D, Schmotzer H, Chon J, et al.: Dynamic support of the human longitudinal arch. Clin Orthop 316:165–172, 1995.

92. Kitaoka H, Ahn T, Luo Z, et al.: Stability of the arch of the foot. Foot Ankle Int 1:644–648, 1997.

93. Gefen A: The *in vivo* elastic properties of the plantar fascia during the contact phase of walking. Foot Ankle Int 24:238–244, 2003.

94. Pfeffer G, Bacchetti P, Deland J, et al.: Comparison of custom and prefabricated orthoses in the initial treatment of proximal plantar fasciitis. Foot Ankle Int 20:214–221, 1999.

95. Sarrafian S: Functional characteristics of the foot and plantar aponeurosis under tibiotalar loading. Foot Ankle 8:4–18, 1987.

96. Cavanagh PR, Rodgers MM, Iiboshi A: Pressure distribution under symptom-free feet during barefoot standing. Foot Ankle 7:262–276, 1987.

97. Kelly VE, Mueller MJ, Sinacore DR: Timing of peak plantar pressure during the stance phase of walking. A study of patients with diabetes mellitus and transmetatarsal amputation. J Am Podiatr Med Assoc 90:18–23, 2000.

98. Morag E, Cavanagh PR: Structural and functional predictors of regional peak pressures under the foot during walking. J Biomech 32:359–370, 1999.

99. Cavanagh PR, Lafortune MA: Ground reaction forces in distance running. J Biomech 13:397–406, 1980.

100. Perry J: Anatomy and biomechanics of the hind foot. Clin Orthop 177:7–15, 1983.

101. MacConaill M, Basmajian J: Muscles and Movement: A Basis for Human Kinesiology. Baltimore, Williams & Wilkins, 1969.

102. Hunt AE, Smith RM, Torode M: Extrinsic muscle activity, foot motion and ankle joint moments during the stance phase of walking. Foot Ankle Int 22:31–41, 2001.

103. Gadeberg P, Andersen H, Jakobsen J: Volume of ankle dorsiflexors and plantar flexors determined with stereological techniques. J Appl Physiol 86:1670–1675, 1999.

104. Czerniecki J: Foot and ankle biomechanics in walking and running. Am J Phys Med Rehabil 67:246–252, 1988.

105. Klein P, Mattys S, Rooze M: Moment arm length variations of selected muscles acting on talocrural and subtalar joints during movement: An *in vitro* study. J Biomech 29:21–30, 1996.

106. Kalin P, Hirsch B: The origins and function of the interosseous muscles of the foot. J Anat 152:83–91, 1987.

107. Powers C, Marfucci R, Hampton S: Rearfoot posture in subjects with patellofemoral pain. J Orthop Sports Phys Ther 22:155–160, 1995.

108. Wen DY, Puffer JC, Schmalzried TP: Lower extremity alignment and risk of overuse injuries in runners. Med Sci Sports Exerc 29:1291–1298, 1997.

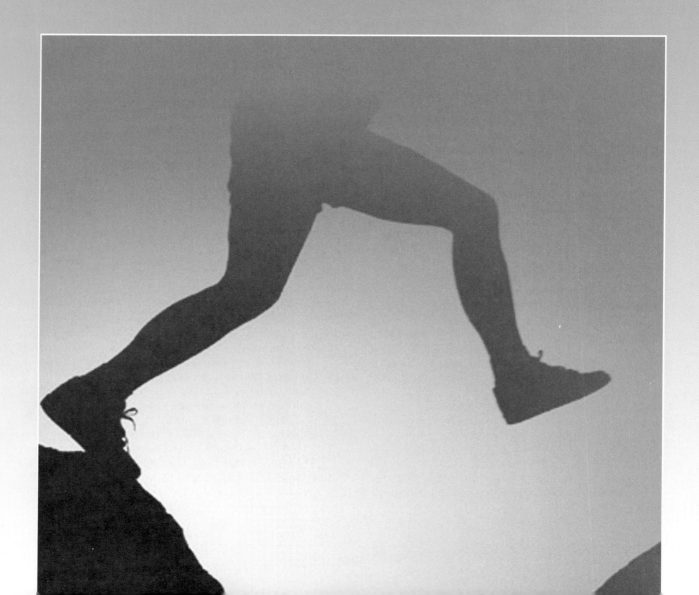

Posture

Cynthia C. Norkin, PT, EdD

◆ Introduction

In this chapter, the focus is on how the various body structures are integrated into a system that enables the body as a whole to maintain a particular posture. We will use our knowledge of individual joint and muscle structure and function as the basis for determining how each structure contributes to the equilibrium and stability of the body in the optimal standing posture We will consider the internal and external forces acting on the body in relation to standing, sitting, and lying postures, and we will explore how these forces will affect the patient in the following case. Throughout the chapter, we will include discussions in relation to a patient's ability to function without many of the normal postural control mechanisms and the internal lower extremity forces necessary to maintain his body in the standing posture, as well as potential problems that he might have in the sitting and lying postures

13-1	**Patient Case**

Dave Nguyen, a 19-year-old college varsity ice hockey player, was injured during a game when two members of the opposing team checked him against the boards. The impact of the collision knocked all three players down onto the ice, with Dave on the bottom and the other players on top. Dave sustained fractures of two thoracic vertebrae (T9 and T10) and a complete spinal cord injury (SCI) which resulted in paraplegia (muscle paralysis in both lower extremities). He has functioning lower abdominal and lower erector spinae muscles but no function in his hip or lower extremity muscles.

When we first meet Dave, his surgically repaired vertebral fractures have healed, and he is medically cleared to begin an aggressive rehabilitation program.

Dave's main goal at this point is to become independent as soon as possible, including being able to walk again. He admits that his legs probably will not regain their function, but he is determined to be able to get around with crutches.

His youth, his good physical condition, and the fact that he is used to the discipline required for participation in a varsity sport should be helpful in the rehabilitation process.

◆ Static and Dynamic Postures

Posture can be either static or dynamic. In static posture, the body and its segments are aligned and maintained in certain positions. Examples of static postures include standing, sitting, lying, and kneeling. Dynamic posture refers to postures in which the body or its segments are moving—walking, running, jumping, throwing, and lifting. An understanding of static posture forms the basis for understanding dynamic posture. Therefore, the static postures of standing and sitting are emphasized in this chapter. The dynamic postures of walking and running are discussed in Chapter 14.

The study of any particular posture includes kinetic and kinematic analyses of all body segments. Humans and other living creatures have the ability to arrange and rearrange body segments to form a large variety of postures, but the sustained maintenance of erect bipedal stance is unique to humans. The erect standing posture allows persons to use their upper extremities for the performance of large and small motor tasks. If the upper extremities need to be engaged by the use of crutches, canes, or other assistive devices to maintain the erect posture, an important human attribute is either severely compromised or lost.

Case Application 13-1: **Predicted Rehabilitation Progression**

Initially our patient, Dave, will be able to attain a standing posture on a tilt table, which will provide support for his entire body. He will progress to standing in the parallel bars, on which he can use his upper extremities to provide support. Standing will not be as much of a problem as walking, but he will have to learn how to transfer from wheelchair to standing and to maintain the standing posture before he can attempt walking. Later he will progress to walking in the parallel bars and finally will be able to use crutches. Walking for any extended length of time or distance may not be a realistic goal for Dave because of the high energy cost involved when walking with crutches with his extent of lower extremity paralysis.

Erect bipedal stance gives us freedom for the upper extremities, but in comparison with the quadrupedal posture, erect stance has certain disadvantages. Erect bipedal stance increases the work of the heart; places increased stress on the vertebral column, pelvis, and lower extremities; and reduces stability. In the quadrupedal posture, the body weight is distributed between the upper and lower extremities. In human stance, the body weight is borne exclusively by the two lower extremities. The human species' base of support (BoS), defined by an area bounded posteriorly by the tips of the heels and anteriorly by a line joining the tips of the toes, is considerably smaller than the quadrupedal BoS (Fig. 13-1). The human's center of gravity (CoG) is the point where the mass of the body is centered and will be referred to in this chapter as the center of mass (CoM). The position of the CoM is not fixed and changes in different postures such as sitting and kneeling, with movements of the extremities or trunk, and when a person is carrying something.[1] When a person is wearing a leg cast on one leg, the CoM moves lower and towards the casted leg. In the sitting posture, the CoM of the body above the seat is located near the armpits.[2] In the young child in the standing posture, the CoM is located within the body about at the level of the 12th vertebra. As the child becomes less "top heavy," the CoM moves lower to a location in the standing adult at about the level of the second sacral segment in the midsagittal plane. The adult position of the CoM is relatively distant from the BoS. Despite the instability caused by a small BoS and a high CoM, maintaining stability in the static erect standing posture

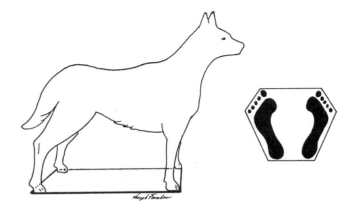

▲ **Figure 13-1** ■ A comparison between the base of support in quadripedal stance and bipedal stance. Note the small BoS and high CoM in the human figure, in comparison with the dog's relatively large BoS and low CoM.

requires only low levels of muscle activity. Passive tension in the joint capsules, muscles, and ligaments are able to provide some of the forces needed to counteract gravity.

Postural Control

Although only a relatively small amount of muscular activity is required to maintain a stable erect standing posture, the control of posture is complex and is a part of the body's motor control system. The main focus of this text is not on the motor control aspects of human function; however, a discussion of some features of postural control is necessary for an understanding of postural stability in standing.

Postural control, which can be either static or dynamic, refers to a person's ability to maintain stability of the body and body segments in response to forces that threaten to disturb the body's equilibrium. According to Horak and associates,[3] the ability to maintain stability in the erect standing posture is a skill that the **central nervous system** (**CNS**) learns, using information from passive biomechanical elements, sensory systems, and muscles. The CNS interprets and organizes inputs from the various structures and systems and selects responses on the basis of past experience and the goal of the response. **Reactive**[3] (**compensatory**[4]) responses occur as reactions to external forces that displace the body's CoM. **Proactive**[3] (**anticipatory**[4]) responses occur in anticipation of internally generated destabilizing forces such as raising arms to catch a ball or bending forward to tie shoes.

Major Goals and Basic Elements of Control

The major goals of postural control in the standing position are to control the body's orientation in space, maintain the body's CoM over the BoS, and stabilize the head with regard to the vertical so that the eye gaze is appropriately oriented. According to DiFabio and Emasithi,[5] stabilizing the head with regard to the vertical is the primary goal of postural regulation. Maintenance and control of posture depend on the integrity of the CNS, visual system, vestibular system, and musculoskeletal system. In addition, postural control depends on information received from receptors located in and around the joints (in joint capsules, tendons, and ligaments), as well as on the soles of the feet. The CNS must be able to detect and predict instability and must be able to respond to all of this input with appropriate output to maintain the equilibrium of the body. Furthermore, the joints in the musculoskeletal system must have a range of motion (ROM) that is adequate for responding to specific tasks, and the muscles must be able to respond with appropriate speeds and forces.

■ **Absent or Altered Inputs and Outputs**

When inputs are altered or absent, the control system must respond to incomplete or distorted data, and thus the person's posture may be altered and stability compromised. Alteration or absence of inputs may occur for a number of reasons, including, among others, the absence of the normal gravitational force in weightless conditions during space flight or decreased sensation in the lower extremities.

Example 13-1

Astronauts aboard the U.S. Space Shuttle Discovery in June 1985 assumed a position in space in which the neck, hip, and knee were flexed significantly more than they were in preflight. They maintained the same flexed posture initially when they returned to earth.[6] Another group of astronauts exhibited changes in multijoint coordination that was attributed to a reweighting of inputs to the vestibular system in the gravity-eliminated condition.[7] The postural changes that have been observed in astronauts upon their return to earth are thought to be due to alterations in tactile, articular, vestibular, and proprioceptive inputs used in postural control.[6,7]

A more common example of altered inputs occurs when a person attempts to attain and maintain an erect standing posture when a foot has "fallen asleep." Attempts at standing may result in a fall because input regarding the position of the foot and ankle, as well as information from contact of the "asleep" foot with the supporting surface, is missing.

Another instance in which inputs may be disturbed is after injury. A disturbance in the kinesthetic sense about the ankle and foot after ankle sprains has been implicated as a cause of poor balance or loss of stability.[8] Forkin and colleagues,[9] in a study of gymnasts 1 to 12 months after an ankle sprain, found that these individuals were less able to detect passive ROM in the previously injured ankle than they were in the uninjured ankle. The gymnasts in the study also reported that they believed that they were less stable in the standing posture than before their injury. Sometimes ankle sprains are followed by chronic functional instability.[10]

In addition to altered inputs, a person's ability to maintain the erect posture may be affected by altered outputs such as the inability of the muscles to respond appropriately to signals from the CNS. In sedentary elderly persons, muscles that have atrophied through disuse may not be able to respond with either the appropriate amount of force to counteract an opposing force or with the necessary speed to maintain stability. In persons with neuromuscular disorders, both agonists and antagonists may respond at the same time, thus reducing the effectiveness of the response.

Case Application 13-2: **Missing Inputs and Outputs**

Dave is missing some of the inputs and outputs necessary for normal postural control. He is not able to receive input for standing postural control either from receptors located around his ankle, knee, and hip joints or from the soles of his feet. He is unable to provide output in response to signals from the CNS because his lower extremity muscles are paralyzed. Consequently, we must look at other aspects of postural control because Dave will have to rely on other mechanisms to monitor and maintain a standing posture. His vestibular and visual systems are intact and able to provide input. Proprioceptive input from his trunk and upper extremities is also intact, and they are able to provide input and output.

■ Muscle Synergies

Although static posture is emphasized in this chapter, the term static can be misleading, especially with regard to standing posture, because the maintenance of standing posture is the result of dynamic control mechanisms. Postural control researchers have suggested that for any particular task such as standing on a moving bus, standing on a ladder, or standing on one leg, many different combinations of muscles may be activated to complete the task. A normally functioning CNS selects the appropriate combination of muscles to complete the task on the basis of an analysis of sensory inputs. Dietz[11] suggested that afferent input from Golgi tendon organs in the leg extensors signals changes in the projection of the body's CoM with regard to the feet. Variations in an individual's past experience and customary patterns of muscle activity will also affect the response. Allum and coworkers[12] suggested that proprioceptive input from the hip or trunk may be more important than input from the legs in signaling and initiating responses. According to these authors, muscle activation is based primarily on input from the hip and trunk proprioceptors. A second level of input includes cues from the vestibular system and proprioceptive input from all body segments.

Monitoring of muscle activity patterns through **electromyography** (**EMG**) and determinations of muscle peak torque and power outputs are some of the methods used to study postural responses during perturbations of upright postural stability. A **perturbation** is any sudden change in conditions that displaces the body posture away from equilibrium.[3] The perturbation can be sensory or mechanical. A **sensory perturbation** might be caused by altering of visual input, such as might occur when a person's eyes are covered unexpectedly. **Mechanical perturbations** are displacements that involve direct changes in the relationship of CoM to the BoS. These displacements may be caused by movements of either body segments or the entir body.[12] Even breathing can displace the CoM. Perturbations in standing that result from respiratory movements of the rib cage are counterbalanced by movements of the trunk and lower limbs. As detemined by EMG, muscle activity in the trunk and hip muscles provides a counterbalance to motions of the rib cage.[13]

One method of studying how people respond to naturally occuring perturbations is to produce mechanical perturbations experimentally by placing subjects on a movable platform. The platform can be moved forward, backward, or from side to side. Some platforms can be tipped, and the velocity of platform motion can be varied. The postural responses to perturbations caused by either platform movement or by pushes and pulls are reactive or compensatory responses in that they are involuntary reactions. These postural responses are referred to in the literature as either synergies[3] or strategies.[4] Therefore, in this text, the terms will be used interchangeably. The synergies are task specific and appear to vary with a number of factors, including the amount and direction of motion of the supporting surface; width and compliance of the supporting surface and the location, magnitude, and velocity of the perturbing force; and initial posture of the individual at the time of the perturbation.

Fixed-Support Synergies

Horak and associates[3] described synergies as centrally organized patterns of muscle activity that occur in response to perturbations of standing postures. **Fixed-support synergies** are patterns of muscle activity in which the BoS remains fixed during the perturbation and recovery of equilibrium. Stability is regained through movements of parts of the body, but the feet remain fixed on the BoS. Two examples of fixed-support synergies are the ankle synergy and the hip synergy.

The **ankle synergy** consists of discrete bursts of muscle activity on either the anterior or posterior aspects of the body that occur in a distal-to-proximal pattern in response to forward and backward movements of the support platform, respectively. Forward motion of the platform results in a relative displacement of the line of gravity (LoG) posteriorly and would be similar to starting to fall backward in a free-standing posture (Fig. 13-2A). The group of muscles that responds to the perturbation is activated in an attempt to restore the LoG to a position within the BoS. Bursts of muscle activity occur in the ankle dorsiflexors, hip flexors, abdominal muscles, and possibly the neck flexors. The tibialis anterior muscle contributes to the restoration of stability by pulling the tibia anteriorly, and hence the body forward, so that the LoG remains or centers within the BoS (see Fig. 13-2B). Backward motion of the platform results in a relative displacement of the LoG anteriorly and is similar to starting to fall forward in a free-standing posture. The muscles responds in an attempt to restore the LoG to a position within the BoS (Fig. 13-3A). Bursts of activity in the plantarflexors, hip extensors, trunk extensors, and neck extensors are used to restore the LoG over the BoS (see Fig. 13-3B).

The **hip synergy** consists of discrete bursts of muscle activity on the side of the body opposite to the ankle pattern in a proximal-to-distal pattern of activation.[14] Maki and McIlroy[4] suggested that the fixed-support hip synergy may be used primarily in situations in which **change-in-support strategies** (**stepping** or **grasping synergies**) are not available.

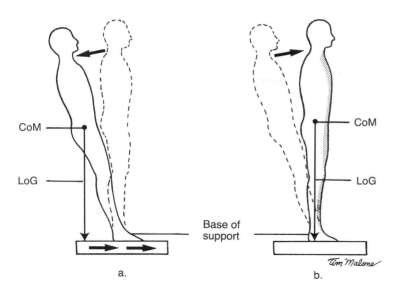

a. b.

◄ **Figure 13-2** ■ Perturbation of erect stance equilibrium caused by forward horizontal platform movement. **A.** Anterior (forward) movement of the platform causes posterior (backward) movement of the body and, as a consequence, displacement of the body's CoM posterior to the base of support. **B.** Use of the ankle strategy (activation of the flexors at the ankle, hip, trunk, and possibly neck) is necessary to bring the body's CoM back over the base of support and reestablish stability.

CONCEPT CORNERSTONE 13-1: *Summary of Fixed Support Strategies*

Ankle Strategies

Perturbations

Forward translation of support surface (backward motion of the body)	Backward translation of support surface*(forward motion of the body)

Muscles Distal to Proximal Response

Tibialis anterior	Gastrocnemius
Quadriceps femoris	Hamstrings
Abdominals (neck flexors)[5]	Paraspinals (neck extensors)[5]

Hip Strategies

Perturbations

Forward translation of support surface (backward motion of the body)	Backward translation of support surface* (forward motion of the body)

Muscles Proximal to Distal Response

Abdominals	Paraspinals
Quadriceps femoris	Hamstrings
Tibialis anterior	Gastrocnemius

*Increasing the velocity of backward platform translations may lead to a mixed ankle-and-hip strategy.[14]

Change-in-Support Strategies

The change-in-support strategies include **stepping** (forward, backward, or sidewise) and **grasping** (using one's hands to grab a bar or other fixed support) in response to shifts in the BoS. Stepping and grasping differ from fixed-support synergies because stepping/grasping

moves or enlarges the body's BoS so that it remains under the body's CoM (Fig. 13-4).[15,16] Previously, it was thought that the stepping synergy was used only as a last resort, being initiated when ankle and hip strategies were insufficient to bring and maintain the CoM over the BoS.[15,17] However, Maki and McIlroy suggested that change-in-support strategies are common responses to perturbations among both the young and the old.[4] Furthermore, these authors observed that change-in-support synergies are the only synergies that are successful in maintaining stability in the instance of a large perturbation.[4] Comparisons of the stepping strategies used by the young and the old show that the younger subjects have a tendency to take only one step, whereas the elderly subjects have a tendency to take multiple steps that are shorter and of less height than those of their younger counterparts.[4,18] However, no differences are apparent in the speed at which the young and the elderly initiate the change-in-support stepping strategy. Luchies and associates[19] found that older subjects lifted their feet just as quickly as did the younger subjects. However, Wojcik and associates found distinct age and gender differences in the magnitudes of joint torques in the stepping extremity that were used to regain balance.[20] Van Wegen and colleagues determined that in quiet standing, the older person's center of pressure (CoP) is located closer to edge of the BoS than in younger subjects.[21] Therefore, the older individuals may have less time to react to a perturbation before exceeding stability limits.

Dave cannot respond to a perturbation by moving his lower extremities; therefore, not only does he need to develop alternative strategies for dealing with perturbations but also he needs to try to avoid sudden perturbations of his standing posture.

Head-Stabilizing Strategies

Two head-stabilizing strategies have been described by DiFabio and Emasithi.[5] These proactive strategies differ

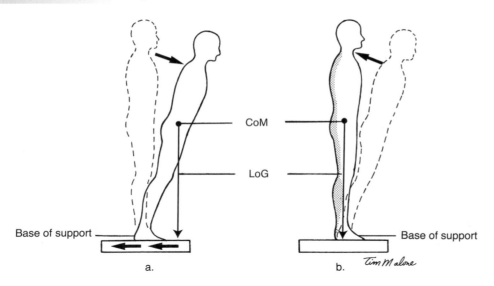

◄ **Figure 13-3 ■** Perturbation of erect stance equilibrium caused by backward horizontal platform movement. **A.** Posterior movement of the platform causes anterior movement of the body and, as a consequence, displacement of the body's CoM anterior to the base of support. **B.** Use of the ankle strategy (activation of the extensors at the ankle, hip, back, and possibly neck) is necessary to bring the body's CoM over the base of support and reestablish stability.

from the previously described reactive strategies because head-stabilizing strategies occur in anticipation of the initiation of internally generated forces caused by changes in position from sitting to standing. The head-stabilizing strategies are used to maintain the head during dynamic tasks such as walking, in contrast to ankle and hip strategies, which are used to maintain the body in a static situation. The authors described the following two strategies for maintaining the vertical stability of the head: **head stabilization in space (HSS)** and **head stabilization on trunk (HST)**.[5] The HSS strategy is a modification of head position in anticipation of displacements of the body's CoG. The anticipatory adjustments to head position are independent of trunk motion. The HST strategy is one in which the head and trunk move as a single unit.

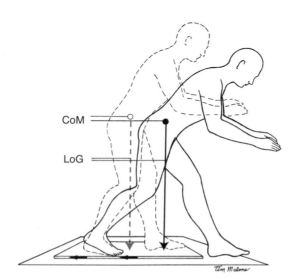

▲ **Figure 13-4 ■** Perturbation of erect stance equilibrium caused by backward platform movement. The person in this illustration is using a stepping strategy to keep from falling forward in response to backward movement of the platform. Stepping forward brings the body's CoM over a new base of support.

Continuing Exploration: **Recent Evidence on the Nature of Postural Control**

Although in the past muscle synergies have been considered fairly automatic responses to perturbations, some evidence suggests that postural control, instead of requiring only a minimal amount of attention, appears to require a significant amount of attention,[22–24] especially the sensory integration aspects.[25] The amount of attention required varies according to the complexity of the postural task (such as bending the trunk backward while standing with the feet close together), the age of the individual, balance abilities, and the type of secondary task (such as a math problem) being performed.[23,24,26] Postural challenges appear to influence reaction time for task performances in both young and old, but under some conditions, older individuals also demonstrate an increase in postural sway.[23,25]

◆ Kinetics and Kinematics of Posture

The muscle strategies described in response to perturbations are examples of the active internal forces employed to counteract the external forces that affect the equilibrium and stability of the body in the erect standing posture. The following section examines the effects of both external and internal forces on the body in the standing posture. The **external forces** that will be considered are **inertia, gravity,** and **ground reaction forces (GRFs)**. The **internal forces** are produced by muscle activity and passive tension in ligaments, tendons, joint capsules, and other soft tissue structures. The sum of all of the external and internal forces and torques acting on the body and its segments must be equal to zero for the body to be in equilibrium. Stability is maintained by keeping the body's CoM over the BoS and the head in a position that permits gaze to be appropriately oriented.

Inertial and Gravitational Forces

In the erect standing posture, little or no accleration of the body occurs, except that the body undergoes a constant swaying motion called **postural sway** or **sway envelope**.[16] The extent of the sway envelope for a normal individual standing with about 4 inches between the feet can be as large as 12° in the sagittal plane and 16° in the frontal plane.[16] The inertial forces that may result from this swaying motion usually are not considered in the analysis of forces for static postures.[27] However, in a postural study using laser technology, Aramaki and colleagues investigated angular displacements, angular velocity and acceleration around the hip and ankle joints.[28] Naturally, inertial forces must be considered in postural analysis of all dynamic postures such as walking, running, and jogging in which the forces needed to produce acceleration or a change in the direction of motion are important for understanding the demands on the body.[29]

Ground Reaction Forces

Whenever the body contacts the ground, the ground pushes back on the body. This force is known as the **GRF,** and the vector representing it is known as the ground reaction force vector (**GRFV**). The GRF is a composite (or resultant) force that represents the magnitude and direction of loading applied to one or both feet. The GRF is typically described as having three components: a vertical component force (along the y-axis), and two force components directed horizontally. One of the two horizontal forces is in a medial-lateral direction (along the x-axis) , whereas the other horizontal force is in an anterior-posterior direction (along the z-axis) on the ground. The composite or resultant GRFV is equal in magnitude but opposite in direction to the gravitational force in the erect static standing posture. The GRFV indicates the magnitude and direction of loading applied to the foot. The point of application of the GRFV is at the body's CoP, which is located in the foot in unilateral stance and between the feet in bilateral standing postures. If a person were doing a handstand, the CoP would be located between the hands. The CoP, like the CoG, is the theoretical point where the force is considered to act, although the body surface that is in contact with the ground may have forces acting over a large portion of its surface area. The path of the CoP that defines the extent of the sway envelope can be determined by plotting the CoP at regular intervals when a person is standing on a force plate system (Fig. 13-5). Much of the research on postural control uses the pattern of displacements of the CoP to evaluate the effects of attentional demands and perturbations on standing posture.

The GRFV and the LoG have coincident action lines in the static erect posture. The LoG represents the force of gravity-on-person and is generally equal in magnitude to and in the same direction as the force of person-on-ground. The GRF is a more common name for the force of ground-on-person. In equilibrium dur-

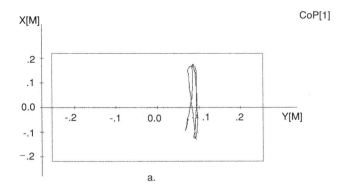

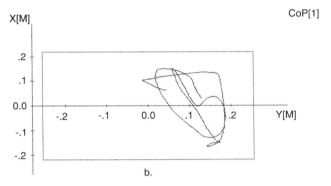

▲ **Figure 13-5** ▪ Path of the center of pressure (CoP) in erect stance. **A.** A CoP tracing plotted for a person standing on a force plate. The rectangle represents the outline of the force plate. The tracing shows a normal rhythmic anterior-posterior "sway envelope" during approximately 30 seconds of stance. **B.** A CoP tracing showing relatively uncontrolled postural sway. (CoP tracings courtesy of Leonard Elbaum, Director of Research at the Physical Therapy Laboratory, Florida International University, Miami, Florida. Data were collected with an Advanced Material Technology, Inc. (AMTI), Force Platform, Newton, Massachusetts. Analysis and display software were provided by Ariel Life Systems, Inc., La Jolla, California.)

ing static stance, we would expect the force of gravity-on-person (represented by the LoG) to be equal in magnitude and opposite in direction to the GRF represented by the GRFV. In many dynamic postures, the intersection of the LoG with the supporting surface may not coincide with the point of application of the GRFV. The horizontal distance from the point on the supporting surface where the LoG intersects the ground and the CoP (where the GRFV acts) indicates the magnitude of the external moment that must be opposed to maintain a posture and keep the person from falling.

The technology required to obtain GRFs, the CoP, and muscle activity may not be available to the average evaluator of human function. Therefore, in the following sections, a simplified method of analyzing posture will be presented with the use of diagrams and with the combined action of the LoG and the GRFV as a reference.

Coincident Action Lines

In an ideal erect posture, body segments are aligned so that the torques and stresses on body segments are minimized and standing can be maintained with a minimal amount of energy expenditure. The coincident action lines formed by the GRFV and the LoG serve as a reference for the analysis of the effects of these forces on body segments (Fig. 13-6). When the LoG and the GRFV coincide, as they do in static posture, it is possible to assess the effects at each joint by using one or the other. However, the reader should be aware that the horizontal forces are not being considered separately. We will use the LoG in the remainder of this chapter. The location of the LoG shifts continually (as does the CoP) because of the postural sway. As a result of the continuous motion of the LoG, the moments acting around the joints are continually changing. Receptors in and around the joints of lower body segments and on the soles of the feet detect these changes and relay this information to the CNS.

Case Application 13-3: **Information from Knee and Ankle Receptors**

Dave will not be able to access information from receptors in his knee and ankle, even though the receptors around these joints are able to transmit the information to the lower spinal cord below the injury. The information cannot go up the spinal cord beyond the level of the injury because of the disruption in the cord at the T10 vertebral level. Under normal conditions, the CNS would analyze the inputs and make an appropriate output response to maintain postural stability.

Sagittal Plane

The effect of **external** forces on body segments in the sagittal plane during standing is determined by the location of the LoG in relation to the axis of motion of body segments. When the LoG passes directly through a joint axis, no **external** gravitational torque is created around that joint. However, if the LoG passes at a distance from the axis, an external gravitational moment is created. This moment will cause rotation of the superimposed body segments around that joint axis unless it is opposed by a counterbalancing **internal** moment (an **isometric** muscle contraction). The **magnitude** of the gravitational moment of force increases as the distance between the LoG and the joint axis increases. The **direction** of the external gravitational moment of force depends on the location of the LoG in relation to a particular joint axis. If the LoG is located *anterior* to a **particular** joint axis, the gravitational moment will tend to cause anterior motion of the proximal segment of the body supported by that joint. If the LoG is *posterior* to the joint axis, the moment will tend to cause motion of the proximal segment in a posterior direction . In a postural analysis, external gravitational torques producing sagittal plane motion of the proximal joint segment are referred to as either *flexion* or *extension moments*.

Example 13-2

If the LoG passes anterior to the ankle joint axis, the external gravitational moment will tend to rotate the tibia (proximal segment) in an anterior direction (Fig. 13-7). Anterior motion of the tibia on the fixed foot will result in dorsiflexion of the ankle. Therefore, the

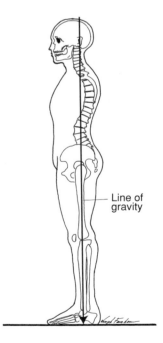

▲ **Figure 13-6** ■ Location of the combined action line formed by the ground reaction force vector (GRFV) and the line of gravity (LoG) in the optimal standing posture.

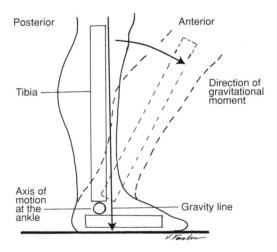

▲ **Figure 13-7** ■ The anterior location of the LoG in relation to the ankle joint axis creates an external dorsiflexion moment. The arrow indicates the direction of the dorsiflexion moment. The dotted line indicates the direction in which the tibia would move if the dorsiflexion moment were unopposed.

moment of force is called a **dorsiflexion moment.** An internal **plantarflexion moment** of equal magnitude will be necessary to oppose the external dorsiflexion moment and establish equilibrium.

Example 13-3

If the LoG passes anterior to the axis of rotation of the knee joint, the gravitational moment will tend to rotate the femur (proximal segment) in an anterior direction (Fig. 13-8). An anterior movement of the femur will cause extension of the knee. Therefore, the moment of force is called an **extension moment.** An internal **flexion moment** of equal magnitude will be necessary to balance the external extension moment.

Case Application 13-4: **Tilt Table Standing**

> After his injury, Dave's first exposure to the standing posture will be on a tilt table. Standing in the tilt table will provide compression on Dave's bones and joints and will get him used to the upright position. Wide straps across his legs and trunk will hold Dave to the table and provide the necessary counterbalancing forces to oppose the external gravitational moments.

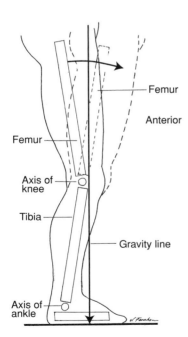

▲ **Figure 13-8** ■ The anterior location of the LoG in relation to the knee joint axis creates an external extension moment. The arrow indicates the direction of the extension moment. The dotted line indicates the direction in which the femur would move if the extension moment were unopposed.

◆ Optimal Posture

Because the force of gravity is constantly acting on the body, an ideal standing posture would be one in which the body segments were aligned vertically and the LoG passed through all joint axes. Normal body structure makes such an ideal posture impossible to achieve, but it is possible to attain a posture that is close to the ideal. In an optimal standing posture, the LoG is close to, but not through, most joint axes. Therefore, the external gravitational moments are relatively small and can be balanced by internal moments generated by passive capsular and ligamentous tension, passive muscle tension (stiffness), and a small but continuous amount of muscle activity.

Slight deviations from the optimal posture are to be expected in a normal population because of the many individual variations found in body structure. However, deviations from an optimal standing posture that are large enough to cause excessive strain in passive structures and to require high levels of muscle activity need to be identified, and remedial action must be taken. If faulty postures are habitual and assumed continually on a daily basis, the body will not recognize these faulty postures as abnormal, and over time, structural adaptations such as ligamentous and muscle shortening or lengthening will occur.

◆ Analysis of Standing Posture

Observational analysis of posture in the sagittal plane involves locating body segments in relation to the LoG. A **plumb line,** or line with a weight on one end, dropped from the ceiling and passing through the external auditory meatus of the ear may be used to represent the LoG. Evaluators of posture should be able to determine whether a body segment or joint deviates widely from the normal optimal postural alignment by using their observational skills. A skilled observational analysis can yield basic information about an individual's posture that can be used either for developing a treatment regimen for the correction of poor posture or to decide whether a more sophisticated analysis such as radiography is warranted.

 CONCEPT CORNERSTONE 13-2: *Effects of Anterior and Posterior Gravitational Moments on Body Segments*

If the LoG passes anterior to the head, vertebral column, or joints of the lower extremities, the gravitational moment will tend to force the segment of the body superior to the joint in an anterior direction. Conversely, when the LoG passes posterior to the joints the body, the gravitational moment will tend to force the body segment that is superior to the joint in a posterior direction.

Sagittal Plane Alignment and Analysis

■ Ankle

In the optimal erect posture, the ankle joint is in the neutral position, or midway between dorsiflexion and plantarflexion. The LoG passes slightly anterior to the lateral malleolus and, therefore, anterior to the ankle joint axis.[30,31] The anterior position of the LoG in relation to the ankle joint axis creates an **external dorsiflexion moment** that must be opposed by an **internal plantarflexion moment** to prevent forward motion of the tibia. In the neutral ankle position, there are no ligamentous checks capable of counterbalancing the external dorsiflexion moment; therefore, activation of the plantarflexors creates the internal plantarflexion moment that is necessary to prevent forward motion of the tibia. The soleus muscle contracts and exerts a posterior pull on the tibia and in this way is able to oppose the dorsiflexion moment (Fig. 13-9). If the force that the muscle can exert is less than the gravitational moment, the tibia will move the ankle into dorsiflexion and the soleus muscle will undergo an eccentric contraction while trying to oppose the forward motion of the tibia.

EMG studies have demonstrated that soleus[32,33] and gastrocnemius[33] activity is fairly continuous in normal subjects during erect standing. This activity suggests that these muscles are exerting a minimal but constant internally generated plantarflexion torque about the ankles to oppose the normal external gravitational dorsiflexion moment. Ankle joint muscles that have shown inconsistent activity in EMG recordings during standing are the tibialis anterior, peroneal, and tibialis posterior muscles.[34] It is possible that these muscles may be helping to provide transverse stability in the foot during postural sway rather than acting to oppose the external dorsiflexion at the ankle joint.

■ Knee

In optimal posture, the knee joint is in full extension, and the LoG passes anterior to the midline of the knee and posterior to the patella. This places the LoG just anterior to the knee joint axis (see Figs. 13-8 and 13-9). The anterior location of the gravitational line in relation to the knee joint axis creates an **external extension moment**.[35] The counterbalancing **internal flexion moment** created by passive tension in the posterior joint capsule and associated ligaments is usually sufficient to balance the gravitational moment and prevent knee hyperextension. However, a small amount of activity has been identified in the hamstrings. Activity of the soleus muscle may augment the gravitational extension moment at the knee through its posterior pull on the tibia as it acts at the ankle joint. In contrast, activity of the gastrocnemius muscle may tend to oppose the gravitational extension moment because the muscle crosses the knee posterior to the knee joint axis.

Case Application 13-5: **How to Oppose External Gravitational Moments in Standing Posture without Muscle Activity**

When Dave progresses from standing on the tilt table to standing in the parallel bars, he will need some means of opposing the external gravitational moments affecting his lower extremities. He has no musculature capable of resisting the external dorsiflexion moment at the ankle and no tilt table straps to help him maintain the standing posture. Therefore, one or more forces will have to be found to substitute for the internal plantarflexor moment that would have been applied by activity in his plantarflexors. Orthoses (braces) at his ankles and the push of the parallel bars or crutches on his head and trunk (HAT) will be able to provide the necessary opposing forces.

All orthoses apply forces to the body that can be used to either resist motion or to protect a body part.[36] Orthoses are based on a three-point pressure system with one force acting in one direction and two forces directed in the opposite direction. The type of orthoses that Dave will use are knee-ankle-foot orthoses (KAFOs), which are deemed sufficient for low thoracic lesions (T9 to T12).[37] These orthoses have standard double metal uprights, posterior thigh bands, plates under the sole of the foot, and anterior knee flexion pads (Fig. 13-10). Locking joints are positioned at the knee and ankle; they are locked when the person is standing but can be unlocked to allow for sitting. There are locks at the ankle and knee to keep the knee and ankle stabilized during standing and to allow knee flexion when sitting.

When Dave is standing, the knee pads on his KAFOs will provide posteriorly directed external forces to oppose the gravitational dorsiflexion moments. The pads and locks at the knee will maintain the knees in

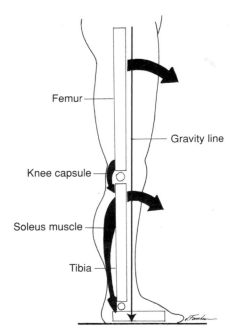

▲ **Figure 13-9** ■ The external extension moment acting around the knee joint is balanced by an internal opposing moment created by passive tension in the posterior joint capsule. The external dorsiflexion moment at the ankle is counterbalanced by an internal moment created by activity of the soleus muscle.

Femur

Gravity line

Knee capsule

Soleus muscle

Tibia

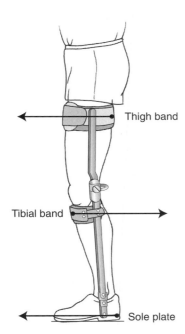

▲ **Figure 13-10** ■ Features of the KAFO. The KAFO's sole plate attachment at the foot and posterior thigh band provide anteriorly directed forces, and the tibial pad below the knee provides a posteriorly directed force.

extension in the event that the LoG passes behind the knee joint axis. The metal uprights will help to support the weight of the body. Anteriorly directed external forces coming from the posterior calf pads and sole plates under the shoe will help ensure that his knees do not go into excessive hyperextension.

■ **Hip and Pelvis**

In optimal posture, according to Kendall and McCreary,[38] the hip is in a neutral position and the pelvis is level with no anterior or posterior tilt (Fig. 13-11A). In a level pelvis position, lines connecting the symphysis pubis and the anterior-superior iliac spines

(ASISs) are vertical, and the lines connecting the ASISs and posterior-superior iliac spines (PSISs) are horizontal.[38] In this optimal position, the LoG passes slightly posterior to the axis of the hip joint, through the greater trochanter.[30,31,35,39] However, during postural sway, the LoG may pass anterior to the hip joint axis, and contraction of the hip exterior may be required. The posterior location of the gravitational line in relation to the hip joint axis creates an external extension moment at the hip that tends to rotate the pelvis (proximal segment) posteriorly on the femoral heads[40] (see Fig. 13-11B). EMG studies have shown activity of the iliopsoas muscle during standing,[41] and it is possible that the iliopsoas is acting to create an internal flexion moment at the hip to prevent hip hyperextension. If the gravitational extension moment at the hip were allowed to act without muscular balance, as in a so-called relaxed or swayback posture,[38] hip hyperextension ultimately would be checked by passive tension in the iliofemoral, pubofemoral, and ischiofemoral ligaments. In the swayback standing posture, the LoG drops farther behind the hip joint axes than in the optimal posture (Fig. 13-12). Therefore, the swayback posture does not require any muscle activity at the hip but causes an increase in the tension stresses on the anterior hip ligaments, which could lead to adaptive lengthening of these ligaments if the posture becomes habitual. Also, because of the diminished demand for hip extensor activity, the gluteal muscles may be weakened by disuse atrophy if the swayback posture is habitually adopted.[42] The relaxed standing or sway posture may also increase the magnitude of the gravitational torque at other joints in the body.

Case Application 13-6: **Swayback Posture** [38, 42]

Although a swayback posture is considered to be a poor posture because of its stress on anterior hip ligaments, Dave has to adopt a swayback standing posture in order to ensure that the LoG remains well behind his hip joints and in front of his knee and ankle joints. In this posture, he does not need to have any hip extensors or any brac-

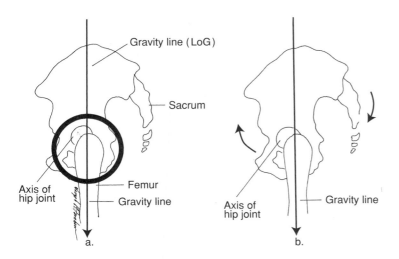

◄ **Figure 13-11** ■ The location of the LoG in relation to the axis of the hip joint. **A.** The LoG passes through the greater trochanter and posterior to the axis of the hip joint. **B.** The posterior location of the LoG creates an external extension moment at the hip, which tends to rotate the pelvis posteriorly on the femoral heads. The arrows indicate the direction of the gravitational moment.

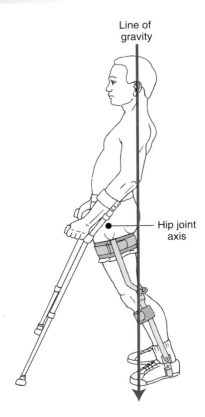

Line of gravity

Hip joint axis

▲ **Figure 13-12** ■ In the swayback posture, the LoG passes well posterior to the hip joint axis, which eliminates the need for activity of the hip extensor muscles. The pelvis is posteriorly rotated, and the hips are hyperextended.

ing at the hip to keep his hip in extension. The KAFOs allow him to balance his weight over his feet with his hips hyperextended (see Fig. 13-12).

■ Lumbosacral and Sacroiliac Joints

The average lumbosacral angle measured between the bottom of the L5 vertebra and the top of the sacrum (S1) is about 30° but can vary between 6° and 30°.[43,44] Anterior tilting of the sacrum increases the lumbosacral

angle and results in an increase in the shearing stress at the lumbosacral joint and may result in an increase in the anterior lumbar convexity in standing (Fig. 13-13A).

Continuing Exploration: **Controversy regarding Relationship between Sacral Inclination and Lumbar Lordosis**

However, the nature of the relationship between sacral inclination and lumbar lordosis remains controversial. Youdas and associates,[45] in a study of 90 male and female subjects, found only a weak association between lumbar lordosis and sacral inclination. On the other hand, Korovessis and coworkers,[46,47] using x-ray evaluations of erect posture, found that the sacral inclination correlated strongly with both thoracic kyphosis and lumbar lordosis.[46]

In the optimal posture, the LoG passes through the body of the fifth lumbar vertebra and close to the axis of rotation of the lumbosacral joint. Gravity therefore creates a very slight extension moment at L5 to S1 that tends to slide L5 and the entire lumbar spine down and forward on S1. This motion is is opposed primarily by the anterior longitudinal ligament and the iliolumbar ligaments. Bony resistance is provided by the locking of the lumbosacral zygapophyseal joints. When the sacrum is in the optimal position, the LoG passes slightly anterior to the sacroiliac joints. The external gravitational moment that is created at the sacroiliac joints tends to cause the anterior superior portion of the sacrum to rotate anteriorly and inferiorly, whereas the posterior inferior portion tends to move posteriorly and superiorly (see Fig. 13-13B). Passive tension in the sacrospinous and sacrotuberous ligaments provides the internal moment that counterbalances the gravitational torque by preventing upward tilting of the lower end of the sacrum.[43]

■ The Vertebral Column

There is considerable variation among individuals, as can be seen in Table 13-1, but the average values are fairly close to one another in the studies presented. In the optimal configuration, the curves of the vertebral column should be fairly close to average or normal con-

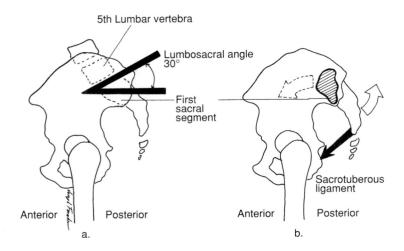

5th Lumbar vertebra

Lumbosacral angle 30°

First sacral segment

Anterior   Posterior

a.

Sacrotuberous ligament

Anterior   Posterior

b.

◀ **Figure 13-13** ■ **A.** The average lumbosacral angle in optimal erect posture is about 30°. **B.** The gravitational moment tends to rotate the superior portion of the sacrum anteriorly and inferiorly. Consequently, the inferior portion tends to thrust posteriorly and superiorly. Passive tension in the sacrotuberous ligament prevents the upward motion of the inferior sacral segment.

Table 13-1	Variations in Spinal Curves in the Sagittal Plane in Standing Posture: Mean Values in Degrees					
	Hardacker et al[48]	Lord et al[49]	Jackson and McManus[50]*	Jackson et al[51]†	Jackson and Hales[52]‡	Gelb et al[53]
	20–70 yrs n=100 Mean (SD)	21–83 yrs n=109 Mean (SD)	20–65 yrs n=100 Mean (SEM)	26–75 yrs n=20 Mean (SD)	20–63 yrs n=75 Mean (SD)	40–70 yrs n=100 Mean (SD)
Cervical	−40 (10)					
Thoracic	49 (11)		42 (9)	43 (9)	46 (11)	
Lumbar	−60 (12)	−49 (15)	−61 (12)	−62 (13)	−63 (12)	−64 (10)

* Ranges: thoracic curve 22 to 68° and lumbar curve −88 to −31°
† Ranges: thoracic curve 23 to 61° and lumbar curve −81 to −38°
‡ Ranges: thoracic curve 22 to 75° and lumbar curve was −90 to −35°

figuration described in Chapter 4. The optimal position of the plumb line LoG is through the midline of the trunk (Fig. 13-14).

Continuing Exploration: **Controversy regarding Location of the LoG above the Fifth Lumbar Vertebra**

The location of the LoG in relation to the vertebral column above the fifth lumbar level is controversial. Cailliet[54] reported that the LoG transects the vertebral bodies at the level of T1 and T12 vertebrae and at the odontoid process of the C2 vertebra. Duval-Beaupere et al.,[39] using x-ray examinations of the vertebral columns of 17 young adults, found that the LoG in these individuals was located anterior to the anterior aspect of the T8 to T10 vertebrae. According to Bogduk,[43] the LoG passes anterior to L4 and thus anterior to the lumbar spine in many individuals. In this instance, a flexion moment that would tend to pull the thorax and upper lumbar spine anteriorly would be present. Activity of the erector spinae would be necessary to counteract the moment and maintain the body in equilibrium.

According to Cailliet's frame of reference, the LoG will pass posterior to the axes of rotation of the cervical and lumbar vertebrae, anterior to the thoracic vertebrae, and through the body of the fifth lumbar vertebra. In this situation, the gravitational moments tend to increase the natural curves in the lumbar, thoracic, and cervical regions. Moreover, according to Cailliet,[54] the maximal gravitational torque occurs at the apex of each curve at C5, T8, and L3, because the apical vertebrae are farthest from the LoG and the moment arms are longest at these points. However, as Table 13-2 shows, there is considerable individual variation in the apices for both thoracic and lumbar curves, but the means are similar among investigators. Cailliet's apices are within the ranges shown in the table.

According to Kendall and McCreary,[38] the LoG passes through the bodies of the lumbar and cervical vertebrae and anterior to the thoracic vertebrae in the optimal posture. In this instance, the stress on the supporting structures would be greatest in the thoracic area, where the LoG would pass at a greatest distance from the vertebrae. Stress in the lumbar and cervical regions would be comparatively less because the LoG passes close to or through the joint axes of these regions.

Although not confirming either Cailliet's or Kendall and McCreary's hypotheses, EMG studies have shown that the longissimus dorsi, rotatores, and neck extensor muscles exhibit intermittent electrical activity during normal standing.[56] This evidence suggests that ligamentous structures and passive muscle tension are unable to provide enough force to oppose all external gravitational moments acting around the joint axes of the upper vertebral column. In the lumbar region, where minimal muscle activity appears to occur, passive tension in the anterior longitudinal ligament and passive tension in the trunk flexors apparently are sufficient to balance the external gravitational extension moment.

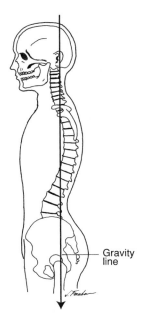

Gravity line

▲ **Figure 13-14** ■ Location of the LoG in relation to the trunk.

Table 13-2	Variations in Apices of Thoracic and Lumbar Curves in the Sagittal Plane in Standing Posture		
Author	Vendantam et al.[55]	Jackson and McManus[50]	Gelb et al.[53]
Subjects	10–18 yr n = 88	20–65 yr n = 100	40–70 plus yr n = 100
	Mean Range	Mean	Mean Range
Thoracic apex	T6 T3–T9	T7–78	T7 T5 disk–T10 disk
Lumbar apex	L4 L2–L5		L4 L2–L5

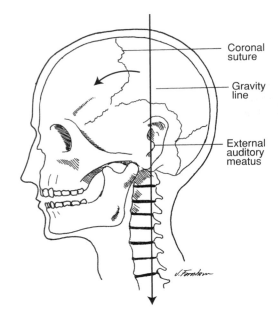

▲ **Figure 13-15** ■ The anterior location of the LoG in relation to the transverse axis for flexion and extension of the head creates an external flexion moment.

■ Head

The LoG in relation to the head passes slightly anterior to the transverse (frontal) axis of rotation for flexion and extension of the head and creates an external flexion moment (Fig. 13-15). This external flexion moment, which tends to tilt the head forward, may be counteracted by internal moments generated by tension in the ligamentum nuchae, tectorial membrane, and posterior aspect of the zygapophyseal joint capsules and by activity of the capital extensors.[54] Ideally, a plumb line extending from the ceiling should pass through the external auditory meatus of the ear, and the head should be directly over the body's CoM at S2.[54,57]

Continuing Exploration: Configuration of the Cervical Spine in Standing

In a lateral radiographic study of the spines of 100 standing men and women between 20 and 70 years of age, plumb lines extending from the odontoid process to C7 fell within a relatively narrow range of 16.8 mm anterior to the center of C7. The greatest lordosis was at C1 to C2 (−31.9; standard deviation [SD] = 7.0), with little lordosis found in the rest of the cervical spine. On average, the occiput-C1 segment was kyphotic, and a segmental kyphosis of 5° or greater was present in 39% of the total group, although no total kyphosis (occiput to C7) was present. In this study, as cervical lordosis increased, thoracic kyphosis increased also.[48]

In a study in which they used slightly different reference points on radiographs, Visscher et al. identified the following two types of cervical spine configurations in 54 men and women students standing in a neutral position: a lordotic curvature and a predominately straight spine with an occasional high lordosis and low kyphosis.[58]

■ Alignment of Body Segments in the Sagittal Plane

Table 13-3 shows the relationship of the LoG to various body segments in the sagittal plane. However, the reader must realize that the swaying motion that occurs in the normal erect posture will change the position of the LoG in relation to individual joint axes. The CoP also will move during swaying. For example, if the amount of forward sway is large enough, the LoG may move from the optimal posterior location in relation to the hip joint axis to a position anterior to the hip joint axis. The CoP will move anteriorly toward the toes. The resulting external flexion moment at the hip created by the change in position of the LoG may be counteracted by activity of the hip extensors, which will move the LoG and CoP posteriorly. On the other hand, increased activity in the soleus muscles rather than in the hip extensors might be used to bring the entire body and thus the LoG back into a position posterior to the hip joint axis. Some independent motion may occur in each leg, and relative motion may occur between body segments in response to postural sway.[57]

If your body is suddenly thrust forward, either by someone bumping into you or by a sudden backward movement of the supporting surface, a large and forceful movement of the LoG will occur. Consequently, flexion moments will be created at the neck and head; cervical, thoracic, and lumbar spines; hip; and ankle. To counteract these moments, the neck, back, hip extensor, and ankle plantarflexor muscles may have to contract. The CNS responds with activation of a muscle or pattern of muscles that will counteract the inertial and flexion moments, bring the LoG back over the CoM, and reestablish static erect equilibrium and stability. Furthermore, individual variations in the curves and apices will cause changes not only in external gravitational moments but also in the amount of internal counterforce that is necessary.

Table 13-3	Alignment in the Sagittal Plane in Standing Posture			
Joints	Line of Gravity	External Moment	Passive Opposing Forces	Active Opposing Forces
Atlanto-occipital	Anterior Anterior-to-transverse axis for flexion and extension	Flexion	Ligamentum nuchae and alar ligament; the tectorial, atlantoaxial, and posterior atlanto-occipital membranes	Rectus capitus posterior major and minor, semi-spinalis capitus and cervicis, splenius capitis and cervicis, and inferior and superior oblique muscles.
Cervical	Posterior	Extension	Anterior longitudinal ligament, anterior anulus fibrosus fibers, and zygapophyseal joint capsules	Anterior scaleni, longus capitis and colli
Thoracic	Anterior	Flexion	Posterior longitudinal, supraspinous, and interspinous ligaments Zygapophyseal joint capsules and posterior anulus fibrosus fibers	Ligamentum flavum, longissimus thoracis, iliocostalis thoracis, spinalis thoracis, and semispinalis thoracis
Lumbar	Posterior	Extension	Anterior longitudinal and iliolumbar ligaments, anterior fibers of the anulus fibrosus, and zygapophyseal joint capsules	Rectus abdominis and external and internal oblique muscles
Sacroiliac joint	Anterior	Nutation	Sacrotuberous, sacrospinous, iliolumbar, and anterior sacroiliac ligaments	Transversus abdominis
Hip joint	Posterior	Extension	Iliofemoral ligament	Ilipsoas
Knee joint	Anterior	Extension	Posterior joint capsule	Hamstrings, gastrocnemius
Ankle joint	Anterior	Dorsiflexion		Soleus, gastrocnemius

Deviations from Optimal Alignment in the Sagittal Plane

Minimizing energy expenditure and stress on supporting structures is one of the primary goals of any posture. Any change in position or malalignment of one body segment will cause changes to occur in adjacent segments, as well as changes in other segments, as the body seeks to adjust or compensate for the malalignment (closed-chain response to keep the head over the sacrum).[58] Large changes from optimal alignment increase stress or increase force per unit area on body structures. If stresses are maintained over long periods of time, body structures may be altered. Muscles may lose sarcomeres if held in shortened positions for extended periods. Such adaptive shortening may accentuate and perpetuate the abnormal posture, as well as prevent full ROM from occurring. Muscles may add sarcomeres if maintained in a lengthened position, and as a consequence, the muscle's length-tension relationship will be altered. Shortening of the ligaments will limit normal ROM, whereas stretching of ligamentous structures will reduce the ligament's ability to provide sufficient tension to stabilize and protect the joints. Prolonged weight-bearing stresses on the joint surfaces increase cartilage deformation and may interfere with the nutrition of the cartilage. As a result, the joint surfaces may become susceptible to early degenerative changes. The following sections illustrate how deviation from normal alignment of one or two body segments causes changes in other segments and increases the amount of energy required to maintain erect standing posture. Postural problems may originate in any part of the body and cause increased stresses and strains in throughout the musculoskeletal system. Postures that represent an attempt to either improve function or normalize appearance are called **compensatory postures**.[59] Evaluators of posture need not only to identify the deviation but also to determine the cause of the deviation, compensatory postures, and possible effects of the deviation on bones, joints, ligaments, and muscles supporting the affected structures.

■ Foot and Toes

Claw Toes

Claw toes is a deformity of the toes characterized by hyperextension of the metatarsophalangeal (MTP) joint, combined with flexion of the proximal interphalangeal (PIP) and distal interphalangeal (DIP) joints.[60-62] The abnormal distribution of weight may result in callus formation under the heads of the metatarsals or under the end of the distal phalanx. Sometimes the proximal phalanx may subluxate dorsally on the metatarsal head (Fig. 13-16A).[60] Calluses may develop on the dorsal aspects of the flexed phalanges from constant rubbing on the inside of shoes. In essence, this deformity reduces the area of the BoS and, as a result, may increase postural sway and decrease stability in the standing position.

A few of the many suggested etiologies for this condition are as follows: the restrictive effect of

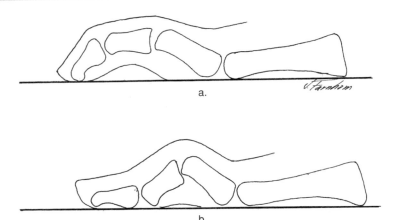

a.

b.

◀ **Figure 13-16** ■ Claw toes and hammer toes.
A. The drawing of claw toes shows hyperextension at the
metatarsophalangeal joint and flexion of the interphalangeal joints. **B.** Hammer toes are characterized by
hypertension of the metatarsophalangal and distal interphalangeal joints and by flexion of the proximal interphalangeal joints.

shoes, a cavus-type foot, muscular imbalance, ineffectiveness of intrinsic foot muscles, neuromuscular disorders, and age-related deficiencies in the plantar structures.

Valmassy[61] suggested that the claw toe deformity is actually the same condition as hammer toe because the only difference in the conditions is that a claw toe deformity affects all toes (second through fifth), whereas hammer toe usually affects only one or two toes.

Hammer Toes

In general, hammer toe is described as a deformity characterized by hyperextension of the MTP joint, flexion of the PIP joint, and hyperextension of the DIP joint (see Fig. 13-16B). Callosities (painless thickenings of the epidermis) may be found on the superior surfaces of the PIP joints over the heads of the first phalanges as a result of pressure from the shoes. The tips of the distal phalanges also may show callosities as a result of abnormal weight-bearing.[61,62] The flexor muscles are stretched over the MTP joint and shortened over the PIP joint. The extensor muscles are shortened over the MTP joint and stretched over the PIP joint. If the long and short toe extensors and lumbrical muscles are selectively paralyzed, the instrinsic and extrinsic toe flexors acting unopposed will buckle the PIP and DIP joints and cause a hammer toe.

■ Knee

Flexed Knee Posture

In the flexed-knee standing posture, which can result from knee flexion contractures, the LoG passes posterior to the knee joint axes. The posterior location of the LoG creates an external flexion moment at the knees that must be balanced by an internal extension moment created by activity of the quadriceps muscles in order to maintain the erect position. The quadriceps force required to maintain equilibrium at the knee in erect stance increases from zero with the knee extended to 22% of a maximum voluntary contraction (MVC) with the knee in 15° of flexion. A rapid rise in

the amount of quadriceps force is required between 15° and 30° of knee flexion. When the knee reaches 30° of flexion, the necessary quadriceps force rises to 51% of a MVC.[63] The increase in muscle activity needed to maintain a flexed knee posture subjects the tibiofemoral and patellofemoral joints to greater-than-normal compressive stress and can lead to fatigue of the quadriceps femoris and other muscles if the posture is maintained for a prolonged period.

Other consequences of a flexed-knee erect standing posture are related to the ankle and hip. Because knee flexion in the upright stance is accompanied by hip flexion and ankle dorsiflexion, the location of the LoG also will be altered in relation to these joint axes. At the hip, the LoG may pass anterior to the hip joint axes, creating an external flexion moment. Activity of the hip extensors may be necessary to create an internal extensor moment to balance the external flexion moment acting around the hip. Increased soleus muscle activity may be required to create an internal plantarflexion moment to counteract the increased external dorsiflexion moment at the ankle (Fig. 13-17). The additional muscle activity subjects the hip and ankle joints to greater-than-normal compression stress. Overall, the increased need for quadriceps, gastrocnemius, soleus and, perhaps, hip extensor activity appears to substantially increase the energy requirements for stance.

Case Application 13-7: **Sitting from Standing**

Dave needs to make sure that that the LoG does not pass anterior to the hip joint, because his hip extensors are paralyzed and unable to counteract a flexion moment at the hip. When he is going to sit down, he needs to make sure that he reaches back for the armrests on the wheelchair or other chair so that he can control the flexion moment at the hip when his trunk begins to flex in preparation for sitting. Therefore, development of his upper extremity strength is of utmost importance in his being able to control the lowering of his body into the chair.

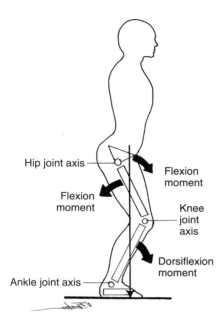

▲ **Figure 13-17** ■ Gravitational moments in a flexed-knee posture. External flexion moments are present, acting around the hip, knee, and ankle joints. The external flexion moments are opposed by internal extension moments acting at the hip and knee and by a plantarflexion moment at the ankle.

Hyperextended Knee Posture (Genu Recurvatum)

The hyperextended knee posture (Fig. 13-18) is one in which the LoG is located considerably anterior to the knee joint axis. The anterior location of the LoG causes an increase in the external extensor moment acting at the knee, which tends to increase the extent of hyper-

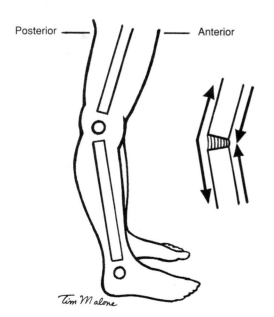

▲ **Figure 13-18** ■ In a hyperextended knee posture, the anterior aspect of the knee is subjected to abnormal compressive forces, whereas the posterior aspect is subjected to abnormal tensile forces. Note the limitation of dorsiflexion at the ankle.

extension and puts the posterior joint capsule under considerable tension stress. A continual adoption of the hyperextended knee posture is likely to result in adaptive lengthening of the posterior capsule and of the cruciate ligaments and, consequently, in a more unstable joint. The anterior portion of the knee joint surfaces on the femoral condyles and anterior portion of the tibial plateaus will be subject to abnormal compression and therefore are subject to degenerative changes of the cartilaginous joint surfaces. The length-tension relationship of the anterior and posterior muscles also may be altered, and the muscles may not be able to provide the force necessary to provide adequate joint stability and mobility.

Hyperextension at the knee is usually caused either by limited dorsiflexion at the ankle or by a fixed plantarflexion position of the foot and ankle called **equinus.** It may also be the result of habits formed in childhood in which the child or adolescent always elects to stand with hips and knees hyperextended in the relaxed or swayback standing posture.

Case Application 13-8: **Knee Hypertension**

> Although our patient, Dave, needs to stand in a swayback posture, he has some protection from knee hyperextension because of the anteriorly directed counterforce provided by the posteriorly placed thigh and calf pads on his KAFOs. However, we need to check for excessive knee hyperextension because Dave will not be aware of his knee joint position or be able to feel pain from his knee.

■ Pelvis

Excessive Anterior Pelvic Tilt

In a posture in which the pelvis is excessively tilted anteriorly, the lower lumbar vertebrae are forced anteriorly. The upper lumbar vertebrae move posteriorly to keep the head over the sacrum, thereby increasing the lumbar anterior convexity (lordotic curve). The LoG is therefore at a greater distance from the lumbar joint axes than is optimal and the extension moment in the lumbar spine is increased. The posterior convexity of the thoracic curve increases and becomes kyphotic to balance the lordotic lumbar curve and maintain the head over the sacrum. Similarly, the anterior convexity of the cervical curve increases to bring the head back over the sacrum (Fig. 13-19). Table 13-4 illustrates the changes that may result from an excessive anterior tilt.

In the optimal posture in erect standing, the lumbar disks are subject to tension anteriorly and compression posteriorly. A greater diffusion of nutrients into the anterior than into the posterior portion of the disk occurs in the optimal erect posture.[64] Increases in the anterior convexity of the lumbar curve during erect standing increases the compressive forces on the posterior annuli and may adversely affect the nutrition of the

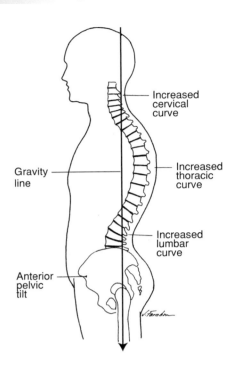

Increased
cervical
curve

Gravity
line

Increased
thoracic
curve

Increased
lumbar
curve

Anterior
pelvic
tilt

▲   **Figure 13-19** ■ An excessive anterior pelvic tilt results in an increase in the lumbar anterior convexity. To compensate for the increased lumbar convexity, there is an increase in the posterior convexity of the thoracic region and an increase in the anterior convexity of the cervical curve.

posterior portion of the intervertebral disks. Also, excessive compressive forces may be applied to the zygapophyseal joints.[65]

■ Vertebral Column

Lordosis and Kyphosis

The term lordosis refers to the normal sagittal plane anteriorly convex curves in the cervical and lumbar regions of the vertebral column. The term kyphosis refers to the normal sagittal plane posteriorly convex curves in the thoracic and sacral regions of the vertebral column.[66] Sometimes an abnormal increase in the normal posterior convexity may occur, and this abnormal condition also may be called a kyphosis.[67,68] This condition may develop as a compensation for an increase in the normal lumbar curve, as seen in Figure 13-19, or the kyphosis may develop as a result of poor postural habits or ostoporosis. Dowager's hump is an easily recognizable excessively kyphotic condition that is found most often in postmenopausal women who have osteoporosis.[60] The anterior aspect of the bodies of a series of vertebrae collapse as a result of osteoporotic weakening. The vertebral body collapse causes an immediate lack of anterior support for a segment of the thoracic vertebral column, which bends forward, causing an increase in the posterior convexity (the hump) and an increase in compression on the anterior aspect of the vertebral bodies (Fig. 13-20A). The LoG passes at a greater distance from the thoracic spine, and the gravitational moment arm increases. Compression

Table 13-4	Possible Effects of Malalignment on Body Structures			
Deviation	Compression	Distraction	Stretching	Shortening
Excessive anterior tilt of pelvis	Posterior aspect of vertebral bodies Interdiskal pressure at L5 to S1 increased	Lumbosacral angle increased Shearing forces at L5 to S1 Likelihood of forward slippage of L5 on S1 increased	Abdominal muscles	Iliopsoas, lumbar extensors
Excessive lumbar lordosis	Posterior vertebral bodies and facet joints Interdiskal pressures increased Intervertebral foramina narrowed	Anterior annulus fibers	Anterior longitudinal ligament	Posterior longitudinal ligament Interspinous ligaments Ligamentum flavum Lumbar extensors
Excessive dorsal kyphosis	Anterior vertebral bodies Intradiskal pressures increased	Facet joint capsules and posterior annulus fibers	Dorsal back extensors Posterior ligaments Scapular muscles	Anterior longitudinal ligament Upper abdominal muscles Anterior shoulder girdle musculature
Excessive cervical lordosis	Posterior vertebral bodies and facet joints Interdiskal pressure increased Intervertebral foramina narrowed	Anterior annulus fibers	Anterior longitudinal ligament	Posterior ligaments Neck extensors

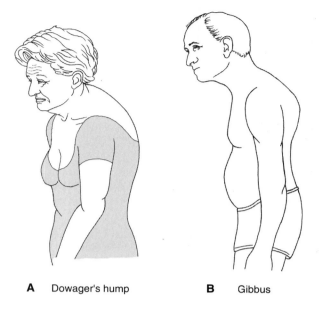

A Dowager's hump B Gibbus

▲ **Figure 13-20** ■ A. Dowager's hump. B. Gibbus deformity.

on the anterior aspects of the vertebral bodies and anterior annulus increases, and the posterior aspect (convexity of the curve) is subjected to tensile stresses in the fibers of the posterior annulus and apophyseal joint capsules.

Diseases such as tuberculosis or ankylosing spondylosis also may cause abnormal increases in the posterior convexity of the thoracic region. A **gibbus** or **humpback deformity** may occur as a result of tuberculosis, which causes vertebral fractures (see Fig. 13-20B). Gibbus or humpback deformity is easily recognized by the gibbus

(hump), which forms a sharp posterior angulation in the upper thoracic vertebral column.

■ **Head**

Forward Head Posture

A forward head posture is one in which the head is positioned anteriorly and the normal anterior cervical convexity is increased with the apex of the lordotic cervical curve at a considerable distance from the LoG in comparison with optimal posture. The constant assumption of a forward head posture causes abnormal compression on the posterior zygapophyseal joints and posterior portions of the intervertebral disks and narrowing of the intervertebral foramina in the lordotic areas of the cervical region. The cervical extensor muscles may become ischemic because of the constant isometric contraction required to counteract the larger than normal external flexion moment and maintain the head in its forward position. The posterior aspect of the zygapophyseal joint capsules may become adaptively shortened, and the narrowed intervertebral foramen may cause nerve root compression. In addition, the structure of the temporomandibular joint may become altered by the forward head posture, and as a result, the joint's function may be disturbed. In the forward head posture, the scapulae may rotate medially, a thoracic kyphosis may develop, the thoracic cavity may be diminished, vital capacity can be reduced, and overall body height may be shortened. Other possible effects of habitual forward head posture, including adverse effects on the temperomandibular joint, are presented in Table 13-5. Dave will need to be aware of his head and neck posture because most of the time he will be working and/or relaxing in a seated posture.

Table 13-5	Forward Head Posture	
Deviation	Structural Components	Long-Term Effects on Structural Function
Forward head	Anterior location of LoG causes an increase in the flexion moment, which requires constant isometric muscle tension to support head Stretch of suprahyoid muscles pulls mandible posteriorly into retrusion	Muscle ischemia, pain, and fatigue and possible protrusion of nucleus pulposus Retruded mandible position causes compression and irritation of retrodiskal pad and may result in inflammation and pain Reduction in range of motion
Increase in cervical lordosis	Narrowing of intervertebral foramen and compression of nerve roots Compression of zygapophyseal joint surfaces and increase in weight-bearing Compression of posterior annulus fibrosus Adaptive shortening of the posterior ligaments Adaptive lengthening of anterior ligaments Increase in compression on posterior vertebral bodies at apex of cervical curve	Damage to spinal cord and/or nerve roots leading to paralysis Damage to cartilage and increased possibility of arthritic changes; adaptive shortening and possible formation of adhesions of joint capsules with subsequent loss of ROM Changes in collagen and early disk degeneration; diminished ROM at the intervertebral joints Decrease in cervical flexion ROM Decrease in cervical extension ROM and decrease in anterior stability Osteophyte formation
Medial rotation of the scapula	Adaptive lengthening of upper posterior back muscles Adaptive shortening of anterior shoulder muscles	Increase in dorsal kyphosis and loss of height Decrease in vital capacity and ROM of shoulder and arm

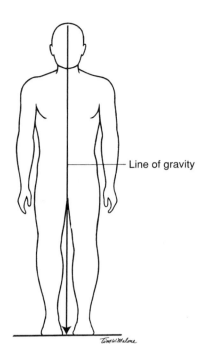

Line of gravity

▲ **Figure 13-21** ■ In anterior view of the human body, the LoG, in optimal posture, divides the body into two symmetrical parts.

Frontal Plane Optimal Alignment and Analysis

In an anterior view, the LoG bisects the body into symmetrical halves (Fig. 13-21). The head is straight, with no tilting or rotation evident. The LoG bisects the face into equal halves. The eyes, clavicles, and shoulders should be level (parallel to the ground). In a posterior view, the inferior angles of the scapulae should be parallel and equidistant from the LoG. The waist angles and gluteal folds should be equal, and the ASIS and PSIS should lie on a line parallel to the ground, as well as being equidistant from the LoG. The joint axes of the hip, knee, and ankle are equidistant from the LoG, and the gravitational line transects the central portion of the vertebral bodies. When postural alignment is optimal, little or no muscle activity is required to maintain medial-lateral stability. The gravitational torques acting on one side of the body are opposed by equal torques acting on the other side of the body (Tables 13-6 and 13-7).

Deviations from Optimal Alignment in the Frontal Plane

Any asymmetry of body segments caused either by movement of a body segment or by a unilateral postural deviation will disturb optimal muscular and ligamentous balance. Symmetrical postural deviations, such as bilateral **genu valgum** (**knock knee**), that disturb the optimal vertical alignment of body segments cause an abnormal distribution of weight-bearing or compressive forces on one side of a joint and increased tensile forces on the other side. The increased gravitational torques that may occur require increased muscular activity and cause ligamentous stress.

■ Foot and Toes

Pes Planus (Flat Foot)

An evaluation of standing posture from the anterior-posterior aspect should include a careful evaluation of the feet. Normally the plumb line should lie equidistant from the malleoli, and the malleoli should appear to be of equal size and directly opposite from one another. When one malleolus appears more prominent or lower than the other and calcaneal eversion is present, it is possible that a common foot problem known as **pes planus,** or **flat foot,** may be present. Calcaneal eversion

Table 13-6	Alignment in the Coronal Plane in the Standing Posture: Anterior Aspect	
Body Segment	**LOG Location**	**Observation**
Head	Passes through middle of the forehead, nose and chin.	Eyes and ears should be level and symmetrical.
Neck/shoulders		Right and left angles between shoulders and neck should be symmetrical. Clavicles also should be symmetrical.
Chest	Passes through the middle of the xyphoid process.	Ribs on each side should be symmetrical.
Abdomen/hips	Passes through the umbilicus (navel).	Right and left waist angles should be symmetrical.
Hips/pelvis	Passes on a line equidistant from the right and left anterior superior iliac spines. Passes through the symphysis pubis.	Anterior superior iliac spines should be level.
Knees	Passes between knees equidistant from medial femoral condyles.	Patella should be symmetrical and facing straight ahead.
Ankles/feet	Passes between ankles equidistant from the medial maleoli.	Malleoli should be symmetrical, and feet should be parallel. Toes should not be curled, overlapping, or deviated to one side.

Table 13-7	Alignment in the Coronal Plane in the Standing Posture: Posterior Aspect	
Body Segment	LoG Location	Observation
Head	Passes through middle of head.	Head should be straight with no lateral tilting. Angles between shoulders and neck should be equal.
Arms		Arms should hang naturally so that the palms of the hands are facing the sides of the body.
Shoulders/spine	Passes along vertebral column in a straight line, which should bisect the back into two symmetrical halves.	Scapulae should lie flat against the rib cage, be equidistant from the LoG, and be separated by about 4 inches in the adult.
Hips/pelvis	Passes through gluteal cleft of buttocks and should be equidistant from posterior superior iliac spines.	The posterior superior iliac spines should be level. The gluteal folds should be level and symmetrical.
Knees	Passes between the knees equidistant from medial joint aspects.	Look to see that the knees are level.
Ankles/feet	Passes between ankles equidistant from the medial malleoli.	The heel cords should be vertical and the malleoli should be level and symmetrical.

of 5° to 10° is normal in toddlers, but by 7 years of age, no calcaneal eversion should be present.[61]

Flat foot, which is characterized by a reduced or absent medial arch, may be either rigid or flexible. A rigid flat foot is a structural deformity that may be hereditary. In the rigid flat foot, the medial longitudinal arch is absent in non–weight-bearing, toe-standing, and normal weight-bearing situations. In the flexible flat foot, the arch is reduced during normal weight-bearing situations but reappears during toe-standing or non–weight-bearing situations.

In either the rigid or flexible type of pes planus, the talar head is displaced anteriorly, medially, and inferiorly. The displacement of the talus causes depression of the navicular bone, tension in the plantar calcaneonavicular (spring) ligament, and lengthening of the tibialis posterior muscle (Fig. 13-22). The extent of flat foot may be estimated by noting the location of the navicular bone in relation to the head of the first metatarsal. Normally, the navicular bone should be intersected by the Feiss line (Fig. 13-23). If the navicular bone is depressed, it will lie below the Feiss line and may even rest on the floor in a severe extent of flat foot. Flat foot results in a relatively overmobile foot that may require muscular contraction to support the osteoligamentous arches during standing. It also may result in increased weight-bearing on the second through fourth metatarsal heads with subsequent plantar callus formation, especially at the second metatarsal. Weight-bearing pronation in the erect standing posture causes medial rotation of the tibia and may affect knee joint function.

Dave has depressed navicular bones on both feet. Do you think that this condition will be a problem for him? Can you think of a possible remedy if it is a problem?

Pes Cavus

The medial longitudinal arch of the foot, instead of being low (as in flat foot), may be unusually high. A high arch is called **pes cavus** (Fig. 13-24). Pes cavus is a more stable position of the foot than is pes planus. The weight in pes cavus is borne on the lateral borders of the foot, and the lateral ligaments and the peroneus longus muscle may be stretched. In walking, the cavus foot is unable to adapt to the supporting surface because the subtalar and transverse tarsal joints tend to be near or at the locked supinated position.

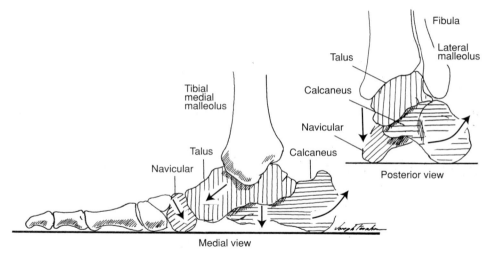

◀ **Figure 13-22** ■ In pes planus ("flat foot"), there is displacement of the talus anteriorly, medially, and inferiorly; depression and pronation of the calcaneus; and depression of the navicular bone.

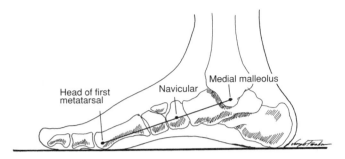

▲ **Figure 13-23** ■ In the normal foot, the medial malleolus, the tuberosity of the navicular bone, and the head of the first metatarsal lie in a straight line called the Feiss line.

■ Knees

Genu valgum (**knock knee**) is considered to be a normal alignment of the lower extremity in children from 2 to 6 years of age.[69] However, by about 6 or 7 years of age, the physiologic valgus should begin to decrease, and by young adulthood, the extent of valgus angulation at the knee should be only about 5° to 7°. In genu valgum, the mechanical axes of the lower extremities are displaced laterally. If the extent of genu valgum exceeds 30° and persists beyond 8 years of age, structural changes may occur. As a result of the increased external torque acting around the knee, the medial knee joint structures are subjected to abnormal tensile or distraction stress, and the lateral structures are subjected to abnormal compressive stress (Fig. 13-25A). The patella may be laterally displaced and therefore predisposed to subluxation.

The foot also is affected as the gravitational torque acting on the foot in genu valgum tends to produce pronation of the foot with an accompanying stress on the medial longitudinal arch and its supporting structures, as well as abnormal weight-bearing on the posterior medial aspect of the calcaneus (valgus torque). Additional related changes may include flat foot, lateral tibial torsion, lateral patellar subluxation, and lumbar spine contralateral rotation.[60]

Genu varum (**bowleg**) is a condition in which the knees are widely separated when the feet are together and the malleoli are touching (see Fig. 13-25B). Some extent of genu varum is normal at birth and during infancy up to 3 or 4 years of age.[62,70] Physiologic bowing is symmetrical and involves both the femur and the

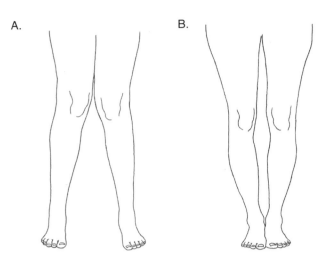

▲ **Figure 13-25** ■ **A.** In genu valgum ("knock knee"), the medial aspect of the knee complex is subjected to tensile stress, and the lateral aspect is subjected to compressive stress. **B.** In genu varum ("bowleg"), the lateral aspect of the knee complex is subjected to tensile stress, and the medial aspect of the knee complex is subjected to compressive stress.

tibia. Cortical thickening on the medial concavity of both the femur and tibia may be present as a result of the increased compressive forces,[70] and the patellae may be displaced medially. Some of the more commonly suggested cause of genu varum are vitamin D deficiency, renal rickets, osteochondritis, or epiphyseal injury.

Squinting or **cross-eyed patella** (patella that faces medially) is a tilted/rotated position of the patella in which the superior medial pole faces medially and the inferior pole faces laterally (Fig. 13-26A). This abnormal patella position may be present in one or both knees and may be a sign of either increased femoral torsion (excessive femoral anteversion)[61] or medial tibial rotation.[60] The Q-angle may be increased in this condition, and patella tracking may be adversely affected. **Grasshopper-eyes patella** refers to a high, laterally displaced position of the patella in which the patella faces upward and outward (see Fig. 13-26B). An abnormally long patella ligament may be responsible for the higher than normal position of the patella (**patella alta**). Femoral retroversion or lateral tibial torsion may be responsible for the rotated position of the patella. Grasshopper-eyes patella leads to abnormal patella tracking and a decrease in the stability of the patella.

■ Vertebral Column

Scoliosis

Another segment of the body that requires special consideration when posture is evaluated from the anterior or posterior view is the vertebral column. Normally, when viewed from the posterior aspect, the vertebral column is vertically aligned and bisected by the LoG. The structures on either side of the column are symmetrical. The LoG passes through the midline of the occiput, through the spinous processes of all vertebrae, and directly through the gluteal cleft. In an optimal

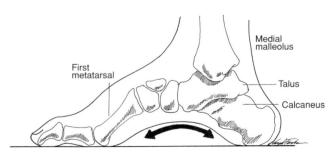

▲ **Figure 13-24** ■ Pes cavus.

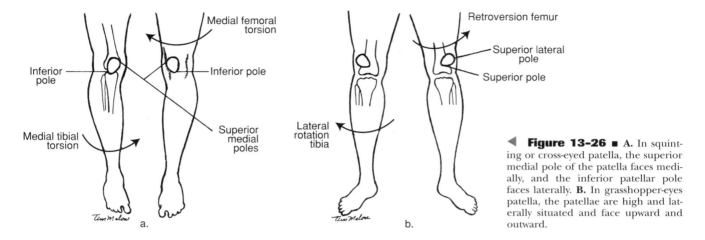

◀ **Figure 13-26** ■ **A.** In squinting or cross-eyed patella, the superior medial pole of the patella faces medially, and the inferior patellar pole faces laterally. **B.** In grasshopper-eyes patella, the patellae are high and laterally situated and face upward and outward.

posture, the vertebral structures, ligaments, and muscles are able to maintain the column in vertical alignment with little stress or energy expenditure. If one or more of the medial-lateral structures fails to provide adequate support, the column will bend to the side. The lateral bending will be accompanied by rotation of the vertebrae because lateral flexion and rotation are coupled motions below the level of the second cervical vertebra.

Consistent lateral deviations of a series of vertebrae from the LoG in one or more regions of the spine may indicate the presence of a lateral spinal curvature in the frontal plane called a **scoliosis** (Fig. 13-27). There are two classifications of curves: **functional curves** and **structural curves**. Functional curves are called nonstructural curves in that they can be reversed if the cause of the curve is corrected. These curves are the result of correctable imbalances such as a leg length discrepancy or a muscle spasm. Structural curves, as the name implies, involve changes in bone and soft tissue structures.

Although scoliosis is usually identified as a lateral curvature of the spine in the frontal plane, the deformity also occurs in the transverse (as vertebrae rotate) and sagittal planes (as the column buckles). Idiopathic scolioses are catagorized by age at onset : **infantile** (0 to 3 years), **juvenile** (4 to 10 years) and **adolescent** (older than 10 years).[70] The adolescent idiopathic scoliosis (**AIS**) type makes up the majority of all scolioses[71,72] and affects up to 4% of schoolchildren worldwide.[72] The term idiopathic means that the cause of the condition is unknown. The curves in scoliosis are named according to the direction of the convexity and location of the curve. If the curve is convex to the left in the cervical area, the curve is designated as a left cervical scoliosis. If more than one region of the vertebral column is involved, the superior segment is named first (e.g., left cervical, right thoracic). A double major curve is present when there are two structural curves of the same size. A triple curve includes three regions of the vertebral column. The curve shown in Figure 13-27 is a structural curve called a right thoracic, left lumbar scoliosis. In a study of 606 AIS cases, the most prevalent (51%) type of curve was the main thoracic curve with its apex

located between the body of T2 and the disk between T11 and T12.[73]

Investigators have postulated that AIS may result from a dysfunction in the vestibular system,[74] a disturbance in control of the muscle spindle,[75] an inherited connective tissue disorder,[76] subcortical brain stem abnormalities,[77–80] developmental instability,[81,82] melatonin production abnormality, growth hormone secretion, and platelet abnormalities.[83] Furthermore, in a recent study, Chan and associates found a genetic locus

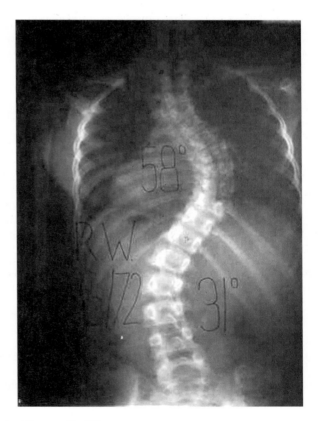

▲ **Figure 13-27** ■ A lateral curvature of the vertebral column that is convex to the right in the thoracic region and convex to the left in the lumbar region. Note the rotation of the vertebra and asymmetry of the rib cage.

for AIS.[72] Lidstrom and coworkers[84] found differences in postural sway in 100 children aged 10 to 14 years; 35 of the children were siblings of scoliotic patients, and 65 were control subjects. This is another finding that suggests the possibility of a genetic component as the causative agent. Nault and associates[80] found a decrease in standing stability among 43 girls diagnosed with scoliosis in comparison with 28 girls without scoliosis. Sway areas, as measured by variations in the CoP and CoM, were larger in the scoliotic group than in the nonscoliotic group. As of this writing, however, no evidence has been presented that unequivocally points to a single etiology for adolescent idiopathic scoliosis,[85] and Ahn et al.[83] suggested that the etiology is multifactorial. Despite the ambiguity surrounding the cause or causes of adolescent idiopathic scoliosis, the effects of unequal torques on the structures of the body are dramatic and can be devastating to those affected. AIS involves changes in the structure of the vertebral bodies, transverse and spinous processes, intervertebral disks, ligaments, and muscles. Asymmetrical growth and development of the vertebral bodies lead to **wedging** of the vertebrae. Growth on the compressed side (concavity) is inhibited or slower than on the side of the convexity of the curve.

The following example depicts a hypothetical series of events for AIS. The first step in the process is unknown because researchers have been unable to identify the supporting structure involved in the initial failure. Therefore, it is just as possible that the sequence of events begins with a developmental disturbance that results in asymmetrical growth of the vertebrae rather than a failure in the muscular or ligamentous support system, as suggested in the model.

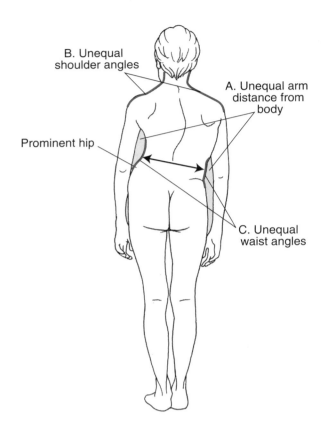

▲ **Figure 13-28** ■ A lateral curvature of the vertebral column that is convex to the right in the thoracic region and convex to the left in the lumbar region.

Example 13-4

Hypothetical Series of Events in Adolescent Idiopathic Scoliosis (Fig. 13-28)

1. possible failure of support as a result of a defect in muscular and/or ligamentous support systems during a period of rapid growth
2. creation of an external lateral flexion moment
3. deviation of the vertebrae with rotation
4. compression of the vertebral body on the side of the concavity of the curve
5. inhibition of growth of vertebral body on the side of the concavity of the curve in a still immature spine
6. wedging of the vertebra in a still immature spine
7. head out of line with sacrum
8. compensatory curve
9. adaptive shortening of trunk musculature on the concavity
10. stretching of muscles, ligaments, and joint capsules on the convexity

---

These changes may progress to produce a severe deformity as growth proceeds unless intervention occurs at the appropriate time. Deformities can interfere with breathing and the function of other internal organs, as

well as being cosmetically unacceptable. Observation combined with periodic follow-up to watch for curve progression is indicated for curves of less than 25°. Bracing is used for flexible curves between 25° and 40°.[70] Adolescents whose vertebral columns are still immature and who have curves between 25° and 40° are considered to be at high risk because curves of this extent tend to progress.[86] Bracing is successful in preventing additional progression of the curve in 70% to 80% of the cases in which it is used.[86] Curves that have progressed beyond 40° may necessitate surgical intervention to prevent further progression. If a curvature is recognized early in its development, then measures may be instituted either to correct the curve or to prevent its increase.[87] However, some curves may progress even after surgery.[88]

According to the second phase of the 1988 Utah study in which a visual assessment (scoliosis screening) of 3000 college-aged women (19 to 21 years of age) was performed in 34 states and 5 foreign countries, 12% of this population had a previously undetected lateral deviation of the spine.[89] In consideration of the fact that AIS may be progressive in some cases and lead to a considerable amount of deformity without treatment, early recognition is important. The vertebral deviations in scoliosis cause asymmetrical changes in body structures, and several of these changes may be detected through simple observation of body contours either at home or in the schools. Usually, home or school screening programs are designed for identification of the fol-

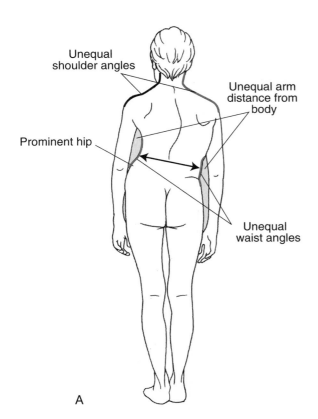

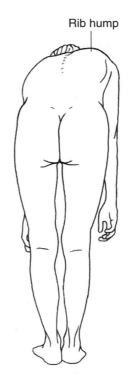

◀ **Figure 13-29** ■ Typical changes in body contours used in scoliosis screening programs. **A.** Uneven waist angles or difference in arm to body space and unequal shoulder height or unequal scapula levels. **B.** A rib hump during forward trunk flexion.

lowing: unequal waist angles, unequal shoulder levels or unequal scapulae (see Fig. 13-29A), rib hump, and obvious lateral spinal curvature (see Fig. 13-29B). The American Academy of Orthopedic Surgeon's Patient Service Brochure on scoliosis, which is available online, recommends that parents check their children's spines for any assymetry in body contours beginning at age 8 years. If the parents observe any postural asymmetries in their child, they should inform the child's physician.[90] The American Physical Therapy Association's (APTA's) pamphlet on scoliosis (also available online) suggests that home screening should take place every 6 months for both boys and girls starting at age 9 years and continue until the child is 14 years of age.[91]

Analysis of Sitting Postures

The overall goal for sitting posture is the same as the goal for standing posture: to attain a stable alignment of the body that can be maintained with the least expenditure of energy and the least stress on body structures. In our analysis of standing posture, we saw that moments at the spine and extremity joints were created when the LoG was at a distance from either a portion of the vertebral column or the axes of the extremity joints. The greater the distance that the LoG was from the joint axes, the larger the moment that was created and, as a result, the more muscle activity and/or passive tension in ligaments and joint capsules that was required to maintain equilibrium and a stable posture. The necessary increase in muscle activity resulted in more energy expenditure and increased

loads on body structures. Our patient, Dave, will have to spend a great deal of time in the sitting position in a wheelchair, and so we will have to consider the effects of prolonged sitting as well as the type of wheelchair that he will need.

In a way, sitting postures are more complex than standing postures. The same gravitational moments as in standing posture must be considered, but, in addition, we must consider the contact forces that are created when various portions of the body interface with various parts of chairs, such as head, back, and foot rests, and seats. The location and amount of support provided to various portions of the body by the chair or stool may change the position of the body parts and thus the magnitude of the stresses on body structures.

Example 13-5

The use of a lumbar support can help to maintain the normal lumbar lordotic curve and reduce the compressive stress on the spine in comparison with sitting without a lumbar support.[92]

There are many different sitting postures, but we will direct our attention to the **active erect sitting posture,** which is defined in this chapter as an unsupported posture in which a person attempts to sit up as straight as possible. A consideration of **muscle activity, interdiskal pressures,** and **seat interface pressures** in the active erect sitting posture will be compared to forces in **relaxed erect, slumped,** and **slouched** sitting and to erect standing postures. In addition, we will discuss how these forces may affect Dave.

Muscle Activity

The LoG passes close to the joint axes of the head and spine in active erect sitting posture. (Fig. 13-30A and B). In the slumped posture, the LoG is more anterior to the joint axes of the cervical, thoracic, and lumbar spines than it is in either active or relaxed erect sitting (see Fig. 13-30C). Therefore, we would expect that more muscle activity would be required in the slumped posture than in the other sitting postures. In contrast to these expectations, researchers have found that maintaining an active erect sitting posture requires not only a greater number of trunk muscles but also an increased level of activity in some of these muscles than in both relaxed erect and slumped postures. O'Sullivan and associates[93] used EMG to monitor activity in the superficial lumbar multifidus, thoracic erector spinae, and internal oblique abdominal muscles in erect and slumped sitting postures. These authors found a significantly greater amount of activity in these muscles in erect sitting than in slumped sitting.

The **flexion relaxation (FR) phenomenon** may provide a possible reason why the slumped sitting posture requires less muscle activity than does the active erect sitting posture. Flexion relaxation is a sudden cessation of muscular activity, as manifested by electrical silence of the back extensors during trunk flexion in either sitting or standing postures. In a study by Callaghan and Dunk, FR occurred in the thoracic erector spinae muscles (thoracic components of the longissimus thoracis and iliocostalis lumborum) in 21 of 22 subjects in slumped sitting and relaxed erect sitting but not in active erect sitting. Muscle activity in the lumbar erector spinae remained the same in both postures. The authors postulated that the passive tissues were able to assume the load in the relaxed erect and slumped postures and that was why the thoracic erector spinae muscles ceased their activity.[94]

Muscle activity in the active erect sitting posture is also greater than in both relaxed erect and slouched sitting. In relaxed erect sitting, the LoG is only slightly anterior from its position in active erect sitting. In the slouched posture, the LoG is posterior to the spine and hips, but body weight is being supported by the back of the chair, and so less muscle activity is required than in active erect posture (Fig. 13-31).[95]

Case Application 13-9: **Strengthening of Trunk Muscle for Sitting and Transfers**

Dave's trunk muscles are not paralyzed but are weakened from the surgery and subsequent bed rest. Therefore, one goal that we will have for Dave is to strengthen his trunk muscles so that he will be able to maintain his stability in sitting as well as in transfer and other daily living activities. (Individuals with a SCI below T3 may use the latissimus dorsi and lower trapezius muscles to help maintain stability in sitting, but it appears that Dave will not need these muscles to help in sitting.)[96]

■ **Muscle Activity in Sitting versus Standing Postures**

The amount of muscle activity employed to maintain a particular posture affects the amount of interdiskal

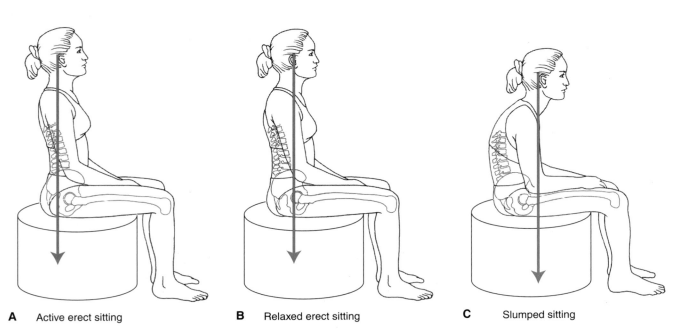

A   Active erect sitting   **B**   Relaxed erect sitting   **C**   Slumped sitting

▲ **Figure 13-30** ■ **A.** In the active erect sitting position, the LoG is close to the axes of rotation of the head, neck, and trunk. **B.** In the relaxed erect sitting posture, the LoG still is relatively close to those axes of rotation. **C.** In the slumped position, the LoG is relatively distant from the axes of rotation of the head, neck, and trunk.

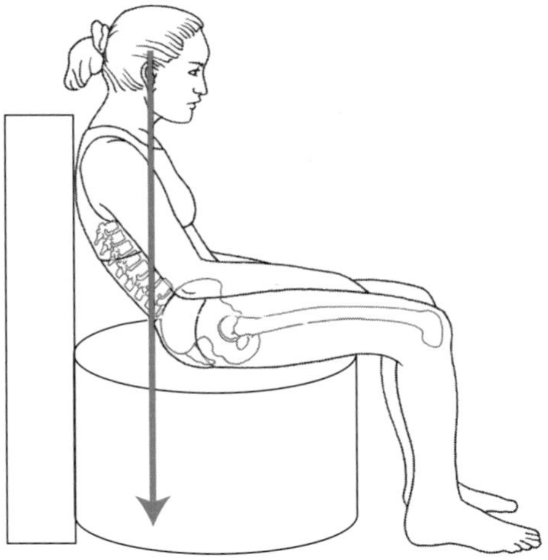

▲ **Figure 13-31** ■ In the slouched sitting posture, the LoG is at a distance from the axes of rotation at the head, neck, and trunk, but the back of the chair is providing support in lieu of muscle support.

pressure and energy expenditure. Increases in muscle activity cause increases in interdiskal pressures and decreases in muscle activity are accompanied by decreases in interdiskal pressures. Callaghan and McGill[97] noted that the upper and lower erector spinae muscles shifted to higher levels of activity during active erect sitting than during standing. This increase in muscle activity has been attributed in part to the differences in the extent of lumbar lordosis observed between sitting and standing. Sitting forces the pelvis into a posterior tilt and, as a result, causes a reduction in the lumbar curve in comparison with that observed in standing.[92] In one radiographic study of 109 patients, the average lumbar curve (L1 to S1) was 15° less in active erect sitting than was an average lumbar curve of 49° in the same population in standing posture.[49] The LoG would be farther away from the apex of the joint axes of the lumbar vertebrae in a flexed or more kyphotic lumbar spine than in a lordotic lumbar spine. Therefore, one would expect that more muscle activity would be required to maintain the active erect sitting posture than to maintain standing. However, the results of the following study raise questions about a more kyphotic lumbar spine's being responsible for all of the increase in muscle activity in active erect sitting versus standing.

Continuing Exploration: **Muscle Activity and Lumbar Lordosis in Standing and Sitting Postures**

When the lordotic lumbar curve in standing was replicated in unsupported active erect sitting in 30 subjects, the EMG activity level of the extensor muscles was significantly higher than in standing.[98] It thus appears from this study that the loss of lordosis in the sitting posture is not totally responsible for the greater amount of muscle activity observed in erect sitting than in standing.

Many variables need to be considered, and it is possible that investigators either did not employ identical conditions in their research or did not consider all of the variables that might affect muscle activity in erect sitting versus erect standing. For instance, something as simple as changing from a hard seat to a soft seat will decrease the amount of activity in the internal and external oblique muscles.[99] Supporting one's arms on a table when using both hands for data entry[100] can reduce the load on the left and right trapezius and erector spinae muscles in comparison with working with unsupported arms.

Interdiskal Pressures and Compressive Loads on the Spine

Direct determinations of interdiskal pressures have been made through the insertion of pressure sensitive sensors or transducers[101–104] into one or more intervertebral disks. Indirect determinations of interdiskal pressures have used measurements of spinal shrinkage (creep)[105–108] and calculation of compressive forces based on information obtained from EMGs about muscle activity.[98,99]

Active erect sitting requires co-contractions of trunk extensors (erector spinae muscles) and flexors (abdominal muscles), which cause higher pressures in the disk between L4 and L5 than does slumped sitting. One of the most well-known studies in which direct interdiskal pressure measurements in erect sitting were compared with pressures in erect standing and other postures was by Nachemson,[101] who reported that there was a 40% increase in pressures in the disk between L4 and L5 in erect sitting in comparison with erect standing. However, the results of some studies[102–104] in which advanced sensor technology was used suggest that interdiskal pressures/loads on the spine in active erect sitting are either only slightly higher than[102] or equal to[103] pressures in erect standing (Fig. 13-32).

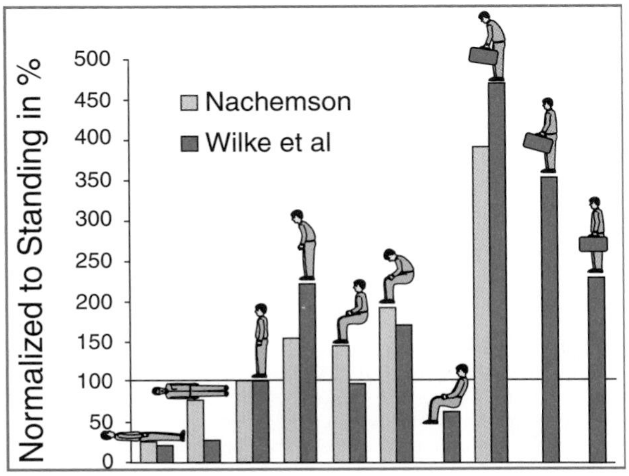

▲ **Figure 13-32** ■ Interdiskal pressures in different sitting and standing positions. (From Wilke H-J, Neef P, Caimi M, et al.: New *in vivo* measurements of pressures in the intervertebral disc in daily life. Spine 24:755, 1999. Reprinted with permission from Lippincott Williams & Wilkins.)

Continuing Exploration: **Comparison of Interdiskal Pressures in Standing and Sitting**

One of the problems in interpreting the results of investigations is that it is not always possible to determine whether the researchers are referring to active erect sitting or relaxed erect sitting. Undoubtedly, the controversy will continue until enough additional studies are performed to either confirm or deny Nachemson's findings. Some researchers agree that interdiskal pressures in relaxed or slouched sitting postures are lower than in erect standing.[102,103] Wilke and colleagues reported that the interdiskal pressure at the disk between L4 and L5 disk in relaxed erect sitting was 0.46 MPa, in comparison with 0.50 MPa in relaxed standing.[102] Straightening the back to attain an active erect sitting posture increased interdiskal pressures by approximately 10% to 0.55 MPa.[102] Rohlmann and associates found that bending moments on an internal spinal fixation device were, on average, 13% lower for relaxed erect sitting than for relaxed erect standing[103] (Fig. 13-33).

The results of spinal shrinkage measurements comparing sitting and standing work lend some support to the findings that, in general, loads in sitting are less than in standing. Leivseth and Drerup[106] showed that shrinkage of the lumbar spine in sitting (1.73 mm) was much less than the shrinkage in standing (4.16 mm). In a comparison of spinal shrinkage between 2 hours of relaxed sitting versus 2 hours work in standing, there actually was a gain in stature in the lumbar spine in the relaxed sitting position. Working in a standing position caused a reduction in height of 0.8 mm per lumbar disk, in comparison with 0.3 mm for work in a sitting position.[106] In another study of spinal shrinkage, van Dieen and colleagues[105] found that a larger stature gain occurred when a person spent 2 hours working in

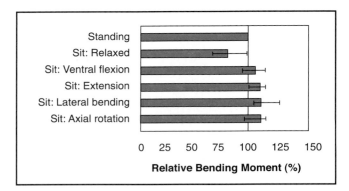

▲ **Figure 13-33** ■ A comparison of average relative bending moments in internal fixation devices from 10 patients in different sitting positions. Values are related to the corresponding value for standing. Note that bending moment in relaxed sitting is less than the bending moment in standing, but the erect sitting (shown as extension) bending moment is greater than in standing. (From Rohlmann A, Graichen F, Bergmann G: Loads on an internal spinal fixation device during physical therapy. Phys Ther 82:49, 2002. Reprinted with permission from the American Physical Therapy Association.)

dynamic chairs than in chairs with fixed seats and backs. Although dynamic chairs may be more desirable than fixed chairs, the task being performed had greater effects on spinal stature than did the type of chair.

Very few studies have investigated either the contriution of soft tissue deformation to measurements of total height loss or the shrinkage of the cervical spine. In an investigation of the soft tissue contribution to total seated height, one group of researchers found that deformation of muscle and fat below the sacrum contributed 28% to 30% at 5 and 10 minutes of loading, respectively. Soft tissue deformation always contributed a small amount to total height loss, but early in the loading cycle, height loss mostly occurred in the spine, whereas at the end of the loading cycle, the loss was a combination of spine and soft tissue.[107] Cervical spine shrinkage was investigated after 1 hour of television watching in a sitting position in the following three different head/neck positions: neutral, 20° of flexion, and 40° of flexion. The neutral head position had no effect on spinal shrinkage, in contrast to the head held at a 40° angle, when the most cervical shrinkage (approximately 1 mm) occurred in 1 hour.[108]

After a literature review, Harrison and colleagues[92] concluded that the lowest lumbar interdiskal pressures and lowest EMG readings are produced by seat back inclinations between 110° and 130°, combined with a lumbar support that protrudes 5 cm from the back of the seat back and a posterior seat inclination of 5°. The use of armrests produces further reductions.[92]

Seat Interface Pressures

Pressure is force per unit area and is measured in pascals (Pa or N/m^2 [pounds per square inch]). The pressure caused by contact forces between the person's body and the seat is referred to as the **seat interface pressure**. Pressure mapping techniques using sensor-containing mats that can be placed on the seat of a chair are used to measure average and maximum seat interface pressures (Fig. 13-34A and B). **Average seat interface pressure** is the mean of pressure sensor values, and the **maximum seat interface pressure** is the highest individual sensor value.[109]

Studies have shown that individuals with physical disabilities (myelomeningocele and paraplegia) have significantly higher seat interface pressures than do people without such disabilities.[110,111] The higher maximum seat interface pressures observed in individuals with SCI than in healthy individuals have been attributed to asymmetrical ischial loading resulting from spinal/pelvic deformities and atrophy of soft tissue over the ischiae. Kernozek et al. studied peak interface pressures in a group of 75 elderly persons with different body mass indices (BMIs). Peak seat interface pressures were found to be highest in the thin elderly persons (ones with the lowest BMI), who had the least amount of soft tissue over the ischiae.[112] These individuals probably had a smaller contact area with more concentration of pressure than did individuals with a greater

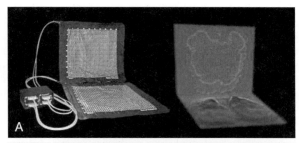

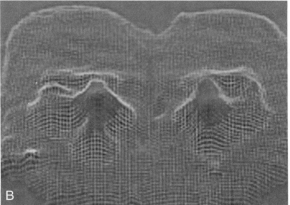

▲ **Figure 13-34** ■ **A.** Tactilus seat pad sensor used for mapping seat pressures. **B.** Three-dimensional image of the pressure distribution, which shows where highest pressures are located. (Courtesy of Sensor Products, Inc., 188 Rt. 10, Suite 307, East Hanover, NJ 07936.)

body mass with increased surface contact area and better pressure distribution. The fact that seat interface pressure has been found to be a good indicator of subcutaneous stress (with the latter being higher than the former)[113] demonstrates the importance of minimizing seat interface pressure. Changes in the position of the body, position of the chair, and the type of seat cushion employed can be employed to minimize the interface pressure.[114]

Case Application 13-10: **Need to Minimize Seat Interface Pressure**

Minimizing seat interface pressure is an extremely important consideration for our patient, Dave, who may have to spend a great deal of his time in a wheelchair. A reduction in seat interface pressures reduces the risk of developing pressure sores, which are caused by unrelieved pressure and shearing forces. When soft tissue is compressed between the seat and bony prominences (such as the ischial spines) for an extended period of time, the external pressure is higher than capillary blood flow pressure. The higher external pressure leads to ischemia (decrease in blood flow) and may lead to death of cells and tissue. Shear pressure (the horizontal force component) also may cause obstruction of blood flood and tissue death. Dave is at high risk because he has lost muscle bulk in his buttocks as a result of the paralysis affecting his hip extensor muscles.

■ **Effects of Changes in Body Posture**

Changes in the posture of the body such as forward and lateral trunk flexion can be effective means of reducing seat interface pressures in individuals like Dave who must spend long periods of time in a wheelchair.[111] Vaisbuch et al.[110] compared maximum seat interface pressures in different body positions (neutral, recline, tilt, lean forward, and lateral flexion) in a group of 15 nondisabled children and in a group of 15 children with myelomeningocele. Maximum pressures for the myelomeningocele group were significantly higher than those found in the nondisabled group for the neutral and lean forward positions. The disabled group experienced significantly lower maximum seat interface pressures in the forward and lateral flexed positions than in the neutral position. Hobson[111] compared seat interface pressure and shear in 10 healthy subjects and in 12 persons with SCIs. The individuals with SCIs had maximum seat interface pressures that, depending on which of the eight positions were assumed in the wheelchair, were 6% to 46% higher than the pressures found in the healthy group. Maximum seat interface pressures could be reduced from neutral position values by 9% when the trunk was flexed forward to 50° and reduced on the unweighted side by 30% to 40% when the trunk was laterally flexed to 15° (Fig. 13-35).

Case Application 13-11: **Pressure-Reducing Activities**

The performance of seat interface pressure–reducing activities is an essential activity for our patient. Dave

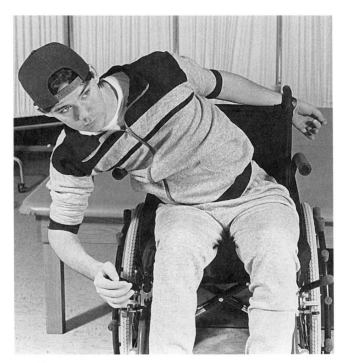

▲ **Figure 13-35** ■ The patient is able to relieve interface pressure by leaning to the side. Leaning is recommended every few minutes.

must be able to maintain stability while performing activities to alleviate pressure and be able to develop sufficient upper extremity strength to elevate his body vertically by performing push-ups on the armrests of his wheelchair. He needs to understand why these activities are important so that he will be motivated to perform them on a continual basis while he is in the wheelchair.

■ Effects of Alterations in the Position of the Chair

Alterations in the angulation of the chair's back rest in combination with footrest and seat inclinations are another method utilized to reduce seat interface pressure.

Continuing Exploration: **Positioning to Reduce Seat Interface Pressure**

Reclining the backrest posteriorly by 30° from 0° has been found to significantly reduce average seat interface pressure (but not maximum seat interface pressure). Supporting a person's feet on blocks of wood to produce 90° of flexion at the hips, knees, and ankles caused an increase in the average seat interface pressure.[109] In another study, the maximum seat interface pressure was observed to be significantly lower when sitting with a 0° backrest inclination when the feet were on the floor rather than when legs were supported on a rest.[115] Hobson[111] found that a recline of the back rest to 120° reduced the neutral backrest position values by 12%. Full body tilt to 20° reduced seat interface pressure values by 11%.

Also, cushions of various compositions and depths are used to reduce seat interface pressures. Materials used in the composition of cushions include synthetic materials, air, water, and gels of various kinds. Cushion thicknesses up to 8 cm have been found to be successful in reducing maximum subcutaneous stress inferior to the ischial tuberosity, but increasing the thickness beyond 8 cm failed to cause an additional decrease in seat interface pressure.[113]

The selection of an appropriate cushion for Dave's wheelchair will be extremely important, and different materials will need to be tried. Ideally, we should map the seat interface pressure in order to customize his seating.

◆ Analysis of Lying Postures

Interdiskal Pressures

In general, interdiskal pressures are less in lying postures than in standing and sitting postures. Wilke and colleagues[104] measured interdiskal pressures over a 24-hour period from a pressure transducer implanted in the nucleus pulposus of the nondegenerated disk between L4 and L5 of a 45-year-old healthy man.

Interdiskal pressures in supine lying (0.10 MPa) were less than in either lying prone (0.11 MPa) or lying on the side (0.12 MPa), and in all of these postures the interdiskal pressure was less than in sitting and standing postures. Lying prone with the back extended and supported on one's elbows had the largest interdiskal pressure (0.25 MPa) among the lying postures tested and was only slightly less than in slouched sitting (0.27 MPa). Rohlmann and associates conducted a study of the bending moments on spinal fixation devices in 10 patients. Movements in the lying posture such as lifting an extended arm or leg in the supine and prone positions did not raise the bending moments above bending moments in standing (Fig. 13-36). However, when the patients raised both extended legs in the supine position, peak bending moments exceeded the moments in the standing posture.[101]

Surface Interface Pressures

In order for pressure-relieving surfaces to be effective, they should be able to reduce the interface pressure below capillary closing pressure (12 mm Hg). Otherwise, blood flow may be compromised, and this may result in tissue breakdown. Also, a uniform pressure distribution over the entire available surface is desirable to prevent sections of increased pressure over certain areas. Examples of some pressure-reducing mattress surfaces include foam, air, gas, water, and gel. Other pressure-relieving surfaces include movable surfaces, usually powered by a motor or pump, which can alternatively inflate and deflate.[116]

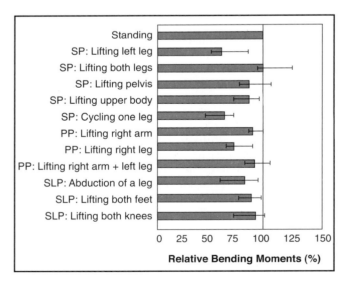

▲ **Figure 13-36** ■ Bending moments that occurred when body parts were moved as they might be in an exercise program when the body is positioned in the supine lying position (SP), prone position (PP), and side-lying position (SLP). The bending moments are compared with the moments in standing. (From Rohlman, A, Graichen, F, Bergmann, G: Loads on an internal spinal fixation device during physical therapy. Physical Theraphy 82:48, 2002. Reprinted with permission from the American Physical Therapy Association.)

Case Application 13-12: **Risk of Pressure Sore Development**

> We need to be concerned about lying postures because of the danger of developing pressure sores. Dave is at risk for skin breakdown because his lower extremity muscles may have atrophied, with an accompanying loss of protective soft tissue over bony prominences. In the supine lying posture, the areas at risk are the backs of his heels and head, his lower vertebral spine, and the sacrum. In the side-lying posture, the areas at risk are his malleoli and the heads of the femur and fibula.

◆ Effects of Age, Pregnancy, Occupation, and Recreation on Posture

Age

■ Infants and Children

Postural control in infants develops progressively during the first year of life, from control of the head to control of the body in a sitting posture and then to control of the body in a standing posture. Stability in a posture, or the ability to fix and hold a posture in relation to gravity, must be accomplished before the child is able to move within a posture. The child learns to maintain a certain posture, usually through co-contraction of antagonist and agonist muscles around a joint, and then is able to move in and out of the posture (sitting to standing and standing to sitting). Once stability is established, the child proceeds to controlled mobility and skill. Controlled mobility refers to the ability to move within the posture—for example, weight shifting in the standing posture. Skill refers to performance of activities such as walking, running, and hopping, which are dynamic postural activities.[117]

According to Woollacott,[118] by the time a child reaches 7 to 10 years of age, postural responses to platform perturbations are less variable and also comparable with those of adults in patterns of muscle activity and timing of responses. Responses of children younger than 7 years of age included greater coactivation of agonists and antagonists and slower response times for muscle activation than in either adults or older children.[118] Newell and colleagues[119] investigated CoP motion (postural sway) in different age groups from 3 years to 92 years of age. The young adult group of students in their 20s had the least amount of movement of the CoP; the individuals in the youngest and oldest groups had the greatest amount of CoP motion.

The erect standing posture in infancy and early childhood differs somewhat from postural alignment in adults, but by the time a child reaches the age of 10 or 11 years, postural alignment in the erect standing position should be similar to adult alignment.[120] However, poor postural alignment in a 7- or 8-year-old child can be recognized because it is similar to poor postural alignment in adults. For example, the poor posture may include forward head, kyphosis, lordosis, and hyperextended knees.[120]

The following two studies investigated the effects of age and gender on the thoracic and lumbar curves. Widhe[121] monitored 90 Swedish boys and girls over a 10-year period, examining them first at 5 to 6 years of age and again at 15 to 16 years of age. Between the first and second measurements, both thoracic kyphosis and lumbar lordosis increased by 6° (Table 13-8). Sagittal mobility decreased in the thoracic region by 27° (9° in flexion and 18° in extension). Lumbar flexion decreased by 9° and extension by 5°. In the second study, 847 Finnish boys and girls were examined annually from ages 10.8 years to 13.8 years. The normal thoracic kyphosis was greater and the normal lumbar lordosis less in boys than in girls both at the beginning and at each annual examination.[122] Mean thoracic kyphosis increased and mean lumbar lordosis decreased with increasing age. Despite wide variations, thoracic kyphosis was between 20° and 40° and lordosis was between 20° and 50° in both genders.[122]

■ Elderly

Postural alignment in elderly people may show a more flexed posture than in the young adult; however, many elderly individuals in their 70s and 80s still demonstrate a close-to-optimal posture. Hardacker and colleagues found that cervical lordosis increased with increasing age[48] (Fig. 13-37). Hammerberg and Wood[123] in a study of the radiographic profiles of 50 elderly individuals 70 to 85 years of age showed an average kyphosis angle of 52°, with a range of 29° to 79°, and an anterior position

Table 13-8	Age Variations in Spinal Curves in the Sagittal Plane in Standing Posture: Values in Degrees					
	Widhe[121]*		Vendantam et al.[55]†	Gelb et al.[53]	Hammerberg and Wood[123]	
	5–6 yr n = 90 Mean (SD)	15–16 yr n = 90 Mean (SD)	10–18 yr n = 88 Mean (SD)	40–49 yr n = 27 Mean (SD)	70–85 yr n = 50 Mean	Range
Thoracic	29 (9)	35 (8)	38 (10)		52	29–79
Lumbar	−31 (8)	−38 (7)	−64 (10)	−68 (11)	−57	−96 to −20

*Widhe measured the thoracic curve from a point between the spinous processes of T2 and T3 to T12. The lumbar curve was measured from a point between T11 and T12 to a point between S1 and S2. The same 90 subjects were measured at different ages.
†Vendantam et al. measured the thoracic curve from T3 to T12 and the lumbar curve from T12 to S1.

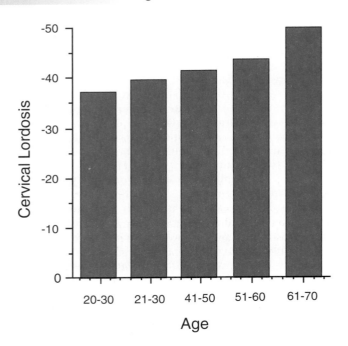

▲ **Figure 13-37** ■ The graph indicates that for the 100 volunteers in the study, the mean cervical lordosis increased with increasing age. (From Hardacker JW, Shuford RF, Capicotto PN, et al.: Radiographic standing cervical segmental alignment in adult volunteers without neck symptoms. Spine 22:1477, 1997. Reprinted with permission from Lippincott Williams & Wilkins.)

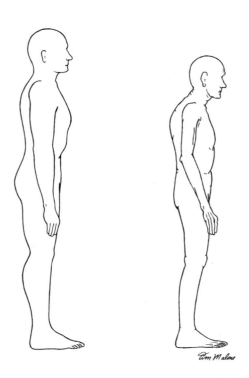

▲ **Figure 13-38** ■ Changes in posture as a result of aging.

of C7. The LoG passed, on average, 40 mm anterior to the posterosuperior corner of S1. Gelb and colleagues[53] in a study of 100 middle-aged and older volunteers (average age of 57 years) noted that as age increased, the LoG was located more anteriorly with a loss of lumbar lordosis and an increase in thoracic and thoracolumbar kyphosis. However, the mean values of 34° for thoracic kyphosis and 64° for lumbar lordosis values fell within normally accepted ranges for younger populations. No correlations were found between age and kyphosis either in the thoracic region or at the thoracolumbar junction. Only the loss of lumbar lordosis at the proximal levels showed the strongest correlation with age.[53] The flexed posture observed in some elderly persons is probably due to a number of factors, some of which may relate to aging processes (Fig. 13-38). Conditions such as osteoporosis may affect posture in elderly persons. Osteoporosis (abnormal rarefaction of bone) weakens the vertebral bodies and makes them liable to fracture. After the collapse of a series of the anterior portions of the weakened vertebrae, the normal posterior convexity of the thoracic curve increases (kyphosis). In kyphosis, the anterior trunk flexor muscles shorten as the posteriorly located trunk extensors lengthen. Teramoto and coworkers[124] evaluated the effects of kyphosis in subjects from 20 to 90 years of age. The authors found that the extent of kyphosis significantly decreased lung volume and maximal inspiratory pressure in the elderly subjects.

The ROM at the knees, hips, ankles, and trunk may be restricted because of muscle shortening and disuse atrophy. Furthermore, as voluntary postural response times in elderly people appear to be longer than in young people, elderly persons may elect to stand with a wide BoS to have a margin of safety. Postural responses of older adults, aged 61 to 78 years, to platform perturbations show differences in timing and amplitude and include greater coactivation of antagonist and agonist muscles in comparison with younger subjects, aged 19 to 38 years. Iverson and associates,[125] who tested noninstitutionalized men 60 to 90 years of age on two types of balance tests that involved one-legged stance, found that balance time and torque production decreased significantly with age. In some of the tests, the authors found that torque production was a significant predictor of balance time; that is, the greater the torque production, the longer the balance time. These authors also found that men who exercised five to six times per week had greater torque production than did men who exercised less frequently. This finding suggests that high levels of fitness and activity may have beneficial effects on the aging person's ability to perform one-legged balancing activities that are needed for activities of daily living such as walking.[125]

Case Application 13-13: **Osteoporosis Risk**

Osteoporosis may be a problem for Dave even before any significant aging because of the lack of weight-bearing on his his lower extremities. However, if Dave happens to enter one of the newer rehabilitation programs that employ treadmill walking for spinal cord–injured patients, osteoporosis may not be as much of a problem. It even may be possible that Dave might be able to gain back muscle strength in his legs and be able to walk with minimal assistance.[126,127]

Another aging consideration for Dave will be a decrease in the thickness of the skin that occurs with normal aging, including reductions in collagen, elastin, proteoglycan, and water content. Therefore, Dave will have to be extremely careful with his skin as he ages, because his skin is already at risk.

Pregnancy

Normal pregnancies are accompanied by weight gain, an increase in weight distribution in the breasts and abdomen, and softening of the ligamentous and connective tissue. The location of the woman's CoG changes because of the increase in weight and its distribution anteriorly. Consequently, postural changes in pregnancy include an increase in the lordotic curves in the cervical and lumbar areas of the vertebral column, protraction of the shoulder girdle, and hyperextension of the knees. Franklin and Conner-Kerr[128] compared postural evaluations of 12 pregnant volunteers in their first trimester with evaluations of the same women in their third trimester. These investigators found changes in lumbar angle, head position, and anterior pelvic tilt. The lumbar angle increased by an average of 5.9°, the anterior pelvic tilt increased by an average of 4°, and the head become more posterior as pregnancy progressed from the first through the third trimesters.[128] These changes in posture represent adaptations that help to maintain the CoM centered over the BoS. Softening of ligamentous and connective tissues, especially in the pelvis, sacroiliac joints, pubic symphyses, and abdomen change the support and protection offered by these structures and predispose pregnant women to strains in supporting structures.[129] Many women experience backache during pregnancy, and all of the women in the study by Franklin and Conner-Kerr complained of backache.[128]

Continuing Exploration: **Effects of Pregnancy on Sitting and Standing Postures**

Gilleard and coworkers,[130] however, did not find any significant effects of pregnancy on upper body posture of nine pregnant women during sitting and quiet standing in films taken at intervals during gestation and at 8 weeks post partum. A flattening of the thoracolumbar curve was observed in some subjects in the sitting posture as pregnancy progressed. No significant differences were found between the postpartum group and a control group in the cervical or thoracic spines, but the postpartum group stood with more thoracolumbar flexion than did the control group.

Occupation and Recreation

Each particular occupational and recreational activity has unique postures and injuries associated with these postures. Bricklayers, surgeons, carpenters, and cashiers assume and perform tasks in standing postures for a majority of the working day. Others, such as secretaries, accountants, computer operators, and receptionists, assume sitting postures for a large proportion of the day. Performing artists often assume asymmetrical postures while playing a musical instrument, dancing, or acting. Running, jogging, and long-distance walking are dynamic postures with which very specific injuries are associated.

Different sitting postures and their effects on intradiskal pressures in the lumbar spine have been analyzed.[131] Wheelchair postures and the effects of different degrees of anterior-posterior and lateral pelvic tilt on the vertebral column and trunk muscle activity in sitting postures in selected work activities also have been investigated.[132] A large portion of the research suggests that many back problems are preventable because they result from mechanical stresses produced by prolonged static postures in the forward stooping or sitting positions and the repeated lifting of heavy loads.

Many of the injuries sustained during both occupational and recreational activities belong to the category of "overuse injuries." This type of injury is caused by repetitive stress that exceeds the physiologic limits of the tissues. Muscles, ligaments, and tendons are especially vulnerable to the effects of repetitive tensile forces, whereas bones and cartilage are susceptible to injury from the application of excessive compressive forces. A random sample of professional musicians in New York revealed that violin, piano, cello, and bass players were frequently affected by back and neck problems.[133] In a larger study involving 485 musicians, the authors found that 64% had painful overuse syndromes. The majority of problems were associated with the musculotendinous unit, and others involved bones, joints, bursae, and muscle. String players experienced shoulder and neck problems caused by the maintenance of abnormal head and neck positions, whereas flute players had shoulder problems associated with maintaining an externally rotated shoulder position that has to be assumed for prolonged periods during performances and practices.[134] Peripheral nerve disorders, including thoracic outlet syndrome, ulnar neuropathy at the elbow, and carpal tunnel syndrome, also appear to be common playing-related disorders.[135,136]

Case Application 13-14: **Succeptibility to Overuse Injuries**

Dave will be succeptible to the same type of upper extremity overuse injuries that are incurred by any sitting worker performing a repetitive task such as data entry. If he chooses to use a hand-propelled wheelchair as his main method of transportation, he could be at risk for shoulder, elbow, and wrist overuse injuries. If he is able to use crutches, he may incur shoulder and wrist overuse injuries.

Each occupational and recreational activity requires a detailed biomechanical analysis of the specific postures involved to determine how abnormal and excessive stresses can be relieved. Sometimes the analysis involves not only a person's posture but also features of the work-site such as chair or table height, weight of objects to be lifted or carried, and weight and shape of a musical instrument or tool. Intervention may involve a combination of modifications of the environment, adaptations of the instrument or tools, and modifications of posture.

Case Application 13-15: **Future Progression from Static to Dynamic Postures**

We have identified some of the problems that may face our patient, Dave, in static postures. He will now progress from static sitting and standing postures to walking. Because he is a former athlete, we hope that he may want to participate in activities such as wheel-chair basketball or in wheelchair marathons. However, the treatment of SCI is changing dramatically, and Dave may not be confined to a wheelchair. Advances in treatment are helping some individuals regain sufficient muscle strength to be able to walk without braces, and we hope that Dave will be able to benefit from these new treatment programs.[126,127]

Summary

In this chapter, we introduced the basic aspects of postural control and analyzed normal postural alignment in the erect standing position. Also, we discussed some of the internal and external forces affecting sitting and lying postures primarily in relation to how they may affect our patient, Dave. The kinematic and kinetic information provided in this chapter and previous chapters forms the basis for the analysis of static posture as well as the dynamic posture of gait.

Study Questions

1. What is a "sway envelope"?
2. Is quadriceps muscle activity necessary to maintain knee extension in static erect stance? Explain your answer.
3. Is activity of the abdominal muscles necessary to keep the pelvis level in static standing posture? Explain your answer.
4. How does the lumbar curve change from standing to sitting, and what effect does the change have on interdiskal pressures?
5. In which areas of the vertebral column would you expect to find the most stress in the erect standing posture? Why?
6. For the erect standing posture, identify the type of stresses that would be affecting the following structures: apophyseal joints in the lumbar region, apophyseal joint capsules in the thoracic region, anulus fibrosus in L5 to S1, anterior longitudinal ligament in the thoracic region, and the sacroiliac joints.
7. What effect might tight hamstrings have on the alignment of the following structures during erect stance: pelvis, lumbosacral angle, hip joint, knee joint, and the lumbar region of the vertebral column?
8. How would you describe a typical idiopathic lateral curvature of the vertebral column?
9. Describe the moments that would be acting at all body segments as a result of an unexpected forward movement of a supporting surface. Describe the muscle activity that would be necessary to bring the body's LoG over the CoP.
10. Identify the changes in body segments that are commonly used in scoliosis screening programs.
11. Explain how our patient manages to stand when he lacks lower extremity musculature and elements of postural control.
12. How do postural responses to perturbations of the erect standing posture in elderly persons compare with responses of children who are 1 to 6 years of age?
13. Compare a flexed lumbar spine posture with an extended posture in terms of the nutrition of the disks and stresses on ligaments and joint structures.
14. What is the relationship between the GRFV, LoG, and CoM in the erect static posture?
15. Explain how a hallux valgus deformity develops.
16. Describe the effects of a forward head posture on the zygapophyseal joints and capsules, intervertebral disks, vertebral column ligaments, and muscles.
17. Explain the possible effects on body structures in a young person with a double major curve (right thoracic, left lumbar)
18. Explain how changes in body position affect seat interface pressures.
19. Compare interdiskal pressures in erect standing with erect, slumped, and relaxed sitting.
20. Compare interdiskal pressures in sitting postures with pressures in lying postures.

References

1. Panjabi MM, White AA: Biomechanics in the Musculosketal System. Philadelphia, Churchill Livingstone, 2001.
2. Nordin M, Frankel VH: Basic Biomechanics of the Musculoskeletal System, 3rd ed. Philadelphia, Lippincott Williams & Wilkins, 2001.
3. Horak FB, Henry SM, Shumway-Cook A: Postural perturbations: New insights for treatment of balance disorders. Phys Ther 77:517, 1997.
4. Maki BE, McIlroy WE: The role of limb movements in maintaining upright stance: The "change- in-support strategy." Phys Ther 77:489, 1997.
5. DiFabio RP, Emasithi A: Aging and the mechanisms underlying head and postural control during voluntary motion. Phys Ther 77:458, 1997.
6. Clement G, Lestienne F: Adaptive modifications of postural attitude in conditions of weightlessness. Exp Brain Res 72:381,1988.
7. Speers RA, Paloski WH, Kuo AD: Multivariate changes in coordination of postural control following spaceflight. J Biomech 31:883, 1998.
8. Garn SN, Newton RA: Kinesthetic awareness in subjects with multiple ankle sprains. Phys Ther 68: 1667, 1988.
9. Forkin DM, Koczur C, Battle R, et al.: Evaluation of kinesthetic defects indicative of balance control in gymnasts with unilateral chronic ankle sprains. J Orthop Sports Phys Ther 23:245, 1996.
10. Bernier JN, Perrin DH: Effect of coordination training on proprioception of the functionally unstable ankle. J Orthop Sports Phys Ther 27:264, 1998.
11. Dietz V: Evidence for a load receptor contribution to the control of posture and locomotion. Neurosci Biobehav Rev 22:495, 1998.
12. Allum JH, Bloem BR, Carpenter MG, et al.: Proprioceptive control of posture: A review of new concepts. Gait Posture 8:214, 1998.
13. Hodges PW, Gurfinkel VS, Brumagne S, et al.: Coexistence of stability and mobility in postural control: Evidence from postural compensation for respiration. Exp Brain Res 144:293, 2002.
14. Runge CF, Shupert CL, Horak FB, et al.: Ankle and hip postural strategies defined by joint torques. Gait Posture 10:161, 1999.
15. Horak FB: Measurement of movement patterns to study postural coordination. Proceedings of the 10th Annual Eugene Michels Research Forum, American Physical Therapy Association Section on Research, New Orleans, LA, 1990.
16. Nashner LM: Sensory, neuromuscular, and biomechanical contributions to human balance. Proceedings of the 10th Annual Eugene Michels Research Forum, American Physical Therapy Research Association Section on Research, New Orleans, LA, 1990.
17. Keshner, EA: Reflex, voluntary and mechanical processes in postural stabilization. Proceedings of the Proceedings of the 10th Annual Eugene Michels Research Forum, American Physical Therapy Research Association Section on Research, New Orleans, LA, 1990.
18. Luchies CW, Alexander NB, Schultz AB, et al.: Stepping responses of young and old adults to postural disturbances: Kinematics. J Am Geriatr Soc 42:506, 1994.
19. Luchies CW, Wallace D, Pazdur R, et al.: Effects of age on balance assessment using voluntary and involuntary step tasks. J Gerontol A Biol Med Sci 54:M140, 1999.
20. Wojcik LA, Thelen DG, Schultz AB, et al.: Age and gender differences in peak lower extremity joint torques and ranges of motion used during single-step balance recovery from a forward fall. J Biomech 34:67, 2001.
21. Van Wegen EEH, van Emmerik REA, Riccio GE: Postural orientation: Age-related changes in variability and time-to-boundary. Hum Mov Sci 21:61, 2002.
22. Hunter MC, Hoffman MA: Postural control: Visual and cognitive manipulations. Gait Posture 13:41, 2001.
23. Rankin JK, Woollacott MH, Shumway-Cook A, et al.: Cognitive influence on postural stability: A neuromuscular analysis in young and older adults. J Gerontol 55:M112, 2000.
24. Melzer I, Benjuya N, Kaplanski J: Age-related changes in postural control: Effect of cognitive tasks. Gerontology 47:189, 2001.
25. Redfern MS, Jennings JR, Martin C, et al.: Attention influences sensory integration for postural control in older adults. Gait Posture 14:211, 2001.
26. Woollacott M, Shumway-Cook A : Attention and the control of posture and gait: A review of an emerging area of research. Gait Posture 16:1, 2002.
27. Schenkman M: Interrelationship of neurological and mechanical factors in balance control. Proceedings of the Proceedings of the 10th Annual Eugene Michels Research Forum, American Physical Therapy Research Association Section on Research, New Orleans, LA, 1990.
28. Aramaki Y, Nozaki D, Masani K, et al.: Reciprocal angular acceleration of the ankle and hip joints during quiet standing in humans. Exp Brain Res 136:463, 2001.
29. Rogers M: Dynamic biomechanics of normal foor and ankle during walking and running. Phys Ther 68:1822, 1988.
30. Cailliet R: Soft Tissue Pain and Disability, 3rd ed. Philadelphia, FA Davis, 1996.
31. Danis CG, Krebs DE, Gill-Body KM, et al.: Relationship between standing posture and stability. Phys Ther 78:502, 1998.
32. Carlsoo S: The static muscle load in different work positions: An electromyographic study. Ergonomics 4:193, 1961.
33. Soames RW, Atha J: The role of antigravity muscles during quiet standing in man. Appl Phys 47: 159, 1981.

34. Gray ER: The role of the leg muscles in variations of the arches in normal and flat feet. Phys Ther 49:1084, 1969.

35. Kagaya H, Sharma M, Kobetic R, et al.: Ankle, knee, and hip moments during standing with and without joint contractures: Simulation study for functional electrical stimulation. Am J Phys Med Rehabil 77:49, 1998.

36. Edelstein JE, Bruckner J: Orthotics: A Comprehensive Clinical Approach. Thorofare, NJ, Slack, Inc., 2002.

37. Schmitz TJ: Traumatic spinal cord injury. In O'Sullivan SB, Schmitz TJ (eds): Physical Rehabilitation: Assessment and Treatment, 4th ed. Philadelphia, FA Davis, 2001.

38. Kendall F, McCreary EK: Muscles: Testing and Function, 4th ed. Baltimore, Williams & Wilkins, 1983.

39. Duval-Beaupere G, Schmidt C, Cosson P: A barycentremetric study of the sagittal shape of spine and pelvis: The conditions required for an economic standing position. Ann Biomed Eng 20:451, 1992.

40. Don Tigny RL: Dysfunction of the sacroiliac joint and its treatment. J Orthop Sports Phys Ther 1:1,1979.

41. Basmajian JV: Muscles Alive, 4th ed. Baltimore, Williams & Wilkins, 1978.

42. Sahrmann SA: Diagnosis and Treatment of Movement Impairment Syndromes. St. Louis, CV Mosby, 2002.

43. Bogduk N: Clinical Anatomy of the Lumbar Spine and Sacrum, 3rd ed. New York, Churchill Livingstone, 1997.

44. Cailliet R: Low Back Pain Syndrome, 5th ed. Philadelphia, FA Davis, 1995.

45. Youdas JW, Garrett TR, Harmsen S, et al.: Lumbar lordosis and pelvic inclination of asymptomatic adults. Phys Ther 76:1066, 1996.

46. Korovessis PG, Stamatakis MV, Baikousis AG: Reciprocal angulation of vertebral bodies in the sagittal plane in an asymptomatic Greek population. Spine 23:700, 1998.

47. Korovessis P, Stamatakis M, Baikousis A: Segmental roentgenographic analysis of vertebral inclination on sagittal plane in asymptomatic versus chronic low back pain patients. J Spinal Disord 12:131, 1999.

48. Hardacker JW, Shuford RF, Capicotto PN, et al.: Radiographic standing cervical segmental alignment in adult volunteers without neck symptoms. Spine 22:1472, 1997.

49. Lord MJ, Small JM, Dinsay JM, et al.: Lumbar lordosis: Effects of sitting and standing. Spine 22:2571, 1997.

50. Jackson RP, McManus AC: Radiographic analysis of sagittal plane alignment and balance in standing volunteers and patients with low back pain matched for age, sex and size. Spine 19:1611, 1994.

51. Jackson RP, Kanemura T, Kawakami N, et al.: Lumbopelvic lordosis and pelvic balance on repeated standing lateral radiographs of adult volunteers and untreated patients with constant low back pain. Spine 25:575, 2000.

52. Jackson RP, Hales C: Congruent spinopelvic alignment on standing lateral radiographs of adult volunteers. Spine 25:2808, 2000.

53. Gelb DE, Lenke LG, Bridwell KH, et al.: An analysis of sagittal spinal alignment in 100 asymptomatic middle and older aged volunteers. Spine 20:1351, 1995.

54. Cailliet R: Neck and Arm Pain, 3rd ed. Philadelphia, FA Davis, 1991.

55. Vendantam R, Lenke LG, Keeney JA, et al.: Comparison of standing sagittal spinal alignment in asymptomatic adolescents and adults. Spine 23:211, 1998.

56. Morris JM, et al.: An electromyographic study of intrinsic muscles of the back in man. J Anat 96: 509,1962.

57. Mizrabi J: Biomechanics of unperturbed standing balance. In Dvir Z (ed): Clinical Biomechanics. Philadelphia, Churchill Livingstone, 2000.

58. Visscher CM, de Boer W, Naeije M: The relationship between posture and curvature of the cervical spine. J Manipulative Physiol Ther 21:388, 1998.

59. Riegger-Krugh C, Keysor JJ: Skeletal malalignments of the lower quarter: Correlated and compensatory motions and postures. Phys Ther 23:164, 1996.

60. Magee DJ: Orthopedic Physical Assessment, 4th ed. Philadelphia, WB Saunders, 2002.

61. Valmassy RL: Clinical Biomechanics of the Lower Extremities. St. Louis, CV Mosby, 1996.

62. Myerson MS, Shereff MJ: The pathological anatomy of claw and hammer toes. J Bone Joint Surg Am 71:45, 1989.

63. Perry J, Antonelli D, Ford W: Analysis of knee-joint forces during flexed-knee stance. J Bone Joint Surg Am 57:961, 1975.

64. Adams MA, Hutton WC: The effect of posture on the diffusion into lumbar intervertebral discs. J Anat 147:121, 1986.

65. Adams MA, Hutton WC: The effect of posture on the lumbar spine. J Bone Joint Surg Br 47:625, 1985.

66. Williams PL (ed): Gray's Anatomy, 38th ed. New York, Churchill Livingstone, 1995.

67. Taber's Cyclopedic Medical Dictionary, 17th ed. Philadelphia, FA Davis, 1993.

68. Mosby's Pocket Dictionary of Medicine, Nursing and Allied Health. St. Louis, CV Mosby, 1990.

69. Cailliet R: Knee Pain and Disability, 3rd ed. Philadelphia, FA Davis, 1992.

70. Jeong GK, Errico TJ: Adolescent idiopathic scoliosis. Medscape Orthop Sports Med 6(1), 2002.

71. Edgar M: A new clarification of adolescent idiopathic scoliosis. Lancet 27:270, 2002.

72. Chan V, Fong GC, Luk KD, et al.: A genetic locus for adolescent idiopathic scoliosis linked to chromosome 19p13.3. Am J Hum Genet 71:401, 2002.

73. Lenke LG, Betz RR, Clements D, et al.: Curve prevalence of a new classification of operative adolescent idiopathic scoliosis: Does classification correlate with treatment? Spine 27:604, 2002.

74. Jensen GM, Wilson KB: Horizontal postrotatory nystagmus response in female subjects with adolescent idiopathic scoliosis. Phys Ther 59: 10,1979.

75. Yekutiel M, Robin GC, Yarom R: Proprioceptive function in children with adolescent scoliosis. Spine 6:560, 1981.

76. Miller NH, Mims B, Child A, et al.: Genetic analysis of structural elastic fiber and collagen genes in familial adolescent idiopathic scoliosis. J Orthop Res 14:994, 1996.

77. Dretakis EK, Paraskevaidis CH, Zarkadoulas V, et al.: Electroencephalographic study of schoolchildren with adolescent idiopathic scoliosis. Spine 13:143, 1988.

78. Geissele AE, Kransdorf MJ, Geyer CA, et al.: Magnetic resonance imaging of the brain stem in adolescent idiopathic scoliosis. Spine 16:761, 1991.

79. Machida M, Dubousset J, Imamura Y, et al.: Pathogenesis of idiopathic scoliosis: SEP's in chicken with experimentally induced scoliosis and in patients with idiopathic scoliosis. J Pediatr Orthop 14:329, 1994.

80. Nault M-L, Allard P, Hinse S, et al.: Relations between standing stability and body posture parameters in adolescent idiopatic scoliosis. Spine 27: 1911, 2002.

81. Goldberg CJ, Dowling FE, Fogarty EE, et al.: Adolescent idiopathic scoliosis as developmental instability. Genetica 96:247, 1995.

82. Goldberg CJ, Fogarty EE, Moore DP, et al.: Scoliosis and developmental theory: Adolescent idiopathic scoliosis. Spine 22:2228, 1997.

83. Ahn UM, Ahn NU, Nallamshetty L, et al.: The etiology of adolescent idiopathic scoliosis. Am J Orthop 31:387, 2002.

84. Lidstrom J, Friberg S, Lindstrom L, et al.: Postural control in siblings of scoliosis patients and scoliosis patients. Spine 13:1070, 1988.

85. Murray DW, Bulstrode CJ: The development of adolescent idiopathic scoliosis. Eur Spine J 5:251, 1996.

86. Roach JW: Adolescent idiopathic scoliosis. Orthop Clin North Am 30:353, 1999.

87. Winter RB, Moe JH: A plea for routine school examination of children for spinal deformity. Minn Med 57:419, 1974.

88. Delorme S, Labelle H, Aubin C-E: The crankshaft phenomenon: Is Cobb angle progression a good indicator in adolescent idiopathic scoliosis? Spine 27:E145, 2002.

89. Francis RS: Scoliosis screening of 3,000 college-aged women: The Utah study. Phase 2. Phys Ther 68:1513,1988.

90. AAOS Online Service Patient Education Brochures: Scoliosis. Available at http://orthoinfo. aaos.org/.

91. American Physical Therapy Association: APTA Scoliosis Brochure. Available at www.apta.org/ptandbody/showcontent.cfm?content.

92. Harrison DD, Harrison SO, Croft AC, et al.: Sitting biomechanics part Review of the literature. J Manipulative Physiol Ther 22:594, 1999.

93. O'Sullivan PB, Grahamslaw KM, Kendell M, et al.: The effect of different standing and sitting postures on trunk muscle activity in a pain-free population. Spine 27:1238, 2002.

94. Callaghan JP, Dunk NM : Examination of the flexion relaxation phenomenon in erector spinae muscles during short duration slumped sitting. Clin Biomech 17:353, 2002.

95. Andersson GBJ, Ortengren R, Schultz A: Analysis and measurement of the loads on the lumbar spine during work at a table. J Biomech 13: 513,1980.

96. Seelen HA, Vuurman EF: Compensatory muscle activity for sitting posture during upper extremity task performance in paraplegic persons. Scand J Rehabil 23:89, 1991.

97. Callaghan JP, McGill SM: Low back joint loading and kinematics during standing and unsupported sitting. Ergonomics 44:280, 2001.

98. Betz U, Bodem F, Hopf C, et al.: [Function of back extensor muscles in upright standing position and during sitting with identical back posture—An electromyography study.] Z Orthop Ihre Grenzgeb 139:147, 2001.

99. Snijders CJ, Bakker MP, Vleeming A, et al.: Oblique abdominal muscle activity in standing and sitting on hard and soft seats. Clin Biomech (Bristol, Avon) 10:73, 1995.

100. Aaras A, Fostervold KI, Ro O, et al.: Postural load during VDU work: A comparison between various work postures. Ergonomics 40:1255, 1997.

101. Nachemson AL: Disc pressure measurements. Spine 6:93, 1981.

102. Wilke H-J, Neef P, Hinz B, et al.: Intradiscal pressures together with anthropometric data—A data set for the validation of models. Clin Biomech (Bristol, Avon) 16(Suppl 1):S111, 2001.

103. Rohlmann A, Graichen F, Bergmann G: Loads on an internal spinal fixation device during physical therapy. Phys Ther 82:44, 2002.

104. Wilke H-J, Neef P, Caimi M, et al.: New *in vivo* measurements of pressures in the intervertebral disc in daily life. Spine 24:755, 1999.

105. van Dieen JH, de Looze MP, Hermans V: Effects of dynamic office chairs on trunk kinematics, trunk extensor EMG and spinal shrinkage. Ergonomics 44:739, 2001.

106. Leivseth G, Drerup B : Spinal shrinkage during work in a sitting posture compared to work in a standing posture. Clin Biomech 12:409, 1997.

107. Kanlayanaphotporn R, Trott P, Williams M, et al.: Contribution of soft tissue deformation below the sacrum to the measurement of total height loss in sitting. Ergonomics 44:685, 2000.

108. Bonney RA, Corlett EN: Head posture and loading of the spine. Appl Ergon 33:415, 2002.

109. Stinson MD, Poter-Armstrong A, Eakin P: Seat-interface pressure: A pilot study of the relationship to gender, body mass index and seating position. Arch Phys Med Rehabil 84:405, 2003.

110. Vaisbuch N, Meyer S, Weiss PL: Effect of seated posture on interface pressure in children who are

able-bodied and who have myelomeningocele. Disabil Rehabil 22:749, 2000.

111. Hobson DA: Comparative effects of posture on pressure and shear at the body-seat interface. J Rehabil Res Develop 29:21, 1992.

112. Kernozek TW, Wilder PA, Amundson A, et al.: The effects of body mass index on peak-interface pressure of institutionalized elderly. Arch Phys Med Rehabil 83:868, 2002.

113. Regan R : Seat-interface pressures on various thicknesses of foam wheelchair cushions: A finite modeling approach. Arch Phys Med Rehabil 83: 872, 2002.

114. Defloor T, Grypdonck MH: Sitting posture and prevention of pressure ulcers. Appl Nurs Res 12:136, 1999.

115. Goosens RHM, Snijders CJ: Design criteria for the reduction of shear forces in beds and seats. J Biomech 28:225, 1994.

116. Gutierrez A: Pressure lessons. Rehab Manag 15: 44, 2002.

117. O'Sullivan SB: Motor control assessment. In O'Sullivan SB, Schmitz TJ (eds): Physical Rehabilitation: Assessment and Treatment, 4th ed. Philadelphia, FA Davis, 2001.

118. Woollacott M: Postural control mechanisms in the young and old. Proceedings of the American Physical Therapy Association (APTA) Forum, APTA, Alexandria, VA, 1990.

119. Newell KM, Slobounov SM, Slobounova ES, et al.: Short-term non-stationarity and the development of postural control. Gait Posture 6:56, 1997.

120. Connolly B: Postural applications in the child and adult. In Kraus S (ed): Clinics in Physical Therapy, Vol 11. New York, Churchill Livingstone, 1988.

121. Widhe T: Spine: Posture, mobility and pain. A longitudinal study from childhood to adolesence. Eur Spine J 10:118, 2001.

122. Nissinen M : Spinal posture during pubertal growth. Acta Paediatr 84:308, 1995.

123. Hammerberg EM, Wood KB: Sagittal profile of the elderly. J Spinal Disord Tech 16:44, 2003.

124. Teramoto S, Suzuki M, Matsuse T, et al.: [Influence of kyphosis on the age-related decline in pulmonary function.] Nippon Ronen Igakkai Zasshi 35:23, 1998.

125. Iverson BD, Gossman MR, Shaddeau SA, et al.: Balance performance, force production, and activity levels in noninstitutionalized men 60 to 90 years of age. Phys Ther 70:348, 1990.

126. Field-Fote EC: Spinal cord control of movement: Implications for locomotor rehabilitation following spinal cord injury. Phys Ther 80:477, 2000.

127. Behrman AL, Harkema SJ: Locomotor training after human spinal cord injury: A series of case studies. Phys Ther 80:688, 2000.

128. Franklin ME, Conner-Kerr T: An analysis of posture and back pain in the first and third trimesters of pregnancy. J Orthop Sports Phys Ther 28:133, 1998.

129. Gleeson PB, Pauls JA: Obstetrical physical therapy: Review of literature. Phys Ther 68:1699, 1988.

130. Gilleard WL, Crosbie J, Smith R: Static trunk posture in sitting and standing during pregnancy and early postpartum. Arch Phys Med Rehabil 83: 1739, 2002.

131. Andersson GBJ, Ortengren R, Schultz A: Analysis and measurement of the loads on the lumbar spine during work at a table. J Biomech 13:513, 1979.

132. Borello-France DF, Burdett RG, Gee ZL: Modification of sitting posture of patients with hemiplegia using seat boards and backboards. Phys Ther 68:67, 1988.

133. Brody JE: For artists and musicians creativity can mean illness and injury. New York Times, October 17, 1989.

134. Lockwood AH: Medical problems of performing artists. N Engl J Med 320:221, 1989.

135. Lederman RJ: Neuromuscular and musculoskeletal problems in instrumental musicians. Muscle Nerve 27:549, 2003.

136. Joubrel I, Robineau S, Petrilli S, et al.: [Musculoskeletal disorders in instrumental musicians: Epidemiological study.] Ann Readapt Med Phys 44:72, 2001.

◆ Introduction

In human locomotion (ambulation, gait), the reader is given the opportunity to discover how individual joints and muscles function in an integrated manner both to maintain upright posture and to produce motion of the body as a whole. Knowledge of the kinematics and kinetics of normal ambulation provides the reader with a foundation for analyzing, identifying, and correcting abnormalities in gait.

Human locomotion, or gait, may be described as a translatory progression of the body as a whole, produced by coordinated, rotatory movements of body segments.[1] The alternating movements of the lower extremities essentially support and carry along the head, arms, and trunk (HAT).[2] HAT constitutes about 75% of total body weight, with the head and arms contributing about 25% of total body weight and the trunk contributing the remaining 50%.[3] Walking is probably the most comprehensively studied of all human movements, and the variety of technologies, coupled with the diversity of disciplinary perspectives, has produced a complex and sometimes daunting literature. Nevertheless, the biomechanical requirements of the movement that explain gait are logical and easily understood if the detail is not permitted to cloud comprehension. The purpose of this chapter is to provide this comprehension of gait that will serve as the foundation for analysis of normal walking and of gait deviations.

General Features

In early gait analysis, investigators used cinematographic film. Until about 20 years ago, sophisticated analysis required frame-by-frame hand-digitizing of markers that had been placed on body landmarks. These data were coupled with knowledge of the center of pressure (CoP) of the foot-floor forces derived from a force platform to give complete, if simplified, kinetic information. This is referred to as the **inverse dynamic approach** with link segment mechanics. Electrogoniometers fastened to joints were also commonly used to describe joint motion and still have applications.[4] Similarly, electromyography (EMG) has been used for many decades, although the expectation that it would be possible to convert those signals to force values in simple, useful ways has not been fulfilled. The past two decades have witnessed an explosion of technical advancements in motion analysis whose greatest virtue is the ability to collect and process large amounts of data. As with the development of any science, the knowledge available far exceeds its current applications. A modern gait laboratory (Fig. 14-1) includes some kind of motion analysis system that gives precise marker locations that are subsequently used to model

a several-segment body with joint centers and centers of mass. One or more force platforms provide simultaneous foot-floor forces. EMG systems provide simultaneous information from surface or, sometimes, indwelling electrodes. An excellent and engaging report of the evolution of clinical gait analysis, including motion analysis and EMG, can be found in Sutherland's articles.[5,6]

To understand gait, let us first identify the fundamental purposes. Winter[7] proposed the following five main tasks for walking gait:

1. maintenance of support of the HAT: that is, preventing collapse of the lower limb
2. maintenance of upright posture and balance of the body
3. control of the foot trajectory to achieve safe ground clearance and a gentle heel or toe landing
4. generation of mechanical energy to maintain the present forward velocity or to increase the forward velocity
5. absorption of mechanical energy for shock absorption and stability or to decrease the forward velocity of the body

The professional staff at Rancho Los Amigos National Rehabilitation Center in California identified three main tasks in walking: (1) weight acceptance (WA), (2) single-limb support, and (3) swing limb advancement.[8] Although worded differently, these concepts correspond to Winter's first three tasks. However, the body moves only because energy is generated by means of concentric contraction of muscle groups. In fact, normal walking at a constant velocity requires small bursts of energy from three muscle groups at two important times in the gait cycle. Likewise, unless energy is removed with each step through eccentric muscle contractions, the velocity of walking would continue to increase.

14-1	**Patient Case**

Marlene Brown is a 63-year-old woman who sustained a stroke 15 days ago and shows right hemiparesis of her arm and leg. She has been in a rehabilitation unit for 10 days and is making good progress walking, although she is ambulating at only 0.20 m/sec. She has weakness in several muscle groups of her lower limb, notably the ankle plantarflexors, ankle dorsiflexors, knee extensors, and hip flexors, with distal muscles more affected than proximal ones. Particularly troublesome is the inability to clear her foot during the swing phase of gait. She uses a cane with a large base (a four-point cane) in her unaffected hand for stability. What will you expect to be the main difficulties with her gait, and what will you attempt to change with rehabilitation?

■ **Gait Initiation**

Gait initiation may be defined as a stereotyped activity that includes the series or sequence of events that occur from the initiation of movement to the beginning of the gait cycle. Gait initiation begins in the erect stand-

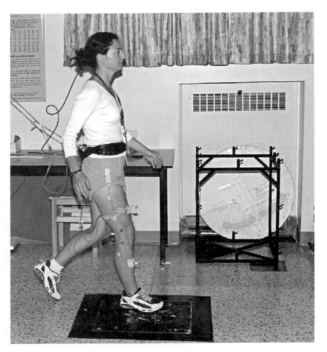

▲ **Figure 14-1** ■ A modern gait laboratory.

ing posture with an activation of the tibialis anterior and vastus lateralis muscles, in conjunction with an inhibition of the gastrocnemius muscle. Bilateral concentric contractions of the tibialis anterior muscle (pulling on the tibias) results in a sagittal torque that inclines the body anteriorly from the ankles. Initially, the CoP is described as shifting either posteriorly and laterally toward the swing foot (foot that is preparing to take the first step)[9] or posteriorly and medially toward the supporting limb.[10] Abduction of the swing hip occurs almost simultaneously with contractions of the tibialis anterior and vastus lateralis muscles and produces a coronal torque that propels the body toward the support limb. According to Elble and colleagues,[9] the support limb hip and knee flex a few degrees (3° to 10°), and the CoP moves anteriorly and medially toward the support limb. This anterior and medial shift of the CoP frees the swing limb so that it can leave the ground. The gait initiation activity ends when either the stepping or swing extremity lifts off the ground[9] or when the heel strikes the ground.[10] The total duration of the gait initiation phase is about 0.64 second.[8] A healthy individual may initiate gait with either the right or left lower extremity, and no changes will be seen in the pattern of events.

Case Application 14-1: **Avoiding Instability in Initiation of Gait**

Patients with hemiplegia (one-sided paralysis), like Ms. Brown, demonstrate a considerable difference between gait initiation that begins with a step by the affected leg and gait initiation that begins with a step by the nonaf-

fected leg. The time when the affected leg initiates gait the pattern of events is practically the same as in a non-affected person, but when the person with paralysis attempts gait initiation with the nonaffected leg, the pattern of events is erratic, and stability is seriously threatened[10].

◆ Kinematics

Phases of the Gait Cycle

Gait has been divided into a number of segments that make it possible to describe, understand, and analyze the events that are occurring. A **gait cycle** spans two successive events of the same limb, usually initial contact (also called heel contact or heel strike) of the lower extremity with the supporting surface. During one gait cycle, each extremity passes through two major phases: a **stance phase,** when some part of the foot is in contact with the floor, which makes up about 60% of the gait cycle,[11] and a **swing phase,** when the foot is not in contact with the floor, which makes up the remaining 40%[11,12] (Fig. 14-2). There are two periods of **double support** occurring between the time one limb makes initial contact and the other one leaves the floor at toe-off. At a normal walking speed, each period of double support occupies about 11% of the gait cycle, which makes a total of approximately 22% for a full cycle.[13] The body is thus supported by only one limb for nearly 80% of the cycle. The approximate value of 10% for each double-support phase is usually used. The approximate value of 10% for each double-support

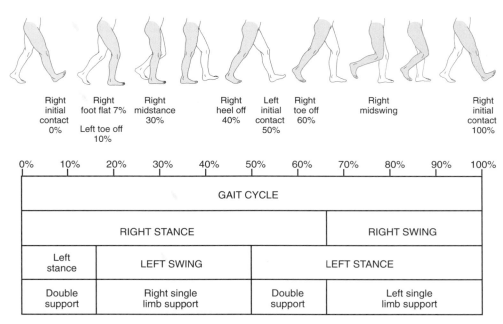

▲ **Figure 14-2** ■ A gait cycle spans the period between initial contact of the reference extremity (right) and the successive contact of the same extremity. This figure shows the gait cycle with major events: stance and swing phases for each limb and periods of single and double support. The stance phase constitutes 60% of the gait cycle, and the swing phase constitutes 40% of the cycle at normal walking speeds. Increases or decreases in walking speeds alter the percentages of time spent in each phase.

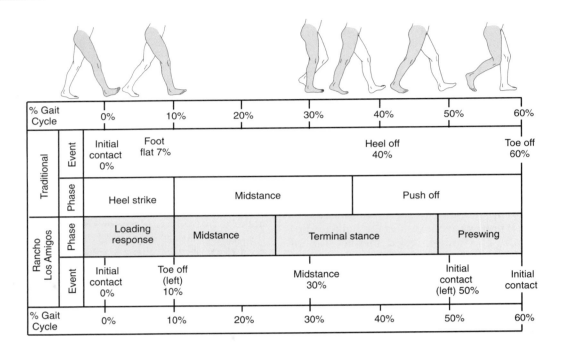

▲ **Figure 14-3** ■ The stance phase of a gait cycle of the right lower limb with comparisons between traditional and Rancho Los Amigos terminologies. The events that delimit subphases are shown for each terminology and expressed as percentages of full gait cycle. FF, foot flat; HO, heel-off; IC, initial contact; IC(L), initial contact of left (contralateral) limb; MS, midstance.

phase is usually assigned to each of the two double-support periods.

The two most common terminologies for the further division of these major phases into sub phases are shown in Figures 14-3 and 14-4, where one will be referred to as traditional (T), and one derived from Rancho Los Amigos (RLA). Both terminologies define "events" that mark the start and end of defined subphases.

Figure 14-3 identifies the events delimiting the major phases in both terminology conventions as **initial contact** (T and RLA) or **heel contact** or **heel strike** (T)

and **toe-off** (RLA and T). In both conventions, the gait cycle is divided into percentiles that will be used to clarify events and phases. Values for normal walking appear in the figures.

■ **Events in Stance Phase**

1. *Heel contact* or *heel strike* (T) refers to the instant at which the heel of the leading extremity strikes the ground (Fig. 14-5). The word "strike" is actually a misnomer inasmuch as the horizontal velocity reduces to about 0.4 m/sec and only 0.05 m/sec vertically.[14] *Initial contact* (T and RLA) refers to the instant the foot of the leading extremity strikes the ground.[8] In normal gait, the heel is the point of contact. In abnormal gait, it is possible for the whole foot or the toes, rather than the heel, to make initial contact with the ground. The term initial contact will be used in referring to this event.

2. *Foot flat* (T) in normal gait occurs after initial contact at approximately 7% of the gait cycle (Fig. 14-6). It is the first instant during stance when the foot is flat on the ground.

3. *Midstance* (T) is the point at which the body weight is directly over the supporting lower extremity (Fig. 14-7), usually about 30% of the gait cycle.

4. *Heel-off* (T) is the point at which the heel of the reference extremity leaves the ground (Fig. 14-8), usually about 40% of the gait cycle.

5. *Toe-off* (T and RLA) is the instant at which the toe of the foot leaves the ground (Fig. 14-9), usually about 60% of the gait cycle.

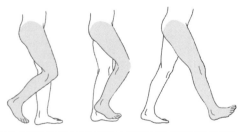

	Early swing 60-75%	Midswing 75-85%	Late swing 85-100%
Traditional	Early swing 60-75%	Midswing 75-85%	Late swing 85-100%
Ranchos Los Amigos	Initial swing 60-73%	Midswing 73-87%	Terminal swing 87-100%

▲ **Figure 14-4** ■ The swing phase of a gait cycle of the right lower limb with comparisons between traditional and Rancho Los Amigos terminologies. Differences are insignificant.

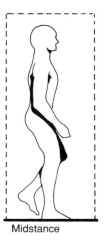

Midstance

▲ **Figure 14-7** ■ Midstance is the point at which the body weight passes directly over the supporting lower extremity.

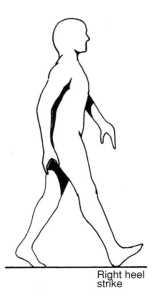

Right heel strike

▲ **Figure 14-5** ■ Initial contact refers to the instant at which any part of the reference extremity contacts the supporting surface. If the heel is first, it may be referred to as heel contact or heel strike. Right heel strike in the diagram constitutes the beginning of the stance phase of gait for the right lower extremity.

■ **Subphases of Stance Phase**

1. *Heel strike phase* (T) begins with initial contact and ends with foot flat and occupies only a small percentage of the gait cycle (see Fig. 14-3).
2. *Loading response* (RLA), or WA, begins at initial contact and ends when the contralateral extremity lifts off the ground at the end of the double-support phase[8] and occupies about 11% of the gait cycle (see Fig. 14-3).
3. *Midstance phase* (T) begins with foot flat at 7% of the

gait cycle and ends with heel-off at about 40% of the gait cycle. *Midstance phase* (RLA) begins when the contralateral extremity lifts off the ground at about 11% of the gait cycle and ends when the body is directly over the supporting limb at about 30% of the gait cycle, which makes it a much smaller portion of stance phase than the T midstance phase.
4. *Terminal stance* (RLA) begins when the body is directly over the supporting limb at about 30% of the gait cycle and ends a point just before initial contact of the contralateral extremity at about 50% of the gait cycle.
5. *Push-off phase* (T) begins with heel-off at about 40% of the gait cycle and ends with toe-off at about 60% of the gait cycle (see Fig. 14-2).
6. *Preswing* (RLA) is the last 10% of stance phase and begins with initial contact of the contralateral foot (at 50% of the gait cycle) and ends with toe-off (at 60%).

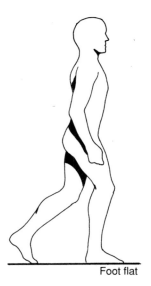

Foot flat

▲ **Figure 14-6** ■ Foot flat occurs immediately after initial contact and is defined as the point at which the foot is flat on the ground.

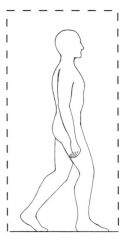

▲ **Figure 14-8** ■ Heel-off is the point at which the heel of the reference extremity (right extremity in the diagram) leaves the supporting surface.

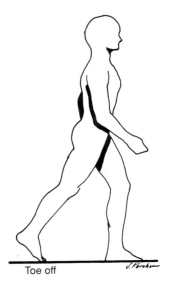

Toe off

▲ **Figure 14-9** ■ Toe-off is defined as the point in which only the toe of the reference extremity (right extremity) is touching the ground.

■ Swing Phase

1. *Acceleration,* or *early swing phase* (T), begins once the toe leaves the ground and continues until midswing, or the point at which the swinging extremity is directly under the body (see Fig. 14-3).
2. *Initial swing* (RLA) begins when the toe leaves the ground and continues until maximum knee flexion occurs.
3. *Midswing* (T) occurs approximately when the extremity passes directly beneath the body, or from the end of acceleration to the beginning of deceleration. *Midswing* (RLA) encompasses the period from maximum knee flexion until the tibia is in a vertical position.
4. *Deceleration* (T), or *late swing phase,* occurs after midswing when limb is decelerating in preparation for heel strike. *Terminal swing* (RLA) includes the period from the point at which the tibia is in the vertical position to a point just before initial contact.

For most purposes, including patient report writing, it is preferable to refer to events as occurring in early, middle, or late stance phase or in early, middle, or late swing phase, and this will be the practice in this chapter. For detailed description or quantitative analysis, more specific events and phases may be needed, but it is most important that the student grasp the overall picture and understand the major events of gait, which can become buried in excessive terminology.

 CONCEPT CORNERSTONE 14-1: *Normative Values for Time and Distance Gait Variables*

The following mean and standard deviation (SD) or range of mean values for time and distance variables for normal gait are derived from the classic work of Finley and Cody,[15] who surreptitiously measured the gait of 1100 pedestrians, and from Kadaba et al.,[16] Oberg et al.,[17] and colleagues of Ranchos Los Amigos National Rehabilitation Center[8] who obtained gait laboratory measurements (Table 14-1).

Gait Terminology

Time and distance are two basic parameters of motion, and measurements of these variables provide a basic description of gait. **Temporal variables** include stance time, single-limb and double-support time, swing time, stride and step time, cadence, and speed. The **distance variables** include stride length, step length and width, and degree of toe-out. These variables, derived in classic research of over 30 years ago, provide essential quantitative information about a person's gait and should be included in any gait description.[8,15–18] Each variable may be affected by such factors as age, sex, height, size and shape of bony components, distribution of mass in body segments, joint mobility, muscle strength, type of clothing and footgear, habit, and psychological status. However, a discussion of all the factors affecting gait is beyond the scope of this text.

Stance time is the amount of time that elapses during the stance phase of one extremity in a gait cycle.

Single-support time is the amount of time that

Characteristic	Male: Mean (SD)	Female: Mean (SD)	Source
Speed of walking in meters per second (m/sec)	1.37 (0.22)	1.23 (0.22)	Finley and Cody[15]
	1.37 (0.17)	1.32 (0.16)	RLA[8]
	Range of means, 1.22–1.32	Range of means, 1.10–1.29	Oberg et al.[17]
	1.34 (0.22)	1.27 (0.16)	Kadaba et al.[16]
Length of one stride in meters (m)	1.48 (0.18)	1.27 (0.19)	Finley and Cody[15]
	1.48 (0.15)	1.32 (0.13)	RLA[8]
	Range of means, 1.23–130	Range of means 1.07–1.19	Oberg et al.[17]
	1.41 (0.14)	1.30 (0.10)	Kadaba et al.[16]
Step cadence in steps per minute	110 (10)	116 (12)	Finley and Cody[15]
	111 (7.6)	121 (8.5)	RLA[8]
	Range of means, 117–121	Range of means, 122–130	Oberg et al.[17]
	112 (9)	115 (9)	Kadaba et al.[16]

Table 14-1 Normative Values for Time and Distance Variables

elapses during the period when only one extremity is on the supporting surface in a gait cycle.

Double-support time is the amount of time spent with both feet on the ground during one gait cycle. The percentage of time spent in double support may be increased in elderly persons and in those with balance disorders. The percentage of time spent in double support decreases as the speed of walking increases.

Stride length is the linear distance between two successive events that are accomplished by the *same* lower extremity during gait.[11] In general, stride length is determined by measuring the linear distance from the point of one heel strike of one lower extremity to the point of the next heel strike of the same extremity (Fig. 14-10). The length of one stride is traveled during one gait cycle and includes all of the events of one gait cycle. Stride length also may be measured by using other events of the same extremity, such as toe-off, but in normal gait, two successive heel strikes are usually used. A stride includes two steps, a right step and a left step. However, stride length is not always twice the length of a single step, because right and left steps may be unequal. Stride length varies greatly among individuals, because it is affected by leg length, height, age, sex, and other variables. Stride length can be normalized by dividing stride length by leg length or by total body height. Stride length usually decreases in elderly persons[12,13,19] and increases as the speed of gait increases.[20] The length of one stride is traveled during one gait cycle.

Stride duration refers to the amount of time it takes to accomplish one stride. Stride duration and gait cycle duration are synonymous. One stride, for a normal adult, lasts approximately 1 second.[21] Complex fluctuations in stride duration during slow, normal, and fast walking have been identified as being statistically correlated with variations in stride duration thousands of strides earlier. These fluctuations appear to be a characteristic of normal gait.[22]

Step length is the linear distance between two successive points of contact of *opposite* extremities. It is usually measured from the heel strike of one extremity to the heel strike of the opposite extremity (see Fig. 14-10). A comparison of right and left step lengths will provide an indication of gait symmetry. The more equal the step lengths, the more symmetrical is the gait. Variability in step length is at a minimum when the ratio of step length to step rate is about 0.006 m/step or at a person's preferred walking speed.[23]

Step duration refers to the amount of time spent during a single step. Measurement usually is expressed as seconds per step. When there is weakness or pain in an extremity, step duration may be decreased on the affected side and increased on the unaffected (stronger) or less painful side.

Cadence is the *number* of steps taken by a person per unit of time. Cadence may be measured as the number of steps per second or per minute, but the latter is more common:

$$\text{Cadence} = \text{number of steps/time}$$

A shorter step length will result in an increased cadence at any given velocity.[20] Lamoreaux found that when a person walks with a cadence between 80 and 120 steps per minute, cadence and stride length had a linear relationship.[11] As a person walks with increased cadence, the duration of the double-support period decreases. When the cadence of walking approaches 180 steps per minute, the period of double support disappears, and running commences. A step frequency or cadence of about 110 steps per minute can be considered as "typical" for adult men; a typical cadence for women is about 116 steps per minute.[3] Sometimes authors report values that refer to stride cadence, which is exactly half the step cadence.

Walking velocity is the rate of linear forward motion of the body, which can be measured in meters or centimeters per second, meters per minute, or miles per hour. Scientific literature favors meters per second. The term velocity implies that direction is specified, although this is frequently not included, and the more correct term **walking speed** should be used if direction is not reported. In instrumented gait analyses, walking velocity is used, inasmuch as the velocities of the segments involve specification of direction:

$$\text{Walking velocity (meters/second)} = \text{distance walked (meters)/time (seconds)}$$

Women tend to walk with shorter and faster steps than do men at the same velocity.[20] Increases in velocity up to 120 steps per minute are brought about by increases in both cadence and stride length, but above 120 steps per minute, step length levels off, and speed increases are achieved with only cadence increases.

Speed of gait may be referred to as slow, free, and fast. **Free speed** of gait refers to a person's normal walking speed; **slow** and **fast** speeds of gait refer to speeds slower or faster than the person's normal comfortable

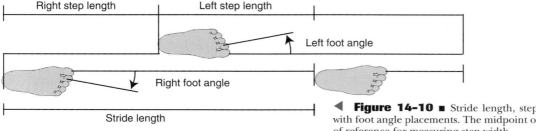

◀ **Figure 14-10** ■ Stride length, step length, and width shown with foot angle placements. The midpoint of the heel is used as a point of reference for measuring step width.

walking speed, designated in a variety of ways. There is a certain amount of variability in the way an individual elects to increase walking speed. Some individuals increase stride length and decrease cadence to achieve a fast walking speed. Other individuals decrease the stride length and increase cadence.

Step width, or width of the walking base, may be found by measuring the linear distance between the midpoint of the heel of one foot and the same point on the other foot (see Fig. 14-10). Step width has been found to increase when there is an increased demand for side-to-side stability, such as occurs in elderly persons and in small children. In toddlers and young children, the center of gravity is higher than in adults, and a wide base of support is necessary for stability. In the normal population, the mean width of the base of support is about 3.5 inches and varies within a range of 1 to 5 inches.

Degree of toe-out represents the angle of foot placement (FP) and may be found by measuring the angle formed by each foot's line of progression and a line intersecting the center of the heel and the second toe. The angle for men normally is about 7° from the line of progression of each foot at free speed walking (see Fig. 14-10).[12] The degree of toe-out decreases as the speed of walking increases in normal men.[12]

Power generation is accomplished when muscles shorten (concentric contraction). They do positive work and add to the total energy of the body. Power is the work or energy value divided by the time over which it is generated. The power of muscle groups performing gait is calculated through an inverse dynamic approach. The power generated or absorbed across a joint is the product of the net internal moment and the net angular velocity across the joint.[24] If both are in the same direction (flexors flexing, extensors extending, for example), positive work is being accomplished by energy generation. The most important phases of power generation and absorption have been designated by joint (H = hip, K = knee, A = ankle) and plane (S = sagittal, F = frontal, T = transverse).[25]

Power absorption is accomplished when muscles perform a lengthening (eccentric) contraction. They do negative work and reduce the energy of the body. If joint motion and moment are in opposite directions, negative work is being performed through energy absorption.

Case Application 14-2: **Effects on Time and Distance Gait Variables**

Ms. Brown walks with a speed of 0.20 m/sec and a cadence of 25 steps per minute. It is evident even on visual inspection that double-support time is considerably longer than normal on both steps. Stance phase is more than 60% of the gait cycle on her affected side, but she spends an even greater proportion of time in stance on the unaffected side. Her left step length (unaffected side) is shorter than her right (affected side), but her stride lengths are equal. Why? If you understand that a person walking in a straight line

must have equal stride lengths but may have unequal step lengths, you understand the concepts of steps and strides.

Joint Motion

Another way in which gait may be described is through measuring the trajectories of the lower extremities and the joint angles. Sophisticated equipment—at first, stroboscopic photography; then cinematography and electrogoniometers; and, more recently, many types of computerized motion analysis systems—have provided comprehensive information about joint angles and limb trajectories in normal and abnormal gait.[5,6,26–28] The most valuable analyses express findings in joint angle plots, frequently three-dimensional.

Less sophisticated and less objective methods are used in observational gait analysis, whereby an observer makes a judgment as to whether a particular joint angle or motion varies from a norm. Usually observational gait analysis is used to hypothesize causes of deviations and direct treatment objectives. One disadvantage of the observational method of analysis is that it requires a great deal of training and practice to be able to identify the particular segment of gait in which a particular joint angle deviates from a norm while a person is walking. Videotaping with slow playback can improve this greatly. Another disadvantage of observational gait analysis methods is that they frequently have low reliability, although recent reports have identified some variables and conditions under which reliability is satisfactory.[29]

■ Sagittal Plane Joint Angles

The approximate range of motion (ROM) needed in normal gait and the time of occurrence of the maximum flexion and extension positions for each major joint may be determined by examining the joint angle profiles in Figures 14-11 and 14-12. The standard deviation bars (dotted lines) around the mean profile (solid lines) give an indication of how much person-to-person variation exists, demonstrating that 67% of subjects' values fell within the range shown. Results reported in gait studies vary with age, gender, and walking speed of subjects and with the method of analysis. Data presented here were derived from three-dimensional analyses.[24] For simplicity, the mean value shown in the figures will be referred to in the text, taken to the nearest 5°, and, to remind the reader that these are not fixed values, the "approximately" sign (~) will be used. In the anatomical position, the hip, knee, and ankle are at approximately 0°. Flexion for the hip and knee and dorsiflexion for the ankle are given positive values, and extension and plantarflexion are given negative values.

From the appearance of, first, the hip in Figure 14-11, it can be seen that the hip achieves maximum flexion (~+20°) around initial contact at 0% of the gait cycle and its most extended position (~−20°) at about 50% of the gait cycle, between heel-off and toe-off. The knee is straight (0°) at initial contact and nearly straight

JOINT ANGLES
SAGGITAL PLANE

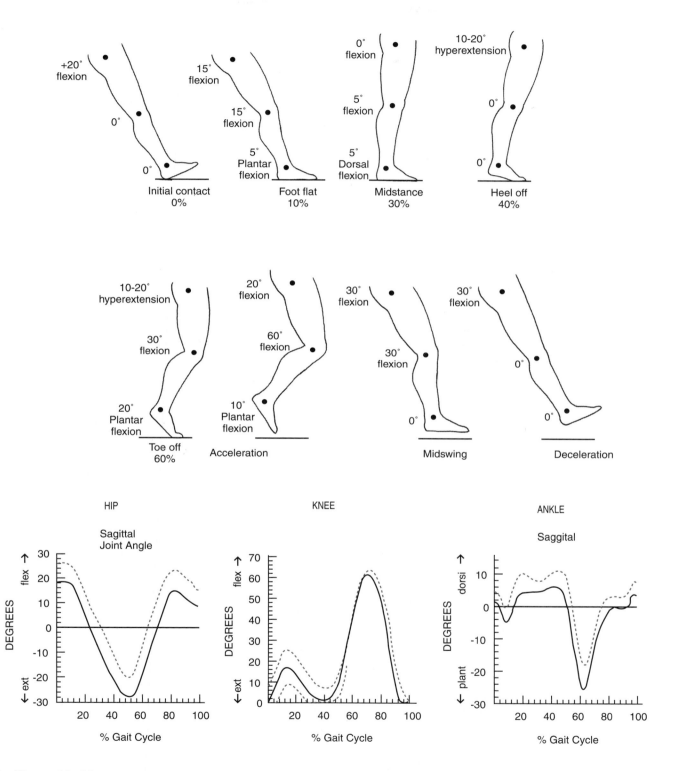

▲ **Figure 14-11** ■ Joint angles in degrees at the hip, knee, and ankle angles in the sagittal plane. The dotted lines in the angle diagrams represent the standard deviation values, and the solid lines represent the mean values. (Joint angle diagrams redrawn from Winter DA, Eng JJ, Isshac MG: A review of kinetic parameters in human walking. In Craik RL, Otis CA [eds]: Gait Analysis: Theory and Application, pp 263-265. St. Louis, Mosby–Year Book, 1994, with permission from Elsevier.)

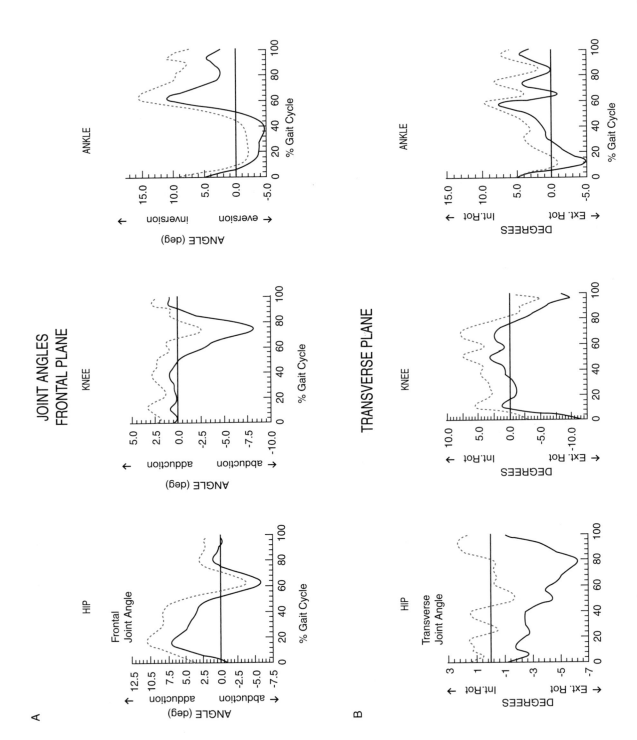

▲ **Figure 14-12** ■ **A.** Joint angles in degrees in the frontal plane at the hip, knee, and ankle. **B.** Transverse plane hip knee and ankle motion in degrees. (Joint angle diagrams for the frontal and transverse planes redrawn from Winter DA, Eng JJ, Isshac MG: A review of kinetic parameters in human walking. In Craik RL, Otis CA [eds]: Gait Analysis: Theory and Application, pp 263-265. St. Louis, Mosby–Year Book, 1994, with permission from Elsevier.)

again just before heel-off at 40% of the gait cycle. During the swing phase, the hip reaches its maximum flexion of ~+60° at ~70% of the gait cycle. (Note that a small knee flexion phase occurring at 10% of the gait cycle peaks at ~+15°.) The ankle reaches maximum dorsiflexion of ~+7° at approximately heel-off at about 40% of the gait cycle and reaches maximum plantarflexion (−25°) at toe-off (60%).

 CONCEPT CORNERSTONE 14-2: *Hip, Knee, and Ankle Range of Motion Needed for Normal Walking*

For normal walking, we need a hip ROM from approximately 20° of extension to 20° of flexion, a knee range from straight (0°) to 60° flexion, and an ankle range from 25° of plantarflexion to 7° dorsiflexion. If these joint ranges are not available, a gait pattern would be expected to show considerable deviation from the norm.

■ **Frontal Plane Joint Angles**

During the first 20% of stance, the pelvis or the contralateral side drops about 5°, which results in adduction of the hip (see Fig. 14-12A). The hip abducts smoothly to about 5° of abduction, peaking about toe-off, then returns to neutral at initial contact. The knee remains more or less neutral, except for a brief abduction peaking at about 7° in midswing, and then returns to neutral.[28] From the figure, it can be seen that the ankle everts from about 5° of inversion to 5° of eversion in early stance and inverts about 15° during push-off.

■ **Transverse Plane Joint Angles**

The hip, knee, and ankle show a great deal of variability in profiles. With regard to the laboratory (global) coordinates, the hip externally rotates until approximately midswing and then internally rotates to near neutral before initial contact (see Fig. 14-12B). The knee joint remains relatively neutral throughout most of the gait cycle but externally rotates in late stance until about foot flat. The ankle has three rapid reversals of rotation from about 40% of the gait cycle until initial contact and reaches a point of maximum external rotation at about foot flat.

Case Application 14-3: **Effects on Joint Angle Patterns**

An examination of videotaped joint angles reveals that Ms. Brown has no knee flexion phase in early stance, and she tends to fully extend her knee in midstance. She has minimal ability to dorsiflex her ankle and has difficulty clearing the floor with her affected limb as a result of poor dorsiflexion and because she does not bend her knee more than a few degrees during swing phase. Instead, she tends to lift her pelvis ("hike") to clear her foot during swing on the affected side. Her affected hip does not extend beyond neutral. How do Ms. Brown's joint angle profiles vary from the normal in stance and swing phases?

Saunders' "Determinants" of Gait

Another way of looking at gait using "determinants" was first described by Saunders and coworkers in 1953.[30] The "determinants" were supposed to represent adjustments made by the pelvis, hips, knees, and ankles that help to keep movement of the body's center of mass to a minimum. By decreasing the vertical and lateral excursions of the body's center of mass it was thought that energy expenditure would be less and gait more efficient. The determinants are pelvic rotation in the transverse plane of about 8°, which is thought to flatten the arc of the passage of the center of mass; lateral pelvic tilt in the frontal plane, in which the pelvis drops on the side of the swing leg, which is thought to keep the peak of the rise lower than if it did not drop; knee flexion in stance phase, which should keep the center of mass from rising as much as it would have to if the body had to pass over a completely extended knee; interaction of the movements of the foot, knee, and ankle, which may work together to minimize the excursion of the center of mass; and physiologic valgus of the knee, which is said to reduce side-to-side movement of the center of mass in frontal plane. Although still useful as descriptors of gait, biomechanical analyses that were not available at Saunders' time do not support these factors as guiding principles of walking (see the following Continuing Exploration).

Continuing Exploration: **Problems with Saunders' "Determinants" Theory**

The premise upon which the classic "determinants" theory of Saunders[30] was based is erroneous: that the energy costs of the body are reflected in the movement of the center of mass. Movements of limbs in opposite directions tend to cancel each other and do not appear as energy costs, despite the fact that energy is required both to accelerate and to decelerate them. Furthermore, energy conservation between potential and kinetic types, which is discussed later in the chapter, was not considered. Authors more than two decades ago[31] and recently[32] concluded that energy conservation of the HAT segment is very high in normal walking, and that lower limb movement dominates the energy picture. Other research also questions the influence of the "determinants" on the excursion of the HAT.[33,34] In summary, Saunders' theory of the determinants of walking probably should be abandoned.

◆ Kinetics

Ground Reaction Force

When a person takes a step, forces are applied to the ground by the foot and by the ground to the foot. These forces are equal in magnitude but opposite in direction. We are usually more interested in the forces being applied to the foot, which are termed ground reaction forces (GRFs). GRFs are described by using a cartesian coordinate system with forces expressed along vertical, anteroposterior, and mediolateral axes.[3] The vector sum of the force components in each direction is a single expression of the ground reaction force (GRFV), which has a typical pattern from initial contact to toe-off. In the vertical direction, the magnitudes are low at first but increase to values that are greater than body weight both in early stance and again in late stance, with lower values at midstance. These fluctuations are expressions of the vertical acceleration and deceleration of the body through the stride. In the anteroposterior direction, the GRF is directed posteriorly against the foot that is making initial contact and prevents the foot from slipping forward. It reaches a maximum magnitude of about 20% of body weight. At midstance, the force becomes neutral, but as the body enters the second half of stance phase, the vector is directed anteriorly against the foot, enabling the person to push off. The mediolateral forces are small in magnitude and are variable across individuals. The usefulness of the GRFs in understanding gait, particularly in the sagittal plane, is discussed later in the chapter.

Center of Pressure

The CoP of the foot on the supporting surface moves along a path during gait and produces a characteristic pattern (Fig. 14-13). The pattern for normal individuals during barefoot walking differs from the patterns in which various types of footgear are used.[35] In barefoot walking, the CoP starts at the posterolateral edge of the heel at the beginning of the stance phase and moves in a nearly linear manner through the midfoot area, remaining lateral to the midline, and then moves medially across the ball of the foot with a large concentration along the metatarsal break. The CoP then moves to second and first toes during terminal stance.

Kinetic Analysis

A kinetic analysis is performed to understand the forces acting on the joints, the moments produced by the muscles crossing the joints, and the energy requirements of gait. Most commonly, a link-segment model is used with an inverse dynamic approach. This means that we look at the body as a model made up of several parts (segments). We approach the analysis segment by segment from distal to proximal, using newtonian mechanics. Figure 14-14 shows a simple four-segment gait model (foot, lower leg, thigh, half of HAT) with one side of the body considered. We must know the positions of body markers in motion analysis technology, and we will place these at joint centers. We also need to know all of the external forces acting on the body, and for the walking person, these are **inertia, gravity,** and the GRF.[3] The magnitude, direction, and point of application of the GRF on the foot is usually determined through the use of a force platform.[36] The inertial force is proportional to the acceleration of the segment.

Continuing Exploration: **Understanding How the Kinetics of Gait Are Studied**

The three equations on which the solutions are based for a two-dimensional analysis are simple: for each segment, the following three are applied:

$$\Sigma F_x = ma_x \quad (1)$$
$$\Sigma F_y = ma_y \quad (2)$$
$$\Sigma M_0 = I\alpha \quad (3)$$

where
Σ means "the sum of all of the"
F_x = forces in the designated x direction, in this case horizontal, in newtons (N)

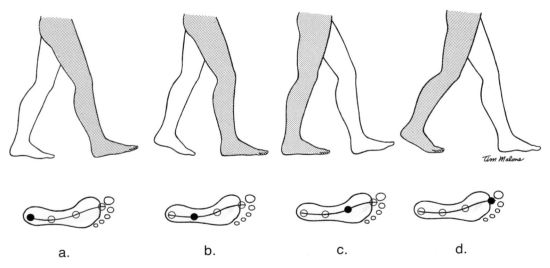

a.   b.   c.   d.

▲ **Figure 14-13** ■ A center of pressure (CoP) pathway is shown by the position of the black dot at initial contact (**A**), at foot flat (**B**), just before heel-off (**C**), and just before toe-off (**D**).

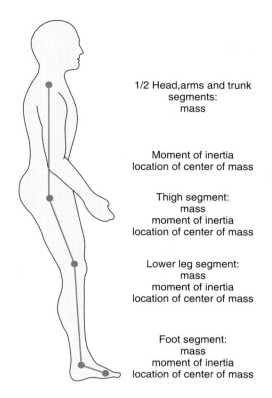

F_y = forces in the designated y direction, in this case vertical, in N

a_y = acceleration of the center of mass derived from position and time data, in m/sec^2

M_0 = moment about selected point 0, the center of mass, in newton-meters (N·m), largely attributable to muscle activity, with ligaments, tendons, joint capsules, and bony components involved to a lesser extent

I = moment of inertia, derived from anthropometric tables, in kg·m^2

α = angular acceleration of segment derived from segment position and time data, in radians per second squared (rad/sec^2)

If we refer to Figure 14-15 with reference to the foot segment, equation (1) says that that the sum of all forces in the x direction (see convention in the figure) must equal the product of the mass of the foot and its acceleration in the x direction. Equation (2) says that the sum of all forces in the y direction (see convention in the figure) must equal the product of the mass of the foot and its acceleration in the y direction. Equation (3) says the sum of the moments about any designated center (we are choosing the center of mass) must equal the product of the moment of inertia (which can be visualized as the resistance to rotation) and the angular acceleration of the segment. Figure 14-15 shows that there are three things we do not know: the X force at the ankle (F_{AX}), the Y force at the ankle (F_{AY}), and the moment around the ankle (M_A). Foot floor forces are designated F_{FX} and F_{FY}. There is no moment about free end of the segment.

Note that, having three equations, we can solve for only three unknowns and cannot calculate the muscle moments on opposite sides of the joint if there is co-contraction. Applying these three equation results in numbers for the X force at the ankle, the Y force at the

▲ **Figure 14-14** ■ Simple four-segment link segment model of half a human body for use in gait studies. For each segment identified, the mass, moment of inertia, and location of the center of mass should be known for applications.

m = mass of the segment, derived from anthropometric tables, in kilograms (kg)

a_x = acceleration of the center of mass in the x direction, derived from position and time data, in meters per second squared (m/sec^2)

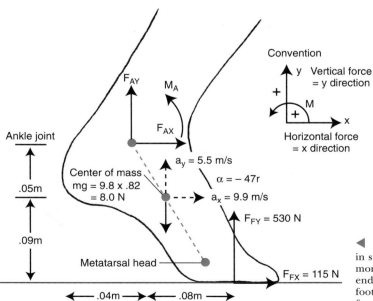

◀ **Figure 14-15** ■ Free body diagram of the foot segment in stance shown with proximal joint (ankle) and all forces and moments acting on the segment. No moment is present at free end of the segment. Known forces and their location are mass of foot and foot-floor force. Unknown forces are joint reaction forces on the ankle and net moment at the ankle joint.

Table 14-2	Input Data and Net Moment and Forces Derived from Example Shown in Figure 14-15				
Given Information			Calculated Information		
Term	Value	Term	Calculated from		Value
Body mass	56.7 kg	Mass of foot	Proportion body mass		0.822 kg
Gravitational constant	9.8	Moment of inertia	Proportion segment length, radius of gyration		0.0026 kg/m^2
Center of mass: acceleration x	9.9 m/s	Force at ankle: F_{ax}	$\Sigma F = ma_x$ $F_{ax} + 115 = m(9.9)$		-107 N
acceleration y	5.5 m/s				
Foot-floor force: x direction	115 N (to right)	Force at ankle: F_{ay}	$\Sigma F = ma_y$ $F_{ay} + 530 - 0.822(9.8) = m$ (9.9)		-517 N
y direction	530 N (upward)	Moment at ankle	$\Sigma M = I\alpha$ $M_{a} + (107)(0.05) +$ $(517)(0.04) + 115(0.09)$ $+ 530(0.08) =$ $.0026(-47.15)$		-78.7 N

Data from Winter DA: Biomechanics and Motor Control of Human Movement, 2nd ed. New York, John Wiley & Sons, 1990.
Calculations performed about center of mass of foot.

ankle, and the moment at the ankle (Table 14-2). *In other words, we are finding out what forces and moments had to have been acting at the ankle in order that the foot with that particular mass and moment of inertia move with those particular linear and angular accelerations.* Now we simply progress up the body segment by segment and solve for the more proximal joint. Larger numbers of segments and three-dimensional analyses are more complex than this, but the principles are the same.

Internal and External Forces, Moments, and Conventions

Internal moments are moments generated by the muscles, joint capsules, and ligaments to counteract the external forces acting on the body. External forces such as the GRF produce external moments about the joints. For example, when the weight is on the forefoot in late stance phase, an internal ankle plantarflexor moment produced by the calf muscle will oppose the external dorsiflexion moment caused by the GRF and other external forces that are tending to dorsiflex the foot. Although some academicians use the external moment convention, we are going to use the internal moment convention in this chapter. The word "internal" will be used frequently for ease of reading.

■ Moment Conventions

Different authors use different conventions to display internal moments on figures, but they usually indicate the direction of the moment by the words "flexor/extensor," "abductor/adductor," or "internal/external rotator." The moment profiles presented here display the following internal moments as positive: ankle plantarflexor, knee extensor, and hip extensor.

■ Sagittal Plane Moments

The sagittal plane joint angles described previously yield the moment profiles for the hip, knee, and ankle (Fig. 14-16).

Before examining the details of joint moments, let us consider the concept of the support moment. An examination of the moments acting at the lower extremity show that for most of stance phase, the algebraic sum of all internal moments acting at the hip, knee, and ankle is a positive or extensor internal moment (Fig. 14-17). Winter[7] called this quantification of the total limb synergy a **support moment,** and he found the extensor support moment to be consistent for all walking speeds for both normal individuals and persons with disabilities. The internal extensor moment keeps the leg from collapsing during the stance phase. Because hip and knee moments may vary considerably among individuals as long as the net moment remains an internal extensor moment, the body can vary how it accomplishes its support. If ankle plantarflexors are deficient, the hip extensors and/or the knee extensors can compensate. If contraction of the knee extensors causes pain, the hip extensor and/or ankle plantarflexors can compensate. The support moment changes from a net internal extensor to a net internal flexor moment in late stance (55% to 60% of the gait cycle) that continues into swing. In late swing, a net internal extensor moment appears again, presumably to assist in the final positioning of the limb for heel contact.[7,37]

The support moment provides a backdrop to understand the joint moment profiles for each joint. In Figure 14-16, observe that hip extension provides all of the positive moment in early stance, but it is soon joined by an internal knee extensor moment. Remember that the moment identifies only the potential of the muscle group to support; it does not mean

Internal Moments
SAGITTAL PLANE

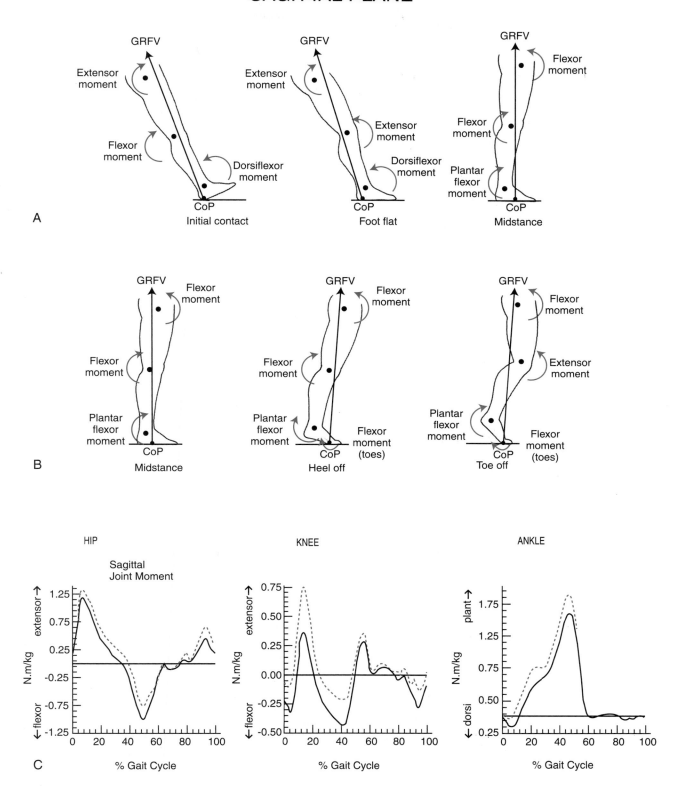

▲ **Figure 14-16** ■ Patterns of internal moments in the sagittal plane at the hip, knee, and ankle with center of pressure (CoP) and ground reaction force vectors (GRFVs). The dotted lines represent the standard deviations, and the solid lines represent the mean values. (Diagrams of internal moments redrawn from Winter DA, Eng JJ, Isshac MG: A review of kinetic parameters in human walking. In Craik RL, Otis CA [eds]: Gait Analysis: Theory and Application, pp 263-265. St. Louis, Mosby–Year Book, 1994, with permission from Elsevier.)

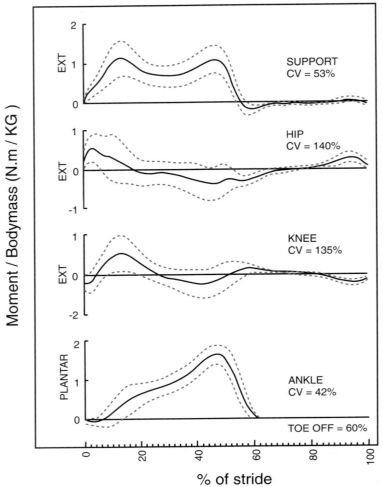

Moment of Force-Natural Cadence (N = 19)

Moment / Bodymass (N.m / KG)

SUPPORT
CV = 53%

HIP
CV = 140%

KNEE
CV = 135%

ANKLE
CV = 42%

TOE OFF = 60%

% of stride

◀ **Figure 14-17** ■ Typical pattern of sagittal plane moments at the hip, knee, and ankle, shown with their algebraic sum, the support moment. (Redrawn from Winter DA: The Biomechanics and Motor Control of Human Gait: Normal, Elderly and Pathological, 2nd ed. Waterloo, Ontario, Waterloo Biomechanics, 1991, with permission from David A. Winter.)

that muscle shortening or lengthening is occurring. If, for example, the net internal moment is caused by the knee extensors, the knee may be flexing (eccentric contraction) or extending (concentric contraction) or remaining unchanged (isometric contraction). There is increasing support by the ankle plantarflexors as stance phase proceeds until they become the only support in most of late stance. During swing phase, moments are very small, as would be expected.

■ **Frontal Plane Moments**

Large internal abduction moments of similar shapes occur at the hip and knee, and a smaller one occurs at the ankle. These are provided largely by ligament forces across the knee and ankle joints and are necessary, inasmuch as the center of mass of the body is considerably medial to the point of support on the foot. There appears to be some active component at the knee, however (either muscular or passive spring related), inasmuch as some power generation is evident in Figure 14-18.

■ **Transverse Plane Moments**

Transverse plane internal moments tend to be small at each of the hip, knee, and ankle joints and follow similar shapes.

Case Application 14-4: **Difficulty in Developing an Adequate Support Moment**

Ms. Brown has low levels of activation of her ankle plantarflexors, knee extensors, and, to a lesser extent, hip extensors. This will make it difficult for her to develop an adequate support moment. This is no doubt the reason that she thrusts her knee backward to gain knee stability. We know that she has smaller deficits at the hip than at the ankle, and so we would encourage hip extension in early stance to assist with the support moment, as well as trying to stimulate the knee extensors. During this early poststroke period, we would expect some natural increase in force-generating capability of the muscles and be prepared to take advantage of it by

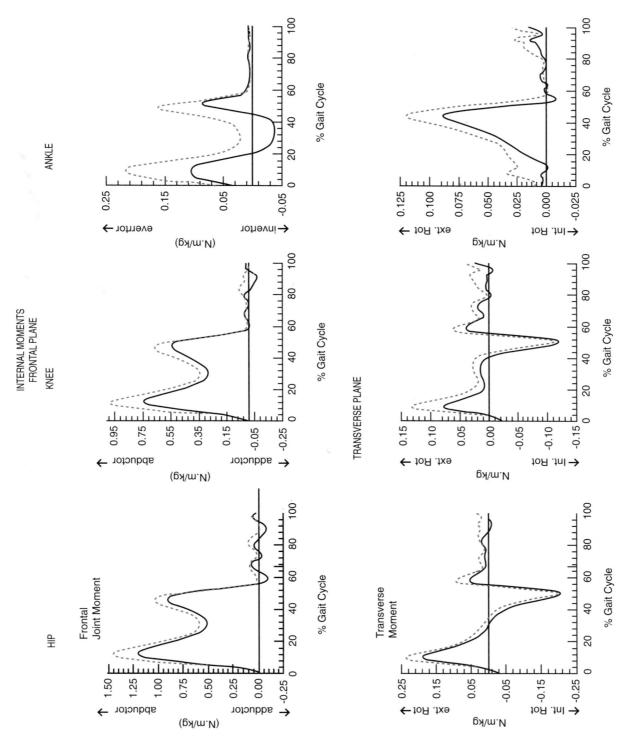

▲ **Figure 14-18** ■ Patterns of internal moments in the frontal plane at the hip, knee, and ankle. The dotted lines represent the standard deviation, and the solid lines indicate the mean values. (Redrawn from Winter DA, Eng JJ, Isshac MG: A review of kinetic parameters in human walking. In Craik RL, Otis CA [eds]: Gait Analysis: Theory and Application, pp 263-265. St. Louis, Mosby–Year Book, 1994, with permission from Elsevier.)

strengthening during functional movements. If over time she is unable to provide enough support, an ankle orthosis would provide a passive extensor moment, but there may be energy costs to doing this.

Continuing Exploration: **Kinematics and Kinetics of the Foot and Ankle**

Specific descriptions of the biomechanics of the foot during gait have been hindered by the use of the terms "pronation" (a composite of dorsiflexion, eversion, and abduction [external rotation]) and "supination" (a composite of plantarflexion, inversion, and adduction [external rotation]). Usually, the foot movement is described as consisting of pronation early in stance, followed by progressive supination. However, three-dimensional analyses of the lower leg and foot, modeling the foot as a rearfoot segment and a forefoot segment, have provided more insight into its behavior during stance.[38,39] Specifically, the rearfoot segment everts with regard to the lower leg early in stance and inverts during push-off. Three very small net moment torques (not exceeding 0.10 Nm/kg) are evident in the frontal plane through stance at the ankle until about 20% of the cycle when an internal evertor moment dominates, followed by an internal invertor moment until near 50% of the cycle. Thereafter, until toe-off, an internal evertor moment dominates. In the transverse plane, the rearfoot segment externally rotates, (abducts) in early stance, followed by smooth internal rotation (adduction) through push-off. The forefoot segment adds considerably to dorsiflexion during early stance and midstance and shows a few degrees of inversion in the frontal plane in early stance, thereafter remaining neutral until push-off, when it once again inverts a few degrees. In the transverse plane, the forefoot rotates externally (abducts) a few degrees in early stance and internally rotates (adducts) during push-off.

Energy Requirements

The main objective of locomotion is to move the body through space with the least expenditure of energy. Energy is the capacity to do work, and both work and energy are expressed in the same units, **joules (J)**. Work is performed by the application of force, which produces accelerations and decelerations of the body and its segments. Muscles use metabolic energy to perform mechanical work by converting metabolic energy into mechanical energy.

The overall metabolic cost incurred during locomotion may be measured by assessing the body's oxygen consumption per unit of distance traveled. If a long distance is traveled but only a small amount of oxygen is consumed, the metabolic cost of that particular gait is low. Oxygen consumption for a person walking at 4 to 5 km/hour averages 100 mL/kg body weight per minute. The highest efficiency is attained when the least amount of energy is necessary to travel a unit of distance. When asked to walk at a comfortable speed, people choose the speed at which they are most efficient, and if the speed of walking increases above this, the energy cost per unit of distance walked increases.[31] Also as described previously, as the speed of walking decreases below free walking speed, the energy cost increases. The probable causes will be apparent when we examine energy costs from a biomechanical rather than a metabolic perspective.

Mechanical Energy of Walking

Muscles perform work on the parts of the body in order that they change their height or change their translational and/or rotational velocity. All energy added to the body by means of concentric muscle contractions results in increases in velocity of some part or parts, increases in height, or both. In other words, energy is generated and **positive work** is done on the body. All energy taken away from the body by means of eccentric contractions results in decreases in velocity of some part or parts, lowering of the part or parts, or both. Another way of saying this is that energy is absorbed and **negative work** is done on the body.

There are two common ways of analyzing work and energy in movement analysis of the human body during gait. The first is usually referred to as the kinematic approach. The other is usually referred to as the mechanical power analysis. Both methods use biomechanical models that can be simple or complex, and both must make a number of simplifying assumptions. Although these are the most commonly used approaches, other investigators have developed models by using a theoretical dynamical systems perspective,[40] pursuing the notion that motor pattern development in locomotion is driven by the underlying dynamics of the task and the dynamic resources available to the person.

Mechanical Energy: Kinematic Approach

The total energy of a body of several "segments" at a given instant in time is the sum of the potential energy and two forms of kinetic energy, translational (linear) and rotational, of each segment. **Translational energy** refers to energy related to the linear velocity of a segment in space. **Rotational energy** is due to the rotational velocity of a segment in space. **Potential energy** is the quantity of mass, multiplied by the height to which it is raised. In other words, whenever a mass is raised, gravity tends to act on it and make it fall, and therefore the mass has potential energy. The amount of potential energy that an elevated mass possesses is equal to the amount of kinetic energy that was necessary to lift the mass against gravity. When the mass has stopped elevating or is at its peak, kinetic energy is transformed into potential energy. When the mass falls, the potential energy is transformed back into kinetic energy as the mass accelerates.

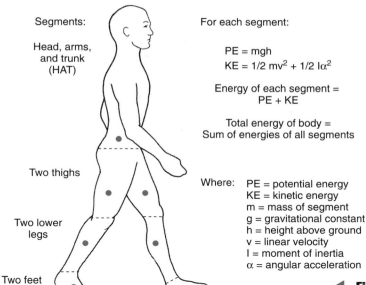

Segments:

Head, arms, and trunk (HAT)

Two thighs

Two lower legs

Two feet

For each segment:

$$PE = mgh$$
$$KE = 1/2\ mv^2 + 1/2\ I\alpha^2$$

Energy of each segment =
PE + KE

Total energy of body =
Sum of energies of all segments

Where: PE = potential energy
KE = kinetic energy
m = mass of segment
g = gravitational constant
h = height above ground
v = linear velocity
I = moment of inertia
α = angular acceleration

◀ **Figure 14–19** ■ Seven-segment model illustrating determination of energy at an instant in time, kinematic approach.

Figure 14-19 is a model of the segmental energies of a simple 7-segment body, and Figure 14-20 shows the potential and kinetic energy levels of the HAT, and their sum.[41] Rotational kinetic energy is neglected because it is very small for the HAT. The low potential energy at initial contact of each foot at 0% and 50% of the gait cycle, respectively, reflects the low position of the body at initial contact. At approximately midstance of each foot, the body reaches its highest position, or maximum potential energy. Examination of the kinetic energy levels for each instant in time reveals that not only is the pattern nearly the "mirror image" of the potential energy but also the magnitudes of the changes are quite similar. At initial contact, the body has the lowest potential energy but is moving the fastest, and as it moves into midstance, the potential energy rises and is exchanged for kinetic energy. In this way there are great energy savings, as can be seen in the top curve, which is the sum of potential and kinetic components. It is also apparent that if kinetic energy does not match potential energy in magnitude—that is, if the person walks much more slowly or much more quickly—conservation would be reduced. Figure 14-21 shows the same total energy curve for the HAT above the total energy curves for each of the two limbs. When the limb curves are added to the HAT curve, yielding the top curve, it is apparent that no energy savings occur between the two limbs and that savings between the HAT and the limbs is modest. Furthermore, the limbs are larger contributors to the total energy costs than is the HAT. Now it is clear why Saunders' determinants theory is inadequate[30]: most of the cost of walking is involved in moving the limbs, not the trunk, despite the greater mass of the trunk.

The segment-by-segment mechanical energy approach has given some important insight into the total costs and the patterns of exchange and transfer between and within body segments that occur during walking. Note, however, that this analysis does not tell us which muscle groups produced the energy, which absorbed it, or when these events occurred. For this we need a mechanical power and work analysis.

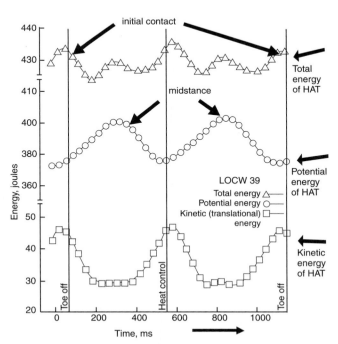

▲ **Figure 14–20** ■ Potential and kinetic energy levels of the head, arms, and trunk (HAT) segment, and their sum for one stride in gait.(Redrawn from Winter DA, Quanbury AO, Reimer GD: Analysis of instaneous energy of normal gait. J Biomech 9:253-257, 1976, with permission from Elsevier.)

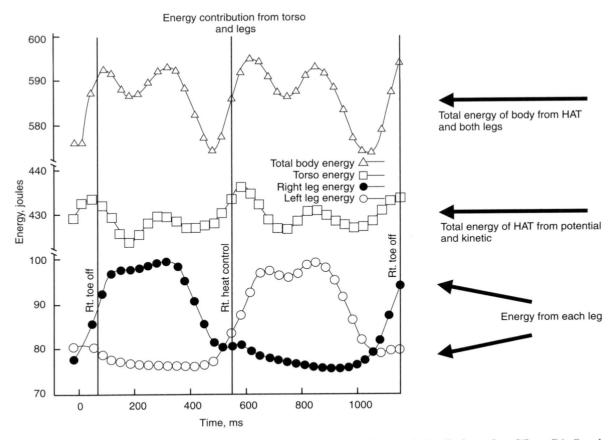

▲ **Figure 14-21** ■ Total energy curve shown with that of the HAT and those of the two limbs. (Redrawn from Winter DA, Quanbury AO, Reimer GD: Analysis of instaneous energy of normal gait. J Biomech 9:253-257, 1976, with permission from Elsevier.)

Continuing Exploration: **Kinematic Approach to Energy**

For simplicity, let us assume that markers are placed immediately over joint centers. The only kinetic information needed is knowledge of the masses of each segment, and these are usually calculated as a percentage of the person's body weight from anthropometric tables.[42] The velocities of the centers of mass of the segments are derived from position data. The locations of the centers of mass are determined from anthropometric tables. Note in Figure 14-19 that two constants are needed: g, the gravitational constant of 9.8 m/sec, and I, the moment of inertia, which is derived from anthropometric tables. The total energy of the body at a given instant in time is calculated as the sum of potential and kinetic energy of each of the involved parts. The difference between the energy levels for one segment at two successive instants in time is the total energy cost of moving the segment over that time interval. Note that the net result may be positive or negative (denoting positive or negative work). The absolute (positive and negative) changes for all segments can be added together algebraically to give the changes for the whole body.

This statement contains a simplifying assumption that is satisfactory for simple models: if the energy level of one segment is increasing while another is decreasing, then energy is being transferred between them.

Case Application 14-5: **Effects of an Ankle-Foot Orthosis**

Recall that Ms. Brown hiked up her affected side (lifted hip and pelvis) in order to clear her foot during swing phase. This has been shown to have a serious energy cost[43] as the full weight of the upper body is raised and lowered, and there are no opportunities for savings by kinetic-potential exchange. Because the inability to adequately dorsiflex her foot appeared to be part of the problem, a light and, it is hoped, temporary ankle foot orthosis was prescribed. This also assisted with her inability to provide sufficient support during stance. She gained the ability to bend her knee in later stance, thus avoiding excessive hip hiking. Watch for possible drawbacks while you read the section on power and work. If the orthosis does not permit any ankle plantarflexion during push-off, she will lose the energy that would otherwise be provided by plantarflexor generation.

Mechanical Power and Work

Power (P) profiles across the hip, knee, and ankle are compared with joint angle and major muscle activity profiles in Figures 14-22 to 14-24. P is measured in watts (W), equivalent to joules per second (J/sec), or newton-meters per second (Nm/sec).[24] Power values are normalized by dividing the power in watts by the subject's weight in kilograms to make it possible to compare across subjects. A summary of the phases of power generation and absorption and of the muscle groups responsible during stance phase appear in Table 14-3 for initial contact to midstance and in Table 14-4 for midstance to toe-off. In the sagittal plane (see Fig. 14-22), a burst of positive work (energy generation) occurs as the hip extensors contract concentrically during early stance (H1-S), while the knee extensors perform negative work (energy absorption) by acting eccentrically (K1-S) to control knee flexion during the same period.[31] Negative work is performed by the plantarflexors (A1-S) as the leg rotates over the foot during the period of stance from foot flat to about 40% of the gait cycle. However, a small amount of positive work is done by the knee extensors at the beginning of this period (K2-S), extending the knee after foot flat.[31] Positive work of the plantarflexors at push-off (late stance, ~40% to 60% of the gait cycle) and hip flexors at pull-off (late stance and in early swing, ~50% to 75% of the gait cycle) increases the energy level of the body. During this 40% to 60% of the gait cycle when energy is being generated from A2-S and H3-S, simultaneous absorption is occurring by knee extensors (K3-S). In late swing, negative work is performed by the knee flexors (K4) as they work eccentrically to decelerate the leg in preparation for initial contact.

Inman estimated that the positive energy generated by the hip muscles during concentric muscle action for normal men walking at a cadence of 109 steps per minute is approximately double the amount of energy absorbed by the hip muscles during eccentric muscle action,[3] but data suggest that the ratio is even larger.[14] At the ankle, the positive energy generated by concentric muscle action during a single gait cycle is almost triple that of the energy absorbed by eccentric muscle action.[3] The knee, in contrast to the hip and ankle, absorbs more energy through eccentric muscle action during a gait cycle than it generates.[3] At slow and normal speeds of walking in healthy subjects, the hip flexors and extensors contribute about 25% of the total concentric work. The ankle plantarflexors contribute about 66%, and the knee extensors contribute about 8%.[32] Clearly, the ankle plantarflexors are of primary importance in walking (see Continuing Exploration: On the Existence of "Rockers" and "Push-off").

In the frontal plane (see Fig. 14-23), an initial period of absorption by the hip abductors is followed by two small bursts of positive work in the remainder of stance. These bursts provide fine control of the mediolateral position of the center of mass of the body. At the knee, there is a very small generation pattern during the first half of stance, followed by a small absorp-

tion (both caused by abductor structures). The ankle power pattern shows minor fluctuations and a small and somewhat inconsistent absorption burst during push-off.

In the transverse plane (see Fig. 14-24), the hip powers are small and somewhat inconsistent, as can be seen by the large standard deviation of the profiles. The power profiles at the knee are also very small, with one consistent negative burst during early stance. This appears to result from passive structures resisting external rotation of the knee. At the ankle, the power is minuscule and inconsistent.

Continuing Exploration: **Understanding Power and Work in Gait**

Examination of power plots helps explain the muscles responsible for gait and its phases. When slow or inefficient gait is a problem, knowledge of the sources of power enables a health practitioner to assist the client compensate for deficiencies. Note that the scales used for power vary, and this must be taken into account when assessing the work (the area under the power curve). In Figure 14-22, identify the joint around which the largest amount of positive work (above zero line) is performed in the sagittal plane. It is apparent that the burst denoted A2-S (S denoting burst in the sagittal plane) is the largest, and this occurs at the ankle. Without more information, one cannot know whether the ankle plantarflexors are flexing or the dorsiflexors are dorsiflexing, but either moment or angle profiles reveal that the first is correct. The second largest burst of positive power, denoted H1-S, is an internal hip extensor moment with hip extension occurring in early stance. The third burst, H3-S, occurs near A2-S. It is caused by an internal hip flexor moment and hip flexion at the end of stance and the beginning of swing and may be called "pull-off."

The knee is not of major importance in energy generation. However, there is a small phase, denoted K2-S, in which the knee extensors extend the knee after the knee flexion phase of early stance. K2-S can be important in pathologies such as cerebral palsy when other sources of energy are not available.

Unless gait velocity is increasing, energy has to be systematically removed. The knee accomplishes this at K1-S (knee flexion with an internal knee extensor moment) and K3-S (small internal knee extensor moment in late stance occurring while the knee is flexing quite quickly). The latter may represent inefficiency in gait.[44] K4-S (knee flexor absorption with knee extension) occurs before initial contact. Note that, as with all absorption phases, the dominating moment is opposite to the movement that is occurring: in this case, an internal flexor moment while knee extension is occurring.

Let us now examine the periods during which simultaneous positive and negative work normally occur, which, if excessive, represents inefficiency. K1-S and A1-S are negative bursts of negative work con-

Text continues on p. 542

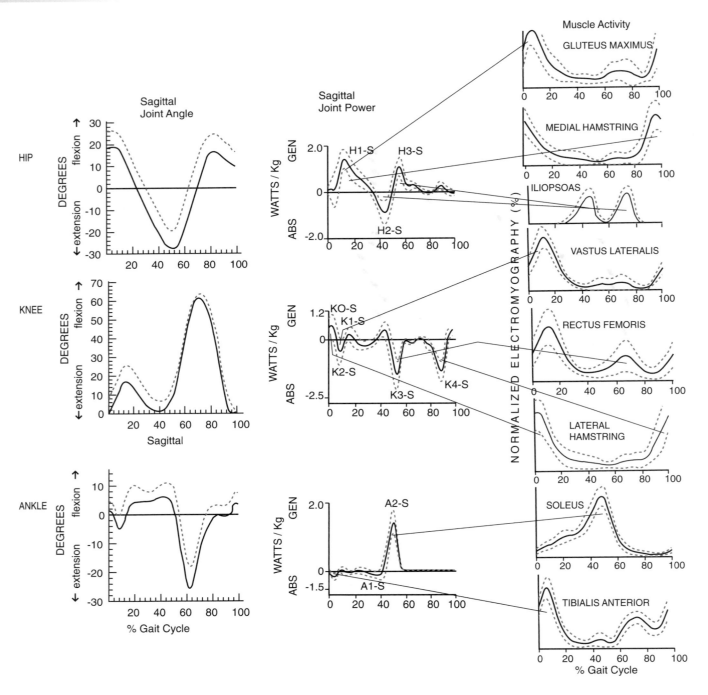

▲ **Figure 14-22** ■ Joint angles and joint powers in the sagittal plane, and EMG profiles of representatives of major contributors to joint powers of hip, knee, and ankle during adult gait. (Angle profiles redrawn from Winter DA, Eng JJ, Isshac MG: A review of kinetic parameters in human walking. In Craik RL, Otis CA [eds]: Gait Analysis: Theory and Application, pp. 263-265. St. Louis, Mosby–Year Book, 1994, with permission from Elsevier. Power profiles redrawn from Eng JJ, Winter DA: Kinetic analysis of the lower limbs during walking: What information can be gained from a three dimensional model? J Biomech 28:753, 1995, with permission from Elsevier. Muscle activity redrawn from Winter DA: The Biomechanics and Motor Control of Human Gait: Normal, Elderly and Pathological, 2nd ed. Waterloo, Ontario, Waterloo Biomechanics, 1991, with permission from David A. Winter. Iliopsoas muscle activity redrawn from Bechtol CO: Normal human gait. In American Academy of Orthopaedic Surgeons: Atlas of Orthotics, p 141. St. Louis, CV Mosby, 1974, with permission from Elsevier.)

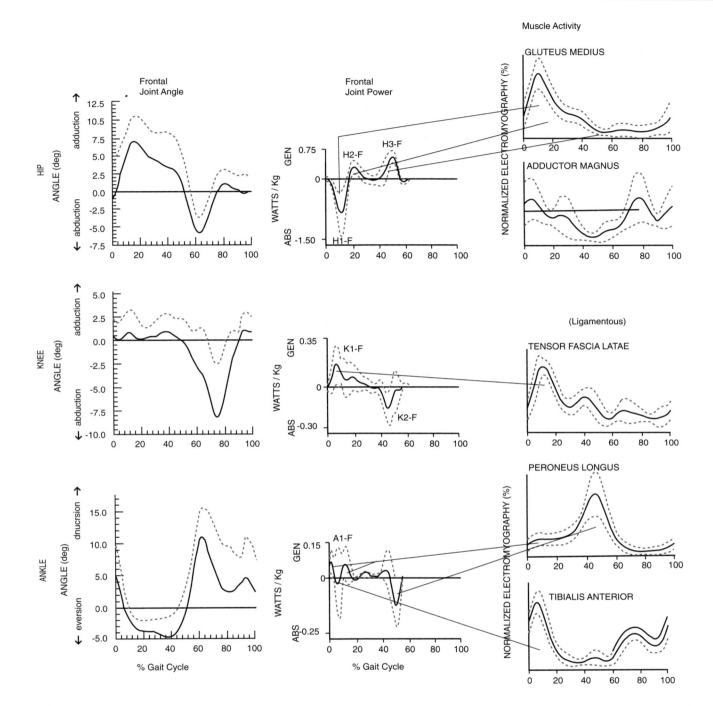

▲ **Figure 14-23** ■ Joint angles and joint powers in the frontal plane, and EMG profiles of representatives of major contributors to joint powers of hip, knee, and ankle during adult gait. (Angle profiles redrawn from Winter DA, Eng JJ, Isshac MJ: A review of kinetic parameters in human walking. In Craik RL, Otis CA [eds]: Gait Analysis: Theory and Application, pp 263-265. St. Louis, Mosby–Year Book, 1994, with permission from Elsevier. Power profiles redrawn from Eng JJ, Winter DA: Kinetic analysis of the lower limbs during walking: What information can be gained from a three dimensional model? J Biomech 28:753, 1995, with permission. Muscle activity redrawn from Winter DA: The Biomechanics and Motor Control of Human Gait: Normal, Elderly and Pathological, 2nd ed. Waterloo, Ontario, Waterloo Biomechanics, 1991. with permission from David A. Winter.)

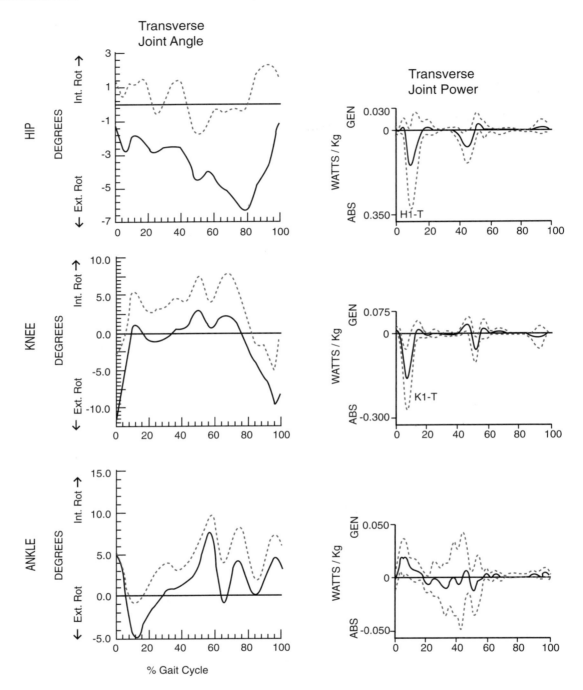

▲ **Figure 14-24** ■ Joint angles and joint powers in the transverse plane of hip, knee, and ankle during adult gait. (Angle profiles redrawn from Winter DA, Eng JJ, Isshac MG: A review of kinetic parameters in human walking. In Craik RL, Otis CA [eds]: Gait Analysis: Theory and Application, pp. 263-265. St. Louis, Mosby–Year Book, 1994, with permission from Elsevier. Power profiles redrawn from Eng JJ, Winter DA: Kinetic analysis of the lower limbs during walking: What information can be gained from a three dimensional model? J Biomech 28:753, 1995, with permission from Elsevier.)

(Heel Strike)

Table 14-3   Summary of Gait Characteristics from Initial Contact to Midstance:

Sagittal Plane Analysis

Joint	Motion	Ground Reaction Force	(What mm is doing) Internal Moment	Power	Major Muscle Activity
Hip	Extends from +20°–+30° to 0°	Anterior to posterior *(causes ↑)* *(causes ↓)*	Extensor to neutral	Generation (hip extensors) *Concentric*	Gluteus maximus Hamstrings
Knee	Flexes from 0° to +15°, then extends +15° to +5°	Anterior to posterior to anterior *(causes ↑)*	Flexor, then extensor then flexor	Generation (knee flexors) Absorption (knee extensors) *neg. work eccentric ✓* Generation (knee extensors) Absorption (knee flexors)	Hamstrings Quadriceps Hamstrings Gastrocnemius
Ankle	Plantarflexes from 0° to −5°, then dorsiflexes to +5°	Posterior to anterior	Dorsiflexor, then plantarflexor	Absorption (dorsiflexors) Generation (plantarflexors)	Tibialis anterior Soleus Gastrocnemius

Frontal Plane Analysis

Joint	Motion	Ground Reaction Force	Moment	Power	Major Muscle Activity
Hip	Adduction from neutral to +5°, then abduction to 3°	Medial	Abductor	Absorption (hip abductors) Generation (hip abductors)	Gluteus medius
Knee	Small variation around neutral	Medial	Abductor	Small generation (knee abductors)	Tensor fasciae latae
Ankle	Everts from 5° inversion to 5° eversion	Medial	Very small everter then neutral or small inverter	Small generation (everters) Very small absorption (inverters) Small generation (everters)	Peroneus longus Peroneus brevis Tibialis anterior

Transverse Plane Analysis

Joint	Motion	Moment	Power	Major Muscle Activity
Hip	Externally rotates a few degrees	External rotator	Absorption (internal rotators)	Tensor fasciae latae Gluteus medius Gluteus minimus (Ligamentous)
Knee	From several degrees of external rotation, rotates internally to neutral	Very small external rotator	Small absorption (external rotators)	
Ankle	Externally rotates from +5° internal rotation to −5° external rotation, then to neutral	External rotator	Extremely small	—

Redrawn from Eng JJ, Winter DA: Kinetic analysis of the lower limbs during walking: What information can be gained from a three dimensional model? J Biomech 28:753, 1995; and from Winter DA, Eng JJ, Isshac MG: A review of kinetic parameters in human walking. In Craik RL, Otis CA (eds): Gait Analysis: Theory and Application. St. Louis, Mosby–Year Book, 1994.
Values are for young males.

Table 14-4	Summary of Gait Characteristics from Midstance to Toe-off

Sagittal Plane Analysis

Joint	Motion	Ground Reaction Force	Moment	Power	Major Muscle Activity
Hip	Extends from 0° to −20° extension, then begins to flex	Posterior *causes /*	Flexor *We need to Create ✓*	Absorption (flexors) *neg. work controlled by hip flexors* Generation (flexors)	Iliopsoas Rectus femoris Iliopsoas Rectus femoris
Knee	From +5° extends a few degrees, then flexes to about +45°	Posterior	Flexor, then extensor	Absorption (extensors) Small generation (knee flexors) Large absorption (extensors)	Vastus Gastrocnemius Rectus femoris
Ankle	From +5° dorsiflexion, dorsiflexes a few more degrees, then rapidly plantarflexes to −25°	Anterior	Plantarflexor	Very small absorption (plantarflexors) Large generation (plantarflexors)	Soleus Gastrocnemius Soleus Gastrocnemius

Frontal Plane Analysis

Joint	Motion	Ground Reaction Force	Moment	Power	Major Muscle Activity
Hip	From +3° smoothly abducts to −5°	Medial	Abductor	Generation (abductors)	Gluteus medius
Knee	Neutral, then abducts to a few degrees −3°	Medial	Abductor	Absorption (abductors)	Tensor fasciae latae, ligaments
Ankle	−5°	Medial	Inverter, then everter	Very small generation Absorption (evertors)	Peroneus longus Peroneus brevis

Transverse Plane Analysis

Joint	Motion	Moment	Power
Hip	From −3°, externally rotates a few more degrees	Internal rotator	Very small absorption (external rotators)
Knee	Remains near neutral	Internal rotator	Very small absorption (ligamentous)
Ankle	From neutral, rotates about 7°, then back to neutral	External rotator	Variable

Redrawn from Eng JJ, Winter DA: Kinetic analysis of the lower limbs during walking: What information can be gained from a three dimensional model J Biomech 28:753, 1995; and from Winter DA, Eng JJ, Isshac MG: A review of kinetic parameters in human walking. In Craik RL, Otis CA (eds): Gait Analysis: Theory and Application. St. Louis, Mosby–Year Book, 1994.
Values are for young males.

current with H1-S, which is positive. K3-S is negative work occurring concurrently with both H3-S and A2-S. Values that are above normal represent excessive inefficiency and usually result in slower walking speeds.

Case Application 14-6: **Continuing Gait Problems**

It was noted that Ms. Brown tended to fully extend her knee in midstance and then flexed her knee only a few degrees during swing phase. A power analysis of Ms. Brown's affected limb, if available, would have shown a severely reduced A2-S and H3-S and virtual absence of an H1-S energy burst. The first two would be apparent to the therapist as no firm push-off[29] and no rapid hip flexion. This meant that Ms. Brown would be unable to push off strongly (A2-S) or pull off strongly (H3-S), because both actions require knee flexion. Every attempt was made during gait training to gain knee control in midstance, not permitting it to fully extend. Strong push-off and strong "pull-off" then could be encouraged.

Because the hip extensors on the affected side were among the least affected muscles, Ms. Brown was encouraged to exploit H1-S, the "push from behind" in early stance. Stronger activity of A2-S, H1-S, and H3-S on the unaffected side, especially later in stages of rehabilitation, would be encouraged to provide interlimb compensation for the reduced activity on the affected side. Gait speed would increase to the degree that these efforts are effective.

Continuing Exploration: **On the Existence of "Rockers" and "Push-Off"**

There has been some controversy concerning these two terms. Orthopedic literature frequently refers to three "rockers" as characterizing the kinematics of the foot and ankle during stance phase. The "first rocker" or "initial rocker" occurs from initial contact until foot flat and has a fulcrum about the heel (heel pivot). The "second rocker" or "midstance rocker" is described as occurring between foot flat and heel-off and has a fulcrum about the ankle joint. The "third rocker" or "terminal rocker" occurs between heel-off and toe-off (push-off), with the leg rotating about the forefoot. Although not incorrect, it is preferable that standard terminology be used.

Before kinetic link segment analysis was common, there were objections to the term "push-off." It was thought that the second peak in the vertical floor reaction force resulted from changes in body alignment, rather than an increasing force resulting from plantarflexor contraction. However, the work of Winter[45] and others[44,46,47] shows that push-off not only exists but is normally responsible for a major portion of the work of walking. It is clear that a person with no ankle plantarflexion (hence no power generation at the ankle) can walk, however. Some compensation can be provided by H1-S and H3-S from both limbs, although people with rigid ankle foot orthoses or inflexible prostheses usually walk more slowly than normal.

Zajac and colleagues and other researchers using similar models have shown that the energy produced by the soleus muscle in late stance is delivered to the trunk to accelerate it forward, but the increase in trunk energy is more than that produced by the soleus muscle.[47,48] It appears that the soleus, rectus femoris, and gastrocnemius work synergistically to ensure forward acceleration of the trunk. These studies show that muscles not only generate and absorb energy but, in many cases, serve to redistribute energy.

Muscle Activity

Muscle activity can be identified by EMG, a technique in which the electrical activity generated by an active muscle is recorded. There is a great deal of information about EMG, the varieties of techniques that can be used, and the patterns obtained during gait.[24,49–53] EMG is often used in conjunction with force plates, goniometry, and/or motion analysis systems to link the muscle activity with other events during the gait cycle. The EMG record provides information about when only particular muscles are acting and the relative level, or profile, of their activity. It does not tell why the muscles are acting or how much force the muscles are generating. The reader is encouraged to follow the developing literature on muscle function that is derived from elaborate mathematical simulations that involve modeling precise muscle geometry and anthropometrics.[46–48] Although this work has just begun, it is already challenging conventional assumptions about the function of muscles.

EMG studies of gait are used to augment the understanding provided by a link segment analysis, to validate theoretical models that attempt to explain why muscles are needed for certain functions, and in theoretical models developed to explain the muscle activity found by EMG.[53] The EMG reported in the section that follows is derived from the work of Winter.[14]

The muscle work of gait can be simplified by anticipating the muscle groups that must be functioning for specific purposes and then adding detailed variations when the general pattern is clear. Muscle work is logical, and the reader already knows that two major features are going to determine its patterns: **the need to provide a support moment through stance** and **the need to generate energy to move.**

Let us follow the logic of what muscle work is likely to be needed for the support moment (see Fig. 14-17) and compare results with Figures 14-25, 14-26, and 14-27. The support moment is made up of some combination of **hip extensors, knee extensors,** and **ankle plantarflexors.** We already have discussed the fact that the **hip extensors** produce an internal extensor moment early in stance; next, **knee extensors** produce an internal knee extensor moment, and then internal **flexor moments** are produced at both the hip and knee before the knee and hip bend in late stance in preparation for swing phase. While these two muscle groups are flexing the segmented system, the **ankle plantarflexors** take the lead and provide support. We should not be surprised, then, to find activity in the hip extensors (**hamstrings**) early in stance and knee extensors (**quadriceps**) almost immediately after, followed by a smoothly increasing contraction of the **ankle plantarflexors** (**soleus, medial,** and **lateral gastrocnemius muscles** and other minor contributors) that continues until mid-push-off and then declines and ceases at about 60% of the cycle.

Now let us look for the muscle work that is responsible for the main bursts of positive work, relating muscle work shown in Figures 14-25 to 14-27 to power profiles shown in Figures 14-22 to 14-24. In the sagittal plane, we note that the **hip extensors (gluteus maximus, medial hamstring,** and **lateral hamstring muscles)** are active in early stance (H1-S); indeed, they were serving the function of providing support during that period. The small energy-generating K2-S that peaks in early stance is reflected in activation of the **quadriceps (vastus medialis, vastus lateralis,** and **rectus femoris**

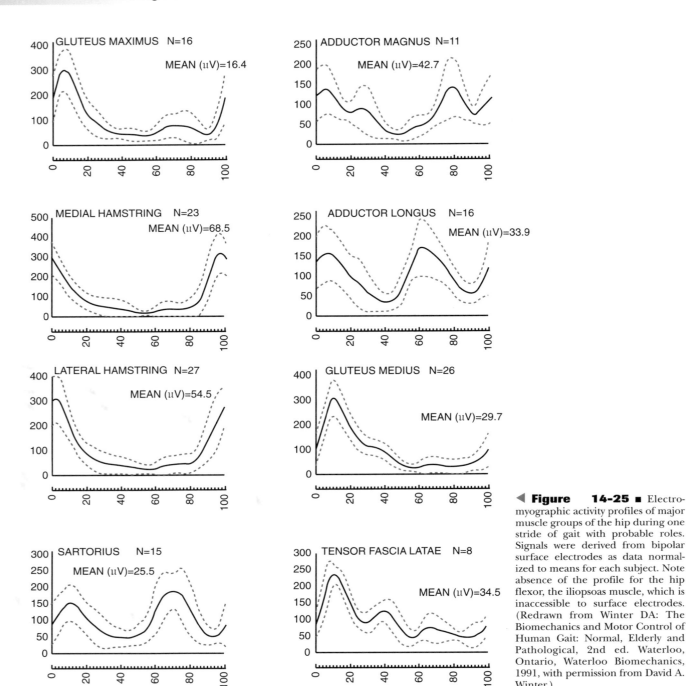

◀ **Figure 14-25** ■ Electromyographic activity profiles of major muscle groups of the hip during one stride of gait with probable roles. Signals were derived from bipolar surface electrodes as data normalized to means for each subject. Note absence of the profile for the hip flexor, the iliopsoas muscle, which is inaccessible to surface electrodes. (Redrawn from Winter DA: The Biomechanics and Motor Control of Human Gait: Normal, Elderly and Pathological, 2nd ed. Waterloo, Ontario, Waterloo Biomechanics, 1991, with permission from David A. Winter.)

muscles). Recall that the largest contribution to the work of walking comes from the **ankle plantarflexors** (largely **soleus, medial,** and **lateral gastrocnemius muscles**). These muscles work eccentrically (lengthening) from early stance until about 40% of the gait cycle, when they overcome the dorsiflexing moment of the foot-floor force (GRF; see later discussion) and produce a burst of concentric activity (A2-S) ending at toe-off, at about 60% of the gait cycle. A similar sequence of first eccentric and then concentric activity occurs in the **hip flexors** (**iliopsoas** and **rectus femoris muscles**). First they lengthen, producing an energy-absorbing

contraction as the hip extends (H2-S); then the muscle force overcomes the opposing force and begins to act concentrically, causing an energy-generating "pull-off " phase (H3-S). The **iliopsoas** muscle is the major hip flexor, but it is inaccessible to surface electrodes. However, the **rectus femoris** muscle is the only quadriceps muscles that crosses the hip and whose activity in late stance is known to correlate with that of iliopsoas. We can see **rectus femoris** activity peaking around 70% of the cycle, reflecting the hip-flexor function.

Now let us look at the major energy-absorbing phases and the muscle groups that are responsible.

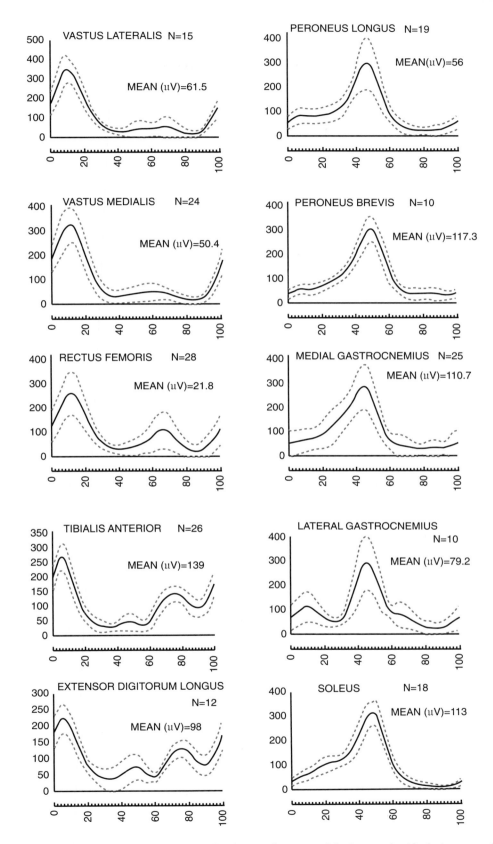

▲ **Figure 14-26** ■ Electromyographic activity profiles of major muscle groups of the knee and ankle during one stride of gait with probable roles. Signals were derived from bipolar surface electrodes as data normalized to means for each subject. (Redrawn from Winter DA: The Biomechanics and Motor Control of Human Gait: Normal, Elderly and Pathological, 2nd ed. Waterloo, Ontario, Waterloo Biomechanics, 1991, with permission from David A. Winter.)

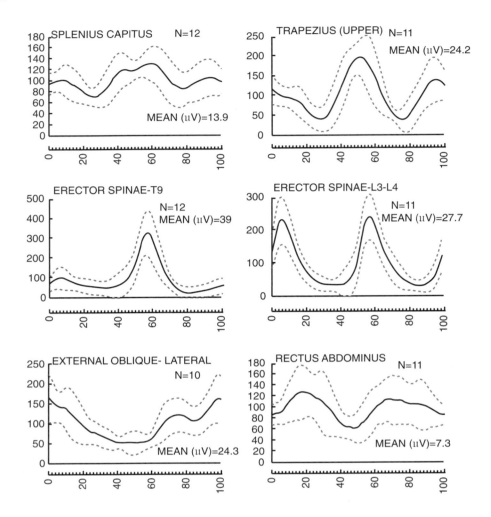

▲ **Figure 14-27** ■ Electromyographic activity profiles of major muscle groups of the trunk during one stride of gait with probable roles. Signals were derived from bipolar surface electrodes as data normalized to means for each subject. (Redrawn from Winter DA: The Biomechanics and Motor Control of Human Gait: Normal, Elderly and Pathological, 2nd ed. Waterloo, Ontario, Waterloo Biomechanics, 1991, with permission from David A. Winter.)

K1-S, occurring before 20% of the cycle, is the eccentric phase of the **knee extensors** (**vastus lateralis, medialis, intermedius** and **rectus femoris**), which precedes its concentric K2-S energy-generating phase. We have discussed H2-S, the eccentric action of the **hip flexors** (**iliopsoas** and **rectus femoris**), during midstance and late stance. Note that the **knee extensor** and the **hip extensor** muscles begin their contraction at the end of swing phase, although at this time the dominant moments are being provided by the knee flexors; in other words, there is a period of co-contraction that is invisible to a link segment analysis but evident from EMG. K3-S is a small energy-absorbing internal knee extensor moment occurring while the knee is flexing rapidly (~50% to 70% of cycle), and this is reflected in low levels of contraction of the **vastus muscles,** particularly the **rectus femoris,** which, because it crosses both hip and knee, is active at that time as a **hip flexor** (H3-S). K4-S, energy absorption of the **knee flexors** at

the end of swing, is reflected in EMG records as activation of the **medial** and **lateral hamstrings**. Note that the **gastrocnemius** muscles, which cross the knee as well as the ankle, also begin activity in late swing phase. At the ankle, A1-S absorption through much of early stance and midstance is attributable to **ankle plantarflexor** activity, which we have already discussed.

Now let us see whether we have missed any major EMG features by deducing muscle activity from support moment and power profiles. First, in the sagittal plane, the **ankle dorsiflexors** (**tibialis anterior, extensor digitorum longus,** and **extensor hallucis longus muscles**) are active eccentrically across the ankle before foot flat to lower the foot to the floor, are active again to hold the foot at a neutral angle during swing phase, and show varying but small levels of activity at other times of the cycle, probably positioning the foot. In the frontal plane, the activity of hip abductor **gluteus medius,** along with gluteus minimus and tensor fasciae latae muscles (not shown), controls the lateral drop of the pelvis on the side of the swinging leg, closely mimicking the pattern of the vasti.[49] Activity of these muscles diminishes during midstance and ceases when the opposite limb has contacted the ground.[12]

Adductor longus and **brevis muscles,** acting in both frontal and sagittal planes, show two fairly equal peaks of activity at ~10% and 65% to 80% of the gait cycle. The first is concurrent with the **hip abductors** and may be providing stabilization; the second is early in swing, providing hip flexion to assist **iliopsoas** and **rectus femoris muscles.** Further information can be found in the literature.[49,51,52] Trunk muscle activity is discussed in a later section.

Ground Reaction Force: Sagittal Plane Analysis

Before full dynamic biomechanical gait analyses were common, attempts were made to link in a visual way the static information from the GRF to the joint positions during gait. There are errors in this kind of analysis because dynamic factors are not included, but during stance phase, these are minimal. Also, they cause less error nearer the force platform. Small errors are produced at the ankle that become larger at the hip, especially at times of push-off and initial contact.[54] If they are used to attempt to reconcile with the internal moment profiles of Figures 14-28 to 14-30, however, they can add important understanding and helpful visualization of normal gait for stance phase of gait (inasmuch as, of course, there is no GRF during swing phase). The general sequence of the most common pattern of GRFV for stance phase is shown in Figure 14-31 (initial contact to midstance) and Figure 14-32 (midstance to toe-off). These should be related to internal moment profiles appearing in Figure 14-28 to 14-30. The analyses included show the location of the GRF in relation to the joints of the lower extremities. The location of the GRFV, joint positions, and muscle activity that were used to create the illustrations were derived from published studies on normal human walking.[3,8,55] Three examples of practical applications will illustrate this process, and the reader is encouraged to attempt others independently.

Example 14-1

In the period of gait from initial contact to the end of midstance, the ankle moves from the neutral position at initial contact to 15° of plantarflexion by the end of loading response and to 10° of dorsiflexion by the end of midstance. The GRFV changes from a location posterior to the ankle joint at initial contact to an anterior position in midstance (see Fig. 14-31). Therefore, at initial contact and during loading response (heel strike to foot flat), there is an external plantarflexion moment, and the ankle is moving in a direction of plantarflexion. An eccentric contraction of the **dorsiflexors** controls the motion, and negative work is done. Note that

this period of energy absorption is so small in magnitude that it does not appear on power profiles. It is, however, functionally important.

Example 14-2

The GRFV tending to flex the hip (external flexion moment) and extend the knee (external extension moment) at initial contact (see Fig. 14-31) is consistent with the opposition provided by an internal hip extensor moment (**hamstrings** and **gluteus maximus**) and internal knee flexor moment (**hamstrings**) shown in Figure 14-28.

Case Application 14-7: **Internal Hip and Knee Flexors**

At heel-off (~40% of gait cycle), the GRFV tending to extend the hip and knee (see Fig. 14-32) is consistent with the opposition provided by the internal hip flexor moment (**iliopsoas** and **rectus femoris muscles**) and the internal knee flexor moment (**gastrocnemius muscles**) (see Fig. 14-28). Consider the effects of a larger than normal tendency to extend the knee, which occurred, for example, when Ms. Brown thrust her knee back into full extension in an effort to gain knee stability (Fig. 14-33). Because the knee flexors that are active at that time (**gastrocnemius muscles**) did not overcome this excessive moment, Ms. Brown had difficulty flexing the knee, which prevented flexion of both the hip and the ankle and reduced the opportunity to generate work from the ankle at A2-S and the hip at H3-S. Avoiding this "knee locking" in stance by rigorous encouragement of knee flexion at the end of stance and by temporary use of an ankle-foot orthosis was important in Ms. Brown's gait reeducation.

 CONCEPT CORNERSTONE 14-3: *What Gait Information Is Important?*

Given the availability of information about walking, it is often not clear what information is helpful for any given situation. First, it is important to determine why you want the information. Usually the reasons include one or more of the following: (1) to gain an understanding of normal or pathological gait; (2) to assist movement diagnosis and identify specific causes of pathological gait; (3) to inform treatment selection; and (4) to evaluate the effectiveness of treatment. Second, you may ask what gait measures are important for the situation. For example, if you want to know whether energy costs are decreased with provision of an ankle orthosis, a measure of self-selected speed of walking may be sufficient. If you want to know which muscle groups could be exploited to gain increased walking speed in treating a person with a neurological condition, you would want to see a power analysis. If you wished to know whether a new ankle-foot orthosis really did return energy during push-off, you would also want a power analysis. If you

Text continues on p. 551

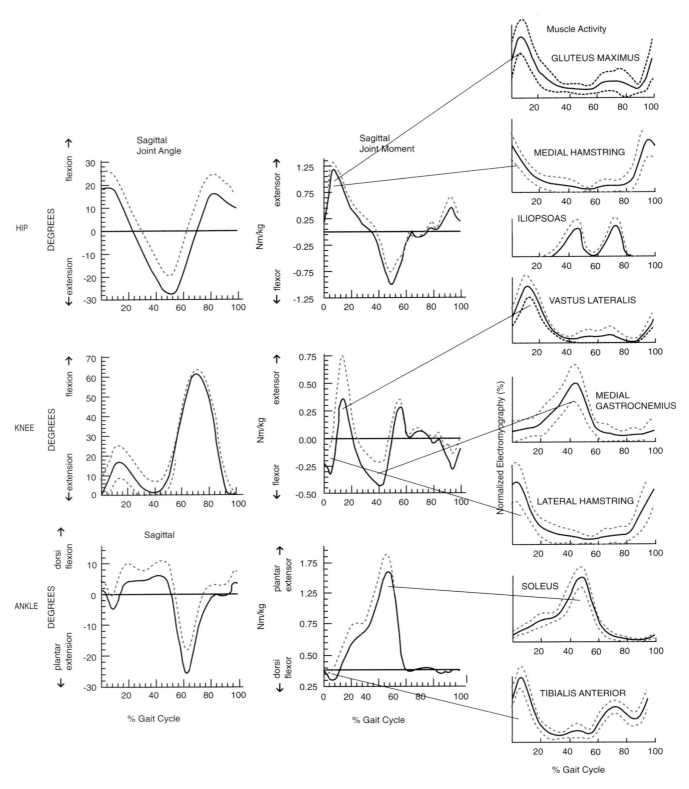

▲ **Figure 14-28** ■ Joint angles and net joint moments in the sagittal plane, and EMG profiles of representatives of major contributors to joint moments of hip, knee, and ankle during adult gait. (Angle and moment profiles redrawn from Winter DA, Eng JJ, Isshac MG: A review of kinetic parameters in human walking. In Craik RL, Otis CA [eds]: Gait Analysis: Theory and Application, pp 263-265. St. Louis, Mosby–Year Book, 1994, with permission from Elsevier. Muscle activity redrawn from Winter DA: The Biomechanics and Motor Control of Human Gait: Normal, Elderly and Pathological, 2nd ed. Waterloo, Ontario, Waterloo Biomechanics, 1991, with permission from David A. Winter. Ilopsoas muscle activity redrawn from Bechtol CO: Normal human gait. In American Academy of Orthopaedic Surgeons: Atlas of Orthotics, p 141. St. Louis, CV Mosby, 1974, with permission from Elsevier.)

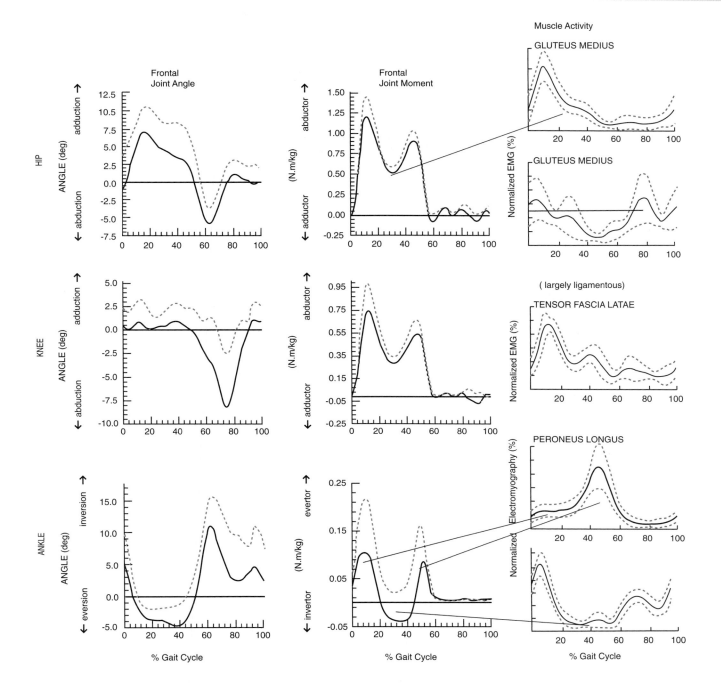

▲ **Figure 14-29** ■ Joint angles and net joint moments in the frontal plane, and EMG profiles of representatives of major contributors to joint moments of hip, knee, and ankle during adult gait. (Angle and moment profiles redrawn from Winter DA, Eng JJ, Isshac MG: A review of kinetic parameters in human walking. In Craik RL, Otis CA [eds]: Gait Analysis: Theory and Application, pp 263-265. St. Louis, Mosby–Year Book, 1994, with permission from Elsevier. Muscle activity redrawn from Winter DA: The Biomechanics and Motor Control of Human Gait: Normal, Elderly and Pathological, 2nd ed. Waterloo, Ontario, Waterloo Biomechanics, 1991, with permission from David A. Winter.)

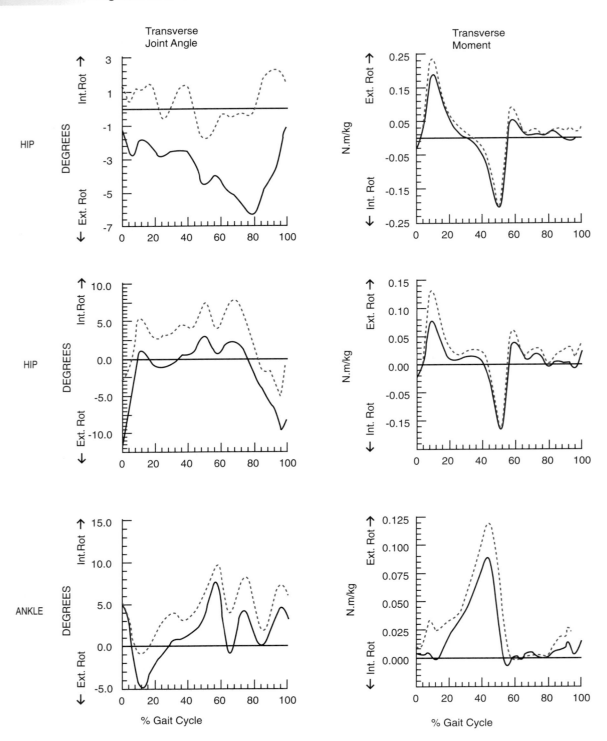

▲ **Figure 14-30** ■ Joint angles and net joint moments in the transverse plane, and EMG profiles of representatives of major contributors to joint moments of hip, knee, and ankle during adult gait. (Angle and moment profiles redrawn from Winter DA, Eng JJ, Isshac MG: A review of kinetic parameters in human walking. In Craik RL, Otis CA [eds]: Gait Analysis: Theory and Application, pp 263-265. St. Louis, Mosby–Year Book, 1994, with permission from Elsevier. Muscle activity redrawn from Winter DA: The Biomechanics and Motor Control of Human Gait: Normal, Elderly and Pathological, 2nd ed. Waterloo, Ontario, Waterloo Biomechanics, 1991, with permission from David A. Winter.)

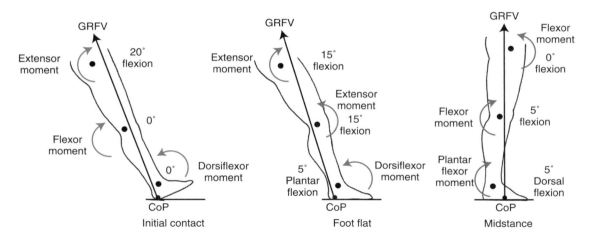

▲ **Figure 14-31** ■ Diagram of joint positions with center of pressure (CoP), ground reaction force vector (GRFV), and **internal net moments** of force for gait cycle events of initial contact, foot flat, and midstance.

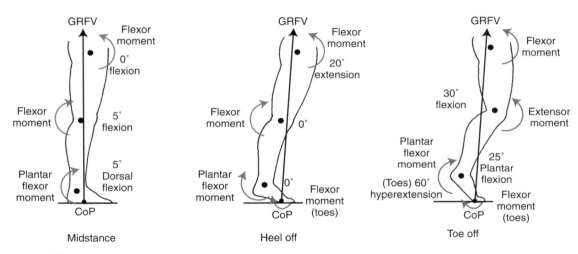

▲ **Figure 14-32** ■ Diagram of joint positions with center of pressure (CoP), ground reaction force vector (GRFV), and **internal net moments** of force for gait cycle events of midstance, heel-off, and toe-off.

wanted to determine whether surgery to realign the tibia and fibula was successful in decreasing a varus or valgus moment on the knee, you would want a moment analysis in the frontal plane. There is a tendency for power analyses to be more useful in neurological conditions and moment analyses in musculoskeletal conditions, particularly those involving pain.

Kinematics and Kinetics of the Trunk and Upper Extremities

Trunk

The trunk remains essentially in the erect position during normal free-speed walking on level ground, varying only $1\frac{1}{2}°$.[56] Krebs and coworkers[57] found that a flexion peak of low amplitude occurred near each

heel strike and an extension peak of low amplitude occurred during single limb support. Winter explained[14] that at initial contact, the forward acceleration of the HAT is quite large and acts at a distance from the hip joint, thus producing an unbalancing moment that acts strongly to cause flexion of the trunk during WA. However, an almost equal and opposite internal moment is provided by the hip extensors (which we have seen before in their role in support and in energy generation at H1-S). In the frontal plane, a similar situation exists. The center of mass of the HAT, always being medial to the hip joint, exerts a considerable moment that is balanced primarily by an internal hip abductor moment from the supporting limb and is assisted by the medial acceleration of the hip.

The biomechanical models used previously in the chapter do not distinguish between the pelvis and the

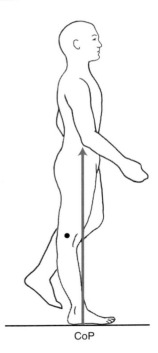

▲ Figure 14-33 ■ GRFV passing excessively anterior to knee joint center, making it difficult for the person to flex the knee.

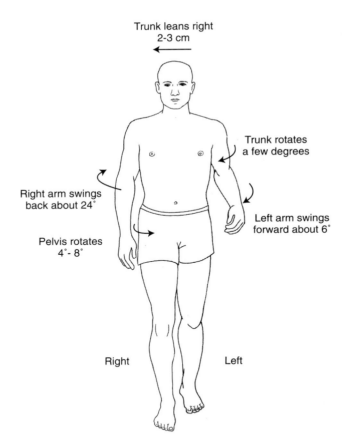

▲ Figure 14-34 ■ Pelvis, trunk, and arm motion. Note that the trunk and arms rotate in a direction opposite to that of the pelvis.

trunk. In the sagittal plane, the pelvis moves sinusoidally up and down 4 or 5 cm with each step, the low point coinciding with initial contact of each foot and the high point coinciding with midstance. In the frontal plane, the pelvis translates from side to side about the same amount toward the standing limb and rotates downward about 5° toward the swinging limb on each side. In the transverse plane, looking at it from above, it rotates 4° to 8° counterclockwise during swing phase of the right limb, goes through neutral position about midstance, then continues rotating the same amount in preparation for left foot initial contact. When the pelvis rotates counterclockwise, preparing for initial contact of the right foot, the trunk rotates clockwise with regard to the pelvis to keep it directed forwards. The amount of transverse rotation of the trunk during gait is slight and occurs primarily in a direction opposite to the direction of pelvic rotation (Fig. 14-34). As the pelvis rotates forward with the swinging lower extremity, the thorax on the opposite side rotates forward as well. Actually, the thorax undergoes a biphasic rotation pattern with a reversal directly after liftoff of the stance leg. The thorax is rotated backward during double support and then slowly rotates forward during single support. This trunk motion helps prevent excess body motion and helps counterbalance rotation of the pelvis. Krebs and coworkers found that at a free speed of gait, transverse rotation reached a maximum of 9° at 10% of the cycle after each heel strike.[57] In a study of treadmill walking, Stokes and associates[58] found that the movements and interactions of the trunk and pelvis were extremely complex when translatory and rotatory movements of the trunk

were considered along with anterior and posterior pelvic tilting, lateral pelvic tilting, and rotation. Mediolateral translations of the trunk occur as side-to-side motions (leans) in relation to the pelvis. For example, the trunk is leaning or moving to the right from right heel strike to left toe-off, at which point the trunk begins a lean to the left until right toe-off. The average total ROM that occurs during the mediolateral trunk leans is about 5.4 cm.[58] Hirasaki and coworkers[59] used a treadmill and a video-based motion analysis system to study trunk and head movements at different walking speeds. These authors found that the relationship between walking speed and head and trunk movements was the most linear in the range of walking speeds from 1.2 to 1.8 m/sec. At velocities above and below this range, head and trunk movements were less well coordinated.

EMG profiles and probable functional roles are shown for some trunk muscles in Figure 14-27. Recent EMG studies on the trunk muscles during gait have shown that there are subgroups of subjects showing similar patterns of muscle activity. White and McNair,[60] using a cluster analysis, demonstrated that there were two patterns of activity for the **internal oblique, external oblique,** and **rectus abdominis muscles.** In the **lumbar erector spinae,** there were three patterns of activity observed. In the **rectus abdominis** and **external oblique muscles,** most subjects had very low levels of activity throughout the gait cycle, but the **internal oblique** and **erector spinae muscles** had more distinct bursts, usually occurring close to initial contact. Other authors have shown two periods of activity[61] for the **erector spinae muscle:** one at initial contact and the second at toe-off. The **erector spinae muscle** is thought to be active to oppose the unbalancing moment that acts strongly to cause flexion of the trunk during WA.

Upper Extremities

Detailed kinetics of the upper extremity during normal gait have not been reported, although extensive mapping of EMG was classically performed several decades ago.[61,62] Although the lower extremities are moving alternately forward and backward, the arms are swinging rhythmically. However, the arm swinging is opposite to that of the legs and pelvis but similar to that of the trunk (see Fig. 14-34). The right arm swings forward with the forward swing of the left lower extremity while the left arm swings backward. This swinging of the arms provides a counterbalancing action to the forward swinging of the leg and helps to decelerate rotation of the body, which is imparted to it by the rotating pelvis. The total ROM at the shoulder is not very large. At normal free velocities, the ROM is only approximately 30° (24° of extension and 6° of flexion).

The normal shoulder motion is the result of the combined effects of gravity and muscle activity. During the *forward* portion of arm swinging, the following medial rotators are active: **subscapularis, teres major,** and **latissimus dorsi muscles.** In *backward* swing, the **middle** and **posterior deltoid muscles** are active throughout, and the **latissimus dorsi** and **teres major muscles** are active only during the first portion of backward swing.[61] The **supraspinatus, trapezius,**[61] and **posterior** and **middle deltoid muscles**[61] are active in both backward and forward swing. It is interesting to note that little or no activity was reported in the **shoulder flexors** in these studies.[61,62] It appears that during forward swing, the **medial rotators** are acting eccentrically to control external rotation of the arm at the shoulder as the **posterior deltoid** acts eccentrically to restrain the forward swing. The **latissimus dorsi** and **teres major muscles,** as well as the **posterior deltoid,** may then act concentrically to produce the backward swing. The role of the **middle deltoid** is unclear, although it has been suggested that it functions to keep the arm abducted so that it may clear the side of the body.[37] Activity in all muscles increases as the speed of gait increases.[61]

Recent work supports neuronal coordination of arm and leg movement during locomotion. Deitz and colleagues[63] and Wannier and colleagues[64] reported the behaviors of the arm to leg corresponding to a system of two coupled oscillators. Results were compatible with the assumption that the proximal arm muscles are associated with the swinging of the arms during gait as a residual function of quadripedal locomotion.

◆ Stair and Running Gaits

Stair Gait

Ascending and descending stairs is a basic body movement required for performing normal activities of daily living such as shopping, using public transportation, or simply getting around in a multistory home or building. Although many similarities exist between level-ground locomotion and stair locomotion, the difference between the two modes of locomotion may be significant for a patient population. The fact that a patient has adequate muscle strength and joint ROM for level-ground walking does not ensure that the patient will be able to walk up and down stairs. Stair walking represents additional stress over level-ground walking and may reveal differences that are not apparent in level-ground walking.[65]

Krebs and coworkers[57] found that trunk ROM during level-ground gait was similar to trunk ROM during stair descent but differed from trunk ROM during stair ascent in all planes. The maximum ROM of trunk flexion in relation to the room during stair ascent was at least double the amount of trunk flexion found in either stair descent or in level-ground walking.[57]

Locomotion on stairs is similar to level-ground walking in that stair gait involves both swing and stance phases in which forward progression of the body is brought about by alternating movements of the lower extremities. Also, in both stair and level-ground gait, the lower extremities must balance and carry along HAT. McFayden and Winter (using step dimensions of 22 cm for the stair riser and 28 cm for the tread) performed a sagittal plane analysis of stair gait.[66] These investigators collected kinetic and kinematic data for one subject during eight trials. The stair gait cycle for stair ascent presented in Figure 14-35 is based on data from McFayden and Winter's study.[66] The net internal moments of the hip, knee, and ankle during stair

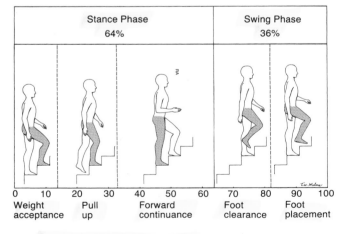

**Stair Gait Cycle
Ascent**

Stance Phase 64%			Swing Phase 36%	

0	10	20	30	40	50	60	70	80	90	100
Weight acceptance		Pull up		Forward continuance			Foot clearance		Foot placement	

▲ **Figure 14-35** ■ Stair gait cycle.

Table 14-5 | Sagittal Plane Analysis of Stair Ascent (Fig. 14–39): Stance Phase–Weight Acceptance (0%–14% of Stance Phase) through Pull-Up (14%–32% of Stance Phase)

Joint	Motion	Muscle	Contraction
Hip	Extension: 60°–30° of flexion	Gluteus maximus Semitendinosus Gluteus medius	Concentric
Knee	Extension: 80°–35° of flexion	Vastus lateralis Rectus femoris	Concentric
Ankle	Dorsiflexion: 20°–25° of dorsiflexion Plantarflexion: 25°–15° of dorsiflexion	Tibialis anterior Soleus Gastrocnemius	Concentric Concentric

ascent and descent can be compared with those during level-ground walking. The internal knee extensor moment in both stair ascent and descent was approximately three times larger than that of level-ground walking, but the ankle moments were approximately the same. Powers were largely generative in stair ascent and absorptive in descent for all joints.

The investigators divided the stance phase of the stair gait cycle into the three subphases and the swing phase into two subphases. The subdivisions of the stance phase are WA, pull-up (PU), and forward continuance (FCN). The subdivisions of the swing phase are foot clearance (FCO) and foot placement (FP). As can be seen in Figure 14-35, WA comprises approximately the first 14% of the gait cycle and is somewhat comparable to the heel strike throughout the loading phase of walking gait. However, in contrast to walking gait, the point of initial contact of the foot on the stairs is usually located on the anterior portion of the foot and travels posteriorly to the middle of the foot as the weight of the body is accepted. The PU portion, which extends from approximately 14% to 32% of the gait cycle, is a period of single-limb support. The initial portion of PU is a time of instability, inasmuch as all of the body weight is shifted onto the stance extremity when it

is flexed at the hip, knee, and ankle. During this period, the task is to pull the weight of the body up to the next stair level. The knee extensors are responsible for most of the energy generation required to accomplish PU. The FCN period is from approximately 32% to 64% of the gait cycle and corresponds roughly to the midstance through toe-off subdivisions of walking gait. In the FCN period, the greatest amount of energy is generated by the ankle plantarflexors.

Some of the data regarding joint ROM and muscle activity for ascending stairs that was collected by McFayden and Winter[66] are presented in Tables 14-5, 14-6, and 14-7. The tables demonstrate differences between level-ground gait and stair gait in regard to joint ROM, as well as some differences in the muscle activity required.

 CONCEPT CORNERSTONE 14-4: *Differences between Level-Ground Gait and Stair Gait*

Table 14-6 shows that considerably more hip and knee flexion are required in the initial portion of stair gait than are required in normal level-ground walking. Therefore, a patient would require a greater ROM for stair climbing (the same stair dimensions

Table 14-6 | Sagittal Plane Analysis of Stair Ascent (Fig. 14–39): Stance Phase–Pull-Up (End of Pull-Up) through Forward Continuance (32%–64% of the Stance Phase of Gait Cycle)

Joint	Motion	Muscle	Contraction
Hip	Extension: 30°–5° flexion	Gluteus maximus Gluteus medius Semitendinosus	Concentric and isometric
	Flexion: 5° to 10°–20° of flexion	Gluteus maximus Gluteus medius	Eccentric
Knee	Extension: 35°–10° of flexion	Vastus lateralis	Concentric
		Rectus femoris	
	Flexion: 5° to 10°–20° of flexion	Rectus femoris Vastus lateralis	Eccentric
Ankle	Plantarflexion: 15° of dorsiflexion to 15°–10° of plantarflexion	Soleus Gastrocnemius	Concentric
		Tibialis anterior	Eccentric

Table 14-7	Sagittal Plane Analysis of Stair Ascent (Fig. 14-39): Swing Phase (64%–100% of Gait Cycle)–Foot Clearance through Foot Placement			
Joint	Motion		Muscle	Contraction
Hip	Flexion: 10°–20° to 40°–60° of flexion		Gluteus medius	Concentric
	Extension: 40°–60° of flexion to 50° of flexion			
Knee	Flexion: 10° of flexion to 90°–100° of flexion		Semitendinosus	Concentric
	Extension: 90°–100° of flexion to 85° of flexion		Vastus lateralis	Concentric
			Rectus femoris	
Ankle	Dorsiflexion: 10° of plantarflexion to 20° of dorsiflexion		Tibialis anterior	Concentric and isometric

and slope) than for normal level-ground walking. Naturally muscle activity and joint ROMs will change if stairs of dimensions other than the ones investigated by McFayden and Winter are used.[66]

Ascending stairs involves a large amount of positive work that is accomplished mainly through concentric action of the rectus femoris, vastus lateralis, soleus, and medial gastrocnemius muscles. Descending stairs is achieved mostly through eccentric activity of the same muscles and involves energy absorption. The support moments during stair ascent, stair descent, and level-ground walking exhibit similar patterns; however, the magnitude of the moments is greater in stair gait, and, consequently, more muscle strength is required. Kirkwood et al.[67] found that the maximum peak internal abductor moment at the hip occurred during descending stairs.

Running Gait

Running is another locomotor activity that is similar to walking, but certain differences need to be examined. As in the case of stair gait, a patient who is able to walk on level ground may not have the ability to run. Running requires greater balance, muscle strength, and ROM than does normal walking. Greater balance is required because running is characterized not only by a considerably reduced base of support but also by an absence of the double-support periods observed in normal walking and the presence of float periods in which both feet are out of contact with the supporting surface (Fig. 14-36). The walking gait cycle presented in Figure 14-37 can be used to compare the gait cycle in walking with running gait. The percentage of the gait cycle spent in float periods will increase as the speed of running increases. Muscles must generate greater energy both to raise HAT higher than in normal walking and to balance and support HAT during the gait cycle. Muscles and joint structures also must be able to absorb more energy to accept and control the weight of HAT.

For example, in normal level-ground walking, the magnitudes of the GRFs at the CoP at initial contact are approximately 70% to 80% of body weight and rarely exceed 120% of body weight during the gait cycle.[68,69] However, during running, the GRFs at the CoP have been shown to reach 200% of body weight and increase to 250% of body weight during the running cycle.

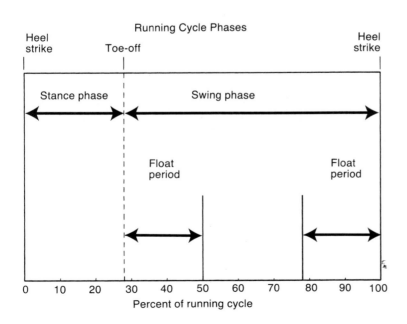

Figure 14-36 ■ Running gait cycle.

Walking Cycle Phases

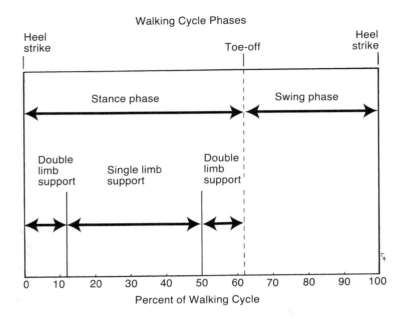

◀ **Figure 14-37** ■ Walking gait cycle.

Furthermore, the knee is flexed at about 20° when the foot strikes the ground. This degree of flexion helps to attenuate impact forces but also increases the forces acting at the patellofemoral joint. The base of support in running is considerably less than in walking. A typical base of support in walking is about 2 to 4 inches, whereas in running, both feet fall in the same line of progression, and so the entire center of mass of the body must be placed over a single support foot. To compensate for the reduced base of support, the functional limb varus angle increases. Functional limb varus angle is the angle between the bisection of the lower leg and the floor.[70] According to McPoil and Cornwall,[70] the functional limb varus angle increases about 5° during running in comparison with walking.

■ Joint Motion and Muscle Activity

Joint Motion

The ROM varies according to the speed of running and among different researchers. Comparisons in joint angles, moments, and powers between walking and running are shown in Figure 14-38.[71] At the beginning of the stance phase of running, the hip is in about 45° of flexion at heel strike and extends during the remainder of the stance phase until it reaches about 20° of hyperextension just after toe-off.[70] The hip then flexes to reach about 55° to 60° of flexion in late swing. Just before the end of the swing phase, the hip extends slightly to 45° to 50° in preparation for heel strike.[58] The knee is flexed to about 20° to 40° at heel strike and continues to flex to 60° during the loading response. Thereafter, the knee begins to extend, reaching 40° of flexion just before toe-off. During the swing phase and initial float period, the knee flexes to reach a maximum of approximately 125° to 130° in the middle of the swing phase. In late swing, the knee extends to 40° in preparation for heel strike.[69] In Figure 14-38, note

these differences in joint angles from level-ground walking. At each joint, the maxima for running exceed those of walking. In the case of the hip, only flexion range is increased. The knee range in running is not very different from that in walking, but it takes place in approximately 25° more flexion. The ankle has greatly increased dorsiflexion and modestly increased plantarflexion.

The ankle is in about 10° of dorsiflexion at heel strike and rapidly dorsiflexes to reach about 25° to 30° dorsiflexion. The rapid dorsiflexion is followed immediately by plantarflexion, which continues throughout the remainder of the stance phase and into the initial part of the swing phase. Plantarflexion reaches a maximum of 25° in the first few seconds of the swing phase. Throughout the rest of the swing phase, the ankle dorsiflexes to reach about 10° in late swing in preparation for heel strike.[69]

The reference extremity begins to medially rotate during the swing phase. At heel strike, the extremity continues to medially rotate and the foot pronates. Lateral rotation of the stance extremity and supination of the foot begins as the swing leg passes the stance limb in midstance. The ROM in the lower extremities needed for running, in comparison with the ROM required for normal walking, is presented in Table 14-8. The largest differences in the total ROM requirements between the two activities appear to be at the knee and hip joints. At the knee joint, up to an additional 90° of flexion is required for running versus walking. At the hip joint running requires about twice the amount of motion that was needed for normal walking.

Muscle Activity

The **gluteus maximus** and **gluteus medius** muscles are active both at the beginning of the stance phase and at the end of the swing phase. The **tensor fasciae latae** muscle is also active at the beginning of stance and at

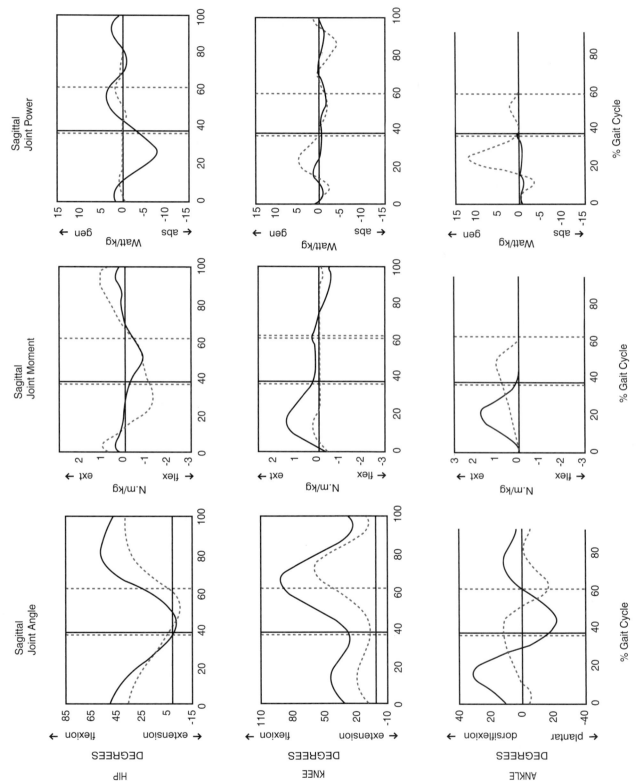

▲ **Figure 14-38** ■ Sagittal plane joint angles, moments, and powers for running (solid line) and walking (dotted line). Joint angles are plotted with flexion and dorsiflexion positive. Moments are internal moments normalized to body mass, plotted with extensor and plantarflexor positive. Powers are normalized to body mass, plotted with generation positive and absorption negative. The vertical solid line near 40% of gait cycle represents toe-off for running; the vertical dotted line near 60% of gait cycle represents toe-off for walking. (Joint angles, moments, and powers for running redrawn from Novacheck TF: The biomechanics of running. Gait Posture 7:77-95, 1998, with permission from Elsevier.)

557

Table 14-8	Average Peak ROM at the Hip, Knee and Ankle: Comparison between Running[69-71] and Walking[8, 71]			
Running		**Walking**		
Hip joint		Hip joint		
Flexion	55°–65°	Flexion	30°	
Extension	10°–20°	Extension	0°–20°	
Knee joint		Knee joint		
Flexion	80°–130°	Flexion	40°–50°	
Extension	0°–5°	Extension	0°	
Ankle joint		Ankle joint		
Dorsiflexion	10°–30°	Dorsiflexion	10°	
Plantarflexion	20°–30°	Plantarflexion	20°	

the end of swing but also is active between early and midswing. The **adductor magnus** muscle shows activity for about 25% of the gait cycle from late stance through the early part of the swing phase. Activity in the **iliopsoas** muscle occurs for about the same percentage of the gait cycle as the adductor longus muscle, but iliopsoas activity also occurs during the swing phase from about 35% to 60% of the gait cycle.

The **quadriceps** muscle acts eccentrically during the first 10% of the stance phase to control knee flexion when the knee is flexing rapidly. The quadriceps ceases activity after the first part of stance, and no activity occurs until the last 20% of the swing phase, when concentric activity begins to extend the knee (to 40° of flexion) in preparation for heel strike. The **medial hamstrings** are active at the beginning of stance and through a large part of swing. For example, the medial hamstrings are active from 18% to 28% of the stance phase, from about 40% to 58% of initial swing, and for the last 20% of swing. During part of this time, the knee is flexing and the hip is extending, and the hamstrings may be acting to extend the hip and to control the knee. During initial swing, the hamstrings are probably acting concentrically at the knee to produce knee flexion, which reaches a maximum at midswing. In late swing, the hamstrings may be contracting eccentrically to control knee extension and to reextend the hip.

A comparison of walking and running muscle activity at the ankle shows that in walking, **gastrocnemius** muscle activity begins just after the loading response at about 15% of the gait cycle and is active to about 50% of the gait cycle (just before toe-off). In running, gastrocnemius muscle activity begins at heel strike and continues through the first 15% of the gait cycle, ending at the point at which activity begins in walking. The gastrocnemius muscle becomes active again during the last 15% of swing.

The **tibialis anterior** muscle activity occurs in both stance and swing phases in walking and running. However, the total period of activity of this muscle in walking (54% of the gait cycle) is less than it is in running, in which it shows activity for about 73% of the gait cycle. The difference in activity of the tibialis anterior muscle between walking and running is due partly to

the differences in the length of the swing phases in the two types of gait. The swing period in walking gait is approximately 40% of the total gait cycle, whereas in running gait, the swing phase constitutes about 62% of the total gait cycle. Most of the activity in the tibialis anterior muscle during both walking and running gait is concentric or isometric action that is necessary to clear the foot in the swing phase of gait. The longer swing phase in running accounts for at least part of the difference in tibialis anterior activity between walking and running gaits. Tibialis anterior activity in the first half of the stance phase in running gait accounts for the remainder of the difference in activity in this muscle.

■ **Moments, Powers, and Energies**

In Figure 14-38, note the differences in internal moments and powers from walking. In all joints, the moments are greatly increased, particularly the knee extensor moment in early stance. Similarly, all the power generators are greatly increased in running. The chief generators are, again, A2, H3, and H1, but an additional source, K2, is now important. Note that the knee extensors in early stance (K2) are important in running. The absorption phases typical of walking are increased at all joints in running.

In walking, potential and kinetic energy of the HAT are out of phase, which results in considerable energetic savings. In running, these savings cannot occur, but two other methods of gaining efficiency are present. First, there are storage and return of elastic potential energy by the stretch of elastic structures, particularly tendons. Second, there is transfer of energy from one body segment to another by two-joint muscles acting as "energy straps."[71]

Summary

As a result of the efforts of many investigators, our present body of knowledge regarding human locomotion is extensive. However, gait is a complex subject, and further research is necessary to standardize methods of measuring and defining kinematic and kinetic variables, to develop inexpensive and reliable methods of analyzing gait in the clinical setting, and to augment the limited amount of knowledge available regarding kinematic and kinetic variables in the gaits of children and elderly persons that would form databases for movement pathologies.

Standardization of equipment and methods used to quantify gait variables, as well as standardization of the terms used to describe these variables, would help eliminate some of the present confusion in the literature and make it possible to compare the findings of various researchers with some degree of accuracy. Some standardization has been provided by the manufacturers of motion analysis systems; as a result, investigators using similar systems tend to use the same conventions. At the present time, inexpensive, quantitative, and reliable clinical methods of evaluating gait are limited to time and distance variables of step length, step duration, stride length, cadence, and velocity.[72] These measures provide a simple means for objective assessment of a patient's status and for detecting overall change, but they provide virtually no help in determining treatment. Increases in step length and decreases in step duration may be used to document a patient's progression toward a more normal gait pattern; however, a normal gait pattern may not be appropriate for many patients. Although many movement practitioners feel that it is best to aim for normal gait during early stages of rehabilitation, it is also important to identify the means by which a person can use the flexibility of the human body to compensate for deficiencies.[24,44] Automated gait analysis computer programs can provide the clinician with information about all of the kinematic and kinetic gait parameters related to a particular subject or patient. However, the researcher or clinician must have sufficient knowledge of the kinematics and kinetics of normal gait to interpret and use the information for the benefit of the patient.

◆ Effects of Age, Gender, Assistive Devices, and Orthoses

Age

Adult gait has been the focus of numerous studies, but the gait of young children has not received the same amount of attention. The relatively few studies of children's gait that have been conducted have shown that the age at which independent ambulation begins is extremely variable among individuals and that this variability continues throughout the developmental stages of walking. Cioni and coworkers[73] found that for 25 full-term infants, the age at which independent walking (ability to move 10 successive steps without support) was attained varied between 12.6 and 16.6 months. In the first stage of independent walking, none of the 25 toddlers had heel strike, reciprocal arm swinging, or trunk rotation. However, 4 months after attainment of independent walking, 11 of the 25 children had heel strike, and 16 of the 25 had reciprocal arm swinging and trunk rotation.

The toddler has a higher center of mass than does the adult and walks with a wider base of support, a decreased single-leg support time, a shorter step length, a slower velocity, and a higher cadence in comparison with normal adult gait. A study of 3- and 5-year-old children showed that some relationships between these variables were similar to the relationships found in adult gaits.[74] For example, as a group, the 3- and 5-year-old children showed significant increases in stride length adjusted for leg length, step length, and cadence from a slow to a free speed and from a free to a fast speed of gait. However, 5-year-olds differed from 3-year-olds in that they had less variability in step length adjusted for height at slow and free speeds.[74] In a study that included children from 6 to 13 years of age, Foley

and associates[75] reported that the ROMs for flexion and extension of the joints of the lower extremities were almost identical to the values obtained for adults. However, linear displacements, velocities, and accelerations were found to be consistently larger for these children than they were for adults.[75] Cadence, stride length, stride time, and other distance and temporal variables have been found to show variability until the child reaches 7 or 8 years of age. A gait pattern that is similar to normal adult gait is demonstrated by children from 8 to 10 years of age.

Sutherland and colleagues,[76] who studied 186 children from 1 to 7 years of age, suggested that the following five gait parameters could be used as indicators of gait maturity: duration of single-limb support, walking velocity, cadence, step length, and the ratio of pelvic span to ankle spread (indicative of base of support). Increases in all of these parameters except for cadence are indicative of increasing gait maturity. In Sutherland and colleagues' study, the duration of single-limb stance increased from about 32% in 1-year-olds to 38% in 7-year-olds (normal mean adult value is 39%). Walking velocity also increased steadily, whereas cadence decreased with age.[76] Beck et al.[77] found that time and distance measures and GRF measurements depended on speed of gait and age of the child. Increases in height and age were the major factors in determining changes in time and distance measures with age. Average stride length was 76% of the child's height at a walking speed of 104 m/sec, regardless of a child's age. According to Beck, after 5 years of age, an adult pattern in the GRF emerged.[77]

Studies involving young children are difficult to perform and often complicated by the fact that the child's musculoskeletal and nervous systems are in various stages of development. However, Sutherland and colleagues attempted to provide evaluators with guidelines for assessing children's gait by developing a group of prediction regions for the kinematic motion curves in normal gait. A test of the prediction regions indicated that they were capable of detecting a high percentage of abnormal motion and therefore could be used as an initial screen to identify deficits in lower extremity function in children.[78]

In contrast to the dearth of gait studies of young children, the effects of aging on gait have been and continue to be the object of many studies.[17,37,79,80] Some of this interest in elderly gait has been prompted by the large number of hip fractures and falls experienced by elderly persons. Fifty percent of elderly people who were able to walk before a hip fracture are not able to either walk or live independently after the fracture. Furthermore, it is estimated that an elderly person experiences at least two falls per year.[81] Therefore, many studies are directed toward determining what constitutes normal elderly gait and whether falls are caused by deficits in motor functioning or control or by other deficits that may accompany normal aging.

The use of different age groups and levels of activity (sedentary versus active groups) among investigators has made it difficult to draw definitive conclusions about the effects of normal aging. Despite some variations in the literature, gait speed and step or stride length have frequently been reported to be reduced in elderly persons, and stance phase and double-support times increased. Some investigators have found that elderly persons, in comparison with younger groups, demonstrate a decrease in natural walking speed, shorter stride and step lengths, longer duration of double-support periods, and smaller ratios of swing to support phases.[17,79] Himann and associates[79] found that between 19 and 62 years of age, there was a 2.5% to 4.5% decline in the normal speed of walking per decade for men and women, respectively. After age 62, there was an accelerated decline in normal walking speed: that is, a 16% and 12% decline in walking speed for men and women, respectively.[79] Winter and associates[37] compared fit and healthy elderly subjects with young adults and found that the natural cadence in the elderly subjects was no different from that in young adults but that the stride length of the elderly subjects was significantly shorter and the period of double support was longer in the elderly subjects than in young adults. Blanke and Hageman[80] compared 12 young men, age 20 to 32 years, with 12 elderly men, age 60 to 74 years, and found no effects of aging in regard to step length, stride length, velocity, and vertical and horizontal excursions of the body's center of mass. However, the ability to generalize Blanke and Hageman's findings is low because of the small size of their sample. Kerrigan and associates[82] found that comfortable walking speed and stride length were significantly slower than in young adults. In a study of fit healthy elderly people, Winter[14] found reduced stride length and a significant increase in stance time, which is consistent with attempting to increase stability. He also reported significantly higher horizontal heel velocity at initial contact, which was surprising because the speed was lower than for the young subjects. This increases the potential for slip-induced falls.

Differences in kinetic parameters of gait have also been reported. Lee and Kerrigan[83] found significant differences in kinetic parameters between a group of elderly persons who fell and an elderly control group. Analysis of data demonstrated significantly greater peak torques in the falling group for hip flexion, hip adduction, knee extension, knee varum, ankle dorsiflexion, and ankle eversion ($P < 0.003$ in each comparison). Also, ankle plantarflexion torque was significantly decreased in the falling group ($P = 0.001$). Joint powers showed different absorption at the knee and ankle in the falling group. Kerrigan and associates[82] also found that older persons, in comparison with younger persons, had reduced plantarflexion power generation, reduced plantarflexion ROM, peak hip extension ROM, and increased anterior pelvic tilt. The authors suggested that subtle hip flexion contractures and concentric plantarflexor weakness might be causes of the joint changes in elderly people.

Mueller and coworkers found that plantarflexor peak torque and ankle dorsiflexion were interrelated.[84] These authors suggested that walking speed and step length might be improved by increasing ankle flexor peak torque and dorsiflexion ROM.[84] Bohannon and colleagues[85] found that hip flexor strength was one of the variables that predicted gait speed. These authors did not test plantarflexor strength. Lord and associates[86] conducted an exercise program for women 60 years of age and older. After the program, the authors found significant increases in cadence and stride length, as well as reductions in stance time, swing time, and stance duration. Connelly and Vandervoort[87] measured the effects of detraining (which involved a decline in quadriceps muscle strength) on walking in a group of elderly persons with a mean age of 82.8 years. Strength values measured 1 year after the training program had declined 68.3%, and the speed of self-selected gait declined by 19.5%.

Winter[14] also reported that push-off work by the ankle plantarflexors was lower at the same time that absorption by the knee extensors was higher. Although several causal explanations are possible, these adaptations both are conducive to a safer gait pattern. Note, however, that the increased absorption by the knee extensors would also produce a less efficient gait.

Walking is considered to be a measure of independence, and faster walking speed is associated with increased levels of independence. A speed that is faster than comfortable walking is needed in many instances to cross a street. Walking in conjunction with exercise is also considered important to help prevent bone loss in the proximal femur.[67] Although differences of opinion have been found regarding gait speed in elderly people, the consensus of opinion appears to be that, in general, elderly persons select a free speed that is slower than the free speed gait of young people; however, as was shown previously, a slow gait requires a greater consumption of energy.

Although the particulars vary, it is clear that there are both kinematic and kinetic differences in the gait of elderly people. These can stem from two sources: early degeneration of strength and/or balance control system or adaptation to make gait safer. It is likely that both are responsible.

Gender

The research regarding gender differences in gait is fraught with the same difficulties as found in gait research with regard to age. Variations among methods, technologies, and subjects used in various studies make it difficult to come to many conclusions regarding the effects of gender. When differences in height, weight, and leg length between the genders are considered, gender differences are not very great. Oberg and associates[88] found significant differences between men and women for knee flexion/extension at slow, normal, and fast speeds at midstance and swing. They found a significant increase in joint angles as gait speed increased. For example, the knee angle at midstance increased from 15° to 24° in men and from 12° to 20° in women. However, Oberg and coworkers looked at only the knee and hip. In another study, the authors looked at velocity, step length, and step frequency.[17] Gait speed was found to be slower in women than in men (118 to 134 cm/sec for men and 110 to 129 cm/sec for women), and step length was smaller in women than in men. Kerrigan and associates[89] found that women had significantly greater hip flexion and less knee extension during gait initiation, a greater internal knee flexion moment in preswing, and greater peak mechanical joint power absorption at the knee in preswing. Kinetic data were normalized for both height and weight. These authors also found that women had a greater stride length in proportion to their height and that they walked with a greater cadence than did their male counterparts.[89]

Assistive Devices

Walking without the use of assistive devices (crutches, canes, and walkers) is preferred by most people. However, such devices often are necessary either after a lower-extremity fracture, when the healing bone is unable to bear full body weight, or as a more permanent adjunct for a balance, to compensate for muscle deficiencies or for joint pain. Recall that a very small force at the hand is needed to produce a large balancing moment about the standing leg because of the long perpendicular distance from the point of application of the force on the hand to the hip joint center. This may be responsible for the popularity of walkers for elderly persons, even when they appear to put little weight on them. Canes have typically been used on the side contralateral to an affected lower extremity to reduce forces acting at the affected hip, the reason being that a lower abductor muscle force on the affected side would be necessary to balance the weight of the upper body during single-limb stance if an upwardly directed force was provided by the hand on a cane at some distance from the hip joint center. Krebs and coworkers[90] tested the effect of cane use on reduction of pressure through the use of an instrumented femoral head prosthesis that quantified contact pressures at the acetabular cartilage. The prosthetic head contained 13 pressure-sensing transducers, which were deflected by 0.00028 mm/MPa pressure from opposing acetabular cartilage. The magnitude of acetabular contact pressure was reduced by 28% on one transducer and by 40% on another transducer in cane-assisted gait in comparison with unaided gait. The reduction in pressure at the hip coincided with reductions in EMG amplitude in comparison with the same pace in unaided gait trials. The authors concluded that the use of a cane on the contralateral side apparently allows the person to increase the base of support and to decrease muscle and GRF forces acting at the affected hip. The hip muscle abductor force was reduced, and gluteus maximus activity was reduced approximately 45%. The maximum GRF during cane-assisted gait occurs between heel strike and midstance.

Recall that Ms. Brown used a four-point cane on her unaffected side, because her arm was also affected.

For her the most important objective was to gain balance and stability, not to reduce joint forces.

Orthoses

The function of orthoses in gait is to alter the mechanics of walking. They are used to support normal alignment, to prevent unwanted motion, to help prevent deformity, to reduce unwanted forces or moments,[91–93] and, more recently, to augment joint power.[94] Although a full discussion is beyond the scope of this book, the student can deduce the effects of various types of devices with knowledge of the mechanics of gait. In all cases, the wish is to reduce or prevent unwanted movement or undesirable forces while permitting as normal mechanics as possible. For example, one may wish to limit ankle plantarflexion in a child with cerebral palsy. However, in so doing, one would prefer not to completely inhibit the active energy-generating activity of the ankle plantarflexors (A2) during push-off. Formerly relying on solid ankles, more recent hinged orthoses prevent excessive plantarflexion by use of a posterior stop but permit the ankle to move into dorsiflexion in late stance, and the child is able to generate some power through the plantarflexion that follows. Attempts have also been made to make use of mechanical characteristics of a leaf-spring design to return energy to the foot during push-off. Although good in concept, designs to date have failed to show return of energy.[94]

Case Application 14-8: Gait Status at Discharge

Recall that Ms. Brown was prescribed an ankle-foot orthosis to assist with providing an adequate support moment during stance phase and to prevent foot drop and the resulting energy-costly hip hiking. However, if the orthosis was rigid, it would make it impossible for her to achieve any A2-S push-off during late stance. Two options were considered: (1) a hinged orthosis that permitted unlimited dorsiflexion but had a stop beyond 10° of plantarflexion, thus allowing limited push-off, and (2) a flexible ankle-foot orthosis that narrowed posterior to the ankle, thus permitting a limited range of both dorsiflexion and plantarflexion. Because it was hoped that use of the device would be temporary, the latter was chosen. Gait reeducation included progressive training without the orthosis as strength was gained, and at discharge, Ms. Brown used her orthosis only for outdoor use. As her stability improved, she was able to progress from a four-point cane to a straight cane. When she was discharged from outpatient treatment, she was walking at 0.55 m/sec.

⬥ Abnormal Gait

Both quantitative and qualitative evaluations of gait are useful for assessors of human function. The most important quantitative variable is gait speed, which has been shown to be related to all levels of disablement.[95]

An individual's gait pattern may reflect not only physical or psychological status but also any defects or injuries in the joints or muscles of the lower extremities. In assessing an abnormal gait, it is helpful to classify the cause or causes of deviations into one or more of the following four causal categories: structural impairment, functional impairment, functional pain, or compensation/adaptation. Definitions and examples follow.

Structural Impairment

These are structural malformations that are congenital, caused by injury, or caused by structural changes occurring secondary to these.

A common structural abnormality is leg length discrepancy. Kaufman and coworkers[96] undertook a study to determine the magnitude of limb length inequality that would result in gait abnormalities. Many minor limb inequalities are found in the general population but many of these do not necessitate any particular treatment or intervention because they do not have any significant effects on normal gait. The authors concluded that a limb length discrepancy of 2.0 cm resulted in an asymmetrical gait and had the potential for causing changes in articular cartilage. Song and colleagues[97] evaluated neurologically normal children who had limb discrepancies of 0.8% to 15.8% of the length of the long extremity (0.6 to 11.1 cm). The compensatory strategies observed were equinus position of the ankle and foot of the short limb (toe walking), vaulting over the long limb, increased flexion of the long limb, and circumduction of the long limb. Children who used toe walking had a greater vertical translation of the body's center of mass during gait than did normal controls.

Structural problems may be implicated in running injuries. Increases in the Q-angle, tibial torsion, and pronation of the foot may contribute causes to patellofemoral syndromes. In running, stresses are greater than in walking, and so there is an accompanying increase in the likelihood of injury. In a survey of the records of 1650 running patients between the years 1978 and 1980, 1819 injuries were identified.[98] The knee was the site most commonly injured in running, and patellofemoral pain was the most common complaint.

At the foot, pes cavus and pes planus cause alterations in weight and may cause abnormal stresses at the hip or knee. In pes cavus, the weight is borne primarily on the hindfoot and metatarsal regions, and the midfoot provides only minimal support.[99] In running, the metatarsals bear a disproportionate share of the weight. In pes planus, the weight is borne primarily by the midfoot rather than being distributed among the hindfoot, lateral midfoot, metatarsals, and toes, as it is in the normal walking foot. The propulsive phase of gait is severely compromised.

Disturbances in the normal gait pattern usually cause increases in the energy cost of walking because the normal patterns of transformation from potential to kinetic energy and redistribution between segments are disturbed. Increases in muscle activity used to compensate for these disturbances may lead to increases in the amount of oxygen that is consumed. In a comparison between patients who had an ankle fusion and patients who had a hip fusion, oxygen consumption for patients with the hip fusion was 32% greater than normal and greater than in patients with the ankle fusion.[100]

Functional Impairment

This group includes all causes in which the timing and/or amplitude of muscle activity is abnormal.

Certain disease conditions such as **Parkinson's disease** produce characteristic gaits that are easily recognized by a trained observer. The parkinsonian gait is characterized by an increased cadence, shortened stride, lack of heel strike and toe-off, and diminished arm swinging. The muscle rigidity that characterizes this disease interferes with normal reciprocal patterns of movement.[101]

When the plantarflexors, which are the major source of mechanical energy generation in gait, are unable to generate sufficient power, muscles at other joints must provide more energy than in normal gait.[3] For example, Winter[102] found that individuals with below-knee amputations used the gluteus maximus, semitendinosus, and knee extensor muscles as energy generators to compensate for loss of the plantarflexors. Olney and associates[32] found that in children who had unilateral plantarflexor paralysis, the involved plantarflexors produced only 33% of the energy generation, in comparison with the 66% produced in normal gait.

Paralysis or paresis of the plantarflexors (gastrocnemius, soleus, flexor digitorum longus, tibialis posterior, plantaris, and flexor hallucis longus muscles) results in a **calcaneal gait** pattern.[103] This pattern is characterized by greater than normal amounts of ankle dorsiflexion and knee flexion during stance and a shorter-than-normal step length on the affected side. The abnormal amount of knee flexion and the fact that the soleus muscle is not pulling the knee into extension necessitate a higher level of quadriceps activity to stabilize the knee during the stance phase. The period of single-limb support is shortened because of the difficulty of stabilizing the tibia and the knee. Step length is shorter than normal because the normal push-off segment of gait is eliminated. The normal heel-off and progression to toe-off are changed into a rather abrupt liftoff of the entire foot. The asymmetry of this type of gait pattern is obvious through observation and a comparison of right and left step lengths.

Sometimes an isolated weakness or paralysis of a single muscle will produce a characteristic gait. For example, a unilateral paralysis of the gluteus medius results in a typical gait pattern called a **gluteus medius gait.** The characteristics of this gait pattern can be deduced by reviewing the function of the gluteus medius during normal gait. Normally, the gluteus medius stabilizes the hip and pelvis by controlling the drop of the pelvis during single-limb support, especially during the first part of the stance phase. If gluteus medius activity on the side of the stance leg is absent, the pelvis, accompanied by the trunk, will fall excessively on the swing side, which results in a loss of balance. To prevent the trunk and pelvis from falling to the unsupported side and to maintain HAT over the stance leg, the individual compensates by laterally bending the trunk over the stance leg. The trunk motion enables the person to maintain balance by keeping the center of mass over the base of support and allows the swing leg to be lifted high enough to clear the ground. The trunk motion reduces the moment arm of gravity, thus reducing the need for hip abductor contraction and the concomitant compression caused by the hip abductors. The lateral trunk lean characterizes the gluteus medius gait. The use of an assistive device such as a cane on the side opposite to the paralyzed muscle reduces the need for the lateral trunk lean. The use of a cane decreases the energy required in a gluteus medius gait, although it remains above that of normal gait.

The gluteus maximus in normal gait provides for stability in the sagittal plane and for restraint of forward progression. This muscle helps to counteract the external flexion moment at the hip in the early part of stance and restrains the forward movement of the femur in late swing in normal gait. When the gluteus maximus is paralyzed, the trunk must be thrown posteriorly at heel strike, to prevent the trunk from falling forward when there is an external flexion moment at the hip. The backward lean is typical of a **gluteus maximus gait.**

The quadriceps is normally active at initial contact throughout early stance when there is an external flexion moment acting at the knee. It is common for people with patellar pain to inhibit quadriceps contraction. Its function is easily compensated for if a person has normal hip extensors and plantarflexors. The gluteus maximus and soleus muscles pull the femur and tibia, respectively, posteriorly, which results in knee extension. Additional compensation may be accomplished by forward trunk bending and a rapid plantarflexion after initial contact. The forward shifting of the weight creates an external extension moment at the knee (at initial contact and during the loading response period). It also places the knee in hyperextension and eliminates the need for quadriceps activity. If both the quadriceps and the gluteus maximus are paralyzed, a person may compensate for the loss by pushing the femur posteriorly with his or her hand at initial contact. The arm supports the trunk; it prevents hip flexion and also thrusts the knee into extension.

CONCEPT CORNERSTONE 14-5: *Paralysis of Dorsiflexors*

The normal functions of the dorsiflexors in gait are (1) to maintain the ankle in neutral so that the heel strikes the floor at initial con-

tact; (2) to control the external plantarflexion moment at heel strike; (3) to dorsiflex the foot in initial swing; and (4) to maintain the ankle in dorsiflexion during midswing and terminal swing. If these functions are absent, the following would be expected to occur: (1) the entire foot or the toes would strike the floor at initial contact; (2) entry into stance phase would be abrupt; (3) the amount of flexion at the hip and knee would have to increase to clear the foot in initial swing; and (4) a method of either shortening the swing leg or lengthening the stance would have to be found to clear the plantarflexed joint.

In patients with bilateral lower extremity paralysis, walking usually involves the use of long leg braces and crutches. In this form of gait, the trunk and upper extremity muscles must perform all of the work of walking, and the energy cost of walking is much greater than normal. A form of electrical stimulation called functional neuromuscular stimulation (FNS) is currently being used to activate the paralyzed lower extremity muscles so that these muscles can generate energy for walking. However, the energy cost of FNS walking is still well above that of normal gait.[104]

■ **Pain**

This group includes all causes of variations that are attributable primarily to pain. All overuse injuries fall into this category.

Iliotibial band syndrome and popliteal tendonitis[104] experienced by runners are common. Plantar fasciitis, caused by repetitive stretching of the planter fascia between its origin at the plantar rim of the calcaneous and its insertion into the metatarsal heads, is a common overuse syndrome seen in young athletes.[105] Many gait variations can be seen in osteoarthritis.[106]

Pain also appears to be a factor leading to an increase in oxygen consumption. As pain increases, oxygen consumption has been found to increase.[107]

■ **Adaptation/Compensation**

This group includes all causes of variations that occur when one lower extremity has a structural or functional impairment and the other (normal) extremity compensates by adapting its gait pattern. The human body is remarkable in its ability to compensate for losses or disturbances in function. Most of the compensations that are made are performed unconsciously, and if the disturbance is slight, such as occurs in excessive pronation of the foot, the individual may not be aware that the gait pattern is in any way unusual. However, most compensations will result in an increase in energy expenditure over the optimal amount and may result in excessive stress on other structures of the body.

Asymmetries of the lower extremities that result in gait adaptations may have structural or functional primary causes, such as contractures of soft tissues around the joints, bony ankylosis, and muscle weakness or spasticity.

Example 14-3

One might see excessive plantarflexion during stance phase in a limb that is normal. The primary cause could be in the other limb: for example, an inability to clear the toes in swing phase as a result of inadequate knee flexion. The excessive plantarflexion would be an adaptation.

Example 14-4

A somewhat different example of adaptation could result from a knee flexion contracture. When the affected extremity is weight-bearing, the normal extremity will be proportionately too long to swing through in a normal manner. A method of equalizing leg lengths is necessary for the swing leg to swing through without hitting the floor. Excessive plantarflexion during push-off of the affected side, described previously, would be one means. In this case, there is no structural or functional abnormality in the adaptive movement. Alternatively, the person could increase the amount of flexion at the hip, knee, and ankle of the unaffected side. Again, the limb showing the adaptation has no structural or functional impairment. Other methods that produce relative shortening of the swinging leg are hip hiking, or circumduction of the leg. Each of these compensations makes it possible to walk, although they increase the energy requirements above normal levels.

Many compensations for inadequate power generation have been identified.[44] For example, persons with hemiparesis resulting from stroke frequently show greater than normal power generation from ankle plantarflexors at push-off (A2-S) of the unaffected limb (interlimb compensation) or in hip extensors in early stance (H1-S) on the affected side (intralimb compensation).

Summary

The objectives of gait analysis are to identify deviations from normal and their causes. Once the cause has been determined, it is possible to take corrective action aimed at improving performance, eliminating or diminishing abnormal stresses, and decreasing energy expenditure. Sometimes the corrective action may be as simple as using a lift in the shoe to equalize leg lengths or developing an exercise program to increase strength or flexibility at the hip, knee, or ankle. In other instances, corrective action may require the use of assistive devices such as braces, canes, or crutches. However, an understanding of the complexities of abnormal gait and the ability to detect abnormal gait patterns and to determine the causes of these deviations must be based on an understanding of normal structure and function. The study of human gait, like the study of human posture, illustrates the interdependence of structure and function and the large variety of postures and gaits available to the human species.

Study Questions

1. The stance phase constitutes what percentage of the gait cycle in normal walking? How does an increase in walking speed affect the percentage of time spent in stance?
2. What percentage of the gait cycle is spent in double support? How is double support affected by increases and decreases in the walking speed?
3. Describe the subdivisions of the stance and swing phases of the walking gait cycle, using the traditional terminology.
4. How do the traditional phases of gait used to describe walking gait compare with the RLA terms? Describe the similarities and differences between the terms.
5. Maximum knee flexion occurs during which period of the gait cycle?
6. What are the approximate values of maximum flexion and extension required for normal gait at the knee, hip, and ankle?
7. How does the total range of motion required for normal gait at the knee, hip, and ankle compare with the range of motion required for running and stair gait?
8. What is the difference between an internal moment and an external moment?
9. What is the concept of the support moment, and what major muscle groups are responsible?
10. What moments are acting at the ankle, knee, and hip at initial contact? Answer the same question with regard to different gait events: foot flat, midstance, heel-off, toe-off.
11. What is largely responsible for the abductor moment at the knee in stance phase?
12. What are the roles of the hamstrings in normal gait? Do they contribute to support and/or to power?
13. What are the major muscle groups that contribute to the positive work of walking, and when in the gait cycle do their contributions occur?

14. Why does walking faster than normal and walking slower than normal usually result in increased energy costs?
15. Why do long double-support times usually result in increased energy costs?
16. What is the role of the tibialis posterior muscle during walking gait?
17. What is the function of the plantarflexors during walking gait?
18. Describe the transverse rotations in the frontal plane at the pelvis, femur, and tibia during walking gait.
19. Describe the motion of the rearfoot segment with respect to the lower leg in stance phase in the frontal plane.
20. What are the functions of the dorsiflexors in normal walking gait?
21. How is the swinging motion of the upper extremities related to movements of the trunk, pelvis, and lower extremities during walking gait?
22. Compare muscle action in walking gait with muscle action in running gait.
23. Explain what would happen in walking and running if a person's plantarflexors were weak. What compensations might you expect?

◆ References

1. Steindler A: Kinesiology. Springfield, IL, Charles C Thomas, 1955.
2. Winter DA: Energy assessments in pathological gait. Physiother Can 30:183, 1978.
3. Rose J, Gamble JG (eds): Human Walking, 2nd ed. Philadelphia, Williams & Wilkins, 1994.
4. Rowe PJ, Myles CM, Walker C, et al.: Knee joint kinematics in gait and other functional activities measured using flexible electrogoniometry: How much knee motion is sufficient for normal daily life? Gait Posture 12:143, 2000.
5. Sutherland DH: The evolution of clinical gait analysis. Part I: Kinesiological EMG. Gait Posture 14:61, 2001.
6. Sutherland DH: The evolution of clinical gait analysis. Part II: Kinematics. Gait Posture 16:159, 2002.
7. Winter DA: Biomechanics of normal and pathological gait: Implications for understanding human locomotor control. J Motor Behav 21:337, 1989.
8. Pathokinesiology Service and Physical Therapy Department at Rancho Los Amigos National Rehabilitation Center: Observational Gait Analysis. Downey, CA, Los Amigos Research and Education, Inc., 2001.
9. Elble RJ, Cousins R, Leffler K, et al.: Gait initiation by patients with lower-half parkinsonism. Brain 119:1705, 1996.
10. Hesse S, Reiter F, Jahnke M, et al.: Asymmetry of gait initiation in hemiparetic stroke subjects. Arch Phys Med Rehabil 78:719, 1997.
11. Lamoreaux LW: Kinematic measurements in the study of human walking. Prosthet Res 69:3, 1971.
12. Murray MP: Gait as a total pattern of movement. Am J Phys Med 46:1, 1967.
13. Murray MP, Drought AB, Kory RC: Walking patterns of normal men. J Bone Joint Surg Am 46:335, 1964.
14. Winter DA: The Biomechanics and Motor Control of Human Gait: Normal, Elderly and Pathological, 2nd ed. Waterloo, Ontario, Waterloo Biomechanics, 1991.
15. Finley FR, Cody KA: Locomotive characteristics of urban pedestrians. Arch Phys Med Rehabil 51:423, 1970.
16. Kadaba MP, Ramakrishnan HK, Wootten ME: Measurement of lower extremity kinematics during level walking. J Orthop Res 8: 383, 1990.
17. Oberg T, Karznia A, Oberg K: Basic gait parameters: Reference data for normal subjects 10–79 years of age. J Rehabil Res Dev 30:210, 1993.
18. Drillis R: The influence of aging of the kinematics of gait. In The Geriatric Amputee (National Academy of Sciences–National Research Council [NAS-NRC] Publication No. 919). Washington, DC, NAS-NRC, 1961.
19. Crowinshield RD, Brand RA, Johnston RC: Effects of walking velocity and age on hip kinematics and kinetics. Clin Orthop 132:140, 1978.
20. Larsson LE, Odenrick P, Sandlund B, et al.: The phases of stride and their interaction in human gait. Scand J Rehabil Med 12:107, 1980.
21. Wernick J, Volpe RG: Lower extremity function. In Valmassy RI (ed): Clinical Biomechanics of the Lower Extremities. St. Louis, CV Mosby, 1996.
22. Hausdorff JM, Purdon PL, Peng CK, et al.: Fractal dynamics of human gait: Stability of long-range correlations in stride interval fluctuations. J Appl Physiol 80:1448, 1996.
23. Sekiya N, Nagasaki H, Ito H, et al.: Optimal walking in terms of variability in step length. J Orthop Sports Phys Ther 26:266, 1997.
24. Winter DA, Eng JJ, Isshac MG: A review of kinetic parameters in human walking. In Craik RL, Otis CA (eds): Gait Analysis: Theory and Application. St. Louis, Mosby–Year Book, 1994.
25. Eng JJ, Winter DA: Kinetic analysis of the lower limbs during walking: What information can be gained from a three dimensional model? J Biomech 28:753, 1995.

26. Soderberg GL, Gavel RH: A light emitting diode system for the analysis of gait. Phys Ther 58:4, 1978.

27. Herschler C, Milner M: Angle-angle diagrams in the assessment of locomotion. Am J Phys Med 59:3, 1980.

28. Lafortune MA, Cavanagh PR, Sommer HJ 3rd, et al.: Three-dimensional kinematics of the human knee during walking. J Biomech 25:347, 1992.

29. McGinley JL, Goldie PA, Greenwood KM, et al.: Accuracy and reliability of observational gait analysis data: Judgments of push-off in gait after stroke. Phys Ther 83:146, 2003.

30. Saunders JB, Inman VT, Eberhart HD: The major determinants in normal and pathological gait. J Bone Joint Surg Am 35:543, 1953.

31. Winter DA: Analysis of instantaneous energy of normal gait. J Biomech 9:253, 1976.

32. Olney SJ, MacPhail HE, Hedden DM, et al.: Work and power in hemiplegic cerebral palsy gait. Phys Ther 70:431, 1990.

33. Childress DS, Gard SA: Investigation of vertical motion of the human body during normal walking [abstract]. Gait Posture 5:161, 1997.

34. Gard SA, Childress DS: The influence of stance-phase knee flexion on the vertical displacement of the trunk during normal walking. Arch Phys Med Rehabil 80:26, 1999.

35. Katoh Y, Chao EY, Laughman RK, et al.: Biomechanical analysis of foot function during gait and clinical applications. Clin Orthop 177:23, 1983.

36. Smidt G: Methods of studying gait. Phys Ther 54:1, 1974.

37. Winter DA, Patla AE, Frank JS, et al.: Biomechanical walking pattern changes in the fit and healthy elderly. Phys Ther 70: 340, 1990.

38. Hunt AE, Smith RM, Torode M, et al.: Intersegment foot motion and ground reaction forces over the stance phase of walking. Clin Biomech (Bristol, Avon) 16:592, 2001.

39. Rattanaprasert U, Smith R, Sullivan M, et al.: Three-dimensional kinematics of the forefoot, rearfoot, and leg without the function of tibialis posterior in comparison with normals during stance. Clin Biomech (Bristol, Avon) 14:14, 1999.

40. Holt KG, Obusek JP, Fonseca ST: Constraints on disordered locomotion. A dynamical systems perspective on spastic cerebral palsy. Hum Mov Sci 15:177, 1996.

41. Winter DA, Quanbury AO, Reimer GD: Analysis of instantaneous energy of normal gait. J Biomech 9:253, 1976.

42. Winter DA: Biomechanics and Motor Control of Human Movement, 2nd ed. New York, John Wiley & Sons, 1990.

43. Olney SJ, Monga TN, Costigan PA: Mechanical energy of walking of stroke patients. Arch Phys Med Rehabil 67:92, 1986.

44. Olney SJ, Richards C: Hemiparetic gait following stroke. Part I: Characteristics. Gait Posture 4:136, 1996.

45. Winter DA: Energy generation and absorption at the ankle and knee during fast, natural and slow cadences. Clin Orthop 175:147, 1983.

46. Zajac FE, Neptune RR, Kautz SA: Biomechanics and muscle coordination of human walking. Part I: Introduction to concepts, power transfer, dynamics and simulations. Gait Posture 16:215, 2002.

47. Zajac FE, Neptune RR, Kautz SA: Biomechanics and muscle coordination of human walking. Part II: Lessons from dynamical simulations and clinical implications. Gait Posture 17:1, 2003.

48. Anderson FC, Pandy MG: Individual muscle contributions to support in normal walking. Gait Posture 17:159, 2003.

49. Shiavi R: Electromyographic patterns in adult locomotion: A comprehensive review. J Rehabil Res Dev 22:85, 1985.

50. Bechtol CO: Normal human gait. In American Academy of Orthopaedic Surgeons: Atlas of Orthotics. St. Louis, CV Mosby, 1974.

51. Kadaba MP, Ramakrishnan HK, Wootten ME, et al.: Repeatability of kinematic, kinetic and electromyographic data in normal adult gait. J Orthop Res 7:849, 1989.

52. Kleissen RFM, Litjens MCA, Baten CTM, et al.: Consistency of surface EMG patterns obtained during gait from three laboratories using standardized measurement technique. Gait Posture 6:200, 1997.

53. Winter DA, Yack HJ: EMG profiles during normal walking: Stride to stride and inter-subject variability. Electroenceph Clin Neurophys (Ireland) 67: 402, 1987.

54. Wells RP: The projection of the ground reaction force as a predictor of internal joint moments. Bull Prosthet Res 10–35:15, 1981.

55. Cerny K: Pathomechanics of stance: Clinical concepts for analysis. Phys Ther 64:1851, 1984

56. Thorstensson A, Nilsson J, Carlson H, et al.: Trunk movements in human locomotion. Acta Physiol Scand 121:9, 1984.

57. Krebs DE, Wong D, Jevsevar D, et al.: Trunk kinematics during locomotor activities. Phys Ther 72:505, 1992.

58. Stokes VP, Andersson C, Forssberg H: Rotational and translational movement features of the pelvis and thorax during adult human locomotion. J Biomech 22:43, 1989.

59. Hirasaki E, Moore ST, Raphan T, et al.: Effects of walking velocity on vertical head and body movements during locomotion. Exp Brain Res 127:117, 1999.

60. White SG, McNair PJ: Abdominal and erector spinae muscle activity during gait: The use of cluster analysis to identify patterns of activity. Clin Biomech 17:177, 2002.

61. Basmajian JV: Muscles Alive, 4th ed. Baltimore, Williams & Wilkins, 1979.

62. Hogue RE: Upper extremity muscle activity at different cadences and inclines during normal gait. Phys Ther 49:9, 1969.

63. Dietz V, Fouad K, Bastiaanse CM: Neuronal coordi-

nation of arm and leg movements during human locomotion. Eur J Neurosci 14:1906, 2001.

64. Wannier T, Bastiaanse C, Colombo G, et al.: Arm to leg coordination in humans during walking, creeping and swimming activities. Exp Brain Res 141:375, 2001.

65. Andriacchi TP, Galante JO, Fermier RW: The influence of total knee-replacement design on walking and stair-climbing. J Bone Joint Surg Am 64:1328, 1982.

66. McFayden BJ, Winter DA: An integrated biomechanical analysis of normal stair ascent and descent. J Biomech 21:733, 1988.

67. Kirkwood RN, Culham EG, Costigan P et al.: Hip moments during level walking, stair climbing and exercise in individuals aged 55 years and older. Phys Ther 79:360, 1999.

68. Nuber GW: Biomechanics of the foot and ankle during gait. Clin Sports Med 7:1, 1988.

69. Mann RA: Biomechanics of running. In D'Ambrosia RD, Drez D (eds): Prevention and Treatment of Running Injuries, 2nd ed. Thorofare, NJ, Slack, Inc., 1989.

70. McPoil TG, Cornwall MW: Applied sports biomechanics in running. In Zachezewski, JE, Quillen S, Magee D (eds): Athletic Injuries and Rehabilitation. Philadelphia, WB Saunders, 1996.

71. Novacheck TF: The biomechanics of running. Gait Posture 7:77, 1998.

72. Norkin C: Gait analysis. In O'Sullivan S, Schmitz TJ (eds): Physical Rehabilitation Assessment and Treatment, 4th ed. Philadelphia, FA Davis, 2001.

73. Cioni G, Duchini F, Milianti B, et al.: Differences and variations in the patterns of early independent walking. Early Hum Dev 35:193, 1993.

74. Rose-Jacobs, R: Development of gait at slow, free, and fast speeds in 3 and 5 year old children. Phys Ther 63:1251, 1983.

75. Foley CD, Quanbury AO, Steinke T: Kinematics of normal child locomotion—A statistical study based upon TV data. J Biomech 12:1, 1979.

76. Sutherland DH, Olshen R, Cooper L, et al.: The development of mature gait. J Bone Joint Surg Am 62:336, 1980.

77. Beck RJ, Andriacchi TP, Kuo KN, et al.: Changes in the gait patterns of growing children. J Bone Joint Surg Am 63:1452, 1981.

78. Sutherland DH, Kaufman KR, Campbell K, et al.: Clinical use of prediction regions for motion analysis. Dev Med Child Neurol 38:773, 1996.

79. Himann JE, Cunningham DA, Rechnitzer PA, et al.: Age-related changes in speed of walking. Med Sci Sports Exerc 20:161, 1988.

80. Blanke DJ, Hageman PA: Comparison of gait of young men and elderly men. Phys Ther 69:144, 1989.

81. Rothstein JM, Roy SH, Wolf SL: The Rehabilitation Specialist's Handbook, 2nd ed. Philadelphia, FA Davis, 1998.

82. Kerrigan DC, Todd MK, Della Croce U, et al.: Biomechanical gait alterations independent of speed in the healthy elderly: Evidence for specific limiting impairments. Arch Phys Med Rehabil 79:317, 1998.

83. Lee LW, Kerrigan C: Identification of kinetic differences between fallers and non-fallers in the elderly. Am J Phys Med Rehabil 78:243, 1999.

84. Mueller MJ, Minor SD, Schaaf JA, et al.: Relationship of plantar-flexor peak torque and dorsiflexion range of motion to kinetic variables during walking. Phys Ther 75:684, 1995.

85. Bohannon RW, Andrews AW, Thomas MW: Walking speed: Reference values and correlates for older adults. J Orthop Sports Phys Ther 24:86, 1996.

86. Lord SR, Lloyd DG, Nirui M, et al.: The effect of exercise on gait patterns in older women: A randomized controlled trial. J Gerontol A Biol Sci Med Sci 51:M64, 1996.

87. Connelly DM, Vandervoort AA: Effects of detraining on knee extensor strength and functional mobility in a group of elderly women. J Orthop Sports Phys Ther 26:340, 1997.

88. Oberg T, Karsznia A, Oberg K: Joint angle parameters in gait: Reference data for normal subjects, 10–79 years of age. J Rehabil Res Dev 31:199, 1994.

89. Kerrigan DC, Todd MK, Della Croce U: Gender differences in joint biomechanics during walking: Normative study in young adults. Am J Phys Med Rehabil 77:2, 1998.

90. Krebs DE, Robbins CE, Lavine L, et al.: Hip biomechanics during gait. J Orthop Sports Phys Ther 28:51, 1998.

91. Crenshaw SJ, Pollo FE, Calton EF: Effects of lateral-wedged insoles on kinetics at the knee. Clin Orthop 375:185, 2000.

92. Finger S, Paulos LE: Clinical and biomechanical evaluation of the unloading brace. J Knee Surg 15:155, 2002.

93. Maly MR, Culham EG, Costigan PA: Static and dynamic biomechanics of foot orthoses in people with medial compartment knee osteoarthritis. Clin Biomech (Bristol, Avon) 17:603, 2002.

94. Ounpuu S, Bell KJ, Davis RB 3rd, et al.: An evaluation of the posterior leaf spring orthosis using joint kinematics and kinetics. J Pediatr Orthop 16:378, 1996.

95. Teixeira-Salmela LF, Nadeau S, Mcbride I, et al.: Effects of muscle strengthening and physical conditioning training of temporal, kinematic and kinetic variables during gait in chronic stroke survivors. J Rehabil Med 33:53, 2001.

96. Kaufman KR, Miller LS, Sutherland DH: Gait asymmetry in patients with limb-length inequality. J Pediatr Orthop 16:144, 1996.

97. Song KM, Halliday SE, Little DG: The effect of limb-length discrepancy on gait. J Bone Joint Surg Am 79:1690, 1997.

98. Clement DB, Taunton JE, Smart GW, et al.: A survey of overuse running injuries. Phys Sportsmed 9:5, 1981.

99. Scranton PE, McMaster JH: Momentary distribution of forces under the foot. J Biomech 9:45, 1976.

100. Waters RWL, Barnes G, Husserl T, et al.: Comparable energy expenditure after arthrodesis of the hip and ankle. J Bone Joint Surg Am 70:1032, 1988.
101. Scandalis TA, Bosak A, Berliner JC, et al.: Resistance training and gait function in patients with Parkinson's disease. Am J Phys Med Rehabil 80:38, 2001.
102. Winter, DA: Biomechanics of below knee amputee gait. J Biomech 21:361, 1988.
103. Perry J: Kinesiology of lower extremity bracing. Clin Orthop 102:18, 1974.
104. Marsolais EB, Edwards BG: Energy costs of walking and standing with functional neuromuscular stimulation and long leg braces. Arch Phys Med Rehabil 69:243, 1988.
105. Taunton JE, Clement DB, Smart GW, et al.: Non-surgical management of overuse knee injuries in runners. Can J Sport Sci 12:11, 1987.
106. Teixeira LF, Olney SJ: Relationships between alignment, kinematic and kinetic measures of the knee of osteoarthritic elderly subjects in level walking. Clin Biomech 11:126, 1996.
107. Gussoni M, Margonato V, Ventura R, et al.: Energy cost of walking with hip impairment. Phys Ther 70:295, 1990.

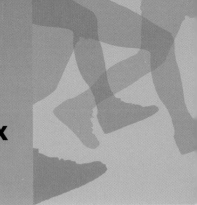

Index

Note: Page numbers followed by the letter f refer to figures; those followed by the letter t refer to tables.